THE AIDS KNOWLEDGE BASE

A TEXTBOOK ON HIV
DISEASE FROM THE
UNIVERSITY OF CALIFORNIA,
SAN FRANCISCO,
AND THE SAN FRANCISCO
GENERAL HOSPITAL

THE
AIDS
KNOWLEDGE
BASE

A TEXTBOOK ON HIV
DISEASE FROM THE
UNIVERSITY OF CALIFORNIA,
SAN FRANCISCO,
AND THE SAN FRANCISCO
GENERAL HOSPITAL

EDITED BY
P.T. COHEN, M.D., Ph.D.
MERLE A. SANDE, M.D.
PAUL A. VOLBERDING, M.D.

THE MEDICAL PUBLISHING GROUP
A Division of the Massachusetts Medical Society

WALTHAM, MASSACHUSETTS
1990

The full text of the *AIDS Knowledge Base* is also available in online and CD-ROM formats. For additional information, please contact the Department of Customer Services, Massachusetts Medical Society, 1440 Main Street, Waltham, MA 02154 USA. Tel: 1 (800) 843-6356 (in Massachusetts, (617) 893-3800 ext. 1199). FAX: (617) 893-0413.

Library of Congress Cataloging-in-Publication Data

The AIDS knowledge base: a textbook on HIV disease from the
   University of California, San Francisco, and the San Francisco
   General Hospital/edited by P.T. Cohen, Merle A. Sande, and Paul A.
   Volberding.
      p.   cm.
   ISBN 0-910133-30-1. — ISBN 0-910133-31-X (soft)
   1. AIDS (Disease)   I. Cohen, P.T. (Philip T.), 1940–   .
II. Sande, Merle A., 1939–   . III. Volberding, Paul A.
IV. University of California, San Francisco. V. San Francisco
General Hospital (Calif.).
   [DNLM: 1. Acquired Immunodeficiency Syndrome.   WD 308 A288345]
RC607.A26A3478 1990
616.97'92 — dc20
DNLM/DLC
for Library of Congress   89-13838
                                                              CIP

Printed in the United States of America
10 9 8 7 6 5 4 3

This book was produced by the Electronic Production Department of the Massachusetts Medical Society. Printed and bound by Edwards Brothers, Inc., Ann Arbor, Michigan. Cover design by Emily Stuart. Cover photograph courtesy of Ewing Galloway/E.P. Jones Co. Index prepared by Grace Olken Sheldrick/Wordsworth Associates.

Foreword

This book version of the *AIDS Knowledge Base* evolved as a response to the catastrophic HIV epidemic. In a process that has often been difficult and painful, and that promises to continue for some time, San Francisco General Hospital has confronted most of the medical, ethical, legal, social, political, and fiscal problems created by the epidemic. We have benefited beyond description from the efforts of a responsive and motivated community, and from the example and teaching of our courageous patients. We have made some mistakes and have learned a great deal. Many authors from San Francisco General Hospital and the University of California, San Francisco, along with several from other institutions, have created the *AIDS Knowledge Base* to make this process easier for others. We hope this book places our experience in perspective and contributes to our goal of widely distributing easily accessible, up-to-date information formulated to be useful for solving real problems posed by HIV disease.

We have taken advantage of the tools of microcomputer technology, electronic publishing, and telecommunications to gain control of the rapidly expanding and evolving body of information about HIV disease and its consequences. The *Knowledge Base* existed first as a searchable online database, continually updated and available since October 1987 from BRS Information Technologies. The second form of the *AIDS Knowledge Base* makes use of compact disk (CD-ROM) technology, which allows presentation of large databases on microcomputer systems. The *AIDS Knowledge Base* has been available since June 1988 on CD-ROM as part of *Compact Library: AIDS* from the Medical Publishing Group of the Massachusetts Medical Society.

Although these electronic media have many advantages in presenting, searching, and managing information, computer technology is new, unfamiliar, and inaccessible to many. Traditional "hardcopy" textbooks have their own advantages, including permanence, tangibility, and familiarity. To distribute the *AIDS Knowledge Base* as widely as possible we have produced this "hardcopy" textbook. We have used the text of the electronic version, adding figures and graphs to enhance the presentation.

Producing the *AIDS Knowledge Base* and maintaining its currency has required a great investment of time and effort by the authors, editors, and publisher. We have undertaken the work in the belief that the information is important and useful. We welcome comments from users of this book and other forms of the *AIDS Knowledge Base*.

P.T. Cohen, M.D., Ph.D.
Merle A. Sande, M.D.
Paul A. Volberding, M.D.

January 5, 1990

Acknowledgements

Many people have contributed to this project and deserve acknowledgement beyond what can be expressed here. First and foremost are our authors and our associate editors Donald Abrams, J. Louise Gerberding, Phil Hopewell, Michael McGrath, Dennis Osmond, and Constance Wofsy.

In San Francisco, during initial development, Karen Heller patiently and ably managed the *AIDS Knowledge Base* project with the effective editorial assistance of Eleanor Haas. Jan Zita Grover, the project's managing editor since October 1987, has overseen the editing and day-to-day operation of the project, has been actively involved in community efforts to combat HIV disease, has kept up with AIDS developments reported in the lay press, and has provided many useful suggestions on content and perspective. Craig Seligman capably handled many routine yet demanding aspects of day-to-day operations.

In Massachusetts, at the Medical Publishing Group, Rob Stuart, our editor, was an endless source of good ideas, constructive suggestions, and accommodation as deadlines drew near. Joe Elia provided effective oversight, mature guidance, and humor when needed. Dave Roh and Gary Mancini capably handled hardware and software development connected with the project. Emily Stuart coaxed the text into an elegant design. Anna Sabasteanski, Barbara Wetherington, and Tom Howes pushed desktop technology to its limits for our project. Our proofreaders, Doug Brandt and Susan Karcz, queried, and queried again until we got things right. Bart Rubenstein, Wendy Faxon, and Carolyn Ferris had the job of making all of us believe that this project made sense economically as well as medically.

We thank them all.

CONTRIBUTORS

Sharone Abramowitz, M.D.
Assistant Clinical Instructor, Department of Psychiatry, UCSF; Behavioral Medicine Faculty, Department of Internal Medicine, Primary Care Division, Highland Hospital, Oakland, California.

Donald I. Abrams, M.D.
Associate Professor of Clinical Medicine, Assistant Director, AIDS Activities, SFGH; UCSF.

A.J. Ammann, M.D.
Director, Clinical Research, Genentech, Inc.; Adjunct Professor, Pediatrics, UCSF Medical Center.

James R. Arden, M.D.
Assistant Professor in Residence, Anesthesia, UCSF.

Peter S. Arno, Ph.D.
Department of Epidemiology and Social Medicine, Montefiore Medical Center/Einstein College of Medicine, Bronx, New York.

Jay Baer, M.D.
Assistant Professor of Psychiatry, Tufts University School of Medicine.

Timothy G. Berger, M.D.
Chief of Dermatology, SFGH; Assistant Clinical Professor, UCSF.

Alicia Boccellari, Ph.D.
Director, Neuropsychology Service, Assistant Clinical Professor of Psychology, Department of Psychiatry, SFGH; UCSF School of Medicine.

Gail Bolan, M.D.
Clinical Instructor, Department of Medicine, UCSF; Director, STD Control, San Francisco Department of Public Health.

Victoria A. Cargill, M.D.
Assistant Professor of Medicine, Case Western Reserve University School of Medicine, Cleveland, Ohio.

Richard E. Chaisson, M.D.
Director, AIDS Service, Johns Hopkins Hospital; Assistant Professor of Medicine and Epidemiology, Johns Hopkins Schools of Medicine and Hygiene and Public Health.

Melvin D. Cheitlin, M.D.
Associate Chair of Cardiology and Professor in Residence, Cardiology, SFGH.

David Chernoff, M.D.
Associate Director, UCSF AIDS Clinic; Assistant Chief, Department of Medicine, UCSF.

Matt Coles, J.D.
Adjunct Assistant Professor of Law, Hastings College of Law, University of California; Staff Lawyer, American Civil Liberties Union of Northern California.

P.T. Cohen, M.D., Ph.D.
Associate Clinical Professor of Medicine, UCSF; Division of General Internal Medicine and Department of Emergency Medicine, SFGH.

Molly Cooke, M.D.
Associate Professor of Clinical Medicine, UCSF; Chair, Ethics Committee, SFGH.

Suzanne Crowe, M.B.B.S., F.R.A.C.P.
Head of AIDS Research Unit, MacFarlane Burnet Centre for Medical Research, Fairfield Hospital, Melbourne, Australia.

James Dilley, M.D.
Assistant Clinical Professor of Psychiatry, UCSF; Director, UCSF AIDS Health Project.

Elizabeth Donegan, M.D.
Assistant Clinical Professor, Laboratory Medicine; Chief, Blood Bank; UCSF.

W. Lawrence Drew, M.D., Ph.D.
Director, Microbiology, Infectious Disease, Mt. Zion Hospital and Medical Center; Associate Professor of Medicine and Laboratory Medicine, UCSF School of Medicine.

Kim S. Erlich, M.D.
Consultant in Infectious Diseases, Seton Medical Center, Daly City, California.

Michael P. Federle, M.D.
Chairman, Radiology Department, University of Pittsburgh.

Scott L. Friedman, M.D.
Assistant Professor of Medicine, UCSF School of Medicine; Attending Gastroenterologist, SFGH.

Gayling Gee, R.N., M.S.
Director, Outpatient Nursing, SFGH;
Assistant Clinical Professor, School of
Nursing, UCSF.

J. Louise Gerberding, M.D.
Assistant Professor, Department of
Medicine, UCSF, SFGH; Project Director,
AIDS Health Care Worker Program,
Medical Service, SFGH.

Philip C. Goodman, M.D.
Associate Professor, Departments of
Radiology and Medicine, UCSF, SFGH.

Jesse Green, Ph.D.
Department of Health Policy Research,
New York University Medical Center,
New York.

Deborah Greenspan, B.D.S.
Associate Clinical Professor of Oral
Medicine, Department of Stomatology,
UCSF.

Moses Grossman, M.D.
Professor of Pediatrics, UCSF; Chief of
Pediatrics, SFGH.

J.Z. Grover, Ph.D.
Senior Editor, Project Coordinator, the
AIDS Knowledge Base, UCSF, SFGH.

Karen S. Heller, M.A.
Research Associate, Medical Anthropology
Program, UCSF.

Marc Hellerstein, M.D., Ph.D.
Assistant Professor of Medicine, Division
of Endocrinology, Metabolism, and
Nutrition, SFGH; Assistant Professor,
Department of Nutritional Sciences,
University of California, Berkeley.

S.R. Hernandez, M.D.
Clinical Instructor of Medicine, UCSF;
Chief of Health Resources and Services
Branch, AIDS Office, San Francisco
Department of Public Health.

David M. Heyer, M.D.
Hematology/Oncology Fellow, UCSF.

Ernesto O. Hinojos, M.P.H.
Assistant Education Director, Campaign
Development, San Francisco AIDS
Foundation.

Harry Hollander, M.D.
Director, AIDS Clinic; Assistant Professor
of Clinical Medicine, UCSF.

Philip C. Hopewell, M.D.
Professor of Medicine, UCSF; Chief, Chest
Service, SFGH.

Michael H. Humphreys, M.D.
Chief, Division of Nephrology, SFGH;
Professor of Medicine, UCSF.

Mark A. Jacobson, M.D.
Clinical Professor of Medicine in
Residence, Division of Infectious Disease
and Clinical Pharmacology, Department of
Medicine, UCSF; Medical Service, SFGH.

James O. Kahn, M.D.
Assistant Clinical Professor of Medicine,
UCSF; Principal Investigator, AIDS
Activities Division, SFGH.

Elizabeth Kantor, M.D.
Associate Clinical Professor of Medicine
and Medical Director, SF County Jails; San
Francisco Department of Public Health,
SFGH; UCSF Department of Medicine.

Lawrence D. Kaplan, M.D.
Assistant Clinical Professor of Medicine,
UCSF; AIDS Activities Division, SFGH.

Farzad Khayam-Bashi, B.S.
Research Associate, SFGH; Research
Associate, UCSF.

Eileen Lemus, M.A.
Visiting Nurse in Hospice; Coordinator of
Hospice Services, SFGH.

Gifford S. Leoung, M.D.
Assistant Clinical Professor, UCSF School
of Medicine; AIDS Activities Division,
SFGH.

Alan Lifson, M.D., M.P.H.
Chief, Research Branch, AIDS Office, San
Francisco Department of Public Health;
Assistant Clinical Professor of Medicine,
UCSF.

Jeannee Parker Martin, R.N., M.P.H.
Director, Hospice Programs; Visiting
Nurses and Hospice of San Francisco,
Pacific Presbyterian Medical Center.

Gandis G. Mazeika, B.S.
Research Associate, SFGH; Research
Associate, UCSF.

Michael S. McGrath, M.D., Ph.D.
Assistant Professor of Medicine, AIDS
Activities Division; Director, AIDS
Immunobiology Research Laboratory,
SFGH.

John Mills, M.D.
Professor of Medicine, Microbiology and
Laboratory Medicine, UCSF; Chief,
Division of Infectious Diseases, SFGH.

Herbert Ochitill, M.D.
Assistant Professor of Psychiatry, UCSF.

James J. O'Donnell, M.D.
Professor and Vice Chairman, Department
of Ophthalmology, UCSF; Director of
Ocular Complications of AIDS Clinic,
SFGH.

Dennis Osmond
Specialist, Department of Epidemiology
and Biostatistics; Project Director, SFGH
Cohort Study.

Lauren Poole, R.N., M.S.
Project AWARE, SFGH, UCSF.

Marcia Quackenbush, M.S.
Coordinator of Training, UCSF AIDS
Health Project.

Catherine Reinis-Lucey, M.D.
Assistant Clinical Professor of Medicine,
University of Texas Health Sciences Center
at San Antonio.

George W. Rutherford, M.D.
Director, AIDS Office, San Francisco
Department of Public Health; Assistant
Clinical Professor, Departments of
Pediatrics and Epidemiology and
International Health, UCSF.

Merle A. Sande, M.D.
Professor and Vice Chairman, School of
Medicine, UCSF; Chief, Medical Services,
SFGH.

Gisela F. Schechter, M.D., M.P.H.
Director, San Francisco Tuberculosis
Clinic, Department of Public Health, City
and County of San Francisco; Assistant
Clinical Professor of Medicine, UCSF.

Patricia Schoenfeld, M.D.
Clinical Professor of Medicine, UCSF;
Medical Director, Renal Center, SFGH.

Jerome Schofferman, M.D.
Chief, Pain Management Programs,
Spinecare Medical Group, Daly City,
California; formerly Medical Director,
Hospice of San Francisco.

Peter M. Small, M.D.
Chief Medical Resident, SFGH, UCSF.

Mark D. Smith, M.D., M.B.A.
Instructor in Medicine and Associate
Director, AIDS Services, Johns Hopkins
University School of Medicine.

Yuen T. So, M.D., Ph.D.
Assistant Professor of Neurology, UCSF;
Attending Physician, SFGH.

C. Daniel Sooy, M.D.
Assistant Professor, Department of
Otolaryngology, UCSF; Director,
Otolaryngology Clinic, SFGH.

Linda M. Udall, M.P.H.
Assistant Director, AIDS Office, San
Francisco Department of Public Health.

Paul A. Volberding, M.D.
Associate Professor of Medicine, and
Director, Center for AIDS Research,
UCSF; Chief, Medical Oncology, and
Director, AIDS Program, SFGH.

Judith C. Wilber, Ph.D.
Viral and Rickettsial Disease Laboratory,
California Department of Health Services;
Assistant Clinical Professor, Department of
Laboratory Medicine, UCSF.

Constance B. Wofsy, M.D.
Professor of Clinical Medicine, UCSF;
Co-Director of AIDS Activities and
Assistant Chief, Infectious Diseases, SFGH.

Roberta J. Wong, Pharm.D.
Assistant Clinical Professor of Pharmacy,
UCSF School of Pharmacy; Drug
Information Pharmacist, UCLA Medical
Center, Los Angeles, California.

THE AIDS KNOWLEDGE BASE

*A Textbook on HIV Disease from the
University of California, San Francisco,
and the San Francisco General Hospital*

1

EPIDEMIOLOGY AND TRANSMISSION OF HIV INFECTION

EDITOR Dennis Osmond

2

TESTING FOR HUMAN IMMUNODEFICIENCY VIRUS

EDITOR   *Paul A. Volberding, M.D.*

3

HUMAN IMMUNODEFICIENCY VIRUS AND PATHOGENESIS OF AIDS

EDITOR   *Michael S. McGrath, M.D., Ph.D.*

4

NATURAL HISTORY, CLINICAL SPECTRUM, AND GENERAL MANAGEMENT OF HIV INFECTION

EDITORS   Paul A. Volberding, M.D., and P.T. Cohen, M.D., Ph.D.

CLINICAL MANIFESTATIONS OF HIV INFECTION

EDITORS   Donald I. Abrams, M.D., and P.T. Cohen, M.D., Ph.D.

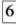
6

INFECTIONS ASSOCIATED WITH AIDS

EDITORS   *Constance B. Wofsy, M.D., and Merle A. Sande, M.D.*

MALIGNANCIES ASSOCIATED WITH AIDS

EDITOR   Paul A. Volberding, M.D.

11

PUBLIC EDUCATION AND PREVENTION STRATEGIES

EDITOR   P.T. Cohen, M.D., Ph.D.

12

ETHICAL ISSUES RELATED TO AIDS

EDITOR   *Molly Cooke, M.D.*

THE
AIDS
KNOWLEDGE
BASE

A TEXTBOOK ON HIV
DISEASE FROM THE
UNIVERSITY OF CALIFORNIA,
SAN FRANCISCO,
AND THE SAN FRANCISCO
GENERAL HOSPITAL

EPIDEMIOLOGY

AND

TRANSMISSION

OF

HIV

INFECTION

EDITOR

Dennis Osmond

1.1

Epidemiology of HIV Infection

Definitions and Codes for HIV Infection and AIDS

Dennis Osmond

Persons infected with the human immunodeficiency virus (HIV)[1-4] may have a variety of manifestations, ranging from asymptomatic infection to severe immunodeficiency and life-threatening secondary infectious diseases or cancers. Various means are now used to describe and assess patients with these manifestations and to describe their signs, symptoms, and laboratory findings. The Centers for Disease Control (CDC) surveillance definition of AIDS has proved to be extremely valuable and reliable for some epidemiologic studies and clinical assessment of patients with the more severe manifestations of disease. However, more inclusive definitions and classifications of HIV infection are needed for optimum patient care, health planning, and public health control strategies, as well as for epidemiologic studies and special surveys. A broadly applicable, easily understood classification system should also facilitate and clarify communication about this disease.

The classification system described in this chapter has been proposed by the CDC.[5] The system is meant to provide a means of grouping patients according to the clinical presentation of disease. It does not imply any change in the definition of AIDS used by the CDC for national reporting.

■ DEFINITION OF HIV INFECTION

The most specific diagnosis of HIV infection is by direct identification of the virus in host tissues by virus isolation. However, the techniques for isolating HIV currently lack sensitivity for detecting infection and are not readily available. For public health purposes, patients with repeatedly reactive screening tests for HIV antibody (e.g., enzyme-linked immunosorbent assay) in whom antibody is also identified by the use of supplemental tests (e.g., Western blot, immunofluorescence assay) should be considered both infected and infective.[6-8]

Although HIV infection is identified by isolation of the virus or, indirectly, by the presence of antibody to the virus, a presumptive clinical diagnosis of HIV infection has been made in some situations in the absence of positive virologic or serologic test results. There is a very strong correlation between the clinical manifestations of AIDS as defined by the CDC and the presence of HIV antibody.[9-12] Most persons whose clinical illness fulfills the CDC surveillance definition for AIDS will have been infected with the virus.[10-12]

■ CLASSIFICATION SYSTEM

This system classifies the manifestations of HIV infection into four mutually exclusive groups, designated by Roman numerals I through IV (Table 1). The classification system applies only to patients diagnosed as having HIV infection. Classification in a particular group is not explicitly intended to have prognostic significance, nor to designate severity of illness. However, classification in the four principal groups, I through IV, is hierarchical in that persons classified in a particular group should not be reclassified in a preceding group if clinical findings resolve, since clinical improvement may not accurately reflect changes in the severity of the underlying disease.

TABLE 1. SUMMARY OF CLASSIFICATION SYSTEM FOR HIV INFECTION

GROUP I.   Acute infection
GROUP II.   Asymptomatic infection*
GROUP III.   Persistent generalized lymphadenopathy*
GROUP IV.   Other disease
  Subgroup A.   Constitutional disease
  Subgroup B.   Neurologic disease
  Subgroup C.   Secondary infectious diseases
    Category C-1.   Specified secondary infectious diseases listed in the CDC surveillance definition for AIDS†
    Category C-2.   Other specified secondary infectious diseases
  Subgroup D.   Secondary cancers**
  Subgroup E.   Other conditions

---

* *Patients in Groups II and III may be subclassified on the basis of a laboratory evaluation.*
† *Includes those patients whose clinical presentation fulfills the definition of AIDS used by the CDC for national reporting.*

Group I includes patients with transient signs and symptoms that appear at the time of, or shortly after, initial infection with HIV as identified by laboratory studies. All patients in Group I should be reclassified in another group after resolution of this acute syndrome.

Group II includes patients who have no signs or symptoms of HIV infection. Patients in this category may be subclassified based on whether hematologic or immunologic laboratory studies have been done and whether results are abnormal in a manner consistent with the effects of HIV infection.

Group III includes patients with persistent generalized lymphadenopathy, but without findings that would lead to classification in Group IV. Patients in this category may be subclassified based on the results of laboratory studies in the same manner as patients in Group II.

Group IV includes patients with clinical symptoms and signs of HIV infection other than or in addition to lymphadenopathy. Patients in this group are assigned to one or more subgroups based on clinical findings. These subgroups are:

  A.   constitutional disease

  B.   neurologic disease

  C.   secondary infectious diseases

  D.   secondary cancers

  E.   other conditions resulting from HIV infection.

There is no a priori hierarchy of severity among subgroups A through E, and these subgroups are not mutually exclusive.

Definitions of the groups and subgroups are as follows.

Group I. Acute HIV Infection.   Defined as a mononucleosis-like syndrome, with or without aseptic meningitis, associated with seroconversion for HIV antibody.[13,14] Antibody seroconversion is required as evidence of initial infection; current viral isolation procedures are not adequately sensitive to be reliable for demonstrating the onset of infection.

Group II. Asymptomatic HIV Infection.   Defined as the absence of signs or symptoms of HIV infection. To be classified in Group II, patients must have had no previous signs or symptoms that would have led to classification in Groups III or IV. Patients whose clinical findings caused them to be classified in Groups III or IV should not be reclassified in Group II if those clinical findings resolve.

Patients in this group may be subclassified on the basis of a laboratory evaluation. Laboratory studies commonly indicated for patients with HIV infection include, but are not limited to, a complete blood count (including differential white blood cell count) and a platelet count. Immunologic tests, especially T lymphocyte helper and suppressor cell counts, are also an important part of the overall evaluation. Patients whose test results are within normal limits, as well as those for whom a laboratory evaluation has not yet been completed, should be differentiated from patients whose test results are consistent with defects associated with HIV infection (e.g., lymphopenia, thrombocytopenia, or decreased number of helper T lymphocytes).

Group III. Persistent Generalized Lymphadenopathy (PGL).   Defined as palpable lymphadenopathy (lymph node enlargement of 1 cm or greater) at two or more extrainguinal sites persisting for more than three months in the absence of a concurrent illness or condition other than HIV infection to explain the findings. Patients in this group may also be subclassified on the basis of a laboratory evaluation, as is done for asymptomatic patients in Group II. Patients with PGL whose clinical findings caused them to be classified in Group IV should not be reclassified in Group III if those other clinical findings resolve.

Group IV. Other HIV Disease.   The clinical manifestations of patients in this group may be designated by assignment to one or more subgroups (A through E) listed below. Within Group IV, subgroup classification is independent of the presence or absence of lymphadenopathy. Each subgroup may include patients who are minimally symptomatic, as well as patients who are severely ill. Increased specificity for manifestations of HIV infection, if needed for clinical purposes or research purposes or for disability determinations, may be achieved by creating additional divisions within each subgroup.

Subgroup A. Constitutional disease.   Defined as one or more of the following: fever persisting more than one month, involuntary weight loss of greater than 10 percent of baseline, or diarrhea persisting more than one month; and the absence of a concurrent illness or condition other than HIV infection to explain the findings.

Subgroup B. Neurologic disease.   Defined as one or more of the following: dementia, myelopathy, or peripheral neuropathy; and the absence of a concurrent illness or condition other than HIV infection to explain the findings.

Subgroup C. Secondary infectious diseases.   Defined as the diagnosis of an infectious disease associated with HIV infection or at least moderately indicative of a defect in cell-mediated immunity. Patients in this subgroup are divided further into two categories.

Category C-1.   Includes patients with symptomatic or invasive disease due to 1 of 12 specified secondary infectious diseases listed in the surveillance definition of AIDS: *Pneumocystis carinii* pneumonia, chronic cryptosporidiosis, toxoplasmosis, extraintestinal strongyloidiasis, isosporiasis, candidiasis (esophageal, bronchial, or pulmonary), cryptococcosis, histoplasmosis, mycobacterial infection with *Mycobacterium avium* complex or *M. kansasii*, cytomegalovirus infection, chronic mucocutaneous or disseminated herpes simplex virus infection, or progressive multifocal leukoencephalopathy.

Category C-2.   Includes patients with symptomatic or invasive disease due to one of six other specified secondary infectious diseases: oral hairy leukoplakia, multidermatomal herpes zoster, recurrent salmonella bacteremia, nocardiosis, tuberculosis, or oral candidiasis (thrush).

Subgroup D. Secondary cancers.   Defined as the diagnosis of one or more kinds of cancer known to be associated with HIV infection as listed in the surveillance definition of AIDS and at least moderately indicative of a defect in cell-mediated immunity: Kaposi's sarcoma, non-Hodgkin's lymphoma (small, noncleaved lymphoma or immunoblastic sarcoma), or primary lymphoma of the brain.

Category C-1 and Subgroup D, it should be noted, include those patients with one or more of the infectious diseases or specified cancers fulfilling the definition of AIDS as used by the CDC for national reporting.

Subgroup E. Other conditions in HIV infection.   Defined as the presence of other clinical findings or diseases, not classifiable above, that may be attributed to HIV infection or may be indicative of a defect in cell-mediated immunity. Included are patients with chronic lymphoid interstitial pneumonitis. Also included are those patients whose signs or symptoms could be attributed either to HIV infection or to another coexisting disease not classified elsewhere, and patients with other clinical illnesses, the course or management of which may be complicated or altered by HIV infection. Examples include patients with constitutional symptoms not meeting the criteria for subgroup IV-A, patients with infectious diseases not listed in subgroup IV-C, and patients with neoplasms not listed in subgroup IV-D.

■ CDC AIDS CASE DEFINITION FOR SURVEILLANCE: 1987 REVISION

As opposed to the CDC's definition of HIV infection, we now explore its definition for cases of AIDS, the syndrome occupying the far end of the spectrum of problems caused by HIV. The first surveillance definition of an AIDS case used by the CDC was published in *Morbidity and Mortality Weekly Report* in September 1982[15]:

> *A case of a disease at least moderately predictive of a defect in cell-mediated immunity occurring in a person with no known cause for diminished resistance to that disease.*

This general definition of AIDS included a list of specific diseases and qualifications as well as a list of disqualifying conditions that were considered possible causes of non-AIDS-related diminished resistance. After 1982, the definition underwent minor revisions.[16-19] A more substantive revision took place in June 1985, when additional diseases were added to the case definition. At the same time, results from HIV antibody tests and viral cultures began to be employed, thereby increasing the specificity with which AIDS-related diseases could be identified.[20] Even so, the CDC has estimated that its 1985 revisions resulted in reclassification of less than one percent of previously reported cases.[20]

1987 CHANGES IN CDC DEFINITION

In August 1987, the CDC published a major revision of the adult case definition for surveillance, broadening the definition in three ways.[21]

Changes in Adult Case Definition

1. Inclusion of HIV encephalopathy and HIV wasting syndrome.

2. Inclusion of diagnoses made presumptively with laboratory evidence for HIV infection.

3. Elimination of exclusions due to other causes of immunodeficiency with laboratory evidence for HIV infection.

Changes in Pediatric Case Definition

1. Inclusion of multiple or recurrent serious bacterial infections.

2. Inclusion of lymphoid interstitial pneumonia or pulmonary lymphoid hyperplasia in children under 13 years old.

1987 CDC ADULT AND PEDIATRIC CASE DEFINITION FOR SURVEILLANCE PURPOSES

Based on this latest revision, the following are the CDC criteria for defining AIDS in adult and pediatric cases.

For national reporting, a case of AIDS is defined as an illness characterized by one or more of the following "indicator" diseases, depending on the status of laboratory evidence of HIV infection, as shown below.

I. **Without Laboratory Evidence of HIV Infection**
   If laboratory tests for HIV were not performed or gave inconclusive results and the patient had no other cause of immunodeficiency as listed in Section I.A. below, then any disease listed in Section I.B. indicates AIDS if it was diagnosed by a definitive method.

   A. Causes of immunodeficiency that disqualify diseases as indicators of AIDS in the absence of laboratory evidence for HIV infection:

      1. High-dose or long-term systemic corticosteroid therapy or other immunosuppressive or cytotoxic therapy <3 months before the onset of the indicator disease.

      2. Any of the following diseases diagnosed <3 months after diagnosis of the indicator disease: Hodgkin's disease, non-Hodgkin's lymphoma (other than primary brain lymphoma), lymphocytic leukemia, multiple myeloma, any other cancer of lymphoreticular or histiocytic tissue, or angioimmunoblastic lymphadenopathy.

      3. A genetic (congenital) immunodeficiency syndrome or an acquired immunodeficiency syndrome atypical of HIV infection, such as one involving hypogammaglobulinemia.

B. Indicator diseases diagnosed definitively:

      1. Candidiasis of the esophagus, trachea, bronchi, or lungs.

      2. Cryptococcosis, extrapulmonary.

      3. Cryptosporidiosis with diarrhea persisting >1 month.

      4. Cytomegalovirus disease of an organ other than liver, spleen, or lymph nodes in a patient >1 month of age.

      5. Herpes simplex virus infection causing a mucocutaneous ulcer that persists longer than one month; or bronchitis, pneumonitis, or esophagitis for any duration affecting a patient >1 month of age.

      6. Kaposi's sarcoma affecting a patient <60 years of age.

      7. Lymphoma of the brain (primary) affecting a patient <60 years of age.

      8. Lymphoid interstitial pneumonia or pulmonary lymphoid hyperplasia (LIP/PLH complex) affecting a child younger than 13 years of age.

      9. *Mycobacterium avium* complex or *M. kansasii* disease, disseminated (at a site other than or in addition to lungs, skin, or cervical or hilar lymph nodes).

     10. *Pneumocystis carinii* pneumonia.

     11. Progressive multifocal leukoencephalopathy.

     12. Toxoplasmosis of the brain affecting a patient >1 month of age.

II. **With Laboratory Evidence of HIV Infection**

Regardless of the presence of other causes of immunodeficiency (Section I.A., above), in the presence of laboratory evidence of HIV infection, any disease listed above (Section I.B.) or below (Sections II.A. or II.B.) indicates a diagnosis of AIDS.

A. Indicator diseases diagnosed definitively:

      1. Bacterial infections, multiple or recurrent (any combination of at least two within a two-year period), of the following types affecting a child <13 years of age: septicemia, pneumonia, meningitis, bone or joint infection, or abscesses of an internal organ or body cavity (excluding otitis media or superficial skin or mucosal abscesses) caused by haemophilus, streptococcus (including pneumococcus), or other pyogenic bacteria.

      2. Coccidioidomycosis, disseminated (at a site other than or in addition to lungs or cervical or hilar lymph nodes).

      3. HIV encephalopathy (also called "HIV dementia," "AIDS dementia," or "subacute encephalitis due to HIV").

      4. Histoplasmosis, disseminated (at a site other than or in addition to lungs or cervical or hilar lymph nodes).

5. Isosporiasis with diarrhea persisting >1 month.

6. Kaposi's sarcoma at any age.

7. Lymphoma of the brain (primary) at any age.

8. Other non-Hodgkin's lymphoma of B-cell or unknown immuno-logic phenotype and the following histologic types:

 a. Small noncleaved lymphoma (either Burkitt or non-Burkitt type).

 b. Immunoblastic sarcoma (equivalent to any of the following, al-though not necessarily all in combination: immunoblastic lymphoma, large-cell lymphoma, diffuse histiocytic lymphoma, diffuse undifferentiated lymphoma, or high-grade lymphoma.

 [Note: Lymphomas are not included here if they are of T-cell immunologic phenotype or their histologic type is not described, or is described as "lymphocytic," "lymphoblastic," "small cleaved," or "plasmacytoid lymphocytic."]

9. Any mycobacterial disease caused by mycobacteria other than *M. tuberculosis,* disseminated (at a site other than or in addition to lungs, skin, or cervical or hilar lymph nodes).

10. Disease caused by *M. tuberculosis*, extrapulmonary (involving at least one site outside the lungs, regardless of whether there is concurrent pulmonary involvement).

11. Salmonella (nontyphoid) septicemia, recurrent.

12. HIV wasting syndrome (emaciation, "slim disease").

B. Indicator diseases diagnosed presumptively:

[Note: Given the seriousness of diseases indicative of AIDS, it is generally important to diagnose them definitively, especially when therapy that would be used may have serious side effects or when definitive diagnosis is needed for eligibility for antiretroviral therapy. Nonetheless, in some situations, a patient's condition will not permit performance of definitive tests. In other situations, accepted clinical practice may be to diagnose presumptively based on the presence of characteristic clinical and laboratory abnormalities.]

1. Candidiasis of the esophagus.

2. Cytomegalovirus retinitis with loss of vision.

3. Kaposi's sarcoma.

4. Lymphoid interstitial pneumonia or pulmonary lymphoid hyper-plasia (LIP/PLH complex) affecting a child <13 years of age.

5. Mycobacterial disease (acid-fast bacilli with species not identified by culture), disseminated (involving at least one site other than or in addition to lungs, skin, or cervical or hilar lymph nodes).

6. *Pneumocystis carinii* pneumonia.

7. Toxoplasmosis of the brain affecting a patient >1 month of age.

III. With Laboratory Evidence against HIV Infection

With laboratory test results negative for HIV infection, a diagnosis of AIDS for surveillance purposes is ruled out unless:

A. All the other causes of immunodeficiency listed above in Section I.A. are excluded; AND

B. The patient has had either

    1. *Pneumocystis carinii* pneumonia diagnosed by a definitive method; OR

    2. **a.** any of the other diseases indicative of AIDS listed above in Section I.B. diagnosed by a definitive method; AND

        b. a T-helper/inducer (CD4) lymphocyte count <400/cubic mm.

■ LABORATORY EVIDENCE FOR OR AGAINST HIV INFECTION

What follows is an attempt to sort out the laboratory-based indications for or against infection with HIV.

LABORATORY EVIDENCE FOR INFECTION

When a patient has disease consistent with AIDS:

a. a serum specimen from a patient >15 months of age, or from a child <15 months of age whose mother is not thought to have had HIV infection during the child's perinatal period, that is repeatedly reactive for HIV antibody by a screening test (e.g., enzyme-linked immunosorbent assay [ELISA]), as long as subsequent HIV-antibody tests (e.g., Western blot, immunofluorescence assay), if done, are positive; OR

b. a serum specimen from a child <15 months of age, whose mother is thought to have had HIV infection during the child's perinatal period, that is repeatedly reactive for HIV antibody by a screening test (e.g., ELISA), plus increased serum immunoglobulin levels and at least one of the following abnormal immunologic test results:

- reduced absolute lymphocyte count

- depressed CD4 (T-helper) lymphocyte count

- decreased CD4/CD8 (helper/suppressor ratio) as long as subsequent antibody tests (e.g., Western blot, immunofluorescence assay), if done, are positive; OR

c. a positive test for HIV serum antigen; OR

d. a positive HIV culture confirmed by both reverse transcriptase detection and a specific HIV-antigen test or in situ hybridization using a nucleic acid probe; OR

e. a positive result on any other highly specific test for HIV (e.g., nucleic acid probe of peripheral blood lymphocytes).

LABORATORY EVIDENCE AGAINST INFECTION

A nonreactive screening test for serum antibody to HIV (e.g., ELISA) without a reactive or positive result on any other test for HIV infection (e.g., antibody, antigen, culture), if done.

INCONCLUSIVE EVIDENCE (NEITHER FOR NOR AGAINST INFECTION)

a. a repeatedly reactive screening test for serum antibody to HIV (e.g., ELISA) followed by a negative or inconclusive supplemental test (e.g., Western blot, immunofluorescence assay) without a positive HIV culture or serum antigen test, if done; OR

b. a serum specimen from a child <15 months of age, whose mother is thought to have had HIV infection during the child's perinatal period, that is repeatedly reactive for HIV antibody by a screening test, even if positive by a supplemental test, without additional evidence for immunodeficiency as described above (in I.b.) and without a positive HIV culture or serum antigen test, if done.

■ DEFINITIVE DIAGNOSTIC METHODS FOR DISEASES INDICATIVE OF AIDS

The following methods have been designated as definitive by the CDC for diagnosis of diseases indicative of AIDS.[23]

TABLE 2.

DISEASES	DEFINITIVE DIAGNOSTIC METHODS
Cryptosporidiosis	Microscopy (histology or cytology)
Cytomegalovirus	Microscopy (histology or cytology)
Isosporiasis	Microscopy (histology or cytology)
Kaposi's sarcoma	Microscopy (histology or cytology)
Lymphoma	Microscopy (histology or cytology)
Lymphoid pneumonia or hyperplasia	Microscopy (histology or cytology)
Pneumocystis carinii pneumonia	Microscopy (histology or cytology)
Progressive multifocal leukoencephalopathy	Microscopy (histology or cytology)
Toxoplasmosis	Microscopy (histology or cytology)
Candidiasis	Gross inspection by endoscopy or by microscopy (histology or cytology) on a specimen obtained directly from the tissues affected (including scrapings from the mucosal surface), not from a culture
Coccidioidomycosis, cryptococcosis, herpes simplex virus, and histoplasmosis	Microscopy (histology or cytology), culture, or detection of antigen in a specimen obtained directly from the tissues affected or a fluid from those tissues
Tuberculosis	Culture
Other mycobacteriosis	Culture
Salmonellosis	Culture
Other bacterial infection	Culture

continued on next page

continued from previous page

TABLE 2.

DISEASES	DEFINITIVE DIAGNOSTIC METHODS
HIV encephalopathy (dementia)*	Clinical findings of disabling cognitive and/or motor dysfunction interfering with occupation or activities of daily living, or loss of behavioral developmental milestones affecting a child, progressing over weeks to months, in the absence of a concurrent illness or condition other than HIV infection that could explain the findings. Methods to rule out such concurrent illnesses and conditions must include cerebrospinal fluid examination and either brain imaging (computed tomography or magnetic resonance) or autopsy.
HIV wasting syndrome*	Findings of profound involuntary weight loss >10 percent of baseline body weight plus either chronic diarrhea (at least two loose stools per day for >30 days) or chronic weakness and documented fever (for >30 days, intermittent or constant) in the absence of a concurrent illness or condition other than HIV infection that could explain the findings (e.g., cancer, tuberculosis, cryptosporidiosis, or other specific enteritis).

* *For HIV encephalopathy and HIV wasting syndrome, the methods of diagnosis described here are not truly definitive, but are sufficiently rigorous for surveillance purposes.*

■ SUGGESTED GUIDELINES FOR PRESUMPTIVE DIAGNOSIS OF DISEASES INDICATIVE OF AIDS

The following guidelines for presumptive diagnosis of diseases indicative of AIDS have been established by the CDC in its 1987 revisions.[24]

Candidiasis of esophagus

Recent onset of retrosternal pain on swallowing, and oral candidiasis diagnosed by the gross appearance of white patches or plaques on an erythematous base or by the microscopic appearance of fungal mycelial filaments in an uncultured specimen scraped from the oral mucosa.

Cytomegalovirus retinitis

A characteristic appearance on serial ophthalmoscopic examinations (e.g., discrete patches of retinal whitening with distinct borders, spreading in a centrifugal manner, following blood vessels, progressing over several months, frequently associated with retinal vasculitis, hemorrhage, and necrosis). Resolution of active disease leaves retinal scarring and atrophy with retinal pigment epithelial mottling.

Mycobacteriosis

Microscopy of a specimen from stool or normally sterile body fluids or tissue from a site other than lungs, skin, or cervical or hilar lymph nodes, showing acid-fast bacilli of a species not identified by culture.

Kaposi's sarcoma

A characteristic gross appearance of an erythematous or violaceous plaque-like lesion on skin or mucous membrane. Presumptive diagnosis of Kaposi's sarcoma should not be made by clinicians who have seen few cases of it.

Lymphoid interstitial pneumonia

Bilateral reticulonodular interstitial pulmonary infiltrates present on chest x-ray for >2 months with no pathogen identified and no response to antibiotic treatment.

Pneumocystis carinii *pneumonia*

(a) A history of dyspnea on exertion or nonproductive cough of recent onset (within the past three months); and (b) chest x-ray evidence of diffuse bilateral interstitial infiltrates or gallium scan evidence of diffuse bilateral pulmonary disease; and (c) arterial blood gas analysis showing an arterial oxygen partial pressure of <70 mm Hg or a low respiratory diffusing capacity (<80 percent of predicted values) or an increase in the alveolar-arterial oxygen tension gradient; and (d) no evidence of a bacterial pneumonia.

Toxoplasmosis of the brain

(a) Recent onset of a focal neurologic brain abnormality consistent with intracranial disease or a reduced level of consciousness; and (b) brain-imaging evidence of a lesion having a mass effect (on computed tomography or magnetic resonance imaging) or the radiographic appearance of which is enhanced by injection of contrast medium; and (c) serum antibody to toxoplasmosis or successful response to therapy for toxoplasmosis.

■ EQUIVALENT TERMS AND INTERNATIONAL CLASSIFICATION OF DISEASE (ICD) CODES FOR AIDS-INDICATIVE LYMPHOMAS

The CDC has defined the following terms and codes to describe lymphomas indicative of AIDS in patients with antibody evidence for HIV infection.[25] Many of these terms are obsolete or equivalent to one another.

TABLE 3. ICD-9-CM (1978)

CODES	TERMS
200.0	**Reticulosarcoma** lymphoma (malignant): histiocytic (diffuse) reticulum cell sarcoma: pleomorphic cell type or not otherwise specified
200.2	**Burkitt's tumor or lymphoma** malignant lymphoma, Burkitt's type

TABLE 4.   ICD-O (ONCOLOGIC HISTOLOGIC TYPES 1976)

CODES	TERMS
9600/3	**Malignant lymphoma, undifferentiated cell type** non-Burkitt's or not otherwise specified
9601/3	**Malignant lymphoma, stem-cell type** stem-cell lymphoma
9612/3	**Malignant lymphoma, immunoblastic type** immunoblastic sarcoma, immunoblastic lymphoma, or immunoblastic lymphosarcoma
9632/3	**Malignant lymphoma, centroblastic type** diffuse or not otherwise specified, or germinoblastic sarcoma: diffuse or not otherwise specified
9633/3	**Malignant lymphoma, follicular center cell, non-cleaved** diffuse or not otherwise specified
9640/3	**Reticulosarcoma, not otherwise specified** malignant lymphoma, histiocytic: diffuse or not otherwise specified reticulum cell sarcoma, not otherwise specified malignant lymphoma, reticulum cell type
9641/3	**Reticulosarcoma, pleomorphic cell type** malignant lymphoma, histiocytic, pleomorphic cell type reticulum cell sarcoma, pleomorphic cell type
9750/3	**Burkitt's lymphoma or Burkitt's tumor** malignant lymphoma, undifferentiated, Burkitt's type malignant lymphoma, lymphoblastic, Burkitt's type

REFERENCES

1. Gallo RC, Salahuddin SZ, Popovic M, et al. Frequent detection and isolation of cytopathic retroviruses (HTLV-III) from patients with AIDS and at risk for AIDS. Science 1984; 224:500-3.
2. Barre-Sinoussi F, Chermann JC, Rey F, et al. Isolation of a T-lymphotropic retrovirus from a patient at risk for acquired immune deficiency syndrome (AIDS). Science 1983; 220:868-71.
3. Levy JA, Hoffman AD, Kramer SM, et al. Isolation of lymphocytopathic retroviruses from San Francisco patients with AIDS. Science 1984; 225:840-2.
4. Coffin J, Haase A, Levy JA, et al. Human immunodeficiency viruses. Science 1986; 232:697.
5. Centers for Disease Control. Current trends: classification system for human T lymphotropic virus type III/lymphadenopathy associated virus infections. MMWR 1986; 35:334-9.
6. Centers for Disease Control. Antibodies to a retrovirus etiologically associated with acquired immuno-deficiency syndrome (AIDS) in populations with increased incidences of the syndrome. MMWR 1984; 33:377-9.
7. Centers for Disease Control. Update: Public Health Service workshop on human T-lymphotropic virus type III antibody testing — United States. MMWR 1985; 34:477-8.
8. Centers for Disease Control. Additional recommendations to reduce sexual and drug abuse-related transmission of human T lymphotropic virus type III/lymphadenopathy-associated virus. MMWR 1986; 35:152-5.
9. Selik RM, Haverkos HW, Curran JW. Acquired immune deficiency syndrome (AIDS) trends in the United States, 1978-1982. Am J Med 1984; 76:493-500.
10. Sarngadharan MG, Popovic M, Bruch L, et al. Antibodies reactive with human T-lymphotropic retro-viruses (HTLV-III) in the serum of patients with AIDS. Science 1984; 224:506-8.
11. Safai B, Sarngadharan MG, Groopman JE, et al. Seroepidemiological studies of human T-lymphotropic retrovirus type III in acquired immunodeficiency syndrome. Lancet 1984; 1:1438-40.
12. Laurence J, Brun-Vezinet F, Schutzer SE, et al. Lymphadenopathy associated viral antibody in AIDS. Immune correlations and definition of a carrier state. N Engl J Med 1984; 311:1269-73.
13. Ho DD, Sarngadharan MG, Resnick L, et al. Primary human T-lymphotropic virus type III infection. Ann Intern Med 1985; 103:880-3.
14. Cooper DA, Gold J, Maclean P, et al. Acute AIDS retrovirus infection. Definition of a clinical illness associated with seroconversion. Lancet 1985; 1:537-40.

15. Centers for Disease Control. Update on acquired immune deficiency syndrome (AIDS) — United States. MMWR 1982; 31:507-14.

16. Jaffe HW, Bregman DJ, Selik RM. Acquired immune deficiency syndrome in the United States: first 1,000 cases. J Infect Dis 1983; 148:339-45.

17. Jaffe HW, Selik RM. Acquired immune deficiency syndrome: is disseminated aspergillosis predictive of underlying cellular immune deficiency? J Infect Dis 1984; 149:829.

18. Selik RM, Haverkos HW, Curran JW. Acquired immune deficiency syndrome (AIDS) trends in the United States, 1978-1982. Am J Med 1984; 76:493-500.

19. Centers for Disease Control. Update: acquired immunodeficiency syndrome (AIDS) — United States. MMWR 1984; 32:688-91.

20. Centers for Disease Control. Revision of the case definition of acquired immunodeficiency syndrome for national reporting — United States. MMWR 1985; 34:373-5.

21. Centers for Disease Control. Revision of the CDC surveillance case definition of acquired immuno-deficiency syndrome. MMWR 1987; 36(Suppl 1):3S-15S.

22. Centers for Disease Control. Revision of the CDC surveillance case definition for acquired immuno-deficiency syndrome. Appendix I. Laboratory evidence for and against HIV infection. MMWR 1987; 36:10S.

23. Centers for Disease Control. Revision of the AIDS surveillance case definition for acquired immuno-deficiency syndrome. Appendix II. Definitive diagnostic methods for diseases indicative of AIDS. MMWR 1987; 36:11S-12S.

24. Centers for Disease Control. Revision of the CDC surveillance case definition for acquired immuno-deficiency syndrome. Appendix III. Suggested guidelines for presumptive diagnosis of diseases indicative of AIDS. MMWR 1987; 36:13S-14S.

25. Centers for Disease Control. Revision of the AIDS surveillance case definition for acquired immuno-deficiency syndrome. Appendix IV. Equivalent terms and international classification of disease (ICD) codes for AIDS-indicative lymphomas. MMWR 1987; 36:15S.

1.1.2

Numbers and Demographic Characteristics of U.S. Cases

Dennis Osmond

The tables in this document are from data released by the Centers for Disease Control (CDC) in their monthly surveillance reports. They therefore include only manifestations of human immunodeficiency virus (HIV) infection that meet the CDC definition of AIDS for surveillance purposes. Since the CDC began monitoring the epidemic in 1981, the race, age, and sex distributions of adult AIDS cases have not changed significantly over time.[1] However, the distribution of reported diseases has changed. The frequency with which *Pneumocystis carinii* pneumonia is reported has increased, whereas the frequency of Kaposi's sarcoma has declined from 21 percent of diagnoses before 1985 to 10 percent during 1987.[1] Proportions of cases attributed to known risk groups also have not changed over time, with the exception of transfusion associated cases, which have risen from a fraction of one percent to over two percent for the year ending March 2, 1987.[1] The apparent increase noted in August 1986 in cases attributed to heterosexual contact (4 percent of all cases compared with 2 percent in July 1986) is due to a revision of that category, which added Haitian cases from the "None of the above/other" category. The combined percent in the two categories, "Heterosexual contact" and "Undetermined," has remained about 7 percent since early in the epidemic.

Geographic distribution of cases by risk group is disproportionate. A preponderance of reported cases in intravenous drug users (IVDUs) is from New York and New Jersey. In New York nearly 30 percent of reported cases are in IVDUs, whereas in San Francisco only 1 percent of cases are among heterosexual IVDUs.[2] Distribution of cases by racial or ethnic group is also disproportionate. Blacks and Hispanics account for 43 percent of all AIDS cases, but make up only 18 percent of the U.S. population.[3,4] Distribution of disease type by risk group is also disproportionate. Kaposi's sarcoma is reported primarily in homosexual men and infrequently in IVDUs.

The category of homosexual or bisexual men includes men who also admit drug use. Currently, 8 percent of all cases are in this category. In the tables of cases by risk group, the groups are listed hierarchically; that is, a case with more than one characteristic is listed only in the first group.

TABLE 1.   UNITED STATES AIDS CASES REPORTED TO THE CDC AS OF 1-30-89 BY DISEASE GROUP

DISEASE GROUP	CASES (%)	DEATHS (%)
PCP	50,670 (60)	29,730 (59)
Other opportunistic diseases	26,867 (32)	15,056 (56)
Kaposi's sarcoma	7,448 (9)	3,796 (51)
Total	84,985 (100)	48,582 (57)

Source: Centers for Disease Control. AIDS Weekly Surveillance Report, January 30, 1989.

TABLE 2.   UNITED STATES AIDS CASES REPORTED TO THE CDC AS OF 10-31-89 BY RACE/ETHNICITY

RACE/ETHNICITY	CASES	PERCENT
White, not Hispanic	63,293	56
Black, not Hispanic	30,643	27
Hispanic	17,199	15
Asian/Pacific Islander	687	1
Indian/Alaskan Native	150	0
Other/Unknown	269	0
Total	112,241	100

Source: Centers for Disease Control. HIV/AIDS Surveillance Report, November 1989.

TABLE 3.   UNITED STATES AIDS CASES REPORTED TO THE CDC AS OF 10-31-89 BY AGE

AGE	CASES	PERCENT
Males		
Under 5	810	1
5–12	229	0
13–19	352	0
20–24	4,159	4
25–29	15,960	16
30–34	24,773	24
35–39	22,344	22
40–44	14,214	14
45–49	8,105	8
50–54	4,671	5
55–59	2,947	3
60–64	1,529	2

continued on next page

continued from previous page

TABLE 3.   UNITED STATES AIDS CASES REPORTED TO THE
CDC AS OF 10-31-89 BY AGE

AGE	CASES	PERCENT
65 or older	1,271	1
Male Subtotal	**101,364**	**100**
Females		
Under 5	756	7
5–12	113	1
13–19	87	1
20–24	700	6
25–29	2,098	19
30–34	2,778	26
35–39	1,926	18
40–44	938	9
45–49	435	4
50–54	275	3
55–59	212	2
60–64	180	2
65 or older	379	3
Female Subtotal	**10,877**	**100**
Total	**112,241**	

Source: Centers for Disease Control. HIV/AIDS Surveillance Report, November 1989.

TABLE 4.   UNITED STATES AIDS CASES REPORTED TO THE
CDC AS OF 10-31-89 BY PATIENT GROUPS
(ADULTS/ADOLESCENTS)

PATIENT GROUPS	CASES	PERCENT
Homosexual or bisexual men	67,096	61
Intravenous (IV) drug abuser	22,822	21
Homosexual male and IV drug abuser	7,749	7
Hemophilia/coagulation disorder	1,034	1
Heterosexual cases	5,242	5
Transfusion, blood/components	2,708	2
Undetermined	3,682	3
Total	**110,333**	**100**

Source: Centers for Disease Control. HIV/AIDS Surveillance Report, November 1989.

TABLE 5. UNITED STATES AIDS CASES REPORTED TO THE CDC AS OF 10-31-89 BY SEXUAL COMPOSITION OF PATIENT GROUP (ADULTS/ADOLESCENTS)

PATIENT GROUPS BY SEX	MALES (%)	FEMALES (%)
Homosexual or bisexual men	67,096 (67)	
Intravenous (IV) drug abuser	17,635 (18)	5,187 (52)
Homosexual male and IV drug abuser	7,749 (8)	
Hemophilia/coagulation disorder	1,007 (1)	27 (0)
Heterosexual cases	2,160 (2)	3,082 (31)
Transfusion, blood/components	1,687 (2)	1,021 (10)
Undetermined	2,991 (3)	691 (7)
Total	**100,325 (91)**	**10,008 (9)**

Source: Centers for Disease Control. HIV/AIDS Surveillance Report, November 1989.

TABLE 6. UNITED STATES AIDS CASES REPORTED TO THE CDC AS OF 10-31-89 BY PATIENT GROUP (PEDIATRIC)

PATIENT GROUP	N	PERCENT
Hemophilia/coagulation disorder	103	5
Parent with/at risk of AIDS	1,541	81
Transfusion, blood/components	206	11
Undetermined	58	3
Total	**1,908**	**100**

Source: Centers for Disease Control. HIV/AIDS Surveillance Report, November 1989.

REFERENCES

1. Centers for Disease Control. AIDS weekly surveillance report — United States AIDS Program. 1987 (March 2):1-5.
2. San Francisco Department of Public Health. Acquired immunodeficiency syndrome (AIDS) monthly surveillance report. Cases reported through March 31, 1987.
3. Centers for Disease Control. HIV/AIDS Surveillance Report, July 1989.
4. Department of Commerce, Bureau of the Census. Population by Race, 1980 Census.

International Epidemiology of AIDS

Dennis Osmond

■ EUROPE

A IDS cases following the CDC case definition have been reported to the World Health Organization (WHO) European Collaborating Centre from all the countries of Western Europe and most countries of Eastern Europe. The surveillance data below are from the World Health Organization and the totals include persons from the Caribbean islands and Africa who were diagnosed in Europe.

TABLE 1. EUROPEAN REGION
AIDS CASES REPORTED TO WHO BY COUNTRY BASED ON
REPORTS RECEIVED THROUGH 31/10/89

COUNTRY	1979–1986 CASES	1987 CASES	RATE (a)	1988 CASES	RATE (b)	1989 CASES	LAST REPORT	CUMUL. CASES
Albania	0	0	0.0	0	0.0	0	31/03/89	0
Austria	55	85	1.1	117	1.6	75	30/09/89	332*
Belgium	242	104	1.1	120	1.2	53	30/06/89	519
Bulgaria	1	2	0.0	0	0.0	0	31/03/89	3
Czechoslovakia	6	2	0.0	4	0.0	5	30/06/89	17
Denmark	142	98	1.9	124	2.4	106	30/09/89	470*
Finland	17	7	0.1	17	0.3	5	30/06/89	46
France	1923	1982	3.6	2486	4.5	758	30/06/89	7149
German Dem. Republic	1	5	0.0	5	0.0	3	30/06/89	14
Germany Fed. Rep.	1063	995	1.6	1134	1.9	680	30/09/89	3872*
Greece	35	53	0.5	82	0.8	56	30/06/89	226
Hungary	1	7	0.1	9	0.1	11	30/09/89	28*
Iceland	4	0	0.0	6	2.5	2	30/06/89	12
Ireland	17	20	0.6	37	1.0	26	30/06/89	100
Israel	43	14	0.3	20	0.5	8	30/06/89	85
Italy	665	1012	1.8	1660	2.9	821	30/06/89	4158
Luxembourg	6	3	0.8	4	1.1	5	30/06/89	18
Malta	5	2	0.6	7	2.0	0	31/03/89	14
Monaco	0	1	3.7	3	11.1	0	31/12/88	4
Netherlands	243	235	1.6	290	2.0	215	30/09/89	983*
Norway	35	35	0.8	30	0.7	29	10/10/89	129*
Poland	1	2	0.0	2	0.0	17	30/09/89	22*
Portugal	52	50	0.5	82	0.8	122	30/09/89	306*

continued on next page

continued from previous page

TABLE 1. EUROPEAN REGION
AIDS CASES REPORTED TO WHO BY COUNTRY BASED ON
REPORTS RECEIVED THROUGH 31/10/89

COUNTRY	1979–1986 CASES	1987 CASES	RATE (a)	1988 CASES	RATE (b)	1989 CASES	LAST REPORT	CUMUL. CASES
Romania	2	1	0.0	7	0.0	0	31/03/89	10
San Marino	0	0	0.0	0	0.0	1	30/06/89	1
Spain	610	822	2.1	1499	3.9	455	30/06/89	3386
Sweden	101	77	0.9	82	1.0	80	30/09/89	340*
Switzerland	254	221	3.4	332	5.1	189	31/08/89	996*
Turkey	3	8	0.0	9	0.0	4	30/06/89	24
UK	792	604	1.1	678	1.2	575	30/09/89	2649†
USSR	1	4	0.0	2	0.0	0	30/06/89	7
Yugoslavia	8	18	0.1	39	0.2	29	29/09/89	94*
Total for the Region	6328	6469	0.8	8887	1.1	4330		26,014

(a) Rate: Reported cases/100,000 population
(b) 1988 Reporting generally incomplete
* *Updated report*
† *UK has revised its previous report of 2651 cases to 2649.*
  Source: World Health Organization

■ EUROPEAN AND UNITED STATES CASES COMPARED

AIDS cases in Western Europe have an epidemiologic pattern similar to that seen in the United States. The majority of cases are among homosexual or bisexual men, followed by intravenous drug users (IVDU), who represent between 15 percent and 20 percent of all cases. As in the United States, there is considerable regional variation in the distribution of cases by risk group. In most of Northern Europe, as in the western U.S., homosexual or bisexual men account for the majority of cases. In Southern Europe, as in the eastern U.S., IVDUs account for a much larger proportion of reported cases. In Italy and Spain, heterosexual IVDUs account for more than 50 percent of all cases. Cases among those with a hemophilia/coagulation disorder are more prevalent in Europe (4 percent of all cases versus 1 percent in the U.S). European cases without known risk factors accounted for 8 percent versus 3 percent in the U.S.[1] This difference may be due to persons from Africa or the Caribbean who were diagnosed in Europe and counted in the WHO surveillance.

A comparison of disease characteristics of European cases also shows them to be similar to U.S. cases. *Pneumocystis carinii* pneumonia is the most common opportunistic infection in both Europe and the U.S. and the other major manifestations of HIV disease, with some variation, are seen with frequencies approximating the clinical picture in the U.S.[1]

Cases that appear to have been AIDS have been identified retrospectively in Europe as early as 1977[2,3]; however, these cases were in persons who probably were infected in Africa. They were Europeans who had worked in Africa or Africans who had emigrated to Europe. (The CDC reports 82 cases before 1981 in the U.S.)

■ CANADA, AUSTRALIA, AND NEW ZEALAND

The epidemiologic pattern of AIDS in these countries is very similar to the pattern in the U.S. and Western Europe with the majority of cases seen in homosexual or bisexual men. The epidemic was manifested early in Australia, which continues to be among the countries reporting the largest numbers of cases.[6]

TABLE 2.

COUNTRY	CUMULATIVE NUMBER OF CASES (10/31/89)	1988 CASE RATE*
Canada	2867	2.9
Australia	1498	2.9
New Zealand	144	1.1

*   *1988 Cases/100,000 population*   *1988 Reporting generally incomplete*
    Source: World Health Organization

■ ASIA AND THE PACIFIC ISLANDS

Only a few cases of AIDS have been reported from Asia and the Pacific Islands; the first cases were attributed to the use of blood products from the United States. The recently noted rapid rise in HIV seroprevalence among prostitutes in Bangkok may signal the beginning of significant heterosexual spread in Asia.[7]

TABLE 3. SOUTHEAST ASIA REGION
AIDS CASES REPORTED TO WHO BY COUNTRY BASED ON
REPORTS RECEIVED THROUGH 31/10/1989

COUNTRY	1979–1986 CASES	1987 CASES	RATE (a)	1988 CASES	RATE (b)	1989 CASES	LAST REPORT	CUMUL. CASES
Bangladesh	0	0	0.0	0	0.0	0	30/09/89	0*
Bhutan	0	0	0.0	0	0.0	0	30/09/89	0*
Burma (see Myanmar)								
Dem. P. Rep. of Korea	0	0	0.0	0	0.0	0	30/09/89	0*
India	5	4	0.0	19	0.0	4	30/09/89	32*
Indonesia	0	1	0.0	2	0.0	3	01/10/89	6*
Maldives	0	0	0.0	0	0.0	0	30/09/89	0*
Mongolia	0	0	0.0	0	0.0	0	15/09/89	0*
Myanmar	0	0	0.0	0	0.0	0	30/09/89	0*
Nepal	0	0	0.0	2	0.0	0	30/10/89	2*
Sri Lanka	0	1	0.0	2	0.0	0	31/12/88	3
Thailand	2	6	0.0	4	0.0	13	30/09/89	25*
Total for the Region	7	12	0.0	29	0.0	20		68

(a) Rate: Reported cases/100,000 population   *(b) 1988 Reporting generally incomplete*
*   *Updated report*
    Source: World Health Organization

TABLE 4. WESTERN PACIFIC REGION
AIDS CASES REPORTED TO WHO BY COUNTRY BASED ON
REPORTS RECEIVED THROUGH 31/10/1989

COUNTRY	1979–1986 CASES	1987 CASES	RATE (a)	1988 CASES	RATE (b)	1989 CASES	LAST REPORT	CUMUL. CASES
Australia	384	365	2.3	463	2.9	286	04/10/89	1498*
Brunei Darussalam	0	0	0.0	1	0.4	0	01/06/89	1
China	1	1	0.0	1	0.0	0	30/09/88	3
Cook Islands	0	0	0.0	0	0.0	0	08/09/87	0
Fiji	0	0	0.0	0	0.0	2	21/06/89	2
French Polynesia	0	1	0.5	6	3.3	1	17/07/89	8
Hong Kong	4	5	0.1	7	0.1	6	25/07/89	22*
Japan	25	34	0.0	31	0.0	18	26/09/89	108*
Kiribati	0	0	0.0	0	0.0	0	18/01/88	0
Malaysia	1	1	0.0	2	0.0	6	31/07/89	10
Mariana Islands	0	0	0.0	0	0.0	0	05/08/87	0
New Caledonia	0	0	0.0	2	1.3	0	01/08/88	2
New Zealand	33	30	0.9	37	1.1	44	14/09/89	144
Papua New Guinea	0	1	0.0	7	0.2	5	28/06/89	13
Philippines	3	9	0.0	8	0.0	6	31/07/89	26
Republic of Korea	0	1	0.0	3	0.0	0	10/09/88	4
Samoa	0	0	0.0	0	0.0	0	18/10/88	0
Singapore	2	2	0.1	6	0.2	3	26/07/89	13
Solomon Islands	0	0	0.0	0	0.0	0	08/09/87	0
Taiwan, China	1	0	0.0	0	0.0	0	26/01/86	1
Tonga	0	1	1.0	0	0.0	0	01/08/88	1
Tuvalu	0	0	0.0	0	0.0	0	08/09/87	0
Vanuatu	0	0	0.0	0	0.0	0	25/01/89	0
Viet Nam	0	0	0.0	0	0.0	0	08/09/87	0
Total for the Region	454	451	0.0	574	0.0	377		1856

(a) Rate: Reported cases/100,000 population
(b) 1988 Reporting generally incomplete
*   *Updated report*
   Source: World Health Organization

■ CARIBBEAN

AIDS in the Caribbean, particularly in Haiti, has a distinct epidemiologic profile — predominantly heterosexual spread — which is similar to the pattern
seen in Africa and in contrast to the U.S./European pattern of predominantly
homosexual spread (see Figure 1.1.3.a). Intravenous drug use is reported much
less frequently in the Caribbean cases than it is in U.S./European cases.[11]

■ HAITI

Haiti was a focus of particular attention early in the epidemic because many of
the first cases recognized in the U.S. were among Haitian immigrants living in
East Coast cities. These individuals had no apparent high-risk factors for infection.[9,11] As a consequence, Haitians with AIDS were listed as a separate risk
group by the Centers for Disease Control until 1985, when the CDC began to

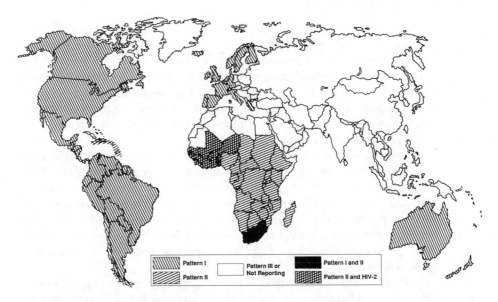

Figure 1.1.3.a   Three infection patterns of HIV-1 are apparent worldwide. Pattern I is found in North and South America, Western Europe, Scandinavia, Australia, and New Zealand. In these areas about 90 percent of the cases are homosexual males or users of intravenous drugs. Pattern II is found in Africa, the Caribbean, and some areas of South America; the primary mode of transmission in these regions is heterosexual sex and the number of infected females and males is approximately equal. Pattern III is typical of Eastern Europe, North Africa, the Middle East, Asia, and the Pacific (excluding Australia and New Zealand); there are relatively few cases and most of them have had contact with pattern-I or pattern-II countries. HIV-2 infection is most common in West Africa and Cape Verde. Adapted from *Scientific American* 1988; 259(4):84.

list cases in Haitian immigrants with others that did not have an identified risk factor. Haitian cases in the U.S. among persons born in Haiti and without a known risk for infection are now included among the cases attributed to heterosexual contact.

AIDS appeared as a new disease in Haiti at approximately the same time as in the United States.[8,9] No evidence exists that AIDS originated in Haiti. Reports from clinicians in Haiti and the incidence of AIDS in recent immigrants (compared with earlier Haitian immigrants to the United States) indicate that the disease is new to Haiti. Recent immigrants have a 40-fold higher incidence of AIDS than earlier immigrants.[10] There is no evidence that Haitians have any special susceptibility to AIDS.

Malnutrition was suspected as an etiologic factor in Haitian immigrants with AIDS, but clinical evidence did not support malnutrition as the primary source of immunosuppression.[11] Subsequently, heterosexual transmission was suspected as a major route of spread. A case–control study of AIDS cases in Haiti identified the number of heterosexual contacts as a risk factor[12]; a similar study of cases among Haitians in the United States found sexual contact with a heterosexual prostitute and a history of gonorrhea as risk factors.[13] One report of a cluster of three cases suggested male-to-female-to-male transmission.[14]

Sexual practices (both homosexual and heterosexual), blood transfusion, and intravenous drug use have been reported, and intramuscular injection of medications with unsterile needles has been suggested, as routes of transmission of HIV in Haiti.[12,13,15] Homosexuality (38 percent of male cases in one series in Haiti[15]) is reported much less frequently among Haitians with AIDS who moved to the United States.[13] This lower incidence of homosexuality may be due to underreporting, since investigators in Haiti found that they were able to identify risk factors in 65 percent of patients after undertaking a systematic evaluation with a standard questionnaire; risk factors were identified in only 20 percent before the procedures were improved.[15] Male cases outnumber female in Haiti by about 3 to 1,[10] versus the 14-to-1 ratio in the United States and the less than 2-to-1 ratio in Africa. Heterosexual transmission is more common in Haiti than in the United States; homosexual transmission is reported more often in Haiti than in Africa.

Clinically, Haitians with AIDS exhibit the same underlying deficiency in cellular immunity as seen in Americans and Europeans with AIDS. As in Africans with AIDS, disease presentations include a higher incidence of candida, cryptosporidium, and isospora infections and a much lower incidence of pneumocystis pneumonia (7 percent incidence of pneumocystis in 131 cases in Haiti versus 71 percent in 80 non-Haitian cases from New York City). Like AIDS in Africa, AIDS in Haiti reflects exposure to different common pathogens than those reported in the United States.

Although Haiti has reported the largest number of cases among Caribbean countries (2041 cases), followed by the Dominican Republic with 856, the case rate per 100,000 is lower than in several other Caribbean countries. The table below gives reported cases and case rates as of October 31, 1989.

■ LATIN AMERICA

The pattern of AIDS in Latin America is similar to the U.S. pattern: a majority of cases are homosexual or bisexual men and the highest incidence rate is in the major cities. Brazil has reported the largest number of cases in Latin America. As in Europe, the epidemic in Latin America appears to be two or three years behind the U.S. epidemic.

TABLE 5. AMERICAN REGION (INCLUDING THE CARIBBEAN AND LATIN AMERICA) AIDS CASES REPORTED TO WHO BY COUNTRY BASED ON REPORTS RECEIVED THROUGH 31/10/1989

COUNTRY	1979–1986 CASES	1987 CASES	RATE (a)	1988 CASES	RATE (b)	1989 CASES	LAST REPORT	CUMUL. CASES
Anguilla	0	0	0.0	3	30.0	0	31/03/89	3
Antigua Barbuda	2	1	1.2	0	0.0	0	31/03/89	3
Argentina	69	72	0.2	174	0.6	27	31/03/89	342
Bahamas	86	90	36.7	93	38.0	39	31/03/89	308
Barbados	31	24	9.5	15	5.9	14	31/03/89	84
Belize	1	6	3.4	4	2.3	0	30/09/88	11
Bermuda	51	21	36.8	28	49.1	13	30/06/89	113
Bolivia	3	2	0.0	11	0.2	0	30/09/88	16
Brazil	1469	1971	1.5	2936	2.2	1411	02/09/89	7787*
British Virgin Is.	0	0	0.0	1	10.0	0	31/03/89	1
Canada	1093	755	3.0	748	2.9	271	08/08/89	2867
Cayman Islands	2	1	5.9	1	5.9	0	31/12/88	4
Chile	23	45	0.4	55	0.5	26	30/06/89	149*
Colombia	81	107	0.4	120	0.4	0	30/09/88	308
Costa Rica	20	23	0.9	50	1.9	13	31/03/89	106

continued on next page

continued from previous page

TABLE 5. AMERICAN REGION (INCLUDING THE CARIBBEAN AND LATIN AMERICA) AIDS CASES REPORTED TO WHO BY COUNTRY BASED ON REPORTS RECEIVED THROUGH 31/10/1989

COUNTRY	1979–1986 CASES	1987 CASES	RATE (a)	1988 CASES	RATE (b)	1989 CASES	LAST REPORT	CUMUL. CASES
Cuba	0	27	0.3	24	0.2	0	31/12/88	51
Dominica	0	6	6.9	0	0.0	0	31/12/88	6
Dominican Republic	115	294	4.6	292	4.6	155	31/03/89	856
Ecuador	11	19	0.2	15	0.2	0	30/06/88	45
El Salvador	7	16	0.3	48	1.0	0	31/12/88	71
French Guiana	74	29	33.0	28	31.8	19	30/06/89	150
Grenada	3	5	4.8	3	2.9	0	31/12/88	11
Guadeloupe	45	37	11.1	40	12.0	0	31/12/88	122
Guatemala	18	16	0.2	13	0.2	0	31/12/88	47
Guyana	0	14	1.5	36	3.8	6	31/03/89	56
Haiti	795	477	8.1	687	11.6	82	31/03/89	2041
Honduras	15	66	1.5	130	3.0	39	31/03/89	250
Jamaica	11	33	1.4	30	1.3	22	31/03/89	96
Martinique	20	19	5.8	19	5.8	0	31/12/88	58
Mexico	793	838	1.1	714	0.9	6	31/03/89	2351
Montserrat	0	0	0.0	0	0.0	0	31/12/88	0
Nicaragua	0	0	0.0	2	0.1	1	31/03/89	3
Panama	18	12	0.6	54	2.5	0	31/12/88	84
Paraguay	1	7	0.2	1	0.0	3	31/03/89	12
Peru	9	60	0.3	68	0.3	19	31/03/89	156
Saint Lucia	3	7	4.9	1	0.7	6	31/03/89	17
Saint Vincent	3	5	4.5	6	5.4	3	31/03/89	17
St. Christopher Nevis	1	0	0.0	17	37.0	0	31/12/88	18
Suriname	4	5	1.3	2	0.5	0	30/09/88	11
Trinidad and Tobago	149	82	6.9	105	8.9	65	31/03/89	401
Turks and Caicos Is.	3	3	30.0	1	10.0	0	31/12/88	7
Uruguay	8	9	0.3	28	0.9	6	31/03/89	51
USA	38,194	25,196	10.5	28,326	11.8	15,592	12/10/89	107,308*
Venezuela	88	101	0.6	127	0.7	0	31/12/88	316
Total for the Region	**43,319**	**30,501**	**4.6**	**35,056**	**5.3**	**17,838**		**126,714**

(a) *Rate: Reported cases/100,000 population*
(b) *1988 Reporting generally incomplete*
*   *Updated report*
    Source: World Health Organization

REFERENCES

1. AIDS surveillance in Europe. Paris: World Health Organization Collaborating Centre on AIDS, 1987; 13:1-26.
2. Bygbjerg IC. AIDS in a Danish surgeon (Zaire, 1976). Lancet 1983; 1:925.
3. Vandepitte J, Verwilghen R, Zachee P. AIDS and cryptococcosis (Zaire 1977). Lancet 1983; 1:925-6.
4. Piot P, Quinn TC, Taelman H, et al. Acquired immunodeficiency syndrome in a heterosexual population in Zaire. Lancet 1984; 2:65-9.

5. Biggar RJ. The AIDS problem in Africa. Lancet 1986; 1:79-82.

6. Statistics from the World Health Organization and the Centers for Disease Control. AIDS 1988; 2:323-5.

7. Mann JM, Chin J, Piot P, Quinn TC. The international epidemiology of AIDS. Scientific American 1988; 259:82-89.

8. Goedert JJ, Blattner WA. The epidemiology of AIDS and related conditions. In: DeVita VT, Hellman S, Rosenberg SA, eds. AIDS: etiology, diagnosis, treatment, and prevention. Philadelphia: J.B. Lippincott, 1985.

9. Pitchenik AE, Fischl MA, Dickinson GM, et al. Opportunistic infections and Kaposi's sarcoma among Haitians: evidence of a new acquired immunodeficiency state. Ann Intern Med 1983; 98:277-84.

10. Hardy AM, Allen JR, Morgan WM, et al. Incidence of AIDS in selected population groups. JAMA 1985; 253:265.

11. Centers for Disease Control. Update on acquired immunodeficiency syndrome (AIDS) — United States. MMWR 1982; 31:507-14.

12. Pape JW, Liautaud B, Thomas F, et al. The acquired immunodeficiency syndrome in Haiti. Ann Intern Med 1985; 103:674-8.

13. Castro KG, Fischl SH, Landesman SH, et al. Risk factors for AIDS among Haitians in the United States [Abstract]. Atlanta: International Conference on Acquired Immunodeficiency Syndrome, 1985; 45.

14. Dournon E, Penalba C, Saimot AG, et al. AIDS in a Haitian couple in Paris. Lancet 1983; 1:1187.

15. Pape JW, Liautaud B, Thomas F, et al. Risk factors associated with AIDS in Haiti. Am J Med Sci 1986; 291:4-7.

1.1.4

AIDS in Africa

Dennis Osmond

This chapter considers transmission routes, geographic distribution, and the probable origin of HIV in Africa. It also surveys seroprevalence rates, describes typical disease presentations, and discusses the epidemiology of HIV-2.

The epidemiology of AIDS in Africa is strikingly different from its epidemiology in Western countries, although the underlying defect in cellular immunity is the same.[1] African isolates of HIV-1 do not differ significantly from European and American isolates.[2,3] African patients infrequently report homosexuality or intravenous drug use — the risk factors seen in most Western patients. Instead, the distribution by sex of African cases is nearly equal.[4] The male-to-female case ratio is reported as 1.1 to 1 in Zaire, 1.9 to 1 in Rwanda, and 1.5 to 1 among Central Africans treated in Belgium.[5-7] These figures contrast strikingly with the 19 to 1 ratio seen in the United States. Africa's distinct epidemiologic pattern implies heterosexual transmission among people in sexually active age groups as the primary mode of spread. Although insects have been suspected as vectors of transmission, the age distribution of cases argues instead for sexual transmission as the dominant mechanism.[4] No direct evidence of insect transmission has been reported.

In addition to the sexual case ratio, several other observations support heterosexual transmission as the primary mechanism of spread. Both the number of heterosexual partners and contact with female prostitutes appear as risk factors in studies of male African patients.[5,6,8] This correlates with serological studies of female prostitutes, which report a high seroprevalence for antibody to HIV in regions that also have a high male seroprevalence rate.[9-11]

AIDS may have originated in Africa and been present there for some time before its spread, but in epidemic form it appears to be new to Africa as well as to the West. Clinicians working in Africa since the 1960s have reported AIDS as a strikingly new disease.[4] Recent increases of an aggressive form of Kaposi's sarcoma (KS) similar to that seen in Western AIDS patients are reported in Zambia and Uganda.[13]

AIDS was not diagnosed in Africans treated in Europe before the late 1970s, although it is now spreading among Africans treated both in Europe and on the African continent. Just as recent cultural changes (e.g., gay liberation, relaxed heterosexual sexual mores, and post-1960 increases in intravenous drug use) in the U.S. may have amplified the spread of HIV, events of the past few decades in Africa have probably played a major role in the epidemic there. Several factors contributed to the rapid spread of HIV in Africa: (1) the growth of urban centers and the accompanying influx of young persons from the countryside, (2) the growth of female prostitution, (3) the movement of armies (paralleling the historic spread of syphilis in Europe), and (4) the disruption of health services.

■ **GEOGRAPHIC DISTRIBUTION OF HIV IN AFRICA**

Although AIDS has appeared in all Western countries, it is still strongly concentrated within a few geographic areas. Strong geographic variation is also a feature of AIDS in Africa. Researchers report that the incidence is highest in the countries of Central Africa: Zaire, Rwanda, Uganda, and Zambia. As of early 1988, Congo and Burundi also reported a high number of cases. In 1984, the incidence of AIDS was estimated at 17 per 100,000 in Kinshasa, Zaire, and 80 per 100,000 in Kigali, Rwanda. In 1986, the annual incidence in Kinshasa was estimated at 55 to 100 per 100,000.[5,6,28] Among East African nations, Kenya and Tanzania follow in the number of cases. Some cases have been reported from South Africa, but the prevalence of infection there appears low when compared with Central and East Africa. A few cases have been reported from West Africa — particularly cases resulting from HIV-2 infection.

Socioeconomic conditions may explain the reportedly high urban seroprevalence and low rural seroprevalence in Zaire and Rwanda — countries in which young people flock to the cities seeking work, in contrast to high rural rates in western Tanzania and southwestern Uganda — regions through which a major trans-African highway passes.[16,18,25]

■ **ORIGINS OF HIV IN AFRICA**

Serological studies have not established that AIDS originated in Africa. Nevertheless, the most plausible current theory is that HIV arose in Africa, perhaps mutating from a less pathogenic human virus, or crossing over from an animal population, before becoming a human pathogen.

Two of the earliest known AIDS cases, recognized retrospectively, are linked to Zaire. In 1976, AIDS-like diseases were diagnosed in Europe in a Danish surgeon who visited Zaire and, in 1977, in a Zairian living in Belgium.[14,15] By reviewing medical case reports from the pre-AIDS era that meet the current CDC surveillance definition for AIDS, researchers have identified possible AIDS cases from as far back as 1962 in Central Africa.[29] Overall, the number of cases identified retrospectively is probably a better reflection of the quality and preservation of different countries' medical records than an accurate picture of the earliest occurrences of AIDS worldwide. Records alone are probably not adequate to establish when and where the earliest cases were diagnosed in Africa.

The isolation of a new human immunodeficiency virus in Africa, HIV-2, and the identification of structurally similar simian immunodeficiency viruses from African macaque and green monkeys (STLV-IIImac and STLV-IIIagm), strengthen the inference that HIV originated in Africa. Stored African serum specimens dating back to 1959 have tested positive for HIV-1,[30] although sera considered positive by Western blot have profiles atypical of seropositive sera from the West.[4]

■ **DIFFICULTIES IN ASSESSING PREVALENCE OF AIDS IN AFRICA**

The magnitude of the AIDS problem in Africa is difficult to estimate. No reliable count of African AIDS cases is available. Surveillance is practically and logistically difficult in many parts of Africa, and until recently, many African countries did not report cases to the World Health Organization (WHO). The CDC definition of AIDS that is used for surveillance in North and South America, Europe, and Australia is not adequate for African AIDS, because the clinical manifestations of HIV-related illness differ from those in Western countries and because laboratory evidence of HIV infection is usually absent. Accurate diagnosis is often difficult because clinical facilities are limited. Presumptively diagnosing Kaposi's sarcoma as AIDS is complicated by the endemic form of KS that occurs in African adults under 60 — a form that may become generalized, and is known to have a noncutaneous, aggressive form.[12] A surveillance definition specific to African conditions has been proposed and is being evaluated.[31]

■ SEROPREVALENCE OF HIV IN AFRICA

Seroprevalence studies in Africa show high rates of infection in the population, especially in urban Central Africa: 3 percent to 28 percent in Rwanda,[8,9,18] 20 percent in Uganda,[20] 3 percent to 12 percent in Zaire,[19] and 2 percent to 8 percent in Kenya.[10] These figures represent a range from relatively low seropositivity among blood donors and medical personnel to high seropositivity among clients of sexually transmitted disease (STD) clinics, who are presumably more sexually active. Such high rates are alarming — and become even more so if extrapolated to the larger population of Central and East Africa. However, given the concentration of AIDS cases in limited geographic areas in both Africa and the West, caution in extrapolating seroprevalence data is probably appropriate.

TABLE 1. PREVALENCE OF HIV ANTIBODY IN AFRICANS (1983–1985)

	PERCENT HIV-ANTIBODY POSITIVE
CENTRAL AFRICA	
Rwanda[8,9,18]	3 to 28
Rwanda prostitutes[9,11]	75 to 88
Zaire[19]	3 to 12
Uganda[20]	20
EAST AFRICA	
Kenya[10]	2 to 8
Kenya prostitutes[10]	56
SOUTH AFRICA	
South Africa[21]	0 to 0.3
Malawi[21]	15
Zambia[19,21]	2 to 18
WEST AFRICA	
Senegal[22]	4
Senegal prostitutes[22]	7
Nigeria[23]	0

The highest rates have been reported among prostitutes from Central Africa. High seroprevalence rates are also reported in East African prostitutes. These seroprevalence data are consistent with the theory that African AIDS began in Central Africa, spread next to East Africa and more recently to South Africa, with little spread (so far) to West Africa.

■ DISEASE PRESENTATION

Typical disease presentation in Africa is different from that in the United States and Europe. African patients seen in European hospitals have shown some differences from patients seen in Africa, but these differences are attributable to the quality of diagnosis and treatment available in different medical facilities.[17] In African patients, a mononucleosis-like syndrome and a chronic lymphadenopathy syndrome (pathologically characterized by nonreactive hyperplasia) are similar to the syndromes seen in Western patients.[4] African patients present more frequently with weight loss and diarrhea[24,32] — a typical presentation includes general malaise and an itchy maculopapular rash.[24,25,32] *Toxoplasma gondii*, salmonella, and mycobacterial infections are also reported more frequently in African patients.[24]

In African patients seen in Europe, the most common opportunistic infections, seen with about equal frequency (14 percent to 25 percent), are cryptococcosis, toxoplasmosis, candidiasis, tuberculosis, and cryptosporidiosis.[40] *Pneumocystis carinii* pneumonia (PCP), the most frequent opportunistic infection in U.S. patients, diagnosed in 64 percent of patients, is reported in only 26 percent of African patients, approximately as frequently as cryptosporidiosis.[17] This difference in reported PCP cannot be attributed to inadequate diagnosis in Africa, since it is reported in only 14 percent of African cases diagnosed in European hospitals.[40] Presumably the differences in these rates of opportunistic infections result from differences in the prevalence of these pathogens in Africa.

In Uganda, the characteristic disease presentation is known as "slim disease," named for the extreme wasting the patients experience.[25] Typical presentation includes weight loss, persistent diarrhea, malaise, and an itchy macupapular rash. Thirty-four of 42 patients in Kampala, Uganda, were seropositive for antibody to human immunodeficiency virus (HIV) and biopsy proven Kaposi's sarcoma was found in 3 of 29.[25] T-lymphocyte counts were not reported in these 42 patients. Clinicians report "slim disease" as a new syndrome, not seen before 1982. No single opportunistic infection or agent other than HIV has been associated with "slim disease." This disease is clearly associated with infection by HIV and, although differing somewhat from typical cases of African AIDS reported in Zaire and Rwanda, it appears to be another manifestation of the syndrome.

Kaposi's sarcoma is endemic in Central Africa, and it usually affects older men and takes an indolent course. More aggressive forms of KS, particularly among children, were also recognized prior to 1980.[12,26] African patients with the endemic form of KS are consistently seronegative for antibody to HIV.[20,24] Recently, an atypical, aggressive form of KS strongly associated with HIV infection has appeared in Uganda and Zambia.[20] These reports indicate that the historic form of KS was not associated with an AIDS-related virus infection, and provide more evidence that AIDS is a new phenomenon in Africa, as well as in the West.

■ RISK FACTORS FOR HIV TRANSMISSION

African AIDS patients rarely give a history of homosexuality, intravenous drug use, hemophilia, or blood transfusion.[5,6,8,11] The inference of heterosexual transmission as the primary mode of infection is supported by reports of clustered AIDS cases among heterosexual partners,[4,5] and by studies that identify the number of heterosexual contacts and sexual contacts with prostitutes as risk factors.[5,6,8,9] Studies of infected children under two years old indicate high rates of vertical transmission.[33] Homosexuality is a taboo subject in many parts of Africa and may be underreported by patients, but the large number of female cases would be unlikely if male homosexual activity were a major mode of transmission. In sexual behavior studies, HIV-seropositive subjects regularly practiced vaginal–penile intercourse. Other types of sexual behavior were rare.[9,10] Homosexuality has not been noted among African AIDS patients treated in Europe.

Sexually transmitted diseases are even more strongly associated with HIV infection in Africa than among homosexual men in Western countries.[10,16] Genital ulcers in particular have been implicated as a possible cofactor facilitating transmission.[34] Other sexually transmitted diseases have also been associated with infection in Africa as well as in the West.[10,35] A statistically significant higher prevalence of STDs has been reported in HIV antibody-seropositive as compared with seronegative prostitutes.[10] Gonorrhea, genital ulcers, and a reactive serologic test for syphilis were all significantly more prevalent in the seropositive women. HIV antibody was also associated with STDs in the two years preceding the test in young males and blood donors in Rwanda.[16] Previous STDs may facilitate infection with HIV either through damage to mucosal or epithelial tissue or through activation of lymphocytes or macrophages, which are the target cells for infection. On the other hand, this association may not be causal or it may be that infection with HIV predisposes to other sexually transmitted diseases. A history of STDs has also been reported as a risk factor for HIV infection in homosexual men in the United States.

In the West, transfusion-associated cases will continue to be limited largely to infections acquired before widespread antibody screening of donated blood (mid-1985). The cost of screening has left much of the African blood supply unprotected, however, so transfusion-associated HIV infection will continue to be a problem in Africa.[36] At least one case of apparent transmission via blood transfusion has been reported.[41] A 17-year-old female required transfusion of six units of whole blood for postpartum bleeding and six months later developed lymphadenopathy, other ARC symptoms, and esophageal candidiasis. She and one of her blood donors were found to be HIV-antibody positive.

In addition to transfusion-related transmission, several other routes of nonsexual transmission have been proposed to explain the spread of AIDS in Africa. The virus is known to be transmitted among intravenous drug users who share needles; thus, practices unusual in the United States and Europe, but common in Africa, that might spread infection by analogous routes have come under suspicion. Scarification rituals, clitoridectomy, the use of unsterile needles for intramuscular injection of medicines, insect or animal vectors, and poor sanitation have been proposed as potential risk factors.[6,7] However, case reports indicate that almost all AIDS patients in Africa are sexually active young and middle-aged adults,[4] a demographic pattern inconsistent with primarily nonsexual routes of transmission. This pattern raises difficulties for theories proposing nonsexual routes of parenteral transmission. If, for example, mosquitoes were a vector for infection, cases would be expected from all age groups. Poor sanitation might be expected to produce clusters of cases within families or particular parts of a city. Ritual scarification, if a route of transmission, should result in a pattern of cases within a few years after the age of the rites among those tribes who practice scarification. None of these patterns has been observed. Cases occur among tribes who do not practice scarification.[27] Studies examining scarification as a risk factor have failed to find an association.[5,10] Insect vectors have not been identified. Frequency of unsterile injections has also not been found to be a risk factor,[5,6,10,16,27] although it cannot be ruled out, since a history of intramuscular injections is frequently reported.[10] Although these practices may still play some role in the spread of infection in Africa, they seem unlikely to be significant modes of transmission.

Heterosexual transmission may occur more readily in Africa than in the United States and Europe because of differences in social patterns, sexual mores, and hygienic habits. Use of barrier contraception is very rare.[10,16] In some urban areas of Central Africa, young men postpone marriage and have a

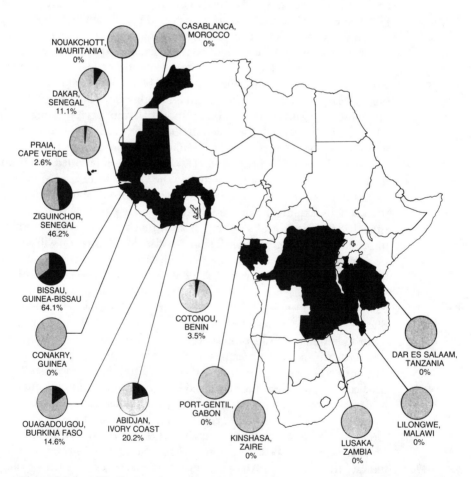

Figure 1.1.4.a Distribution of HIV-2 in Africa was established by serological testing of female prostitutes, who constitute a high-risk group. The seroprevalence rates (the fraction of individuals who tested positive for HIV-2) are given for 15 cities in 14 countries where the test was administered. The virus appears to be limited to West Africa. Adapted from *Scientific American* 1988; 259(4):70.

high frequency of sexual contact with prostitutes.[16] If these behavior patterns are much more frequent in Africa than in the West, and African urban prostitutes are a reservoir of infection, the potential for heterosexual transmission may remain greater in Africa than in the industrial countries.

■ EPIDEMIOLOGY OF HIV-2

HIV-2, a retrovirus distinct from HIV-1, has been isolated from West African patients with AIDS (in Cape Verde and Guinea-Bissau), raising a number of questions that cannot yet be answered about the interrelation of the two viruses[37] (see Figure 1.1.4.a). HIV-2 has been reported in several AIDS cases in Europe. Recently in the U.S., a case of AIDS associated with HIV-2 infection was reported in a recent West African immigrant.[38]

The core proteins of HIV-2 are similar to those of HIV-1, but its envelope proteins cross-react with those of SIV-1 (STLV-III). A serological survey of 4248 individuals from six countries of West Africa used antibodies to the HTLV-IV isolate that cross-react with SIV-1 and HIV-2, and found high rates of seroprevalence in prostitutes and low rates in hospital patients.[39] These results have been interpreted as indicating that HIV-2 is less pathologic than HIV-1, but controversy persists on this point. The lack of reactivity of HIV-2 with HIV-1 ELISAs will necessitate the development of immunoassays for use in population screening and securing blood supplies that can detect both viruses.

TABLE 2. AFRICAN REGION
AIDS CASES REPORTED TO WHO BY COUNTRY BASED ON REPORTS RECEIVED THROUGH 31/10/1989

COUNTRY	1979–1986 CASES	1987 CASES	RATE (a)	1988 CASES	RATE (b)	1989 CASES	LAST REPORT	CUMUL. CASES
Algeria	3	5	0.0	5	0.0	0	26/03/88	13
Angola	9	32	0.4	63	0.7	0	31/12/88	104
Benin	3	6	0.1	18	0.4	9	31/03/89	36
Botswana	7	9	0.8	33	3.1	0	31/03/89	49
Burkina Faso	10	21	0.3	394	5.0	130	31/03/89	555
Burundi	269	652	13.8	1054	22.3	0	31/12/88	1975
Cameroon	21	20	0.2	33	0.3	4	31/03/89	78
Cape Verde	2	16	4.8	0	0.0	7	31/07/89	25
Central African Rep.	254	178	6.9	230	8.9	0	31/12/88	662
Chad	2	2	0.0	7	0.1	3	30/06/89	14
Comoros	0	0	0.0	1	0.2	0	28/02/89	1
Congo	250	1000	57.5	0	0.0	0	31/12/87	1250
Cote d'Ivoire	118	132	1.3	0	0.0	0	20/11/87	250
Equatorial Guinea	0	1	0.3	1	0.3	1	27/06/89	3
Ethiopia	2	17	0.0	62	0.1	112	31/08/89	193*
Gabon	13	4	0.4	10	1.0	8	30/06/89	35
Gambia	13	22	3.0	27	3.6	0	31/12/88	62
Ghana	26	35	0.3	266	2.1	594	31/08/89	921*
Guinea	0	4	0.1	29	0.5	19	31/05/89	52
Guinea-Bissau	0	29	3.3	29	3.3	18	18/05/89	76

continued on next page

continued from previous page

TABLE 2.   AFRICAN REGION
AIDS CASES REPORTED TO WHO BY COUNTRY BASED ON
REPORTS RECEIVED THROUGH 31/10/1989

COUNTRY	1979–1986 CASES	1987 CASES	RATE (a)	1988 CASES	RATE (b)	1989 CASES	LAST REPORT	CUMUL. CASES
Kenya	274	1223	6.0	2817	13.8	1690	30/06/89	6004
Lesotho	1	1	0.1	2	0.1	4	15/09/89	8*
Liberia	0	2	0.1	0	0.0	0	11/03/88	2
Madagascar	0	0	0.0	0	0.0	0	01/02/89	0
Malawi	144	860	12.0	1582	22.2	0	30/06/88	2586
Mali	6	23	0.3	0	0.0	0	14/01/88	29
Mauritania	0	0	0.0	0	0.0	0	31/07/88	0
Mauritius	0	1	0.1	1	0.1	2	05/10/89	4*
Mozambique	1	3	0.0	23	0.2	18	14/09/89	45*
Niger	0	17	0.3	26	0.4	13	31/03/89	56
Nigeria	0	10	0.0	3	0.0	22	02/08/89	35*
Reunion	0	1	0.2	12	2.2	22	25/09/89	35*
Rwanda	705	295	4.8	267	4.4	35	28/02/89	1302
Sao Tome & Principe	0	0	0.0	1	0.9	1	14/04/89	2
Senegal	6	60	0.9	115	1.8	26	04/08/89	207
Seychelles	0	0	0.0	0	0.0	0	20/04/89	0
Sierra Leone	0	3	0.1	12	0.3	6	30/06/89	21
South Africa	46	38	0.1	86	0.3	74	31/07/89	244
Swaziland	1	6	0.9	7	1.1	0	16/06/88	14
Togo	0	2	0.1	15	0.5	6	22/06/89	23
Uganda	911	1789	11.5	4072	26.3	603	15/04/89	7375
United Rep. Tanzania	699	909	4.0	2550	11.2	0	31/12/88	4158
Zaire	0	335	1.1	0	0.0	0	30/06/87	335
Zambia	288	345	4.9	1057	15.1	202	01/05/89	1892
Zimbabwe	0	119	1.4	202	2.4	827	30/09/89	1148*
Total for the Region	4084	8227	1.8	15,112	3.4	4456		31,879

(a) *Rate: Reported cases/100,000 population*

(b) *1988 Reporting generally incomplete*

* *Updated report*

Source: World Health Organization

REFERENCES

1. Clumeck N, Sonnet J, Taelman H, et al. Acquired immunodeficiency syndrome in African patients. N Engl J Med 1984; 310:492-7.
2. Brun-Vezinet F, Rouxioux C, Montagier L, et al. Prevalence of antibodies to lymphadenopathy associated retrovirus in African patients with AIDS. Science 1985; 226:453-6.
3. McCormick JB, Krebs JW, Mitchell SW, et al. Isolation of human immunodeficiency virus from African AIDS patients and from persons without AIDS or IgG antibody to human immunodeficiency virus. Am J Trop Med Hyg 1987; 36:102-6.
4. Biggar RJ. The AIDS problem in Africa. Lancet 1986; 1:79-83.

5. Piot P, Quinn TC, Taelman H, et al. Acquired immunodeficiency syndrome in a heterosexual population in Zaire. Lancet 1984; 2:65-9.

6. Van de Perre P, Rouvroy D, Lepage P, et al. Acquired immunodeficiency syndrome in Rwanda. Lancet 1984; 2:62-5.

7. Clumeck N, Sonnet J, Taelman H, et al. Acquired immunodeficiency syndrome in Belgium and its relation to Central Africa. Ann NY Acad Sci 1984; 437:264-9.

8. Clumeck N, Van De Perre, Carael M, et al. Heterosexual promiscuity among African patients with AIDS. N Engl J Med 1985; 313:182.

9. Van de Perre P, Clumeck N, Carael M, et al. Female prostitutes: a risk group for infection with human T-cell lymphotropic virus type III. Lancet 1985; 2:524-7.

10. Kreiss JK, Koech D, Plummer FA, et al. AIDS virus infection in Nairobi prostitutes. N Engl J Med 1986; 314:414-8.

11. Clumeck N, Robert-Guroff M, Van de Perre P, et al. Seroepidemiological studies of HTLV-III antibody prevalence among selected groups of heterosexual Africans. JAMA 1985; 254:2599-2602.

12. Hutt MS. The epidemiology of Kaposi's sarcoma. Antibiot Chemother 1981; 29:3-8.

13. Bayley AC. Aggressive Kaposi's sarcoma in Zambia, 1983. Lancet 1984; 1:1318-20.

14. Bygbjerg IC. AIDS in a Danish surgeon (Zaire, 1976). Lancet 1983; 1:925.

15. Vandepitte J, Verwilgen R, Zachee P. AIDS and cryptococcosis (Zaire, 1977). Lancet 1983; 1:925-6.

16. Carael M, Van de Perre P, Akingeneye E, et al. Socio-cultural factors in relation to HTLV-III/LAV transmission in urban areas in central Africa [Abstract]. Brussels: International Symposium on African AIDS, 1985.

17. Taelman H, Sonnet J. Clinical and biological profile of African AIDS [Abstract]. Brussels: International Symposium on African AIDS, 1985.

18. Van de Perre P, Kanyamupira JB, Carael M, et al. HTLV-III/LAV infection in central Africa [Abstract]. Brussels: International Symposium on African AIDS, 1985.

19. Biggar RJ, Gigase PL, Melbye M, et al. ELISA HTLV-III retrovirus antibody reactivity associated with malaria and immune complexes in healthy Africans. Lancet 1985; 2:520-3.

20. Bayley AC, Downing RG, Cheingsong-Popov R, et al. HTLV-III seroepidemiology distinguishes atypical and endemic Kaposi's sarcoma in Africa. Lancet 1985; 1:359-61.

21. Sher R. Seroepidemiological studies of HTLV-III/LAV infection in southern African countries [Abstract]. Brussels: International Symposium on African AIDS, 1985.

22. Barin F, M'Boup S, Denis F, et al. Serological evidence for virus related to simian T-lymphotropic retrovirus III in residents of West Africa. Lancet 1985; 2:1387-9.

23. Okpara RA, Williams E, Schneider J, et al. Antibodies to human T-cell leukemia virus types I and III in blood donors from Calabar, Nigeria. Ann Intern Med 1986; 104:132.

24. Biggar RJ, Melbye M, Kestems L, et al. Kaposi's sarcoma in Zaire is not associated with HTLV-III infection. N Engl J Med 1984; 311:1051-2.

25. Serwadda D, Mugerwa RD, Sewankambo NK, et al. Slim disease: a new disease in Uganda and its association with HTLV-III infection. Lancet 1985; 2:849-52.

26. Davies JNP, Lother F. Kaposi's sarcoma in African children. In: Ackerman LV, Murray JF, eds. Symposium on Kaposi's sarcoma. Unio international contra cancrum. Vol. 13. Basel: Karger, 1962:81-6.

27. Hutt MSR. Kaposi's sarcoma. Br Med Bull 1984; 40:355-8.

28. Mann JM, Francis H, Quinn T, et al. Surveillance for AIDS in a central African city: Kinshasa, Zaire. JAMA 1986; 255:3255-9.

29. Sonnet J, Michaux J-L, Zech F, et al. Early AIDS cases originating from Zaire and Burundi (1962-1976). Scand J Infect Dis 1987; 19:511-7.

30. Nahmias AJ, Weiss J, Yao X, et al. Evidence for human infection with an HTLV III/LAV-like virus in Central Africa, 1959. Lancet 1986; 1:1279-80.

31. Colebunders R, Mann JM, Francis H, et al. Evaluation of a clinical case-definition of acquired immunodeficiency syndrome in Africa. Lancet 1987; 1:492-4.

32. Bernan TY. HIV infection in developing countries: emerging clinical pictures in Africa [Abstract]. The Global Impact of AIDS Conference. London: World Health Organization, 1988; 21.

33. Mann JM, Francis H, Davachi F, et al. Risk factors for human immunodeficiency virus seropositivity among children 1-24 months old in Kinshasa, Zaire. Lancet 1986; 2:654-7.

34. Piot P, Mann JM. Transmission patterns of LAV/HTLV-III: Evidence for heterosexual transmission. Second International Conference on AIDS. Paris, 1986; 107.

35. Quinn TC, Piot P, McCormick JB, et al. Serologic and immunologic studies in patients with AIDS in North America and Africa. The potential role of infectious agents as cofactors in human immunodeficiency virus infection. JAMA 1987; 257:2617-21.

36. Fleming AF. The prevention of transmission of HIV by blood transfusion in developing countries [Abstract]. The Global Impact of AIDS Conference. London: World Health Organization, 1988; 53.

37. Clavel F, Guetard D, Brun-Vezinet F, et al. Isolation of a new retrovirus from West African patients with AIDS. Science 1986; 233:343-6.

38. Centers for Disease Control. AIDS due to HIV-2 infection—New Jersey. MMWR 1988; 37:33-5.

39. Kanki PJ, M'Boup S, Ricard D, et al. Human T-lymphotropic virus type 4 and the human immunodeficiency virus in West Africa. Science 1987; 236:827-31.

40. Biggar RJ, Bouvet E, Ebbesen P, et al. Clinical features of AIDS in Europe. Eur J Cancer Clin Oncol 1984; 20:165-7.

41. Van de Perre P, Munyambuga D, Zissis G, et al. Antibody to HTLV-III in blood donors in central Africa. Lancet 1985; 1:336-7.

Growth of the Epidemic in the U.S.: Rates for Incidence and Mortality

Dennis Osmond

■ GROWTH OF THE AIDS EPIDEMIC

In May 1981, five cases of *Pneumocystis carinii* pneumonia (PCP) in previously healthy young homosexual men from Los Angeles were reported.[1] At about the same time, 26 cases of Kaposi's sarcoma (KS) in homosexual men were reported from New York and San Francisco.[2] By the fall of 1981, over 100 cases had been reported to the Centers for Disease Control (CDC). In September of 1982, a definition for surveillance of the new syndrome was published by the CDC.[3] Retrospective search of records subsequently identified patients with AIDS as early as 1978. The CDC recognizes 9 cases diagnosed prior to 1979, 12 in 1979, and 49 in 1980.[4]

In February 1983, five years after the first cases were diagnosed, the first 1000 cases had been reported.[5] The second 1000 cases were reported in the next six months and the third 1000 were reported five months later in December 1983.[6] Although cases have now been reported from every state, the majority of cases have continued to be reported from the cities identifying the earliest cases. As of January 30, 1989, 42 percent of total cases are reported from five standard metropolitan statistical areas (SMSA): New York (21 percent), San Francisco (8 percent), Los Angeles (7 percent), Houston (3 percent), and Newark, N.J. (3 percent).[4]

■ DOUBLING TIME

The rate of growth of the epidemic is reflected in the length of time required to double the number of reported cases. When the epidemic curve was steepest in 1982 and 1983, the doubling time was approximately six months. It is now more than one year (see Table 1).[7,15]

TABLE 1. DOUBLING TIME FOR REPORTED CASES FROM 1981 THROUGH 1987

DATE	CUMULATIVE CASES REPORTED	DOUBLING TIME (MONTHS)
September 1981	129	—
January 1982	220	5

continued on next page

continued from previous page

TABLE 1. DOUBLING TIME FOR REPORTED CASES FROM 1981 THROUGH 1987

DATE	CUMULATIVE CASES REPORTED	DOUBLING TIME (MONTHS)
June 1982	439	6
December 1982	878	6
July 1983	1,756	7
February 1984	3,512	8
December 1984	7,025	9
October 1985	14,049	11
December 1986	28,098	13
December 1987	49,006	15+

Table 2 shows the growth of the epidemic by year within each risk group.[7,16]

TABLE 2. UNITED STATES AIDS CASES REPORTED BY YEAR BY PATIENT GROUP

Patient Group	CASES REPORTED BY JANUARY OF:							
	1982	1983	1984	1985	1986	1987	1988	1989
Homosex/bisex men/IV drug users	16	66	211	418	599	2260	3858	5874
Homosex/bisex men/no IV drug use	178	473	1341	2939	5669	19,079	33,369	50,325
IV drug abusers	22	138	392	785	1429	4951	8877	16,151
Hemophilia/coagulation disorder	0	7	10	38	69	252	519	773
Heterosexual cases	1	10	18	53	100	1110	2058	3589
Transfusion, blood/components	0	6	28	56	171	544	1206	2044
Undetermined	3	28	76	131	348	918	1580	2662
Born outside U.S.*	7	48	85	114	144	—	—	—
Subtotal	227	776	2161	4534	8529	29,114	51,467	81,418
Pediatric	0	16	35	48	132	422	789	1346
Total	227	792	2196	4582	8661	29,536	52,256	82,764

*   *This category was eliminated by the CDC in August 1986 and integrated with heterosexual cases.*

■ INCIDENCE RATES

Incidence rates can be calculated for reported cases meeting the CDC surveillance definition of AIDS. The definition represents the most severe consequences of infection. There is no surveillance for less severe manifestations, called AIDS-related complex (ARC), lesser AIDS, or pre-AIDS, terms that have no generally agreed-upon definition. In addition, the surveillance definition does not include other diseases that may be a consequence of human immunodeficiency virus (HIV) infection, such as tuberculosis, Hodgkin's lymphoma, and central nervous system (CNS) pathology. Incidence rates for reported cases thus underrepresent the total impact of HIV infection.

The reporting of patients meeting the CDC definition of AIDS appears complete enough to make reported cases a reliable numerator for calculating rates.[8] Different denominators are chosen to calculate rates, and range from the population at large to specific AIDS risk groups. With the United States population as denominator, the cumulative rate for all cases reported since June 1, 1981, is 9 cases per 100,000 (U.S. Census data).[4] The annual rate for 1985 is 4 per 100,000. Since June 1, 1981, for the New York City SMSA, the cumulative rate is 69 per 100,000; for the San Francisco SMSA, 66 per 100,000. Clearly, rates that use the entire population as a denominator greatly underrepresent the impact of the epidemic on the principal risk groups. Because reliable data are not available on the size of the two principal risk groups, homosexual men and intravenous drug users, estimated or surrogate denominators are used to calculate approximate rates.

Incidence Rates in Homosexual Men. Rates have been calculated for homosexual men using census data on never-married adult males (single men) as the denominator.[6,9] These denominators exclude the estimated 10 percent to 20 percent of homosexual men who have been married[10] but include all heterosexual adult men who have not been married. Rates derived from them will approximate the true rate only in areas in which a high proportion of single men are homosexual.

In the United States, the annual rate of AIDS cases reported in homosexual men in 1985, using never-married men 15 years or older as the denominator, was 25.1 per 100,000 population.[6] The cumulative rate at the end of 1985 was 47.6 per 100,000.

In San Francisco, the annual rate of AIDS cases in 1985, using never-married men 20 years or older as the denominator, was 658 per 100,000; the cumulative rate was 1412 per 100,000 or almost 1.5 percent of the population of single men 20 or older.[9] Earlier analysis of incidence in census tracts from neighborhoods of San Francisco with high proportions of homosexual men estimated the cumulative incidence in homosexual men in San Francisco at 770 per 100,000 at the end of 1983.[9] Extrapolating that estimate to cases reported through the end of 1985 gives an estimated cumulative incidence of 3392 per 100,000, or approximately 3 percent of homosexual men in San Francisco. This estimate accords well with the 4 percent diagnosed with AIDS in a clinic cohort being followed prospectively in San Francisco.[11]

Incidence Rates in Other Risk Groups. Annual national incidence rates (January 1985 through January 1986) have been calculated for intravenous drug users (191 per 100,000), adult transfusion recipients (9 per 100,000), and type A and B hemophilia patients (477 per 100,000).[6] It should be kept in mind that the denominator for the number of intravenous drug users is an estimate, and that the number of transfusion recipients represents survivors six months post-transfusion (estimated to be 60 percent) over a six-year period. The denominator for hemophiliacs is probably the most reliable of those used in these calculations.

■ MORTALITY RATES

The proportion of deaths to reported cases has increased somewhat since early in the epidemic, when the number of prevalent cases exceeded the mortalities (see Table 3).[12] Currently, 57 percent of reported cases are known dead. Prognosis varies with the presenting disease. Patients with Kaposi's sarcoma have the best survival rate and patients with both Kaposi's sarcoma and pneumocystis pneumonia have the worst.

TABLE 3. MORTALITY BY DISEASE GROUP
(AS OF FEBRUARY 20, 1989)

DISEASE GROUP	CASES (%)	DEATHS (%)
PCP	51,960 (60)	30,534 (59)
Other opportunistic diseases	27,719 (32)	15,579 (56)
Kaposi's sarcoma	7509 (9)	3863 (51)
Total	87,188 (100)	49,976 (57)

Source: Centers for Disease Control. AIDS Weekly Surveillance Report, February 20, 1989.

As seen in Table 4,[12] long-term survival is low.

TABLE 4. CASE FATALITY RATE BY YEAR OF
DIAGNOSIS (AS OF MAY 31, 1989)

CASES DIAGNOSED	CASE FATALITY RATE (%)	
	ADULTS/ ADOLESCENTS	CHILDREN
Before 1981	82	67
1981	92	83
1982	90	78
1983	91	78
1984	86	76
1985	84	70
1986	75	65
1987	58	53
1988	35	33

continued on next page

continued from previous page

TABLE 4. CASE FATALITY RATE BY YEAR OF
DIAGNOSIS (AS OF MAY 31, 1989)

CASES DIAGNOSED	CASE FATALITY RATE (%)	
	ADULTS/ ADOLESCENTS	CHILDREN
1989	17	29
Total	58	55

Source: Centers for Disease Control. HIV/AIDS Surveillance Report, June 1989.

Actual mortality may be somewhat higher due to incomplete follow-up. A follow-up mortality study of 165 patients diagnosed in San Francisco found that the median survival of 75 patients with Kaposi's sarcoma was 21 months and among 90 patients with opportunistic infection (mostly pneumocystis pneumonia), 9 months.[13] Among patients with opportunistic infections, survival at 21 months was zero. In a follow-up report of 1007 patients from New York City, median survival for KS alone was 30 months; for KS and opportunistic infection (OI), 15 months; for KS and PCP, 14 months; for KS, PCP, and OI, 11 months; for PCP and OI, 10 months; PCP alone, 8 months; and OI alone, 4 months.[14]

REFERENCES

1. Gottlieb MS, Schroff R, Schanker HM, et al. *Pneumocystis carinii* pneumonia and mucosal candidiasis in previously healthy homosexual men: evidence of a new acquired cellular immunodeficiency. N Engl J Med 1981; 305:1425-31.

2. Centers for Disease Control. Kaposi's sarcoma and pneumocystis pneumonia among homosexual men — New York City and California. MMWR 1981; 30:305-8.

3. Centers for Disease Control. Update on acquired immunodeficiency syndrome (AIDS) — United States. MMWR 1982; 31:507-14.

4. Centers for Disease Control. Weekly surveillance report, January 30, 1989.

5. Jaffe HW, Bregman DJ, Selik RM. Acquired immunodeficiency syndrome in the United States: the first 1,000 cases. J Infect Dis 1984; 148:339-45.

6. Hardy AM, Allen JR, Morgan WM, Curran JW. The incidence rate of acquired immunodeficiency syndrome in selected populations. JAMA 1985; 253:215-20.

7. Centers for Disease Control. Update: acquired immunodeficiency syndrome — United States. MMWR 1986; 35:757.

8. Chamberland ME, Allen J, Monroe JM, et al. Acquired immunodeficiency syndrome in New York City: evaluation of an active surveillance system. JAMA 1985; 254:383-7.

9. Moss AR, Bacchetti P, Osmond D, et al. Incidence of the acquired immunodeficiency syndrome in San Francisco, 1980-1983. J Infect Dis 1985; 152:152-61.

10. Bell AP, Weinberg MS. Homosexualities. New York: Simon and Schuster, 1978.

11. Echenberg D, Rutherford G, O'Malley P, et al. Update: acquired immunodeficiency syndrome in the San Francisco cohort study, 1978-1985. MMWR 1985; 34:573-5.

12. Centers for Disease Control. Weekly surveillance report, January 30, 1989.

13. Moss AR, McCallum G, Volberding PA, et al. Mortality associated with mode of presentation in the acquired immunodeficiency syndrome. J Natl Cancer Inst 1984; 73:1281-4.

14. Rivin BE, Monroe JM, Habschman BP, et al. AIDS outcome: a first follow-up. N Engl J Med 1984; 311:857.

15. Centers for Disease Control. Weekly surveillance report, February 15, 1988.

16. Centers for Disease Control. Weekly surveillance report, February 1, 1988.

Progression to AIDS in Persons Testing Seropositive for Antibody to HIV

Dennis Osmond

T his chapter describes what is currently known about progression rates from HIV infection to full-blown AIDS in various risk groups. It discusses what has been learned from cohort studies of HIV-positive persons, draws some conclusions about incubation period and predictors of high rates of progression, and describes progression studies of homosexual men with lymphadenopathy and members of other risk groups in detail. Possible cofactors for progression from HIV infection to AIDS are briefly considered.

■ PROGRESSION TO AIDS FOLLOWING HIV INFECTION

The pathogenesis of HIV infection shows a high degree of variability, ranging from development of AIDS and death within a year of infection to an absence of any disease manifestations many years after infection. The proportion of HIV-infected persons developing AIDS is still not known; however, recent data from prospective studies suggest that a very high proportion of seropositive persons will ultimately develop disease.

Two parameters can be used to characterize progression from the HIV-seropositive, asymptomatic state: progression rate and incubation period. Progression rate is the percentage of HIV seropositives diagnosed with AIDS as defined by the Centers for Disease Control (CDC) over a stated period of time. Incubation period is defined as the time (expressed as a median or mean) from seroconversion to diagnosis of CDC-defined AIDS.

PROGRESSION RATES FROM COHORT STUDIES OF HIV SEROPOSITIVES

Data from several prospective studies with varying lengths of follow-up have provided a basis for minimum estimates of the progression rate to AIDS among HIV seropositives.[1-6,24,25] These studies report progression rates much higher than the early estimates.

Table 1 shows rates of progression to AIDS that have been reported for HIV seropositive subjects from different risk groups. The percentages are based on the product–limit (Kaplan–Meier) method of survival analysis; they are estimates that take into account differing lengths of follow-up for different individuals and may differ from raw percentages calculated directly from the numbers cited in the table.

TABLE 1.   PROPORTION OF SEROPOSITIVES PROGRESSING
TO AIDS*

HOMOSEXUAL MEN	FOLLOW-UP	NUMBER	% PROGRESSING
Manhattan[2]	36 months	44	34
Washington[2]	36 months	42	17
San Francisco[1]	120 months	121	54
San Francisco[36]	56 months	288	33
4 U.S. cities[4]	60 months	1523	21
HEMOPHILIA PATIENTS			
Hershey, Pa.[24]	96 months	577	29
Pittsburgh, Pa.[25]	90 months	79	27
United Kingdom[32]	96 months	104	31
IV DRUG USERS			
New York City[33]	30 months	288	12
Newark, N.J.[34]	60 months	148	20
DONORS OF INFECTED BLOOD			
United States[5]	84 months	71	36
Sweden[6]	60 months	48	29

*   *Table compiled by the author.*

Several studies suggest that the annual progression rate increases with time postinfection. Although transfusion cases, especially infants, have developed AIDS in the first year following infection, progression to clinical AIDS in healthy adults is rare during the first two years after seroconversion. A long-term retrospective study of 121 seropositive men who participated in the hepatitis B vaccine trial in San Francisco shows an actuarial progression rate of 54 percent at 10 years after infection[1] and an increasing progression rate after 5 years of follow-up. Only 18 percent of these 121 men had no signs or symptoms of HIV disease.

At four and one-half years of follow-up, a study of 288 HIV-seropositive men at San Francisco General Hospital found a 33 percent rate of progression to AIDS.[36] Although dates of seroconversion are unknown, it is possible to estimate, based on seroconversion rates in San Francisco during the early 1980s, that most of these men had been infected for one to three years on average before enrollment in the study. The rate of progression to AIDS has been approximately 7 percent per year for each of the last three years of study. Extrapolating this annual rate, 50 percent of seropositives will have developed AIDS by 7 to 8 years of study, or an estimated 9 to 10 years past infection. A median incubation period of 9 to 10 years is consistent both with recent estimates of the incubation period (see below) and with the long-term follow-up of 121 men cited above.

In the SFGH Cohort Study an additional 20 percent to 25 percent of subjects are projected to progress to symptomatic HIV disease in the next three years. Men with symptomatic HIV disease have a high probability of eventually progressing to AIDS — the two-year rate of progression from symptomatic HIV disease to AIDS in this study is 50 percent. Most subjects not developing clinical disease developed laboratory abnormalities strongly predictive of eventual progression to disease. These results suggest that most HIV seropositives will eventually progress to AIDS.

Estimated progression rates from some cohorts in Table 1 may be biased in the direction of overestimating clinical disease by recruitment that overrepresents symptomatic seropositives. On the other hand, bias in the opposite direction may be present because of subjects lost to follow-up. The lower rate in Table 1 reported from the large four-city cohort (Los Angeles, Baltimore, Chicago, and Pittsburgh — the MACS study) may reflect recruitment of subjects more recently infected than subjects in other prospective studies. Evidence from studies with estimated five-year progression rates suggests that 20 percent to 30 percent is a lower limit for five-year progression.[1,3] The evidence also suggests that progression rates are not significantly different in the different populations at risk.

■ INCUBATION PERIOD

The incubation period from HIV infection until emergence of AIDS has proved to be much longer than previously thought — a recent non-parametric estimate from San Francisco data found a median of 9.8 years[35] and other recent studies are consistent with this estimate (see Figure 1.1.6.a). The very long incubation period has slowed understanding of the natural history of HIV

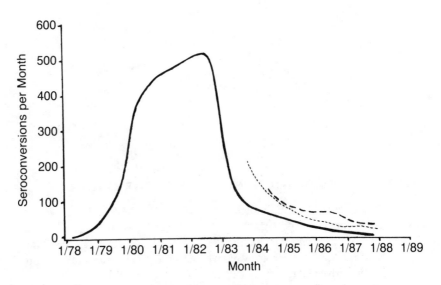

Figure 1.1.6.a HIV-1 antibody seroconversion rates in three San Francisco prospective studies of homosexual men: the hepatitis B vaccine trial (solid line), the San Francisco Men's Health Study (long dashes), and the San Francisco General Hospital Study (short dashes). Adapted from *Nature* 1989; 338:252.

infection. Prospective clinical studies of HIV seropositive individuals are ongoing in several countries. Most of these were not started until 1983 or 1984, so their data are from limited follow-up periods. As follow-up times lengthen, more events associated with HIV infection can be characterized.

Cases with the shortest incubation periods appeared first, and thus were overrepresented in the estimates made early in the epidemic. Of these cases, transfusion recipients were overrepresented because their date of infection could be most easily established. Many transfusion recipients were either neonates or of average older age and in poorer health than members of other risk groups. Early in the epidemic, the average incubation period was consequently estimated at one to two years — an estimate that has subsequently grown steadily longer.[23,26,35] An 8- to 10-year mean incubation period appears more in accord with the picture emerging from prospective studies of homosexual men.[1]

Progression rates are very low in the first two years after infection and increase thereafter. In the incubation distribution estimated by Bacchetti and Moss from San Francisco,[35] the following proportions progress to AIDS annually.

TABLE 2.   ESTIMATED PROBABILITIES OF DEVELOPING AIDS BY YEAR FOLLOWING SEROCONVERSION

YEAR	PROBABILITY OF AIDS (%)
1	0.2
2	0.7
3	2.2
4	4.3
5	6.1
6	7.3
7	8.2
8	8.1
9	7.4
10	6.7

■ PREDICTORS OF HIGH RATES OF PROGRESSION

In addition to the high rates of progression to AIDS and ARC, HIV seropositive men under prospective study show a steady worsening of laboratory values that are in themselves predictive of progression to AIDS (see Figures 1.1.6.b and 1.1.6.c). The progressive worsening of such values in asymptomatic HIV seropositives suggests that disease progression rates will ultimately be higher than those reported to date. Loss of CD4 (T-helper) lymphocytes, accompanied by a reversal of the CD4/CD8 (helper/suppressor) ratio, was recognized early as a characteristic of HIV infection. A low CD4 count is a predictor of

Correlation of Several Tests and Three-Year Progression Rates to AIDS

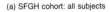

(a) SFGH cohort: all subjects

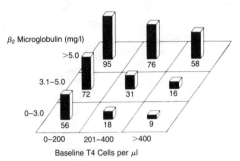

(b) SFGH cohort: subjects *without* detectable p24 antigen

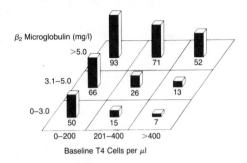

(c) SFGH cohort: subjects *with* detectable p24 antigen

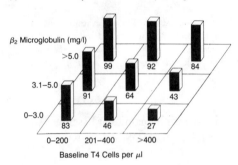

Figure 1.1.6.b Three-year progression rates to AIDS in the San Francisco General Hospital (SFGH) cohort by CD4 count, serum β_2-microglobulin level, and presence of HIV-p24 antigen. (a) All subjects, (b) subjects *without* detectable p24 antigen, and (c) subjects *with* detectable p24 antigen. Number in square is the percentage progressing to AIDS. Adapted from *AIDS* 1989; 3:58.

progression to disease, as is a low helper/suppressor ratio or a low proportion of CD4 lymphocytes.[4,7]

Other laboratory markers are also strongly predictive of probable development of AIDS. The presence of serum HIV p24 antigen is predictive; so too is the absence or reduction in titer of the complementary p24 antibody.[27,28] Increased levels of serum β_2-microglobulin and of neopterin (measured in serum or urine) are also prognostic for AIDS. The San Francisco General Hospital follow-up study of HIV seropositive men has defined a five-factor multivariate model for predicting progression to AIDS.[3] The following are independent predictors of the risk of developing AIDS.

- Serum level of β_2-microglobulin >3.0 microgram/ml
- T4 count < 200 cells/cubic mm
- T4 lymphocytes < 25 percent of total lymphocytes
- Presence of p24 antigen
- Hematocrit < 40

This model is a strong predictor of the probability of progression to AIDS within the next 24 months. Subjects with two or more of these abnormalities had a 57 percent three-year progression rate to AIDS, compared with a 7

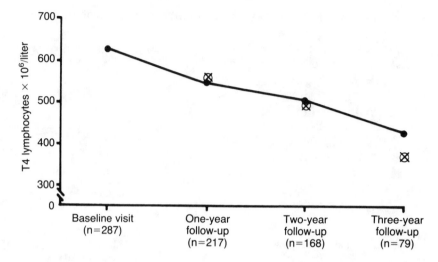

Figure 1.1.6.c   Median T4 lymphocytes ×10⁶/liter at successive follow-up examinations in subjects who had not yet developed AIDS-defining conditions. The progressive loss of T4 lymphocytes in this group suggests that they will eventually develop AIDS. ●=raw medians (observed values); ⊗=median changes from baseline. Adapted from *British Medical Journal* 1988; 296:749.

percent three-year progression in subjects with no abnormalities at baseline. All subjects with four or more abnormalities progressed to AIDS within two years.

■ LYMPHADENOPATHY SYNDROME AND PROGRESSION TO AIDS

Rates of progression have also been reported for homosexual men with lymphadenopathy syndrome. These reports suggest that lymphadenopathy syndrome is not a predictor of rapid progression to AIDS. Although cohorts of patients defined by clinical signs and symptoms may not be comparable to cohorts defined by antibody status alone, data from cohorts of antibody-positive men show no correlation between lymphadenopathy and measures of immunosuppression, or between presence of lymphadenopathy and probabilities of progression to AIDS.[29] Reported rates of progression to AIDS (in Table 3 below) show about the same range as those for asymptomatic HIV-seropositive persons in Table 1.[9-12]

TABLE 3.   PROPORTION OF HOMOSEXUAL MEN WITH LYMPHADENOPATHY PROGRESSING TO AIDS*

HOMOSEXUAL MEN	FOLLOW-UP PERIOD	N AIDS/N	% PROGRESSING
San Francisco[9]	60 months	47/143	36†
Atlanta[10]	20 months	5/78	6
New York[11]	52 months	12/42	29
Atlanta[12]	52 months	14/75	29†

*   *Table compiled by the author.*
†   *Derived through Kaplan–Meier survival analysis.*

■ COFACTORS FOR PROGRESSION TO AIDS IN INFECTED PERSONS

Prospective data have identified age as a cofactor for progression to AIDS. Seropositive men over age 35 have a higher progression rate than those under 35,[3] but sexual behavior or other infections have not been associated with higher progression rates. An analysis of age and AIDS incidence rates corroborates age as a cofactor for progression.[31] Progression to symptomatic HIV disease may be influenced by coinfection with other viruses such as CMV, EBV, or HBV, or HTLV-I. Coinfection with the human T-lymphotropic virus type I has been reported to increase the rate at which HIV seropositives develop AIDS.[34] A number of other possible cofactors have been proposed: infection with more than one strain of HIV; prior or coinfection with enteric parasites; exposure to allogenic antigens, such as semen and blood; malnutrition; and use of immunotoxic or mutagenic drugs.[2,13-16] Other host determinants of immune response and the size or route of the original inoculum of HIV may also affect the outcome of infection.

Because Kaposi's sarcoma (KS) is predominantly identified in homosexual men, cofactors for KS have been sought that are more common in homosexual men than in the other risk groups. Potential cofactors for KS that have drawn the most attention are CMV infection,[17,18] the use of amyl and butyl nitrites ("poppers") as recreational drugs,[5,19-21] the human leukocyte antigen (HLA) type DR5,[22] and other sexually transmitted agents. Given present knowledge, the evidence for any of these as a cofactor in KS must be regarded as speculative.

REFERENCES

1. Lifson A, Hessol NA, Rutherford GW, et al. The natural history of HIV infection in a cohort of homosexual and bisexual men: clinical manifestations, 1978-1989. V International Conference on AIDS. Montreal, 1989:T.A.O.32.
2. Goedert JJ, Biggar RJ, Weiss SH, et al. Three-year incidence of AIDS in five cohorts of HTLV-III infected risk group members. Science 1986; 231:992-5.
3. Moss AR, Bacchetti P, Osmond D, et al. Seropositivity of HIV and the development of AIDS or AIDS related condition: three year follow up of the San Francisco General Hospital cohort. Br Med J 1988; 296:745-50.
4. Phair J, Munoz A, Kingsley L, et al. Incidence of AIDS in homosexual men developing HIV infection. IV International Conference on AIDS. Stockholm, 1988; 1:4093.
5. Ward J, Perkins H, Pepkowitz S, et al. Dose response or strain variation may influence disease progression in HIV-infected blood recipients. IV International Conference on AIDS. Stockholm, 1988; 2:7711.
6. Giesecke J, Scalia-Tomba G, Berglund O, et al. Incidence of symptoms and AIDS in 146 Swedish haemophiliacs and blood transfusion recipients infected with human immunodeficiency virus. Br Med J 1988; 297:99-102.
7. Goedert JJ, Biggar RJ, Melbye M, et al. Effect of T4 count and cofactors on the incidence of AIDS in homosexual men infected with human immunodeficiency virus. JAMA 1987; 257:331-4.
8. Goedert JJ, Biggar RJ, Weiss SH, et al. Three-year incidence of AIDS in five cohorts of HTLV-III infected risk group members. Science 1986; 231:992-5.
9. Abrams DI, Kirn DH, Feigal DW, Volberding P. Lymphadenopathy: update of a 60-month prospective study [Abstract]. Washington, D.C.: III International Conference on Acquired Immunodeficiency Syndrome, 1987.
10. Fishbein DB, Kaplan JE, Spira TJ, et al. Unexplained lymphadenopathy in homosexual men: a longitudinal study. JAMA 1985; 254:930-5.
11. Mathur-Wagh U, Mildvan D, Senie RT. Follow-up at 4.5 years on homosexual men with generalized lymphadenopathy. N Engl J Med 1985; 311:1542-3.
12. Kaplan JE, Spira TJ, Fishbein DB, et al. Lymphadenopathy syndrome in homosexual men. JAMA 1987; 257:335-7.
13. Goedert JJ, Blattner WA. The epidemiology of AIDS and related conditions. In: DeVita VT, Hellman S, Rosenberg SA, eds. AIDS: etiology, diagnosis, treatment and prevention. Philadelphia: J.B. Lippincott, 1985:1-30.

14. Curran JW, Morgan WM, Hardy AM, et al. The epidemiology of AIDS: current status and future prospects. Science 1985; 229:1352-7.

15. Archer DL, Glinsmann WH. Enteric infections and other cofactors in AIDS. Immunology Today 1985; 6:292-5.

16. Schecter MT, Boyko WJ, Jeffries E, et al. The Vancouver lymphadenopathy AIDS study: 4. Effects of exposure factors, cofactors and HTLV-III seropositivity on number of helper T cells. Can Med Assoc J 1985; 113:286-92.

17. Mintz L, Drew WL, Miner RC, et al. Cytomegalovirus infection in homosexual men: an epidemiologic study. Ann Intern Med 1983; 99:326.

18. Giraldo G, Bethe E, Henle W, et al. Antibody patterns to herpesviruses in Kaposi's sarcoma. II. Serological association of American Kaposi's sarcoma with cytomegalovirus. Int J Cancer 1978; 22:126.

19. Jorgensen MA, Lawesson SO. Amyl nitrite and Kaposi's sarcoma in homosexual men. N Engl J Med 1982; 307:893-4.

20. Osmond D, Moss AR, Bacchetti P, et al. A case-control study of risk factors for AIDS in San Francisco [Abstract]. Atlanta: International Conference on Acquired Immunodeficiency Syndrome, 1985; 24.

21. Haverkos HW, Pinsky PF, Drotman DP, et al. Disease manifestations among homosexual men with acquired immunodeficiency syndrome: a possible role of nitrites in Kaposi's sarcoma. J Sex Trans Dis 1985; 12:203-8.

22. Friedman-Kien AE, Laubenstein LJ, Rubenstein P, et al. Disseminated Kaposi's sarcoma in homosexual men. Ann Intern Med 1982; 96:693.

23. Lui KJ, Lawrence DN, Morgan WM, et al. A model-based approach for estimating the mean incubation period of transfusion-associated acquired immunodeficiency syndrome. Proc Natl Acad Sci 1986; 83:3051-5.

24. Goedert JJ, Eyster ME, Friedman RM, Gail MH. AIDS rates, markers and cofactors. IV International Conference on AIDS. Stockholm, 1988; 1:4144.

25. Jason J, Lui K-J, Ragni MV, et al. Risk of developing AIDS in HIV-infected cohorts of hemophiliac and homosexual men. JAMA 1989; 261:725-7.

26. Medley GF, Anderson RM, Cox DR, Billard L. Incubation period of AIDS in patients infected via blood transfusion. Nature 1987; 328:719-21.

27. Wiley JA, Rutherford GW, Moss AR, Winkelstein W. Age and cumulative incidence of AIDS among seropositive homosexual men in high incidence areas of San Francisco [Abstract]. Washington, D.C.: Third International Conference on Acquired Immunodeficiency Syndrome, 1987; 206.

28. Weber JN, Clapham PR, Weiss RA, et al. Human immunodeficiency virus infection in two cohorts of homosexual men: neutralising sera and association of anti-gag antibody with prognosis. Lancet 1987; 1:119-22.

29. Osmond D, Chaisson R, Moss A, et al. Lymphadenopathy in asymptomatic patients seropositive for HIV. N Engl J Med 1987; 317:246.

30. Allain JP. LAV infection by blood and blood derivatives. In: Gluckman JC, Vilmer E, eds. Acquired immunodeficiency syndrome. Paris: Elsevier, 1986:167-71.

31. Lange JM, Paul DA, Huisman HG, et al. Persistent HIV antigenaemia and decline of HIV core antibodies associated with transition to AIDS. Br Med J 1986; 293:1459-62.

32. Lee CA, Miller EJ, Griffiths PD, et al. HIV disease in a cohort of 104 haemophiliacs. IV International Conference on AIDS. Stockholm, 1988; 2:7733.

33. Selwyn PA, Hartel D, Schoenbaum EE, et al. Clinical progression of HIV-related disease in intravenous drug users (IVDU) in a prospective cohort study: 1985-1989. V International Conference on AIDS. Montreal, 1989:Th.A.O.24.

34. Weiss SH, French J, Holland B, et al. HTLV-I/II co-infection is significantly associated with risk for progression to AIDS among HIV+ intravenous drug abusers. V International Conference on AIDS. Montreal, 1989:Th.A.O.23.

35. Bacchetti P, Moss AR. Incubation period of AIDS in San Francisco. Nature 1989; 338:251-3.

36. Moss AR, Bacchetti P, Osmond DH, et al. Progression to AIDS in the San Francisco General Hospital Cohort Study. V International Conference on AIDS. Montreal, 1989:T.A.O.31.

Prevalence of Infection
and Projections
for the Future

Dennis Osmond

Because of the long incubation period from HIV infection to AIDS, many more individuals are infected with the virus than diagnosed with AIDS. The average length of the incubation period is now estimated at over 8 years, with a reported range of 4 months to 10 years.[1] The number of persons who are likely to be diagnosed with AIDS in the next few years is largely determined by the number of persons who are already infected. Widely differing estimates of HIV seroprevalence in the United States have appeared in the literature. Serologic studies estimate the incidence of HIV within specific risk groups. Screening of special populations, such as blood donors and military recruits, is a source of nationwide data, but extrapolating an estimate from this data for the entire U.S. population remains uncertain.

■ EARLIEST EVIDENCE OF HIV INFECTION IN THE U.S.

AIDS was first recognized as a new clinical syndrome in the United States in 1981. The first cases of *Pneumocystis carinii* pneumonia and Kaposi's sarcoma were diagnosed among homosexual men. Looking back at earlier reports, researchers have identified cases appearing to fit the AIDS surveillance definition as early as the 1950s and 1960s.[36] Frozen tissue and serum samples were available for one of these possible early AIDS cases — a 15-year-old black male from St. Louis who was hospitalized in 1968 and died of an aggressive, disseminated Kaposi's sarcoma.[37] His tissue and serum specimens were HIV antibody-positive on Western blot and antigen positive on ELISA. This appears to be the first confirmed case of HIV infection in the U.S.

■ HIV SEROPREVALENCE IN RISK GROUPS

Seroprevalence studies of homosexual men, intravenous drug users (IVDUs), and hemophiliacs show a high prevalence of HIV antibody in these groups.[1,2,4-12] Retrospective testing of stored sera has documented that rapid seroconversion occurred in all three groups during the early 1980s. Annual rates of seroconversion in homosexual men were very high during 1981–1984. The studies below show seroconversion rates during that period as averaging between 10 percent and 15 percent a year.

HOMOSEXUAL MEN

In 1984, two studies randomly sampled homosexual men in San Francisco neighborhoods with high proportions of single men and found that approxi-

TABLE 1.

LOCATION	FOLLOW-UP PERIOD	N CONVERTING/N	ANNUAL RATE (%)
San Francisco[6]	1978–1984	239/360	10
New York City[13]	1982–1983	4/29	14
New York City[2]	1978–1984	121/277	5.5–10.6
Vancouver[14]	1982–1984	14/130	15
Denmark[15]	1982–1983	4/34	12

mately 40 percent of the subjects were seropositive.[4,5] At the same time, two studies of homosexual men recruited from sexually transmitted disease (STD) clinics in San Francisco — men presumably more sexually active than average — both showed that nearly 70 percent of the subjects were antibody-positive.[4,6] Also in 1984, a smaller study from a private medical practice in Manhattan reported that 36 percent of those studied were positive, a result similar to the neighborhood studies in San Francisco.[16] Ongoing follow-up of the San Francisco neighborhood cohorts shows that approximately 50 percent of subjects are now seropositive (Osmond D: unpublished data). Because the incidence curves for San Francisco, New York City, and Los Angeles have paralleled each other from the beginning of the epidemic, the San Francisco estimate that 50 percent of its homosexual population is infected probably also applies to the homosexual populations of Manhattan and West Los Angeles.[17] Closely comparable prevalence rates for Los Angeles have been reported from the Multicenter AIDS Cohort Study.[30] In San Francisco, a prospective study of HIV seronegative homosexual men has observed a dramatic reduction in the seroconversion rate; the seroconversion rate of 10 percent to 20 percent per year in the early 1980s was down to less than 1 percent per year in 1987–88.[35]

Prevalence data in other U.S. cities come primarily from studies of homosexual men tested in STD clinics. Rates are therefore likely to be higher than the community-wide average. Seroprevalence ranged from 12 percent among homosexual men in STD clinics in New Mexico to 70 percent in a Philadelphia STD clinic.[30] The Centers for Disease Control (CDC) estimates that 20 percent to 25 percent of exclusively homosexual men are infected. The infected homosexual male population has been estimated at 0.5 to 0.65 million, but the CDC concedes that there is a very wide margin of error in estimating the size of the population at risk.[30]

Intravenous Drug Users (IVDUs). IVDUs in both the United States and Europe show rapid rates of seroconversion that are similar to those seen in homosexual men during the early 1980s. The IVDU seroconversion rates began to climb one to two years after those for homosexual men.[8-11,18,19] Strong geographic variation is an important feature of the seroprevalence rates among IVDUs. Half or more than half of IVDUs have been infected in the high-incidence areas of New York City and northern New Jersey.[8] In 1984, one drug detoxification program in New York City found a 58 percent prevalence of antibodies to HIV.[8] A retrospective New York study found seropositivity increased from 9 percent in 1978 to 50 percent in 1982.[20] In 1984, in a survey of over 900 IV drug users in northern New Jersey who lived within five miles of

New York City, 50 percent were found to be positive.[21] The number of IVDUs in the United States is estimated at 750,000.[22]

Outside of the New York–New Jersey region, seroprevalence among IVDUs has tended to be much lower, ranging from 0 percent to 44 percent.[30] In most U.S. cities not on the East Coast, rates are in the 0 percent to 10 percent range. In San Francisco, the rates are between 10 percent and 20 percent.[23] Why the epidemic has reached an advanced stage in some areas of the East Coast and has stayed in an early stage in many interior and West Coast cities remains unclear. Similar differences are observed in Europe, where, for example, HIV infection spread very rapidly through IVDUs in Edinburgh but not in those from nearby Glasgow.

Hemophiliacs.   The highest seropositive rates have been found in hemophiliacs. Between 64 percent and 90 percent of hemophiliacs receiving factor VIII have been reported as infected with HIV.[10,26,27] Studies of stored sera show a rapid increase in antibody prevalence from 1981 to 1983.[11,12] These studies also show differences in HIV infection depending on the type of factor administered and the severity of the disorder. The CDC estimates that 70 percent of all hemophiliacs in the United States receiving factor VIII (hemophilia A) and 35 percent of those receiving factor IX (hemophilia B) are now seropositive.[30] The number of hemophiliacs in the United States is estimated at 14,467.[21]

Prevalence among Persons with No Known Risk Factor.   Nationwide serologic data are available from ongoing screening in selected populations, including blood donors, Job Corps applicants, and both military applicants and military personnel. While these data are useful in monitoring the spread of the epidemic, they are difficult to interpret because risk-factor information is not available from the individuals screened. In addition, the degree and reasons for self-deferral are not known in populations tested repeatedly in cross-sectional studies. Besides these nationwide data, screening has been conducted in some states among childbearing women, in prenatal clinics, at STD clinics, and at sentinel hospitals. Recent data on seroprevalence rates are shown in Table 2.[30,34]

Very little risk-factor information is available from these studies, but the CDC has investigated small samples of tested individuals and found that 80 percent to 90 percent have one or more established risk factors for HIV infection. By assuming that 15 percent of positives from these seroprevalence studies (Table 2) are without risk factors, the CDC estimates a national seroprevalence among the 142 million adult Americans without known risk factors at 0.21 per 1000 — an estimated 30,000 infected without known risk factors.

TABLE 2.   SEROPREVALENCE OF HIV INFECTION IN SELECTED U.S. POPULATIONS

POPULATION	DATE	NO. TESTED	%HIV+
Blood donors — all Red Cross	1985–87	12.6 million	0.2/1000
Blood donors — first time	1985–87	NA*	0.4/1000
Military applicants — U.S.	1985–88	1.5 million	1.4/1000
Military applicants — N.Y.C.	1985–86	9,498	10.3/1000

continued on next page

continued from previous page

TABLE 2. SEROPREVALENCE OF HIV INFECTION IN SELECTED U.S. POPULATIONS

POPULATION	DATE	NO. TESTED	%HIV+
Job Corps applicants	1987	25,000	3.3/1000
Childbearing women — Mass.	1986–87	30,708	2.1/1000
Childbearing women — N.Y.C.	1986–87	1,192	23.0/1000
Sentinel hospitals — midwest (4)	1986–87	8,668	3.2/1000

*   NA = *not available.*

This would suggest that the spread of HIV infection is still primarily confined to identified risk groups, but the striking feature of the seroprevalence data in the table above is that rates are an order of magnitude greater in New York City, where they are in the 1 percent to 3 percent range, than in the rest of the country, where they are in the 0.1 percent to 0.3 percent range. Even within states there is a large urban differential; for example, in the Massachusetts study of childbearing women, seroprevalence averaged 8 per 1000 for urban hospitals and 0.9 per 1000 for suburban and rural hospitals.[30] These high urban rates may portend the next major expansion of the epidemic among inner-city populations.

■ ESTIMATES OF SEROPREVALENCE IN THE UNITED STATES

Estimates of HIV seroprevalence for the entire U.S. population range from 0.5 million to 3 million. These projections have generated intense controversy in both the scientific and popular literature.[29-33] In June 1986 the U.S. Public Health Service (PHS) estimated 1 to 1.5 million infected.[32] In November 1987 they left that number essentially unchanged in their revised estimate of 945,000 to 1.4 million.[30] The PHS estimate is derived by extrapolating average rates of infection in the risk groups to estimates of the population sizes of those groups. Another approach estimated that in 1987 the total number should have risen from 0.5 to 0.8 million infected persons, based on rates of progression from HIV infection to AIDS that were derived from cohort studies of seropositive persons.[33] There is a wide margin of error in all estimates of national seroprevalence, but 0.5 million can probably be taken as a lower limit.

■ PROJECTIONS FOR THE FUTURE

Predictions of the number of cases of AIDS that will occur in the future are based upon estimates of both the number of persons currently infected and the rate at which infected persons progress to AIDS. As the follow-up times of prospective studies of infected persons lengthen, estimates of the rate of progression to AIDS improve. Seroprevalence surveys are also rapidly expanding the data available on the prevalence of HIV infection, but overall estimates of the number of persons infected in the United States remain uncertain and projections of future cases therefore also remain uncertain.

Data from prospective studies of HIV-seropositive individuals suggest that the majority, if not all, will eventually develop AIDS, but that the median time from infection to AIDS may be close to 10 years. Estimates of the number currently infected in the United States range from 0.5 million to 3 million.

Projection methods that apply progression rates to the number of persons infected in the country are hampered by the wide uncertainty about the prevalence of infection (see Figure 1.1.7.a). Methods that fit a mathematical function to the distribution of cases to date in order to extrapolate that function into the future are limited by the implicit assumption that the future distribution will be similar to that of the past. This method may work well for the short term (one or two years), but it becomes more dubious when extrapolations are made beyond that point.

The U.S. Public Health Service has used this curve-fitting method to estimate that a cumulative total of 270,000 AIDS cases will occur by 1991.[1] As of mid-1989 the cumulative total exceeded 100,000. Cases in 1989 appear to be

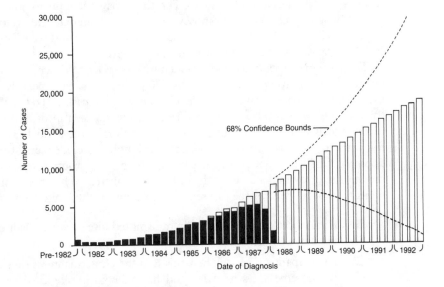

Figure 1.1.7.a   Quarterly incidence of AIDS in the U.S. is projected through 1992 by extrapolating pre-1987 trends. Actual cases reported to the Centers for Disease Control in Atlanta through March 31, 1988 (*solid portion of bars*), account for about 90 percent of the total projected. Adapted from *Scientific American* 1988; 259(4):81.

falling below the CDC projections for 1989, but because the lag time in reporting cases averages several months and may be lengthening, it will not be clear for some time whether the estimate for 1989 is too high. The projected 1991 cumulative total of 270,000, however, will not occur unless there are substantial increases in the number of cases in the very near future. So far the 1989 increases do not appear large enough to justify the 1991 projections.

Trends and the Future of the Epidemic in the United States.   Estimates of the prevalence of infection in homosexual men in the cities where the epidemic first appeared in the United States find approximately 50 percent seropositive. Surveys of self-reported sexual behavior in homosexual men in San Francisco have shown substantial change to "safe sex" practices,[39,40] and rates for rectal and pharyngeal gonorrhea in males declined 59 percent in Manhattan between 1980 and 1983.[41] A similar decline occurred in San Francisco in rectal gonorrhea and syphilis rates.[42] Prospective studies of homosexual men in San Francisco report seroconversion rates of 1 percent to 2 percent per year or less since 1984, a considerable reduction from the 10 percent to 15 percent seen in the early 1980s. All these data suggest the epidemic spread of HIV infection among homosexual men has greatly slowed in the high incidence cities. Since homosexual men still account for nearly three fourths of all cases, the large reduction in seroconversion rates will be followed by a substantial downturn in the number of AIDS cases seen in this population. In San Francisco, surveillance data suggest the beginning of a levelling off or downturn in the number of homosexual male cases. The number of cases among homosexual men in San Francisco did not increase between the first and second six months of 1987 and was slightly lower in the first six months of 1988 (671 cases) than in either half of 1987 (699 and 693 cases).[9]

These San Francisco data suggest that the number of cases of AIDS may level off among homosexual men in New York and Los Angeles in the near future — if it has not already done so. This trend may not apply to other urban centers, where spread among homosexual men began later and trends for rates of progression to AIDS are probably one to three years behind New York, San Francisco, and Los Angeles in the epidemic.

The epidemic among homosexual men may be slowing down, but the epidemic among intravenous drug users is still rapidly increasing, especially in East Coast cities. Heterosexual cases in the U.S. are also increasing. To what extent these trends will cancel out or whether the increases seen in drug users and heterosexuals will be large enough to continue to raise the annual case count for years to come is difficult to predict. Although the epidemic still has the potential for further devastating expansion among the groups already at risk, much larger growth depends on the potential for increased heterosexual transmission. Two models for the future of the epidemic in the United States exist.

1. The African Model: a sexually transmitted disease spread bidirectionally between males and females.

2. The Hepatitis B Model: hepatitis B in the United States is transmitted in the same ways as AIDS and has an epidemiologic pattern very similar to the pattern seen in AIDS, with endemic infection in the principal risk groups and relatively little spread outside those groups.

The African Model.   If heterosexual transmission is to become a major route of spread in the U.S., five years into the epidemic signs of its increasing contribution to new cases should have appeared. Such signs have not yet been seen. The proportion attributed to heterosexual transmission has remained nearly constant. Nonetheless, the relatively small proportion attributed to heterosexual transmission could be more an artifact of the very rapid spread of the epidemic in the principal risk groups than an indication of the potential for heterosexual spread. In industrialized countries, intravenous drug users (IVDUs) are the source of the majority of heterosexual transmission cases. If the African pattern is to occur in the United States and Europe, it most likely will be seen as increased heterosexual transmission in the population of IVDUs in the major urban centers, and in populations already at risk for sexually transmitted diseases (poor, inner city, minority).

The Hepatitis B Model.   AIDS cases are now being reported in the United States in numbers approaching the number of cases of hepatitis B, approximately 1350 AIDS cases per month compared with 2000 hepatitis B cases. Hepatitis B appears more readily transmitted than the human immunodeficiency virus (HIV), at least in the nosocomial setting; but on the other hand, a higher percentage of persons infected with HIV may become infectious carriers than the 5 percent to 10 percent estimated for hepatitis B.[45] As these differences probably influence the relative rates of transmission of HIV and hepatitis B in opposite directions, it is too early to tell whether HIV will spread more extensively than hepatitis B. Hepatitis B, which in the United States has stayed primarily within the major risk groups, has a different epidemiologic pattern in the Third World, where in some countries it is one of the most significant health problems and is transmitted both sexually and perinatally.[45]

There are major cultural differences between Africa and the United States and Europe that may continue to shape the epidemic differently in Africa. The pattern of AIDS may be analogous to the pattern of hepatitis B and it may, like hepatitis B, continue to follow different courses in the Third World and in the industrialized countries.

REFERENCES

1. Medley GF, Anderson RM, Cox DR, Billard L. Incubation period of AIDS in patients infected via blood transfusion. Nature 1987; 328:719-21.

2. Lui KJ, Darrow WW, Rutherford GW. A model-based estimate of the mean incubation period for AIDS in homosexual men. Science 1988; 240:1333-5.

3. Kalbfleisch JD, Lawless JF. Estimating the incubation period for AIDS patients. Nature 1988; 333:504-5.

4. Moss AM, Osmond DH, Bacchetti P, et al. One-year follow-up of men exposed to AIDS in San Francisco [Abstract]. Atlanta: International Conference on the Acquired Immunodeficiency Syndrome, 1985; 83.

5. Anderson RE, Levy JA. Prevalence of antibodies to AIDS associated retrovirus in single men in San Francisco. Lancet 1985; 1:217.

6. Jaffe HW, Darrow WW, Echenberg DF, et al. The acquired immunodeficiency syndrome in a cohort of homosexual men: a six year follow-up study. Ann Intern Med 1985; 103:210-4.

7. Collier AC, Barnes RC, Handsfield HH. Prevalence of antibody to LAV/HTLV-III among homosexual men in Seattle. Am J Public Health 1986; 76:564-5.

8. Spira TJ, Des Jarlais DC, Marmor M, et al. Prevalence of antibody to lymphadenopathy-associated virus among drug detoxification patients in New York. N Engl J Med 1984; 311:467-8.

9. Robertson JR, Bucknall AB, Welsby PD, et al. Epidemic of AIDS related virus (HTLV-III/LAV) infection among intravenous drug abusers. Br Med J 1986; 292:527-9.

10. Goedert JJ, Sarngadharan MG, Eyster ME, et al. Antibodies reactive with human T cell leukemia viruses (HTLV-III) in the serum of hemophiliacs receiving factor VIII concentrate. Blood 1985; 65:492-5.

11. Gurtler LG, Wernicke D, Eberle J, et al. Increase in prevalence of anti-HTLV-III in haemophiliacs. Lancet 1984; 2:1275-6.

12. Eyster ME, Goedert JJ, Sarngadharan MG, et al. Development and early natural history of HTLV-III antibodies in patients with hemophilia. JAMA 1985; 253:2219.

13. Goedert JJ, Biggar RJ, Winn D, et al. Determinants of retrovirus (HTLV-III) antibody and immunodeficiency conditions in homosexual men. Lancet 1984; 2:711-5.

14. Jeffries E, Willoughby KB, Boyko W, et al. The Vancouver lymphadenopathy-AIDS study: 2. Seroepidemiology of HTLV-III antibody. Can Med Assoc J 1985; 132:1373-7.

15. Melbye M, Biggar R, Ebbesen P, et al. Seroepidemiology of HTLV-III antibody in Danish homosexual men: prevalence, transmission, and disease outcome. Br Med J 1984; 289:573-5.

16. Marmor M, El-Sadr W, Zolla-Pazner S, et al. HTLV-III seropositivity and its relationship to disease in a prospective study of homosexual males [Abstract]. Atlanta: International Conference on Acquired Immunodeficiency Syndrome, 1985; 27.

17. Enstrom JE. AIDS among homosexual men in California. Lancet 1986; 1:975-6.

18. Angarano G, Pastore G, Monno L, et al. Rapid spread of HTLV-III infection among drug addicts in Italy. Lancet 1985; 2:1302.

19. Kitchen LW, Barin F, Sullivan JL, et al. Aetiology of AIDS antibodies to human T-cell leukaemia virus (type III) in haemophiliacs. Nature 1984; 312:367-9.

20. Novick D, Kreek MJ, Des Jarlais DC, et al. Abstract of clinical research findings: therapeutic and historical aspects. In: Harris LS, ed. Problems of drug dependence, 1985. Proceedings of the 47th Annual Scientific Meeting, the Committee on Problems of Drug Dependence, Inc. NIDA research monograph 67. Washington, D.C.: NIDA, 1986:318.

21. Weiss SH, Ginzburg HM, Goedert JJ, et al. Risk for HTLV-III exposure and AIDS among parenteral drug abusers in New Jersey [Abstract]. In: The International Conference on Acquired Immunodeficiency Syndrome: Abstracts. Philadelphia: The American College of Physicians, 1985.

22. Hardy AM, Allen JR, Morgan WM, et al. The incidence rate of acquired immunodeficiency syndrome in selected populations. JAMA 1985; 253:215-20.

23. Chaisson RE, Moss AK, Onishi R, et al. Human immunodeficiency virus infection in heterosexual intravenous drug users in San Francisco. Am J Public Health 1987; 77:169-72.

24. D'Aguilla R, Williams AB, Kleber HD, et al. Prevalence of HTLV-III infection among New Haven, Connecticut, parenteral drug abusers in 1982–1983. N Engl J Med 1986; 314:117-8.

25. Mortimer PP, Vandervelde EM, Jesson WJ, et al. HTLV-III antibody in Swiss and English intravenous drug abusers. Lancet 1985; 2:449-50.

26. Melbye M, Biggar RJ, Chermann JC, et al. High prevalence of lymphadenopathy virus (LAV) in European hemophiliacs. Lancet 1984; 2:40-1.

27. Ramsey RB, Palmer EL, McDougal JS, et al. Antibody to lymphadenopathy-associated virus in hemophiliacs with and without AIDS. Lancet 1984; 2:397-8.

28. Curran JW, Morgan WM, Hardy AM, et al. The epidemiology of AIDS: current status and future prospects. Science 1985; 229:1352-7.

29. Sivak SL, Wormser GP. How common is HTLV-III infection in the United States? N Engl J Med 1985; 313:1352.

30. Centers for Disease Control. Human immunodeficiency virus infection in the United States: a review of current knowledge. MMWR 1987; 36:Suppl 6:1S-48S.

31. Rees M. The sombre view of AIDS. Nature 1987; 326:343-5.

32. U.S. Department of Health and Human Services, Public Health Service. Coolfont report: a PHS plan for prevention and control of AIDS and AIDS virus. Pub Health Rep 1986; 101:341-8.

33. Osmond D, Moss AR. The prevalence of HIV infection in the United States: a reappraisal of the Public Health Service estimate. In: Volberding P, Jacobson M, eds. 1989 Clinical AIDS review (in press).

34. Burke DS, Brundage JF, Bernier W, et al. Demography of HIV infections among civilian applicants for military service in four counties in New York City. NY State J Med 1987; 87:262-4.

35. Winkelstein W Jr, Wiley JA, Padian NS, et al. The San Francisco Men's Health Study: continued decline in HIV seroconversion rates among homosexual/bisexual men. Am J Public Health 1988; 78:1472-4.

36. Huminer D, Rosenfeld JB, Pitlik SD. AIDS in the pre-AIDS era. Rev Infect Dis 1987; 9:1102-8.

37. Garry RF, Witte MH, Gottlieb AA, et al. Documentation of an AIDS virus infection in the United States in 1968. JAMA 1988; 260:2085-7.

38. U.S. Public Health Department. PHS plan for prevention and control of AIDS and the AIDS virus. Public Health Reports 101 (July -August 1986):341-8.

39. Bye L. Designing an effective AIDS prevention campaign strategy for San Francisco: results from the first probability sample of an urban gay male community. San Francisco, California: Research and Decisions Corporation, 1984.

40. McKusick ML, Horstman W, Coates TJ. AIDS and sexual behavior reported by gay men in San Francisco. Am J Public Health 1985; 75:493-6.

41. Centers for Disease Control. Declining rates of rectal and pharyngeal gonorrhea among males — New York City. MMWR 1984; 33:295-7.

42. Rectal gonorrhea in San Francisco, October 1984-September 1986. San Francisco Epidemiologic Bulletin 1986; 2:12.

43. AIDS Office, San Francisco Department of Public Health. Acquired Immunodeficiency Syndrome (AIDS) Monthly Surveillance Report. Cases reported through 3/31/87.

44. Moss AR, Bacchetti P, Osmond D, et al. Incidence of the acquired immunodeficiency syndrome in San Francisco, 1980-1983. J Infect Dis 1985; 152:152-61.

45. Vyas GN, Cohen SN, Schmid R, eds. Viral hepatitis. Philadelphia: Franklin Institute Press, 1978.

46. Lindan C, Rutherford GW, Payne S, et al. Decline in rate of new AIDS cases among homosexual and bisexual men in San Francisco. V International Conference on AIDS. Montreal, 1989:W.A.P.24.

AIDS and HIV Infection in Prisoners: Epidemiology

Elizabeth Kantor, M.D.

Prisoners represent a group at high risk for AIDS because of the casual connection between IV drug use and criminal incarceration. No precise count exists of AIDS cases in prisons and jails. Brief incarceration often prevents identification or diagnosis of the affected inmates. Sick inmates may leave the institution for diagnosis and treatment and may not return. In addition, no national system for reporting prison cases exists in the United States; the Centers for Disease Control (CDC) surveillance information does not include individuals' custody status. However, independent surveys have been performed by the American Civil Liberties Union and the National Institute of Justice in the United States, and by the Council of Europe in 17 countries.[1,2,5-7]

There are more than 750,000 prisoners in the United States. As of October 1, 1987, a survey of 50 state prison systems, the federal prison system, and 31 large urban jail systems revealed a total of 1964 past and current AIDS cases. Of these cases, 421 were current.[6] Numbers of AIDS cases have been gathered annually from these institutions for three consecutive years.[1,5] Although the incidence of AIDS in the United States as a whole has increased 79 percent (1985–86) and 61 percent (1986–87), AIDS cases in the U.S. correctional institutions surveyed increased 61 percent and 59 percent in the corresponding years — less than in the general community.[1,5,6]

The incidence of AIDS in American prisoners parallels the incidence of AIDS in intravenous drug users (IVDUs). New York, New Jersey, and Pennsylvania share 62.3 percent of U.S. prison AIDS cases; in these states, AIDS associated with intravenous drug abuse (IVDA) is most prevalent.[6] As of May 8, 1988, 95 percent of the 532 reported AIDS deaths in New York state prisons were found in inmates with histories of IVDA.[8] In California prisons, 39 AIDS deaths had been identified by May 8, 1988; about 80 percent of these inmates reported intravenous drug use (Khouri N: personal communication). AIDS in California is still largely a disease of homosexual men, and is much less common among prisoners than in New York. Figures are available for the racial breakdown of prison AIDS cases in New York State. A much larger proportion of patients are nonwhite than in the general community: 45.3 percent Hispanic, 42.6 percent black, and 12.1 percent white. This reflects the racial distribution of IVDUs in the New York area.[8]

It has been my experience that in prison systems where HIV tests are regularly performed, AIDS diagnoses are not always made according to strict CDC case definition (i.e., an HIV-positive inmate with a pneumonia that improves on trimethoprim/sulfamethoxazole is given an AIDS diagnosis, although pneumocystis is never histologically identified).

In 202 New York State prisoners, the survival time from date of diagnosis until death fell far below that of New York City nonprisoner AIDS patients, even when both groups were matched for risk group and race.[8] HIV seropositivity rates among prisoners in the United States have been determined in limited, blind epidemiologic studies. This information has also been routinely gathered in several prison systems that perform mandatory HIV antibody tests on all inmates. Prisons that test and screen, whose seroprevalence rates are available, have been those with the lowest incidence of AIDS. New York, New Jersey, Florida, and Texas prisons, which report the majority of cases but do not screen inmates, may be predicted to have much higher rates of seropositivity than those of the U.S. prison systems listed in Table 1.

Studies of prisoners in New York and New Jersey have provided data that contributed to the early understanding of AIDS epidemiology; specifically, the long incubation period between exposure and illness in IVDUs with AIDS and the association of low leukocyte counts with subsequent development of AIDS.[3,4]

HIV seropositivity rates in U.S. and European prisons and jails are listed below in Table 1.

TABLE 1.   RESULTS OF PRISON EPIDEMIOLOGIC STUDIES AND MASS SCREENING

EPIDEMIOLOGIC STUDIES (BLINDED)

Prison	Number Tested	Category	#HIV+	%HIV+
Michigan	571	New inmates	5	0.9 (ref. 6)
New York	494	New inmates 1/88	84	17.4 (ref. 12)
Washington	342	Clinic patients	0	0 (ref. 9)
Wisconsin	997	All new inmates 1986	3	0.3 (ref. 9)

MASS SCREENING

Prison	Number Tested	Category	#HIV+	%HIV+
Alabama	400	Unspecified 1987	7	1.7 (ref. 9)
Colorado	5112	All new inmates	43	0.8 (ref. 6)
Idaho	163	All new inmates 1987	0	0 (ref. 6)
Iowa	1925	All new inmates 1/9/87	7	0.4 (ref. 6)
Maryland	785	All new inmates 1985	55	7.0 (ref. 9)
Missouri	1540	All new inmates	6	0.4 (ref. 6)
Nebraska	812	All new inmates	2	0.2 (ref. 6)
Nevada	6021	All new inmates	81	1.3 (ref. 6)
	3820	All current in. 8/85	96	2.5 (ref. 6)
Oklahoma	2308	All new inmates	10	0.4 (ref. 6)
	9820	All current in. 6/87	41	0.4 (ref. 6)
South Dakota	1025	All new inmates	1	0.1 (ref. 6)
	982	All current in. 7/87	2	0.2 (ref. 6)
West Virginia	300	Current inmates 87	2	0.6 (ref. 6)
US Federal — all	9640	New inmates 6/10/87	240	2.5 (ref. 6)
US Federal — all	5100	Upon release 6/12/87	103	2.6 (ref. 6)
US Federal — all	29193	Unspecified 4/88	843	2.9 (ref. 10)

continued on next page

continued from previous page

TABLE 1. RESULTS OF PRISON EPIDEMIOLOGIC STUDIES AND MASS SCREENING

RISK-GROUP SCREENING

Prison	Number Tested	Category	#HIV+	%HIV+
Alabama	770	Sex offenders, homosexuals, pregnant women, IVDUs	11	1.4 (ref. 6)
Nebraska	127	Unspecified, voluntary 1987	0	0 (ref. 9)
New Hampshire	128	Homosexuals, IVDUs	5	3.9 (ref. 6)
Orange County, Calif.	978	Female prostitutes	28	2.9 (ref. 6)
Hennepin County, Minn.	526	Homosexuals, IVDUs	10	1.9 (ref. 6)
Kansas	150	Unspecified	6	4.0 (ref. 6)
Harris County, Tex.	526	Unspecified	175	33.3 (ref. 6)

EUROPEAN EPIDEMIOLOGIC STUDIES

Prison	Number Tested	Category	#HIV+	%HIV+
Fresnes, France	500	New inmates	—	12.6 (ref. 7)
Amsterdam, Neth.	?	Unspecified	—	11 (ref. 7)
Bern, Switz.	?	Unspecified	—	11 (ref. 7)
Denmark	291	Two-month study	14	4.7 (ref. 11)

MASS SCREENING

Prison	Number Tested	Category	#HIV+	%HIV+
Italy	30392	All new inmates (voluntary)	5106	16.8 (ref. 7)
Luxembourg	324	All new entries	7	2.1 (ref. 7)
Portugal	8307	All prisoners	4	0.1 (ref. 11)
Belgium	7102	All inmates 1986	91	1.3 (ref. 7)

RISK-GROUP SCREENING

Prison	Number Tested	Category	#HIV+	%HIV+
Spain	26309	All identified	6777	26 (ref. 7)
Cyprus	222	All identified	—	0 (ref. 11)
Greece	3843	Unspecified	4	0.1 (ref. 11)
France	113	IVDUs 1986	68	61 (ref. 7)

By the end of 1986, only two European countries reported significant numbers of AIDS cases among prisoners: 22 in Spain and 10 in Italy.[7] A sample of 113 incarcerated French IVDUs was found to have an HIV seropositivity rate of 61 percent in 1986.[7] This suggests that a dramatic rise in AIDS cases will be seen soon in these prisons. Few American studies of HIV in IVDUs have approached this rate of seropositivity.[7] In Europe, as in the U.S., IVDUs are the population at risk in the prisons.

REFERENCES

1. Hammett TM. AIDS in correctional facilities. Rockville, Md.: U.S. Department of Justice, 1986.
2. Vaid U. AIDS in prison. American Civil Liberties Union National Prison Project Journal 1985; 6:1-5.

3. Hanrahan JP, Wormser GP, Reilley AA, et al. Prolonged incubation of AIDS in intravenous drug abusers: epidemiological evidence in prison inmates. J Infect Dis 1984; 150:263-6.

4. Wormser GP, Krupp LB, Hanrahan JP, et al. Acquired immunodeficiency syndrome in male prisoners. New insights into an emerging syndrome. Ann Intern Med 1983; 98:297-303.

5. Hammett TM. 1986 Update: AIDS in correctional facilities. Rockville, Md.: U.S. Department of Justice, 1987.

6. Hammett TM. AIDS in correctional facilities; issues and options. Third edition. Rockville, Md.: U.S. Department of Justice, 1988.

7. Harding TW. AIDS in prison. Lancet 1987; 2:1260-3.

8. Gido RL, Gaunay W. Update: acquired immune deficiency syndrome; a demographic profile of New York State inmate mortalities 1981–1986. NY State Commission of Correction, 1987.

9. Human immunodeficiency virus infection in the United States. A review of current knowledge. MMWR 1987; 36(Suppl 6):32-3.

10. Quarterly report to the Domestic Policy Council on prevalence and rate of spread of HIV and AIDS infection in the United States. MMWR 1988; 37:225.

11. Harding TW. Health problems facing prison administrations. Strasbourg: Counseil de l'Europe Eighth Conference of Directors of Prison Administration, 1987.

12. Truman BI, Morse D, Mikl J, et al. HIV seroprevalence and risk factors among prison inmates entering New York State prisons [Abstract]. Stockholm: IV International Conference on AIDS 1988; 311.

AIDS and HIV Infection in Prostitutes: Epidemiology

Constance B. Wofsy, M.D.

E arly in the AIDS epidemic, it was suggested that prostitutes would be the means by which AIDS would spread into the heterosexual community in the United States. In point of fact, since the beginning of the AIDS epidemic, between 20 percent and 30 percent of reported AIDS cases have been in heterosexuals, primarily heterosexual IV drug users.[1] The bulk of heterosexual transmission cases have been in sexual partners of men and women with AIDS, ARC, or in AIDS risk groups. There has been little confirmation that human immunodeficiency virus (HIV) infection is particularly prevalent in prostitutes, that female prostitutes constitute a significant means of viral transmission, or that sexual activity per se constitutes a high-risk activity for prostitutes and their clients.

The prevalence of HIV in American and European non-IV-drug-using prostitutes is low. The principal risk among prostitutes appears to lie instead with IV drug use; existing studies suggest that prostitutes who use IV drugs are at the same risk for HIV exposure as other IV drug users in the same geographic area.

However, prostitutes and others with sexual partners whose sexual and drug-using behaviors are unknown should be presumed to be at risk and deserve special educational efforts, both for their personal safety and for the safety of their partners.

■ EVIDENCE LINKING HIV AND PROSTITUTION IN AFRICA

In 1983, clusters of AIDS cases in Kinshasa, Zaire, in Central Africa, indicated a male-to-female ratio of 1:1 and first suggested bidirectional spread of HIV within Central Africa.[2] African female prostitutes were thought to be at particular risk, since 4 out of 9 women with AIDS diagnosed in Rwanda in 1983 considered themselves prostitutes.[2] At the same time, 17 men in Rwanda, all middle to upper-middle class, were diagnosed with AIDS, and 11 of these 17 reported contact with prostitutes but denied other risk behaviors. These studies confirmed that men with AIDS had higher numbers of regular female sexual contacts, including contacts with female prostitutes.[3]

In 1985, Belgian researchers working in Zaire stated that "in Central Africa, infection with HTLV-III or lymphadenopathy-associated virus is linked to heterosexual promiscuity and female prostitution."[4] In their study, 24 percent of 40 African women with AIDS were prostitutes who did not have histories of addiction to oral or intravenous drugs. Compared with 81 percent of 58 male AIDS patients, only 34 percent of 58 control males had visited a prostitute. However, the patients reported a mean of 32 sexual partners per year versus 3 partners per year by the control males. Unspecified cofactors were suspected to play a role in the acquisition of viral infection and expression of disease.[4] Further studies in Central Africa confirm the greater prevalence of HIV antibody in African female prostitutes and male customers of prostitutes than in controls.[6,7]

In 1985, Kreiss studied 90 female prostitutes in Nairobi, Kenya, East Africa.[7] Prevalence of HIV was high and related to socioeconomic status of the prostitute. Sixty percent of low socioeconomic prostitutes were infected versus 31 percent of higher class prostitutes, in contrast to 8 percent of all clinic patients and 2 percent of medical personnel. The avenue of exposure in these women was thought to be contact with males from Central Africa, suggesting a pattern for geographical spread of the infection within Africa.

All sexual contact in Kreiss's study was reported to be vaginal without use of condoms. Among the lower socioeconomic class prostitutes, sexually transmitted diseases (STDs) were found in over 40 percent, and there was a strong correlation between seropositivity and venereal disease. Venereal disease is widespread in Africa.[8] The role of venereal disease as a cofactor in HIV infection in Africa is supported by recent studies linking HIV transmission to ulcerative venereal diseases.[19]

Caution should be used in extrapolating data from Central and East Africa. In contrast, only 1 of 98 prostitutes (1 percent) tested in Accra, Ghana (West Africa), was seropositive.[9] Such regional variations make accurate general suppositions about AIDS in prostitutes difficult, if not impossible.

■ PROSTITUTES AND AIDS: UNITED STATES AND EUROPE

In the United States and Europe, studies of prostitutes and HIV infection have largely been seroprevalence surveys done in jails, sexually transmitted disease clinics, red-light districts, or other sites where prostitutes congregate.[10-17] Personal IV drug use has been strongly associated with seropositivity (see Table 1) though IV drug use has not always been recognized and treated as an independent cofactor.

TABLE 1. HIV ANTIBODY IN FEMALE PROSTITUTES

SITE	SOURCE	NUMBER TESTED	PERCENT POSITIVE	PERCENT IVDU‡	% OF HIV+ IVDU
Seattle	Jail	92	5	unk§ (ref. 9)	
Miami	AIDS clinic	25	40	unk	80 (ref. 9)
Amsterdam	Addicts	52	23	All	unk (ref. 10)
Germany*	NA	1	unk	unk (ref. 11)	
Germany†	NA	20–50	unk	unk (ref. 11)	
Greece*	NA	6	unk	unk (ref. 12)	
Italy	Clinic	24	0	58	NA (ref. 13)
London	STD clinic	50	0	6	NA (ref. 14)
Paris	Street prostitutes	56	0	0	NA (ref. 15)
San Francisco	Various	87	4	42	100 (ref. 16)

*   *Registered prostitutes.*
†   *Unregistered prostitutes, train station.*
‡   *IVDU = intravenous drug user.*
§   *unk = unknown.*

■ CDC'S SEVEN-CITY STUDY OF U.S. PROSTITUTES

Recently, the Centers for Disease Control (CDC) has coordinated a large, multi-center, ongoing, cross-sectional study of women engaged in prostitution in seven U.S. cities: Atlanta, Colorado Springs, Las Vegas, Los Angeles, Miami, Newark/Jersey City/Paterson, and San Francisco.[18] The subjects were recruited from STD clinics, drug treatment programs, jails, and through community outreach.

Eight hundred thirty-five women met the inclusion criteria for the study. Forty-seven of the 62 seropositive women (76 percent) gave a history of IV drug use. Intravenous drug use had a strong correlation with seropositivity (see Table 2).

TABLE 2.   RISK FACTORS FOR HIV ANTIBODY IN FEMALE
PROSTITUTES AND FOR AIDS IN WOMEN, BY RACE OR
ETHNIC GROUP — SELECTED CITIES, UNITED STATES,
MARCH 10, 1987

	FEMALE PROSTITUTES*		WOMEN WITH AIDS†	
	HIV ab+/tested	% +	No.	% of Total
Black or Hispanic IV drug user	31/124	25.0	108	43.0
Other, unknown	12/156‡	7.7	143	57.0
Total	43/280	15.4	251	100.0
White or other IV drug user	16/157	10.2	26	53.1
Other, unknown	3/127§	2.4	23	46.9
Total	19/284	6.7	49	100.0

* Analysis restricted to the 564 study participants (of 835 tested) who answered the question regarding IV drug abuse.

† Includes 46 women who were born in countries where heterosexual transmission is believed to play a major role, who were reported to CDC as meeting the surveillance case definition for AIDS, and who were residents of one of the seven research sites.

‡ Odds ratio = 4.0; 95% confidence interval = 2.0 to 8.2.

§ Odds ratio = 4.7; 95% confidence interval = 1.3 to 16.5.

Reprinted with permission of the Centers for Disease Control and MMWR 1987; 36:11.

The prevalence of HIV among prostitutes appears to parallel the cumulative incidence of AIDS in all women in the seven research sites (see Table 3), which suggests that prostitutes' risk factors are similar to those of other women in these regions. Where there is a high prevalence of HIV seropositivity among women as a whole, e.g., northern New Jersey, there is a parallel incidence (57.1 percent) of seropositivity among female prostitutes (see Table 3).

TABLE 3. HIV ANTIBODY IN FEMALE PROSTITUTES AND
REPORTED AIDS CASES IN WOMEN — SELECTED CITIES,
UNITED STATES, MARCH 10, 1987

| | FEMALE PROSTITUTES* | | WOMEN WITH AIDS† | |
	HIV ab+/tested	% +	No.	Cases/ 1,000,000
Eastern United States				
Atlanta	1/92	1.1	8	12.5
Miami	47/252	18.7	100	145.3
Newark/Jersey City/Paterson	32/56	57.1	143	526.2
Western United States				
Colorado Springs	1/71	1.4	1	9.6
Las Vegas	0/34	0.0	1	16.0
Los Angeles	8/184	4.3	26	21.7
San Francisco	9/146	6.2	21	71.9

* *Includes 45 women (>16 years of age) from Miami and one from Newark who were born in countries where heterosexual transmission is believed to play a major role.*

† *Rate based on the number of females (>16 years of age) reported as residing in the urban area or place of study. Bureau of the Census, 1980 census of population.*

Reprinted with permission of the Centers for Disease Control and MMWR 1987; 36:11.

Bivariate analyses of characteristics associated with HIV seropositivity yielded markedly different results among the seven geographic sites. In San Francisco (117 women), the correlates of HIV seropositivity, in order of magnitude, were seromarker for syphilis (0.45); race — black or Latina (0.34); and months injecting drugs (0.17).

Although over 80 percent of prostitutes in the seven-city study reported that at least one of their sexual partners had employed condoms during the past five years and 4 percent reported condom use with each vaginal exposure over the same time, condom use was much less frequent with husbands or boyfriends (16 percent) than with clients (78 percent).[18] The effectiveness of barrier protection when used is suggested by the zero seropositivity of 22 prostitutes all of whose partners always used condoms compared with the 11 percent HIV seropositivity among 546 prostitutes who had unprotected vaginal exposure (p = 0.10 after controlling for IV drug use).[18]

REFERENCES

1. Centers for Disease Control, Center for Infectious Diseases. AIDS Weekly Surveillance Report, July 28, 1986:1.

2. Piot P, Taelman H, Minlangu KB, et al. Acquired immunodeficiency syndrome in a heterosexual population in Zaire. Lancet 1984; 2:65-9.

3. Van De Perre P, Lepage P, Kestelyn P, et al. Acquired immunodeficiency syndrome in Rwanda. Lancet 1984; 2:62-4.

4. Clumeck N, Van De Perre P, Carael M, et al. Heterosexual promiscuity among African patients with AIDS. N Engl J Med 1985; 313:182.

5. Van De Perre P, Carael M, Robert-Guroff M, et al. Female prostitutes: a risk group for infection with human T-cell lymphotropic virus type III. Lancet 1985; 2:524-7.

6. Clumeck N, Robert-Guroff M, Van De Perre P, et al. Seroepidemiological studies of HTLV-III antibody prevalence among selected groups of heterosexual Africans. JAMA 1985; 254:2599-2602.

7. Kreiss JK, Koech D, Plummer FA, et al. AIDS virus infection in Nairobi prostitutes; spread of the epidemic to East Africa. N Engl J Med 1986; 314:414-8.

8. Biggar RJ. The AIDS problem in Africa. Lancet 1986; 1:79-82.

9. Neequaye AR, Neequaye J, Mingle JA, Adjei DO. Preponderance of females with AIDS in Ghana. Lancet 1986; 2:978.

10. Centers for Disease Control. Heterosexual transmission of human T-lymphotropic virus type III/lymphadenopathy associated virus. MMWR 1985; 34:561-3.

11. Buning EC, Coutinho RA, van Brussel GHA, et al. Preventing AIDS in drug addicts in Amsterdam. Lancet 1986; 1:1435.

12. James JJ, Morgenstern MA, Hatten JA. HTLV-III/LAV antibody-positive soldiers in Berlin. N Engl J Med 1986; 314:55.

13. Papaevangelou G, Roumeliotou-Karayannis A, Kallinikos G, Papoutsakis G. LAV/HTLV-III infection in female prostitutes. Lancet 1985; 2:1018.

14. Tirelli U, Vaccher E, Carbone A, et al. Serological studies in Rwanda, Athens, Seattle, and Miami suggest that prostitutes are an important human reservoir of HTLV-III. Lancet 1985; 2:1424.

15. Barton SE, Underhill GS, Gilchrist C, et al. HTLV-III antibody in prostitutes. Lancet 1985; 2:1424.

16. Brenky-Faudeux D, Fribourg-Blanc A. American studies suggest that prostitutes are at high risk of AIDS. Lancet 1985; 2:1424.

17. Cohen JB, Hauer LB, Poole LE, et al. Prevalence of AIDS antibody and associated risk factors in a prospective study of 400 San Francisco prostitutes and other sexually active women [Abstract]. Paris: Proceedings of the International Conference on AIDS, 1986:111.

18. Centers for Disease Control. Antibody to human immunodeficiency virus in female prostitutes. MMWR 1987; 36:157-61.

19. Simonsen JN, Cameron DW, Gakinya MN, et al. Human immunodeficiency virus infection among men with sexually transmitted diseases. Experiences from a center in Africa. N Engl J Med 1988; 319:274-8.

1.2

Transmission of HIV Infection

Transmission of HIV in Body Fluids

Harry Hollander, M.D.

This chapter reviews the frequency and significance of human immunodeficiency virus (HIV) in body fluids other than blood. As shown in Table 1, the virus has been isolated from semen,[1,2] saliva,[3] tears,[4] cerebrospinal fluid (CSF),[5,14,15,19] breast milk,[6] amniotic fluid,[16] urine,[7] vaginal/cervical secretions,[8-10] and bronchoalveolar fluid.[18]

TABLE 1.   FREQUENCY OF HIV ISOLATION FROM
BODY FLUIDS*

BODY FLUIDS	HEALTHY SERO-POSITIVES	ARC/LAN	AIDS	CONDITION NOT SPECIFIED
Semen[1,2]	1/1	NA†	2/2	4/19
Saliva[3]	4/24	4/48	1/29	3/34
Tears[4]	NA†	0/1	1/6	NA†
CSF[5]	NA†	3/3	10/11	NA†
CSF[14,15]	7/10	11/12	20/29	6/13
Breast milk[6]	3/4	NA†	NA†	NA†
Urine[7]	NA†	NA†	NA†	1/5
Vaginal/cervical secretions[8,9,10]	6/11	6/16	0/1	—
Amniotic fluid[16]	1/1	—	—	—
Bronchoalveolar lavage fluid[18]	—	—	—	2/30

*   *Compiled from references 1-11; 15-18.*
†   *NA = not available.*

Other fluids not yet systematically studied include aqueous and vitreous humor, gastrointestinal, and sweat. In general, the source of virus in fluids other than blood is lymphocytes, although extracellular virus has been shown on occasion, most notably in cerebrospinal fluid. Thus, it is likely that all fluids that can be contaminated by lymphocytes will eventually be shown to harbor the virus. As a rule, however, virus seems to be found more frequently in blood than in other fluids. Cerebrospinal fluid is an important exception. Several cases demonstrate that finding virus in nonplasma fluids does not necessarily predict viremia, although the reverse can also be true. Whether fluids from AIDS patients are less frequently infected than fluids from healthy HIV-seropositive individuals or from ARC patients is unknown. One saliva study suggests that viral recovery may well be easier early in the course of HIV disease.[7] However, a more recent study does not corroborate this observation and emphasizes the rarity of viral recovery from saliva.[11]

Although virus is theoretically transmissible via these fluids, no cases of HIV transmission by external body fluids other than semen have been documented. Of course, isolation of virus from amniotic fluid provides important confirmatory evidence for the ease of perinatal in utero transmission. Since the virus causes no pathology in the glands secreting the fluids, its biologic significance in them is unclear.

The presence of virus in cerebrospinal fluid, however, has pathologic implications. Although the fluid's proximity to the central nervous system does not appear to be a factor in HIV's transmissibility, it may explain the neurologic dysfunction seen in many patients with AIDS-related illness. Chronic syndromes such as subacute encephalitis[12] and vacuolar myelopathy[13] have eluded explanation and probably represent direct HIV neuropathic effect. Acute aseptic meningitis with virus-positive CSF has also been reported.[14] Cerebrospinal fluid is unusual because its extralymphocytic pathologic effects are not seen in other infected body fluids. Also unique is the ability of HIV to exist in high titer in cell-free cerebrospinal fluid.[5] This may be further evidence that neural cells, not lymphocytes, are the site of viral replication and shedding.

Thus, isolation of HIV from a variety of sites has supported existing epidemiologic conclusions about routes of transmission while raising new concerns. Isolation of HIV from cerebrospinal fluid has added support to the concept of HIV neurotropism and has shed light upon some heretofore unexplained neurologic syndromes. The time-course and frequency of cerebrospinal fluid infection need to be established, since these will affect efforts to treat the virus directly.

REFERENCES

1. Zagury D, Bernard J, Leibowitch J, et al. HTLV-III in cells cultured from semen of two patients with AIDS. Science 1984; 226:449-51.

2. Ho DD, Schooley RT, Rota TR, et al. HTLV-III in the semen and blood of a healthy homosexual man. Science 1984; 226:447-8.

3. Groopman JE, Salahuddin SZ, Sarngadharan MG, et al. HTLV-III in saliva of people with AIDS-related complex and healthy homosexual men at risk for AIDS. Science 1984; 226:447-8.

4. Fujikawa LS, Palestine AG, Nussenblatt RB, et al. Isolation of human T-lymphotropic virus type III from the tears of a patient with the acquired immunodeficiency syndrome. Lancet 1985; 2:529-30.

5. Levy JA, Shimabukuro J, Hollander H, et al. Isolation of AIDS-associated retroviruses from cerebrospinal fluid and brain of patients with neurological symptoms. Lancet 1985; 2:586-8.

6. Thiry L, Sprecher-Goldberger S, Jonckheer T, et al. Isolation of AIDS virus from cell-free breast milk of three healthy virus carriers. Lancet 1985; 2:891-2.

7. Levy JA, Kaminsky LS, Morrow WJW, et al. Infection by the retrovirus associated with the acquired immunodeficiency syndrome: clinical, biological, and molecular features. Ann Intern Med 1985; 103:694-9.

8. Vogt MW, Witt DJ, Craven DE. Isolation patterns of the human immunodeficiency virus from cervical secretions during the menstrual cycle of women at risk for the acquired immunodeficiency syndrome. Ann Intern Med 1987; 106:380-2.

9. Vogt MW, Craven DE, Crawford DF, et al. Isolation of HTLV-III/LAV from cervical secretions of women at risk for AIDS. Lancet 1986; 1:525-7.

10. Wofsy CB, Cohen JB, Hauer LB, et al. Isolation of AIDS associated retrovirus from genital secretions of women with antibodies to the virus. Lancet 1986; 1:527-9.

11. Ho DD, Byington R, Schooley RT, et al. Infrequency of isolation of HTLV-III virus from saliva in AIDS. N Engl J Med 1985; 313:1606.

12. Shaw GM, Harper ME, Hahn BH, et al. HTLV-III infection in brains of children and adults with AIDS encephalopathy. Science 1985; 227:177-81.

13. Petito CK, Bradford AN, Cho ES, et al. Vacuolar myelopathy pathologically resembling subacute combined degeneration in patients with the acquired immunodeficiency syndrome. N Engl J Med 1985; 312:874-9.

14. Ho DD, Rota TR, Schooley RT, et al. Isolation of HTLV-III from cerebrospinal fluid and neural tissues of patients with neurologic syndromes related to the acquired immunodeficiency syndrome. N Engl J Med 1985; 313:1493-7.

15. Hollander H, Levy JA. Neurologic abnormalities and recovery of human immunodeficiency virus from cerebrospinal fluid. Ann Intern Med 1987; 106:692-5.

16. Mundy DC, Schinazi RF, Gerber AR, et al. Human immunodeficiency virus isolated from amniotic fluid. Lancet 1987; 2:459-60.

17. McArthur JC. Neurologic manifestations of AIDS. Medicine (Baltimore) 1987; 66:407-37.

18. Dean NC, Golden JA, Evans LA, et al. Human immunodeficiency virus recovery from bronchoalveolar lavage fluid in patients with AIDS. Chest 1988; 93:1176-9.

19. Hollander H. Cerebrospinal fluid normalities and abnormalities in individuals infected with human immunodeficiency virus. J Infect Dis 1988; 158:855-8.

Sexual Transmission of HIV Infection: Overview

Dennis Osmond

It is now clear that both homosexual and heterosexual activity play major roles in the transmission of HIV infection worldwide. In the United States and Europe, over two thirds of all persons with AIDS are homosexual men. In Africa, most cases appear to result from heterosexual transmission of HIV. However, several important questions about the frequency and routes of sexual transmission are unanswered.

The potential for transmission by different sexual practices is not well understood. The relative efficiency of transmission from male to female versus female to male is still uncertain. Variations in the infectiousness of seropositive individuals remain unexplained. A better understanding of the role that cofactors play in increasing susceptibility to infection is needed. Slowing the rate of sexual transmission poses the greatest challenge to AIDS prevention since (as with historic attempts to control syphilis) it raises difficult social and political issues.

■ ROUTES OF SEXUAL TRANSMISSION

HIV has been isolated from blood, semen, vaginal secretions, urine, cerebrospinal fluid (CSF), saliva, tears, and breast milk of infected individuals. Except for CSF, HIV in nonblood fluids is primarily found in lymphocytes, although extracellular virus has been occasionally found.[1] Transmission could theoretically occur from sexual behavior involving contact with any of these fluids, but the concentration of HIV found in saliva and tears is extremely low. Moreover, no cases of HIV infection have been traced to saliva or tears. Virus is found in greater concentration in semen than in vaginal secretions, which supports the hypothesis that transmission occurs more readily from male to female than from female to male.[2]

In an animal experiment, a chimpanzee was infected vaginally with HIV by a viral swab. Attempts to orally infect a second chimpanzee by repeated viral swabs of oral mucosa failed.[3] A male rhesus monkey was infected with simian immunodeficiency virus (SIV) by inoculating the urethra with a swab.[22] In humans, a close analogy to experimental infection occurred when 4 of 8 women seroconverted after being inseminated by a seropositive donor; this demonstrates that infection can occur via the vagina even without the presence of trauma or a predisposing condition facilitating viral entry.[4]

Among homosexual men, the receptive partner in anal intercourse is at high risk, although seroconversions have also occurred among men reporting only insertive anal intercourse. The efficiency of transmission to the receptive partner in anal intercourse may be explained by the fact that HIV enters the bloodstream through tears in the rectal mucosa. Recent evidence suggests that HIV directly infects bowel epithelial cells — another possible mechanism of transmission via anal-receptive intercourse.[5]

Most studies have not found a risk of HIV infection among men reporting only oral intercourse, but some uncertainty has been introduced into the study of risk factors by reports of the potentially long latency period from HIV infection to seroconversion.[23,24] Most studies of risk factors have relied on examining sexual behavior in a period from some months to a year before seroconversion. For some individuals, the relevant risk behavior may have occurred more than a year before seroconversion, and atypical individual case reports are likely to select individuals with unusually long latency periods before seroconversion. This may explain why occasional reports describe seroconversion among men with a self-reported history of recent sexual behavior restricted to oral intercourse. In contrast, prospective data from a large cohort study of homosexual men found no seroconverters among men practicing only oral intercourse.[25]

Male-to-female infection occurs through vaginal or anal intercourse, and female-to-male infection through vaginal intercourse. Two case reports (one of female-to-female and one of male-to-male transmission) attribute infection and seroconversion to exposing broken skin or oral mucosa to infected blood during sexual activities.[6,7]

■ COFACTORS

Rates of sexual transmission may differ among individuals, between homosexuals and heterosexuals, among risk groups, and in different parts of the world (e.g., Africa and the United States) because of the presence of cofactors that influence susceptibility to infection. A history of other sexually transmitted diseases (STDs) is associated with risk of HIV infection in a number of studies in both Western and African countries.[8-11] An STD may increase susceptibility to infection by causing genital lesions that facilitate viral entry or by increasing the number of target cells for HIV (activated lymphocytes or monocytes). Genital ulcers in particular have been identified as a risk factor in Africa.[8,9] In studies conducted in African STD clinics, these ulcers are often caused by *Hemophilus ducreyi* infection (chancroid), which is seen much less frequently in Western countries. Syphilis and herpes simplex infection — STDs that can cause genital ulceration — have also been reported as possible cofactors of infection.[11,12] Viral infections that do not cause genital lesions but result in activation of target cells, such as cytomegalovirus (CMV) and Epstein–Barr virus (EBV) infection, are also theoretical cofactors.[26] Because high-risk sexual behaviors are strongly correlated with both HIV and other STD infections, other STDs have frequently been interpreted as cofactors for HIV infection. In addition to genital lesions, lack of circumcision in males and the use of oral contraceptives in females have been reported as cofactors in African studies.[19,20] There is evidence that age is a cofactor for progression to disease, but age has not been shown to influence susceptibility to infection.

■ INFECTIVITY

DNA studies indicate that HIV infection is lifelong and that all persons testing positive for HIV antibody or antigen are potentially infectious. Studies of sexual partners of infected individuals, however, find wide variation in seropositivity, ranging from 10 percent to 20 percent in the spouses of HIV-infected hemophiliacs to 40 percent to 75 percent in partners of individuals with AIDS; this suggests a wide variation in infectivity of the HIV-infected individual as well. Some of the variation is probably due to differences in sexual practices and number of sexual contacts, but behavior alone does not appear to explain these variations. Studies have found individuals who were infected by a single unprotected sexual contact while others have remained seronegative after hundreds of unprotected sexual contacts.[12] This variation could be caused by varying susceptibility to infection, by changing degrees of infectiousness in an HIV-infected individual over time, by differences in strains of HIV, or by some combination of all of these possibilities.

Variation in the virus itself is theoretically a factor in transmission, but the substantial variation in the envelope of HIV-1 isolates has not yet been related to infectivity. Differences in the relative infectiousness of HIV-1 and HIV-2 have not yet been determined.

The percent of peripheral mononuclear cells infected by HIV is quite low — roughly 1 in 10,000 to as few as 1 in 100,000. The relatively small number of infected cells may help explain the variation in infection rates. Infection may occur via infected cells or via free virus. Currently, HIV can be detected in blood specimens from seropositive individuals by lymphocyte culture, by enzyme immunoassay of serum or plasma for the HIV p24 major core antigen, or by hybridization of HIV RNA or proviral DNA. The probability of a positive result by culture or antigen detection correlates with the clinical status of the person tested: virus is found more frequently in AIDS and ARC patients than in asymptomatic seropositives.[13,14]

If infectivity varies in a seropositive individual over time (increasing, for example, when the individual becomes antigenemic), then transmission rates could be complicated by length of time infected. Since the different major risk groups in the United States have probably been infected on average for different lengths of time, under this hypothesis transmission rates would be expected to differ by risk group.

Indirect evidence of a correlation between the disease-status of the index partner and the risk of infection in regular sexual partners is seen in both male-to-female partner studies and female-to-male studies. Seropositivity rates tend to be higher in the partners of patients with AIDS or ARC than in partners of asymptomatic seropositives.[15,16,27] After controlling for the duration of the sexual relationship and the frequency of contact, a study of male sexual partners of homosexual men who developed AIDS found that transmission was more frequent when sexual contact took place up to or after the diagnosis of AIDS.[14] In a study of the spouses of hemophiliacs, seroconversion was associated with a declining CD4/CD8 ratio in the seropositive male partner.[16] An African study of both male and female spouses of AIDS, ARC, and asymptomatic HIV seropositives found a trend of increasing infectivity in the index partners with ARC or AIDS.[18] A U.S. study of male and female spouses reported a correlation between seroconversion of the spouses and HIV p24 antigenemia in the index subjects.[21] Other studies, however, have not found an association between the clinical condition of the infected patient and infection in the sexual partner,[12,17] so this hypothesis remains open to question.

Factors other than those considered above may affect transmission. Some individuals may be unusually resistant to HIV infection, although markers for resistance have not yet been demonstrated. Variation in transmissibility remains the most significant unexplained aspect of HIV infection.

REFERENCES

1. Hollander H, Levy JA. Neurologic abnormalities and recovery of human immunodeficiency virus from cerebrospinal fluid. Ann Intern Med 1987; 106:692-5.

2. Wofsy CB, Cohen JB, Hauer LB, et al. Isolation of AIDS- associated retrovirus from genital secretions of women with antibodies to the virus. Lancet 1986; 1:527-9.

3. Fultz PN, McClure HM, Daugharty H, et al. Vaginal transmission of human immunodeficiency virus (HIV) to a chimpanzee. J Infect Dis 1986; 154:896-900.

4. Stewart GJ, Tyler JP, Cunningham AL, et al. Transmission of human T-cell lymphotrophic virus type III (HTLV-III) by artificial insemination by donor. Lancet 1985; 2:581-5.

5. Nelson JA, Wiley CA, Reynolds-Kohler C, et al. Human immunodeficiency virus detected in bowel epithelium from patients with gastrointestinal symptoms. Lancet 1988; 1:259-62.

6. Donovan B, Tindall B, Cooper D. Brachioproctic eroticism and transmission of retrovirus associated with acquired immune deficiency syndrome (AIDS). Genitourin Med 1986; 62:390-2.

7. Marmor M, Weiss LR, Lyden M, et al. Possible female-to-female transmission of human immunodeficiency virus. Ann Intern Med 1986; 105:969.

8. Cameron DW, Plummer FA, Simonsen JN, et al. Female to male heterosexual transmission of HIV infection in Nairobi [Abstract]. Washington, D.C.: III International Conference on AIDS, 1987; 25.

9. Greenblatt RM, Lukehart SA, Plummer FA, et al. Genital ulceration as a risk factor for human immunodeficiency virus infection. AIDS 1988; 2:47-50.

10. Handsfield HH, Ashley RL, Rompalo AM, et al. Association of anogenital ulcer disease with human immunodeficiency virus infection in homosexual men [Abstract]. Washington, D.C.: III International Conference on AIDS, 1987; 206.

11. Moss AR, Osmond D, Bacchetti P, et al. Risk factors for AIDS and HIV seropositivity in homosexual men. Am J Epidemiol 1987; 125:1035-47.

12. Peterman TA, Stoneburner RL, Allen JR, et al. Risk of human immunodeficiency virus transmission from heterosexual adults with transfusion-associated infections. JAMA 1988; 259:55-8.

13. Wittek AE, Phelan MA, Wells MA, et al. Detection of human immunodeficiency virus core protein in plasma by enzyme immunoassay. Association of antigenemia with symptomatic disease and T-helper cell depletion. Ann Intern Med 1987; 107:286-92.

14. Paul DA, Falk LA, Kessler HA, et al. Correlation of serum HIV antigen and antibody with clinical status in HIV-infected patients. J Med Virol 1987; 22:357-63.

15. Osmond D, Bacchetti P, Chaisson RE, et al. Time of exposure and risk of HIV infection in homosexual partners of men with AIDS. Am J Public Health 1988; 78:944-8.

16. Goedert J, Eyster ME, Biggar RJ. Heterosexual transmission of human immunodeficiency virus (HIV): association with severe T-helper lymphocytes in men with hemophilia. AIDS Res Hum Retrovir 1987; 3:355-61.

17. Padian N, Marquis L, Francis DP, et al. Male-to-female transmission of human immunodeficiency virus. JAMA 1987; 258:788-90.

18. Hira S, Wadhawan D, Nkowane B, et al. Heterosexual transmission of HIV in Zambia [Abstract]. IV International Conference on AIDS. Stockholm, 1988; 1:261, 4006.

19. Cameron DW, D'Costa LJ, Ndinya-Achola JO, Piot P, Plummer FA. Incidence and risk factors for female to male transmission of HIV [Abstract]. IV International Conference on AIDS. Stockholm, 1988; 1:275, 4061.

20. Plummer F, Cameron W, Simonsen N, et al. Co-factors in male-female transmission of HIV [Abstract]. IV International Conference on AIDS. Stockholm, 1988; 2:200, 4554.

21. Fischl M, Fayne T, Flanagan S, et al. Seroprevalence and risks of HIV infections in spouses of persons infected with HIV [Abstract]. IV International Conference on AIDS. Stockholm, 1988; 1:274, 4060.

22. Miller CJ, Alexander N, Jennings M, et al. Transmission of simian immunodeficiency virus (SIV) across the genital mucosas of male and female rhesus macaques [Abstract]. IV International Conference on AIDS. Stockholm, 1988; 2:121, 2581.

23. Ranki A, Valle SL, Krohn M, et al. Long latency precedes overt seroconversion in virus infection. Lancet 1987; 2:589-93.

24. Wolinsky S, Rinaldo C, Farzedegan H, et al. Polymerase chain reaction (PCR) detection of HIV provirus before HIV seroconversion [Abstract]. IV International Conference on AIDS. Stockholm, 1988; 1:137, 1099.

25. Kingsley LA, Detels R, Kaslow R, et al. Risk factors for seroconversion to human immunodeficiency virus among male homosexuals. Results from the Multicenter AIDS Cohort Study. Lancet 1987; 1:345-9.

26. Quinn TC, Piot P, McCormick JB, et al. Serologic and immunologic studies in patients with AIDS in North America and Africa. JAMA 1987; 257:2617-21.

27. De Vincenzi I, The European Study Group on Heterosexual Transmission of HIV. Heterosexual transmission of HIV: a European Community multicentre study [Abstract]. IV International Conference on AIDS. Stockholm, 1988; 1:265, 4024.

Homosexual Transmission of HIV

Dennis Osmond

T his chapter reviews what is known about male-to-male and female-to-female sexual transmission of HIV. It particularly draws upon long-term prospective studies of homosexual men in San Francisco.

■ EARLIEST MALE-TO-MALE CASES

The earliest AIDS cases in the U.S. were among a cluster of young homosexual men who were sexual partners or who shared mutual sexual partners.[1] The rapid spread of AIDS among homosexual men in New York, San Francisco, and Los Angeles further implicated sexual transmission in this population. Although AIDS was quickly recognized among other risk groups, homosexual men have accounted for between two thirds and three fourths of all reported AIDS cases in the United States. The U.S. Public Health Service estimates that homosexual men still account for at least two thirds of those infected with HIV and therefore will continue to account for most new AIDS cases for the next several years.[3]

■ MALE-TO-MALE TRANSMISSION

The earliest studies of HIV seroprevalence, as well as the first studies of sexual transmission of HIV, were carried out among homosexual men.[2,4,5,7] Very high rates of seroprevalence (ranging from 21 percent to 71 percent) were found in 1983 and 1984 among homosexual men in several U.S. cities.[6,11,13,14] Two random samples of neighborhoods in San Francisco, carried out six months apart in 1984, found seroprevalence rates of 41 percent and 48 percent.[11,16] During the early 1980's, seroconversion rates among homosexual men in New York, San Francisco, and Los Angeles were extremely high. Estimates from San Francisco suggest that seroconversion was on the order of 10 percent to 20 percent per year between 1980 and 1983.[18] Given the parallel epidemic curves in these cities, rates similar to those in San Francisco probably occur in the other two cities. Recent data from ongoing prospective studies of homosexual men in San Francisco show much lower current seroconversion rates — in the range of 1 percent to 2 percent a year (Moss A, Winkelstein W: personal communication). Corroborative data on the reduction in the rate of HIV transmission in San Francisco are seen in the steadily declining incidence of rectal gonorrhea from 1981 to 1986 reported to the San Francisco Public Health Department.[19] Whether comparable reductions in transmission rates are occurring in other U.S. cities is not yet clear.

Risk-factor studies consistently report that receptive anal intercourse and the number of male sexual partners are the most significant risk factors for transmission in homosexual men.[7-11,13,16] Other reported risk factors fall into one of three groups: (1) other sexual behaviors, (2) history of sexually transmitted disease, and (3) drug-use behavior.

Sexual behaviors other than anal intercourse that have been identified as risk factors include rectal douching,[11,13,16] penetrating the rectum with the hand ("fisting"), sexual contact with partners from cities with a high incidence of AIDS, and sexual contact in bathhouses or clubs. Rectal douching and fisting may cause damage to the rectal mucosa, thus facilitating viral entry, or these behaviors may be markers for probable contact with an infected partner. Risk from sexual contact with men from high-incidence cities or with men in bathhouses occurs in the early stages of an epidemic when there are geographic areas with marked differences in the prevalence of infection as well as marked differences in prevalence among subgroups of homosexual men within a single city. This risk diminishes over time as infection becomes more widespread and more evenly distributed among cities and subpopulations of groups at risk.

The studies cited above did not find independent risk for HIV infection associated with insertive anal intercourse, oral intercourse, or ingestion of semen. Nevertheless, homosexual men who have seroconverted while under prospective study (as well as case reports of seropositive men with atypical sexual histories) show that sexual transmission in homosexual men does occur by routes other than receptive anal intercourse.[12,20] Insertive anal intercourse appears to be the probable source of infection in most instances. No report attributes infection to oral transmission of HIV, although this cannot be ruled out as a possible route of infection. The largest prospective study reported seroconversion in 3 of 344 homosexual men (0.9 percent) who practiced insertive anal intercourse but not receptive anal intercourse over a six-month period, and in none of 147 homosexual men who practiced oral intercourse but neither receptive nor insertive anal intercourse.[12] In one instance, an HIV seroconversion was attributed to manual penetration of the rectum.[21]

One study of the male sexual partners of men with AIDS found greater risk associated with the time of exposure to the infected partner. After controlling for the number of other sexual partners and the number of sexual contacts with the infected partner, risk was found to be greater among those partners who had receptive anal intercourse with the infected partner up to or beyond his diagnosis with AIDS than among those whose last sexual contact preceded the AIDS diagnosis.[20]

Several studies, both in the U.S. and in Africa, have found independent risk associated with a history of sexually transmitted disease. A history of anogenital ulcers, syphilis, giardiasis, gonorrhea, and hepatitis B have all been associated with a higher risk of infection.[11,15,22,23] Risk associated with a history of sexually transmitted disease may be a marker for the probability of contact with an infected partner or it may reflect independent biologic effects predisposing to infection. The particular disease identified as a risk factor varies by study, and the lack of consistency casts some doubt on a hypothesis implicating independent biologic effect. Sexually transmitted diseases that result in genital lesions, and thus facilitate viral entry, are the most likely true cofactors. Among heterosexuals, chancroid (which causes genital ulceration) has been reported as a risk factor in Africa.[24,25]

Intravenous drug use, any use of illicit drugs, and use of amyl or butyl nitrites ("poppers") have been reported as risk factors for HIV infection.[2,11,13,16] The sharing of contaminated drug paraphernalia by intravenous drug users is a known route of HIV transmission. However, based on the infrequency with which it has been found to be a risk factor in studies of HIV infection among homosexual men, intravenous drug use does not appear to account for a very large part of HIV transmission in this population. Any illicit drug use — particularly the use of amyl or butyl nitrite, which are short-acting drugs often used in association with sexual intercourse — may be a marker for a lifestyle offering a high probability of sexual contact with an infectious person. On the other hand, nitrite use may increase susceptibility to infection through a biologic effect such as immunosuppression or vasodilation.

■ FEMALE-TO-FEMALE TRANSMISSION

Two reports of possible female-to-female HIV transmission have appeared in the literature. In the more persuasive of the two, transmission apparently occurred during a four- to six-week period after the woman began a relationship with a seropositive parenteral drug user.[17] Sexual activities were traumatic, resulting in vaginal bleeding, and also occurred during menses. Sexual practices involved digital and oral contact with the vagina and oral contact with the anus. The second case is a seropositive 24-year-old female who denied any heterosexual contact or intravenous drug use, but who had orogenital contact with a number of female partners in the years prior to her positive antibody test.[26]

REFERENCES

1. Centers for Disease Control. A cluster of Kaposi's sarcoma and *Pneumocystis carinii* pneumonia among homosexual male residents of Los Angeles and Orange Counties, California. MMWR 1982; 31:305-7.
2. Marmor M, Laubenstein L, William D, et al. Risk factors for Kaposi's sarcoma in homosexual men. Lancet 1982; 1:1083-6.
3. Centers for Disease Control. Human immunodeficiency virus infection in the United States: a review of current knowledge. MMWR 1987; 36(Suppl 6):1S-48S.
4. Jaffe HW, Choi K, Thomas P, et al. National case-control study of Kaposi's sarcoma and *Pneumocystis carinii* pneumonia in homosexual men. Ann Intern Med 1983; 99:145-5.
5. Melbye M, Biggar R, Ebbesen P, et al. Seroepidemiology of HTLV-III antibody in Danish homosexual men: prevalence, transmission, and disease outcome. Br Med J 1984; 289:573-5.
6. Polk BF, Fox R, Brookmeyer R, et al. Predictors of the acquired immunodeficiency syndrome developing in a cohort of seropositive homosexual men. N Engl J Med 1987; 316:61-6.
7. Goedert J, Biggar R, Winn D, et al. Determinants of retrovirus (HTLV-III) antibody and immunodeficiency conditions in homosexual men. Lancet 1984; 2:711-5.
8. Nicholson J, McDougal J, Jaffe H, et al. Exposure to human T-lymphotropic virus type III/lymphadenopathy-associated virus and immunologic abnormalities in asymptomatic homosexual men. Ann Intern Med 1985; 103:37-42.
9. Jeffries E, Willoughby KB, Boyko W, et al. The Vancouver lymphadenopathy-AIDS study: 2. Seroepidemiology of HTLV-III antibody. Can Med Assoc J 1985; 132:1373-7.
10. Groopman J, Mayer K, Sarngadharan M, et al. Seroepidemiology of human T-lymphotropic virus type III among homosexual men with the acquired immunodeficiency syndrome or generalized lymphadenopathy and among asymptomatic controls in Boston. Ann Intern Med 1985; 102:334-7.
11. Moss AR, Osmond DH, Bacchetti PB, et al. Risk factors for AIDS and HIV seropositivity in homosexual men. Am J Epidemiol 1987; 125:1035-47.
12. Kingsley LA, Detels R, Kaslow R, et al. Risk factors for seroconversion to human immunodeficiency virus among male homosexuals. Lancet 1987; 1:345-9.
13. Stevens CE, Taylor PE, Zang EA, et al. Human T-cell lymphotropic virus type III infection in a cohort of homosexual men in New York City. JAMA 1986; 255:2167-72.
14. Collier AC, Barnes RC, Handsfield HH. Prevalence of antibody to LAV/HTLV-III among homosexual men in Seattle. Am J Pub Health 1986; 76:564-5.
15. Schechter MT, Boyko WJ, Jeffries E, et al. The Vancouver lymphadenopathy-AIDS study: 1. Persistent generalized lymphadenopathy. Can Med Assoc J 1985; 132:273-9.
16. Winkelstein W Jr, Lyman DM, Padian N, et al. Sexual practices and risk of infection by the human immunodeficiency virus. The San Francisco Men's Health Study. JAMA 1987; 257:321-5.
17. Marmor M, Weiss LR, Lyden M, et al. Possible female-to-female transmission of human immunodeficiency virus. Ann Intern Med 1986; 105:969.

18. Winkelstein W Jr, Samuel M, Padian NS, et al. The San Francisco Men's Health Study: III. Reduction in human immunodeficiency virus transmission among homosexual/bisexual men, 1982-86. Am J Public Health 1987; 77:685-9.

19. Pickering J, Wiley JA, Padian NS, et al. Modeling the incidence of acquired immunodeficiency syndrome (AIDS) in San Francisco, Los Angeles, and New York. Mathematical Modeling 1986; 7:661-88.

20. Osmond DH, Bacchetti PB, Chaisson RE, et al. Time of exposure and risk of HIV infection in homosexual partners of men with AIDS. Am J Public Health 1988; 78:944-8.

21. Donovan B, Tindall B, Cooper D. Brachioproctic eroticism and transmission of retrovirus associated with acquired immune deficiency syndrome (AIDS). Genitourin Med 1986; 62:390-2.

22. Carne CA, Weller IV, Sutherland S, et al. Rising prevalence of human T-lymphotropic virus type III (HTLV-III) infection in homosexual men in London. Lancet 1985; 1:1261-2.

23. Handsfield HH, Ashley RL, Rompalo AM, et al. Association of anogenital ulcer disease with human immunodeficiency virus infection in homosexual men [Abstract]. Washington, D.C.: III International Conference on AIDS, 1987:206.

24. Cameron DW, Plummer FA, Simonsen JN, et al. Female to male heterosexual transmission of HIV infection in Nairobi [Abstract]. Washington, D.C.: III International Conference on AIDS, 1987:25.

25. Greenblatt RM, Lukehart SA, Plummer FA, et al. Genital ulceration as a risk factor for human immunodeficiency virus infection. AIDS 1988; 2:47-50.

26. Monzon OT, Capellan JM. Female-to-female transmission of HIV. Lancet 1987; 1:40-1.

Heterosexual Transmission of HIV

Dennis Osmond

Heterosexual transmission of the human immunodeficiency virus (HIV) is suggested by AIDS diagnoses in both males and females who report that their only disease risk is sexual contact with a person with AIDS or a person at risk for AIDS.[1-3] More evidence is available for male-to-female than female-to-male transmission. Serologic studies of female partners of hemophiliacs and other infected males imply male-to-female transmission.[4,5] More direct evidence of the potential for male-to-female infection is found in a report of seroconversion in females artificially inseminated by specimens from an infected male.[6]

In Zaire, AIDS occurs in males and females in a ratio of approximately 1.1 to 1, indirect evidence that female-to-male transmission occurs and that heterosexual transmission may play a major role in spreading the disease in Africa.[7] Studies of central African cases report a high prevalence of antibody in prostitutes and contact with prostitutes as a risk factor for infection.[8-10] Studies of male AIDS cases without known risk, in the United States and Haiti as well as in Africa, have reported the number of heterosexual partners as being a risk factor.[9,11-13] The distribution of the disease in Africa may be a model for its potential distribution in the United States, but there are many unanswered questions about the differences between AIDS in Africa and in the United States.

Cases reported to the Centers for Disease Control (CDC) show little evidence that the rate of heterosexual transmission is increasing in the United States. The 7 percent of total cases either attributed to heterosexual contact (i.e., contact with a person with AIDS or in an AIDS risk group) or classified as having an undetermined risk factor has not changed significantly over time.[14] This constant percentage is the primary evidence that the role of heterosexual transmission in the spread of the virus is still small. However, because of the long incubation period of AIDS, changes in rates of infection may not be reflected in reported cases for several years after they occur.

The 4 percent of cases attributed to heterosexual contact should be considered a conservative estimate. It is likely that the 3 percent with undetermined risk factors includes additional individuals who acquired the virus through heterosexual contact with a person with AIDS or in an AIDS risk group. Of 111 "non-risk" cases available for in-depth interview, 35 percent (39) gave histories of gonorrhea, syphilis, or both. Twenty-six percent of the men (15/57) gave histories of sexual contact with prostitutes.[15]

■ DEMOGRAPHIC CHARACTERISTICS OF CASES

Risk Group of Partner. As of April 25, 1986, according to the CDC, most of the spread in the United States associated with heterosexual contact is found in females, and the majority of it is attributed to contact with intravenous drug users (IVDUs). Of the 253 cases attributed to heterosexual contact, 82 percent (225) are in women and 18 percent (48) are in men. Sixty percent (163) of the heterosexual cases are associated with sexual contact with an IVDU. Among the females, 62 percent (139) are associated with contact with an IVDU, and among the males, 50 percent (24) (CDC surveillance data). A number of reports are still pending investigation. In addition, some males denying any risk factor have admitted to contact with female prostitutes, some of whom may have been IVDUs.[14] These cases are placed in the "no identified risk" (NIR) group. Of the remaining 30 percent of female heterosexual contact cases, 13 (10 percent) are attributed to contact with a recipient of blood or blood products or contact with a male without an identified risk factor, and 28 (20 percent) to contact with a bisexual male. Thus, the ratio of cases attributed to contact with an IVDU versus contact with a bisexual male is 4 to 1. The ratio for cases attributed to contact with an IVDU versus the number of IVDU cases is 1 to 20, and the corresponding ratio for cases attributed to contact with a bisexual male versus homosexual/bisexual cases is 1 to 400.

Racial Distribution. The racial breakdown of heterosexual contact cases is 21 percent white, 48 percent black, and 31 percent Hispanic. The percentage of black and Hispanic cases (combined, 79 percent) is disproportionate to their distribution in the general population and to their distribution among all AIDS cases (combined, 39 percent). This skewedness reflects the distribution of racial groups among IVDUs, where the majority of the cases of heterosexual transmission have originated, and the higher prevalence of infection among non-white IVDUs.[16]

Geographic Distribution. According to Ann Hardy of the Centers for Disease Control, the regional distribution of heterosexual contact cases is as follows: New York, 41 percent (112); New Jersey, 13 percent (36); Florida, 11 percent (29); California, 6 percent (17); Puerto Rico, 4 percent (12); and "other" (23 states and District of Columbia each with fewer than 10 cases each), 25 percent (67). (Source: Ann Hardy, Centers for Disease Control, personal communication.)

The regional distribution is also disproportionate with the distribution of all AIDS cases. Again, this is a result of the association of most heterosexual contact cases with IV drug users and reflects the preponderance of cases from that risk group in the New York and New Jersey area. The concentration of cases in New York and New Jersey is decreasing somewhat as the epidemic among IVDUs spreads. At the end of 1985, cases from those states accounted for 61 percent of IVDU cases versus 54 percent in 1987.

■ MALE-TO-FEMALE TRANSMISSION

Sexual Practices. HIV is transmitted from an infected male to his female sexual partner by vaginal or anal intercourse.[2,3,5,17-21] Transmission may possibly occur via other sexual practices (such as fellatio), but such cases are not well documented, and the risk of oral transmission is far lower than that for vaginal intercourse. Anal intercourse probably represents the greatest risk for male-to-female transmission, because the anal mucosa is more fragile than the vaginal mucosa.

The estimated risk to heterosexuals from anal intercourse is derived primarily from studies of transmission in homosexual men. Vaginal transmission of HIV

— without trauma or other predisposing conditions — was demonstrated when four women seroconverted after receiving artificial insemination from an HIV-infected donor[6] and by the experimental infection of a chimpanzee via a vaginal swab containing an HIV inoculum.[22]

Several studies of homosexual men found evidence that sexual practices that may result in mucosal breaks, such as penetration of the rectum with the hand or fist ("fisting"), may also pose an increased risk for HIV infection, presumably by facilitating viral entry into the bloodstream.

Frequency of Transmission. Although all persons testing seropositive for HIV may be capable of transmitting the virus, studies of the female partners of seropositive males show a wide range of infection rates. The proportion of female partners who test positive ranges from 7 percent in one study of 148 hemophiliac spouses to 74 percent in another study of 38 African AIDS patients.[24,25] The low rates of infection seen in some female-partner studies — particularly in the spouses of hemophiliacs — suggest that HIV is not always transmitted easily from a seropositive male to a female — even after frequent sexual contact over a period of years. Many of the spouses of hemophiliacs practiced vaginal intercourse without barrier contraception for long periods of time (up to several years) before they became aware of their husband's HIV infection. Nonetheless, a high proportion tested negative for HIV. On the other hand, some individuals appear to have been infected after only one or two sexual exposures.[26] Case reports also show that infected males can infect consecutive female partners over a period of years.[27] Theories proposed to account for this extreme variation in transmission rates include: (1) the presence of cofactors in either the male or the female such as other STDs (which facilitate transmission); (2) genetic differences in the host's susceptibility to infection; (3) variations in infectiousness of particular strains of HIV; and (4) changes in the infectiousness of the carrier over time (a factor that may be related to the progression of HIV disease). These theories are not mutually exclusive; combinations may account for the observed differences in transmission rates.

Seroprevalence rates in female partners tend to differ by the risk group under study. Partners of hemophiliacs and transfusion recipients show relatively low rates of infection, for example, whereas the partners of IVDUs have higher rates. Rates among female partners in Africa, many of whom have been partners of AIDS patients, have also been high. A variety of subtle and difficult-to-document factors may influence transmission rates within different risk groups. Because the disease status of the infected partner is thought to be related to the probability of transmission, rates categorized by risk group may be additionally complicated by the disease status of the male partner. The frequency of high-risk sexual practices may also vary by risk group, further complicating comparison of seroprevalence studies in different risk groups. Unreported drug use in the IVDU studies could also account for some transmission in that group. Partners of transfusion recipients may have lower rates because transfusion recipients are, on average, older and sicker and therefore presumably less sexually active than other risk groups. If disease status of the infected partner is related to the probability of transmission, then seroprevalence rates among risk groups may vary because the proportion of symptomatic subjects varies by risk group. For example, most of the hemophiliacs studied have been asymptomatic seropositives, whereas a high proportion of the IVDUs have had symptomatic HIV disease. Not all studies find an association between the disease status of the index partner and the risk of infection.[19] Thus it remains unclear whether differences in transmission rates are due to disease status or other factors.

In African studies, other sexually transmitted diseases (especially STDs such as chancroid) appear to be cofactors. STDs may play a significant role in heterosexual transmission of HIV in Africa. They may also be important in heterosexual transmission in the U.S., although there is less evidence of this in U.S. studies, and infections such as chancroid are far less prevalent here. STDs have also been implicated, by self-reported history and serologic study, as possible cofactors in homosexual men in the U.S. The use of oral contraceptives was also associated with risk for seroconversion in an African study of female prostitutes,[28] but this finding should be regarded as speculative.

Most studies have not reported an association between risk of infection and the number of sexual contacts with the index partner. Given a constant risk, the frequency of unprotected intercourse should be a strong risk factor. The failure to identify frequency of sexual contact as a risk in the majority of transmission studies suggests that variability of infectiousness in the seropositive index partner or variability in the susceptibility of the uninfected partner are significant determinants of transmission risk.

Seroprevalence rates may also differ for methodologic reasons. For example, some partners came to the attention of investigators because they were symptomatic and therefore had a higher probability of testing positive than asymptomatic subjects. Methodologic differences also influence the analysis of risk factors. Most published reports are cross-sectional studies that examine both male and female partners at one point in time. Because of this technique, it is not possible to know for certain which partner was infected first. In the case of hemophiliacs and their wives, the index infection is presumably the male exposed to HIV through infected factor VIII or IX. Likewise, in the case of a seropositive couple, one of whom is a transfusion recipient, the recipient may be presumed infected first; but in a cross-sectional study of seropositive couples from other risk groups, the presence of disease or disease symptoms in one partner and the absence in the other partner is not evidence that the symptomatic partner was infected first. Prospective studies enrolling monogamous couples in which one partner is initially infected and the other is not should provide clearer answers to questions concerning heterosexual transmission. Some prospective data have been reported, but much more information is needed. Tables 1 and 2 summarize cross-sectional and prospective studies of male-to-female transmission.

TABLE 1.   CROSS-SECTIONAL STUDIES OF MALE-TO-FEMALE HIV TRANSMISSION*

RISK GROUP	HIV DISEASE STATUS	# HIV+/ # PARTNERS TESTED	PERCENT	95% CI
Africans	?	28/38	74	60–88[25]
Africans	AIDS	8/12	67	40–94[29]
IVDU	AIDS	41/88	47	37–57[30]
Mixed†	Mixed	38/159	24	18–31[19]
Transfusion recip.	Mixed	10/55	18	0–36[27]
IVDU/NIR‡	AIDS/symp	15/34	44	27–61[31]

continued on next page

continued from previous page

TABLE 1. CROSS-SECTIONAL STUDIES OF MALE-TO-FEMALE HIV TRANSMISSION*

RISK GROUP	HIV DISEASE STATUS	# HIV+/ # PARTNERS TESTED	PERCENT	95% CI
Mixed	AIDS	4/28	14	1–27[18]
Hemophiliacs	Mostly asymp	4/24	17	2–32[32]
Hemophiliacs	Mostly asymp	4/40	10	1–19[33]
Hemophiliacs	Mostly asymp	2/21	10	0–22[4]
Hemophiliacs	Mostly asymp	3/33	9	0–19[23]
Hemophiliacs	Mostly asymp	10/148	7	3–11[24]

* *Compiled by the author.*
† *Mixed: individuals from multiple risk groups.*
‡ *No identified risk.*

TABLE 2. PROSPECTIVE STUDIES OF MALE-TO-FEMALE HIV TRANSMISSION*

PARTNER'S RISK GROUP	HIV DISEASE STATUS	# CONVERTED/ # STUDIED	PERCENT	FOLLOW-UP TIME
Mixed	AIDS	10/24†	42	11–36 mo[18]
Hemophiliacs	AIDS	3/7‡	43	23[33]
Hemophiliacs	Asymp	3/31‡	10	23[33]

* *Compiled by the author.*
† *12/14 having sex and not using condoms seroconverted (males and females combined — sex break-down not given) and of those continuing to have sex with or without condoms 10/16 seroconverted.*
‡ *These are from the same cohort, divided into two groups by the male's disease status.*

■ FEMALE-TO-MALE TRANSMISSION

Female-to-male sexual transmission of HIV is supported by biological plausibility, equal numbers of male and female AIDS cases in some African countries, case reports of males with no risk factors other than heterosexual intercourse, and seroconversion of male sexual partners of infected females that occurred while the couples were being studied prospectively. In the United States, data on female-to-male transmission have been limited because the majority of reported cases have occurred in populations entirely or largely male: homosexual men, hemophiliacs, and intravenous drug users. As a result, studies of heterosexual couples have usually begun with an infected male as the index case. Larger studies of female-to-male transmission have been possible in Africa.

Female-to-male transmission is biologically plausible for a number of reasons: other known sexually transmitted diseases are bidirectional; HIV can be isolated from vaginal secretions[34]; and in an animal model a female monkey has been infected with simian immunodeficiency virus (SIV) with a urethral swab.[37] The most persuasive case reports of female-to-male transmission are (1) those in which the female acquired infection from a transfusion or organ transplant and her male partner (without other known risk factors) subsequently seroconverted[35]; and (2) those in which a sequential chain of male-to-female-to-male transmission was observed.[36] Prospective data on seroconversions among males with seropositive female partners are given below in Table 3.

TABLE 3.   PROSPECTIVE STUDIES OF FEMALE-TO-MALE HIV TRANSMISSION

RISK GROUP	HIV DISEASE STATUS	# HIV+/ # FOLLOWED	PERCENT	FOLLOW-UP
Mixed	AIDS cases	3/8	38	24 mo[40]
African	HIV-positive	23/291	8	11 wk[28]
Mixed	Mixed	0/20	0	24 mo[45]

Frequency of Transmission.   The efficiency of female-to-male transmission relative to male-to-female transmission has significant bearing on the dynamics of the AIDS epidemic. The efficiency remains unclear, however. The disproportionate percentage of female AIDS cases attributed to heterosexual transmission from an infected man is used to argue that male-to-female transmission is much more efficient than the reverse.[39] However, the much larger pool of infected males in high-risk populations results in more cases of male-to-female transmission and valid inferences about the frequency of transmission cannot be made from these cases alone. Prospective studies of the male partners of infected females provide better data; similarly, results from large prospective studies with longer follow-up should eventually improve our information. The limited prospective data now available (discussed below) suggest that the efficiency of transmission may not differ greatly.

Cross-sectional studies of HIV-infected females and their male partners provide data on the proportion of male partners who are seropositive, but often researchers cannot know which partner was infected first. The interpretation of these data is therefore uncertain. Table 4 can be compared with the table on the proportion of HIV-infected female partners in cross-sectional studies found in the section on male-to-female transmission. Like the cross-sectional studies of female partners, these studies show a wide variation in the proportion of infected males and a tendency for higher rates of infection among partners in studies where the index case had been diagnosed with AIDS.

TABLE 4.   CROSS-SECTIONAL STUDIES OF FEMALE-TO-MALE HIV TRANSMISSION

RISK GROUP	HIV DISEASE STATUS	#HIV+/ # PARTNERS TESTED	PERCENT	95% CI
African	AIDS cases	57/78	73	63–83[38]
Mixed	AIDS cases	12/17	71	49–92[40]

continued on next page

continued from previous page

TABLE 4.   CROSS-SECTIONAL STUDIES OF FEMALE-TO-MALE HIV TRANSMISSION

RISK GROUP	HIV DISEASE STATUS	#HIV+/ # PARTNERS TESTED	PERCENT	95% CI
Mostly IVDUs	AIDS cases	7/14	50	24–76[30]
African	HIV-positive	8/29	28	12–44[41]
Not given	HIV-positive	10/65	16	7–25[42]
Mostly IVDUs	Mixed	7/65	11	3–19[43]
Transfused	HIV-positive	2/25	8	0–19[27]
Not given	HIV-positive	2/49	4	0–10[44]
Mixed	Mixed	0/20	0	0–15[45]

The relative efficiency of female-to-male transmission versus male-to-female in cross-sectional studies varies from no evidence of a difference[42] to very substantial differences.[44] For the reasons discussed above, these cross-sectional data should be interpreted cautiously.

Fischl et al. observed that 3 of 8 (38 percent) male partners of females with AIDS seroconverted during a median follow-up of 24 months, compared with 10 of 24 (42 percent) female partners of male AIDS cases during the same period. These rates are nearly identical but have wide confidence intervals.

Although comparing the absolute number of male AIDS cases to female AIDS cases is misleading, national surveillance data make it possible to look at the relative rates for female-to-male and male-to-female transmission. The proportion by sex of cases attributed to heterosexual contact with a high-risk individual can be compared with the proportion of cases attributed to high-risk members of the opposite sex to give a ratio for cases attributed to transmission in each direction. For example, using CDC surveillance data for cases reported between June 1987 and May 1989 (1,094 cases of female partners of IVDUs versus 10,285 male IVDU cases), the proportion of female cases attributed to contact with a male IVDU versus the number of male IVDU cases is 10.6 percent (male-to-female transmission). The corresponding proportion for male cases attributed to contact with female IVDUs is 11.1 percent (female-to-male transmission) (453 male partners of female IVDUs versus 3137 female IVDU cases). The ratio of the two suggests that there may be little difference in the rates of transmission — in fact, female-to-male transmission appears more common. However, this comparison may be substantially biased because it ignores other factors that may affect the rate of differential transmission between the sexes, such as average number of sexual partners and length of time infected. The comparison also assumes that males and females progress to AIDS at about the same rate. Nevertheless, the estimates suggest that the difference in efficiency between male-to-female and female-to-male transmission, if any, may not be very great.

Cofactors for Female-to-Male Transmission.   Other sexually transmitted diseases (STDs) have been associated with female-to-male transmission of HIV. It has been suggested that other STDs, particularly those causing genital ulcers, may act as cofactors facilitating transmission of HIV.[46] Different rates for circumcised and uncircumcised males have been proposed in African data, but conflicting data have appeared in both African and U.S. studies.[47,48]

REFERENCES

1. Centers for Disease Control. Heterosexual transmission of human T-lymphotrophic virus type III/lymphadenopathy associated virus. MMWR 1985; 34:561-3.

2. Pitchenik AE, Shafron RD, Glasser RM, et al. The acquired immunodeficiency syndrome in the wife of a hemophiliac. Ann Intern Med 1984; 100:62-5.

3. Groopman JE, Sarngadharan MG, Salahuddin MS, et al. Apparent transmission of human t-cell leukemia virus type III to a heterosexual woman with the acquired immunodeficiency syndrome. Ann Intern Med 1985; 102:63-6.

4. Kreiss JK, Kitchen LW, Prince HE, et al. Antibody to human t-lymphotrophic virus type III in wives of hemophiliacs: Evidence for heterosexual transmission. Ann Intern Med 1985; 102:623-6.

5. Harris C, Small CB, Klein RS, et al. Immunodeficiency in female sexual partners of men with the acquired immunodeficiency syndrome. N Engl J Med 1983; 308:1181-4.

6. Stewart GJ, Tyler JPP, Cunningham AJ, et al. Transmission of human T-cell lymphotrophic virus type III (HTLV-III) by artificial insemination by donor. Lancet 1985; 2:581-5.

7. Piot P, Quinn TC, Taelman H, et al. Acquired immunodeficiency syndrome in an heterosexual population in Zaire. Lancet 1984; 2:65-9.

8. Clumeck N, Robert-Guroff M, Van de Perre P, et al. Seroepidemiological studies of HTLV-III antibody prevalence among selected groups of heterosexual Africans. JAMA 1985; 254:2599-2602.

9. Van de Perre P, Clumeck N, Carael M, et al. Female prostitutes: a risk group for infection with human T-cell lymphotrophic virus type III. Lancet 1985; 2:524-6.

10. Kriess JK, Koech D, Plummer FA, et al. AIDS virus infection in Nairobi prostitutes. N Engl J Med 1986; 314:414-8.

11. Redfield RR, Markham PD, Salahuddin SZ, et al. Heterosexually acquired HTLV-III/LAV disease (AIDS-related complex and AIDS). JAMA 1985; 254:2094-6.

12. Clumeck N, Van de Perre P, Carael M, et al. Heterosexual promiscuity in African patients with AIDS. N Engl J Med 1985; 313:182.

13. Castro KG, Fischl MA, Landesman SH, et al. Risk factors for AIDS among Haitians in the United States [Abstract]. In: The International Conference on Acquired Immunodeficiency Syndrome: Abstracts 1985. Philadelphia: The American College of Physicians, 1985.

14. Centers for Disease Control. Update: acquired immunodeficiency syndrome — United States. MMWR 1985; 34:561-3.

15. Centers for Disease Control. Update: acquired immunodeficiency syndrome — United States. MMWR 1986; 35:17-20.

16. Chaisson RF, Moss AR, Onishi R, et al. AIDS virus infection in heterosexual intravenous drug users in San Francisco. Am J Public Health (in press).

17. Fischl M, Fayne T, Flanagan S, et al. Seroprevalence and risks of HIV infections in spouses of persons infected with HIV [Abstract]. IV International Conference on AIDS. Stockholm, 1988; 1:274, 4060.

18. Padian N, Marquis L, Francis DP, et al. Male-to-female transmission of human immunodeficiency virus. JAMA 1987; 258:788-90.

19. Melbye M, Ingerslev J, Biggar RJ, et al. Anal intercourse as a possible factor in heterosexual transmission of HTLV-III to spouses of hemophiliacs. N Engl J Med 1985; 312:857.

20. Jason JM, McDougal S, Dixon G, et al. HTLV-III/LAV antibody and immune status of household contacts and sexual partners of persons with hemophilia. JAMA 1985; 255:212-5.

21. Redfield RR, Markham PD, Salahuddin SZ, et al. Frequent transmission of HTLV-III among spouses of patients with AIDS-related complex and AIDS. JAMA 1985; 253:1571-3.

22. Fultz PN, McClure HM, Daugharty H, et al. Vaginal transmission of human immunodeficiency virus (HIV) to a chimpanzee. J Infect Dis 1986; 154:896-900.

23. Jones P, Hamilton PJ, Bird G, et al. AIDS and hemophilia: morbidity and mortality in a well-defined population. Br Med J 1985; 291:695-9.

24. Allain JP. Prevalence of HTLV-III/LAV antibodies in patients with hemophilia and in their sexual partners in France. N Engl J Med 1986; 315:517-8.

25. Taelman H, Bonneux L, Cornet P, et al. Transmission of HIV to partners of seropositive heterosexuals from Africa [Abstract]. III International Conference on AIDS. Washington, D.C., 1987:23.

26. Clumeck N, Hermans P, Taelman H, et al. Clusters of heterosexual transmission of HIV in Brussels [Abstract]. III International Conference on AIDS. Washington, D.C., 1987; 76,TP.82.

27. Peterman TA, Stoneburner RL, Allen JR, et al. Risk of human immunodeficiency virus transmission from heterosexual adults with transfusion-associated infections. JAMA 1988; 259:55-8.

28. Cameron DW, D'Costa LJ, Ndinya-Achola JO, et al. Incidence and risk factors for female-to-male transmission of HIV [Abstract]. IV International Conference on AIDS. Stockholm, 1988; 1:275, 4061.

29. Sewankambo NK, Carswell JW, Mugerwa RD, et al. HIV infection through normal heterosexual contact in Uganda. AIDS 1987; 1:113-6.

30. Steigbigel NH, Maude DW, Feiner CJ, et al. Heterosexual transmission of HIV infection [Abstract]. IV International Conference on AIDS. Stockholm, 1988; 1:274, 4057.

31. Redfield RR. Heterosexual transmission of human T lymphotropic virus type III: syphilis revisited. Mount Sinai J Med 1986; 53:592-7.

32. Goedert JJ, Eyster ME, Biggar RJ, Blattner WA. Heterosexual transmission of human immunodeficiency virus: association with severe depletion of T-helper lymphocytes in men with hemophilia. AIDS Res Hum Retroviruses 1987; 3:355-61.

33. Biberfeld G, Bottiger B, Berntorp E, et al. Transmission of HIV infection to heterosexual partners but not to household contacts of seropositive haemophiliacs. Scand J Infect Dis 1986; 18:497-500.

34. Wofsy CB, Cohen JB, Hauer LB, et al. Isolation of AIDS associated retrovirus from genital secretions of women with antibodies to the virus. Lancet 1986; 1:527-9.

35. L'Age-Stehr J, Schwarz A, Offermann G, et al. HTLV-III infection in kidney transplant recipients. Lancet 1985; 2:1361-2.

36. Calabrese LH, Gopalakrishna KV. Transmission of HTLV-III infection from man to woman to man. N Engl J Med 1986; 314:987.

37. Miller CJ, Alexander N, Jennings M, et al. Transmission of simian immunodeficiency virus (SIV) across the genital mucosas of male and female rhesus macaques [Abstract]. IV International Conference on AIDS. Stockholm, 1988; 2:121, 2581.

38. Hira S, Wadhawan D, Nkowane B, et al. Heterosexual transmission of HIV in Zambia. IV International Conference on AIDS. Stockholm, 1988; 1:4006.

39. Norman C. AIDS trends: projections from limited data. Science 1985; 230:1018-21.

40. Fischl MA, Dickinson GM, Scott GB, et al. Evaluation of heterosexual partners, children, and household contacts of adults with AIDS. JAMA 1987; 257:640-4.

41. Nzila N, Laga M, Kivuvu M, et al. HIV risk factors in steady male sex partners of Kinshasa prostitutes. V International Conference on AIDS. Montreal, 1989:T.A.P.90.

42. Costigliola P, Ricchi E, Marinacci B, et al. Risk factors in heterosexual transmission of HIV. V International Conference on AIDS. Montreal, 1989:T.A.O.19.

43. De Vincenzi I, Ancelle-Park R. Heterosexual transmission of HIV: a European study. II: female-to-male transmission. V International Conference on AIDS. Montreal, 1989:Th.A.O.20.

44. Staszewski S, Rehmet S, Helm EB, Stille W. Co-factors in the heterosexual transmission of HIV in West Germany. V International Conference on AIDS. Montreal, 1989:T.A.O.15.

45. Padian N, Glass S, Marquis L, et al. Heterosexual transmission of HIV in California: results from a heterosexual partners' study. IV International Conference on AIDS. Stockholm, 1988; 1:4020.

46. Greenblatt RM, Lukehart SA, Plummer FA, et al. Genital ulceration as a risk factor for human immunodeficiency virus infection. AIDS 1988; 2:47-50.

47. Bongaarts J, Reining P, Way P, Conant FP. The relationship between male circumcision and HIV infection in African populations [Abstract]. V International Conference on AIDS. Montreal, 1989; T.A.P.86.

48. Surick I, McLaughlin M, Chiasson M, et al. HIV infection and circumcision status [Abstract]. V International Conference on AIDS. Montreal, 1989; T.A.P.89.

Transmission of HIV by Prostitutes and Prevention of Spread

Constance B. Wofsy, M.D.

Despite evidence that some prostitutes in the United States and Europe are infected with human immunodeficiency virus (HIV) (mostly IV drug users), no case has confirmed direct transmission of HIV from a female prostitute to a male partner. The strongest inference has come from Redfield, who reported high levels of heterosexual activity and use of prostitutes by United States servicemen with AIDS. Nine servicemen who denied any other risk activity indicated exposure to female prostitutes (primarily in Germany) as the only other possible risk for exposure to HIV.[1] The extent of HIV infection in German prostitutes was hotly debated in letters to the editor of the *New England Journal of Medicine,* with estimates ranging from 1 percent to 20 to 50 percent.[2-6]

Female-to-male transmission of HIV is strongly implied by the African data and is increasingly established in the United States.[7] The Centers for Disease Control (CDC) report 460 men and 402 women with AIDS as a result of heterosexual exposure as of July 28, 1986. The "less probable heterosexual transmission cases," such as men reporting contacts with a female prostitute as the only possible risk, continue to be included in the "None of the above" category.[8] Of the 32 women with AIDS in the "None of the above" category who had a detailed interview, none acknowledged payment for sex within the five years prior to diagnosis (CDC, personal communication).

The finding of HIV in small quantities in female genital secretions[9,10] and the known presence of virus in blood suggest two potential mechanisms of transmission from menstruating or nonmenstruating women to their male partners. Rectal intercourse does not appear to play a major role in heterosexual transmission.[7]

The best protection against sexual transmission of HIV can be accomplished by the use of a spermicide containing nonoxynol 9 in conjunction with a properly used condom. Condoms of five types prevented passage of HIV across the condom sheath in simulated intercourse done in the laboratory.[11] Condoms also prevent passage of cytomegalovirus[12] and herpesvirus.[13] Hepatitis B virus did not pass across five types of latex, but did penetrate through "natural" condoms.[14] Nonoxynol 9 is HIV viricidal in vitro,[15] but extreme caution must be used in relying on nonoxynol-9 spermicides as sole protection during sexual activity. Prostitutes are more likely than their peers to use condoms with customers, although not necessarily with their own partners or mates (COYOTE, National Task Force on Prostitution, personal communication).[16] Unfortunately, however, possession of condoms may be used by police as evidence of intent to engage in prostitution, and condoms are routinely confiscated from suspected prostitutes who are jailed in some states.

Many female prostitutes have developed educational workshops on techniques to increase the use of condoms by their clients or to refuse to have sex without one. In many instances it is the male partner who is resistant. Condoms do not offer absolute protection. They may be defective, rupture, or come off. If a lubricant is used, it should be water soluble, since petroleum-based lubricants make condoms more susceptible to breakage or leakage.

Persons who are known to have antibody to HIV must be counseled about risks to themselves and to others. Anonymous or semianonymous sexual activity must be avoided. It is important to realize that there are many forms of prostitution, that some individuals choose prostitution as a means of livelihood, and others resort to prostitution as a means of supporting an intravenous drug habit. Referrals to drug rehabilitation, job retraining, and other social service agencies are thus central to decreasing AIDS risk in this population.[1]

The role of male prostitution in transmission of AIDS to predominantly heterosexual men has had little study and is very seldom discussed, probably because of the social implications. Males who frequent male prostitutes may cover up that activity by acknowledging a visit to a female prostitute. It seems probable that exposure to a male prostitute poses a greater risk than exposure to a female prostitute, depending on the baseline rate of infection of homosexuals in that community.

Goals for health-care workers who deal with prostitutes should include:

1. AIDS education and advice given in a nonjudgmental fashion;

2. recognition that intravenous drug use is the major means by which prostitutes acquire HIV; if IV drug use is an issue, every effort should be made to encourage women to join treatment programs and referrals should be readily available;

3. advice to women about categories of men who are at risk for HIV; if a woman's husband, boyfriend, or regular sexual partner uses IV drugs or has other partners, condoms and other protection must be used with him as well as with paying customers;

4. counseling of all women who might be at risk about the danger of transmission of HIV to unborn children and about the advisability of preconception antibody testing done confidentially;

5. the spelling out of risks to males who engage in prostitution and others who may consider themselves "straight"; and

6. making safer sex guidelines readily available.

For the man who has had contact with a female prostitute and is concerned, the following information should be provided: female-to-male transmission does occur, but there is no documentation of direct prostitute transmission at this point. Men who frequent prostitutes or who have frequent and anonymous sexual relations regardless of the exchange of money are a special group to target for education about HIV and risks of infection. If they choose to continue to engage in anonymous sex despite the potential risks, the protective role of condoms must be stressed.

REFERENCES

1. Redfield RR, Markham PD, Salahuddin SZ, et al. Heterosexually acquired HTLV III/LAV disease (AIDS-related complex and AIDS). JAMA 1985; 254:2094-6.

2. James JJ, Morgenstern MA, Hatten JA. HTLV-III/LAV antibody-positive soldiers in Berlin. N Engl J Med 1986; 314:55.

3. Papaevangelou G, Roumeliotou-Karayannis A, Kallinikos G, Papoutsakis G. LAV/HTLV-III infection in female prostitutes. Lancet 1985; 2:1018.

4. Tirelli U, Vaccher E, Carbone A, et al. Serological studies in Rwanda, Athens, Seattle, and Miami suggest that prostitutes are an important human reservoir of HTLV-III. Lancet 1985; 2:1424.

5. Barton SE, Underhill GS, Gilchrist C, et al. HTLV-III antibody in prostitutes. Lancet 1985; 2:1424.

6. Brenky-Faudeux D, Fribourg-Blanc A. American studies suggest that prostitutes are at high risk of AIDS. Lancet 1985; 2:1424.

7. Fischl MA, Dickinson GM, Scott GB, et al. Heterosexual and household transmission of the human T lymphotropic virus type III [Abstract]. Paris: Proceedings of the International Conference on AIDS, 1986:107.

8. Centers for Disease Control, Center for Infectious Diseases. AIDS Weekly Surveillance Report, July 28, 1986:1.

9. Vogt MW, Craven DE, Crawford DF, et al. Isolation of HTLV III/LAV from cervical secretions of women at risk for AIDS. Lancet 1986; 1:525-7.

10. Wofsy CB, Hauer LB, Michaelis BA, et al. Isolation of AIDS associated retrovirus from genital secretions of women with antibodies to the virus. Lancet 1986; 1:527-9.

11. Conant M, Hardy D, Sernatinger J, et al. Condoms prevent transmission of AIDS-associated retrovirus. JAMA 1986; 255:1706.

12. Katznelson S, Drew WL, Mintz L. Efficacy of the condom as a barrier to the transmission of cytomegalovirus. J Infect Dis 1984; 150:155-7.

13. Conant MA, Spicer DW, Smith CD. Herpes simplex virus transmission: condom studies. Sex Transm Dis 1984; 11:94-5.

14. Minuk GY, Bohme CE, Bowen TJ. Condoms and hepatitis B virus infection. Ann Intern Med 1986; 104:584.

15. Hicks DR, Martin LS, Getchell JP, et al. Inactivation of HTLV-III/LAV-infected cultures of normal human lymphocytes by nonoxynol-9 in vitro. Lancet 1985; 2:1422-3.

16. Centers for Disease Control. Antibody to human immunodeficiency virus in female prostitutes. MMWR 1987; 36:157-61.

1.2.6

Transmission of HIV in Intravenous Drug Users

Richard E. Chaisson, M.D.

T ransmission of AIDS by intravenous drug users (IVDUs) became apparent early in the AIDS epidemic when increasing numbers of heterosexual drug addicts in New York and New Jersey were diagnosed with opportunistic infections. These individuals lacked the sexual risk factors present in male homosexuals but reported histories of intravenous drug use and diseases related to drug use. Additionally, non-drug-using female sexual partners of drug addicts were noted to have immunologic abnormalities and frank AIDS, suggesting that sexual transmission from drug addicts was occurring.[1] As the AIDS epidemic has progressed, IVDUs have consistently comprised the second largest risk group among AIDS patients reported to the Centers for Disease Control (CDC). Seventeen percent of all AIDS cases in the United States are attributed to IV drug use; 8 percent of cases occur in homosexual men who also use IV drugs, although the additional risk conferred by IV drug use in these cases is uncertain.[2-4] IVDUs are also responsible for transmission of the human immunodeficiency virus (HIV) to other groups, most notably sexual partners and children of drug addicts. Seventy-six percent of AIDS cases attributed to heterosexual spread involves a sex partner who uses IV drugs, and 59 percent of pediatric AIDS cases have a parent who uses IV drugs (Hardy A: personal communication, June 1986). As the rate of seroconversion among homosexual men declines, IVDUs may account for an increasing proportion of AIDS cases.

■ SEROPREVALENCE OF INFECTION

Isolation of HIV and the development of serologic tests for evidence of infection have permitted population surveys of infection in asymptomatic drug addicts to be carried out. It is now apparent that large numbers of drug addicts throughout the United States and Europe are infected with HIV. It is also apparent that when HIV is introduced into a community of IVDUs, it spreads rapidly to infect a large proportion of individuals who are regular IVDUs (see Fig. 1.2.6.a).

AIDS in IVDUs was first observed in New York City, and early work identified a high prevalence of seropositivity for HIV antibodies among asymptomatic addicts. A survey of 86 IVDUs entering drug detoxification programs in New York City in 1984 revealed a 58 percent prevalence of antibodies to HIV, confirmed by radioimmunoprecipitation assay (RIPA).[5] Additional studies in New York using sera collected from IVDUs in 1983 and 1984 found an antibody prevalence of 33 percent in subjects enrolled in a drug-free treatment program and 70 percent in subjects hospitalized for nonopportunistic infections.[6] This study did not use confirmatory tests for verifying ELISA-positive sera. Retrospective testing of stored sera from IVDUs collected in New York from 1978 to 1982 shows that HIV was present in 1978 and that the prevalence of infection increased markedly during a four-year period. In 1978, 9 percent of sera (1 of 11)

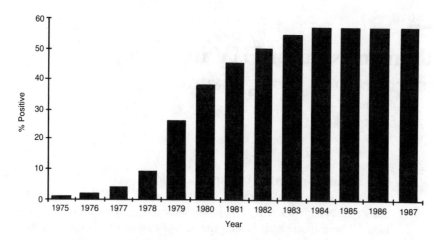

Figure 1.2.6.a   Historical reconstruction of human immunodeficiency virus type 1 seroprevalence among active intravenous drug users in Manhattan, New York City. Reconstruction is based on seroprevalence data for 1978 through 1984 and 1986 through 1987, with acquired immunodeficiency syndrome case data used to estimate seroprevalence for other years. Curve has been smoothed for 1984 through 1987. Adapted from *JAMA* 1989; 261:1010.

tested positive for HIV antibodies; in 1979, 30 percent of sera were positive; and in 1980 and 1982 the proportion of positive sera rose to 40 percent and 50 percent, respectively.[7] Although this study used stored sera from selected addicts enrolled in research protocols unrelated to AIDS, the changing prevalence of seropositivity shows a rapid dispersion of the virus among active IVDUs. A recent survey of 361 addicts with a history of IV drug use since 1978 enrolled in a methadone maintenance program in the Bronx showed that 31 percent had antibodies to HIV.[8]

Northern New Jersey has a high concentration of IVDUs among its AIDS cases, and a seroepidemiologic study of addicts shows a high prevalence of antibodies to HIV, particularly in addicts living in close proximity to New York City. In a survey of over 900 IVDUs undergoing treatment for addiction in 1984, 50 percent of those living within 5 miles of New York City were seropositive compared with only 2 percent of those living more than 100 miles from New York City.[9] Other areas of high prevalence of antibodies in IVDUs include Edinburgh, with a seroprevalence of 51 percent,[10] Milan, where between 30 percent and 50 percent of addicts tested in 1984 and 1985 were seropositive,[11] and Spain, where one study revealed a seroprevalence of 37 percent.[12] Studies in Edinburgh and Milan also show a rapid spread of HIV infection among drug users after initial introduction; the majority of seroconversions in Edinburgh occurred within a two-year period, and in Milan a less than 5 percent prevalence in 1981 increased to 30 percent to 50 percent in 1985.[10,11] Surveys in other metropolitan areas have shown lower prevalences of antibody positivity, including 10 percent in New Haven in 1982,[13] and 10 percent in San Francisco in 1985.[14]

■ **RISK FACTORS FOR INFECTION**

Transmission of HIV in IVDUs occurs primarily through contamination of injection paraphernalia with infected blood. Behaviors that intensify exposure to infected blood increase the risk of infection. Sharing of needles and syringes is common among drug users and is reinforced by legal and economic forces that restrict the availability of sterile equipment. Cultural norms place value on the use of a common vessel for injecting drugs as well. In New York City, the use of "shooting galleries," sites where drugs are sold and injection equipment is rented and shared by customers, is common and is a significant risk factor for seropositivity.[15] Initial exposure to HIV in heterosexual IVDUs in New York probably occurred through needle sharing with homosexual heroin addicts.[16] In a study of heterosexual IV-drug-using AIDS and ARC patients in the Bronx, 57 percent of subjects had a history of sharing needles with homosexual men and 74 percent frequented shooting galleries. In another New York study, the frequency of attendance at shooting galleries was significantly associated with seropositivity, ranging from 35 percent in addicts who never used shooting galleries to 75 percent in addicts injecting in shooting galleries more than 45 times per month.[15]

As would be expected, the frequency of injection has been shown to be a significant risk factor for infection. In New York, the seroprevalence in addicts with no recent needle use is 21 percent; in those who inject 1 to 5 times monthly, 31 percent; in those who inject 6 to 45 times monthly, 47 percent; and in those injecting more than 45 times monthly, the seroprevalence is 61 percent.[15]

Needle sharing, per se, has been identified as a significant risk factor for seropositivity in several studies. In Edinburgh, among addicts whose frequency of needle sharing was known, 30 percent of those never sharing, 56 percent of those sometimes sharing, and 75 percent of those usually sharing were seropositive.[10] In San Francisco, a linear relationship between the number of persons with whom needles were regularly shared and seropositivity was demonstrated; 3 percent of those not sharing regularly, 9 percent of those sharing regularly with one other person, and 15 percent of those sharing regularly with two or more persons were seropositive. A number of other behaviors related to injecting drugs have been studied for effect on seropositivity, yielding mixed results. No strong protective trend has been demonstrated for needle cleaning with either water or alcohol, presumably because of the inconsistency with which this is actually practiced on a day-to-day basis.

Demographic factors are strongly associated with HIV infection for reasons that are not well understood. Members of ethnic minorities are overrepresented among both AIDS cases and HIV infection in IVDUs in the United States. In New York, Hispanics and blacks have a significantly higher seroprevalence than whites.[8] Blacks and Hispanics in San Francisco have an almost threefold greater prevalence of infection than whites.[14] In New Jersey, a higher proportion of AIDS cases attributed to IV drug use occurs in blacks than would be predicted by the proportion of drug users who are black. No behavioral factors have been identified that put minority group members at increased risk, although needle-sharing habits are suspected to play a role. However, in San Francisco, the number of persons with whom needles are regularly shared is greater in whites than in nonwhites.[14] Racial differences in seroprevalence appear to be limited to the United States, although national origin is an important risk factor in some European cities. Differences in seropositivity by sex varies geographically; there is a 13 percent greater seroprevalence among male drug users in New York and no difference in seroprevalence by sex in New Jersey and San Francisco.

Although IVDUs can clearly transmit HIV infection through sexual contact, the primary mode of infection in addicts is needle use and not sexual exposure.

This is shown in several studies of prostitutes that identify IV drug use, not prostitution, as the primary risk factor for infection.[17,18] Almost all seropositive prostitutes identified to date in the United States and Europe have a history of IV drug use, whereas extensive surveys of non-drug-using prostitutes have failed to identify any significant level of infection.[19] In San Francisco, the seroprevalence is the same in female IVDUs with a history of prostitution as in those without a history of prostitution.[14] Studies of heterosexual couples in which one or both partners are IVDUs have shown that heterosexual transmission to a non-drug-using partner is unusual, whereas when both partners use drugs, concomitant infection is common.[20]

REFERENCES

1. Masur H, Michelis MA, Wormser GP, et al. Opportunistic infection in previously healthy women: initial manifestations of a community acquired cellular immunodeficiency. Ann Intern Med 1982; 97:533-9.

2. Centers for Disease Control. Update: acquired immunodeficiency syndrome (AIDS): United States. MMWR 1986; 35:1.

3. Osmond D, Moss AR, Bachetti P, et al. A case control study of risk factors for AIDS in San Francisco [Abstract]. Atlanta: International Conference on AIDS, 1985; 24.

4. Stevens CE, Taylor PE, Zang, et al. Human T cell lymphotropic virus type III infection in a cohort of homosexual men in New York City. JAMA 1986; 255:2167-72.

5. Spira TJ, DesJarlais DC, Marmor M, et al. Prevalence of antibody to lymphadenopathy associated virus among drug detoxification patients in New York. N Engl J Med 1984; 311:467-8.

6. Maayan S, Backenroth R, Rieber E, et al. Antibody to lymphadenopathy associated virus/human T lymphotrophic virus type III in various groups of illicit drug abusers in New York City. J Infect Dis 1985; 152:843.

7. Novick D, Kreek MJ, DesJarlais DC, et al. Abstract of clinical research findings: therapeutic and historical aspects. In: Harris LS, ed. Problems of drug dependence, 1985: Proceedings of the 47th Annual Scientific Meeting, the Committee on Problems of Drug Dependence, Inc. NIDA research monograph 67. Washington, D.C.: NIDA, 1986.

8. Schoenbaum EE, Selwyn PA, Klein RS, et al. Prevalence of and risk factors associated with HTLV-III/LAV antibodies among intravenous drug abusers in methadone programs in New York City [Abstract]. Paris: Proceedings of the International Conference on AIDS, 1986; 111.

9. Weiss SH, Ginzburg HM, Goedert JJ, et al. Risk for HTLV-III exposure and AIDS among parenteral drug abusers in New Jersey [Abstract]. Atlanta: International Conference on AIDS, 1985; 44.

10. Robertson JR, Bucknall ABV, Welsby PD, et al. Epidemic of AIDS related virus (HTLV-III/LAV) infection among intravenous drug abusers. Br Med J 1986; 292:527-9.

11. Ferroni P, Geroldi D, Galli C, et al. HTLV-III antibody among Italian drug addicts. Lancet 1985; 2:52-3.

12. Rodrigo JM, Serra MA, Aguilar E, et al. HTLV-III antibodies in drug addicts in Spain. Lancet 1985; 2:156-7.

13. D'Aquila R, Williams AB, Kleber HD, Williams AE. Prevalence of HTLV-III infection among New Haven, Connecticut, parenteral drug abusers in 1982–1983. N Engl J Med 1986; 314:117-8.

14. Chaisson RE, Onishi R, Moss AR, et al. Human immunodeficiency virus infection in heterosexual intravenous drug users in San Francisco. Am J Public Health 1987; 77:169-72.

15. Cohen H, Marmor M, DesJarlais D, et al. Behavioral risk factors for HTLV-III/LAV seropositivity among intravenous drug abusers [Abstract]. Atlanta: International Conference on AIDS, 1985; 44.

16. Friedland GH, Harris C, Butkus-Small C, et al. Intravenous drug abusers and the acquired immunodeficiency syndrome (AIDS): demographic, drug use, and needle sharing patterns. Arch Intern Med 1985; 145:1413-7.

17. Centers for Disease Control. Heterosexual transmission of human T lymphotrophic type III/lymphadenopathy associated virus. MMWR 1985; 34:561-3.

18. James JJ, Morgenstern MA, Hatten JA. HTLV-III/LAV antibody positive soldiers in Berlin. N Engl J Med 1986; 314:55.

19. Cohen JB, Hauer LB, Poole LE, et al. Prevalence of AIDS antibody and associated risk factors in a prospective study of 400 San Francisco prostitutes and other sexually active women [Abstract]. Paris: Proceedings of the International Conference on AIDS, 1986; 111.

20. Tirelli U, Vaccher E, Carbone A, et al. Heterosexual contact is not the predominant mode of HTLV-III transmission among intravenous drug abusers. JAMA 1986; 255:2289.

Transmission of HIV in Prisoners

Elizabeth Kantor, M.D.

A lthough there is no known evidence of an AIDS case acquired in jail or prison, numerous activities known to occur among prisoners may be responsible for HIV transmission. Reviews from New York State in 1984 and 1987 found that the onset of HIV-related symptoms among inmates ranged from 0 to 84 months after incarceration and occurred in individuals who engaged in high-risk activities "outside."[3,4] To identify transmission of HIV in prison, two groups of Maryland state prison inmates were tested for HIV antibody in 1985: 58 of 787 (7 percent) new inmates and 2 of 137 long-term inmate—volunteers were found to be seropositive. The two are believed to have seroconverted in prison because their continuous incarceration began before the virus was found in the community.[1] No information is available regarding their behavior.

To date, no cases of seroconversion, AIDS, or ARC have occurred among correctional staff that could be attributed to contacts with inmates.[5]

■ RISK ACTIVITIES FOR HIV TRANSMISSION

Sexual activity between male inmates is not uncommon in prisons and jails, but reliable figures on this activity are not available. A Federal Bureau of Prisons study in 1982 reported that 30 percent of federal prison inmates engage in homosexual activity while incarcerated.[2] Homosexual activity in many inmates is limited to the institutional setting and occurs overwhelmingly between consenting men.

The frequency of homosexual rape in jails and prisons is extremely difficult to estimate. Interpersonal dynamics discourage the victim from reporting a rape. He must consider the probability of further suffering and worse injury from his legally prosecuted attacker as well as from his attacker's associates, for these always wield more power in the prison hierarchy. The Federal Bureau of Prisons study reported that 9 percent to 20 percent of federal inmates, especially new or homosexual inmates, are victims of rape.[2]

Incidents of interpersonal violence (including rape and fights involving lacerations, bites, and bleeding in two or more participants) present varying risks for HIV transmission. Fights usually occur among inmates only, although they may involve correctional staff. These are the only risk activities occurring in prisons and jails that do not involve consenting participants.

Intravenous drug users share syringes in prisons and jails because these items are scarce. A handmade syringe may be fashioned from (among other things) the glass found inside a light bulb. Other potential vectors of infection include shared razors, which prisons provide for groups of inmates, as blades are likely to be used as weapons. Inmates have been told that if the common blade is not returned to the guard after use, all prisoners' visits will be canceled. Thus, the guard doesn't need to observe every shaver and no razor blade can be "lost." Prisoners share toothbrushes as well as razors in facilities where they are not issued or where inmates are unable to purchase their own.

Tattooing is a widely practiced prison activity that is usually performed without fresh or sterile instruments. It involves multiple skin punctures with recycled, sharpened, and altered implements; commonly, staples or paper clips are used. Prison wisdom holds that tattooing that causes blood to flow results in the best quality image and is least likely to become infected. Homemade pigment is delivered intradermally rather than through direct puncture. Metal points connected to a battery or other electrical source are capable of producing vibration; these increase the number of skin punctures exponentially, and create a better quality tattoo. As with intravenous drug equipment, "needle" cleaning procedures vary. Water and matches are generally available. Peroxide, alcohol, or bleach may be used by inmates who work in health-care areas or on cleaning assignments.

■ PREVENTION OF TRANSMISSION: INSTITUTIONAL RESPONSES

Education.   Prisoners represent a crucial target population for AIDS education programs. Prisons concentrate individuals who are not easily reached in the community by such programs. The lifestyle of IV drug users doesn't lend itself to getting information about drug-use hazards. Of the local, state, and federal prisons surveyed in the National Institute of Justice study, 97 percent reported educational programs for staff and 96 percent reported educational programs for inmates.[5] As many as 50 percent of American prisoners are functionally illiterate and many are not native English speakers; effective information programs must meet their needs. The generally available informational literature does not reach most inmates or address many of their particular needs. An excellent video, "AIDS: A Bad Way to Die," has been made by New York State prisoners.[6] Another effective and gripping film that provides information and advice specifically for prisoners is "Con to Con" from Georgia State Prison.

In prison, as in the community, education is the only means of overcoming the fear and hysteria produced by AIDS. Unlike the community, however, prison populations — fearful inmates, guards, administrators, or health-care staff — may demand and establish the quarantine of individuals with AIDS or known HIV seropositivity, regardless of those individuals' behavior or wishes. Accurate and adequate information for staff and inmates in the prison setting can reduce fears, and ultimately affect institutional policies that profoundly alter prisoners' lives. All inmates entering prison should be informed in clear, simple terms and in their own language about how to avoid transmission of HIV and other communicable diseases within the institutional setting.

Condoms, Sterile Syringes, Bleach.   Most correctional administrators have not permitted the distribution of condoms to inmates. Although homosexual activity is known to occur, existing statutes make sexual activity in prison a punishable crime, and one that condom distribution would seem to promote. In Britain, where homosexual acts in private are not an offense if both parties have consented and are 21 or older, prison cells are not regarded as places of privacy, thereby making sex between prisoners illegal.[7] Another objection to condoms in institutions is that they are considered contraband — a vehicle for hiding drugs or other illegal things that inmates may swallow after placing them in a condom. Currently, condoms are available only to selected inmates in the New York City Jail on Riker's Island and to inmates in the State Prison of Vermont through the medical staff (accompanied by counseling). In Mississippi, condoms are sold at institutional canteens from vending machines.[5] Inmates in Geneva and Zurich, Switzerland, and other European prisons also have access to condoms.[8,9]

The distribution of sterile syringes to inmates has also been discussed as a means of preventing HIV transmission, but the objection has been raised that the correctional institutions should provide drug-addiction treatment instead.[7]

Education for the intravenous drug user must emphasize that bleach effectively kills HIV and should also provide instruction in cleaning the "works." Bleach is often available in institutions. Informed inmates with access to bleach do use it.

Quarantine.   Quarantine of inmates identified with AIDS and/or HIV seropositivity exists in many prisons and jails. In the United States (and worldwide), some prison systems perform mandatory screening of all inmates for HIV antibody and then segregate seropositives to prevent viral transmission in the institution. Correctional officers have demanded the identification and segregation of HIV seropositives, claiming they can thus protect themselves from transmission. Years of experience and data will be necessary to measure the effectiveness of this practice and to compare transmission rates in institutions that do not impose quarantine.

The alternative to quarantine is education to prevent transmission through consensual activities. Nonconsensual transmission through violence and homosexual rape may be diminished by increasing staff-to-prisoner ratios, decreasing overcrowding, classifying and housing inmates properly, and providing activities for the inmates.[7] Preventing such violence is the ongoing responsibility of the prison wardens.

REFERENCES

1. First AIDS in prison study completed. CDC AIDS Weekly 1986; (January 6):19.
2. Nacci P, Kane T. Sex and sexual aggression in federal prisons. Washington, D.C.: Federal Bureau of Prisons, 1982.
3. Hanrahan JP, Wormser GP, Reilly AA, et al. Prolonged incubation of AIDS in intravenous drug abusers: epidemiological evidence in prison inmates. J Infect Dis 1984; 150:263-6.
4. Gido RL, Gaunay W. Update: acquired immune deficiency syndrome: a demographic profile of New York State inmate mortalities 1981-1986. New York State Commission of Correction, 1987.
5. Hammett TM. AIDS in correctional facilities: issues and options. 3rd ed. Washington, D.C.: National Institute of Justice, 1988.
6. Copies of the videotape are available without charge by sending a blank VHS cassette with self-addressed mailer to Charles Hernandez, Superintendent, Taconic Correctional Facility, 250 Harris Road, Bedford Hills, NY 10507; tel. 914-241-3010.
7. Harding TW. AIDS in prison. Lancet 1987; 2:1260-3.
8. Hornblum A. A Philadelphia AIDS policy. Corrections Today, December 1988.
9. Hornblum A. The condom wars. American Jails, Fall 1988.

Transmission of HIV in Health-Care Workers

J. Louise Gerberding, M.D.

E pidemiologic evidence indicates that human immunodeficiency virus (HIV) is transmitted through sexual contact with infected partners, through direct exposure to contaminated blood or blood products, and through perinatal transmission from infected mothers to their offspring. Other viruses with similar modes of transmission, such as hepatitis B virus, are known to be transmitted to health-care workers through occupational exposures. These risks to health-care workers posed by patients infected with HIV are currently under evaluation in several medical centers in the United States. This chapter reviews case reports and cohort studies related to occupational exposure to HIV among health-care workers.

Over 4000 health-care workers have been enrolled in studies and tested for evidence of HIV infection, including more than 1200 subjects who have sustained accidental parenteral exposures.[1-9,19,20,24,25] Five documented cases of occupational transmission have been demonstrated in study subjects.[4,10,21,24,25] Cumulative evidence from the studies of health-care workers indicates that the magnitude of risk from needlestick exposure to HIV-infected blood carries less than a 1 percent probability of seroconversion. This is at least an order of magnitude less than the risk after similar exposure to hepatitis B.[11,12] One additional study of 265 laboratory workers has identified two infected health-care workers exposed to highly concentrated specimens of HIV in a research laboratory.[22]

As of June 1989, 19 cases of well-documented occupational HIV infection have been reported in the world. Twelve infections were attributed to needlestick exposure to blood containing HIV, one to a deep laceration, four to mucocutaneous contact, and two to percutaneous contact with high-titer virus specimens in research laboratories.

■ CASE REPORTS

1. Direct injection of an aliquot of blood from a female African AIDS patient into a female nurse in Britain during an accidental needlestick resulted in transmission of HIV. Thirteen days after injection, the nurse developed a sore throat, fever, headache, myalgia, facial neuralgia, and lymphadenopathy. Seventeen days after injection, a diffuse, nonpruritic macular rash appeared and persisted for one week. Severe arthralgia without arthritis was also present. The symptoms and signs persisted for 21 days; recovery was complete. Serum drawn 27 days after the injection was negative for antibody to HIV, but specimens on days 49 and 57 were confirmed positive. Epidemiologic investigation did not reveal evidence of other risk factors for HIV; serologic studies for other viral infections known to cause a similar syndrome were negative.[13]

2. A health-care worker sustaining a needlestick contaminated with blood from an AIDS patient who was positive for hepatitis B surface antigen (HBsAg) subsequently developed acute hepatitis B 15 weeks after exposure. Recovery from the hepatitis was uneventful. Fifteen months after exposure, serum was tested for antibody to HIV by indirect fluorescent antibody (IFA) test and was negative; T-cell subsets were normal.[14]

3. A female nurse sustained a deep intramuscular puncture wound with a large-bore needle attached to a syringe containing blood from a patient with AIDS. The nurse was tested for antibody to HIV within 30 days of the exposure; no antibody was detected. Two weeks after the exposure, she developed an acute mononucleosis-like illness that spontaneously resolved. Six months after the exposure, the nurse was retested and had antibody to HIV, although cultures for the virus were negative.[4,10]

4. A female nurse received a superficial needlestick while recapping a needle contaminated with bloody pleural fluid. Three weeks later, she had a viral syndrome consistent with acute HIV infection. She did not have HIV antibody at the time of exposure, but antibody was present by day 68 after the accident.[15]

5. A female nurse in the Caribbean sustaining a superficial needlestick with blood from an infected AIDS patient had a documented seroconversion for antibody to HIV.[16]

6. The mother of a child infected with HIV after a postnatal blood transfusion apparently developed antibody to HIV several months after the child was diagnosed. She had routinely provided skilled nursing care for the child, including handling of diarrheal fluids, without using gloves or other protection against exposure.[17]

7. A female health-care worker was exposed to a patient's blood (later found to be infected with HIV) while applying 20 minutes of compression with her fingertip to a bleeding artery during a resuscitation. The worker had complained of severely chapped hands and was not wearing gloves during the exposure. She later developed a viral syndrome suggestive of acute HIV infection and subsequently developed antibody to HIV.[18]

8. A female worker was splashed while injecting HIV-infected blood into a serum tube. Blood splashed onto her face and into her mouth. She was wearing gloves and prescription glasses at the time of the exposure. The day after the accident, she had no antibody to HIV but was found to be positive for HIV antibody nine months later when donating blood.[18]

9. A female technologist spilled a large volume of blood on her hands and forearms during a malfunction of an apheresis machine. She was not wearing gloves at the time. She had no cutaneous lesions on the exposed areas but did have a chronic dermatitis of her ear, which she may have touched. The patient donating blood was subsequently found to be infected with HIV. Eight weeks after the exposure, the worker developed a viral syndrome suggestive of acute HIV infection. By 12 weeks after exposure, she had developed antibody to HIV.[18]

■ COHORT STUDIES OF HEALTH-CARE WORKERS WITH OCCUPATIONAL EXPOSURE TO HIV

Eighty-five health-care workers in Massachusetts who collectively sustained 33 needlesticks or equivalent injuries from occupational exposure to AIDS and ARC patients were evaluated for antibody to HTLV-III (HIV). None of the workers tested positive.[1]

Two hundred seventy health-care workers at San Francisco General Hospital, none of whom had established risk factors for AIDS and all of whom had intensive exposure to AIDS and ARC patients, including 94 individuals who sustained a total of 327 needlesticks or similar direct inoculations, were tested for antibody to HIV in a prospective study. None of the health-care workers had HIV antibody when first tested; none developed antibody during the 10-month follow-up interval.[2] Since the original report, more than 500 accidental parenteral exposures to HIV have been prospectively evaluated in this population. One infected health-care worker, who seroconverted after a deep needlestick, has been identified.[21]

Three hundred sixty-one health-care workers in New York with frequent exposure to AIDS and ARC patients were tested for antibody to HTLV-III (HIV). Three health-care workers without other risk factors for AIDS were antibody-positive by ELISA and Western blot tests. All three had sustained accidental needlestick exposures before enrollment in the study. Occupational exposure was a possible mode of transmission but could not be proven, since baseline serum obtained before exposure was not available to document seroconversion.[3]

Four hundred fifty-one health-care workers who have sustained needlesticks or other accidental occupational exposures in hospitals throughout the U.S. have been enrolled in the Centers for Disease Control (CDC) Cooperative Needlestick Study. Only two of the health-care workers lacking established risk factors for AIDS have developed antibody to HIV.[7] One of these individuals sustained a deep puncture wound with a large needle attached to a syringe containing blood from an AIDS patient and developed antibody to HIV after the exposure.[4,10] The other belonged in the group of three subjects discussed above[3] for whom baseline serum was unavailable to document seroconversion as a result of occupational exposure. Since the initial publication, two additional infected heath-care workers have been identified in the expanded cohort of the study.[23]

Five hundred thirty-one health-care workers with occupational exposure to patients with AIDS, including 150 individuals with accidental needlestick or mucous membrane exposures, were enrolled in a prospective study at the National Institutes of Health. None of the subjects lacking established risk factors for AIDS has antibody to HIV.[8] Since the time of the original publication, one health-care worker, who was exposed to HIV during a laceration, has seroconverted. None of 246 female health-care workers prospectively followed for 9 to 12 months developed antibody to HIV, despite intensive exposure.[6]

REFERENCES

1. Hirsch MS, Wormser GP, Schooley RT, et al. Risk of nosocomial infection with human T cell lymphotropic virus III (HTLV-III). N Engl J Med 1985; 312:1-4.
2. Gerberding JL, Bryant-LeBlanc CE, Nelson K, et al. Risk of transmitting the human immunodeficiency virus, hepatitis B virus, and cytomegalovirus to health-care workers exposed to patients with AIDS and AIDS-related conditions. J Infect Dis 1987; 156:1-8.
3. Weiss SH, Saxinger WC, Rechtman D, et al. HTLV-III infection among health care workers: association with needlestick injuries. JAMA 1985; 254:2089-93.

4. McCray E, Cooperative Needlestick Group. Occupational risk of the acquired immunodeficiency syndrome among health care workers. N Engl J Med 1986; 314:1127-32.

5. Henderson DK, Saah AJ, Zak BJ, et al. Risk of nosocomial infection with human T cell lymphotropic virus type III/lymphadenopathy associated virus in a large cohort of intensively exposed health care workers. Ann Intern Med 1986; 104:644-7.

6. Kuhls TL, Viker S, Parris NB, et al. Occupational risk of HIV, HBV, and HSV-2 infections in health care personnel caring for AIDS patients. Am J Public Health 1987; 77:1306-9.

7. Flynn NM, Pollet SM, Van Horne JR, et al. Absence of HIV antibody among dental professionals exposed to infected patients. West J Med 1987; 146:439-42.

8. Klein RS, Phelan J, Friedland GH, et al. Prevalence of antibodies to HTLV-III/LAV among dental professionals [Abstract]. New Orleans: Twenty-sixth Interscience Congress on Antimicrobial Agents and Chemotherapy. American Society for Microbiology, 1986:283.

9. Gerberding JL, Nelson K, Greenspan D, et al. Risk to dentists from occupational exposure to human immunodeficiency virus (HIV): Followup [Abstract]. Washington, D.C.: Twenty-seventh Interscience Conference on Antimicrobial Agents and Chemotherapy. American Society for Microbiology, 1987.

10. Stricof RL, Morse DL. HTLV-III/LAV seroconversion following a deep intramuscular needlestick injury. N Engl J Med 1986; 314:1115.

11. West D. The risk of hepatitis B in health care professionals in the United States. Am J Med Sci 1984; 287:26-33.

12. Werner BJ, Grady GF. Accidental hepatitis B surface antigen positive inoculations: Use of e antigen to estimate infectivity. Ann Intern Med 1982; 97:367-9.

13. Anonymous. Needlestick transmission of HTLV-III from a patient infected in Africa. Lancet 1984; 2:1376-7.

14. Hopewell PC, Kaminsky LS, Sande MA. Transmission of hepatitis B without transmission of AIDS by accidental needlestick. N Engl J Med 1985; 312:56-7.

15. Oksenhendler E, Harzic M, Le Roux JM, et al. HIV infection with seroconversion after a superficial needlestick injury to the finger. N Engl J Med 1986; 315:582.

16. Neisson-Vernant C, Arfi S, Mathez D, et al. Needlestick HIV seroconversion in a nurse. Lancet 1986; 2:814.

17. Centers for Disease Control. Apparent transmission of human T lymphotropic virus type III/lymphadenopathy-associated virus from a child to a mother providing health care. MMWR 1986; 35:76-9.

18. Centers for Disease Control. Update: human immunodeficiency virus infections in health care workers exposed to blood of infected patients. MMWR 1987; 36:285-9.

19. McEvoy M, Porter K, Mortimer P, et al. Prospective study of clinical, laboratory, and ancillary staff with accidental exposures to blood or body fluids from patients infected with HIV. Br Med J 1987; 294:1595-7.

20. Joline C, Wormser GP. Update on a prospective study of health care workers exposed to blood and body fluids of acquired immunodeficiency syndrome patients. Am J Infect Control 1987; 15:86.

21. Gerberding JL, Henderson DK. Design of rational infection control policies for human immunodeficiency virus infection. J Infect Dis 1987; 156:861-4.

22. Weiss SH, Goedert JJ, Gartner S, et al. Risk of human immunodeficiency virus (HIV) infection among laboratory workers. Science 1988; 239:68-71.

23. Centers for Disease Control. Recommendations for prevention of HIV transmission in health care settings. MMWR 1987; 36(Suppl 2):1S-18S.

24. Update: acquired immunodeficiency syndrome and human immunodeficiency virus infection among health-care workers. MMWR 1988; 37:229-34, 239.

25. Marcus R. Surveillance of health care workers exposed to blood from patients infected with the human immunodeficiency virus. N Engl J Med 1988; 319:1118-23.

Transmission of HIV in Blood Products

Elizabeth Donegan, M.D.

Transmission of HIV-1 has been documented after transfusion of the following single-donor blood and blood components: whole blood, packed red cells (including washed and buffy-coat poor), fresh-frozen plasma, cryoprecipitated, and platelets.[1,3] Plasma-derived blood products that are manufactured from plasma pooled from 2,000 to 30,000 donors can transmit HIV-1, depending upon the production process.[4] This chapter discusses HIV transmission, incidence, control measures, and future prospects for the safety of U.S. blood products.

■ TRANSFUSION-ASSOCIATED HIV INFECTION: PRE-1985, SINGLE-DONOR COMPONENTS

HIV-1 infection following blood transfusion has been repeatedly documented since the first case report in late 1982.[5-9,11,24] Currently, 3 percent of adult and 12 percent of pediatric AIDS cases reported to the Centers for Disease Control were caused by HIV-infected transfusions. Almost all of these are due to blood transfused before HIV-1 antibody testing became available in March 1985. There are an estimated 12,000 living transfusion recipients.[10] Many remain unaware that they are infected. Ninety percent of recipients transfused with HIV antibody-positive blood are themselves antibody-positive at follow-up.[40] No persistently seronegative HIV-1-infected transfusion recipients have yet been identified. Seroconversion is independent of the type of component transfused (excluding washed red cells, which transmit HIV at a lower rate), the age or sex of the recipient, or the reason for transfusion.[13] HIV-1 transmission does not increase the recipient's mortality rates immediately, but transfusion recipients do develop AIDS at rates comparable to others infected for similar periods of time.[14,15] Currently, the mean progression to AIDS is estimated to be 8.2 years for adult transfusion recipients, with a cumulative prevalence of 20 percent after five years of infection.[26] This prevalence may prove to be overestimated, since it is based primarily on data from recipients who have themselves developed AIDS or who received blood from donors who subsequently developed AIDS.

■ TRANSFUSION FOLLOW-UP PROGRAMS

A variety of programs to locate and test recipients of blood transfused between 1978 and March 1985 have been initiated. Attempted follow-up of all transfusion recipients during this period has met with variable success. The first such program, initiated in Columbus, Ohio (a low-risk area for AIDS), identified only 1 infected recipient out of 2343 persons tested.[16] In San Francisco, however, 2 percent of recipients tested from one hospital were antibody-positive.[17]

"Look-Back" programs have identified larger numbers of infected recipients. These programs focus upon locating and testing recipients of blood from donors who subsequently developed AIDS or who tested HIV antibody-positive. Between 38 percent and 60 percent of living recipients of these donations are antibody-positive.[16]

HIV-1 antibody testing should be considered by all individuals transfused between 1978 and March 1985. Such testing may prevent transmission of HIV-1 to recipients' sexual partners, allow the treatment of asymptomatic individuals, and aid clinicians in diagnosing HIV-related disease.

■ TRANSFUSION-ASSOCIATED HIV: SINGLE-DONOR COMPONENTS SINCE 1985

Transfusion-transmitted HIV-1 has became rare since the beginning of voluntary deferral of donors at risk for HIV-1 infection and the routine HIV antibody testing of all donations.[2,19] Despite these measures, an estimated risk of HIV-1 transmission remains, ranging from 1 in 28,000 to 1 in 100,000 per units of blood transfused.[2,19,20]

Blood-bank screening fails when at-risk persons are not excluded from making donations. Exclusion of donors is voluntary. Interviews with antibody-positive donors reveal that most recognize their risk but fail to self-exclude.[21]

Laboratory screening tests, although more than 99 percent sensitive,[18] may fail because of technical difficulties or errors. Of far greater concern, however, is the inability of current screening tests to detect either recently HIV-1-infected individuals who have not yet developed antibody ("window period")[2] or persistently antibody-negative but HIV-1-infected donors.[22]

Several studies have evaluated laboratory tests that detect HIV-1 p24 antigen. It was hoped that this test, which does not depend upon antibody production, would detect HIV-infected but antibody-negative donors. Unfortunately, both retrospective and prospective studies on blood donors have failed to find any p24 antigen-positive, HIV-1 antibody-negative donors after testing more than 750,000 specimens.[23] A more sensitive method for virus detection, using the polymerase chain reaction, may have application to banked blood. This method of gene amplification, which can detect minute amounts of HIV-1 proviral sequences, has not yet been adapted for testing large numbers of samples at one time.

■ OTHER RETROVIRUSES: HIV-2, HTLV-I/II

HIV-2 infection is rarely reported in the United States, although occasional cases have been reported in Europe.[25,27,28] No transfusion-transmitted HIV-2 cases have been reported in the United States. At present, blood banks do not screen donations for HIV-2. However, current HIV-1 antibody ELISA tests detect 42 percent to 92 percent of HIV-2 infections.[25] ELISA tests that could detect HIV-1 and HIV-2 with equal efficiency are being developed.

Human T-cell leukemia (or T-lymphotropic) virus type I (HTLV-I) is a human retrovirus associated with a variety of clinical syndromes, including an asymptomatic carrier state, neurologic disease (tropical spastic paraparesis, myelopathy), cutaneous lesions, lymphadenopathy, hepatosplenomegaly, hypercalcemia, and adult T-cell leukemia and lymphoma.[29,31,34] Epidemiologic data from endemic areas indicates a long latency period (10 to 30 years) between infection and clinical illness. Transmission is associated with sexual contact, intravenous (IV) drug use, in utero exposure, and receipt of cellular blood products.[29,31,34,36]

HTLV-II (human T-cell leukemia, or T-lymphotropic virus type II) is a human retrovirus whose amino-acid sequence homology and immunologic cross-reactivity link it closely to HTLV-I. This makes serological distinction between HTLV-I and HTLV-II impossible by routine screening assays. HTLV-II has only rarely been associated with human malignancy. Little is known about its long-term effects or geographic origin. A significant proportion of New Orleans IV drug users appear to be infected with it. HTLV-II is probably transmitted by contaminated needles shared during IV drug use. Presumably, contaminated blood products could also transmit it. Because serologic screening of blood products detects both HTLV-I and HTLV-II without distinguishing between them, the viruses are collectively designated and discussed as HTLV-I/II.[46]

As of July 1, 1989, blood donations in the United States are also screened for HTLV-I/II. Depending upon the geographic location of the blood center, from 1 in 1000 to 1 in 4000 volunteer blood donors are antibody-positive for HTLV-I/II.[30,32] HTLV-I/II can be transmitted through cellular blood components (whole blood, packed red cells, platelets, etc.), but they have not been reported to transmit infection through cell-free products (i.e., fresh-frozen plasma, cryoprecipitate). Although in Japan 60 percent of patients receiving cellular products have been reported as infected with HTLV-I/II, evidence in the United States suggests that transmission (60 percent rate) requires that the cellular products have been stored for less than eight days. No transmission is evident when transfusion of components follows storage for longer periods of time.[33,35]

■ HIV-1 TRANSMISSION IN PLASMA-DERIVED BLOOD PRODUCTS

Plasma-pooled products (2,000 to 30,000 donors per lot) carry a greater potential for HIV-1 transmission than single-donor components, depending upon the manufacturing process used. One HIV-1-infected donor can contaminate an entire lot of product if HIV-1 is not neutralized with sufficient heat or by cold ethanol treatment (or both) during production. Albumin and plasma protein (Cohn fractions IV and V) are extracted with the maximum concentration of cold ethanol and then pasteurized. They do not transmit HIV-1. Cohn fraction II products (i.e., immune globulins such as Rh immune globulin, gamma globulin, hepatitis B immune globulin) are treated with somewhat lower concentrations of cold ethanol and cannot be pasteurized without loss of activity. The presence of high-titer antibody to HIV-1 in some lots of hepatitis B immune globulin and isolated recipient-transient (less than six months' duration) low HIV-1 antibody titers has raised questions about the safety of these products. However, there have been no documented cases of HIV-1 disease as a result of their use. Over 4.5 million doses of Rh immune globulin have been given since 1968 with no reported cases of AIDS. Although recipients of hepatitis B immunoglobulin may be transiently HIV-1 antibody-positive, there is no evidence that they are infected.[25,37]

Before 1984, Factor VIII and Factor IX concentrates infected many recipients. Factor concentrates are produced early in the Cohn fractionation procedure. Factor VIII precipitates before cold ethanol is added to the process and Factor IX is produced in Cohn fraction I. Before 1984, factor concentrates were not heat-treated to prevent their hemostatic activity from being lost. As a result, roughly 80 percent of treated hemophilia A patients and 50 percent of treated hemophilia B patients are now HIV-1 antibody-positive.[38,39,41] Early hopes that antibody formation in hemophiliacs was due to inactivated virus have not proven true. Instead, epidemiologic and culture studies suggest that the presence of antibody indicates infection.[42] As of July 1989, 5 percent (1,044 of 20,000) of U.S. hemophiliacs have developed AIDS. Decreasing helper/suppressor ratios and falling absolute T4 cell counts predict that an increasing number of hemophiliacs, particularly older hemophiliacs, will develop AIDS.[43]

Factor concentrates are far safer today, although they are still manufactured from the pooled blood of thousands of donors. Plasma donors are now asked to self-exclude if they are at risk for HIV-1 infection; they are now screened like volunteer blood donors and are tested for HIV-1 antibody. Since 1984, multiple methods for inactivating virus have been developed and applied.[44] Most methods use heat treatment, although some chemical methods are also available. No seroconversions have yet occurred among persons not already infected who are using factor products now on the market. However, 18 cases of seroconversion were reported using dry-heat methods, which are no longer employed.[12,45] The factor VIII gene has recently been cloned. Once recombinant factor concentrates are readily available, they should eliminate transmission of viral infections in factor products.

REFERENCES

1. Donegan E, and the Transfusion Safety Study Group. Comparison of HTLV-I/II with HIV-1 transmission by component type and shelf storage before administration. Accepted for presentation at the American Association of Blood Banks 42nd Annual Meeting, New Orleans, October 21-26, 1989.

2. Ward JW, Holmberg SD, Allen JR, et al. Transmission of human immunodeficiency virus (HIV) by blood transfusions screened as negative for HIV antibody. N Engl J Med 1988; 318:473-7.

3. Natural history of primary infection with LAV in multitransfused patients. By the AIDS-Hemophilia French Study Group. Blood 1986; 68:89-94.

4. Berkman SA, Groopman JE. Transfusion associated AIDS. Transfusion Med Rev 1988; 2:18-28.

5. Ammann AJ, Wara DW, Dritz S, Cowan M, Weintrub P, et al. Acquired immunodeficiency in an infant: possible transmission by means of blood products. Lancet 1983; 1:956-8.

6. Curran JW, Lawrence DN, Jaffe H, Kaplan JE, Zyla LD, et al. Acquired immunodeficiency syndrome (AIDS) associated with transfusion. N Engl J Med 1984; 310:69-75.

7. Peterman TA, Jaffe HW, Feorino PM, et al. Transfusion-associated acquired immunodeficiency syndrome in the United States. JAMA 1985; 254:2913-7.

8. Anderson KC, Gorgone BC, Marlink RG, et al. Transfusion-acquired human immunodeficiency virus infection among immunocompromised persons. Ann Intern Med 1986; 105:519-27.

9. Jaffe HW, Sarngadharan MG, DeVico AL, et al. Infection with HTLV-III/LAV and transfusion-associated acquired immunodeficiency syndrome. Serologic evidence of an association. JAMA 1985; 254:770-3.

10. Peterman TA, Lui KJ, Lawrence DN, Allen JR. Estimating the risk of transfusion-associated acquired immune deficiency syndrome and human immunodeficiency virus infection. Transfusion 1987; 27:371-4.

11. Ward JW, Deppe DA, Samson S, Perkins H, Holland P, et al. Risk of human immunodeficiency virus infection from blood donors who later developed the acquired immunodeficiency syndrome. Ann Intern Med 1987; 106:61-2.

12. Safety of therapeutic products used for hemophilia patients. MMWR 1988; 37:441.

13. Kleinman S, and the Transfusion Safety Study Group. The infectivity of anti-HIV-positive blood components. III International Conference on AIDS. Washington, D.C., 1987; TP.234.

14. Donegan E, Perkins H, Vyas G, and the Transfusion Safety Study (TSS) Group. Mortality in the recipients of blood in the Transfusion Safety Study. Blood 1986; 68:296A.

15. Giesecke J, Scalia-Tomba G, Berglund O, et al. Incidence of symptoms and AIDS in 146 Swedish haemophiliacs and blood transfusion recipients infected with human immunodeficiency virus. Br Med J [Clin Res]1988; 297:99-102.

16. Ng AT, Conway MA, Blanda E, et al. Tracing HIV-1 infected blood recipients: large-scale recipient screening vs. look-back testing. JAMA 1987; 258:201-2.

17. Donegan E, Johnson D, Remedios V, Cohen S. Mass notification of transfusion recipients at risk for HIV infection. JAMA 1988; 260:922-3.

18. Update: serologic testing for antibody to human immunodeficiency virus. MMWR 1988; 36:833-845.

19. Cohen ND, Munoz A, Reitz BA, et al. Transmission of retroviruses by transfusion of screened blood in patients undergoing cardiac surgery. N Engl J Med 1989; 320:1172-6.

20. Kleinman S, Secord K. Risk of human immunodeficiency virus (HIV) transmission by anti-HIV negative blood. Estimates using the lookback methodology. Transfusion 1988; 28:499-501.

21. Cleary PD, Singer E, Rogers TF, et al. Sociodemographic and behavioral characteristics of HIV antibody-positive blood donors. Am J Public Health 1988; 78:953-7.

22. Imagawa DT, Lee MH, Wolinsky SM, et al. Human immunodeficiency virus type 1 infection in homosexual men who remain seronegative for prolonged periods. N Engl J Med 1989; 320:1458-62.

23. FDA advisory committee recommends against the use of HIV antigen test for blood screening. Blood Bank Week 1989; 6:1-6.

24. Human immunodeficiency virus infection in transfusion recipients and their family members. MMWR 1987; 36:137-40.

25. Update: AIDS due to HIV-2 infection. MMWR 1988; 37:33-5.

26. Medley GF, Anderson RM, Cox DR, Billard L. Incubation period of AIDS in patients infected via blood transfusion. Nature 1987; 328:719.

27. Vittecog D, Ferchal F, Chamaret S, et al. Routes of HIV-2 transmission in western Europe. Lancet 1987; 1:1150-1.

28. Courouce AM. HIV-2 in blood donors and in different risk groups in France. Lancet 1987; 1:1151.

29. Minamoto GY, Gold JWM, Scheinberg DA, et al. Infection with human T-cell leukemia virus type 1 in patients with leukemia. N Engl J Med 1988; 318:219-22.

30. Williams AE, Fang CT, Slamon DJ, et al. Seroprevalence and epidemiological correlates of HTLV-I infection in U.S. blood donors. Science 1988; 240:643-6.

31. Larson CJ, Taswell HF. Human T-cell leukemia virus type I (HTLV-I) and blood transfusion. Mayo Clin Proc 1988; 63:869-75.

32. Transfusion Safety Study Group. Antibody to HTLV-I/II among blood donors in four cities of the United States. V International Conference on AIDS. Montreal, 1989; Th.A.P.32.

33. Okochi K, Sato H, Hinuma Y. A retrospective study on transmission of adult T cell leukemia virus by blood transfusion: seroconversion in recipients. Vox Sang 1984; 46:245-53.

34. Kim JH, Durack DT. Manifestations of human T-lymphotropic virus type I infection. Am J Med 1988; 84:919-28.

35. Donegan E, and the Transfusion Safety Study (TSS) Group. Comparison of HTLV-I/II with HIV-1 transmission by component type and shelf storage before administration. AABB Meeting 1989; Presentation.

36. Ehrlich GD, Poiesz BJ. Clinical and molecular parameters of HTLV-I infection. Clin Lab Med 1988; 8:65-84.

37. Sugg U, Schneider W, Kaufmann R, Gurtler L. Safety of immunoglobulin preparations with respect to transmission of human immunodeficiency virus. Transfusion 1987; 27:115.

38. Tedder RS, Uttley A, Cheingsong-Popov R. Safety of immunoglobulin preparation containing anti-HTLV-III. Lancet 1985; 1:815.

39. Ragni MV, Winkelstein A, Kingsley L, et al. 1986 update of HIV seroprevalence, seroconversion, AIDS incidence, and immunologic correlates of HIV infection in patients with hemophilia A and B. Blood 1987; 70:786-90.

40. Donegan E, and the Transfusion Safety Study (TSS) Group. Course of HIV infection in transfusion recipients. IV International Conference on AIDS. Stockholm, 1988; 2:7710.

41. Immunologic and virologic status of multitransfused patients: role of type and origin of blood products. By the AIDS-Hemophilia French Study Group. Blood 1985; 66:896-901.

42. Allain JP. Prevalence of HTLV-III/LAV antibodies in patients with hemophilia and in their sexual partners in France. N Engl J Med 1986; 315:517-8.

43. Gomperts ED, Feorino P, Evatt BL, et al. LAV/HTLV-III presence in peripheral blood lymphocytes of seropositive young hemophiliacs. Blood 1985; 65:1549-52.

44. Eyster ME, Gail MH, Ballard JO, et al. Natural history of human immunodeficiency virus infections in hemophiliacs: effects of T-cell subsets, platelet counts, and age. Ann Intern Med 1987; 107:1-6.

45. Brettler DG, Levine PH. Review: factor concentrates for treatment of hemophilia: which one to choose? Blood 1989; 73:2067-73.

46. Lee H, Swanson P, Shorty VS, et al. High rate of HTLV-II infection in seropositive IV drug abusers in New Orleans. Science 1989; 244:471-5.

HIV Transmission in Transplant Recipients and Artificial Insemination Recipients

Dennis Osmond

This chapter reviews reports of HIV transmission through transplantation and artificial insemination. Transmission by blood and blood products and blood banking policy guidelines are reviewed elsewhere.

■ ESTIMATES OF HIV TRANSMISSION IN TRANSPLANT/ARTIFICIAL INSEMINATION RECIPIENTS

HIV has been transmitted through kidney,[5,6] liver, heart, pancreas,[7] bone,[8] and possibly skin transplants.[9] It has also been transmitted through artificial insemination.[4,10] Because these procedures are less common than blood transfusion, relatively few cases of HIV transmission have been reported through these routes. More than 20 million patients received blood transfusions between 1978 and early 1985, when routine screening of blood for HIV began. During that same period, an estimated 140,000 persons received artificial insemination.[1] The Centers for Disease Control (CDC) has estimated that 12,000 individuals have been infected with HIV through blood transfusions, but there are many uncertainties in this estimate.[11] Estimates for the number of infected transplant and semen recipients are even more difficult to derive because estimates of seroprevalence among organ donors and semen donors are not available.

The current risk of HIV infection from organ/tissue transplant or artificial insemination is unknown. Like the risk from blood transfusion, it depends primarily on the prevalence of HIV-infected donors testing seronegative at the time of donation. In the absence of reliable data, the risk may be considered equal to that of infection through blood transfusion — perhaps 1 in 250,000.[12]

Transmission through artificial insemination is of particular interest because it approximates "experimental" sexual transmission. HIV can be retrieved from mononuclear cells in semen.[2,3] Reports of seroconversion among women undergoing artificial insemination appear to demonstrate HIV transmission from male to female via the vaginal route without trauma, prior conditions favoring viral entry, or prior immunosuppression in the host. However, artificial insemination may not be directly comparable to vaginal intercourse in its potential for infection; during the procedure, semen is deposited directly in the cervix — this is not the case in vaginal intercourse. Whether this changes the probability of infection is unknown. On the other hand, the potential for minor trauma to vaginal tissue from vaginal intercourse may increase the likelihood of infection via that route. In either case, infection rates in women receiving semen from seropositive donors may yield information on rates of sexual transmission.

■ CASE REPORTS

Australian investigators reported eight women who were inseminated with the semen of a donor subsequently found to be HIV antibody-positive.[4] Four of the women became antibody-positive. None of the four gave a history of conditions that might have enhanced viral entry; one woman developed persistent lymphadenopathy. None of the four women reported a mononucleosis-like syndrome (acute HIV infection). Viral isolations were not reported. All four seropositive women were married and neither they nor their husbands had a known risk factor for HIV infection. All four husbands were antibody-negative. Three of the women conceived and gave birth; all three children are healthy and antibody-negative.

The investigators found an inverse correlation between length of storage time for the semen specimens and probability of infection (1 to 4 months of storage in antibody-positive women versus 16 to 17 months of storage in antibody-negative women), suggesting that prolonged storage may reduce the risk of transmission. Perhaps T4 lymphocytes containing virus are not optimally preserved by the technique of glycerol cryopreservation that is used to store these semen specimens.

Although 50 percent (four of eight) of the recipients were antibody-positive and none of their husbands was antibody-positive, conclusions about the relative efficiency of male-to-female and female-to-male transmission should be drawn with caution. This was not a random sampling; antibody status in these women was studied because one of them developed lymphadenopathy syndrome, a marker of HIV infection, which made it very likely that at least one of the four would test positive and that all four were recipients of infectious semen.

A second report found a much lower rate of infection in recipients. Thirty women were identified as receiving semen from a seropositive donor. Of these, 24 were tested and 2 were HIV seropositive (8 percent).[10]

These two studies provide insufficient data for generalization, but it is worth noting that the range of infection rates (8 percent to 50 percent) is similar to that reported in heterosexual partner studies.

REFERENCES

1. Curie-Cohen M, Luttrell L, Shapiro S. Current practice of artificial insemination by donor in the United States. N Engl J Med 1979; 300:585-90.

2. Zagury D, Bernard J, Liebowitch J, et al. HTLV-III in cells cultured from semen from two patients with AIDS. Science 1984; 226:449-51.

3. Ho DD, Schooley RT, Tota TR. HTLV-III in the semen and blood of a healthy homosexual man. Science 1984; 226:451-3.

4. Stewart GJ, Cunningham AL, Driscoll GL, et al. Transmission of human t-cell lymphotropic virus type III (HTLV-III) by artificial insemination by donor. Lancet 1985; 2:581-4.

5. Human immunodeficiency virus infection transmitted from an organ donor screened for HIV antibody — North Carolina. MMWR 1987; 36:306-8.

6. Neumayer HH, Fassbinder W, Kresse S, Wagner K. Human T-lymphotropic virus III antibody screening in kidney transplant recipients and patients receiving maintenance hemodialysis. Transplant Proc 1987; 19:2169-71.

7. Erice A, Rahme F, Sullivan C, et al. Human immunodeficiency virus (HIV) infection in organ transplant recipients (OTRS) [Abstract]. IV International Conference on AIDS, Stockholm, 1988:7756.

8. Transmission of HIV through bone transplantation: case report and public health recommendations. MMWR 1988; 37:597-9.

9. Clarke JA. HIV transmission and skin grafts. Lancet 1987; 1:983.

10. Rekart M. HIV transmission by artificial insemination [Abstract]. IV International Conference on AIDS. Stockholm, 1988:4026.

11. Human immunodeficiency virus infection in transfusion recipients and their family members. MMWR 1987; 36:137-40.

12. Bove JR. Transfusion-associated hepatitis and AIDS: What is the risk? N Engl J Med 1987; 317:242-5.

Transmission of HIV in Households

Alan Lifson, M.D., M.P.H.

Human immunodeficiency virus (HIV) is transmitted primarily through three routes: sexual contact with an infected person, parenteral exposure to infected blood or blood products (including rare occupational exposure and needle-sharing among intravenous drug users), and perinatal exposure.[1] A number of studies provide evidence that HIV is not transmitted through household or other casual contact (see below).

■ TRANSMISSION OF HIV IN HOUSEHOLDS AND SCHOOLS

At least 12 studies in the United States and Europe have evaluated the risk of nonsexually transmitted HIV infection in over 700 household or boarding school contacts between non-HIV-infected persons and persons infected with HIV.[2,3,5-14] Household members have in some cases helped infected persons to bathe, dress, and eat; some have also shared household items (such as eating and drinking utensils) and facilities (such as the kitchen, bath, and toilet) with them. None of these studies have found serologic or virologic evidence of HIV transmission among household members who lack other risks for infection. For example, in one study, 199 of 200 non-sexual household contacts of 85 AIDS patients were negative for HIV serum antibody.[10] The one HIV-positive subject was a child who had probably been infected perinatally. In a study of children living in a French boarding school, half of the hemophiliac children were HIV infected[11]; however, none of the non-hemophiliac children who had lived in the same school for at least a year was seropositive for HIV.

One case of household HIV transmission (associated with major exposures to blood and secretions) occurred in a mother who seroconverted while providing health care for a child who had undergone numerous surgical procedures after birth and who had been infected from a transfusion at three months of age.[4] The mother was closely involved in all aspects of the child's care in and out of the hospital, including drawing blood, removing intravenous lines, changing ostomy bags, inserting rectal tubes, changing nasogastric tubes, and changing surgical dressings. She could not recall an accidental percutaneous exposure. However, she did not use gloves and on numerous occasions her hands became contaminated with blood and feces that often contained blood. It is worth re-emphasizing that this mother's exposure consisted of intensive exposure to blood, stools, and other secretions, unlike the exposures of most household contacts.

The possibility that HIV can be transmitted through a human bite was suggested by a report of two HIV-infected siblings.[17] However, because the history was retrospectively obtained from the mother after both children were known to be seropositive and because the bite did not break the skin or cause bleeding, the exact route of transmission in this family is uncertain. Investigations of other children and of health-care workers have found no evidence that anyone has seroconverted after being bitten by an HIV-infected person.[1,9,18,19]

Studies from Africa have not found any association between HIV transmission and nonsexual, person-to-person contact.[20] In one study from Zaire, 314 household contacts (excluding spouses) of HIV-infected persons and non-infected controls were evaluated. The rate of HIV seropositivity did not differ significantly between study subjects and controls. For adults in case households who were not spouses, the number seropositive was similar to that predicted from age- and sex-specific HIV seroprevalence rates.

■ TRANSMISSION OF HIV IN THE WORKPLACE

If HIV is not transmitted between household members whose exposures are repeated and sometimes prolonged, it is even less likely to be transmitted in the workplace. There is no evidence that blood-borne and sexually transmitted infections such as HIV are transmitted while preparing or serving food and beverages.[15] U.S. Public Health Service guidelines state that HIV-infected workers (including food-service workers) should not be prevented from working solely because they are infected, nor should they be prevented from using telephones, office equipment, toilets, showers, eating facilities, or water fountains used by other workers or the public.[15]

REFERENCES

1. Lifson AR. Do alternate modes for transmission of human immunodeficiency virus exist? A review. JAMA 1988; 259:1353-6.
2. Jason JM, McDougal S, Dixon G, et al. HTLV-III/LAV antibody and immune status of household contacts and sexual partners of persons with hemophilia. JAMA 1986; 255:212-5.
3. Redfield RR, Markham PD, Salahuddin SZ, et al. Frequent transmission of HTLV-III among spouses of patients with AIDS-related complex and AIDS. JAMA 1985; 253:1571-3.
4. Apparent transmission of human T-lymphotropic virus type III/lymphadenopathy-associated virus from a child to a mother providing health care. MMWR 1986; 35:76-9.
5. Kaplan JE, Oleske JM, Getchell JP, et al. Evidence against transmission of human T-lymphotropic virus/lymphadenopathy-associated virus (HTLV-III/LAV) in families of children with the acquired immunodeficiency syndrome. Pediatr Infect Dis 1985; 4:468-71.
6. Lawrence DN, Jason JM, Bouhasin JD, et al. HTLV-III/LAV antibody status of spouses and household contacts assisting in home infusion of hemophilia patients. Blood 1985; 66:703-5.
7. Thomas PA, Lubin K, Enlow RW, Getchell J. Comparison of HTLV-III serology, T-cell levels, and general health status of children whose mothers have AIDS with children of healthy inner city mothers in New York. I International Conference on AIDS, Atlanta, 1985; T-81.
8. Lewin EB, Zack R, Ayodele A. Communicability of AIDS in a foster care setting. I International Conference on AIDS, Atlanta, 1985; T-78.
9. Rogers MF, White CR, Sanders R. Can children transmit HTLV-III/LAV infection? Twenty-sixth Interscience Conference on Antimicrobial Agents and Chemotherapy. New Orleans, 1986.
10. Friedland GH, Saltzman B, Rogers M, et al. Additional evidence for lack of transmission of HIV infection to household contacts of AIDS patients. III International Conference on AIDS, Washington, D.C., 1987; TP.67.
11. Berthier A, Chamaret S, Fauchet R, et al. Transmissibility of human immunodeficiency virus in haemophiliac children living in a private school in France. Lancet 1986; 2:598-601.
12. Fischl MA, Dickinson GM, Scott GB, et al. Evaluation of heterosexual partners, children, and household contacts of adults with AIDS. JAMA 1987; 257:640-4.
13. Peterman TA, Stoneburner RL, Allen JR, et al. Risk of human immunodeficiency virus transmission from heterosexual adults with transfusion-associated infections. JAMA 1988; 259:55-8.
14. Brettler DB, Forsberg AD, Levine PH, et al. Human immunodeficiency virus isolation studies and antibody testing. Household contacts and sexual partners of persons with hemophilia. Arch Intern Med 1988; 148:1299-301.
15. Recommendations for preventing transmission of infection with human T-lymphotropic virus type III/lymphadenopathy-associated virus in the workplace. MMWR 1985; 34:681-6, 691-5.
16. Recommendations for prevention of HIV transmission in health-care settings. MMWR 1987; 36(Suppl 2S):1S-18S.

17. Wahn V, Kramer HH, Voit T, et al. Horizontal transmission of HIV infection between two siblings. Lancet 1986; 2:694.
18. Drummond JA. Seronegative 18 months after being bitten by a patient with AIDS. JAMA 1986; 256:2342-3.
19. Tsoukas C, Hadjis T, Theberge L, et al. Risk of transmission of HTLV-III/LAV from human bites. II International Conference on AIDS, Paris, 1986; poster 211.
20. Mann JM, Quinn TC, Francis H, et al. Prevalence of HTLV-III/LAV in household contacts of patients with confirmed AIDS and controls in Kinshasa, Zaire. JAMA 1986; 256:721-4.

TESTING
FOR
HUMAN
IMMUNODEFICIENCY
VIRUS

EDITOR
Paul A. Volberding, M.D.

2.1

Testing for Human Immunodeficiency Virus

Indications for Use of HIV Antibody Testing

Paul A. Volberding, M.D., and P.T. Cohen, M.D., Ph.D.

Testing for HIV infection is useful for public health and infection-control purposes, for epidemiologic monitoring, and for identifying HIV-infected individuals who may benefit from early medical intervention. Serious issues of confidentiality, public and occupational health and safety, civil rights and liberties, and ethics are involved in approaches to testing. This chapter reviews the background and proposes indications for HIV testing. Technical aspects of tests, including detection of HIV antibody and HIV antigen, culturing of live HIV, and detection of HIV nucleic acid by the polymerase-chain-reaction method, are discussed in other chapters.

Tests for HIV infection may be done for several reasons:

1. benefit to the individual being tested;
2. public health and infection control (for epidemiologic characterization or public health policy-making);
3. benefit of another individual who may have been exposed to infection (such as by a needlestick injury);
4. institutional requirement or policy (such as a requirement for insurance).

Each of these cases will be discussed after considering common issues.

■ GENERAL CONSIDERATIONS

Testing serum for antibodies to HIV is currently the most cost-effective and accurate method of screening for infection.[1,2,12-14] Antibody testing has revealed critical information about the epidemiology of HIV infection, the mechanisms of transmission, and the course of infection in people over time. There is strong and growing evidence that asymptomatic or minimally symptomatic HIV-infected individuals benefit from early diagnosis.[15] Decisions about pregnancy, sexual practices, and career planning may be affected by the antibody test. Thus, there is a strong rationale for voluntary testing — that is, testing for HIV infection with the individual's consent and understanding of the risks and benefits involved.[15,16] There is no strong rationale, however, for a policy of mandatory testing (that is, testing people without their consent) for purposes of controlling the HIV epidemic.

The risk that HIV test results will become known must be recognized by testing counselors, clinicians, public-health policy makers, and above all by individuals who are considering being tested. Unfortunately, persons infected with HIV confront not only fear and pain from knowing they are infected, but also serious social, financial, and emotional problems resulting from unfortunate social and institutional attitudes toward HIV infection. Eviction, job loss, the inability to buy or maintain health insurance, and abandonment by friends and loved ones are examples of some of the unfortunate consequences of being labeled as infected with "the AIDS virus." These are not rare events, and they can occur whenever confidentiality is violated or whenever test results are requested by and released to employers, insurance companies, or others.

Erroneous test results and improper interpretation may occur when tests are performed by inexperienced or inexpert laboratory personnel.[1,2]

Antibody tests may occasionally be falsely positive, even when carried out and interpreted properly.[3] False-positive tests are rare and can usually be identified by additional testing.

The HIV antibody test has limitations. Because an infected individual does not develop antibodies immediately (in most HIV infections, antibodies appear within three to six months after infection), a negative result cannot rule out more recent HIV infection. If recent exposure is suspected, the test must be repeated in six months.

In what are believed to be uncommon situations,[17-20] antibody testing may be insensitive and may require repeated testing or evaluation by additional techniques, such as HIV culture,[21] HIV antigen detection, or the polymerase chain reaction. However, these alternative techniques have not yet proved to be highly specific or sensitive, so their role in HIV detection is still undefined.

■ PREDICTIVE VALUE OF TESTS

The predictive value of HIV antibody tests depends on the prevalence of HIV infection in the population. This concept is crucial to planning testing strategies and interpreting test results. In a population with a very low prevalence of HIV infection, the predictive value of a positive test is very low — that is, a positive test result is very likely to be a false-positive result. Thus, HIV antibody testing of low-prevalence populations (e.g., all applicants for marriage licenses) is likely to produce more false- than true-positive results.

A positive HIV antibody test in a person without apparent risks or in a low-prevalence population should be followed by rigorous retesting of new serum specimens in a laboratory known for its quality control and proficiency.

■ COUNSELING

Testing for evidence of HIV infection should always be accompanied by pre- and post-test counseling. Special expertise and training are required to counsel persons effectively. Because results of tests for HIV infection have profound consequences and raise many questions, individuals should give informed consent for the testing procedure and understand the choices implied by the test results. Counseling issues include advice and information about the test, high-risk behaviors associated with transmission of HIV, consequences of the various results for the individual (pregnancy, employment, insurance) and others (family, lovers, friends), and the need for appropriate follow-up in the event of positive test results. Discussion of equivocal results that require additional tests may be necessary. Even for an individual whose result is negative, counseling may be needed to allay a false sense of security and to promote future preventive behaviors.

Counseling should be provided by personnel who understand these issues, so professionals intending to administer the test should become familiar with them. Institutions where the test is commonly administered should establish a testing service made up of personnel able to do effective counseling.

■ CONFIDENTIALITY AND ANONYMOUS TESTING

Although confidentiality is a goal to be vigorously pursued, it is misleading to suggest that it can be guaranteed. An exception is anonymous testing, where the person being tested is identified in records by a code (such as a number) so that even the person administering the test cannot associate the result with a name. The person tested is then free to divulge or keep secret the test result. Anonymous testing is usually done in a testing program outside of the clinical setting.

While in theory all test results can be kept confidential, in reality, institutional confidentiality may at times be violated in many ways. Some examples include disclosure of results by the person tested; idle gossip among personnel acquainted with a clinical case or a laboratory result; easy access to records by those other than the person ordering the test; wide circulation of information about a case when several consulting services become involved or the case is presented at a conference; inferences drawn from circumstances of treatment by observers such as friends, family members, other patients, or employers; subpoena of records for a legal proceeding; and requirements for reporting diseases to public-health departments.

Anonymous testing ensures confidentiality and may be reasonable if the test result is not expected to be positive and thus require medical management, or if fears of violated confidentiality keep a person from obtaining the test. Anonymous testing cannot be employed when results are to be used for medical management, since clinicians must have documentation of results in the medical record.

■ TESTING TO BENEFIT THE INDIVIDUAL

The potential benefits of testing include:

Test Result Positive:

1. information useful for medical management, including anti-HIV therapy, staging of HIV infection, prophylaxis against certain opportunistic infections, enrollment in new treatment protocols, and other aspects of health maintenance

2. incentive to control behavior that may contribute to progression of disease and worsening of health (e.g., exposure to sexually transmitted diseases and other infections; malnutrition; drug, alcohol, and tobacco use)

3. incentive for modifying sexual and drug-use behaviors that may transmit HIV infection to others

4. ability to make long-term plans that may be altered by HIV infection (e.g., career, health care, personal and sexual relationships, pregnancy)

5. peace of mind when anxiety over not knowing interferes with planning and carrying out daily activities

Test Results Negative:

1. peace of mind that HIV infection is ruled out

2. confirmation that behavior modification to prevent infection works

3. knowledge useful for medical management based on the absence of HIV infection

The risks of a positive test result have been discussed. A possible risk of a negative test result is a false sense of security. This could occur either because the individual was recently infected and had not yet produced detectable HIV antibody or because the individual wrongly assumed that a negative test implied immunity from future infection.

TESTING TO ASSIST MANAGEMENT OF MEDICAL PROBLEMS IN ASYMPTOMATIC PATIENTS

HIV infection is now recognized as a spectrum of disease ranging from an asymptomatic state to full-blown AIDS and severe immunosuppression. Research increasingly indicates that progression to AIDS is the rule rather than the exception. Fortunately, new therapies offer interventions that may slow this progression and significantly help infected persons. To achieve the greatest benefit, however, infected persons must be identified as early as possible. In addition, preventing the spread of HIV infection to others can best be achieved if infected persons recognize their status and its potential risk to others.

Anti-HIV therapy with zidovudine (AZT) is beneficial in asymptomatic patients with T4 lymphocyte counts below 500 cells/cubic mm. For patients with T4 lymphocyte counts below 200 cells/cubic mm, survival is significantly increased by prophylaxis against *Pneumocystis carinii* pneumonia. To derive this benefit, HIV-infected patients must be identified and their T4 counts determined periodically. Knowledge that HIV infection is present changes the recommended management of asymptomatic individuals in several situations, e.g.:

1. the examination of cerebrospinal fluid in asymptomatic persons with syphilis infection of greater than one year's duration[22];

2. the interpretation of a PPD test as positive if it is greater than or equal to 5 mm induration, and administration of tuberculosis prophylaxis with isoniazid[23];

3. the administration of influenza and Pneumovax vaccines and use of inactivated (rather than live) oral polio vaccine.[24-26]

TESTING TO ASSIST MANAGEMENT OF MEDICAL PROBLEMS IN SYMPTOMATIC PATIENTS

The considerations listed above apply to symptomatic HIV-infected patients as well. In many clinical situations, HIV infection is apparent from the history of risk factors and various clinical manifestations of immunosuppression. When the history and presenting signs and symptoms are not diagnostic, an HIV antibody test can confirm or rule out infection. The most recent Centers for Disease Control (CDC) surveillance definition[4] lists a number of conditions considered diagnostic for AIDS only when they are accompanied by laboratory evidence of HIV infection. In these less-clear cases, testing is needed to clarify management options.

Confirmation of a patient's HIV infection influences a number of medical management issues:

1. Infections such as herpes simplex, bacterial sinusitis, or salmonella gastro-enteritis may recur and require long-term suppressive antibiotic therapy.

2. Many clinicians treating malignancies like non-Hodgkin's lymphoma use less immunotoxic treatment regimens in HIV-infected patients than in non-HIV-infected patients.

3. AZT can prolong and improve life in HIV-infected patients, but its toxicity may be considerable. Therefore it is necessary to know that HIV infection underlies whatever syndrome is being treated. This is especially true for patients with equivocal and nonspecific signs, such as chronic weight loss or diarrhea.

TESTING INDIVIDUALS FOR REASONS OTHER THAN MEDICAL MANAGEMENT

Testing for HIV infection can benefit the individual in ways other than for the management of specific medical problems. Examples include:

1. After a known or suspected exposure to HIV (such as a needlestick injury or rape), evidence of infection can be documented or ruled out by an HIV antibody test six months after exposure. A baseline test immediately after exposure is needed for documenting the fact that subsequent seroconversion is related to the exposure.

2. Knowledge of HIV infection usually alters decisions about attempting or terminating pregnancy, seeking health or life insurance, planning careers, and sexual practices.

3. Many individuals seek testing because of fears about possible past exposures (most often sexual contacts). Not infrequently, anxiety builds to a level interfering with the activities of daily living. In such cases, testing (even of low-risk individuals) may be of benefit.

4. Education and prevention strategies to encourage modification of high-risk behavior are presently the most useful approach to controlling the HIV epidemic. Being tested, counseled, and knowing whether or not one is infected may encourage awareness and modification of high-risk behaviors.

PREOPERATIVE HIV TESTING

If surgery were a factor in accelerating HIV disease, then patients might benefit from preoperative screening for evidence of HIV infection, particularly in the case of elective procedures; there are no data, however, to support this hypothesis. Thus, routine preoperative screening is not justified on the grounds of patient benefit.[27] The issue of preoperative screening for the benefit of operating-room personnel is discussed below.

■ TESTING TO BENEFIT PUBLIC HEALTH AND SAFETY

The public benefits of widespread testing for HIV infection include epidemiologic monitoring of the epidemic (to gain information for design of prevention and treatment strategies) and screening of blood and organ donors to ensure safety. There is no evidence that widespread testing to identify HIV-infected individuals helps to control the spread of infection. Prevention and behavior-modification strategies do not require learning the identities of HIV-infected individuals.

If quarantine strategies were useful (e.g., if HIV infection were air- or water-borne, or spread by casual contact), then individuals' rights to privacy and confidentiality might take second place to public safety. Mandatory testing might then be justified. However, extensive evidence[5] indicates that HIV transmission does not occur by casual contact. Instead, only direct inoculation of HIV into blood or mucous membranes (e.g., intravenous drug use with a shared needle), transfusion of contaminated blood products, sexual, or maternal–infant contact have been identified as transmission routes.

Testing to identify individuals for purposes of quarantine is not a defensible goal. Quarantine would require confining all infected individuals for as long as they are infectious — their entire lifetime — presumably so that they could not transmit disease sexually or through intravenous drug use. The CDC estimates that there are between 1 and 1.5 million HIV-infected individuals in the United States. Even assuming that the overwhelming political, moral, ethical, logistical, economic, legal, and sociological problems with such a policy were confronted, quarantine would discourage individuals from cooperating with voluntary testing and would make effective surveillance of the epidemic difficult, if not impossible.

Testing the blood supply has reduced the risk of transfusion-associated HIV infection to a very low level.[13,14] Rarely, a blood product may be infected and escape detection if the donor was recently infected and has not yet produced detectable HIV antibodies. Some persons might be tempted to donate blood to obtain the results of the blood bank's HIV test. This is clearly undesirable because it encourages donation by potentially infected persons. Free, anonymous or confidential alternative testing sites discourage this phenomenon.

■ TESTING ONE INDIVIDUAL FOR THE BENEFIT OF ANOTHER

Knowing that one individual is or is not HIV infected may alter the choices and options of another individual. Some examples include:

1. A police officer is stabbed by a suspect's dirty needle while making an arrest.

2. A nurse receives a puncture wound from a contaminated needle recently used to draw blood from a patient.

3. A surgeon sustains a puncture wound in the finger from a bone sliver in a bloody incision during an orthopedic surgical procedure.

In these cases, tremendous anxiety could be allayed by knowing that the source's blood had tested negative for HIV antibody. Cases where the source does not consent to be tested raise legal issues that are difficult, vary from locale to locale, and must be addressed on a case-by-case basis.

Hospitals, police departments, and other institutions employing personnel at risk for occupational exposure should establish protocols for testing sources of exposure as well as for testing and following-up recipients exposed to HIV.

■ TESTING AN INDIVIDUAL FOR INSTITUTIONAL PURPOSES NOT RELATED TO THE INDIVIDUAL'S WELFARE

In some situations, individuals are asked to submit to a test for HIV infection that cannot benefit them and may even be detrimental. Examples include:

1. routine screening of patients before surgical procedures to identify patients who may be infected;

2. routine mandatory screening as part of a pre-employment health evaluation;

3. routine mandatory screening as part of a qualification for insurance coverage.

■ TESTING OF PREOPERATIVE PATIENTS FOR RISK REDUCTION OF HEALTH-CARE WORKERS

The following discussion assumes that HIV infection is not used as a reason to withhold medical treatment from a patient. This assumption seems fundamental to the ethical and legal responsibilities of licensed health-care workers.

Routine screening of preoperative patients for HIV infection cannot be justified by existing evidence. Screening of selected patients may be useful if known HIV antibody status would lead to a change in medical management.

The issue of screening preoperative patients involves several questions: (1) Is there a sufficient risk to justify the consideration of HIV infection? (2) Are there ways to reduce the risk? (3) Can the results of screening for HIV infection be useful in reducing the risk?

Screening of all preoperative patients has been proposed[6] and discussed.[7,8] Inevitably and with some regularity, surgical gloves and (less frequently) the surgeon's skin are punctured during surgery. Certain types of procedures (e.g., orthopedic procedures where fragmented bone must be manipulated in the wound) theoretically have a higher risk for skin puncture, although studies to date have failed to demonstrate such an increased risk for HIV infection. Similar concerns apply to emergency-room personnel and others involved in invasive and bloody procedures.

Surgeons have a risk for hepatitis B seropositivity that is 1.5 times higher than other physicians.[9] The risk of HIV infection, even after a needlestick exposure to blood from an HIV-infected patient, is less than 1 percent[10] compared to a risk of hepatitis B seroconversion of 25 percent after exposure to hepatitis B–infected blood.[7] The surgeon's risk, however, must be assumed to be cumulative. Prospective studies have not revealed evidence of great risk to surgeons or other health workers, but these studies reveal a few examples of HIV seroconversion, proving that some risk does exist.[10]

The risk of exposure can be reduced by following recommended infection-control precautions.[8] These are effective not only for HIV infection but for hepatitis B and other infectious diseases. Knowing that a patient is HIV antibody-negative may create a false sense of security because individuals may occasionally be infected but not produce antibodies.[8] Moreover, other infectious agents capable of causing fatal diseases (such as hepatitis B virus, HTLV-I, etc.) may be present. Thus infection-control procedures should be followed irrespective of a patient's known HIV antibody status.

In some cases, surgeons change management, based on knowledge of a patient's HIV infection. If alternative surgical procedures are possible, the one with the least risk to operating room personnel should be chosen (less hand-to-hand instrument passing; stapling instead of hand-suturing; electrocautery instead of scalpel cutting).[8] Some of these modifications may, however, prolong operating time, resulting in increased risk to the patient. Thus, testing certain patients may be useful if a pretest plan exists for using the test result to alter management.

Additional data from prospective studies are needed to evaluate risks of specific procedures and practices. To avoid potential ethical and legal issues, institutional protocols and guidelines should be developed for ordering pre-operative testing. Preoperative testing requires pre- and post-test counseling and informed patient consent.

■ TESTING FOR PRE-EMPLOYMENT EVALUATION

At present there is no evidence that HIV testing is useful or reasonable for pre-employment screening. Many HIV-infected individuals have no symptoms and no work limitations. Whether or not a person with HIV infection can work should be evaluated on the basis of his or her specific signs, symptoms, and functional state rather than on the basis of a test for evidence of HIV infection. The mechanisms of HIV transmission make it clear that HIV-infected individuals are not a risk to co-workers or the public unless their job involves a high-risk practice such as sexual intercourse.[5]

■ TESTING FOR INSURANCE AND HEALTH-CARE ELIGIBILITY

Testing is increasingly required for eligibility for such services as health plans or insurance coverage. The issues involved are complex and include fundamental considerations about how such services are funded and controlled and the role of the private versus the public sector. In California, insurance companies are not allowed to use HIV screening tests to determine eligibility. The California state statute is designed in part to ensure that the private sector bears a share of the burden of providing health care for AIDS patients. It is currently being contested by the insurance industry. HIV-infected individuals' loss of private insurance and health benefits places an increasing financial burden on the public sector to provide for their care.[11]

REFERENCES

1. Update: serologic testing for antibody to human immunodeficiency virus. MMWR 1988; 36:833-40.
2. Schwartz JS, Dans PE, Kinosian BP. Human immunodeficiency virus test evaluation, performance and use. JAMA 1988; 259:2574-9.
3. Meyer KB, Pauker SG. Screening for HIV: Can we afford the false positive rate? N Engl J Med 1987; 317:238-41.
4. Centers for Disease Control. Revision of the CDC surveillance case definition for acquired immunodeficiency syndrome. MMWR 1987; 36(Suppl 1S):3S-15S.
5. Friedland GH, Klein RS. Transmission of the human immunodeficiency virus. N Engl J Med 1987; 317:1125-35.
6. Breo D. Dr. Koop calls for AIDS tests before surgery. Am Med News. June 26, 1987:1, 17-21.
7. Hagen MD, Meyer KB, Pauker SG. Routine preoperative screening for HIV. JAMA 1988; 259:1357-9.
8. Centers for Disease Control. Recommendations for prevention of HIV transmission in health-care settings. MMWR 1987; 36(Suppl 2S):3S-18S.
9. Denes AE, Smith JL, Maynard JE, et al. Hepatitis B infection in physicians: results of a nationwide seroepidemiologic survey. JAMA 1978; 239:210-6.
10. Centers for Disease Control. Update: Acquired immunodeficiency syndrome and human immunodeficiency virus infection among health-care workers. MMWR 1988; 37:229-39.
11. Bloom DE, Carliner G. The economic impact of AIDS in the United States. Science 1988; 239:604-10.
12. Burke DS, Brundage JF, Redfield RR, et al. Measurement of the false positive rate in a screening program for human immunodeficiency virus infections. N Engl J Med 1988; 319:961-4.
13. Cohen ND, Munoz A, Reitz BA, et al. Transmission of retroviruses by transfusion of screened blood in patients undergoing cardiac surgery. N Engl J Med 1989; 320:1172-6.

14. MacDonald KL, Jackson JB, Bowman RJ, et al. Performance characteristics of serologic tests for human immunodeficiency virus type 1 (HIV-1) antibody among Minnesota blood donors. Public health and clinical implications. Ann Intern Med 1989; 110:617-21.

15. Rhame FS, Maki DG. The case for wider use of testing for HIV infection. N Engl J Med 1989; 320:1248-54.

16. Lo B, Steinbrook RL, Cooke M, et al. Voluntary screening for human immunodeficiency virus (HIV) infection. Weighing the benefits and harms. Ann Intern Med 1989; 110:727-33.

17. Ranki A, Valle S-L, Krohn M, et al. Long latency precedes overt seroconversion in sexually transmitted human-immunodeficiency-virus infection. Lancet 1987; 2:589-93.

18. Imagawa DT, Lee MH, Wolinsky SM, et al. Human immunodeficiency virus type 1 infection in homsexual men who remain seronegative for prolonged periods. N Engl J Med 1989; 320:1458-62.

19. Farzadegan H, Polis MA, Wolinsky SM, et al. Loss of human immunodeficiency virus type 1 (HIV-1) antibodies with evidence of viral infection in asymptomatic homosexual men. A report from the Multi-center AIDS Cohort Study. Ann Intern Med 1988; 108:785-90.

20. Haseltine WA. Silent HIV infections. N Engl J Med 1989; 320:1487-9.

21. Jackson JB, Coombs RW, Sannerud K, et al. Rapid and sensitive viral culture method for human immunodeficiency virus type 1. J Clin Microbiol 1988; 26:1416-8.

22. Recommendations for diagnosing and treating syphilis in HIV-infected patients. MMWR 1988; 37:600-2, 607-8.

23. Tuberculosis and human immunodeficiency virus infection: recommendations of the Advisory Committee for the Elimination of Tuberculosis (ACET). MMWR 1989; 38:236-50.

24. Pneumococcal polysaccharide vaccine. MMWR 1989; 38:64-8, 73-6.

25. Prevention and control of influenza. Part 1. Vaccines. MMWR 1989; 38:297-8, 303-11.

26. General recommendations on immunization. MMWR 1989; 38:205-14, 219-27.

27. Scannell KA. Surgery and human immunodeficiency virus disease. J Acquir Immune Defic Syndr 1989; 2:43-53.

HIV Antibody Testing: Methodology

Judith C. Wilber, Ph.D.

Most HIV testing involves antibody assays because they are best suited for routine use in blood banks and screening programs.[1] The use of these antibody assays to determine a person's HIV antibody status is based on two assumptions: (1) people who have been infected with HIV produce detectable antibody, and (2) those with detectable HIV antibody are infected with HIV. The enzyme-linked immunosorbent assay (ELISA) is very accurate, but no one should ever be told that his or her ELISA is positive until a supplemental test (such as Western blot (WB) or immunofluorescence assay (IFA)) has been performed. Radioimmunoprecipitation assays (RIPA) are also occasionally used for confirmation. If the test results are inconclusive or if there is any question whatsoever about the results, the tests should be repeated on a new blood specimen.

HIV antibody assays are highly sensitive and specific but have a low predictive value in populations with a very low incidence of HIV infection. That is, when an individual with no risk for HIV infection tests positive for HIV antibody, the result is more likely to be a false positive than a true positive because the occurrence of disease is more rare than the occurrence of a false-positive test. Thus widespread screening of low-risk populations (e.g., military recruits, premarital couples, blood donors) produces many false-positive results and discovers relatively few true positives (and therefore few true HIV infections). For this reason, it is imperative that all HIV-antibody-positive results be confirmed by Western blot or other confirmatory test.

The goals of widespread HIV antibody screening must be evaluated in light of statistical principles of testing. Those who administer HIV antibody tests and those who report results must recognize the potential harm resulting from a false-positive test result. Positive tests must be verified by confirmatory testing before results are reported. Testing should be preceded and followed by counseling. Clinical and laboratory personnel must rigorously enforce the confidentiality of a person's tests results. The performance standards of laboratories that offer HIV antibody testing and the quality of the materials they use for testing must be regularly verified.

HIV antibody assays are performed on serum or plasma. The preferred specimen is 5 to 7 ml of sterile, whole clotted blood; this quantity is sufficient for performing repeat tests as well as any needed supplemental tests. Blood specimens should be refrigerated, but transportation at ambient temperature is not likely to affect test results.[2] Separated serum can be stored frozen or refrigerated.

All the commonly used antibody assays are based on similar principles, but the means of visualizing a positive reaction differs with each method. The following is a description of the methods for determining the presence of HIV antibody.

■ ENZYME IMMUNOASSAY (ENZYME-LINKED IMMUNOSORBENT ASSAY)

ELISA Methodology.   HIV antigen (usually purified viral lysate) is coated onto the wells of a microtiter plate (or onto beads that are then placed in the wells) to form the solid phase of the assay. The patient's serum is placed in the well, allowed to react with the antigen, and then washed away. An indicator conjugate — an anti-human antibody bound to an enzyme — is then placed in the well. If the patient's serum contained HIV-specific antibodies that attached to the antigen, the enzyme antihuman-antibody conjugate will attach to these antibodies and thus to the solid phase as well. Another washing step follows. The enzyme remains attached to the solid phase and is available to catalyze a color-producing reaction when an appropriate substrate is added to the well. The color change is measured with a spectrophotometer. A cutoff absorbance value is calculated from control samples, giving a threshold above which specimens are considered reactive.

ELISA Interpretation.   An initially reactive ELISA test should be repeated in duplicate on the same specimen. If one or both repeat tests are reactive, the ELISA is considered repeatedly reactive. The results of ELISAs should never be reported to a patient, even as a "preliminary result." Laboratory procedural errors (such as inadequate washing and incorrect dilution) may cause falsely reactive tests that are unrelated to the patient's serum. Repeating the procedure in duplicate reduces this source of error. Before the patient or donor is informed of the results, the repeatedly reactive specimens should be confirmed by another type of test. Currently, Western blot or an immunofluorescence assay is used for confirmation.[3]

Specificity, Sensitivity, and Predictive Value of ELISA.   There are seven licensed manufacturers of enzyme immunoassays for antibody to HIV. All of them have clinical trial data and independently published studies showing sensitivity and specificity of over 98 percent; many of them approach 100 percent. This has led to some misconceptions about the meaning of a positive result.

HIV antibody assays are most widely used to screen populations with the least risk of being infected (blood donors, military recruits) and these assays have the lowest predictive value in these populations (i.e., a "positive" result is most likely to be a false positive). Thus, statistically, the majority of positive results in low-risk groups will be false positives. This necessitates confirmatory testing by other methods.

Investigators have attempted to identify factors that cause false reactivity in ELISA. The HIV antigen used for the antibody assays is produced in cultured human T cells. Occasional false-positive assays caused by T-cell antigens have been reported in sera from individuals with autoimmune diseases, a history of multiple pregnancies or multiple transfusions, or antibodies to certain class II histocompatibility antigens (especially HLA-DR4).[4] Because of these problems, manufacturers have developed methods to block reaction with interfering antibodies in these sera. As a result, even in extremely low-prevalence populations, test specificity has been greatly improved. In addition, specimens that are falsely reactive in one test are generally not falsely reactive in another type of assay. This is the reason for doing confirmatory assays (such as immunofluorescence assay or Western blot) on reactive ELISA specimens.

False-positive antibody tests have occurred because of HIV antibody passively transferred to the patient in hepatitis B immune globulin (HBIG) prepared before routine HIV antibody screening of immunoglobulin preparations was introduced.[23]

Recently, the U.S. Army reviewed its test records to determine the false positivity rate.[5] Of 135,000 specimens tested, 15 had been reported as positive by both ELISA and Western blot. These 15 specimens were retested using four different assays. Fourteen were found to be reactive in all the tests and one had been incorrectly called positive based on interpretative criteria for the Western blot that are no longer in use. Based on this study, a false-positive rate of 1 in 135,000 was found in a low-risk population.

In a study screening for HIV antibody in 630,190 units of blood from 290,110 donors, a false-positive rate of no more than 0.0006 percent and a specificity of at least 99.9994 percent were obtained by sequential ELISA and Western blot testing.[24]

These low false-positive rates were obtained with a rigorous algorithm of confirmatory testing to follow up positive results of the initial test. All tests were performed by experienced personnel. It must be emphasized that all laboratories offering HIV antibody testing will not achieve this high standard.

The sensitivity of current-generation ELISAs is close to 100 percent when the antibody is present in peripheral blood. However, these assays do not detect HIV antibody in the earliest stages of infection.[6-9] The time interval between HIV infection and appearance of antibody in the blood is variable.[25] In most patients this period is less than six months after infection, although longer periods of seronegativity — up to 34 months — have been reported.[26,27] Occasional patients have also been reported who are initially HIV-seropositive and who subsequently revert to a seronegative status.[28] There is also a period late in HIV infection when antibody may be undetectable because it has become complexed with excess antigen.

■ WESTERN BLOT (WB)

The immunoelectrophoresis or immunoblot procedure, commonly called the Western blot, gained immediate acceptance as a test for "confirmation" of HIV seropositivity because it was used prominently in the early isolation and characterization of HIV. Only recently have there been standardized commercial reagents available. The limitations of the procedure as a routine clinical assay are largely due to the variety of techniques and interpretations used by different laboratories. Because Western blot detects immune response to specific viral proteins, it is also a useful research tool for studying the course of HIV infection.

Western Blot Methodology. A purified HIV antigen mixture is layered onto an SDS polyacrylamide gel slab and is electrophoresed. These procedures distribute the viral proteins (the HIV antigens) throughout the gel according to molecular weight, with the higher molecular weight proteins forming bands near the top of the gel. The proteins on the gel are then transferred ("blotted") to nitrocellulose paper by another electrophoretic procedure. This paper is then sliced into thin strips, each with the full distribution of viral-protein bands. A single test strip is incubated with a 1:50 or 1:100 dilution of a test sample or a control. The strip is then washed and incubated with a labeled (tagged) antihuman globulin. At this point, the procedure is similar to any other indirect immunoassay. The label is usually an enzyme (horseradish peroxidase or alkaline phosphatase) that will react with a specific colorless substrate to produce an insoluble colored band on the strip wherever there is an antigen—antibody complex.

Reaction with a positive serum sample produces a pattern of bands on the strip that is characteristic of HIV. Many of these bands have been identified as specific viral gene products, designated as follows: the envelope glycoproteins (*env*) gp160, gp120, and gp41; the core proteins (*gag*), p55, p24, and p17; and the polymerase (*pol*) p66, p51, and p31. The numbers correspond to the molecular weight of the gene product in kilodaltons.

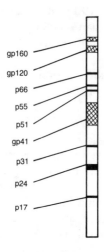

Figure 2.1.2.a   Diagram of the distribution pattern of HIV-1 protein bands separated by the Western blot procedure. The nine principal viral bands are labeled "p" for protein and "gp" for glycoprotein, along with the molecular weight in kilodaltons. The envelope bands (*env*), which appear diffuse, are gp160, gp120, and gp41. The core (*gag*) proteins are p55, p24, and p17; and the polymerase-associated (*pol*) bands are p66, p51, and p31.

Western Blot Interpretation.   Most HIV antibody-positive sera react with all of the bands mentioned above, in which case interpretation is not difficult. However, both very early and very late in HIV infection (i.e., after development of symptoms), the patient may not have detectable antibody to some of the viral antigens. It must therefore be determined which reactive bands make a Western blot positive. The interpretation of Western blot has evolved, so it is important to know the interpretive criteria used by the laboratory that reports a result as "positive." Not all investigators use the same criteria.

The Centers for Disease Control originally required only the presence of p24 and/or gp41 bands to call a test result positive. However, there are fairly common nonspecific reactions of HIV-negative sera with *gag* proteins, especially p24 (alone or in combination with p17 or p55). These may reflect reaction with nonviral cellular material in the antigen preparation or with cross-reacting antibody. However, because p24 can also be the first band to develop after infection, this pattern may also represent a true positive test. We have learned more about the significance of the different viral proteins and their roles, and new recommendations have made the Western blot more specific by requiring other band patterns for a positive result.

In 1987, the FDA licensed a Western blot kit and included extremely stringent requirements for a positive Western blot interpretation. These were based on reaction with specific bands representing three different gene products: p24 (*gag*), p31 (*pol*), and an *env* band — either gp41, gp120, or gp160.[10,11] The specificity of the Western blot using the FDA criteria is extremely high. The disadvantage of such stringent requirements is a loss of sensitivity. Many AIDS patients, for example, lack antibody to p24 and their tests are therefore considered indeterminate. The Association of State and Territorial Public Health

Laboratory Directors Consensus Conference on HIV testing has agreed to define a reactive Western blot as one containing two out of three of the specific bands of p24, gp41, and gp120 or gp160. This guideline takes advantage of the apparent specificity of the envelope bands.[12] Another proposed guideline would require reaction with each of three gene products (as does the FDA guideline), but it does not specify which band is necessary from each group (Dodd R: personal communication).

Since most laboratories will interpret a strip as negative only if it contains no viral bands, there are many specimens with band patterns that do not fit the criteria for either a positive or negative test result. These must be interpreted as indeterminate. An indeterminate pattern may represent a nonspecific reaction or a stage in the progression of HIV disease.

Western Blot Sensitivity and Specificity.   Western blot results can be used to follow HIV disease progression. If proper materials, methods, and interpretive criteria are used, it is both sensitive and specific. However, it is extremely labor-intensive and costly, and until recently, unstandardized. Caution is warranted in choosing the laboratory to perform Western blot assays, for there is great variability in technique and quality. There are commercial sources of Western blot strips, one of which has received FDA approval for use as an aid in interpreting repeatedly reactive HIV ELISA tests on blood donors. While still expensive, commercial preparation of the strips cuts much of the labor involved and will aid in standardizing the procedure.

■ IMMUNOFLUORESCENCE ASSAY (IFA)

The immunofluorescence assay[13,14] for HIV antibody is less technically demanding and much less expensive than Western blot. Because virtually all the antigens present in an infected cell are available for reaction with the test specimen, it is a very sensitive assay. It is a procedure familiar to many laboratories because it is used for detecting antibodies to a wide variety of viral and bacterial antigens.

Immunofluorescence Assay Methodology.   A suspension of a lymphocyte cell culture infected with HIV is spotted on microscope slides, air-dried, and fixed in acetone. Uninfected cells added to the suspension provide a means for detecting nonspecific reactions. (Acetone-fixed slides can be made in large batches and stored frozen or desiccated.) In the assay, diluted test sera are incubated on the cell spots, washed, incubated again with fluorescein-conjugated antihuman globulin, washed again, and then observed for fluorescein fluorescence using a UV microscope.

Typical localized fluorescence of infected cells is seen after reaction with positive sera. Little or no fluorescence is seen with negative sera. Nonspecific reactions (such as those caused by antinuclear antibody) are recognized by observing fluorescence in uninfected cells.

Immunofluorescence Assay Interpretation.   Although the immunofluorescence assay is a relatively simple procedure, interpretation is subjective and requires experience. Its use also requires the ability to grow HIV in cell culture in order to prepare the slides. There are a few commercial sources of prepared slides, for research use only, for HIV immunofluorescence assay. Western blot and immunofluorescence assay are considered to have equal specificity and sensitivity and each may be used to resolve indeterminate reactions with the other technique.

■ RADIOIMMUNOPRECIPITATION

For this method of HIV antibody testing, HIV is cultured in cells with radio-labeled cysteine or glucosamine, or viral proteins are labeled by direct reaction with I-125. The disrupted virus is exposed to the test specimen and specific antigen–antibody complexes are concentrated and isolated by immunoprecipitation. After extensive washing, the precipitate is disrupted and distributed through a polyacrylamide gel by electrophoresis. Antigen–antibody bands are detected by autoradiography.

The radioimmunoprecipitation assay (RIP) is used primarily in research. It is too technically demanding for routine use in clinical laboratories. Radioimmunoprecipitation is especially sensitive for antibodies to the higher molecular-weight major envelope glycoproteins gp160 and gp120, which are missed by some Western blot techniques. Sera from blood donors with probable false-positive Western blot patterns (such as p24 alone) are often negative by RIP. Thus, the technique may be useful in resolving conflicting results from other HIV antibody assays.[15,16]

■ ASSAYS USING SYNTHETIC AND RECOMBINANT ANTIGENS

Specific antigens for use as reagents can be generated synthetically or by recombinant technology. These antigens are theoretically more specific than those purified from HIV culture. Their use minimizes false reactions caused by cross-reactivity with nonviral cellular antigens. However, care must be taken to select antigens that have a broad enough sensitivity to react with antibodies to many strains of HIV. Assays now being evaluated include a nitrocellulose strip containing four recombinant HIV antigens (that mimics a Western blot), and an ELISA using five separate recombinant antigens.[22]

■ RAPID TESTS

Rapid tests incorporating recombinant or synthetic antigens are also being developed. These tests include latex agglutination,[17] red-cell agglutination,[18] and a dip stick.[19] Recently, a rapid latex-agglutination test was approved by the FDA for use in detecting HIV antibody.[21]

These are rapid methods with relatively simple procedures. They will be very useful in field studies and possibly in emergency situations, such as evaluating organ donations from cadavers. However, these tests should be used with as much quality control as the current technology.[20] They should be performed by licensed laboratory personnel trained to interpret each test and to confirm positive tests.

Several issues should be carefully considered in deciding the appropriate uses of rapid tests.[20] The laws and regulations of several states (including New York, New Jersey, and California) require that any HIV antibody test be performed in a licensed clinical laboratory specifically approved for HIV testing. This would not include most doctors' offices, emergency rooms, or people's homes, where rigorous quality control is not possible. A rapid test is not necessarily simple to interpret. Latex agglutination tests can be very difficult to interpret and must be confirmed (if positive) with Western blot or immunofluorescence assay. In fact, this test may not be as sensitive as ELISA and Western blot.[19] Therefore, it has the potential of missing positives (false negatives). Thus, it may be necessary to confirm both its positives and negatives.

Rapid, simple assays that require less equipment than ELISA are important in developing countries where facilities to test for HIV antibody are scarce — even in blood bank screening programs. In the U.S., rapid tests may be useful in emergency settings, but their use should be discussed and carefully defined because of the danger of neglecting the rights of the patient in these situations. Informed patient consent and counseling are necessary in association with any HIV antibody testing.

REFERENCES

1. Wilber JC. Serologic testing of human immunodeficiency virus infection. Clin Lab Med 1987; 7:777-91.

2. Fipps DR, Damato JJ, Brandt B, Burke DS. Effects of multiple freeze thaws and various temperatures on the reactivity of human immunodeficiency virus antibody using three detection assays. J Virol Methods 1988; 20:127-32.

3. Public Health Service guidelines for counseling and antibody testing to prevent HIV infection and AIDS. MMWR 1987; 36:509-15.

4. Kuhnl P, Seidl S, Holzberger G. HLA DR4 antibodies cause positive HTLV-III antibody ELISA results. Lancet 1985; 1:1222-3.

5. Burke DS, Brundage JF, Redfield RR, et al. Measurement of the false positive rate in a screening program for human immunodeficiency virus infections. N Engl J Med 1988; 319:961-4.

6. Laure F, Courgnaud V, Rouzioux C, et al. Detection of HIV-1 DNA in infants and children by means of the polymerase chain reaction. Lancet 1988; 2:538-41.

7. Loche M, Mach B. Identification of HIV-infected seronegative individuals by a direct diagnostic test based on hybridisation to amplified viral DNA. Lancet 1988; 2:418-21.

8. Marx JL. Multiplying genes by leaps and bounds. Science 1988; 240:1408-10.

9. Schumacher RT, Garrett PE, Tegtmeier G, et al. Comparative detection of anti-HIV in early HIV seroconversion. J Clin Immunol 1988; 11:130-4.

10. Hausler WJ Jr. Report of the Third Consensus Conference on HIV testing sponsored by the Association of State and Territorial Public Health Laboratory Directors. Infect Control Hosp Epidemiol 1988; 9:345-9.

11. Human immunodeficiency virus (HIV) BIOTECH/DUPONT HIV Western Blot Kit. Wilmington, Del.; DuPont Company, 1987 (publication number 770557.003) (Western blot kit instruction pamphlet).

12. Lelie PN, van der Poel CL, Reesink HW. Interpretation of isolated HIV anti-p24 reactivity in Western blot analysis. Lancet 1987; 1:632.

13. Gallo D, Diggs JL, Shell GR, et al. Comparison of detection of antibody to the acquired immune deficiency syndrome virus by enzyme immunoassay, immunofluorescence, and Western blot methods. J Clin Microbiol 1986; 23:1049-51.

14. McHugh TM, Stites DP, Casavant CH, et al. Evaluation of the indirect immunofluorescence assay as a confirmatory test for detecting antibodies to the human immunodeficiency virus. Diagn Immunol 1986; 4:233-40.

15. Pinter A, Honnen WJ. A sensitive radioimmunoprecipitation assay for human immunodeficiency virus (HIV). J Immunol Methods 1988; 112:235-41.

16. Tersmette M, Lelie PN, van der Poel CL, et al. Confirmation of HIV seropositivity: comparison of a novel radioimmunoprecipitation assay to immunoblotting and virus culture. J Med Virol 1988; 24:109-16.

17. Quinn TC, Riggin CH, Kline RL, et al. Rapid latex agglutination assay using recombinant envelope polypeptide for the detection of antibody to the HIV. JAMA 1988; 260:510-3.

18. Kemp BE, Rylatt DB, Bundesen PG, et al. Autologous red cell agglutination assay for HIV-1 antibodies: simplified test with whole blood. Science 1988; 241:1352-4.

19. Van de Perre P, Nzaramba D, Allen S, et al. Comparison of six serological assays for human immunodeficiency virus antibody detection in developing countries. J Clin Microbiol 1988; 26:552-6.

20. Heyward WL, Curran JW. Rapid screening tests for HIV infection. JAMA 1988; 260:542.

21. FDA. 5-Minute DNA test for HIV-1 antibodies. FDA Drug Bulletin 1989; 19(February):7-8.

22. Ng VL, Chiang CS, DeBouck C, et al. Reliable confirmation of antibodies to human immunodeficiency virus type 1 (HIV-1) with an enzyme-linked immunoassay using recombinant antigen derived from the HIV-1 *gag*, *pol*, and *env* genes. J Clin Microbiol 1989; 27:977-82.

23. Albersheim SG, Smyth JA, Solimano A, Cook D. Passively acquired human immunodeficiency virus seropositivity in a neonate after hepatitis B immunoglobulin. J Pediatr 1988; 112:915-6.

24. MacDonald KL, Jackson JB, Bowman RJ, et al. Performance characteristics of serologic tests for human immunodeficiency virus type 1 (HIV-1) antibody among Minnesota blood donors. Public health and clinical implications. Ann Intern Med 1989; 110:617-21.

25. Haseltine WA. Silent HIV infections. N Engl J Med 1989; 320:1487-9.

26. Ranki A, Valle S-L, Krohn M, et al. Long latency precedes overt seroconversion in sexually transmitted human-immunodeficiency-virus infection. Lancet 1987; 2:589-93.

27. Imagawa DT, Lee MH, Wolinsky SM, et al. Human immunodeficiency virus type 1 infection in homosexual men who remain seronegative for prolonged periods. N Engl J Med 1989; 320:1458-62.

28. Farzadegan H, Polis MA, Wolinsky SM, et al. Loss of human immunodeficiency virus type 1 (HIV-1) antibodies with evidence of viral infection in asymptomatic homosexual men. A report from the Multi-center AIDS Cohort Study. Ann Intern Med 1988; 108:785-90.

HIV Antigen Testing

Suzanne Crowe, M.B.B.S., F.R.A.C.P., John Mills, M.D., and Michael S. McGrath, M.D., Ph.D.

The current screening test employed to detect HIV (human immunodeficiency virus) infection is the ELISA (enzyme-linked immunosorbent assay), which identifies virus-infected persons indirectly by detecting anti-HIV antibodies. HIV infection is usually confirmed by the Western blot method, which separates antibodies to the various gene products of HIV. One of these genes, the *gag* gene, encodes for a precursor protein, p55, which is processed to core proteins p24, p17, and p15.

Commercial tests are now available that detect HIV p24 antigen in serum, plasma, and cerebrospinal fluid (CSF) of infected individuals, as well as in the supernatant media of viral cultures.[1-3] Perhaps most important, these enzyme immunoassays have clinical applications in evaluating the virologic efficacy of antiretroviral therapy.[3]

■ METHODS OF HIV ANTIGEN DETECTION

Until recently, the only method for HIV antigen detection was by immuno-fluorescent staining of peripheral blood mononuclear cells, using antibody directed against HIV antigens (commonly p24).[4] However, this method is generally not reliable or useful, since less than 0.01 percent of mononuclear cells are infected with HIV.[5]

Newer commercial kits can detect HIV p24 antigen in serum and CSF of infected individuals as well as in culture supernatants. These enzyme immunoassays (Abbott HTLV-III antigen assay and Dupont HIV p24 ELISA) are highly specific and sensitive when compared with reverse transcriptase assays.

The Abbott HTLV-III antigen assay uses a solid-phase antigen capture enzyme immunoassay.[2,6] Human polyclonal anti-HIV antibody adsorbed to polystyrene beads is incubated with the specimen to be tested. After washing the beads, rabbit anti-HIV IgG, labeled with horseradish peroxidase, is used to identify and quantify captured p24 antigen. A standard curve is made by assaying dilutions of a known amount of purified HIV lysate. The quantity of p24 antigen in the test serum can be determined by plotting the value against the reference curve. The sensitivity of this assay is reported as being 10 to 30 pg/ml.[2,6] Specificity can be ascertained by a neutralization assay using pretreated human sera with polyclonal antibody to HIV.[7] This specifically abolishes reactivity of the HIV p24 antigen capture assay. The incidence of false-positive reactions is low, approximately 0.05 percent.[6]

The Dupont HIV p24 ELISA also employs an antigen capture technique. Anti-HIV p24 adsorbed to microtiter plate wells captures any HIV p24 antigen present in the test sera. This captured antigen is then detected by probing with biotinylated anti-HIV p24, followed by streptavidin horseradish peroxidase; color is developed with o-phenylene diamine as substrate. The amount of color generated is proportional to the quantity of HIV p24 antigen captured. This assay is regarded as having sensitivity and specificity similar to the Abbott assay, but there are currently no published data comparing the two assays.

■ HIV P24 ANTIGENEMIA — CLINICAL AND SEROLOGIC ASSOCIATIONS

Tests for antibody to HIV are currently the best and most practical method for identifying HIV infection. However, these tests will be negative during early infection, before the development of specific antibody. Following infection with HIV but prior to seroconversion, circulating viral antigens (specifically HIV p24) are present in the serum of some and possibly all infected individuals. HIV p24 antigenemia is usually transient,[1] appearing as early as two weeks after infection and lasting three to five months.[6] Serum antibody usually appears after HIV p24 antigen, although it has been reported to precede antigen detection in some individuals.[1]

In a study of the sera of 35 homosexual men who were bled serially before and after seroconversion, HIV p24 antigen was detected in 11 individuals. Five of the 11 developed antigen prior to and 6 after seroconversion.[1] While the HIV p24 antigen assay is considered highly specific, the sensitivity may be increased by repeated analyses. Thus it is possible that these six individuals whose antigen was only detectable after seroconversion were antigenemic prior to documented seroconversion.

Once specific antibody to HIV p24 is generated, HIV p24 antigen usually disappears.[6] However, in some individuals persistent antigenemia has been observed, often in association with clinical deterioration and a poor prognosis.[1,8]

Later in the course of HIV infection, a trend toward the reappearance of HIV p24 antigen has been observed. This correlates with the loss of antibody to HIV p24.[9,10] Asymptomatic seropositive individuals generally have a low incidence of circulating HIV p24 (4 percent to 7 percent).[1,4,7,11] However, the incidence of antigenemia in adult patients with persistent generalized lymphadenopathy and ARC (AIDS-related complex) is between 25 percent and 50 percent.[1,4,7,11] In patients with AIDS, the incidence of antigenemia is between 70 percent and 100 percent.[1,4,7,11]

To summarize: in individuals who are followed prospectively, p24 antigenemia is detected early after infection but usually disappears as specific antibody appears. After a variable period, during which time the individual is usually asymptomatic, anti-HIV p24 antibody falls and p24 antigen reappears in the serum. Often at this stage, clinical deterioration occurs and the patient progresses to AIDS.

The decline in antibody against p24 may reflect augmented HIV gene expression and viral replication, with production of an excess of HIV antigen that complexes with specific antibody.[12] In those individuals whose sera contain both anti-HIV p24 and p24 antigen, the titer of the latter is generally low.[6] Another, but simplistic, explanation for decline in antibody level is "exhaustion" of the whole immune response. This is unlikely, however; antibodies directed against other viral components (e.g., envelope glycoproteins) persist in the circulation.[8]

Antigenemia in Children.   The serologic diagnosis of HIV infection in infants born to infected mothers is difficult during the first 6 months of life because of the persistence of maternal antibody (IgG) that crossed the placenta before birth. HIV p24 antigen assays can be useful in detecting infant infection under such circumstances.[4]

In infants infected with HIV, the p24 antigen test is often positive during the early neonatal period. This is presumably a result of the lymphocyte activation that characteristically occurs during the first few weeks of life, associated with viral proliferation and expression.[4] There have been reports of pediatric AIDS cases in which assays for HIV antibody have been negative.[2] In a recent study of 85 children infected with HIV, 9 were antibody negative but had detectable HIV antigen by enzyme immunoassay.[8] Like adult patients, children with AIDS are much more likely to have circulating p24 antigen and a virtual absence of anti-p24 antibody than healthy seropositive children.[8]

HIV Antigens in the CSF.   HIV p24 antigen has been detected in cerebrospinal fluid. This antigen is present transiently in early infection of individuals with and without neurologic symptoms, as well as in cases of adult and child progressive encephalopathy.[1] The presence of HIV antigen in CSF is not merely due to leakage of viral proteins across the blood—brain barrier, for high titers of p24 antigen may be present in serum while antigen is absent from the CSF.[1] The persistence of HIV antigen in CSF is thought to reflect severe central nervous system involvement.[1]

■ CONCLUSIONS

The availability of commercial kits for detection of HIV p24 antigenemia may allow earlier diagnosis of HIV infection, particularly in those patients presenting with symptomatic illness associated with acute HIV infection. p24 antigen detection may also provide prognostic value later in infection as a predictor for the onset of AIDS. However, data supporting this use are scanty.[8]

The potential use of p24 antigen testing extends to blood banks.[13] Current screening methods for detecting anti-HIV antibody identify the majority of infectious donations. Some donations, however, may contain HIV but will be antibody negative prior to the donors' seroconversion. If HIV p24 antigen testing were introduced to supplement existing screening tests, some but not all of post-transfusion HIV infection could be prevented.[13] Even HIV antigen tests are not always positive during this period, however. In addition, cost analysis determinations are needed to assess antigen testing's relative potential benefit versus its expense. Finally, p24 antigen assays are likely to provide a practical and useful means for evaluating the virologic efficacy of antiretroviral therapy.[3]

REFERENCES

1. Goudsmit J, De Wolf F, Lange JMA. Expression of human immunodeficiency virus antigen (HIV-Ag) in serum and cerebrospinal fluid during acute and chronic infection. Lancet 1986; 2:177-80.

2. Borkowsky W, Krasinski K, Paul D. Human immunodeficiency virus infections in infants negative for anti-HIV by enzyme linked immunoassay. Lancet 1987; 1:1168-71.

3. Chaisson RE, Allain J-P, Leuther M, Volberding PA. Significant changes in HIV antigen level in the serum of patients treated with azidothymidine. N Engl J Med 1986; 315:1610-11.

4. Tovo PA, Gabiano C, Riva C, et al. Specific antibody and virus antigen expression in congenital HIV infection. Lancet 1987; 1:1201.

5. Harper ME, Marselle LM, Gallo RC, Wong Staal F. Detection of lymphocytes expressing human T lymphotropic virus type III in lymph nodes and peripheral blood from infected individuals by in situ hybridization. Proc Natl Acad Sci 1986; 83:772-6.

6. Allain J-P, Laurian Y, Paul DA, et al. Serological markers in early stages of human immunodeficiency virus infection in haemophiliacs. Lancet 1986; 2:1233-6.

7. Kenny C, Parkin J, Underhill G, et al. HIV antigen testing. Lancet 1987; 1:565-6.

8. Lange JMA, Paul DA, Huisman HG, et al. Persistent HIV antigenaemia and decline of HIV core antibodies associated with transition to AIDS. Clin Res 1987; 1:119-22.

9. Schupbach J, Haller O, Vogt M, et al. Antibodies to HTLV-III in Swiss patients with AIDS and pre-AIDS and in groups at risk for AIDS. N Engl J Med 1985; 312:265-70.

10. Kalyanaraman VS, Cabradilla CD, Getchell JP, et al. Antibodies to the core protein of lymphadenopathy-associated virus (LAV) in patients with AIDS. Science 1984; 225:321-3.

11. Falk LA, Paul D, Landay A, Kessler H. HIV isolation from plasma of HIV infected persons. N Engl J Med 1987; 316:1547-8.

12. Goudsmit J, Lange JMA, Paul DA, Dawson GJ. Antigenemia and antibody titers to core and envelope antigens in AIDS, AIDS-related complex, and subclinical human immunodeficiency virus infection. J Infect Dis 1987; 155:558-60.

13. Contreras M, Barbara JAJ. Routine tests for HIV antigen. Lancet 1987; 1:807.

HIV Isolation and Cultivation

Michael S. McGrath, M.D., Ph.D.

■ ISOLATION

The human immunodeficiency virus (HIV), a retrovirus, has been isolated from individuals within all groups at risk for developing AIDS and HIV-related syndromes.[1,2] The first isolate was derived from lymphocytes cultured in vitro from an individual with lymphadenopathy syndrome. Because of its unique characteristics, it was identified as a new retrovirus unlike any previously described.[3] Subsequently, many groups have succeeded in culturing and isolating similar HIVs from a variety of sources.[4,5] HIV has been isolated most frequently from human peripheral blood lymphocytes obtained from individuals whose serum contains antibodies that recognize HIV components (these individuals are seropositive). Rarely, HIV may be isolated from seronegative individuals with a history of HIV exposure.[6] HIV has also been isolated from lymph nodes, serum, brain, saliva, semen, breast milk, urine, tears, cerebrospinal fluid, and most recently, cervical secretions.[7] With modified techniques, sensitivities up to 99 percent have been reported for HIV viral culture of peripheral blood mononuclear cells from HIV-1 antibody-positive individuals.[13]

■ CULTIVATION

HIV can be isolated through in vitro cultivation of suspected infected T lymphocytes with the T-cell growth factor, interleukin-2 (IL-2). Fluid suspected of containing free HIV can be added to cultures of normal T lymphocytes, which will replicate to give rise to measurable amounts of progeny virus. The typical cultivation assay employed for routine virus isolation utilizes peripheral blood mononuclear cells from seropositive individuals. These cells are separated from other blood components on a Ficoll–Hypaque gradient, and placed in culture with IL-2 after activation with the T-cell mitogen, phytohemagglutinin (PHA). Supernatants from these cultures are typically analyzed every three to seven days for the presence of reverse transcriptase activity, a marker for infectious HIV.[1,4] The lymphocytes are kept in culture for up to two months, since it is sometimes very difficult to isolate virus from certain cell types that may harbor latent HIV. Because of the long culture time, most laboratories add PHA-activated T cells from unrelated donors at weekly intervals to serve as fresh target cells in which the retrovirus replicates.

HIV can be isolated from the majority of individuals suspected of being infected, especially those who are positive for HIV antibodies.[2] Modifications to improve culture sensitivity have included an improved antigen detection assay to detect virus; eliminating amphotericin B from culture medium; and stimulating donor peripheral blood mononuclear cells with phytohemagglutinin-P for shorter times (two to four days).[13] The percentage of blood samples that will test positive for HIV growth depends on the clinical status of the blood donor. HIV has been isolated from up to 70 percent of AIDS patients with Kaposi's sarcoma and patients with symptomatic, non-AIDS HIV infection. In clinically healthy seropositive gay men and AIDS patients with opportunistic infections, the isolation of infectious HIV is usually less frequent (30 percent to 50 percent), although high sensitivities have been reported.[13] Sixty-five percent of cultures that become positive for HIV reverse transcriptase activity do so within 9 to 15 days of in vitro culture. Up to 85 percent are positive within three weeks.[2] Human immunodeficiency viruses have been isolated up to 60 days after initiating cultures of certain body fluids, especially tears and cervical secretions.[7]

■ IN VITRO CHARACTERISTICS OF HIV-INFECTED CELLS

Upon successful infection of a CD4+ (leu3/T4) T lymphocyte, or expression of viral proteins within a CD4+ T lymphocyte, cultures of HIV-infected cells form multinucleated giant cells. HIV is known to interact with the CD4 molecule on the surface of helper T lymphocytes, and an interaction between an infected cell and an uninfected cell results in the two cells fusing together.[8] This fusion results in the formation of the characteristic multinucleated giant cells observed in HIV cultures. In a culture of peripheral blood lymphocytes containing helper T cells (CD4+), suppressor T cells (CD8+), B lymphocytes, and monocytes, multinucleated giant cells form only between cells that express the CD4 antigen. The level of CD4+ cells in HIV-infected cultures decreases rapidly after the appearance of reverse transcriptase activity and multinucleated giant cells in vitro.[9] Cells that do not express the CD4 antigen (i.e., suppressor T lymphocytes) appear to be unaffected by cultivation with HIV in vitro.[10]

HIV may persist in a latent form in CD4-negative cell populations in cultures. After an initial burst of HIV from CD4+ T cells and their subsequent death, the reverse transcriptase activity in peripheral blood mononuclear cell cultures rapidly decreases. Analysis of these cultures after several months revealed the continued absence of viable CD4+ T cells. However, a very low level of virus expression could be detected.[10] The exact identity of these CD4-negative peripheral blood mononuclear cells is speculative at present, but could represent CD4-positive cells that no longer express the CD4 cell surface marker but are productively infected at a low level. Alternatively, these cells could represent monocytes that have become infected. HIV has also been isolated from a CD4-negative subclone of an HIV-infected CD4+ T lymphoma cell line after induction of a latent form of virus with 5-iodo-2-deoxyuridine.[11]

■ MEASUREMENT OF HIV

The quantity of infectious HIV present in a cell-free culture supernatant can be indirectly determined by in vitro culture methods. A number of T-cell lines have been identified that express HIV antigens within three days to one week after infection with the retrovirus. These cell lines, which include the H9, CEM, and HUT-78 T lymphoma cell lines,[2,4] are permissive for HIV infection, and produce relatively large amounts of this virus in culture over long periods of time. The identification of cell lines that produce HIV retroviruses constitutively has allowed investigators to grow and propagate large amounts of HIV for use in antibody detection systems (e.g., the HIV ELISA). The cultivation of these cell lines with fluid containing HIV results in cell-surface virus antigen expression within one week, which can be identified through cell surface immunofluorescence assays.[2] The dilution that no longer causes immunofluorescence, determined by dilution analysis, roughly correlates with the level of infectious HIV present in a culture supernatant.

In vitro culture of peripheral blood lymphocytes, isolation of HIV, and quantitation of that virus by analysis of reverse transcriptase activity does not reflect the exact quantity of HIV that may be present in cells within culture, or within a person infected with HIV. The most common assay employed for detection and quantitation of HIV in culture supernatants is the reverse transcriptase assay. This assay relies on the HIV reverse transcriptase protein to convert a radioactive DNA precursor (thymidine) to a large form of radioactive DNA that can be quantified. The amount of radioactive DNA produced by this assay correlates directly with the amount of HIV reverse transcriptase activity present in a culture supernatant.

In attempting to quantitate the level of HIV in vivo, lymphocytes suspected of harboring HIV are cultured for long periods of time in vitro, involving large-scale expansion of infected and uninfected lymphocyte populations. The level of reverse transcriptase that may appear in culture supernatants of these cells two weeks after the initiation of culture (or up to six to eight weeks later) does not reflect a quantitative presence of HIV genomes within cells initially present in those cultures. Individuals with full-blown AIDS have very few peripheral blood lymphocytes; yet many other nonlymphoid tissues, such as brain and lymphoid tissues that do not circulate within the blood (e.g., lymph node), may harbor very large amounts of this retrovirus.[12] Therefore, the quantity of reverse transcriptase activity present within a long-term peripheral blood lymphocyte culture is unlikely to reflect the status of disease or the degree to which a person may be infected with HIV. The reverse transcriptase assay may yield useful information in longitudinal antiviral drug trials if a previously positive individual were to become reproducibly negative after therapy.

REFERENCES

1. Salahudden SZ. Isolates of infectious human T cell leukemia/lymphotropic virus type III (HTLV-III) from patients with acquired immunodeficiency syndrome (AIDS) or AIDS related complex (ARC) and from healthy carriers. Proc Natl Acad Sci USA 1985; 82:5530-4.

2. Levy JA, Shimabukuro J. Recovery of AIDS-associated retroviruses from patients with AIDS related conditions and clinically healthy individuals. J Infect Dis 1985; 152:734-8.

3. Barre-Sinoussi F, Chermann JC, Rey R, et al. Isolation of a T-lymphotropic retrovirus from a patient at risk for acquired immune deficiency syndrome (AIDS). Science 1983; 220:868-71.

4. Popovic M, Sarngadharan MG, Read E, Gallo RC. Detection, isolation, and continuous production of cytopathic retroviruses (HTLV-III) from patients with AIDS and pre-AIDS. Science 1984; 224:497-500.

5. Levy JA, Hoffman AD, Kramer SM, et al. Isolation of lymphocytopathic viruses from San Francisco patients with AIDS. Science 1984; 225:840-2.

6. Mayer KH, Stoddard AM, McCusker J, et al. Human T lymphotropic virus type III in high risk, antibody negative homosexual men. Ann Intern Med 1986; 104:194-6.

7. Wofsy CB, Cohen JB, Hauer LB, et al. Isolation of AIDS-associated retrovirus from genital secretions of women with antibodies to virus. Lancet 1986; 1:527.

8. Lifson J, Reyes G, McGrath MS, et al. AIDS retrovirus induced cytopathology: giant cell formation and involvement of CD4 antigen. Science 1986; 232:1123-7.

9. Klatzman D, Barre-Sinoussi F, Nugeyre MT, et al. Selective tropism of lymphadenopathy associated virus (LAV) for helper-inducer T lymphocytes. Science 1984; 225:59-63.

10. Hoxie JA, Haggarty BS, Rackowski JL, et al. Persistent noncytopathic infection of normal human T lymphocytes with AIDS-associated retrovirus. Science 1985; 229:1400-2.

11. Folks T, Powell DM, Lightfoot MM, et al. Induction of HTLV-III/LAV from a nonvirus producing T-cell line: implications for latency. Science 1986; 231:600-3.

12. Gallo RC, Shaw GM, Markham PD. The etiology of AIDS. In: DeVita V, Hellman S, Rosenberg S, eds. AIDS. New York: J.B. Lippincott Co., 1984:31-54.

13. Jackson JB, Coombs RW, Sannerud K, et al. Rapid and sensitive viral culture method for human immunodeficiency virus type 1. J Clin Microbiol 1988; 26:1416-8.

Assays for HIV Nucleic Acid: the Polymerase Chain Reaction

P.T. Cohen, M.D., Ph.D.

Detecting very small specific sequences of HIV DNA or RNA among the relatively large quantity of host nucleic acid is now possible by use of "gene amplification" techniques. These are typified by the polymerase chain reaction (PCR).[1-3] Applications of PCR include assays for HIV proviral DNA and HIV messenger RNA (mRNA). These assays may detect HIV infection when assays for HIV antigen, HIV antibody, and viral culture are not diagnostic.

Mole for mole, HIV nucleic acid is present in infected individuals in relatively small quantities when compared with HIV antigens and HIV antibodies. In addition, on a per-weight basis, HIV DNA and mRNA are a very small fraction of the total DNA and RNA in host cells. Thus, very sensitive assay procedures are required to detect a few infected host cells containing copies of the HIV genome and HIV mRNA from among the many uninfected cells, each with the full complement of host nucleic acid.

PCR and similar nucleic acid amplification techniques have led to dramatic advances in a variety of clinical and research applications. PCR has already proved to be a powerful tool in basic research on HIV. However, many questions remain unanswered about the characteristics and limitations of PCR as a clinical diagnostic test. This is partly because there is no adequate "gold standard" with which to compare PCR's performance in settings in which viral cultures and assays for HIV antigens and antibodies have been negative.

HIV nucleic acid may be the only molecular sign of infection under a number of circumstances: early in the HIV infectious process; during latency, when HIV replication occurs at a very low rate; or during infancy, when maternally-derived HIV antibody from an infected mother is present. HIV infection in any of these situations would be undetectable by screening assays that look for HIV antibody. HIV antigen assays have not yet proved sensitive in these cases. HIV culture techniques might detect infection in these individuals, but culturing the virus has several limitations. It requires two to three weeks, it is relatively costly in material and personnel, it does not lend itself to automation for mass applications, it is vulnerable to interference by an inhibitory factor at any part of the HIV life cycle, and it may be falsely negative too frequently to be a sensitive assay procedure.

■ DESCRIPTION OF THE POLYMERASE-CHAIN-REACTION TECHNIQUE

In its most fundamental form, PCR detects a small, known sequence of designated DNA amid a much larger quantity of DNA (e.g., a single gene or a small HIV-DNA sequence among the entire human genome).[3] This is achieved by selectively and repeatedly making copies of the desired DNA sequence but not of the remainder of DNA in the sample. The desired sequence is reproduced until it is present in a quantity sufficient for detection by conventional assay methods, using specific DNA hybridization probes.

PCR amplifies unique DNA sequences on the order of 100 base pairs in length. For detecting HIV-DNA sequences, the PCR technique involves preparing two oligonucleotides (short single-stranded unique DNA sequences), one for each of the DNA strands. These are called primer oligonucleotides, or "primers." Each of the primers is complementary to a sequence located on one of the DNA strands at the 3′ end of the desired HIV sequence. In the presence of a great molar excess of the primers, the DNA sample is heated to separate the DNA strands. The temperature is then lowered and complementary sequences are hybridized. The primer oligonucleotides hybridize to each strand of the sample DNA, but only at sites at the 3′ end of the desired HIV sequence. Thus, they create two single complementary strands, each with a short double-strand segment where the oligonucleotides have hybridized.

These short double-strand segments serve as primer sites for DNA polymerase. When nucleotide triphosphates and DNA polymerase are added to the reaction, the enzyme synthesizes complementary DNA sequences for each of the strands of the desired HIV sequence. This results in four strands — two with the desired HIV sequence and two complementary to this sequence. These strands may now be heat-separated and allowed to rehybridize with the primer oligonucleotides. They then become templates for additional copies. Multiple cycles of this process lead to exponential reproduction of the desired sequence. A millionfold or more increase in copies of the DNA sequence is possible, resulting in quantities detectable by conventional assays such as hybridization with a specific radioisotope-labeled nucleic-acid probe.

Using a polymerase that is heat-stable eliminates the need to replace heat-denatured polymerase after each amplification cycle.[4] An automated apparatus can process multiple samples through successive timed cycles of heating, cooling, and polymerase synthesis. Results may be obtained in three days.

■ VARIATIONS OF THE POLYMERASE-CHAIN-REACTION ASSAY

HIV mRNA Detected by Reverse Transcription and PCR.   HIV mRNA can be detected by first treating the sample with reverse transcriptase, which synthesizes DNA complementary to the mRNA sequences. PCR is then used with appropriate primers to amplify the resulting complementary DNA. This shows promise as a clinical assay because it detects mRNA (and thus HIV gene expression) in infected cells even when antibody and antigen are not being produced. Differentiation between states in which HIV genes are and are not being expressed allows further characterization of HIV during the so-called latent period. The assay also provides a method for examining gene expression by regulatory genes of the HIV and for determining splice-junction sequences in HIV mRNA.[6,17]

HIV mRNA Detected by PCR with a Transcriptional Step.   HIV RNA can be amplified by coupling PCR with a transcriptional step. Using primer oligonucleotides containing a promoter sequence for a T7 RNA polymerase, the products of several cycles of chain reaction can serve as templates for RNA synthesis by the polymerase. Amplifications of a millionfold or more are reported for this technique.[7,8]

■ CLINICAL APPLICATIONS OF NUCLEIC ACID AMPLIFICATION ASSAYS

Potential clinical applications for PCR include testing of infants and children of HIV-seropositive women, patients in early stages of HIV infection (before antibodies appear), patients who were seropositive but who no longer have detectable antibodies in their blood, and patients on antiviral therapy.

Infants born to HIV-seropositive mothers do not make antibodies early in life but do carry HIV maternal antibodies in their blood. HIV antigen assays have not yet proven sensitive in this setting, possibly because HIV replication is often minimal and little antigen is produced. Several studies report HIV infection detected by PCR assay in such infants when HIV antigen is not detected.[9-12,18,19] However, the performance characteristics of this application of the PCR assay can be determined only by observing these infants over time to see which are truly infected. Large-scale studies for this purpose are in progress.

In adults, the PCR assay has detected HIV nucleic acid after infection but prior to seroconversion.[13,14,20] It has also detected it when antibodies had disappeared from the blood of infected patients.[15] Studies have detected HIV nucleic acid by PCR in blood of patients who tested negative by HIV culture[2] and by HIV-antigen assay.[6]

The PCR assay detected HIV mRNA in seropositive subjects who tested negative by HIV-antigen assay.[6] Theoretically, the mRNA assay can be used to make decisions about antiviral therapy, although many additional data are needed to develop this application for clinical use.

■ LIMITATIONS AND PERFORMANCE CHARACTERISTICS OF THE PCR ASSAY

To date, published data on using PCR to detect HIV infection are scanty and preliminary. The method must still be considered experimental. Sensitivity, specificity, predictive value, and limitations must be worked out before results can be used for patient management or large-scale screening. The following discussion attempts to summarize information from published clinical data.

PCR is most useful in settings where other assays (antibody, antigen, and culture) are ineffective. In these settings, there is no standard assay to compare with the performance of PCR.

The statistical sensitivity or false-negative rate can be crudely estimated from published small studies. These assume that HIV-seropositive patients are infected and should give a positive PCR assay. In three studies, PCR assays were negative for 1 of 18, 4 of 22, and 1 of 5 HIV-seropositive patients.[2,6,15] Taken at face value, these numbers indicate a sensitivity in the range of 80 percent to 94 percent (false-negative rate = 6 percent to 20 percent). Of reported patients who were HIV antibody-positive and HIV culture-negative, 4 of 11 tested negative by the PCR assay,[2] a statistical sensitivity of 64 percent (false-negative rate = 36 percent) for this subgroup. This is a low statistical sensitivity for a screening assay (compared to 99 percent for HIV antibody assays). Presumably, experience and refinement of assay methodology will improve the statistical sensitivity, but published data at this time do not support the assumption that a negative PCR assay alone is sufficient to rule out HIV infection.

TABLE 1. DIAGRAMMATIC ILLUSTRATION OF THE POLYMERASE CHAIN REACTION*

INGREDIENTS

primer oligonucleotides: 5′ − ATGCCGTAT − 3′ and 3′ − CGATATGCGC − 5′

unique desired HIV DNA sequence in large double-stranded DNA molecule

3′ − ∧| |\/\/\/\/\TACGGCATA------------CGATATGCGC\/\/\/\| |\/ − 5′
5′ − \/| |/\/\/\/\ATGCCGTAT + + + + GCTATACGCG/\/\/\/| |∧ − 3′

Step 1: Hybridization of oligonucleotides to a region on each strand flanking the desired sequence.

        5′ − ATGCCGTAT − 3′
3′ − ∧| |\/\/\/\/\TACGGCATA-----------CGATATGCGC\/\/\/\| |\/ − 5′

                3′ − CGATATGCGC − 5′
5′ − \/| |/\/\/\/\ATGCCGTAT + + + + + + GCTATACGCG/\/\/\/| |∧ − 3′

Step 2: Elongation from double-stranded primer sites by DNA polymerase.

                DNA polymerase
    ↓   +
            nucleotide triphosphates
        5′ − ATGCCGTAT + + + + + 3′   → synthesis
3′ − ∧| |\/\/\/\/\TACGGCATA-----------CGATATGCGC\/\/\/\| |\/ − 5′

            synthesis ← 3′-------CGATATGCGC − 5′
5′ − \/| |/\/\/\/\ATGCCGTAT + + + + + GCTATACGCG/\/\/\/| |∧ − 3′

                ↓

        5′ − ATGCCGTAT + + + + + GCTATACGCG − 3′
3′ − ∧| |\/\/\/\/\TACGGCATA--------------CGATATGCGC\/\/\/\| |\/ − 5′

        3′ − TACGGCATA--------------CGATATGCGC − 5′
5′ − \/| |/\/\/\/\ATGCCGTAT + + + + + GCTATACGCG/\/\/\/| |∧ − 3′

Four template strands now exist and can be recycled to create eight strands in the next cycle.

* *Compiled by the author.*

Theoretically, a PCR assay of DNA from peripheral blood cells could be negative when HIV antibody is present: if the quantity of HIV nucleic acid were below the detectable level; if genetic variation made the infecting virus sufficiently different from the primers (unlikely if primers are derived from conserved nucleic acid sequences and several primer pairs are used to maximize assay sensitivity); if only one primer pair were used in the assay; if the patient's HIV antibody test were falsely positive; or if the virus were eliminated from the patient's peripheral blood but not from other tissue.[2]

False-positive PCR assay results are impossible to confirm by currently available techniques because no assay can prove that a patient is uninfected (as opposed to harboring a few molecules of HIV proviral nucleic acid). Lack of clinical evidence for infection is not a useful criterion, because clinical signs or symptoms of infection may not emerge for many years in an infected patient. However, false-positive rates may be inferred by assaying individuals known to lack risk factors for HIV infection. Seronegative controls were negative by PCR assay in all 13[2] and all 9[6] assays in two studies, allowing crude estimation of the false-positive rate at less than 4 percent (statistical specificity greater than 94 percent).

A positive PCR assay in a patient who has not become ill may reflect HIV-DNA that is incapable of initiating viral replication — i.e., a defective HIV proviral genome. Such defective HIV proviruses have been reported.[5] False-positive PCR assay results have been reported in non-HIV assay systems due to contamination of primer materials.[16] Proper controls should identify this problem where it exists.

REFERENCES

1. Kwok S, Mack DH, Mullis KB, et al. Identification of human immunodeficiency virus sequences by using in vitro enzymatic amplification and oligomer cleavage detection. J Virol 1987; 61:1690-4.

2. Ou C, Kwok S, Mitchell SW, et al. DNA amplification for direct detection of HIV-1 in DNA of peripheral blood mononuclear cells. Science 1988; 239:295-7.

3. Mullis KB, Faloona FA. Specific synthesis of DNA in vitro via a polymerase-catalyzed chain reaction. Methods Enzymol 1987; 155:335-50.

4. Saiki RK, Gelfand DH, Stoffel S, et al. Primer-directed enzymatic amplification of DNA with a thermostable DNA polymerase. Science 1988; 239:487-91.

5. Willey RL, Rutledge RA, Dias S, et al. Identification of conserved and divergent domains within the envelope gene of the acquired immunodeficiency syndrome retrovirus. Proc Natl Acad Sci USA 1986; 83:5038-42.

6. Hart C, Schochetman G, Spira T, et al. Direct detection of HIV RNA expression in seropositive subjects. Lancet 1988; 2:596-9.

7. Murakawa GJ, Zaia JA, Spallone PA, et al. Direct detection of HIV-1 RNA from AIDS and ARC patient samples. DNA 1988; 7:287-95.

8. Rossi JJ, Murakawa G, Arnold B, et al. Simultaneous amplification and direct detection of HIV-1, T-cell receptor, and β-actin mRNA sequences from peripheral blood samples [Abstract]. Stockholm: IV International Conference on AIDS 1988; 2:78, A1612.

9. Wolinsky S, Mack D, Yogev R, et al. Direct detection of HIV infection in pediatric patients and their mothers by the polymerase chain reaction (PCR) procedure [Abstract]. Stockholm: IV International Conference on AIDS 1988; 2:87, A1646.

10. Rogers M. Prospective study of virologic parameters for infants born to HIV-seropositive women [Abstract]. Stockholm: IV International Conference on AIDS 1988; 1:87, A7257.

11. Laure F, Courgnaud V, Rouzioux C, et al. Detection of HIV-1 DNA in infants and children by means of the polymerase chain reaction. Lancet 1988; 2:538-41.

12. DeRossi A, Amadori A, Chieco-Bianchi L, et al. Polymerase chain reaction and in-vitro antibody production for early diagnosis of paediatric HIV infection. Lancet 1988; 2:278.

13. Wolinsky S, Rinaldo C, Farzedegan H, et al. Polymerase chain reaction (PCR) detection of HIV provirus before HIV seroconversion [Abstract]. Stockholm: IV International Conference on AIDS 1988; 1:137, A1099.

14. Loche M, Mach B. Identification of HIV-infected seronegative individuals by a direct diagnostic test based on hybridisation to amplified viral DNA. Lancet 1988; 2:418-21.

15. Farzadegan H, Polis MA, Wolinsky SM, et al. Loss of human immunodeficiency virus type 1 (HIV-1) antibodies with evidence of viral infection in asymptomatic homosexual men: a report from the multi-center AIDS cohort study. Ann Intern Med 1988; 108:785-90.

16. Lo YM, Mehal WZ, Fleming KA. False-positive results and the polymerase chain reaction. Lancet 1988; 2:579.

17. Klotman ME, DeRossi A, Buchbinder A, Wong-Staal F. RNA splicing events detected in early in vitro HIV infection using the polymerase chain reaction (PCR) [Abstract]. V International Conference on AIDS. Montreal, 1989; 1:T.C.O.13.

18. Rogers MF, Ou C-Y, Rayfield M, et al. Use of the polymerase chain reaction for early detection of the proviral sequences of human immunodeficiency virus in infants born to seropositive mothers. N Engl J Med 1989; 320:1649-54.

19. Katz SL, Wilfert CM. Human immunodeficiency virus infection of newborns. N Engl J Med 1989; 320:1687-9.

20. Imagawa DT, Lee MH, Wolinsky SM, et al. Human immunodeficiency virus type 1 infection in homosexual men who remain seronegative for prolonged periods. N Engl J Med 1989; 320:1458-62.

How to Tell Patients They Have HIV Disease

Paul A. Volberding, M.D.

T he almost limitless diversity of physician experience and attitudes, as well as patient-to-patient variability in prognosis and social setting, makes the title of this chapter seem at first glance hopelessly naive. Yet, despite the obvious complexities, many common underlying themes permit generalization.

Physicians, for the most part, are members of the dominant culture, whereas HIV-infected patients, with occasional exceptions, come from socially and politically isolated subcultures. While the physicians are usually heterosexual, middle class, nonintravenous drug users, their patients are often homosexual, members of a racial or ethnic minority, or users of intravenous drugs, or sometimes all of these. Despite these differences, HIV-infected patients are almost always young and all share the prognosis of a chronic, disfiguring, transmissible, and ultimately fatal disease. In the end, these shared features should be remembered and stressed by clinicians when informing patients of a diagnosis of HIV disease. This and the principles of honesty, realistic optimism, and practical support should guide the physician in this stressful discussion.

■ HONESTY

The first goal in relaying an HIV disease diagnosis should be to empower the patient to make a subsequent decision by providing sufficient factual information in terms the patient can understand. This takes time, but is rewarded by increased trust between patient and physician. This trust and the active involvement of the patient can help in making the many difficult decisions that characterize the management of HIV disease.

In discussing the diagnosis, the physician must first assess the patient's level of information and degree of anxiety. Many people at high risk already know friends or acquaintances who have died of the disease. Thus, they may know the disease quite well. Still, they may need information as it pertains to their specific case. In choosing the most appropriate language, the physician should couple the needed information with an estimate of the medical sophistication of the patient. In doing this, the physician must remember how emotionally charged this time is for the patient. The first discussion of the diagnosis should be expressed directly, using lay terms in most cases, and should itself be brief. The physician should expect that the patient will "not hear" a detailed description of management options and these should be discussed or reviewed at the next visit, which should be scheduled promptly if the patient is not hospitalized. If the patient has a close friend or family member, that person should be invited to participate in discussing the diagnosis, since someone not so immediately involved can retain more of what is said, and thus help inform and support the patient after visiting the physician.

Medical information given to the newly diagnosed AIDS patient should include the name of the HIV-related diagnosis in medical terms (e.g., *Pneumocystis carinii* pneumonia) as well as a lay description of the disease. The relationship to AIDS should be discussed in explicit terms (e.g., the pneumonia you have means you have AIDS). The immediate management of the clinical problem should be stressed. The physician should not try to diminish the importance of the underlying HIV disease but should avoid speculating about future prognosis and, in particular, should not estimate the patient's survival time.

■ REALISTIC OPTIMISM

The prognosis of HIV disease, while certainly one of limited prospect, is not uniform. It must be stressed to recently diagnosed cases that statistics quoting probability of death are not directly applicable to individual patients. It must also be stressed that our understanding of HIV and its attendant clinical problems are expanding rapidly, and that drugs potentially able to block further damage from this virus infection are being developed and tested rapidly. It can also be said that along with this basic work, we are improving the routine clinical management of HIV-related cancers and infections; again, with the hope of extending survival even in those patients with established AIDS.

In informing the new HIV-infected patient of the diagnosis, the physician has the difficult task of balancing the need for honesty with hope. The physician's tone should be as optimistic as possible without subtracting from the obligation to provide factual data.

■ PRACTICAL SUPPORT

One area that can be addressed by the physician in caring for an HIV-infected patient is that of dealing with the patient's immediate practical needs. A newly diagnosed patient is, in many cases, suffering severe emotional stress and needs to know where to turn for help. Often this help is simply the availability of someone to talk to about the meanings of the diagnosis. HIV disease often affects people who have only a limited array of close friends or family; thus, for many San Francisco AIDS patients, help for this immediate need has come from volunteer, nonprofessional counselling organizations. The talking out of the diagnosis may occur in individual or group meetings. Although not suitable for all new patients, they are helpful for many; the physician should be aware of these resources so that the patient can, in turn, follow through on establishing this connection.

A similar philosophy obtains for practical patient needs. AIDS patients may need housing, emergency financial help, or food. As with counseling, these needs may be met by existing community organizations and, again, it is the physician's responsibility to ensure that appropriate referrals for these agencies are made.

Perhaps the most difficult questions on the mind of a newly diagnosed patient surround death. When will I die? What will it be like? Will it be painful? Will I die alone? To a variable degree, these often unstated questions should be addressed explicitly by the physician. The physician should not speculate about time of death unless this appears imminent, but should reassure the patient that pain will be vigorously controlled and when death is approaching, others, whether family, friends, or medical staff, will be present. This discussion should be conducted in a calm, quiet, non-hurried, and supportive environment. It is not appropriate to discuss these issues with all patients at the time of diagnosis, but they should be dealt with well before death is imminent.

Along with answering questions regarding death, the physician should determine the patient's wishes for medical management in the extreme situation. Should respiratory insufficiency occur, for example, does the patient wish mechanical ventilation? Although these discussions may seem abstract for relatively healthy outpatients and decisions may change, it is vital for the patient to consider these issues in advance, particularly given the frequency of preterminal HIV-related dementia.

A final area to be addressed concerns power of attorney. This, related to the discussion above, is also best conducted in advance. Here, patients can select another individual who is empowered to participate in clinical management decisions with the physician if the patient himself is unable to do so.

3

HUMAN
IMMUNODEFICIENCY
VIRUS
AND
PATHOGENESIS
OF
AIDS

EDITOR

Michael S. McGrath, M.D., Ph.D.

3.1

Characteristics of HIV and Related Viruses

HIV: Overview and General Description

Michael S. McGrath, M.D., Ph.D.

R etroviruses are enveloped RNA viruses characteristically possessing an RNA-dependent DNA polymerase (reverse transcriptase). The family Retroviridae comprises three subfamilies — the Oncovirinae or RNA tumor viruses (including the human T-cell leukemia viruses, HTLV-I and HTLV-II), the nononcogenic, nonpathogenic Spumavirinae, and the Lentivirinae. The human immunodeficiency virus (HIV) is most closely related to the Lentivirinae subfamily of retroviruses but may ultimately be deemed to represent a novel subfamily. Early AIDS virus isolates were termed HTLV-III, LAV, and ARV, but they are all now known to be closely related and are jointly termed HIV. With the recent discovery of another class of AIDS virus in West Africa, initially termed LAV-2,[1] the current AIDS virus terminology recognizes these two main classes of virus as HIV-1 and HIV-2.

TABLE 1. THE FAMILY RETROVIRIDAE*

ONCOVIRINAE	LENTIVIRINAE	SPUMAVIRINAE
avian leukemia virus	visna/maedi	syncytial and foamy viruses of humans, cats, monkeys, and cattle
avian sarcoma virus (Rous)	caprine arthritis	
avian erythroblastosis virus	encephalitis virus	
mouse mammary tumor virus	equine infectious anemia virus	
murine leukemia virus	human immuno-deficiency virus	
murine sarcoma virus	simian T-cell immuno-deficiency virus	
feline sarcoma virus		
bovine leukemia virus		
simian sarcoma virus		
human T-cell leukemia virus I		
human T-cell leukemia virus II		

* *Compiled by the author.*

HIV-infected individuals develop a wide spectrum of disease states ranging from the asymptomatic carrier state to full-blown AIDS. The clinical features of HIV infection range from an acute mononucleosis-like illness to chronic fever, weight loss, malaise, diarrhea, dementia, and lymphadenopathy, and finally to

AIDS in individuals whose cellular immune systems are unable to defend the hosts against opportunistic infections. Dementia and malignancies (primarily Kaposi's sarcoma and high-grade non-Hodgkin's lymphoma) also develop in individuals infected with HIV. Currently, the role HIV plays in the development of this spectrum of diseases is poorly understood.

HIV is a retrovirus that has characteristics in common with another family of human retroviruses, the human T-lymphotropic viruses, but it most closely resembles members of the lentivirus family.[2-4] Human lymphotropic viruses (HTLV) Types I and II are associated with T-lymphocyte transformation, whereas HIV and lentiviruses (i.e., EIA, visna, CAEV) do not cause malignant transformation. Like lentiviruses, a mature HIV in extracellular form is a lipid-encoated vesicle approximately 100 to 120 nm in diameter. It is an RNA virus with a central cylindrical RNA genome 90 nm long, and measuring approximately 45 nm at its narrowest point. HIV, like other lipid-membrane-encoated retroviruses, is extremely sensitive to inactivation with detergent (greater than 0.5 percent), alcohol (greater than 25 percent), heat (greater than 60°C), bleach (10 percent), and formaldehyde (0.37 percent).

HIV is composed of a single positive strand of RNA that is 9300 nucleotide bases in length, along with viral genetic segments encoding both structural and regulatory proteins, and a virus replication promoter region termed the long terminal repeat (LTR). The regulatory gene products have recently been renamed; in the list below, the old terminology is in parentheses. The protein-encoding regions are:

1. the *gag* gene, which encodes the major internal viral structural proteins p17, p24, p15;

2. the *pol* gene, which encodes the reverse transcriptase enzyme (p53, p66), which transcribes viral RNA into DNA, a step required before HIV viral proteins and new viruses can be made. Also encoded in the *pol* gene are a portion of the HIV protease (5′ end) and an endonuclease protein (p31);

3. the *vif* (*sor*) and *nef* (3′ *orf*) genes, which respectively encode proteins of 23,000 and 27,000 molecular weight and effect virus replication by increasing (*vif*) or decreasing (*nef*) virus production;

4. the *tat* gene, which encodes a transactivating genetic element that increases the production of viral and cellular proteins;

5. the *rev* (*art/trs*) gene, which is required for viral protein messenger RNA processing;

6. the envelope gene, which encodes the major virion surface envelope glycoprotein gp160, which then is processed to form a transmembrane segment (gp41) and a glycosylated external segment (gp120);

7. the *vpr* (r) gene, whose function is presently unknown.

HIV-infected cells contain two major forms of virus. A DNA copy of the entire HIV genome may become permanently integrated into the genome of an infected cell (DNA provirus), or the genome may exist as a double-stranded linear DNA copy of the virus that is present in the cytoplasm of infected cells but not integrated into the host genome. The myriad disease processes associated with HIV infection occur through a complex series of interactions between host cell proteins, virion proteins, and nucleic acids.

HIV has been found in only a small fraction of cells in infected individuals. The cell population most profoundly affected by HIV is the helper subset of T lymphocytes that expresses the cell surface CD4 (leu3/T4) molecule. In vitro studies (in situ hybridization) allowing the detection of HIV genes in infected cells have shown that HIV genes are present in 1 in 10,000 to 1 in 1,000,000 lymphocytes in tissues from AIDS and ARC patients. These infected lymphocytes are primarily T lymphocytes, most likely from the CD4-expressing T-helper cell subset. This same in vitro analysis technique has also detected HIV genes in the brains of AIDS patients — most likely in microglial cells, and in macrophages.

The immune system demonstrates both acute and chronic effects after a successful HIV infection.[4,5] The most devastating effect on an HIV-infected individual is the gradual but progressive depletion of helper T lymphocytes, leading to an as-yet-irreversible immunodeficiency state. Although HIV interacts with the same cell population as human T-lymphotropic viruses Type I and II, rather than cause T-helper cell transformation, HIV causes T-helper cell death. In vitro, a major mechanism of T-cell death is through cell–cell fusion, and the formation of multinucleated giant cells, which die within 24 to 48 hours. The HIV envelope glycoprotein gp160, expressed on the surface of an HIV-infected cell, binds with the CD4 (leu3/T4) molecule on an uninfected T cell and initiates fusion.[6] Replication of viral genes within infected cells, and the accumulation of unintegrated HIV DNA have also been implicated as a mechanism for HIV-mediated killing of infected T cells.[7]

In vivo, a series of abnormalities contribute to the profound immunodeficiency that develops in individuals infected with HIV. These include polyclonal B-cell activation and the formation of autoantibodies and immune complexes, impaired processing of foreign antigens and decreased macrophage function, and the decreased induction of killer T lymphocytes, allowing other viruses, parasites, and tumor cells to proliferate more effectively in the HIV-infected individual.

REFERENCES

1. Brun-Vezinet F, Rey MA, Katlama C, et al. Lymphadenopathy-associated virus type 2 in AIDS and AIDS-related patients. Clinical and virological features in four patients. Lancet 1987; 1:128-32.

2. Crowe S, Mills J, McGrath MS. Quantitative immunocytofluorographic analysis of CD4 surface antigen expression and HIV infection of human peripheral blood monocyte/macrophages. AIDS Res Hum Retroviruses 1987; 135-45.

3. Wong-Staal F, Gallo RC. Human T-cell lymphotropic retroviruses. Nature 1985; 317:395-403.

4. Bowen DL, Lane HC, Fauci AS. Immunopathogenesis of the acquired immunodeficiency syndrome. Ann Intern Med 1985; 103:704-9.

5. Lane HC, Fauci AS. Immunologic abnormalities in the acquired immunodeficiency syndrome. Ann Rev Immunol 1985; 103:477-500.

6. Lifson JD, Reyes GR, McGrath MS, et al. AIDS retrovirus induced cytopathology: giant cell formation is mediated by cell-cell fusion involving the CD4 molecule. Science 1986; 232:1132.

7. Levy JA, Kaminsky LS, Morrow WJW, et al. Infection by the retrovirus associated with the acquired immunodeficiency syndrome. Ann Intern Med 1985; 103:694-9.

AIDS Vaccine Development: Role of Neutralizing Antibodies

Michael S. McGrath, M.D., Ph.D.

■ ROLE OF NEUTRALIZING ANTIBODIES

A subpopulation of individuals infected with the human immunodeficiency virus (HIV) has antibodies capable of neutralizing HIV infectivity in vitro. One of the principal mechanisms by which animals protect themselves from a successful retrovirus infection is by inactivating the virus before the infection becomes widespread. This can be accomplished if the animal's serum contains antibodies which, on contact with an infectious retrovirus, prevent infection. These antibodies are called neutralizing antibodies. Investigators have reported the presence of neutralizing antibodies in as few as 10 percent[1] and in as many as 80 percent of persons infected with HIV.[2,3]

The ability to detect neutralizing antibodies in persons infected with HIV is variable. Absence or low titer of neutralizing antibody does not appear to correlate with the severity of the HIV-related disease state. Several investigators have found that a high percentage of AIDS patients express HIV neutralizing antibodies,[2,4] whereas others have found that a low percentage express them.[3] In studies with substantial methodologic differences, neutralization assays were performed with different HIV isolates, target cells for infection, and methods for scoring neutralization, making comparison of results between individual studies difficult.[1-4] Most investigators agreed, however, that if present, neutralizing antibodies are generally present at a low titer — regardless of the subjects from whom they are taken. Currently, no correlation can be made between the level of serum neutralizing antibodies (as measured in vitro) and in vivo protection from progression of HIV-associated disease in an infected person. The HIV envelope glycoprotein, gp120, is the major target for HIV neutralizing antibody.

The most direct experimental evidence implicating the HIV envelope glycoprotein as the target of neutralizing antibodies involves the use of vesicular stomatitis (HIV) pseudotype viruses — viruses containing the vesicular stomatitis virus genome within an HIV envelope. In a standard neutralization assay, these pseudotype viruses, expressing only the HIV envelope proteins, were neutralized in a pattern similar to native HIV.[2] The HIV envelope glycoprotein molecule also mediates the binding of HIV to the CD4 (leu3/T4) molecule on the surface of target T lymphocytes.[6] Monoclonal antibodies directed to determinants on the CD4 molecule inhibit HIV infection of T lymphocytes in vitro, effectively "neutralizing" the HIV by disruption of a T-cell surface interaction.

HIV is related to a class of viruses called lentiviruses,[7] which induce neutralizing antibodies in infected animals. Visna virus, a lentivirus causing central nervous system damage in infected sheep, induces neutralizing antibodies that may be partially protective in vivo. Neutralizing antibody isolated from a sheep soon after visna virus infection will generally not neutralize a visna virus isolate obtained from the same sheep at a later point in time. The presence of neutralizing antibodies in a sheep soon after visna virus infection apparently places the virus under immunologic selective pressure to change its envelope glycoprotein configuration, thereby escaping neutralization.[8,9] This may occur repeatedly in visna virus infected sheep, which eventually die as a result of secondary visna virus-induced disease.

Like the visna virus, different HIV isolates show the greatest heterogeneity in the envelope gene region. Point mutation studies of HIV gp120 reveal that this sequence heterogeneity defines a means by which HIV can escape neutralization.[25] Clearly, for any HIV vaccine to be effective, it must induce immunity to a conserved region common to all HIV isolates — that is, one that would not change in the presence of in vivo neutralizing antibody. Investigators have used site-specific mutagenesis techniques on gp120 and observed that mutations in the second conserved HIV *env* domain rendered HIV noninfectious. The gp120 produced by the mutants did not bind to CD4 molecules in vitro. Thus, it would seem that alterations involving the second conserved domain of HIV gp120 may interfere with an essential early step in the virus's replication process.

HIV undergoes genetic changes both with in vitro cultivation and in vivo as AIDS progresses. A recent study showed that the growth of HIV in the constant presence of a neutralizing antiserum yielded a viral population that was resistant to neutralization by that same antiserum.[26] The sequence of the variant non-neutralizable virus was identical to the parent HIV, with the exception of a single amino acid difference in the variant envelope glycoprotein.

In addition, another study has shown that HIV undergoes extensive variation in vivo. By examining viral isolates from two HIV-seropositive individuals, 17 distinct isolates were observed from one individual and 13 distinct isolates were found in the other.[27] Thus, gp120 may be a very difficult target for a vaccine program that attempts to induce gp120 neutralizing antibodies.

Some neutralizing antibodies do not block gp120–CD4 binding; they block the fusion of the virus with the cell membrane by binding to the transmembrane portion of the HIV gp41. Fusion-inhibiting antibodies have also been elicited by immunization with gp160 and were found to be directed against the central portion of the HIV *env* gp120.[28] The role of HIV gp41 protein may prove to be quite important in vaccination efforts, since in mice antibodies to the p15E transmembrane protein of MuLV were effective in intervening with the course of murine leukemia. However, HIV gp41 and human MHC class II antigen share at least two homologous regions. Thus, antibodies directed against gp41 may react with class II self-antigens, thereby triggering autoimmune pathways and leading to further immunodeficiency.[29] These findings further complicate efforts to develop effective vaccines, but because the specificities of currently identified antibodies that inhibit (neutralize) HIV infection recognize either the HIV envelope protein(s) or the cellular receptor for the envelope glycoprotein, the first vaccine candidates have been those that induced a "neutralizing" anti-envelope immune response in vivo.

Another potential problem is that of "enhancing antibodies," a phenomenon that has been observed in vitro. Enhancing antibodies increase HIV infectivity, probably by forming immune complexes of antibody and HIV particles that can be taken up by Fc receptors on the surface of macrophages, thereby bypassing the CD4 receptor. By facilitating non-CD4-mediated HIV infection of cells, enhancing antibodies may thwart therapy (e.g., with soluble CD4) directed at blocking the combination of HIV and the CD4 receptor. Clearly, to be effective a vaccine must either not elicit production of enhancing antibodies or it must block the action of enhancing antibodies (e.g., by blocking Fc receptors).[35]

■ NON-LIVE VIRUS VACCINES

The first major avenue of investigation for an effective vaccine has been the use of either the complete HIV envelope or the subunits identified by HIV neutralizing antibodies. A number of research groups have now cloned several different HIV genomes and subsegments of those genes. Cloned HIV gene segments can be made into subsegmental pieces of corresponding protein in vitro, depending upon the DNA cloning method employed.[10]

Low-titer HIV neutralizing antibodies have been induced in animals injected with portions of the HIV envelope protein. Native HIV gp120[11] (molecularly cloned and purified by affinity chromatography[12]), gp160,[20] and HIV envelope glycoprotein peptides[13] have induced low-titer neutralizing antibodies to several HIV isolates. Unfortunately, only low levels of neutralizing antibody have been induced in vaccinated animals and immunized chimpanzees. These antibodies were not protective after an infective HIV challenge.[14] In addition, immunized chimpanzees developed only type-specific neutralizing antibodies.[30] Even more disappointing are the recent reports showing the failure of HIV immune globulin to protect chimpanzees against an experimental challenge with HIV, even though the neutralizing antibody levels were approximately 100 times higher than those required to neutralize 100 infectious units of HIV.[31] All of these studies raise questions about how passive or active immunity might be provided prior to HIV infection. At present, the only HIV vaccine currently approved for human trials in the U.S. is molecularly cloned gp160.[20]

■ ROLE OF CELLULAR IMMUNITY

Because HIV can probably be transmitted by both free virus and infected cells (i.e., transfusion), it is likely that a vaccination scheme will also need to induce HIV-specific cellular immunity. This is the type of immunity that is normally required to kill virus-infected cells in vivo; it is mediated wholly or in part by cytotoxic T cells that in this case would specifically recognize and kill HIV- infected cells. Cytotoxic T lymphocytes have been detected in individuals infected with HTLV-I,[15] but cytotoxic T lymphocytes directed against HIV- infected cells have been more difficult to detect. One study showed that MHC-restricted CD3+CD8+ cytotoxic T lymphocytes in the blood of many HIV-infected individuals responded against cells expressing HIV reverse transcriptase. Since the *pol* sequence is highly conserved among different isolates and generates both humoral and cellular immune responses, it may have potential as a broadly cross-reactive vaccine.[32] Clearly, the capacity of a candidate vaccine to stimulate both HIV neutralizing antibody and cytotoxic T cells will need to be tested.

■ EXPERIMENTAL LIVE VIRUS VACCINE

A live virus (vaccinia) recombinant HIV gp160 vaccine has recently been injected into healthy HIV-seronegative humans. Daniel Zagury, a French immunologist,[16] injected himself and a group of Zairian military volunteers with a live virus vaccine. This vaccine uses a strain of vaccinia (cowpox) virus that has been molecularly constructed to contain the entire HIV gp160 gene. When this virus infects cells, these cells express the HIV envelope (and no other HIV proteins) on their surface.

The use of a live virus vaccine for other diseases (i.e., smallpox) has induced both T-cell and antibody-mediated immunity. Zagury's preliminary results indicate that the vaccinia gp160 vaccine can induce some T-cell immunity to HIV. One year after the original vaccination, Zagury reported that HIV-specific humoral and cellular immune responses were induced. High levels of antibodies to the viral *env* gene and neutralizing antibodies against divergent HIV-1 strains (such as HTLV-IIIB and HTLV-IIIRF) were induced with Zagury's complex vaccination scheme. In addition, group-specific cell-mediated immunity and cell-mediated cytotoxicity against infected CD4+ cells were attained after primary vaccinations; these responses were further enhanced by booster immunizations. Skin tests revealed both immediate and delayed hypersensitivity to gp160 in vivo.[33] Unfortunately, the HIV-specific immunity was short-lived and required repeated boosts for reinduction. This type of vaccine has been used in chimpanzees, and although it induced neutralizing antibody and specific T-cell immunity, it failed to protect the animals against infection with HIV.[21,22] Long-term follow-up of vaccinated individuals will be required to determine the level of antibody and T-cell responses induced by this vaccine and to determine its efficacy and safety.

■ ANIMAL MODELS IN VACCINE DEVELOPMENT

The creation of an effective vaccine strategy will require the testing of prospective vaccines in appropriate animal models. Currently, no completely appropriate animal model exists to study the development of AIDS in vivo. Upon infection with HIV, chimpanzees become seropositive for HIV antibodies and experience a transient immunosuppression. However, they do not develop AIDS.[17] Similarly, STLV-III, although antigenically cross-reactive with HIV, does not cause significant immunosuppression or disease in African green monkeys in vivo.[18] Simian AIDS (SAIDS) occurs in rhesus monkeys infected with the type D simian retroviruses SRV-I and SRV-II, but the targets for viral infection and killing are not limited to the CD4 (leu 3/T4) T-cell subset alone, since all lymphocyte subpopulations, macrophages, and neutrophils are infected by these viruses.[19] Currently, the closest animal model of human AIDS is the simian immunodeficiency virus (SIV-1)-infected macaque monkey.[23,24] CD8+ lymphocytes block virus replication in peripheral blood lymphocytes of SIV-infected monkeys, just as they do in HIV-infected humans. In addition, SIV of macaques is morphologically indistinguishable from HIV in humans, sharing CD4+ cell tropism and inducing an AIDS-like disease in rhesus monkeys.[34] Vaccine studies will be forthcoming in the near future.

A new animal model for HIV disease that uses mice with SCID (severe combined immunodeficiency) reconstituted with a human immune system has recently been described.[36] SCID mice were given transplants of both fetal[36] and adult[37] human lymphoid cells and lymphoid-cell precursors; they then develop immune systems with human characteristics. These SCID-Hu mice can be infected with HIV.[38] Further study will determine whether the SCID-Hu mouse will be a useful model system for HIV vaccine development.

REFERENCES

1. Clavel F, Klatzman D, Montagnier L. Deficient LAV_1 neutralizing capacity of sera from patients with AIDS or related syndromes. Lancet 1985; 1:879-80.
2. Weiss RA, Clapham PR, Cheingsong-Popov R, et al. Neutralization of human T-lymphotropic virus type III by sera of AIDS and AIDS-risk patients. Nature 1985; 316:69-72.
3. Robert-Guroff M, Brown M, Gallo RC. HTLV-III-neutralizing antibodies in patients with AIDS and AIDS-related complex. Nature 1985; 316:72-4.
4. Ho DD, Rota TR, Hirsch MS. Antibody to lymphadenopathy-associated virus in AIDS. N Engl J Med 1985; 312:649-50.
5. Allan JS, Coligan JE, Barin F, et al. Major glycoprotein antigens that induce antibodies in AIDS patients are encoded by HTLV-III. Science 1985; 228:1091-3.
6. McDougal JS, Kennedy MS, Sligh JM, et al. Binding of HTLV-III/LAV to T-4+ cells by a complex of the 110,000 viral protein and the T-4 molecule. Science 1986; 231:383-5.
7. Gonda MA, Wong-Staal F, Gallo RC, et al. Sequence homology and morphologic similarity of HTLV-III and visna virus, pathogenic lentivirus. Science 1985; 227:173-7.
8. Clements JE, Pedersen FS, Narayan O, Haseltine WA. Genomic changes associated with antigenic variation of visna virus during persistent infection. Proc Natl Acad Sci USA 1980; 77:4454-8.
9. Narayan O, Griffin DE, Chase J. Antigenic shift of visna virus in persistently infected sheep. Science 1977; 197:576-8.
10. Chang NT, Chanda PK, Barone AD, et al. Expression in *Escherichia coli* of open reading frame gene segments of HTLV-III. Science 1985; 228:93-6.
11. Robey WG, Arthur LO, Matthews TJ, et al. Prospect for prevention of human immunodeficiency virus infection: Purified 120-kDa envelope glycoprotein induces neutralizing antibody. Proc Natl Acad Sci USA 1986; 83:7023-7.
12. Arthur LO, Pyle SW, Nara PL, et al. Serological responses in chimpanzees inoculated with human immunodeficiency virus glycoprotein (gp120) subunit vaccine. Proc Natl Acad Sci USA 1987; 84:8583-7.
13. Chanh TC, Dreesman GR, Kanda P, et al. Induction of anti HIV neutralizing antibodies by synthetic peptides. Embo J 1986; 5:3065-71.
14. Dreesman GR, Chanh TC, Kanda P, et al. Immune response and challenge of chimpanzees immunized with a gp41 synthetic peptide [Abstract]. Washington, D.C.: III International Conference on AIDS, 1987:180.
15. Mitsuya H, Matis LA, Megson M, et al. Generation of an HLA restricted cytotoxic T cell line reactive against cultured tumor cells from a patient infected with human T-cell leukemia/lymphoma virus (HTLV). J Exp Med 1983; 158:994.
16. Zagury D, Leonard R, Fouchard M, et al. Immunization against AIDS in humans. Nature 1987; 326:249-50.
17. Alter HJ, Eichberg JW, Masur H, et al. Transmission of HTLV III infection from human plasma to chimpanzees: an animal model for AIDS. Science 1984; 226:549-52.
18. Kanki PJ, Alroy J, Essex M. Isolation of retrovirus related to HTLV-III/LAV from wild-caught African green monkeys. Science 1985; 230:951.
19. Marx PA, Maul DH, Orbson KG, et al. Simian AIDS: isolation of a type D retrovirus and transmission of the disease. Science 1984; 223:1083-6.
20. Rusche JR, Lynn DL, Robert-Guroff M, et al. Humoral immune response to the entire human immunodeficiency virus envelope glycoprotein made in insect cells. Proc Natl Acad Sci USA 1987; 84:6924-8.
21. Hu SL, Fultz PN, McClure HM, et al. Effect of immunization with a vaccinia-HIV *env* recombinant on HIV infection of chimpanzees. Nature 1987; 328:721-3.
22. Zarling JM, Morton W, Moran PA, et al. T-cell responses to human AIDS virus in macaques immunized with recombinant vaccinia viruses. Nature 1986; 323:344-6.
23. Mayer KH, Falk LA, Paul DA, et al. Correlation of enzyme-linked immunosorbent assays for serum human immunodeficiency virus antigen and antibodies to recombinant viral proteins with subsequent clinical outcomes in a cohort of asymptomatic homosexual men. Am J Med 1987; 83:208-12.

24. Kannagi M, Kiyotaki M, King NW, et al. Simian immunodeficiency virus induces expression of class II major histocompatibility complex structures on infected target cells in vitro. J Virol 1987; 61:1421-6.

25. Lasky LA, Nakamura G, Smith DH, et al. Delineation of a region of the human immunodeficiency virus type 1 gp120 glycoprotein critical for interaction with the CD4 receptor. Cell 1987; 50:975-85.

26. Reitz MS Jr, Wilson C, Naugle C, Gallo RC, Robert-Guroff M. Generation of a neutralization-resistant variant of HIV-1 is due to selection for a point mutation in the envelope gene. Cell 1988; 54:57-63.

27. Saag MS, Hahn BH, Gibons J, et al. Extensive variation of human immunodeficiency virus type-1 in vivo. Nature 1988; 334:440-4.

28. Rusche JR, Javaherian K, McDanal C, et al. Antibodies that inhibit fusion of human immunodeficiency virus-infected cells bind a 24-amino acid sequence of the viral envelope, gp120. Proc Natl Acad Sci USA 1988; 85:3198-202.

29. Golding H, Robey FA, Gates FT III, et al. Identification of homologous regions in human immunodeficiency virus I gp41 and human MHC class II β 1 domain. I. Monoclonal antibodies against the gp41-derived peptide and patients' sera react with native HLA class II antigens, suggesting a role for autoimmunity in the pathogenesis of acquired immune deficiency syndrome. J Exp Med 1988; 167:914-23.

30. Arthur LO, Pyle SW, Nara PL, et al. Serological responses in chimpanzees inoculated with human immunodeficiency virus glycoprotein (gp120) subunit vaccine. Proc Natl Acad Sci USA 1987; 84:8583-7.

31. Eichberg JW, Zarling JM, Alter HJ, et al. T-cell responses to human immunodeficiency virus (HIV) and its recombinant antigens in HIV-infected chimpanzees. J Virol 1987; 61:3804-8.

32. Walker BD, Flexner C, Paradis TJ, et al. HIV-1 reverse transcriptase is a target for cytotoxic T lymphocytes in infected individuals. Science 1988; 240:64-6.

33. Zagury D, Bernard J, Cheynier R, et al. A group specific anamnestic immune reaction against HIV-1 induced by a candidate vaccine against AIDS. Nature 1988; 332:728-31.

34. Kanagi M, Chalifoux LV, Lord CI, Letvin NL. Suppression of simian immunodeficiency virus replication in vitro by CD8+ lymphocytes. J Immunol 1988; 140:2237-42.

35. Homsy J, Meyer M, Tateno M, et al. The Fc and not CD4 receptor mediates antibody enhancement of HIV infection in human cells. Science 1989; 244:1357-60.

36. Mosier DE, Gulizia RJ, Baird SM, Wilson DB. Transfer of a functional human immune system to mice with severe combined immunodeficiency. Nature 1988; 335:256-9.

37. McCune JM, Namikawa R, Kaneshima H, et al. The SCID-Hu mouse: murine model for the analysis of human hematolymphoid differentiation and function. Science 1988; 241:1632-9.

38. Nakikawa R, Kaneshima H, Lieberman M, et al. Infection of the SCID-Hu mouse by HIV-1. Science 1988; 242:1684-6.

HIV Target-Cell Interactions

Farzad Khayam-Bashi, B.S., and Michael S. McGrath, M.D., Ph.D.

The human immunodeficiency virus (HIV) preferentially infects cells that express CD4 (leu-3/T4), the T-cell-identifying molecule, on their surface.[1,2] HIV gains entry into CD4+ T lymphocytes by direct fusion of the virus envelope with the plasma membrane of the cell; this fusion is pH-independent[12] and does not require endocytosis. Macrophages and monocytes are also susceptible to HIV infection and are known to express surface CD4 molecules.[13] In persons who develop AIDS, the infection of CD4+ cells in vivo leads to the gradual but persistent depletion of this T-cell subpopulation.

HIV infection of peripheral blood lymphocytes results in a burst of HIV production from CD4+ T cells. HIV-infected cells form characteristic multinucleated giant cells that die within 24 to 48 hours. In vitro cultures show this virus burst to occur between 5 and 14 days after the initial infection; cultures maintained longer than three to four weeks are devoid of CD4+ cells.[3] HIV infection of certain T-cell lines (Jurkat), with the subsequent expression of HIV *tat* protein, causes an increase in CD4 receptor expression, thus allowing superinfection.[27] T cells can also take up HIV *tat* protein from their environment. *Tat* protein may thus function to transactivate latent virus.[28] In addition, current evidence indicates that HIV replication facilitates the disappearance of the CD4 receptor by causing gp120-receptor complexes, thereby masking the gp120-binding CD4 epitope. CD4 mRNA transcription is also reduced, thereby inhibiting the synthesis of new CD4 receptors.[29] However, it is important to note that the cytopathic effects of HIV correlate primarily with virus production from infected cells and syncytial cells. Syncytial formation is an "early and transitory" phenomenon and correlates poorly with cell killing.[14,15]

The most critical result of HIV infection of a CD4+ T-lymphocyte population is cell death. HIV-associated multinucleated giant cell formation and induction of cellular cytopathology are mediated through CD4-directed cell fusion.[9] This fusion occurs between an HIV-infected T lymphocyte and an uninfected CD4+ lymphocyte. In vitro, this interaction results in cell-to-cell fusion, and leads to a burst of virus production and subsequent cell death after a short time. The effect is completely blocked by antibodies to CD4 as well as by antisera to recombinant HIV gp160 — specifically to a central portion of the envelope (a 24 amino acid sequence).[16] Most if not all CD4+ normal T lymphocytes and the majority of CD4+ T-cell lines tested are permissive for HIV infection and die a short time after in vitro infection. Three T-cell lines have been discovered, however, that are permissive for HIV infection, show a minimal amount of cytopathology, and can replicate infectious HIV at a high level. Although these three in vitro T-lymphoma cell lines, CEM,[4] H9,[5] and HUT-78[6] all express cell-surface CD4 molecules, they are not killed by HIV. One major difference between these cell lines and those killed by HIV is that these three T-lymphoma cell lines contain integrated HIV genomes, but do not accumulate intracytoplasmic double-stranded HIV DNA to the same extent as those killed by the virus. The over-accumulation of intracytoplasmic double-stranded HIV DNA may lead directly to cell death in vitro.[7]

Antibodies to CD4 block HIV infection of T-cell lines and T lymphocytes in vitro.[4,8] Preincubation of human T lymphocytes or T-lymphoma cell lines with antibodies to CD4 determinants blocks HIV infectivity and the development of typical HIV-associated cytopathology in vitro. The use of anti-CD4 has proven effective in vitro, but it is unlikely that anti-CD4 can serve as an effective therapeutic in vivo because these antibodies may lead to the destruction of CD4+ T cells. Similarly, soluble CD4 injected into patients may cause the generation of autoantibodies via an anti-idiotypic mechanism and actually tag CD4+ cells for destruction by the immune system, thus inducing further immunosuppression.[17]

Mutant cell lines, specifically those that become CD4 negative after a productive HIV infection in vitro, are resistant to subsequent HIV infection.[4,9] These data indicate that CD4 plays a critical role in the attachment of the retrovirus. They also show that genetically identical CD4-negative T-cell clones are completely nonpermissive for HIV infection in vitro.

The CD4 molecule mediates the binding of HIV to the surface of T lymphocytes and lymphoma cell lines by interacting with the HIV envelope glycoprotein gp120.[10] Anti-CD4 monoclonal antibodies co-isolate with the CD4 molecule and the envelope glycoprotein of HIV gp120 when both are present in vitro. Similarly, antibodies containing anti-HIV gp120 activity co-isolate the 58 kd molecular weight CD4 molecule. A battery of anti-CD4 monoclonal antibodies have been tested for their ability to block HIV binding and to inhibit gp120-CD4 interactions. Monoclonal antibodies recognizing the OKT4a (leu 3a) epitope most specifically interrupted these interactions.

Purified CD4 interacts with purified HIV gp120 with a high affinity. The strong affinity of HIV gp120 for the cell-surface receptor, CD4 (approximate dissociation constant $= 4 \times 10^{-9}$ M) has led several groups to develop soluble recombinant CD4 molecules as potential inhibitors of HIV binding, virus replication, and syncytial formation.[17] Through mutation studies, the portion of CD4 that interacts with gp120 has been located in the N-terminal one-quarter of the CD4 molecule.[18] MHC class II specific T-cell interactions were uninhibited by CD4 proteins, whereas they virtually ceased when equivalent amounts of anti-CD4 antibodies were present.[19]

Although the mechanism of T-cell depletion is not thoroughly understood, a current and novel theory proposes that a subset of CD4+ gp120-specific class II restricted cytotoxic lymphocyte clones direct their cytolytic activity to uninfected activated CD4+ T cells in reaction to gp120 uptake by the CD4 receptor. It may be that activated CD4+ T cells that respond to common pathogens coinfecting AIDS patients (for example, Epstein–Barr virus or cytomegalovirus) are selectively destroyed by these CD4+ gp120-specific cytotoxic lymphocytes as a consequence of the interaction of gp120 with the CD4 receptor. Recent evidence also indicates that antibodies against a peptide sequence within the HIV *env* protein cross-react with human interleukin-2, leading to the suppressive autoimmune responses that have been observed in AIDS patients.[30] This interaction may delete critical helper T-cell clonal specificities, leaving the individual susceptible to further opportunistic infections.[20]

Many non-T lymphocytes can be productively infected with HIV.[11] Evidence exists that monocytes and macrophages may be productively infected with HIV. It has been suggested that HIV's entry to non-lymphoid cells is mediated by receptors other than CD4, such as Fc receptors on monocytes.[21,31] Mannosyl residues on HIV gp120 are important in HIV-1 pathogenesis, and macrophages have abundant mannose receptors that could be responsible for some HIV-1 binding.[22] HIV may infect progenitor cells of human bone marrow, which may serve as a potential reservoir of HIV.[23,32] Langerhans' cells, which are epidermal antigen-presenting cells, can also be infected by HIV,[23,33] as can natural killer (NK) cells.[24] Some B cells can also be infected with HIV. Despite the presence of Epstein—Barr virus, B-cell lines were demonstrably susceptible to both HIV-1 and HIV-2 infections.[25] Recent evidence also suggests that a subpopulation of cells within the human brain may be infected with HIV.[7,11] Furthermore, recent studies indicate that the neuropathology linked with HIV may result from the *env* gp120 shed from HIV interfering with endogenous neurotropics.[34]

Computerized analysis of secondary structures of HIV-1, HTLV-I, and HTLV-II envelope proteins revealed that the three viruses share only one antigenic epitope, which is composed of amino acids EAL. A similar antigenic epitope is also found in the human and rat brain hormone vasopressin—neurophysin. It is possible that antibodies to the antigenic epitope EAL of HIV may cross-react in AIDS patients with brain vasopressin—neurophysin, leading to a decline in this brain peptide hormone and the onset of symptoms similar to those seen in multiple sclerosis.[26] Molecules mediating HIV binding and productive infection of these various cell populations have yet to be characterized, but CD4 antigenic determinants have been detected on cells other than T lymphocytes, including monocytes and some B-cell lines.

REFERENCES

1. Gallo RC, Wong-Staal F. A human T-lymphotropic retrovirus (HTLV-III) as the cause of the acquired immunodeficiency syndrome. Ann Intern Med 1985; 103:679-89.

2. Montagnier L. Lymphadenopathy-associated virus: from molecular biology to pathogenicity. Ann Intern Med 1985; 103:689-93.

3. Klatzman D, Barre-Sinoussi F, Nugeyre MT, et al. Selective tropism of lymphadenopathy associated virus (LAV) for helper-inducer T lymphocytes. Science 1984; 225:59-63.

4. Dagleish AG, Beverley PCL, Clapham P, et al. The CD4 (T4) antigen is an essential component of the receptor for the AIDS retrovirus. Nature 1984; 312:763-7.

5. Popovic M, Sarngadharan MG, Read E, Gallo RC. Detection, isolation, and continuous production of cytopathic retroviruses (HTLV-III) from patients with AIDS and pre-AIDS. Science 1984; 224:497-500.

6. Levy JA, Hoffman AD, Kramer SM, et al. Isolation of lymphocytopathic viruses from San Francisco patients with AIDS. Science 1984; 225:840-2.

7. Levy JA, Kaminsky LS, Morrow WJW, et al. Infection by the retrovirus associated with the acquired immunodeficiency syndrome. Ann Intern Med 1985; 103:694-9.

8. Klatzman D, Hampagne E, Chamaret S, et al. T-lymphocyte T4 molecule behaves as the receptor for human retrovirus LAV. Nature 1984; 312:767-8.

9. Lifson JD, Reyes GR, McGrath MS, et al. AIDS retrovirus induced cytopathology: giant cell formation is mediated by cell-cell fusion involving the CD4 molecule. Science 1986; 232:1123-7.

10. McDougal JS, Kennedy MS, Sligh JM, et al. Binding of HTLV-III/LAV to T-4+ T cells by a complex of the 110,000 viral protein and the T-4 molecule. Science 1986; 231:383.

11. Levy JA, Shimabukuro J, McHugh T, et al. AIDS associated retroviruses (ARV) can productively infect other cells besides human T helper cells. Virology 1985; 147:441-8.

12. Stein BS, Gowda SD, Lifson JD, et al. pH-independent HIV entry into CD4-positive T cells via virus envelope fusion to the plasma membrane. Cell 1987; 49:659-68.

13. Maddon PJ, McDougal JS, Clapham PR, et al. HIV infection does not require endocytosis of its receptor, CD4. Cell 1988; 54:865-74.

14. Somasundaran M, Robinson HL. A major mechanism of human immunodeficiency virus-induced cell killing does not involve cell fusion. J Virol 1987; 61:3114-9.

15. Leonard R, Zagury D, Desportes I, et al. Cytopathic effect of human immunodeficiency virus in T4 cells is linked to the last stage of virus infection. Proc Natl Acad Sci USA 1988; 85:3570-4.

16. Rusche JR, Javaherian K, McDanal C, et al. Antibodies that inhibit fusion of human immunodeficiency virus-infected cells bind a 24-amino acid sequence of the viral envelope gp120. Proc Natl Acad Sci USA 1988; 85:3198-202.

17. Lasky LA, Nakamura G. Delineation of a region of the human immunodeficiency virus type 1 gp120 glycoprotein critical for interaction with the CD4 receptor. Cell 1987; 50:975-85.

18. Bedinger P, Moriarty A, von Borstel RC II, et al. Internalization of the human immunodeficiency virus does not require the cytoplasmic domain of CD4. Nature 1988; 334:162-5.

19. Hussey RE, Richardson NE, Kowalski M, et al. A soluble CD4 protein selectively inhibits HIV replication and syncytium formation. Nature 1988; 331:78-81.

20. Siliciano RF, Lawton T, Knoll C, et al. Analysis of host-virus interactions in AIDS with anti-gp120 T cell clones: effect of HIV sequence variation and a mechanism for CD4+ cell depletion. Cell 1988; 54:561-75.

21. Weiss RA. Receptor molecule blocks HIV. Nature 1988; 331:15.

22. Robinson WE Jr, Montefiori DC, Mitchell WM. Evidence that mannosyl residues are involved in human immunodeficiency virus type 1 (HIV-1) pathogenesis. AIDS Res Hum Retrovir 1987; 3:265-82.

23. Rappersberger K, Gartner S. Langerhans cells are an actual site of HIV 1 replication. Intervirology 1988; July–August:185-94.

24. Robinson WE Jr, Mitchell WM, Chambers WH, et al. Natural killer cell infection and inactivation in vitro by the human immunodeficiency virus. Hum Pathol 1988; 19:535-40.

25. Monroe JE, Calendar A, Mulder C. Epstein-Barr virus-positive and -negative B-cell lines can be infected with human immunodeficiency virus types 1 and 2. J Virol 1988; 62:3497-500.

26. Becker Y. Multiple sclerosis autoantibodies and antibodies in AIDS may deplete a brain peptide hormone. Med Hypotheses 1988; 26:1.

27. Koka P, Yunis J, Passarelli AL, et al. Increased expression of CD4 molecules on Jurkat cells mediated by human immunodeficiency virus *tat* protein. J Virol 1988; 62:4353-7.

28. Frankel AD, Pabo CO. Cellular uptake of the *tat* protein from human immunodeficiency virus. Cell 1988; 55:1189-93.

29. Salmon P, Olivier R, Riviere Y, et al. Loss of CD4 membrane expression and CD4 mRNA during acute human immunodeficiency virus replication. J Exp Med 1988; 168:1953-69.

30. Bost KL, Pascual DW. Antibodies against a peptide sequence within the HIV envelope protein cross-reacts with human interleukin-2. Immunol Invest 1988; 17:577-86.

31. Pauza CD, Price TM. Human immunodeficiency virus infection of T cells and monocytes proceeds via receptor-mediated endocytosis. J Cell Biol 1988; 107:959-68.

32. Folks TM, Kessler SW, Orenstein JM, et al. Infection and replication of HIV-1 in purified progenitor cells of normal human bone marrow. Science 1988; 242:919-22.

33. Braathen LR. Langerhans cells and HIV infection. Biomed Pharmacother 1988; 42:305-8.

34. Brenneman DE, Westbrook GL, Fitzgerald SP, et al. Neuronal cell killing by the envelope protein of HIV and its prevention by vasoactive intestinal peptide. Nature 1988; 335:639-42.

HIV Stability and Methods for Inactivation

Michael S. McGrath, M.D., Ph.D.

The human immunodeficiency virus (HIV) is stable for long periods of time at room temperature.[1,2] Solutions of HIV were analyzed for presence of infectious particles and reverse transcriptase activity after exposure to different temperatures over a three-week time period. Competent HIV was no longer detectable after three to five hours at 56°C, after 11 days at 37°C, and was barely detectable after 15 days at room temperature (20° to 23°C). HIV solutions that were allowed to dry at room temperature yielded infectious particles upon reconstitution between three and seven days after the initial drying step.[1,2] In contrast to HIV in solution, cell-associated HIV in preparations that were dried and then reconstituted no longer yielded infectious virus 24 hours after drying.

Infectious HIV present in human plasma may copurify with factor VIII during preparation of factor VIII concentrate. HIV was detected in cryoprecipitate prepared from artificially infected human plasma and could be inactivated by heating at 60°C for one half hour.[3] Lyophilized (freeze-dried) Factor VIII concentrate prepared from this HIV infected cryoprecipitate yielded infectious HIV up to 36 hours after heating at 60°C. This experiment showed the marked resistance of dried HIV to heat not characteristic of HIV in solution. Therefore, HIV appears to be most stable in liquid form at room temperature, and is most susceptible to heat inactivation in liquid form. Dried HIV is also very stable and may remain infectious on contaminated needles or laboratory surfaces exposed to infected blood for an extended period of time. This stability emphasizes the importance of decontamination procedures. These procedures should be implemented by laboratories working with or exposed to fluids containing human immunodeficiency viruses.

HIV is inactivated after in vitro exposure to a wide range of detergents, disinfectants, and tissue fixatives.[1,4,5] Table 1 shows the concentration of various substances that have been shown to inactivate HIV in vitro. All substances inactivated infectious HIV within 1 to 30 minutes of exposure; substances 1, 2, and 6 were active within 1 minute.

HIV is insensitive to very high doses of gamma and ultraviolet light irradiation. When HIV preparations were exposed to increasing doses of gamma rays, the lowest dose that resulted in complete inactivation of infectious HIV was 2.5×10^5 rads, or at least ten times more than that normally used for sera and food sterilization.[6] The level of ultraviolet light emitted by the germicidal light present in biohazard laminar flow hoods has no effect on HIV infectivity. An ultraviolet light dose of 5000 J/square meter was required to inactivate HIV in vitro, a level much higher than that attained in operating rooms and laboratories that are exposed to standard germicidal lights for sterilization between use. These observations and those outlined in Table 1 suggest that chemical disinfection is the only quick and reliable method for inactivating surfaces and equipment contaminated by HIV.

TABLE 1.   SUBSTANCES AND CONCENTRATIONS SHOWN TO INACTIVATE HIV IN VITRO

SUBSTANCE	CONCENTRATION
1. Sodium hypochlorite (bleach)	0.2†
(1:10 dilution of bleach = 0.5%)	0.5†
	1.0‡
2. Alcohol (ethanol)	25%†
Isopropyl alcohol	70%*
3. Formalin (0.37% formaldehyde)	1.0%‡
4. Glutaraldehyde	0.0125–1%†
5. Paraformaldehyde	0.5%‡
6. Nonionic detergent, NP-40	0.5%*
7. Quaternary ammonium solutions (disinfectants, normal strength)	0.08%*
8. Sodium hydroxide (NaOH)	0.04M

*   *See reference 1.*
†   *See reference 4.*
‡   *See reference 5.*

REFERENCES

1. Resnick L, Veren K, Salahuddin SZ, et al. Stability and inactivation of HTLV-III/LAV under clinical and laboratory environments. JAMA 1986; 225:1187-91.
2. Barre-Sinoussi F, Nugeyre MT, Chermann JC. Resistance of AIDS virus at room temperature. Lancet 1985; 2:721-2.
3. Levy JA, Mitra GA, Wong MF, Mozen MM. Inactivation by wet and dry heat of AIDS-associated retroviruses during factor VIII purification from plasma. Lancet 1985; 1:1456.
4. Spire B, Barre-Sinoussi F, Montagnier L, Chermann JC. Inactivation of lymphadenopathy-associated virus by chemical disinfectants. Lancet 1984; 2:899-900.
5. Lifson JD, Sasaki DT, Engleman EG. Utility of formaldehyde fixation for flow cytometry and inactivation of the AIDS associated retrovirus. J Immunol Methods 1986; 86:143-9.
6. Spire B, Dormont D, Barre-Sinoussi F, et al. Inactivation of lymphadenopathy-associated virus by heat, gamma rays, and ultraviolet light. Lancet 1985; 1:188-9.

3.1.5

Genetic Heterogeneity
of HIV Isolates

Gandis G. Mazeika, B.S., and Michael S. McGrath, M.D., Ph.D.

The human immunodeficiency virus (HIV) displays an unusual degree of genetic variation.[1] Genetic heterogeneity between individual isolates was documented as early as 1984.[2,4] By 1985, over 130 AIDS viral isolates had been reported in the literature.[2,3] More recently, genetically distinct (though closely related) subsets of HIV have been demonstrated within single, chronically infected individuals.[13,14] This suggests a very rapid rate of spontaneous mutation.

Several types of genetic variation have been documented in HIV, including DNA base insertion, deletion, substitution, and duplication. Such changes are probably the result of errors in reverse transcription (RNA→DNA), forward transcription (DNA→RNA), copy-choice misreading of viral RNA templates, and possibly recombination between different coexisting viral forms. Any of these occurrences may result in altered amino acid sequences in viral proteins.[2,6] The primary mechanism accounting for the remarkable heterogeneity of HIV isolates, however, appears to be the exceptionally high error rate of HIV reverse transcriptase (RT). The error rate of HIV-1 may be as high as 1 in 1700.[26]

The extent of genetic heterogeneity between independent HIV isolates has been assayed by several methods. In one approach, DNA copies of HIV genomes were cloned and then studied by restriction endonuclease mapping and nucleotide sequence analysis.[4,8] Heterogeneity was also demonstrated by nucleic acid hybridization studies using HIV genomic RNA from different isolates.[2] RNA from HIV isolates with a high degree of similarity hybridized more efficiently than those with a more heterogeneous nucleic acid composition.

Among the different HIV-1 strains, the overall extent of divergence in nucleic acid sequence varies from 1 percent to as much as 10 percent[4,5]; variation within individual HIV genes may be greater. The greatest variation in nucleotide sequence occurs within the envelope gene, which codes for gp41 and gp120. The gene sequence coding for gp120 (the viral surface antigen) may differ between independent isolates by as much as 25 percent.[2,3,5-7,16] Even one conservative substitution in gp120 can drastically reduce the ability of cytotoxic T cells or humoral antibodies to recognize virions or antigen-presenting cells or both. This rapid variation helps HIV-1 to evade immunologic surveillance.[15]

Another implication of HIV-1's rapid rate of mutation is the possibility that target-cell tropism may be both refined and broadened during the course of a person's infection. In a recent experiment, five HIV-1 clones isolated from a single patient were assessed. They had distinct host-cell ranges and markedly different infection kinetics and cytopathogenic properties.[27] Though possible initial infection by multiple isolates cannot be ruled out, it is likely that at least some of these clones emerged during the course of infection.

The extent and rapidity of genetic changes during the course of HIV infection suggests that host factors may exert strong selective pressures on the virus, thus selecting strains capable of not only evading immunologic defense but also of infecting specific cell types preferentially, to interact with specific MHC antigens, and to carry out other feints.[8,9,19] Relative viral infectivity has been assessed by comparing the ratios of plaque-forming unit titers to reverse transcriptase activity for given virus/host cell systems.[10] HIV isolates have also been compared by syncytium-inducing activity in cell lines and by susceptibility to neutralization by HIV antibody-positive human sera.[11,12] The fact that genotypic changes occur more rapidly in vivo than during continuous passaging in vitro[13,14,21] supports the theory that selective pressure may play a significant role in causing this variability.

There is preliminary evidence that genotypic variation in HIV-1 is associated with important clinical differences among infected individuals.[19] For example, genotypically distinct forms have been identified in one patient with pronounced central nervous system dysfunction.[22] The forms could be distinguished on the basis of differential replicative activity in macrophages compared with brain glioma explant cultures. In another recent study, viral isolates were obtained at intervals during the course of infection in four individuals. The development of AIDS-related disease correlated with the emergence of HIV-1 variants that were increasingly cytopathic in vitro.[23]

Not all mutations in HIV-1 result in the production of functional, infectious progeny. A cell line has been identified that contains a defective copy of HIV-1 proviral DNA and that produces noninfectious viral particles lacking reverse transcriptase and endonuclease.[17] The defect was traced to a single-point deletion in the *pol* gene, leading to generation of a truncated form of RT.[18] These findings suggest that HIV can exist in integrated but defective forms, with the possibility of reverting to virulent forms through recombinational events at a later time.

In contrast to the marked overall genetic heterogeneity described between independent HIV isolates, portions of the viral genome appear to be highly conserved between different HIVs.[1,5] Both conserved and variable regions of the HIV viral genome may be critical for specific viral functions. The *env* gene, which encodes the envelope glycoprotein, plays a critical role in the pathogenesis of HIV infection. This gene contains segments that display the greatest degree of variation noted between different HIV isolates, but it also contains several conserved regions. One highly conserved region of the envelope gene encodes the region of the envelope glycoprotein that interacts directly with the CD4 (leu 3/T4) cell surface receptor found on T4 lymphocytes and on subsets of macrophages and glial cells.[24,25] Conserved nucleic acid sequences also flank the cleavage site for the transmembrane portion of the envelope glycoprotein p41.[5] The coexistence of both variable and conserved nucleic acid regions in different HIVs has also been observed in other closely related lentiviruses.[6] These constant and variable gene regions may be responsible for the unique target-cell tropism and pathogenesis of disease induced by this class of viruses. An interesting possibility is that the variable regions of gp120 may function as highly immunogenic decoys, directing the immune response away from the CD4-binding domain. The latter domain, which must remain highly conserved, may be found in a cleft or otherwise protected site.

REFERENCES

1. Essex, M. The etiology of AIDS: introduction and overview. In: Kulsted R, ed. AIDS, Papers from Science, 1982-1985. Washington, D.C.: American Association for the Advancement of Science, 1986; 3-7.

2. Levy JA, Kaminsky LS, Morrow WJW, et al. Infection by the retrovirus associated with the acquired immunodeficiency syndrome. Ann Intern Med 1985; 103:694-9.

3. Gallo RC, Wong-Staal F. HTLV-III as the cause of the acquired immunodeficiency syndrome. Ann Intern Med 1985; 103:679-89.

4. Shaw GM, Hahn BH, Arya SK, et al. Molecular characterization of human T cell leukemia (lymphotropic) virus type III in the acquired immune deficiency syndrome. Science 1984; 226:1165-71.

5. Wong-Staal F, Gallo RC. Human T-cell lymphotropic retroviruses. Nature 1985; 317:395-403.

6. Montagnier L. Lymphadenopathy-associated virus: from molecular biology to pathogenicity. Ann Intern Med 1985; 103:689-93.

7. Rabson AB, Martin MA. Molecular organization of the AIDS retrovirus. Cell 1985; 40:447-80.

8. Hahn B, Gonda M, Shaw G, et al. Genomic diversity of the acquired immune deficiency syndrome virus HTLV-III: different viruses exhibit greatest divergence in their envelope genes. Proc Natl Acad Sci USA 1985; 82:4813-7.

9. Hahn BH, Shaw GM, Taylor ME, et al. Genetic variation in HTLV-III/LAV over time in patients with AIDS or at risk for AIDS. Science 1986; 232:1548-53.

10. Harada S, Yamamoto N, Hinuma Y. Clonal analysis of functional differences among strains of human immunodeficiency virus (HIV). J Virol Methods 1987; 18:291-303.

11. Cheng-Mayer C, Homsy J, Evans LA, Levy JA. Identification of human immunodeficiency virus subtypes with distinct patterns of sensitivity to serum neutralization. Proc Natl Acad Sci USA 1988; 85:2815-9.

12. Tersmette M, De Goede RE, Al BJ, et al. Differential syncytium-inducing capacity of human immunodeficiency virus isolates: frequent detection of syncytium-inducing isolates in patients with acquired immunodeficiency syndrome (AIDS) and AIDS-related complex. J Virol 1988; 62:2026-32.

13. Saag MS, Hahn BJ, Gibbons J, et al. Extensive variation of human immunodeficiency virus type-1 in vivo. Nature 1988; 334:440-4.

14. Fisher AG, Ensoli B, Looney D, et al. Biologically diverse molecular variants within a single HIV-1 isolate. Nature 1988; 334:444-7.

15. Siliciano RF, Lawton T, Knall C, et al. Analysis of host-virus interactions in AIDS with anti-gp120 T cell clones: effect of HIV sequence variation and a mechanism for CD4+ cell depletion. Cell 1988; 54:561-75.

16. Gurgo C, Guo HG, Franchini G, et al. Envelope sequences of two new United States HIV-1 isolates. Virology 1988; 164:531-6.

17. Veronese FD, Copeland TD, Oroszlan S, et al. Biochemical and immunological analysis of human immunodeficiency virus *gag* gene products p17 and p24. J Virol 1988; 62:795-801.

18. Gendelman HE, Theodore TS, Willey R, et al. Molecular characterization of a polymerase mutant human immunodeficiency virus. Virology 1987; 160:323-9.

19. Gartner S, Markovits P, Markovitz DM, et al. The role of mononuclear phagocytes in HTLV-III/LAV infection. Science 1986; 232:215-9.

20. Koyanagi Y, Miles S, Mitsuyasu RT, et al. Dual infection of the central nervous system by AIDS viruses with distinct cellular tropisms. Science 1987; 236:819.

21. Shalaby MR, Krowka JF, Gregory TJ, et al. The effects of human immunodeficiency virus recombinant envelope glycoprotein on immune cell functions in vitro. Cell Immunol 1987; 110:140-8.

22. Gallaher WR. Detection of a fusion peptide sequence in the transmembrane protein of human immunodeficiency virus. Cell 1987; 50:327-8.

23. Cheng-Mayer C, Seto D, Tateno M, Levy JA. Biologic features of HIV-1 that correlate with virulence in the host. Science 1988; 240:80-2.

24. Jameson BA, Rao PE, Kong LI, et al. Location and chemical synthesis of a binding site for HIV-1 on the CD4 protein. Science 1988; 240:1335-9.

25. Landau NR, Warton M, Littman DR. The envelope glycoprotein of the human immunodeficiency virus binds to the immunoglobulin-like domain of CD-4. Nature 1988; 334:159-62.

26. Roberts JD, Bebenek K, Kunkel TA. The accuracy of reverse transcriptase from HIV-1. Science 1988; 242:1171-3.

27. Sakai K, Dewhurst S, Ma XY, Volsky DJ. Differences in cytopathogenicity and host cell range among infectious molecular clones of human immunodeficiency virus type 1 simultaneously isolated from an individual. J Virol 1988; 62:4078-85.

Genome Structure: HIV and the Family Retroviridae

Gandis G. Mazeika, B.S., and Michael S. McGrath, M.D., Ph.D.

T he human immunodeficiency virus (HIV) genome displays organizational features similar to those of other retroviruses. Retroviruses can be classified into at least three groups by analyzing the complexity of their genome structure.[1] HIV belongs to the third most complex group (see Figure 3.1.6.a).

■ CHRONIC LEUKEMIA VIRUSES

The simplest genome structure is exhibited by the most commonly occurring retroviruses, the chronic leukemia viruses; these include the following: feline leukemia virus, mouse leukemia virus, avian leukemia virus, and gibbon ape

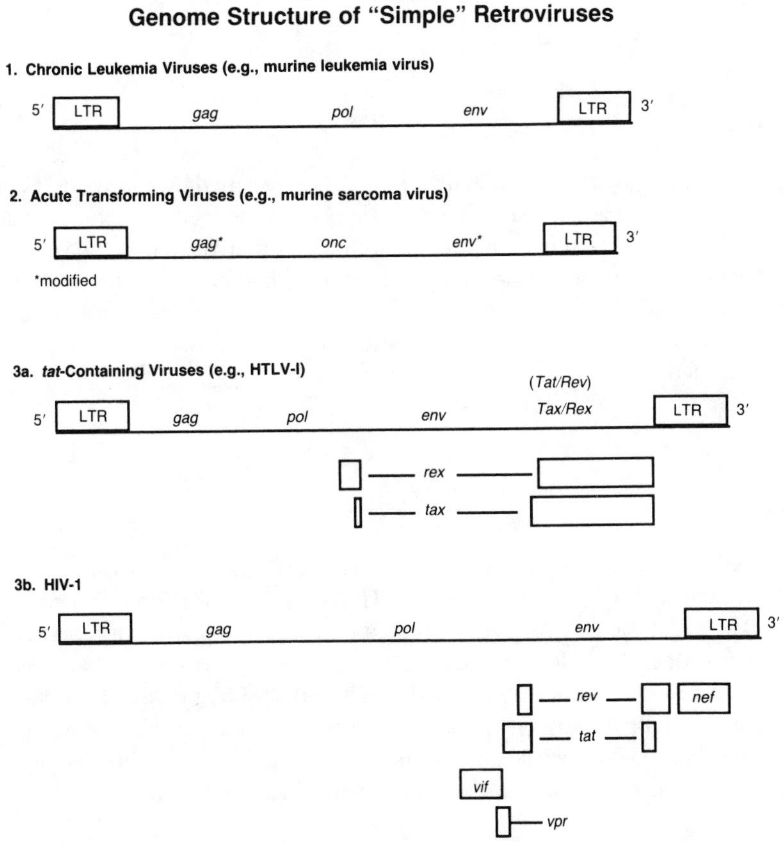

Genome Structure of "Simple" Retroviruses

1. Chronic Leukemia Viruses (e.g., murine leukemia virus)

2. Acute Transforming Viruses (e.g., murine sarcoma virus)
   *modified

3a. *tat*-Containing Viruses (e.g., HTLV-I)

3b. HIV-1

Figure 3.1.6.a

leukemia virus. Their genomes are composed of the three genes required for viral replication: the *gag* gene, for virion internal structural proteins; the *pol* gene, for reverse transcriptase and protease activities; and the *env* gene, for envelope proteins. Like other retroviruses, when integrated into the host genome, both ends are flanked by long terminal repeat (LTR) sequences, which regulate expression of viral genes. In addition, the LTRs may regulate retrovirus integration into the host genome and effect the expression of nearby cellular genes.[1] The leukemias caused by these viruses are monoclonal and have a long latency period (the interval from infection to disease). These viruses may also produce nonmalignant diseases.

■ ACUTELY TRANSFORMING VIRUSES

The second class of retroviruses, the acutely transforming viruses, are generally defective and contain a cell-derived oncogene in addition to the three prototypical viral genes (or portions of them) and LTR sequences contained in the chronic leukemia viruses. Some examples are Rous and murine sarcoma viruses, Abelson leukemia virus, and avian erythroblastosis virus. Oncogene-containing retroviruses may have arisen through a recombinational event between the retroviral and host-cell gene sequences. The resulting transforming virus produces neoplasia with a short latency period. These viruses are rarely isolated in nature and have not been identified in humans.[1]

■ COMPLEX RETROVIRUSES

The third group of retroviral genomes is represented by retroviruses containing one or more additional genes that are not cell-derived. It includes HTLV-I and -II, bovine leukemia virus, and possibly all lentiviruses. All these viruses contain a *tat* gene, which is necessary for viral replication.[2] The *tat* gene encodes a protein that is a transactivator of transcription or translation in infected cells. In addition, it may regulate expression of certain host-cell genes, including the interleukin-2 receptor.[1]

■ HIV

HIV possesses unique features that distinguish it from HTLV-I, -II, and bovine leukemia virus. Genome maps of HTLV-I, -II, and HIV-1 are shown in Table 1. Note that the HIV *tat* gene is located between the *vif* and *env* genes, rather than adjacent to the LTR, as in the HTLV viruses.[4-6] This *tat* gene is not associated with transformation, as it may be in other retroviruses.[1] In addition, HIV possesses five other viral gene sequences that encode specific viral proteins, bringing the total number of HIV-specific genes to nine.[3] The family of retroviruses represented by HIV is the most complex class of retrovirus identified to date.

TABLE 1.   GENOME STRUCTURE OF HTLV-I, -II, AND HIV-1

NAME AND KNOWN DERIVATION	PREVIOUS NAMES	MOLECULAR MASS $\times 10^{-3}$	FUNCTION
HTLV-I and HTLV-II genes:			
tax_1	x-lor,p40x,*tat*$_1$	41,41,42	Transactivator of all viral proteins
tax_2 tat_2	TA	38	
rex_1	pp27x,tel	27	Regulates expression of virion proteins
rex_2		25	
HIV Genes:			
tat (transactivator)	*tat-3*,TA	14	Transactivator of all viral proteins
rev (regulator of viral proteins)	*art,trs*	19,20	Regulates expression of virion proteins
vif (virion infectivity factor)	*sor*,A,P,Q	23	Determines virus infectivity
vpr (R)	R	?	Unknown
nef (negative factor)	3'*orf*,B,E',F	27	Reduces virus expression

REFERENCES

1. Gallo RC, Wong-Staal F. A human retrovirus (HTLV-III) as the cause of the acquired immunodeficiency syndrome. Ann Intern Med 1985; 103:679-89.
2. Chen ISY, Slamon DJ, Rosenblatt JD, et al. The X gene is essential for HTLV replication. Science 1985; 229:54-8.
3. Gallo R, Wong-Staal F, Montagnier L, et al. HIV/HTLV gene nomenclature. Nature 1988; 333:504.
4. Sodroski J, Rosen C, Wong-Staal F, et al. Transacting transcriptional regulation of human T cell leukemia virus type III long terminal repeat. Science 1985; 227:171-3.
5. Arya SK, Guo C, Josephs SF, Wong-Staal F. Transactivator gene of HTLV-III. Science 1985; 229:69-73.
6. Sodroski J, Pataraca R, Rosen C, Wong-Staal F, Hazeltine B. Location of transactivating region of the genome of human T cell lymphotropic virus type III. Science 1985; 229:74-7.

HIV Viral Proteins:
Structure and Function

Gandis G. Mazeika, B.S., and Michael S. McGrath, M.D., Ph.D.

The human immunodeficiency virus (HIV) genome encodes at least seven groups of viral proteins. These groups of proteins include the three classes of polypeptides present in the majority of animal retroviruses:

1. structural, nonenvelope polypeptides encoded by the *gag* gene;

2. enzymes required for virion replication (reverse transcriptase/*rt*) and for cleavage of viral precursor proteins (protease/*pr*), both encoded by the *pol* gene;

3. envelope polypeptides encoded by the *env* gene.

In addition, HIVs possess genes that encode four sets of polypeptides not found in the majority of typical retroviruses (see Figure 3.1.7.a). These include a transactivating regulator of RNA translation (*tat*), a cis-acting downregulator of RNA transcription (*nef*), a regulator that modulates the expression of structural proteins (*rev*), a protein that modulates viral infectivity (*vif*), and two proteins (*vpr, vpu*) whose functions are still unclear. The genomic order of viral genes encoding the initial portion of each of these proteins (5' to 3') is *gag-pr-pol-vif-tat-rev-env-nef*.[1,2]

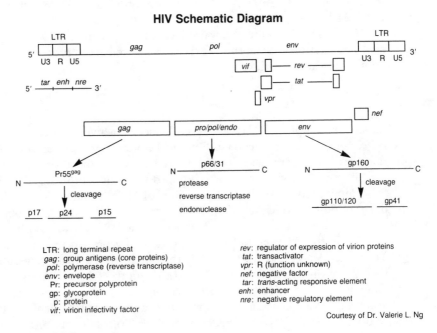

HIV Schematic Diagram

LTR: long terminal repeat
gag: group antigens (core proteins)
pol: polymerase (reverse transcriptase)
env: envelope
Pr: precursor polyprotein
gp: glycoprotein
p: protein
vif: virion infectivity factor

rev: regulator of expression of virion proteins
tat: transactivator
vpr: R (function unknown)
nef: negative factor
tar: *trans*-acting responsive element
enh: enhancer
nre: negative regulatory element

Courtesy of Dr. Valerie L. Ng

Figure 3.1.7.a

EARLY EVENTS IN THE TRANSLATION OF VIRAL STRUCTURAL PROTEINS

Both *gag* and *pol* proteins are initially translated as a single fusion polyprotein, which is noteworthy because, as with other retroviruses, the HIV-1 *gag* and *pol* genes are believed to be in different reading frames.[6] A frameshift may be induced during translation by a stem-loop in the mRNA structure adjacent to the shifting site. The *gag–pol* polyprotein also contains the amino acid sequence of the viral protease.[48] It is unknown whether the polyprotein cleaves itself or whether it must be cleaved by an unassociated protease molecule.

GAG

The *gag* gene encodes three structural proteins that are major constituents of the virion's inner core. During virus replication, these three proteins are synthesized initially as a 55-kilodalton (kd) precursor, processed by the viral protease to an intermediate cleavage product of 40-kd, en route to the final protein products of 17-kd (p17), 24-kd (p24), and 15-kd (p15) in molecular weight.[2,3] p24 is methionine-rich[3] and is phosphorylated[17]; p17, the nucleocapsid protein (NC), is a myristylated phosphoprotein, probably involved in the binding, stabilization, and packaging of viral RNA.[2,49] Evidence from the Moloney Murine Leukemia Virus model suggests that NC is a zinc-binding protein.[49]

HIV *gag* proteins display features both common to and distinct from other retroviruses. HIV p24 is small compared with *gag* proteins of the analogous mammalian type C retrovirus.[4] Immunoprecipitation studies suggest that HIV p24 and the equivalent protein of equine infectious anemia virus (EIAV) share a common epitope. Sera from EIAV-infected horses recognize the p24 of HIV; however, sera from patients with symptomatic HIV disease do not contain antibodies that bind to the EIAV p24.[3] This suggests that the p24 proteins of HIV and EIAV are antigenically related but not identical. In contrast, individuals infected with HTLV-I do not have antibodies that cross-react with the HIV p24.[3]

HIV p17, the amino-terminus product of the *gag* precursor, being myristylated, bears a strong resemblance to the amino-terminal *gag* proteins of all other known human retroviruses.[17]

POL

Reverse transcriptase, RNase H, and endonuclease activities are encoded by the *pol* region of the viral genome. Full biochemical characterization of the endonuclease activity remains to be completed; however, the reverse transcriptase and RNase H activities have been ascribed to a single protein (*rt*).[5,18,19,50] *rt* exists in two active forms: as a homodimer of 66-kd subunits and as a heterodimer of 66-kd and 51-kd subunits.[50] Both 51-kd and 66-kd (p51, p66) proteins have been purified from two independent HIV isolates and have been mapped in the *pol* region of the viral genome by protein sequence analysis. There is evidence, however, that only the p66 form is actually translated and then cleaved into two products, p15 and p51, probably by a cellular protease.[50] Only p66 appears to have polymerase activity, as evidenced by acrylamide gel analysis.[18] RNase H activity is found in p66, and to a lesser extent in p15, the carboxy-terminal cleavage product of p66.[18,19] Both p66 and p51 are highly immunogenic. Antibodies to these proteins are found in 80 percent of HIV-infected patients, regardless of their clinical status.[5]

Human DNA has been shown to contain a wide variety of endogenous retrovirus-related RT coding sequences,[51] which suggests an ancient association between retroviruses and humans.

■ PR

HIV contains protease activity encoded near the 5′ end of the *pol* gene. The protein responsible for this activity, *pr*, has been characterized as 22-kd dimer consisting of two identical 11-kd polypeptides[20,52] and it is known to cleave *gag* and *pol* precursors at a specific nonapeptide sequence. The activity of *pr* is sensitive to inhibitors of aspartic proteases, such as pepstatin,[52,53] suggesting that *pr* belongs to the family of aspartic proteases.

■ ENV

The most important class of proteins required for HIV infectivity is the envelope glycoproteins, which mediate binding of virions to the surface of target cells. These include a large glycoprotein found on the virion surface (SU/gp120) and a smaller transmembrane glycoprotein (TM/gp41) that anchors gp120 to the virion surface.

The gp120 portion of the envelope glycoprotein binds to the CD4 (leu3/T4) molecule on the surface of target T lymphocytes, macrophages, and several other cell types. The active site of gp120 is thought to be in a valley or invagination of the glycoprotein that recognizes a finger-like epitope of CD4.[21-26] The N-linked glycans that stud portions of the surface of gp120 appear to play an important role in CD4-binding.[20,54] Both soluble and virion-associated forms of gp120 bind to CD4, suggesting that the soluble form may participate in immune-system suppression by binding to and blocking recognition of CD4.[27] gp120 is also thought to play a role in early viral replication events[28,29] and may confer resistance to cytolysis in HIV-infected cells.[30] Recent reports suggest that gp120 may be directly toxic to neuronal cells.[55]

Large glycoproteins such as gp120 have been identified only in lentiviruses.[4,7] In contrast, the smaller gp41 closely resembles the transmembrane portion of various viral envelope proteins, including those of mumps, measles, parainfluenza, Sendai and respiratory syncytial viruses.[5,31,32]

The mechanism by which gp120 mediates binding and virus uptake is currently under investigation. Data have been presented showing that binding of HIV to CD4 induces rapid and sustained phosphorylation of CD4, possibly involving protein kinase C. In contrast, soluble gp120 alone was not capable of effecting the same changes.[33] These findings suggest that phosphorylation of CD4 is necessary for infection and that CD4 is activated by the gp120–gp41 complex rather than by gp120 alone. Recent work with truncated and otherwise modified CD4 molecules, however, has demonstrated that the cytoplasmic domain of CD4 is not necessary for virus uptake, suggesting that fusion of viral and cellular membranes is sufficient for infection.[34] These two apparently contradictory reports remain unreconciled.

As with the *gag* proteins, synthesis of the envelope protein involves a number of steps. Initially, the *env* gene is transcribed and translated into a 90-kd polypeptide. This polypeptide is then glycosylated at up to 30 different sites to form a glycoprotein of approximately 160-kd (gp160). gp160 is then cleaved by a cellular protease to form the gp120 and gp41 found in mature virions.[35] While gp120 and gp41 have been isolated from both mature HIV virions and HIV-infected cells, gp160 has been isolated primarily from HIV-infected cells.[2,3,7,8]

■ TAT

The *tat* gene encodes a 14-kd protein that transactivates and increases transcription of DNA in HIV-infected cells.[9,10] The *tat* gene consists of two separate segments that have been mapped to a location in the HIV genome between the *vif* and *nef* regions. It encodes for a 14-kd protein that exists as a metal-linked dimer in infected cells.[36,37] Products of the *tat* gene have been shown to greatly augment the rate of viral protein synthesis in HIV-infected cells, and thus to increase the production of HIV virions. An unusual feature of *tat* is that it is readily taken up by cells and rapidly localizes itself in the nucleus, particularly in the nucleolus.[56] Thus, it is possible that *tat* plays an important role in activating latently infected cells. The effects of *tat* uptake may not be limited to the upregulation of viral replication alone. A recent report that *tat*-transgenic mice develop Kaposi's sarcoma–like lesions suggests that *tat* may stimulate production of endogenous growth factors as well as viral proteins.[57]

The mechanism of action of the *tat* product is controversial. Until recently, it was thought that the HIV *tat* gene encoded a function that was active primarily on the level of protein synthesis (translation from mRNA to protein) in a virus-infected cell.[11] Recent work, however, has demonstrated that the *tat* protein binds to a stem-loop structure in the promoter region of the HIV 5′ long terminal repeat (LTR), and acts as a transcriptional enhancer, possibly functioning by allowing transcription (viral DNA to mRNA) to bypass an early stop codon.[36,38-41,57] These recent findings are more consistent with what is known about the *tat* proteins of the other major class of human retroviruses — the human T lymphotropic viruses (HTLV), which also express a *tat* gene and a protein that increases transcription.

■ REV

The *rev* gene encodes a 20-kd protein that appears to have several important functions, including regulation of transcription and modulation of the relative proportions of structural versus regulatory proteins at the level of transcription.[42] Recent work shows that *rev* is rapidly but transiently phosphorylated by protein kinase C, suggesting that factors affecting protein kinase C activity play an indirect role in HIV regulation.[58]

Recent experiments have shown endogenous sequences in the *env* and *gag* genes that inhibit HIV gene expression. The *rev* protein acts in both *cis* and *trans* forms to relieve repression of gene expression in these genes, either by stabilizing unspliced mRNA transcripts or by assisting in their transport from the nucleus to the cytoplasm, allowing transition to occur.[41,42,44,59,60] These data are supported by the finding that a transfected virus with a defective *rev* gene was only able to synthesize fragments of mRNA not exceeding 1.8 kB in size.[43] Recent work shows that the site of *cis* activity of *rev* is a short segment of mRNA on *env* gene transcripts that is thought to form a stem-loop structure.[59,60] It is unknown if *rev* actually binds to this region. However, deletion or mutation of the region abolishes the production of structural proteins.[60]

▪ NEF

The *nef* protein is a 27-kd polypeptide that downregulates transcription of viral DNA by acting on sequences present in the HIV 5' LTR[45] and may therefore play a role in maintaining viral latency. It is coded for by an open reading frame in the vicinity of the 3' LTR, adjacent to the *env* gene. It is highly antigenic: in a recent study, antibodies to *nef* were found in 60 percent of individuals who had seroconverted to HIV-1 structural proteins.[46]

▪ VIF, VPU, VPR

Little is known yet about these three nonstructural proteins. *vpu* is a 16-kd polypeptide to which antibodies have been found in about one-third of seropositive individuals tested. Preliminary studies suggest that *vpu* may affect the efficiency of viral replication.[47]

The *vif* protein is a 23-kd tryptophan-rich protein that is not essential for virus replication. However, *vif* mutants replicate HIV to a lesser extent than wild-type HIV.[12-14] *vif* is apparently expressed in vivo, judging by the large proportion of HIV-infected individuals with antibodies to *vif* in their sera.

REFERENCES

1. Luria SE, Darnell JE Jr, Baltimore D, Campbell A, eds. General virology. 3rd ed. New York: John Wiley & Sons, 1978; 79-90.
2. Essex M, Allan J, Kanki P, et al. Antigens of human T lymphotropic virus type III/lymphadenopathy associated virus. Ann Intern Med 1985; 103:700-3.
3. Montagnier L. Lymphadenopathy-associated virus: from molecular biology to pathogenicity. Ann Intern Med 1985; 103:689-93.
4. Kramer RA, Schaber MD, Skalka AM, et al. HTLV-III *gag* protein is processed in yeast cells by the virus *pol*-protease. Science 1986; 231:1580-4.
5. Wong-Staal F, Gallo RC. Human T-cell lymphotropic retroviruses. Nature 1985; 317:395-403.
6. Jacks T, Madhani HD, Masiarz FR, Varmus HE. Signals for ribosomal frameshifting in the Rous sarcoma virus *gag-pol* region. Cell 1988; 55:447-58.
7. Robey WG, Safai B, Oroszlan S, et al. Characterization of envelope and core structural gene products of HTLV-III with sera from AIDS patients. Science 1985; 228:593-5.
8. Allan J, Coligen JE, Barin F, et al. Major glycoprotein antigens that induce antibodies in AIDS patients are encoded by HTLV-III. Science 1985; 228:1091-4.
9. Sodroski J, Goh WC, Rosen C, et al. Replicative and cytopathic potential of HTLV-III/LAV with *sor* gene deletions. Science 1986; 231:1549-53.
10. Lee T, Coligan JE, Allan JS, et al. A new HTLV-III/LAV protein encoded by a gene found in cytopathic retroviruses. Science 1986; 231:1546-9.
11. Kan NC, Franchini G, Wong-Staal F, et al. Identification of HTLV-III/LAV *sor* gene product and detection of antibodies in human sera. Science 1986; 231:1553-5.
12. Allan JS, Coligan JE, Lee TH, et al. A new HTLV-III/LAV encoded antigen detected by antibodies from AIDS patients. Science 1985; 230:810-3.
13. Arya SK, Guo C, Josephs SF, Wong-Staal F. Trans-activator gene of human T-lymphotropic virus type III. Science 1985; 229:69-73.
14. Sodroski J, Patarca R, Rosen C, et al. Localization of the trans-activating region of the genome of human T-cell lymphotropic virus type III. Science 1985; 229:74-7.
15. Sodroski J, Goh WC, Dayton A, et al. A second post-translational trans-activator gene required for HTLV-III replication. Nature 1986; 321:412-7.
16. Feinberg MB, Jarrett RF, Aldovini A, et al. HTLV-III expression and production involve complex regulation at the levels of splicing and translation of viral RNA. Cell 1986; 46:807-17.
17. Veronese FD, Copeland TD, Oroszlan S, et al. Biochemical and immunological analysis of human immunodeficiency virus *gag* gene products p17 and p24. J Virol 1988; 62:795-801.
18. Hansen J, Schultze T, Mellert W, Moelling K. Identification and characterization of HIV-specific RNase H by monoclonal antibody. EMBO J 1988; 7:239-43.
19. Starnes MC, Gao W, Ting RYC, Cheng YC. Enzyme activity gel analysis of human immunodeficiency virus reverse transcriptase. J Biol Chem 1988; 263:5132-4.

20. Fenouillet E, Clerget-Raslain B, Gluckman JC, et al. Role of N-linked glycans in the interaction between envelope glycoprotein of human immunodeficiency virus and its CD4 cellular receptor. Structural enzymatic analysis. J Exp Med 1989; 169:807-22.

21. Richardson NE, Brown NR, Hussey RE, et al. Binding site for human immunodeficiency virus coat protein gp120 is located in NH2-terminal region of T4 (CD4) and requires the intact variable-region-like domain. Proc Natl Acad Sci USA 1988; 85:6102-6.

22. Lifson JD, Hwang KM, Nara PL, et al. Synthetic CD4 peptide derivatives that inhibit human immunodeficiency virus infection and cytopathicity. Science 1988; 241:712-6.

23. Bahraoui E, Clerget-Raslain B, Chapuis F, et al. A molecular mechanism of inhibition of HIV-1 binding to CD4+ cells by monoclonal antibodies to gp110. AIDS 1988; 2:165-9.

24. Landau NR, Warton M, Littman DR. The envelope glycoprotein of the human immunodeficiency virus binds to the immunoglobulin-like domain of CD4. Nature 1988; 334:159-62.

25. Peterson A, Seed B. Genetic analysis of monoclonal antibody and HIV binding sites on the human lymphocyte antigen CD4. Cell 1988; 54:65-72.

26. Jameson BA, Rao PE, Kong LI, et al. Location and chemical synthesis of a binding site for HIV-1 on the CD4 protein. Science 1988; 240:1335-9.

27. Shalaby MR, Krowka JF, Gregory TJ, et al. The effects of human immunodeficiency virus recombinant envelope glycoprotein on immune cell functions in vitro. Cell Immunol 1987; 110:140-8.

28. Willey RL, Smith DH, Lasky LA, et al. In vitro mutagenesis identifies a region within the envelope gene of the human immunodeficiency virus that is critical for infectivity. J Virol 1988; 62:139-47.

29. Ho DD, Kaplan JC, Rackauskas IE, Gurney ME. Second conserved domain of gp120 is important for HIV infectivity and antibody neutralization. Science 1988; 239:1021-3.

30. Stevenson M, Meier C, Mann AM, et al. Envelope glycoprotein of HIV induces interference and cytolysis resistance in CD4+ cells: mechanism for persistence in AIDS. Cell 1988; 53:483-96.

31. Gallaher WR. Detection of a fusion peptide sequence in the transmembrane protein of human immunodeficiency virus. Cell 1987; 50:327-8.

32. Gonzalez-Scarano F, Waxham MN, Ross AM, Hoxie JA. Sequence similarities between human immunodeficiency virus gp41 and paramyxovirus fusion proteins. AIDS Res Hum Retroviruses 1987; 3:245-52.

33. Fields AP, Bednarik DP, Hess A, May WS. Human immunodeficiency virus induces phosphorylation of its cell surface receptor. Nature 1988; 333:278-80.

34. Bedinger P, Moriarty A, von Borstel RC II, et al. Internalization of the human immunodeficiency virus does not require the cytoplasmic domain of CD4. Nature 1988; 334:162-5.

35. McCune JM, Rabin LB, Feinberg MB, et al. Endoproteolytic cleavage of gp160 is required for the activation of human immunodeficiency virus. Cell 1988; 53:55-67.

36. Rice AP, Mathews MB. Transcriptional but not translational regulation of HIV-1 by the *tat* gene product. Nature 1988; 332:551-3.

37. Frankel AD, Bredt DS, Pabo CO. *tat* protein from human immunodeficiency virus forms a metal-linked dimer. Science 1988; 240:70-3.

38. Kao SY, Calman AF, Luciw PA, et al. Anti-termination of transcription within the long terminal repeat of HIV-1 by *tat* gene product. Nature 1987; 330:489-93.

39. Falkner FG, Fuerst TR, Moss B. Use of vaccinia virus vectors to study the synthesis, intracellular localization, and action of the human immunodeficiency virus transactivator protein. Virology 1988; 164:450-7.

40. Jakobovits A, Smith DH, Jakobovits EB, Capon DJ. A discrete element 3′ of human immunodeficiency virus 1 (HIV-1) and HIV-2 mRNA initiation sites mediates transcriptional activation by a HIV trans activator. Mol Cell Biol 1988; 8:2555-61.

41. Rice AP, Mathews MB. Trans-activation of the human immunodeficiency long terminal repeat sequences, expressed in an adenovirus vector, by adenovirus E1A 13S protein. Proc Natl Acad Sci USA 1988; 85:4200-4.

42. Rosen CA, Terwilliger E, Dayton A, et al. Intragenic cis-acting *art* gene-responsive sequences of the human immunodeficiency virus. Proc Natl Acad Sci USA 1988; 85:2071-5.

43. Sadaie MR, Benter T, Wong-Staal F. Site-directed mutagenesis of two trans-regulatory genes (*tat-III*, *trs*) of HIV-1. Science 1988; 239:910-3.

44. Malim MH, Hauber J, Fenrick R, Cullen BR. Immunodeficiency virus *rev* trans-activator modulates the expression of viral regulatory genes. Nature 1988; 335:181-3.

45. Ahmad N, Venkatesan S. *nef* protein of HIV-1 is a transcriptional repressor of HIV-1 LTR. Science 1988; 241:1481-5.

46. DeRonde A, Reiss P, Dekker J, et al. Seroconversion to HIV-1 negative regulation factor. Lancet 1988; 2:574.

47. Strebel K, Klimkait T, Martin MA. A novel gene of HIV-1, *vpu*, and its 16-kilodalton product. Science 1988; 241:1221-3.

48. Blundell T, Pearl L. Retroviral proteinases. A second front against AIDS. Nature 1989; 337:596.

49. Gorelick RJ, Henderson LE, Hanser JP, Rein A. Point mutants of Moloney murine leukemia virus that fail to package viral RNA: evidence for specific RNA recognition by a "zinc finger-like" protein sequence. Proc Natl Acad Sci USA 1988; 85:8420-4.

50. Lowe DM, Aitken A, Bradley C, et al. HIV-1 reverse transcriptase: crystallization and analysis of domain structure by limited proteolysis. Biochemistry 1988; 27:8884-9.

51. Shih A, Misra R, Rush MG. Detection of multiple, novel reverse transcriptase coding sequences in human nucleic acids: relation to primate retroviruses. J Virol 1989; 63:64-75.

52. Meek TD, Dayton BD, Metcalf BW, et al. Human immunodeficiency virus 1 protease expressed in *Escherichia coli* behaves as a dimeric aspartic protease. Proc Natl Acad Sci USA 1989; 86:1841-5.

53. Darke PL, Leu CT, Davis LJ, et al. Human immunodeficiency virus protease. Bacterial expression and characterization of the purified aspartic protease. J Biol Chem 1989; 264:2307-12.

54. Mizuochi T, Spellman MW, Larkin M, et al. Carbohydrate structures of the human-immunodeficiency-virus (HIV) recombinant envelope glycoprotein gp120 produced in Chinese-hamster ovary cells. Biochem J 1988; 254:599-603.

55. Brenneman DE, Westbrook GL, Fitzgerald SP, et al. Neuronal cell killing by the envelope protein of HIV and its prevention by vasoactive intestinal peptide. Nature 1988; 335:639-42.

56. Frankel AD, Pabo CO. Cellular uptake of the *tat* protein from human immunodeficiency virus. Cell 1988; 55:1189-93.

57. Vogel J, Hinrichs SH, Reynolds RK, et al. The HIV *tat* gene induces dermal lesions resembling Kaposi's sarcoma in transgenic mice. Nature 1988; 335:606-11.

58. Hauber J, Bouvier M, **Malim MH**, Cullen BR. Phosphorylation of the *rev* gene product of human immunodeficiency virus type 1. J Virol 1988; 62:4801-4.

59. Felber BK, Hadzopoulou-Cladaras M, Cladaras C, et al. *rev* protein of human immunodeficiency virus type 1 affects the stability and transport of the viral mRNA. Proc Natl Acad Sci USA 1989; 86:1495-9.

60. Malim MH, Hauber J, Le S-Y, et al. The HIV-1 *rev* trans-activator acts through a structured target sequence to activate nuclear export of unspliced viral mRNA. Nature 1989; 338:254-7.

Comparison of Human T Lymphotropic Viruses Types I and II and HIV

Farzad Khayam-Bashi, B.S., and Michael S. McGrath, M.D., Ph.D.

The human immunodeficiency virus (HIV) has many characteristics that are similar to those of the human T-lymphoma/leukemia viruses, HTLV-I and HTLV-II.[1] They are all retroviruses and all use a magnesium-requiring reverse transcriptase enzyme for replication. The principal target cell for infection by these viruses is the CD4 (leu3/T-4) T-lymphocyte subpopulation, and all induce multinucleated giant cells within this infected cell population. Their similarities have suggested that these viruses all belong to a common retrovirus family. However, more recent evidence suggests that HIV may be more related to animal lentiviruses than to the HTLVs.[2]

The diseases associated with human retrovirus infection range from malignancies and neurologic disorders to profound immunodeficiency states.[3-5] HTLV-I is the etiologic agent of adult T-cell leukemia (ATL); this neoplasm is an aggressive, high-grade T-cell lymphoma, and is endemic to southern Japan, the Caribbean, Central America, and Central Africa. HTLV-I has also been found in patients with mycosis fungoides and Sezary's syndrome in these endemic areas. HTLV-II was first isolated from a patient with T-cell hairy-cell leukemia,[6] although it has not been directly implicated with the induction of human disease. HIV is the etiologic agent of AIDS.

The different in vivo disease spectra associated with HTLV-I and HIV infection are consistent with their specific behavior in vitro.[1,4,5] HTLV-I has been associated with both T- and B-cell transformation in vitro[7,8] as well as with lymphomas in vivo. In contrast, HIV does not transform lymphocytes, but instead causes profound cytopathic changes in the infected cells. Studies have been conducted to determine if HTLV-I may act as a cofactor for the development of immunosuppression. It has been reported that human peripheral blood leukocytes infected with HIV-1 in vitro can be mitogenically stimulated by noninfectious HTLV-I virions to produce large quantities of HIV-1.[11,12] Both HTLV-I and HIV infections have been reported in a single patient.[18] The patient's recurring polymyositis was attributed to HTLV-I. However, because both HTLV-I and HIV exert their pathologic effects only after long latency periods, the role each virus plays as a direct pathogen is difficult to determine.

The HTLVs and HIV share some similar structural and regulatory proteins. The post-transcriptional regulator (*rex*) of HTLV-I is a positive post-transcriptional regulator for *gag*, *pol*, and *env* protein expression. At high doses, it also acts as an indirect negative regulator of viral transcription. Evidently, *rex* acts in a fashion similar to the *art/trs* of HIV-1.[13] The HTLV types I and II have two nonstructural genes — *tax* and *rex* — that are encoded in overlapping reading frames. These two HTLV regulatory proteins show some similarity to the HIV-1 proteins *tat* and *rev* (or *art/trs*).[14] Recently, investigators have identified and purified a human immunoglobulin enhancer binding protein (NF-kappa B), which is found only in cells that transcribe the immunoglobulin light chain. In vitro, NF-kappa B is capable of activating transcription of HIV-1 promoter.[15] Interestingly, it appears that *tax*, the HTLV-I transactivator, is capable of inducing IL-2 receptor expression through an NF-kappa B-like factor.[16,17] This may prove to be an effective model for explaining the interaction of both HTLV-I and HIV-1 through NF-kappa B-like transcription factors.

Individuals within AIDS risk groups may have antibodies to HTLV-I, HTLV-II, and HIV. Serologic analysis of intravenous drug users[9] and homosexual men[10] has revealed the presence of antibodies to all of the human retroviruses in the sera of a small percentage of individuals. The role that HTLV-I or HTLV-II may play in the pathogenesis of disease within HIV-infected people is currently unknown.

REFERENCES

1. Gallo RC. The human T cell leukemia/lymphotropic retroviruses (HTLV) family: past, present and future. Cancer Res 1985; 45(9 Suppl):4524S-33S.

2. Gonda MA, Wong-Staal F, Gallo RC, et al. Sequence homology and morphologic similarity of HTLV-III and visna virus, a pathogenic lentivirus. Science 1985; 227:173-7.

3. Broder S, Gallo RC. Human T-cell leukemia virus (HTLV): a unique family of pathogenic retroviruses. Ann Rev Immunol 1985; 3:321-36.

4. Wong-Staal F, Gallo RC. The family of human T-lymphotropic leukemia viruses: HTLV-I as the cause of adult T cell leukemia and HTLV-III as the cause of acquired immunodeficiency syndrome. Blood 1985; 65:253-63.

5. Urba GJ, Longo DL. Clinical spectrum of human retroviral induced diseases. Cancer Res 1985; 45(9 Suppl):4637S-43S.

6. Kalyanaraman VS, Sarngadharan MG, Robert-Guroff M, et al. A new subtype of human leukemia virus (HTLV-II) associated with a T-cell variant of hairy cell leukemia. Science 1982; 218:571-3.

7. Koyanagi B, Yamamoto N, Kobayashi N, et al. Characterization of human B-cell lines harbouring both adult T-cell leukemia (ATL) virus and Epstein-Barr virus derived from ATL patients. J Gen Virol 1984; 65:1781-9.

8. Longo D, Gelmann EP, Cossman J, et al. Isolation of HTLV-transformed B-lymphocyte clone from a patient with HTLV-associated adult T-cell leukaemia. Nature 1984; 310:505-6.

9. Robert-Guroff M, Weiss SH, Giron JA, et al. Prevalence of antibodies to HTLV-I, II and III in intravenous drug abusers from an AIDS endemic region. JAMA 1986; 255:3133.

10. Tedder RS, Shanson DC, Jeffries DJ. Low prevalence in the UK of HTLV-I and HTLV-II infection in subjects with AIDS, with extended lymphadenopathy and at risk for AIDS. Lancet 1984; 2:125.

11. Zack JA, Cann AJ, Lugo JP, Chen IS. HIV-1 production from infected peripheral blood T cells after HTLV-I induced mitogenic stimulation. Science 1988; 240:1026-9.

12. Okamoto T, Akagi T, Shima H, et al. Superinduction of trans-activation accounts for augmented human immunodeficiency virus replication in HTLV-I-transformed cells. Jpn J Cancer Res 1987; 78:1297-301.

13. Hidaka M, Inoue J, Yoshida M, Seiki M. Post-transcriptional regulator (*rex*) of HTLV-I initiates expression of viral structural proteins but suppresses expression of regulatory proteins. EMBO J 1988; 7:519-23.

14. Rosenblatt JD, Cann AJ, Slamon DJ, et al. HTLV-II transactivation is regulated by the overlapping *tax/rex* nonstructural genes. Science 1988; 240:919.

15. Kawakami K, Scheidereit C, Roeder RG. Identification and purification of a human immunoglobulin-enhancer-binding protein (NF-kappa B) that activates transcription from a human immunodeficiency virus type 1 promoter in vitro. Proc Natl Acad Sci USA 1988; 85:4700-4.

16. Leung K, Nabel GJ. HTLV-I transactivator induces interleukin-2 receptor expression through an NF-kappa B-like factor. Nature 1988; 333:776-8.

17. Ruben S, Poteat H, Tan TH, et al. Cellular transcription factors and regulation of IL-2 receptor gene expression by HTLV-I *tax* gene product. Science 1988; 241:89-92.

18. Wiley CA, Nerenberg M, Cros D, Soto-Aguilar MC. HTLV-I polymyositis in a patient also infected with the human immunodeficiency virus. N Engl J Med 1989; 320:992-5.

3.1.9

Models for HIV Pathology in Animal Lentiviruses

Suzanne Crowe, M.B.B.S., F.R.A.C.P., and Michael S. McGrath, M.D., Ph.D.

L entiviruses are slowly replicating, pathogenic but nononcogenic retroviruses that until recently were thought to infect only ungulate (hoofed) animals. The prefix lenti was used because of the slow time course of the diseases caused by this group of viruses in animals and humans. The ovine-caprine lentiviruses (visna, maedi, caprine arthritis-encephalitis virus) and the equine infectious anemia virus have similar morphologic properties and exhibit considerable nucleic acid homology.[1] Recently, HIV has been shown to be morphologically similar and to share antigenic determinants and nucleotide sequences with each of the ungulate lentiviruses, particularly with visna.[2-4] These data provide evidence for taxonomic relatedness between HIV and the lentiviruses.

■ GENERAL PATHOLOGIC CHARACTERISTICS

As a group, lentiviruses do not transform the cells they infect (i.e., they are nononcogenic). They replicate at a slow rate within their natural host and cause persistent lifelong infections. Infection is commonly subclinical[5]; however, some infected animals develop slowly progressive inflammatory lesions within target organs, including the central nervous system (CNS), lungs, and joints. The incubation period is generally prolonged (months to years) and symptoms begin insidiously. These features of animal lentivirus infection are shared with human HIV infection.

■ PATHOGENETIC AND IMMUNOLOGIC FEATURES

Monocytes and macrophages are susceptible to infection by all lentiviruses.[6-8] Infection of these cells does not result in cell lysis and this may account in part for the persistent, lifelong infection in the host. Animal lentiviruses will replicate productively at slow rates in mature macrophages within target organs and nonproductively in peripheral blood lymphocytes (PBLs), monocytes, and perhaps other cell lines.[9] Recently, HIV has been shown to infect monocytes and macrophages,[8] as well as CD4+ lymphocytes. Lentiviruses replicate in very few of these infected cells; the majority harbor the virus in a latent form. Active viral replication occurs in only one per hundred or thousand cells.[10] In situ hybridization studies have shown that restriction of replication occurs at the level of transcription of viral DNA.[11] Latently infected cells with a viral genome present as an integrated provirus do not synthesize viral antigens. Restricted gene expression is likely to be the major mechanism retarding virus replication and producing persistent infection and slow disease progression.[10] It is suggested that a latently infected cell, such as the blood monocyte, may transport the virus to tissues including brain and lung, concealing and protecting the virus from immunologic surveillance mechanisms. Once in the tissue, the macrophage may transfer virus to other cells, e.g., choroid plexus cells.[10]

Approximately four to eight weeks after infection, infected animals develop neutralizing antibodies to the envelope glycoproteins and major core proteins of lentiviruses.[7,12] Similarly, humans infected with HIV develop antibodies, including neutralizing antibodies,[13] within three months of infection. Despite the in vitro effectiveness of antibodies in achieving neutralization of virus infectivity, kinetic studies using visna have shown that antibody binding to the visna virus occurs more slowly than binding of virus to target macrophages.[7,14] This kinetic infectious advantage, as well as the potential for direct cell-to-cell spread of virus, suggests that neutralizing antibody would provide little in vivo protection against an invading lentivirus. This coincides with the clinical observation that preexisting antibody does not protect animals against lentivirus infection.

Another factor contributing to the persistence of infection with lentiviruses is the frequent occurrence of spontaneous mutations within the envelope region of the viral genome.[15] Envelope gene mutations are thought to result in the development of mutant lentivirus strains that can escape effective immune surveillance. The phenomenon of antigenic shift has been demonstrated with both visna and EIAV,[15] and most recently, restriction enzyme analysis revealed that different strains of HIV show heterogeneity in the envelope region.[13]

Further analyses must be carried out to determine whether the antigenic and biologic differences noted between different HIV isolates are the result of antigenic drift, or whether individuals with different apparent HIVs have merely been infected with multiple individual HIV species.

■ SPECIFIC ANIMAL MODELS: CLINICAL AND PATHOLOGIC FEATURES

VISNA AND MAEDI

Clinical Features.   Visna, derived from the Icelandic term for wasting, is a slowly progressive neurologic disease originally recognized in Icelandic sheep as an infrequent complication of maedi (Icelandic for shortness of breath).[16] Both diseases are caused by the same virus.

Transmission of the virus occurs via horizontal spread, through contact with infected colostrum or milk, and probably also via droplet transmission. Occasional vertical transmission from mother to offspring has also been documented.[5] Symptoms of visna rarely develop in sheep less than two years of age. Infected animals initially develop ataxia, involving one or both hind limbs, which worsens over ensuing months causing hind-limb paralysis or quadriplegia.[5]

Maedi is the most common clinical manifestation of visna virus infection in adult sheep. Infected sheep develop respiratory distress and a dry cough; cachexia is a prominent feature. Nearly all infected animals die within one year.[5]

Pathology.   Viremia in visna occurs two to four weeks after infection and persists throughout the lifelong illness. Visna virus can be isolated from lymph node, brain, and lung throughout the sheep's life span.[17] However, as with other lentivirus-associated diseases, only minimal quantities of cell-free infectious virus can be obtained from tissue homogenates.[5,17]

Like HIV, visna infects brain, peripheral blood lymphocytes, and monocytes/macrophages.[6,18] Although only about 10 percent of sheep with visna develop overt disease within one year of infection, postmortem studies have revealed that over 80 percent of infected animals have histologic lesions within their central nervous systems (CNS).[12] Two types of pathologic changes have been observed. The most common is an intense accumulation of mononuclear cells distributed as perivascular cuffs or as infiltrates within the neuropil. Less commonly, focal demyelination, meningitis, and choroiditis are evident.[17]

The immune function of visna virus infected sheep is virtually normal and the pathologic lesions of visna are thought to be due to the vigorous antiviral immune response. Immunosuppression of infected sheep with anti-sheep thymocyte serum plus cyclophosphamide lessens the CNS inflammatory response.[19] In contrast, the most common postmortem findings in patients who develop AIDS-associated encephalopathy are cerebral atrophy associated with scattered microglial nodules and minimal inflammation.[18] This lack of inflammatory response in AIDS patients likely reflects depressed immune function, whereas immune mechanisms in sheep with visna are normal. Thus, the pathogenesis of CNS disease in AIDS is probably very different from that in sheep with visna.

CAPRINE ARTHRITIS ENCEPHALITIS

Clinical Features.   Caprine arthritis encephalitis virus (CAEV) infection of goats shares many of the clinical and pathologic features of maedi-visna infection of sheep.[7] Infection results in a chronic inflammatory disease affecting joints, CNS, lungs, and mammary glands. The disease has an insidious onset, is slowly progressive, and results in cachexia, respiratory dysfunction, and chronic arthritis or paralysis.[7] Arthritis is the most common manifestation of infection with CAEV. Arthritis after CAEV infection usually occurs in adult goats and progresses over months to years to a debilitating chronic arthritis, particularly involving the knees. A small percentage of CAEV-infected adult goats develop leukoencephalitis resulting in hind-limb ataxia, which rapidly progresses to quadriplegia and often death.[5,20] The most frequent clinical manifestation of CAEV infection in kids is neurologic disease[21]; but this may occur in older goats as well, in which case the course is more prolonged, similar to sheep with visna. Mild interstitial pneumonia occurs frequently in all CAEV-infected goats.[21]

Pathology.   Autopsy findings usually reveal demyelination within the CNS, as well as a mononuclear inflammatory response within the white matter, which may progress to cavitation.[5,22]

EQUINE INFECTIOUS ANEMIA

Clinical Features.   Equine infectious anemia (EIA) is a chronic, relapsing disease of horses due to infection with EIAV. The initial attack usually occurs within one month of infection and is manifested by fever, anorexia, anemia (due to complement-mediated hemolysis and bone-marrow suppression), and thrombocytopenia.[23] During early stages, infected animals are viremic but do not have detectable antiviral antibodies. The initial attack subsides within one week, but periodic relapses occur that decrease in frequency and intensity over a period of about one year. Eventually most horses become asymptomatic chronic carriers of EIAV with persistence of anti-EIAV antibodies in their sera.[23] Rarely, the disease has a rapidly progressive and fatal course.[24]

Pathogenesis.   EIAV replicates in macrophages and, once infected, the horse remains viremic throughout life.[23] Recurrences of fever and hemolysis result from the development (selection) of antigenic variants of EIAV. Once neutralizing antibody is produced to a variant, virus symptoms remit.[15] Cross-reactivity between EIAV antibodies (directed against p25) and HIV has been reported.[25]

SUMMARY

HIV is a unique nononcogenic retrovirus that may be included within the subfamily Lentivirinae. Although HIV infection results in disease that differs from other lentivirus infections (i.e., profound immunosuppression), there are many similarities between HIV and other members of the Lentivirinae, particularly visna. These similarities include chronic viremia and insidious onset of chronic disease states.

HIV preferentially infects lymphocytes bearing the CD4 differentiation antigen and has recently been shown to infect monocyte/macrophages, a feature shared with the ungulate lentiviruses. HIV has a long incubation period and causes slowly progressive neurologic disease (dementia, encephalopathy), as is seen with visna and caprine leukoencephalitis. Persistent viremia in the presence of neutralizing antibody is a finding common to the Lentivirinae.

Tables 1 and 2 outline many of the unique features of each member of the Lentivirinae family of retroviruses.

TABLE 1.   LENTIVIRUS-ASSOCIATED DISEASE CHARACTERISTICS

	VISNA/MAEDI	CAEV	EIAV	HIV
Disease	wasting paralysis pneumonitis	arthritis leukoencephalitis	anemia	AIDS
Host	sheep	goats	horses	humans
Target Cell	macrophage	macrophage	macrophage	OKT4 lymphocyte macrophage
Primary Organs	brain, lung (joints, mammary glands)	brain (lung, mammary glands)	?	lymphoid organs, brain

TABLE 2.   LENTIVIRUS-ASSOCIATED DISEASE CHARACTERISTICS

	VISNA/MAEDI	CAEV	EIAV	HIV
Persistent viremia	+	+	+	+
Insidious onset of chronic disease	+	+	+	+
Immunosuppression	−	−	−	+
Neutralizing antibody	+	−	+	+
Antigenic shift	+	−	+	?

Ungulate lentivirus infections are of tremendous economic importance; control of these diseases within animal populations has required widespread slaughter. To date no effective vaccine has been developed for any of these lentivirus diseases. Mutations within the region of the envelope gene (visna, EIAV) as well as the identification of genomic variants (HTLV-III, ARV, LAV) have made progress in vaccine development difficult.

REFERENCES

1. Lowry, DR. Transformation and oncogenesis: retroviruses. In: Fields BN, ed. Virology. New York: Raven Press, 1985.

2. Stephens RM, Casey JW, Rice NR. Equine infectious anaemia virus *gag* and *pol* genes: relatedness to visna and AIDS virus. Science 1986; 231:589-94.

3. Gonda MA, Wong-Staal F, Gallo RC, et al. Homology and morphologic similarity of HTLV-III and visna virus, a pathogenic lentivirus. Science 1985; 227:173-7.

4. Chiu IM, Yaniv A, Dahlberg JE, et al. Nucleotide sequence evidence for relationship of AIDS retrovirus to lentivirus. Nature 1985; 317:366-7.

5. Narayan O, Cork L. Lentiviral diseases of sheep and goats: chronic pneumonia, leukoencephalitis and arthritis. Rev Infect Dis 1985; 7:89-98.

6. Gendelman HE, Narayan O, Kennedy-Stoskopf S, et al. Slow virus-macrophage interactions. Lab Invest 1984; 51:547-55.

7. Kennedy-Stoskopf S, Narayan O. Neutralizing antibodies to visna lentivirus: mechanism of action and possible role in virus persistence. J Virol 1986; 59:37-44.

8. Gartner S, Markovits P, Markovitz DM, et al. The role of mononuclear phagocytes in HTLV-III/LAV infection. Science 1986; 233:215-9.

9. Narayan O, Kennedy-Stoskopf S, Sheffer D, et al. Activation of caprine arthritis-encephalitis virus expression during maturation of monocytes to macrophages. Infect Immun 1983; 41:67-73.

10. Haase AT. Pathogenesis of lentivirus infections. Nature 1986; 332:130-6.

11. Haase AT, Stowring L, Narayan O, et al. Slow persistent infection caused by visna virus: role of host restriction. Science 1977; 195:175-7.

12. Petersson G, Nathansen N, Georgssen G, et al. Pathogenesis of visna: I. Sequential virologic, serologic, and pathologic studies. Lab Invest 1976; 35:402-12.

13. Robert-Guroff M, Brown M, Gallo RC. HTLV-III-neutralizing antibodies in patients with AIDS and AIDS-related complex. Nature 1985; 316; 72-4.

14. Griffin DE, Narayan O, Adams RT. Early immune responses in visna, a slow viral disease of sheep. J Infect Dis 1978; 138:340-50.

15. Narayan O, Griffin DE, Chase J. Antigenic shift of visna virus in persistently infected sheep. Science 1976:376-8.

16. Sigrirdsson B, Palsson PA. Visna of sheep. A slow demyelinating infection. Br J Exp Pathol 1958; 39:519-28.

17. Nathanson N, Georgsson G, Palsson PA, et al. Experimental visna in Icelandic sheep: the prototype lentiviral infection. Rev Infect Dis 1985; 7:75-82.

18. Shaw AM, Harper ME, Hahn BH, et al. HTLV-III infection in brains of children and adults with AIDS encephalopathy. Science 1985; 227:177-81.

19. Nathanson N, Panitch H, Palsson PA, et al. Pathogenesis of visna: II. Effect of immunosuppression upon early central nervous system lesions. Lab Invest 1976; 35:444-51.

20. Crawford TB, Adams DS, Cheevers WP, Crok LC. Chronic arthritis in goats caused by retrovirus. Science 1980; 207:997-9.

21. Cork LC, Ladlow WJ, Crawford TB, et al. Infectious leukoencephalomyelitis of goats. J Infect Dis 1974; 129:134-41.

22. Cork LC, Narayan O. The pathogenesis of viral leukoencephalomyelitis arthritis of goats. Lab Invest 1980; 42:596-602.

23. Cheevers WP, McGuire TC. Equine infectious anaemia virus: immunopathogenesis and persistence. Rev Infect Dis 1985; 7:83-8.

24. Charman HP, Bladen S, Gilden RV, Coggins L. Equine infectious anaemia virus: evidence favoring classification as a retrovirus. J Virology 1976; 19:1073-9.

25. Montagnier L. Lymphadenopathy-associated virus: from molecular biology to pathogenicity. Ann Intern Med 1985; 103:689-93.

Relationship Between HIV, the New African Retroviruses HIV-II/HTLV-IV, and the Simian Retroviruses

Suzanne Crowe, M.B.B.S., F.R.A.C.P., and Michael S. McGrath, M.D., Ph.D.

A type D retrovirus, the simian retrovirus type I (SRV-I), is the prototype virus of the simian acquired immune deficiency syndrome (SAIDS) in macaque monkeys. As in HIV infection, the CNS is a reservoir of latent virus.[1] However, this virus's genomic organization and nucleotide sequence differ substantially when compared with HIV.[2]

The animal retrovirus most closely resembling HIV is the simian immunodeficiency virus, SIV (also known as simian T lymphotropic virus, STLV-III). Although this virus has type C morphology (rather than the type D morphology characteristic of HIV), the virus has similar antigenic properties and growth characteristics when compared with HIV. STLV-III infection can also cause clinical features similar to those of HIV.

STLV-III causes an immune deficiency syndrome in captive macaque monkeys.[3] A nonpathogenic variant of STLV-III has also been isolated from healthy African green monkeys (AGM). Antibodies to STLV-III have been detected in the sera of AGMs from Kenya and Ethiopia but not from those in the Caribbean. Because AGMs were first transported to the Caribbean about two hundred years ago, it is likely that infection of these primates with STLV-III occurred within the past two centuries.[4]

Recently, two new human retroviruses have been isolated from individuals in West Africa. These closely related viruses differ in their in vitro cytopathology and their clinical manifestations. HIV-II (also known as LAV-2) has been isolated from AIDS and ARC patients and from asymptomatic individuals from Guinea-Bissau and the Cape Verde Islands.[5-7] HIV-II has been cloned and found to be more closely related to SIV than HIV-I.[8]

Although the core antigens show significant homology, there is wide genetic variation between the envelope glycoproteins of HIV-I and HIV-II. However, HIV-II has similar morphology, cell tropism, and causes similar in vitro cytopathic effects on T-helper lymphocytes.

The second virus, HTLV-IV, has been isolated from healthy prostitutes in Senegal but not from patients with AIDS.[9] This virus is relatively non cytopathic in vitro and is much more closely related to STLV-III than to HIV-II.[10]

The mode of transmission of these human retroviruses in Africa is predominantly via heterosexual contact, parenteral exposure through infected blood transfusions and unsterilized needles, and transmission from infected mothers to their newborn babies. Seroprevalence rates for HIV among healthy blood donors varies from less than 1 percent in the Congo to about 20 percent in

Kigali, Rwanda. Among female prostitutes, seroprevalence varies from 27 percent to 88 percent, depending upon geographic location.[11]

It is likely that all of these human and simian retroviruses have evolved from a common ancestral virus. More detailed genomic comparisons, epidemiologic research, and clinical investigations will increase our understanding of this group of viruses.

REFERENCES

1. Gardner M, Marx P, Maul D, et al. Simian AIDS caused by type D retrovirus [Abstract]. Paris: International Conference on AIDS, 1986; 10.

2. Power MD, Marx PA, Bryant ML, et al. Nucleotide sequence of SRV-I, a type D simian acquired immune deficiency syndrome retrovirus. Science 1986; 231:1567-72.

3. Daniel MD, Letvin NL, Kinp NW, et al. Isolation of T-cell tropic HTLV-III-like retrovirus from macaques. Science 1985; 228:1201-4.

4. Hendry RM, Wells MA, Phelan MA, et al. Prevalence of antibodies to STLV-III agm in African green monkeys from Africa in 1957-62 and 1980-85 and the Caribbean in 1980-85 [Abstract]. Paris: International Conference on AIDS, 1986; 19.

5. Clavel F, Guetard D, Brun-Vezinet F, et al. Isolation of a new human retrovirus from West African patients with AIDS. Science 1986; 233:343-6.

6. Brun-Vezinet F, Katlama C, Roulot D, et al. Lymphadenopathy associated virus type 2 in AIDS and AIDS-related complex. Lancet 1987; 1:128-32.

7. Clavel F, Mansinho K, Chamaret S, et al. Human immunodeficiency virus type 2 infection associated with AIDS in West Africa. N Engl J Med 1987; 316:1180-5.

8. Clavel F, Guyader M, Guetard D, et al. Molecular cloning and polymorphism of the human immune deficiency virus type 2. Nature 1986; 324:691-3.

9. Kanki PJ, Barin F, M'Boup S, et al. New human T-lymphotropic retrovirus related to simian t-lymphotropic virus type III (STLV-III agm). Science 1986; 232:238-43.

10. Kornfeld H, Riedel N, Viglianti GA, et al. Cloning of HTLV-IV and its relation to simian and human immunodeficiency viruses. Nature 1987; 326:610-13.

11. Quinn TC, Mann JM, Curran JW, Piot P. AIDS in Africa: an epidemiologic paradigm. Science 1986; 234:955-63.

3.2

HIV Immunopathogenesis

Immunology of AIDS: Overview

Michael S. McGrath, M.D., Ph.D.

Persons infected with the human immunodeficiency virus (HIV) suffer from a wide spectrum of immunologic abnormalities,[1,2] the most devastating of which is the complete loss of the cellular immune system, resulting in severe opportunistic infections and death.

The immunologic abnormalities associated with HIV infection are thought to be partly the direct result of HIV interactions with specific components of the immune system, and partly the result of activation or inhibition of portions of the immune system by other infectious agents. Virtually all of the components of the immune system are affected, including the controlling elements of the cellular immune system (T cell), the humoral immune system (B cell), as well as other components of the cellular immune system (monocyte/macrophages, natural killer cells).

The most profound and most easily quantitated abnormality in individuals infected with HIV is the gradual but progressive depletion of the CD4 (leu3/T4) expressing T-cell population. This helper T-cell population is normally responsible for inducing effective immune responses in all other T-cell and B-cell compartments.[3] The removal of this one T-cell population contributes to the body's decreased ability to mount cytotoxic T-cell responses to virally infected cells or cancers, to form delayed type hypersensitivity reactions, and, later on in the disease, to make specific antibody responses to new foreign substances that invade an infected individual's body.

Marked abnormalities in mounting specific antibody responses occur in individuals infected with HIV. Early in the development of AIDS, infected individuals exhibit a hypergammaglobulinemia secondary to B-cell activation. Because many B cells become activated through polyclonal B-cell activators (EBV, CMV, and HIV), fewer and fewer B cells are able to respond to immunologic challenges as the disease progresses.[4,5] This polyclonal B-cell activation almost certainly contributes to the finding of autoantibodies in individuals with AIDS and ARC, most notably antibodies directed against lymphocytes and platelets.[6,7] As the disease progresses, fewer and fewer B cells can be recruited into making new immune responses. In vitro analysis of B lymphocytes from AIDS patients has revealed an increased level of spontaneous B-cell proliferation and differentiation. This increased frequency of activated B cells may or may not be related directly to EBV infection. However, it probably does play a role in B-cell transformation, since individuals within AIDS risk groups have an increased incidence of high-grade B-cell lymphomas.[8]

Monocytes and macrophages can be infected by HIV,[3] and as disease severity increases, evidence for marked abnormalities in monocyte/macrophage function in vivo is apparent.[1,2] The mechanisms by which the monocyte/macrophage system becomes affected by the HIV are currently unknown. A wide range of functional abnormalities have been noted, including decreased ability for monocytes from HIV infected individuals to present antigen, a decreased ability of macrophages to phagocytose opsonized bacteria, and immune complexes both in vitro and in vivo. The increased infection rate of AIDS patients with encapsulated bacterial organisms may result from decreased de novo humoral immune responses, as well as an inability for macrophages to phagocytose processed bacteria.

Nonspecific cellular immunity, mediated in part through natural killer (NK) cells, is severely decreased in AIDS patients.[9] Natural killer cells can kill virus-infected cells as well as tumor cells, and are severely decreased in vivo during the AIDS disease progression. The decrease in NK cell activity can be partially reversed in vitro after culturing with the T-cell growth factor interleukin-2 (IL-2). Therefore, suppression of NK cell activity may be related to both decreased NK cell numbers as well as the severe depletion of CD4+ T cells, which produce IL-2 in vivo.

Overall, as the severity of AIDS-associated disease progresses, abnormalities are noted in all of the cellular and humoral immune system components, but the most profound abnormality associated with the death of infected individuals is the loss of the T-cell, antigen specific, cellular immune system. The depletion of the cellular immune system, then, allows the opportunistic infections observed in AIDS patients to occur, and depletes the immune system's ability to successfully rid the body of cancers, including Kaposi's sarcoma and high-grade lymphomas.

REFERENCES

1. Lane HC, Fauci AS. Immunologic abnormalities in the acquired immunodeficiency syndrome. Ann Rev Immunol 1985; 3:477-500.

2. Bowen DL, Lane HC, Fauci AS. Immunopathogenesis of the acquired immunodeficiency syndrome. Ann Intern Med 1985; 704-9.

3. Ho D, Rota TR, Hirsch MS. Infection of monocyte/macrophages by human T lymphotropic virus type III. J Clin Invest 1986; 77:1-4.

4. Pahwa S, Pahwa R, Saxinger C, et al. Influence of the human T lymphotropic virus/lymphadenopathy associated virus and functions of human lymphocytes: evidence of immunosuppressive effects and polyclonal B-cell activation by banded viral and lymphocyte preparations. Proc Natl Acad Sci USA 1985; 82:8198-8202.

5. Ammann AJ, Schiffman G, Abrams DI, et al. B-cell immunodeficiency in acquired immunodeficiency syndrome. JAMA 1984; 251:1447-9.

6. Tomar RH, John PA, Hennig AK, Koster B. Cellular targets of antilymphocyte antibodies in AIDS and LAS. Clin Immunol Immunopathol 1985; 37:37-47.

7. Stricker RB, Abrams DI, Corash C, Shuman M. Target platelet antigen in homosexual men with immune thrombocytopenia. N Engl J Med 1985; 313:1375-80.

8. Levine AM, Meyer PR, Begandy MK, et al. Development of B cell lymphoma in homosexual men: clinical and immunologic findings. Ann Intern Med 1984; 100:7.

9. Rook AH, Masur H, Lane HC, et al. Interleukin-2 enhances the depressed natural killer cell and cytomegalovirus specific cytotoxic activities of lymphocytes from patients with AIDS. J Clin Invest 1983; 72:398-403.

T-Cell Abnormalities

Michael S. McGrath, M.D., Ph.D.

■ QUANTITATIVE ABNORMALITIES

The earliest, most easily identifiable and reproducible finding in individuals with AIDS is an absolute lymphopenia, most specifically in the subpopulation of T cells designated as helper T lymphocytes (CD4, leu3/T4).[1] T cells are normally divided into several subclasses dictated by surface phenotype. These include the CD4+ T-helper cell subset and the CD8 cell populations, which include T-suppressor as well as T-cytotoxic cell subsets.

The CD4+ cell population can be subdivided into two functionally different subpopulations dictated by the expression of the cell surface TQ1/leu8 antigen, which divides the CD4 T-cell subpopulation into helper (TQ1/leu8 –) and inducer (TQ1/leu8 +) subsets. This second CD4+ inducer T-cell subset is the cell population affected earliest during the progression toward AIDS.[2] As the severity of disease increases, patients will typically develop total CD4 cell counts of less than 500 cells per cubic millimeter and T helper/T suppressor ratios of less than 0.85 (normal ratio: approximately 2 to 1). The level of CD4 cells is lowest in individuals with opportunistic infections and highest in symptomatic individuals with ARC and lymphadenopathy syndrome. Patients with Kaposi's sarcoma have variable levels of CD4 cells.

In contrast to their CD4+ T-cell levels, individuals with AIDS express varying levels of CD8+ cells, including increased, normal, or decreased levels. Because CMV and EBV normally may increase CD8+ cell levels,[4] the variable level of the CD8+ cell population may be a secondary rather than a primary finding during the development of AIDS. A detailed analysis of lymphocytes from patients with increased levels of CD8+ cells revealed that the majority of these CD8+ cells did not express the T-cell surface marker Leu-15.[5] This finding suggests that the elevated level of CD8+ cells observed in most AIDS patients are of the cytotoxic CD8+Leu15 – subset. The role that elevated cytotoxic T-cell levels might play in the development of AIDS is currently unknown.

■ FUNCTIONAL ABNORMALITIES

Many functional abnormalities occur in the T-lymphocyte populations of individuals infected with HIV, the most serious consequence of which is death secondary to neoplasms and opportunistic infections. The most direct in vivo test to measure immune function and T-cell response is skin testing. The response of AIDS patients to a series of specific antigens, including PPD, tetanus toxoid, and candida, is markedly depressed, and in severe AIDS there may be an absence of skin test reactivity.[3] Transient skin-test reactivity was restored in an AIDS patient transfused with an identical twin's reactive T lymphocytes; however, this reactivity did not alter the course of disease.[6] Similarly, bone marrow and thymus transplantation have been unsuccessful in restoration of T-cell immunity in AIDS patients.[7]

Many in vitro tests of T-cell function are abnormal in individuals infected with HIV.[3] T lymphocytes isolated from this patient population show an elevated level of spontaneous proliferation; an increased proportion expresses the cell-surface activation antigen DR. The cells do not, however, express interleukin-2 (IL-2) receptors as would be expected of fully antigen-activated T cells. More significantly, lymphocytes isolated from individuals infected with HIV show a markedly decreased responsiveness to mitogens and antigens in vitro. The majority of these patients have low levels of CD4+ T cells, which explains the decreased mitogen responsiveness (to pokeweed, PHA) observed. However, even on a cell- corrected basis, in comparison with normal CD4+ T cells, very little if any antigen-specific responsiveness can be demonstrated to soluble antigen (tetanus toxoid, candida). This antigen unresponsiveness is also translated to the B cell/immunoglobulin system, since CD4+ lymphocytes from AIDS patients will not help (or do so poorly) B cells undergo immunospecific expansion and secretion of immunoglobulin. This feature appears relatively late during the development of AIDS.

The most devastating effect on the immune system of individuals infected with HIV is the decreased generation of effective cytotoxic T lymphocytes. The cytotoxic T-cell subpopulation is responsible for the attack and removal from the body of virally infected and malignant cell populations. During progression from clinical health to AIDS, individuals lose CMV-specific killer T lymphocytes, and in reconstitution experiments those killer cells cannot be induced with CD4+ cells from AIDS patients.[8] The addition of IL-2 to these cytotoxic T-cell populations increases CMV-specific killing. Therefore, it is likely that at least one other major defect in cell-mediated immunity observed in AIDS patients is the result of a decreased level of CD4+ cells capable of producing IL-2. Interleukin-2, in turn, responds to antigen and effectively increases both the amount and efficiency of cytotoxic T-cell killing.

Recently, two groups have reported the existence of HIV-specific cytotoxic T lymphocytes in HIV-infected people. In one study, T cells from 8 of 8 seropositive donors recognized and killed autologous B cells infected with vaccinia virus carrying the HIV envelope gene. Three of 8 killed cells infected by vaccinia carrying the HIV *gag* gene.[11] Another group identified cytotoxic T lymphocytes that killed autologous HIV-infected alveolar macrophages in bronchoalveolar lavage fluids from patients with lymphocytic interstitial pneumonitis.[12] Further studies will be required to determine whether the presence of cytotoxic T lymphocytes recognizing HIV in infected cells is protective in infected individuals.

T cells from individuals infected with HIV show a decreased ability to expand in a clonal fashion.[8] T cells from both helper and suppressor phenotypes (CD4 and CD8) do not clone or expand in a normal fashion in response to IL-2, although there is no gross abnormality in the cells' ability to express the IL-2 receptor. This indicates a potential intrinsic abnormality in T-cell activation in these cell populations.

Natural killer-cell activity is depressed in individuals with AIDS. Natural killer (NK) cells, which mediate killing of virally infected and tumor cells in a nonrestricted fashion in vitro, are decreased in individuals with AIDS.[9] However, the decrease in natural killers is not very consistent and is not highly correlated with disease state. This decreased NK killing ability can be augmented in vitro by the addition of IL-2, although it cannot be corrected to normal. This NK cell-mediated killing augmentation may occur through IL-2 stimulated induction of NK cell cytolytic factors.[10] The effects of decreased NK activity in vivo in this patient population are currently unknown.

Because the most marked abnormality in individuals with AIDS is a decrease in CD4+ cells, it is likely that the majority of effects seen during the progression toward AIDS is the result of decreased T-cell-mediated helper/inducer function rather than active immunosuppression. Evidence to date suggests that the quantitative and qualitative CD4+ cell abnormalities can account for many of the immunologic defects observed in AIDS, whereas very little data support ongoing active immunosuppression mediated through suppressor T-lymphocyte factors.[3,8]

REFERENCES

1. Gottlieb MS, Schroff R, Schanker H, et al. *Pneumocystis carinii* pneumonia and mucosal candidiasis in previously healthy homosexual men: evidence for a new acquired cellular immunodeficiency. N Engl J Med 1981; 305:1425-31.

2. Nicholson JK, McDougal JS, Spira TJ, et al. Immunoregulatory subsets of the T helper and T suppressor cell populations in homosexual men with chronic unexplained lymphadenopathy. J Clin Invest 1984; 73:191-210.

3. Lane HC, Fauci AS. Immunologic abnormalities in acquired immunodeficiency syndrome. Ann Rev Immunol 1985; 3:477-500.

4. Reinherz EL, O'Brien C, Rosenthal P, et al. The cellular basis for viral-induced immunodeficiency: analysis by monoclonal antibodies. J Immunol 1980; 175:1269-76.

5. Stites D, Casavant CH, McHugh TM, et al. Flow cytometric analysis of lymphocyte phenotypes in AIDS using monoclonal antibodies and simultaneous dual immunofluorescence. Clin Immunol Immunopathol 1986; 38:161-77.

6. Lane HC, Masur H, Longo DL, et al. Partial immune reconstitution in a patient with the acquired immunodeficiency syndrome. N Engl J Med 1984; 311:1099-1103.

7. Lane HC, Fauci AS. Immunologic reconstitution in acquired immunodeficiency syndrome. Ann Intern Med 1985; 103:714-8.

8. Bowen DL, Lane HC, Fauci AS. Immunopathogenesis of the acquired immunodeficiency syndrome. Ann Intern Med 1985; 704-9.

9. Rook AH, Masur H, Lane HC, et al. Interleukin-2 enhances the depressed natural killer cell and cytomegalovirus specific cytotoxic activities of lymphocytes from patients with AIDS. J Clin Invest 1983; 72:398-403.

10. Bonavida B, Katz J, Gottlieb M. Mechanism of defective NK cell activity in patients with acquired immunodeficiency syndrome (AIDS) and AIDS related complex. I. Defective trigger on NK cells for NKCF production by target cells and partial restoration by IL-2. J Immunol 1986; 137:1157.

11. Walker BD, Chakrabarti S, Moss B, et al. HIV-specific cytotoxic T lymphocytes in seropositive individuals. Nature 1987; 328:345-7.

12. Plata F, Autran B, Pedroza Martins L, et al. AIDS virus-specific cytotoxic T lymphocytes in lung disorders. Nature 1987; 328:348-51.

B-Cell Abnormalities

Farzad Khayam-Bashi, B.S., and Michael S. McGrath, M.D., Ph.D.

Individuals infected with the human immunodeficiency virus (HIV) exhibit substantial abnormalities in their humoral (B-cell) immune system. These abnormalities include: nonspecific elevation of polyclonal immunoglobulins, increased circulating immune complexes, inability to mount new B-cell-mediated immune responses to new antigens or infectious agents, increased spontaneous B-cell proliferation and differentiation, and inability to respond to specific T-cell signals for antigen-specific proliferation, differentiation, or both.[1,2] Serum paraproteins similar to those in multiple myeloma may occur and should be carefully investigated before treatment, since they may represent protective HIV antibodies.[14] This spectrum of abnormalities in humoral immunity, coupled with defects in the cellular immune system, contributes to the overall immunodeficiency observed in AIDS patients.

Humoral response to new antigens is markedly decreased in patients with AIDS. Immunization of AIDS patients with a potent protein antigen (keyhole limpet hemocyanin), a recall antigen (tetanus toxoid), and a T-cell independent antigen (pneumococcal polysaccharide) resulted in antibody production that was less than 10 percent of the level generated in healthy controls.[1,3] Immunoglobulins are normally produced by mature B lymphocytes (plasma cells), which become activated (proliferate and differentiate) after exposure to antigens or mitogens. B lymphocytes isolated from the peripheral blood of AIDS patients show a decreased proliferative response to the B-cell mitogen *Staphylococcus aureus* and a decreased ability to secrete immunoglobulin in response to pokeweed mitogen.[1]

Decreased mitogen and specific antigenic responsiveness in B cells from AIDS patients suggest that both T-cell and B-cell defects occur during the development of AIDS. These AIDS-related defects may occur secondary to altered T-cell regulation. Recently, however, proteins from disrupted HIV preparations were shown to induce many AIDS-associated B-cell defects in vitro, implying a direct role for HIV protein-mediated immunosuppression in vivo.[4] Because both B and T lymphocytes from AIDS patients are incapable of responding appropriately to neoantigens, the expected increases in titers of antibody to specific infectious agents such as toxoplasma and coccidioides may not occur.[2] This could invalidate diagnostic tests that are based upon measurements of antibody titers to these infectious agents.

High levels of polyclonal immunoglobulins and immune complexes are present in the serum of patients with AIDS and AIDS-related complex (ARC). Peripheral blood B lymphocytes isolated from AIDS patients are polyclonally activated and spontaneously secrete immunoglobulin at levels at least ten times higher than B lymphocytes from uninfected individuals.[1] This polyclonal B-cell activation may occur in HIV-infected persons as a result of concurrent infection[5] with one of the polyclonal B-cell activating viruses, Epstein–Barr virus (EBV) and cytomegalovirus (CMV).[6] Alternatively, HIV proteins may stimulate peripheral blood B lymphocytes directly, causing levels of B-cell activation and immunoglobulin secretion similar to those induced by EBV in vitro.[4] Additional recent evidence suggests that HIV production in monocytes and macrophages induces the synthesis of IL-6, a B-cell stimulatory factor similar to IFN-β-2, which may contribute to polyclonal B-cell activation.[22]

Polyclonally activated B cells may not only contribute directly to the elevated immunoglobulins seen in the serum of AIDS patients but may also produce antilymphocyte,[7] antiplatelet,[8] antinuclear antigen,[9] and antimyelin[10] antibodies; these are associated with a wide spectrum of side effects, including nonspecific immunosuppression, in this patient population. These autoantibodies are likely to contribute directly to the high level of circulating immune complexes frequently found in the serum of HIV-infected individuals[11]; this may inhibit other components of the immune system.

A small subpopulation of HIV-infected patients with hypergammaglobulinemia have serum paraprotein levels similar to those seen in patients with multiple myeloma.[15,16] In the past, other infectious diseases, including malaria, cytomegalovirus infection, and congenital toxoplasmosis,[17,18,19] have been associated with transient paraproteinemia. Recently, a definitive molecular analysis of an AIDS-associated paraprotein revealed it to be polyclonal, with antibody activity directed primarily at HIV protein components.[14] Based on this finding, HIV-infected persons who are producing multiple myeloma-like paraproteins should not be treated for multiple myeloma unless there are overwhelming clinical data to support the diagnosis.

B lymphocytes may be directly infected by HIV. The first long-term in vitro cell line to continuously produce HIV was an EBV-immortalized B-lymphocyte line. A recent study has revealed that the HIV LTR was more efficiently transcribed in a B-cell line than in a T-cell line, presumably because the B lymphocytes had higher levels of NF-kappa B, a cellular-derived enhancer of HIV-1 transcription.[20] Analysis of a series of B-cell lines indicated that the presence of EBV in a B-cell line affected the amount of virus produced by that line. However, the B-cell line did not require previous infection with EBV to become productively infected with HIV.[12] A more recent study has found that EBV-positive and EBV-negative B-cell lines can be infected with both HIV-1 and HIV-2.[21] Evidence exists that HIV-infected B cells are more susceptible to natural killer and lymphokine-activated killer cells than uninfected B cells.[23] There was a direct correlation between HIV infectibility of B-cell lines and the presence of the CD4 (leu3/T4) T-cell surface molecule.[13] As observed with T lymphocytes, apparently only those B lymphocytes expressing the CD4 cell-surface molecule can be infected by HIV, and viral gene expression and replication are more efficient in CD4+ B cells than in CD4+ T cells.[20] This could account for the relative sparing of B cells in AIDS patients, since only rare B cells express the CD4 molecule. However, even those rare B cells harboring HIV can be very important, since the interactions of B and T lymphocytes could provide a direct pathway for viral transfer.

REFERENCES

1. Lane HC, Masur H, Edgar LC, et al. Abnormalities of B cell activation and immunoregulation of patients with the acquired immunodeficiency syndrome. N Engl J Med 1983; 309:453-8.
2. Bowen DL, Lane HC, Fauci AS. Immunopathogenesis of the acquired immunodeficiency syndrome. Ann Intern Med 1985; 103:704-9.
3. Ammann AJ. Schiffman G, Abrams DI, et al. B cell immunodeficiency in acquired immunodeficiency syndrome. JAMA 1984; 251:1447-9.

4. Pahwa S, Pahwa R, Saxinger C, et al. Influence of the human T-lymphotropic virus/lymphadenopathy-associated virus and functions of human lymphocytes: evidence of immunosuppressive effects and polyclonal B-cell activation by banded viral and lymphocyte preparations. Proc Natl Acad Sci USA 1985; 82:8198-202.

5. Quinnan GV, Masur H, Rook AH, et al. Herpes virus infections in the acquired immunodeficiency syndrome. JAMA 1984; 252:72-7.

6. Lane HC, Fauci AS. Immunologic abnormalities in the acquired immunodeficiency syndrome. Ann Rev Immunol 1985; 3:477-500.

7. Tomar RH, John PA, Hennig AK, Kloster B. Cellular targets of antilymphocyte antibodies in AIDS and LAS. Clin Immunol Immunopathol 1985; 37:37-47.

8. Stricker RB, Abrams DI, Corash C, Shuman M. Target platelet antigen in homosexual men with immune thrombocytopenia. N Engl J Med 1985; 313:1375-80.

9. Abrams DI, Lewis BJ, Beckstead JH, et al. Persistent diffuse lymphadenopathy in homosexual men: Endpoint or prodrome? Ann Intern Med 1984; 100:801-8.

10. Lipkin I, Parry G, Kiprov D, Abrams DI. Inflammatory neuropathy in homosexual men with lymphadenopathy. Neurology 1985; 35:1479-83.

11. McDougal JS, Hubbard M, Nicholson JKA, et al. Immune complexes in the acquired immunodeficiency syndrome (AIDS): relationship to disease manifestation risk group and immunologic defect. J Clin Immunol 1985; 5:130-8.

12. Montagnier L, Gruest J, Chamaret S, et al. Adaptation of lymphadenopathy associated virus (LAV) to replication in EBV-transformed B lymphoblastoid cell lines. Science 1984; 225:63-6.

13. Levy JA, Shimabukuro J, McHugh T, et al. AIDS associated retroviruses (ARV) can productively infect other cells besides human T helper cells. Virology 1985; 147:441-8.

14. Ng VL, Hwang KM, Reyes GR, et al. High titer anti-HIV antibody reactivity associated with a paraprotein spike in a homosexual male with AIDS related complex (ARC) Blood 1988; 71:1397-401.

15. Heriot K, Hallquist AE, Tomar RH. Paraproteinemia in patients with acquired immunodeficiency syndrome (AIDS) or lymphadenopathy syndrome (LAS). Clin Chem 1985; 31:1224-6.

16. Papadopoulos NM, Lane HC, Costello R, et al. Oligoclonal immunoglobulins in patients with the acquired immunodeficiency syndrome. Clin Immunol Immunopathol 1985; 35:43-6.

17. Weinberg AG, McCracken GH Jr, LoSpalluto J, Luby JP. Monoclonal macroglobulinemia and cytomegalic inclusion disease. Pediatrics 1973; 51:518-24.

18. Griscelli C, Desmonts G, Gny B, Frommel D. Congenital toxoplasmosis. Fetal synthesis of oligoclonal immunoglobulin G in intrauterine infection. J Pediatr 1973; 83:20-6.

19. Ritzmann SE. Immunoglobulin abnormalities. In: Ritzmann S, Daniel JC, eds. Serum protein abnormalities, diagnostic and clinical aspects. Boston: Little, Brown and Co., 1975:463.

20. Calman AF, Busch MP, Vyas GN, et al. Transcription and replication of human immunodeficiency virus-1 in B lymphocytes in vitro. AIDS 1988; 2:185-93.

21. Monroe JE, Calender A, Mulder C. Epstein-Barr virus-positive and -negative B-cell lines can be infected with human immunodeficiency virus types 1 and 2. J Virol 1988; 62:3497-500.

22. Nakajima K, Martinez-Maza O, Hirano T, et al. Induction of IL-6 (B-cell stimulatory factor-2/IFN-β-2) production by HIV. J Immunol 1989; 142:531-6.

23. Malkovsky M, Philpott K, Dagleish AG, et al. Infection of B lymphocytes by the human immunodeficiency virus and their susceptibility to cytotoxic cells. Eur J Immunol 1988; 18:1315-21.

3.2.4

Monocyte/Macrophages

*Suzanne Crowe, M.B.B.S., F.R.A.C.P., John Mills, M.D.,
and Michael S. McGrath, M.D., Ph.D.*

T he role of the monocyte/macrophage in the pathogenesis of AIDS is receiving increasing attention. It is no longer thought that infection of T-helper lymphocytes with human immunodeficiency virus (HIV) can fully explain the immunologic dysfunction characteristic of AIDS.

Monocyte/macrophages assume a pivotal role within the immune system. Their functions include antigen processing, phagocytosis, antibody-dependent cellular cytotoxicity, tumoricidal activity, and monokine production.[1] HIV infection of monocytes, thereby inducing their dysfunction, could thus contribute to the wide range of immunologic abnormalities seen in AIDS. Because monocyte/macrophages are thought to provide a major contribution to the in vivo reservoir of HIV, the efficacy of potential antiretrovirals on HIV replication within this target-cell population is of particular relevance.

As with other lentivirus infections (including visna and caprine arthritis-encephalitis virus) in which the macrophage is the target of infection,[2,3] HIV-infected macrophages may serve as reservoirs of virus, as well as providing a means of disseminating HIV to other cells.

Several groups have shown that HIV can be recovered from monocyte/macrophages of AIDS patients and that peripheral blood and tissue (brain, alveolar) monocyte/macrophages can be productively infected with HIV.[4-7] One study reported that 12 percent to 58 percent of bronchial alveolar lavage macrophages in patients with lymphocytic interstitial pneumonitis contained HIV antigen.[14] The addition of cytokines, such as Colony Stimulating Factor 1 (CSF1) may increase the susceptibility of monocytes to HIV infection.[15] By cytofluorographic analysis, it has been shown that up to 70 percent of a population of in vitro infected macrophages can be infected with HIV.[8] Of interest is the fact that once infected, these monocyte/macrophages show little cytopathology and thus may survive as an in vivo reservoir of HIV. This is in direct contrast to T lymphocytes, which die rapidly after infection with HIV.[9]

At least a proportion of monocyte/macrophages bear the CD4 molecule on their surface.[8] Although the CD4 molecule is the T-cell receptor for HIV, whether CD4 is the only receptor for HIV on monocyte/macrophages is still unclear. It is possible that other receptors (e.g., Fc receptors) may play a role in HIV infection of these cells. Monocyte/macrophages may become infected by phagocytosis of immune complexes containing HIV, but this route remains speculative. The only mechanism yet proved is HIV attachment to the CD4 receptor.

Individuals infected with HIV have high levels of circulating immune complexes.[10] Normally, immune complexes are removed from the human circulatory system by phagocytosis after macrophage recognition of the Fc portion of an immunoglobulin involved in the complex. Studies on the rate of removal of immune complexes from AIDS patients have shown a marked decrease in efficient removal of both complexes and antibody-coated red blood cells.[11] This decreased phagocytosis of immunoglobulin–antigen complexes may contribute to the observed higher incidence of infection with encapsulated bacterial organisms, which are normally removed efficiently by an intact reticuloendothelial system. In vitro studies of monocytes from AIDS patients have shown decreased chemotactic response to bacterial substances. This diminished response would further inhibit monocyte/macrophage–mediated removal of foreign organisms.[12]

As observed in B-lymphocyte populations in these patients (see B-cell abnormalities), monocytes from AIDS patients appear to be in a preactivated state that results in diminished responsiveness to new antigenic challenges.[13] This adds another mechanism by which the human immune system becomes overwhelmed during the development of AIDS.

REFERENCES

1. Nathan CF, Murray HW, Cohn ZA. The macrophage as an effector cell. N Engl J Med 1980; 303:622-6.
2. Gendelman HE, Narayan O, Kennedy-Stoskopf S, et al. Slow virus-macrophage interactions: characterization of a transformed cell line of sheep alveolar macrophages that express a marker for susceptibility to ovine-caprine lentivirus infections. Lab Invest 1984; 51:547-55.
3. Haase AT. Pathogenesis of lentivirus infections. Nature 1986; 322:130-6.
4. Ho DD, Rota TR, Hirsch MS. Infection of monocyte/macrophages by human T lymphotropic virus type III. J Clin Invest 1986; 77:1712-5.
5. Salahuddin SZ, Rose RM, Groopman JE, et al. Human T lymphotropic virus type III infection of human alveolar macrophages. Blood 1986; 68:281-4.
6. Ruscetti FW, Mikovits JA, Kalyanaraman VS, et al. Analysis of effector mechanisms against HTLV-I and HTLV-III/LAV-infected lymphoid cells. J Immunol 1986; 136:3619-24.
7. Gartner S, Markovits P, Markovitz DM, et al. The role of mononuclear phagocytes in HTLV-III/LAV infection. Science 1986; 233:215-9.
8. Crowe S, Mills J, McGrath MS. Quantitative immunocytofluorographic analysis of CD4 surface antigen expression and HIV infection of human peripheral blood monocyte/macrophages. Res Hum Retroviruses 1987; 3:135-45.
9. Lifson JD, Reyes GR, McGrath MS, et al. AIDS retrovirus induced cytopathology: giant cell formation and involvement of CD4 antigen. Science 1986; 232:1123-7.
10. Lightfoot MM, Folks TM, Sell KW. Analysis of immune complex components isolated from serum of AIDS patients. Fed Proc 1984; 43:1921.
11. Bender BS, Quinn TC, Lawley TJ, et al. Acquired immune deficiency syndrome: a defect in Fc-receptor specific clearance. Clin Res 1984; 32:511.
12. Lane HC, Fauci AS. Immunologic abnormalities in the acquired immunodeficiency syndrome. Ann Rev Immunol 1985; 3:477-500.
13. Smith P, Ohura K, Masur H, et al. Monocyte function in the acquired immunodeficiency syndrome: decreased chemotaxis. J Clin Invest 1984; 74:2121-8.
14. Plata F, Autran B, Martins LP, et al. AIDS virus-specific cytotoxic T lymphocytes in lung disorders. Nature 1987; 328:348-51.
15. Gendelman HE, Orenstein JM, Martin MA, et al. Efficient isolation and propagation of human immunodeficiency virus on recombinant colony-stimulating factor 1-treated monocytes. J Exp Med 1988; 167:1428-41.

3.2.5

Antiviral Drug Therapy for HIV Infection: Rationale

Suzanne Crowe, M.B.B.S., F.R.A.C.P., Michael S. McGrath, M.D., Ph.D., and Paul A. Volberding, M.D.

Several events in the replicative cycle of the human immunodeficiency virus (HIV) are potential targets for antivirals, and numerous antivirals (including interferons alpha and beta, nucleoside analogues, and soluble CD4) have been shown to inhibit HIV replication in vitro. However, difficulties may develop in treating HIV-infected patients. Because HIV is neurotropic, effective drugs must penetrate the brain and cerebrospinal fluid to inhibit replication in those sites. Infection of cells other than CD4-bearing lymphocytes (e.g., monocyte/macrophages) may perpetuate latent HIV infection. For example, ongoing, low-level infection of new target cells mediated by infected monocyte/macrophages may occur without necessarily involving the early stages of HIV's replicative cycle. Fusion of an infected macrophage with a target cell may allow extrachromosomal proviral DNA to pass into uninfected cells and thus bypass the transcription of viral RNA by reverse transcriptase (RT). Therefore, a drug acting at one specific site, such as on the RT, may suppress HIV replication without eradicating infection. Drugs that attack the reservoir of infected cells are needed and GLQ-223 shows promise in initial studies.

The ideal drug for the treatment of HIV infections would have several characteristics. Because HIV infection is chronic, any drug would need to be convenient to take and nontoxic, both for short- and long-term administration. Drugs with half-lives so short that they require continuous parenteral administration, for example, are very unlikely to be effective strategies for broad clinical application. Similarly, drugs associated with substantial subjective toxicities are unacceptable to many patients, particularly those in otherwise good general health. Finally, because HIV infects the central nervous system (CNS) even very early after exposure, the ideal antiretroviral agent must penetrate the CNS to prevent progressive encephalopathy. (The National Institutes of Health's drug development program seeks to establish such important parameters before potential drugs enter clinical trials; for a detailed outline of their 15-step program, see reference 1.)

■ REPLICATION OF HIV

HIV's unique mode of replication has been reviewed by Hirsch.[2] The envelope glycoproteins of HIV mediate attachment of the virus to a specific target-cell receptor, which comprises all or part of the CD4 antigen.[3] This antigen is also present on the surface of monocytes and macrophages and may be responsible for viral attachment in these cells. A truncated form of the CD4 antigen that may serve as a receptor for HIV occurs in neural tissue. HIV enters the target cell by endocytosis or fusion and viral uncoating, then proceeds within the cytoplasm.

Subsequent to infection, the single-stranded viral RNA is transcribed into DNA by the virus-encoded RNA-dependent DNA polymerase (reverse transcriptase). This minus-strand DNA copy (complementary, or cDNA) of the viral RNA serves as a template for synthesis of a plus-strand DNA, forming a linear double-stranded DNA copy (provirus) of the HIV RNA, which then becomes circular and may either be integrated into the host-cell genome or remain extrachromosomal.

The DNA provirus serves as a template for synthesis of viral mRNA, which undergoes modification at the 5′ end by "capping" with methylated guanosine residues, and the 3′ end undergoes polyadenylation. Virus-specific mRNA is then translated on host-cell ribosomes to form viral precursor proteins. These proteins are further processed (e.g., proteolytic cleavage) and glycosylated within the rough endoplasmic reticulum and then transported to the cell surface via the Golgi apparatus. The final stages in the replicative cycle of HIV involve assembly of virions at the plasma membrane with the budding of mature envelope virus particles. The entire replicative process occurs within 48 to 72 hours after HIV attaches itself to susceptible T cells.

TABLE 1. TARGET SITES FOR ANTIVIRAL AGENTS IN THE REPLICATIVE CYCLE OF HIV

TARGET SITE	POTENTIAL AGENTS
Attachment to host-cell receptor (CD4 antigen)	Receptor analogues; dextran sulfate, soluble CD4, AL-721
Transcription of RNA by reverse transcriptase	1. Reverse transcriptase (RT) inhibitors, e.g., ansamycin; phosphonoformate; nucleoside analogs (zidovudine, ddI, ddC) 2. Terminators of DNA chain synthesis, nucleoside analogs (zidovudine)
Translation of mRNA	Prevention of 5′ capping of mRNA, e.g., ribavirin
Processing of viral proteins	Castanospermine, deoxynojirimycin, protease inhibitors
Inactivation of infected-cell ribosome	GLQ-223 (trichosanthin)
Assembly and budding of virus	Alpha and beta interferons, ampligen

■ INHIBITION OF ATTACHMENT TO TARGET-CELL RECEPTOR

Soluble CD4. Several approaches have the potential to inhibit HIV by blocking the attachment of HIV to the surface receptor (CD4 receptor, CD4 antigen) of the target cell.

Soluble CD4 (recombinant soluble CD4, recombinant CD4, rsCD4, rCD4, sCD4, recombinant T4, recombinant soluble T4, rsT4) is a soluble form of the CD4 receptor (the binding site of gp120, the HIV envelope glycoprotein) produced by transfection of mammalian cells with vectors encoding versions of CD4 that lack the transmembrane and cytoplasmic domains. Soluble CD4 inhibits HIV replication and syncytia formation in vitro by competitively inhibiting HIV binding to the CD4 receptor of target cells.[4-9] In vitro sCD4 does not block MHC class II-mediated foreign antigen presentation to T4 lymphocytes and thus does not appear to affect T-cell activation.[6] Phase I trials have not shown toxicity or immunosuppression.[10] Phase II trials are in progress.

Soluble CD4 has a short serum half-life. One experimental approach to this problem is to attach sCD4 to an immunoglobulin Fc fragment.[11] Other theoretical concerns about sCD4 include whether long-term use could induce antibodies capable of triggering autoimmune reactions; whether sCD4 will impair normal immune system functioning by interfering with T-cell activation; and whether sCD4 will select for HIV strains that enter target cells by alternative pathways (e.g., via the Fc receptor of CD4 lymphocytes and the FcRIII receptor of macrophages that in vitro bind HIV complexed with "enhancing antibodies"[18]).

Recombinant soluble CD4-linked toxins of several types are under investigation. CD4-PE (CD4-pseudomonas exotoxin) is a hybrid protein consisting of the first 178 amino acids of the CD4 protein (including the HIV binding site) fused with the second two domains of pseudomonas exotoxin (including membrane translocation and ADP-ribosylation activities).[21] CD4-dgA (soluble CD4-deglycosylated ricin A chain) is a conjugate of sCD4 with the A chain of ricin[22] — a 30-kilodalton enzyme that inactivates the 30S subunit of eukaryotic cells by modifying nucleoside residues of 28S RNA.[23] After reaching the cytoplasm a single molecule of either toxin can be lethal to a cell. In vitro the hybrid molecules are not toxic to uninfected cells, presumably because these do not express the envelope glycoprotein gp120. In vivo studies are in preparation.

Phase I clinical trials in San Francisco and Boston have shown that recombinant soluble CD4 given intravenously, intramuscularly, or subcutaneously is well tolerated.[25,26] No clear evidence of immunologic or antiviral efficacy has been shown yet. Antibodies directed against CD4 have been found in only one individual to date. Further studies with escalating doses are under way to assess safety and pharmacokinetics.

Dextran Sulfate.   Although initial in vitro studies with this sulfated polysaccharide were promising,[27,28] the results of a Phase I/II trial in San Francisco failed to show any clinical immunologic or antiviral efficacy, possibly because the oral dextran sulfate failed to be absorbed.[29] Other sulfated polysaccharides that have shown in vitro antiretroviral efficacy include pentosan polysulfate, heparin, and fucordan.

AL-721.   AL-721 is a brand name for a mixture of lipids composed of neutral glycerides, phosphatidylcholine, and phosphatidylethanolamine in a 7:2:1 ratio. A similar product, EL-721, is derived from egg lecithins. The products alter the structure of lipid-containing membranes, and it was hoped that they would destabilize the cholesterol-rich membrane of HIV, thereby preventing proper binding to CD4 receptors.

An open-labeled dose-ranging trial of AL-721 in patients with persistent generalized lymphadenopathy and symptomatic HIV disease showed that the compound was well tolerated; the chief side effect was a significant increase in serum cholesterol levels. There was no evidence of antiviral or immunologic efficacy.[30]

■ REVERSE TRANSCRIPTASE INHIBITORS

Ansamycin.   Ansamycin (rifabutin) is a derivative of rifamycin S and has activity against *Mycobacterium avium* complex bacteria (MAC).[12] Rifamycin analogues have also demonstrated selective activity against the RT of various retroviruses (HTLV-I, HTLV-II, HIV),[13] but not against cellular DNA polymerase alpha. Currently, trials are under way to examine the efficacy of ansamycin for the treatment of both MAC and HIV infections.

Phosphonoformate.   Trisodium phosphonoformate (foscarnet) acts as an analogue of the pyrophosphate component of nucleoside triphosphates. It inhibits DNA polymerases of herpes viruses and the RT of several animal retroviruses. The RT of HIV in H9 cell culture demonstrates dose-dependent inhibition by phosphonoformate.[14] Immunocompromised patients with cytomegalovirus retinitis are being treated with this drug[15] and clinical trials in patients with HIV infection are under way in the United States and Europe under the sponsorship of Astra Pharmaceutical Company. The major acute side effect is nephrotoxicity; bone and tooth enamel changes have occurred in animals treated for prolonged periods. Unfortunately, penetration of CSF by phosphonoformate is very limited,[16] and oral absorption is poor.

■ TERMINATORS OF DNA SYNTHESIS

Zidovudine (AZT).   Zidovudine (3'-azido-3' deoxythymidine, AZT, formerly called azidothymidine) is a thymidine derivative and analogue discovered in 1964 during a search for anticancer drugs. It was "discarded" because it was inactive against tumor cells. It is phosphorylated intracellularly to the triphosphate form. It then becomes incorporated in the growing DNA strand via the 3' hydroxy group, but prevents the formation of 5' to 3' phosphodiester linkages because the compound lacks a 5' hydroxy group. Viral transcription halts, and synthesis of the growing DNA chain is terminated with production of incomplete, nonfunctional proviral DNA. Zidovudine triphosphate is also a competitive inhibitor of HIV RT. Cellular DNA polymerase alpha is 100-fold less susceptible to inhibition by zidovudine than HIV RT.

Zidovudine has undergone testing in animal models[17] and is used clinically in patients with AIDS and symptomatic HIV infection.[19,31,32] The ability of this drug to cross the blood—brain barrier diminishes the possibility of continued viral replication in neuronal tissue. Another advantage is that it can be given orally, retaining 67 percent bioavailability.

With prolonged use of zidovudine, further side effects have been observed, including nail and mucous-membrane pigmentation, myopathy,[33] and acute meningo-encephalitis associated with reduction in dosage.[34]

Zidovudine is the first agent with clinically beneficial effects on HIV infection, and its testing has been the cause for understandable optimism. It is licensed for use in AIDS patients and symptomatic HIV-infected persons with less than 200 helper T cells. At this stage, it is not clear how long-lasting the effects of zidovudine will be or whether the drug is beneficial to asymptomatic patients. Clinical trial experience is needed to show a favorable therapeutic index. Issues of possible resistance to zidovudine have been raised.[35] In vitro studies show that relative resistance (measured by an increase in the 50 percent inhibitory dose (ID50) and 95 percent inhibitory dose (ID95) appears in nearly all patients with advanced HIV disease after six to nine months of zidovudine treatment. The clinical implications of this study require further consideration.

Studies to evaluate the efficacy of zidovudine (1200 mg/day for 6 weeks) for health-care workers who sustain needlestick injuries or other significant muco-cutaneous exposures have started. However, because the incidence of infection following such exposure is so low, it will require a huge study to assess the drug's efficacy for this purpose.

2′3′Dideoxythymidine; 2′3′Dideoxycytidine (ddC); Dideoxyinosine (ddI).   These are nucleoside analogues with structural similarities to zidovudine. They are generally more potent antiretrovirals than zidovudine but they exhibit less toxicity in vitro.[19,20] Phase I clinical trials of dideoxycytidine (ddC) initially caused concern because of a high frequency of painful axonal neuropathy. Further studies found that this toxicity was largely preventable through dose reduction. Phase II trials of ddC using these lower doses are in progress. Dideoxyinosine (ddI) is also entering Phase II investigation after Phase I trials documented a low rate of toxicity and promising effects on CD4+ cell counts and on laboratory markers for HIV replication. Over 50 percent of patients showed a decrease in serum p24 antigen at the end of the 24-week study.[36] An escalating-dose Phase I study of ddI in patients with AIDS or symptomatic HIV disease showed dose-related anti-HIV efficacy with a sustained decline in serum p24 antigen in six of seven subjects with detectable p24 at entry. Noteworthy toxicity in a minority of patients included convulsions, irritability, and difficulty sleeping.[37]

Ribavirin.   In Phase I studies of oral ribavirin, toxicity was noted, especially anemia. This anemia was dose-limiting in quantities greater than approximately 1200 mg daily. Due to problems with interpretation of data from the initial studies, a repeat Phase I study was performed in patients with symptomatic HIV disease using oral ribavirin (1200 to 1600 mg/day for 12 to 20 weeks). No evidence of virologic or immunologic efficacy was reported.[38]

■ ELIMINATING THE RESERVOIR OF LATENT HIV INFECTION

GLQ-223.   GLQ-223 ("Q," trichosanthin) is a 25-kilodalton, highly positively charged protein from the root of a Chinese cucumber, *Trichosanthes kirilowii*.[39] GLQ-223 has potent HIV inhibitory activity in vitro, including selective killing of HIV-infected cells and selective inhibition of HIV RNA synthesis relative to total cellular RNA synthesis. In part, GLQ-223 appears to work by inactivating ribosomes in HIV-infected cells. In contrast to drugs like zidovudine that block new infection of cells but that do not affect latent HIV, GLQ-223 has the potential to eliminate the reservoir of latent HIV, believed to be mononuclear cells and macrophages. GLQ-223 has been used in China to induce abortion and to treat metastatic choriocarcinoma; reportedly it is well tolerated in doses likely to affect HIV in vivo. For choriocarcinoma, the drug is frequently administered one to two times per week for three weeks. In contrast to many plant proteins, it reportedly does not produce hypersensitivity, even with repeated doses. Both FDA-approved and unapproved trials are in progress in San Francisco.

GLQ-223 is purified from extracts of fresh *T. kirilowii* root using ion exchange chromatography. Impure extracts contain lectins that induce potentially fatal coagulopathies. Because of the promise shown in initial evaluation and the relative ease of obtaining *T. kirilowii*, the potential for harm from unregulated preparations exists. Clinicians should be aware of this and warn their patients about the danger of self-medication with this drug. They should also watch for signs of complications from patients using illicit preparations of trichosanthin.

■ ASSEMBLY AND BUDDING OF VIRUS

Interferons (IFN).   Before HIV was recognized as the etiologic agent of AIDS, trials with alpha interferon (IFN) had commenced in patients with Kaposi's sarcoma, based on these cytokines' antiproliferative activity. When the viral etiology of AIDS was established, the antiviral activity of interferons prompted further studies to evaluate their efficacy against HIV. Recombinant human IFN alpha-A has a dose-related suppressive effect on HIV in vitro.[24] Beta IFN is less active; gamma IFN was ineffective in suppressing HIV replication.[2] How interferons inhibit HIV replication is unclear, but they probably retard the assembly and release of mature virions from the cell surface. Trials to assess alpha IFN in patients with symptomatic HIV infection and AIDS are under way. Toxicity of IFN includes fever, malaise, myalgia, and bone-marrow suppression. Interferons must also be given parenterally and penetrate the CNS poorly.

Inhibitors of Glycosylation: Castanospermine, Deoxynojirimycin.   HIV-1 contains the heavily glycosylated envelope proteins, gp120 and gp41, which function in attaching HIV to the CD4 cell-surface receptor. The glycosylation steps offer potential sites of inhibition. Castanospermine and deoxynojirimycin are plant alkaloids that inhibit α-glucosidase I, an enzyme in the endoplasmic reticulum involved in the trimming of N-linked oligosaccharides attached to glycoproteins.[40,41] In vitro, deoxynojirimycin and castanospermine inhibit cell-to-cell spread and syncytia formation induced by HIV.[42-44] Because toxicity of these compounds is not severe, clinical trials are planned.

Viral Protease Inhibitors.   The *gag* gene product of HIV-1 is processed into several HIV core proteins by a protease encoded near the 5′ end of the *gag–pol* region of the HIV genome.[45,46] The viral protease is essential for HIV's infectivity.[47,48] The protease structure, active site, amino-acid sequence, inhibition characteristics, and substrate specificity show that the protease is a pepsin-like aspartic protease.[49-52] The protease gene has been cloned and expressed in several cellular systems[53,54] and an analogue 99-residue enzyme has been chemically synthesized,[55] allowing testing of compounds for potential inhibitory activity. In vitro inhibition of HIV by protease inhibitors has been reported.[56] Thus protease inhibitors as candidates for clinical trials should emerge from the active research into these systems.

■ INHIBITION OF HIV GENE EXPRESSION

With increased understanding of how HIV regulates its own gene expression, a new approach to anti-HIV therapy has emerged. HIV possesses several regulatory genes that produce proteins capable of causing expression and regulation of HIV RNA. The most potent of these are the *tat* and *rev* genes. In order to make new HIV, these regulatory genes first become transcribed, then translated into the respective regulatory protein. A new focus of antiviral therapy is aimed at blocking transcription and translation of these proteins using HIV *rev* and *tat* sequence-specific antisense oligonucleotides. Matsukura et al.[57] showed in vitro that antisense oligodeoxynucleotides were capable of inhibiting HIV replication and cytopathic effects, presumably by complexing with *rev* and *tat* genes and blocking their expression. With the recent finding that one of the predominant cells infected by HIV is the macrophage,[39] delivery of these antisense oligodeoxynucleotides might be facilitated by encapsulating them in liposomes (LIP).[58,59] The evolution of this new class of viral gene-specific therapeutics is in its formative stage. However, it may eventually play a significant role in inhibiting HIV expression in cells already infected with HIV.

■ ACTIVATION OF ANTIVIRAL DEFENSES

Ampligen.   Enhancement or activation of natural antiviral defenses is another approach for anti-HIV therapies. A candidate drug for this approach is ampligen, a mismatched double-stranded RNA molecule that has been reported to inhibit HIV in vitro[60,61] and in vivo.[62] Structurally, ampligen is poly I–poly C with some inserted uracil residues that serve as sites for RNase cleavage. Reports suggest several mechanisms of action: induction of interferon production, activation of double-stranded RNA-dependent intracellular enzymes, induction of natural killer (NK) cells, and perhaps other immunomodulatory actions. Toxicity in human trials has been limited to flu-like symptoms and flushing. Despite initial promising reports of anti-HIV activity, a Phase II trial failed to demonstrate any impact on progression from symptomatic HIV disease to AIDS.[63] Further trials are under way, and trials of ampligen in combination with other therapies are anticipated.

REFERENCES

1. Broder S. Identification of therapies against the retroviruses. In: De Vita VT Jr, moderator. Developmental therapeutics and the acquired immunodeficiency syndrome. Ann Intern Med 1987; 106:568-71.

2. Hirsch MS. Prospects for chemotherapy of retroviruses. In: Mills J, Corey L, eds. Antiviral chemotherapy: new directions for clinical application and research. San Francisco: Proceedings of the Conference on New Directions in Antiviral Chemotherapy, 1985; 112-7.

3. Dagleish AB, Beverley P, Clapham PR, et al. The CD4 T4 antigen is an essential component for the receptor for the AIDS retrovirus. Nature 1984; 312:763-6.

4. Smith DH, Byrn RA, Marsters SA, et al. Blocking of HIV-1 infectivity by a soluble, secreted form of the CD4 antigen. Science 1987; 238:1704-7.

5. Fisher RA, Bertonis JM, Meier W, et al. HIV infection is blocked in vitro by recombinant soluble CD4. Nature 1988; 331:76-8.

6. Hussey RE, Richardson NE, Kowalski M, et al. A soluble CD4 protein selectively inhibits HIV replication and syncytium formation. Nature 1988; 331:78-81.

7. Deen KC, McDougal JS, Inacker R, et al. A soluble form of CD4 (T4) protein inhibits AIDS virus infection. Nature 1988; 331:82-4.

8. Traunecker A, Luke W, Karjalainen K. Soluble CD4 molecules neutralize human immunodeficiency virus type 1. Nature 1988; 331:84-6.

9. Lifson JD, Hwang KM, Nara PL, et al. Synthetic CD4 peptide derivatives that inhibit HIV infection and cytopathicity. Science 1988; 241:712-6.

10. American Foundation for AIDS Research (AmFAR). Recombinant soluble CD4. AIDS/HIV Experimental Treatment Directory 1988; 2:84-5.

11. Capon DJ, Chamow SM, Mordenti J, et al. Designing CD4 immunoadhesins for AIDS therapy. Nature 1989; 337:525-31.

12. Woodley CL, Kilburn JO. In vitro susceptibility of *Mycobacterium avium* complex and *Mycobacterium tuberculosis* to a spiro-piperidyl rifamycin. Am Rev Resp Dis 1982; 126:586-7.

13. Anand R, Moore J, Srinivasan A, Curran J. Inhibition of HTLV-III/LAV replication by rifabutin [Abstract]. II International Conference on AIDS. Paris, 1986; 26.

14. Sandstrom EG, Kaplan JC, Byington RE, Hirsch MS. Inhibition of human T-cell lymphotropic virus type III in vitro by phosphonoformate. Lancet 1985; 1:1480-2.

15. Walmsley S, Chew E, Fanning MM, et al. Treatment of cytomegalovirus retinitis with tri-sodium phosphonoformate [Abstract]. New Orleans: Twenty-Sixth Interscience Conference on Antimicrobial Agents and Chemotherapy, 1986; 200.

16. Oberg B. Antiviral effects of phosphonoformate (PRA foscarnet sodium). Pharm Ther 1983; 19:387-415.

17. Ruprecht RM, O'Brien L. 3'-Azido-3'deoxythymidine (AZT) prolongs the life of mice infected with murine retroviruses [Abstract]. II International Conference on AIDS. Paris, 1986; 26.

18. Homsy J, Meyer M, Tateno M, et al. The Fc and not CD4 receptor mediates antibody enhancement of HIV infection in human cells. Science 1989; 244:1357-60.

19. Schinazi RF, Chu CK, Feorino P, Sommadosi J-P. 3' Azido 2',3'-dideoxy-5-ethyluridine (CS-85) — a new potent selective anti-HTLV-III/LAV compound [Abstract]. New Orleans: Twenty-Sixth Interscience Conference on Antimicrobial Agents and Chemotherapy, 1986; 296.

20. Mitsuya H, Broder S. Strategies for antiviral therapy in AIDS. Nature 1987; 325:773-8.

21. Chaudhary VK, Mizukami T, Fuerst TR, et al. Selective killing of HIV-infected cells by recombinant human CD4-Pseudomonas exotoxin hybrid protein. Nature 1988; 335:369-72.

22. Till MA, Ghetie V, Gregory T, et al. HIV-infected cells are killed by rCD4-ricin A chain. Science 1988; 242:1166-8.

23. Vitetta ES, Fulton RJ, May RD, et al. Redesigning nature's poisons to create anti-tumor reagents. Science 1987; 238:1098-104.

24. Ho DD, Hartshorn KL, Rota TR, et al. Recombinant human interferon alpha-A suppresses HTLV-III replication in vitro. Lancet 1985; 1:602-4.

25. Kahn J, Davis AJ, Groopman J, et al. Pharmacokinetic studies of recombinant soluble CD4 in patients with AIDS and AIDS-related complex [Abstract]. V International Conference on AIDS. Montreal, 1989:Th.B.O.5.

26. Schooley R, Ho D, Gaut P, et al. Escalating dose tolerance trial of recombinant soluble CD4 in humans [Abstract]. V International Conference on AIDS. Montreal, 1989:ThB.O.6.

27. Baba M, Snoeck R, Pauwels R, De Clercq E. Sulfated polysaccharides are potent and selective inhibitors of various enveloped viruses, including herpes simplex virus, cytomegalovirus, vesicular stomatitis virus, and human immunodeficiency virus. Antimicrob Agents Chemother 1988; 32:1742-5.

28. Mitsuya H, Looney DJ, Kuno S, et al. Dextran sulfate suppression of viruses in the HIV family: inhibition of virion binding to CD4+ cells. Science 1988; 240:646-9.

29. Abrams D, Pettinelli C, Power M, et al. A Phase I/II dose ranging trial of oral dextran sulfate in HIV p24 antigen positive individuals (ACTTG 060): results of a safety and efficacy trial [Abstract]. V International Conference on AIDS. Montreal, 1989:W.B.P.315.

30. Mildvan D, Armstrong D, Antoniskis D, et al. An open-label dose-ranging trial of AL721 in PGL and ARC [Abstract]. V International Conference on AIDS. Montreal, 1989:W.B.P.312.

31. Fischl MA, Richman DD, Grieco MH, et al. The efficacy of azidothymidine (AZT) in the treatment of patients with AIDS and AIDS-related complex. A double-blind, placebo-controlled trial. N Engl J Med 1987; 317:185-91.

32. Richman DD, Fischl MA, Grieco MH, et al. The toxicity of azidothymidine (AZT) in the treatment of patients with AIDS and AIDS-related complex. A double-blind, placebo-controlled trial. N Engl J Med 1987; 317:192-7.

33. Bessen LJ, Greene JB, Louie E, et al. Severe polymyositis-like syndrome associated with zidovudine therapy of AIDS and ARC. N Engl J Med 1988; 318:708.

34. Helbert M, Robinson D, Peddle B, et al. Acute meningo-encephalitis on dose reduction of zidovudine. Lancet 1988; 1; 1249-52.

35. Larder BA, Darby G, Richman DD. HIV with reduced sensitivity to zidovudine (AZT) isolated during prolonged therapy. Science 1989; 243:1731-4.

36. Gottlieb M, Galpin J, Thompkins J, et al. 2',3' dideoxycytidine (ddC) in the treatment of patients with AIDS and ARC [Abstract]. V International Conference on AIDS. Montreal, 1989:Th.B.O.3.

37. Yarchoan R, Thomas RV, Pluda JM, et al. Escalating dose Phase I study of intravenous and oral 2',3' dideoxyinosine (ddI) in patients with AIDS or ARC [Abstract]. V International Conference on AIDS. Montreal, 1989:Th.B.O.4.

38. Roberts RB, Makuch R, Jurica K. Phase I trial of oral ribavirin in high-risk patients for AIDS [Abstract]. V International Conference on AIDS. Montreal, 1989:Th.B.O.1.

39. McGrath MS, Hwang KM, Caldwell SE, et al. GLQ223: an inhibitor of human immunodeficiency virus replication in acutely and chronically infected cells of lymphocyte and mononuclear phagocyte lineage. Proc Natl Acad Sci USA 1989; 86:2844-8.

40. Fennie C, Lasky LA. Model for intracellular folding of the human immunodeficiency virus type 1 gp120. J Virol 1989; 63:639-46.

41. Montefiori DC, Robinson WE Jr, Mitchell WM. Role of protein N-glycosylation in pathogenesis of human immunodeficiency virus type 1. Proc Natl Acad Sci USA 1988; 85:9248-52.

42. Pal R, Kalyanaraman VS, Hoke GM, Sarngadharan MG. Processing and secretion of envelope glycoproteins of human immunodeficiency virus type 1 in the presence of trimming glucosidase inhibitor deoxynojirimycin. Intervirology 1989; 30:27-35.

43. Gruters RA, Neefjes JJ, Tersmette M, et al. Interference with HIV-induced syncytium formation and viral infectivity by inhibitors of trimming glucosidase. Nature 1987; 330:74-7.

44. Tyms AS, Berrie EM, Ryder TA, et al. Castanospermine and other plant alkaloid inhibitors of glucosidase activity block the growth of HIV. Lancet 1987; 2:1025-6.

45. Farmerie WG, Loeb DD, Casavant NC, et al. Expression and processing of the AIDS virus reverse transcriptase in *Escherichia coli*. Science 1987; 236:305-8.

46. Kramer RA, Schaber MD, Skalka AM, et al. HTLV-III*gag* protein is processed in yeast cells by the virus *pol*-protease. Science 1986; 231:1580-4.

47. Kohl NE, Emini EA, Schleif WA, et al. Active human immunodeficiency virus protease is required for viral infectivity. Proc Natl Acad Sci USA 1988; 85:4686-90.

48. Peng C, Ho BK, Chang TW, Chang NT. Role of human immunodeficiency virus type 1-specific protease in core protein maturation and viral infectivity. J Virol 1989; 63:2550-6.

49. Navia MA, Fitzgerald PM, McKeever BM, et al. Three-dimensional structure of aspartyl protease from human immunodeficiency virus HIV-1. Nature 1989; 337:615-20.

50. Weber IT, Miller M, Jaskolski M, et al. Molecular modeling of the HIV-1 protease and its substrate binding site. Science 1989; 243:928-31.

51. Meek TD, Dayton BD, Metcalf BW, et al. Human immunodeficiency virus 1 protease expressed in *Escherichia coli* behaves as a dimeric aspartic protease. Proc Natl Acad Sci USA 1989; 86:1841-5.

52. Darke PL, Leu CT, Davis LJ, et al. Human immunodeficiency virus protease. Bacterial expression and characterization of the purified aspartic protease. J Biol Chem 1989; 264:2307-12.

53. Graves MC, Lim JJ, Heimer EP, Kramer RA. An 11-kDa form of human immunodeficiency virus protease expressed in *Escherichia coli* is sufficient for enzymatic activity. Proc Natl Acad Sci USA 1988; 85:2449-53.

54. Debouck C, Gorniak JG, Strickler JE, et al. Human immunodeficiency virus protease expressed in *Escherichia coli* exhibits autoprocessing and specific maturation of the *gag* precursor. Proc Natl Acad Sci USA 1987; 84:8903-6.

55. Schneider J, Kent SB. Enzymatic activity of a synthetic 99 residue protein corresponding to the putative HIV-1 protease. Cell 1988; 54:363-8.

56. von der Helm K, Gurtler L, Eberle J, Deinhardt F. Inhibition of HIV replication in cell culture by the specific aspartic protease inhibitor pepstatin A. FEBS Lett 1989; 247:349-52.

57. Matsukura M, Shinozuka K, Zon G, et al. Phosphorothioate analogs of oligodeoxynucleotides: inhibitors of replication and cytopathic effects of human immunodeficiency virus. Proc Natl Acad Sci USA 1987; 84:7706-10.

58. Alving CR. Delivery of liposome-encapsulated drugs to macrophages. Pharmacol Ther 1983; 22:407-24.

59. Szoka FC Jr, Chu CJ. Increased efficacy of phosphonoformate and phosphonoacetate inhibition of herpes simplex virus type 2 replication by encapsulation in liposomes. Antimicrob Agents Chemother 1988; 32:858-64.

60. Montefiori DC, Pellegrino MG, Robinson WE Jr, et al. Inhibition of HIV-1 proviral DNA synthesis and RNA accumulation by mismatched dsRNA. Biochem Biophys Res Commun 1989; 158:943-50.

61. Montefiori DC, Mitchell WM. Antiviral activity of mismatched double-stranded RNA against human immunodeficiency virus in vitro. Proc Natl Acad Sci USA 1987; 84:2985-9.

62. Carter WA, Strayer DR, Brodsky I, et al. Clinical, immunological, and virological effects of ampligen, a mismatched double-stranded RNA, in patients with AIDS or AIDS-related complex. Lancet 1987; 1:1286-92.

63. American Foundation for AIDS Research (AmFar). Ampligen. AIDS/HIV Experimental Treatment Directory 1988; 2:26-7.

NATURAL HISTORY, CLINICAL SPECTRUM, AND GENERAL MANAGEMENT OF HIV INFECTION

EDITORS

Paul A. Volberding, M.D., and P.T. Cohen, M.D., Ph.D.

4.1

Natural History and Spectrum of HIV Infection

Clinical Spectrum of HIV Infection

Paul A. Volberding, M.D., and P.T. Cohen, M.D., Ph.D.

H uman immunodeficiency virus (HIV) disease progresses from latent HIV infection (identified only by laboratory evidence in otherwise healthy asymptomatic patients) to severely damaged immunologic function in patients with AIDS (acquired immunodeficiency syndrome). This spectrum will be discussed in terms of (1) the general progression of events from HIV infection to the development of AIDS; (2) nomenclature used to characterize the spectrum; (3) various clinical presentations and characteristics that locate or classify a particular patient within the spectrum; and (4) factors that may influence or predict the rate of disease progression.

■ GENERAL DESCRIPTION OF PROGRESSION OF HIV INFECTION

HIV infection begins when the individual is inoculated with the virus. Inoculation can occur either directly into the bloodstream (as during intravenous drug use with needle sharing, a needlestick injury, or receipt of HIV-contaminated blood products); or by exposure of the broken skin, an open wound, or mucous membranes to HIV-contaminated fluids (as during sexual contact with an HIV-infected partner, or occupational exposure to HIV-contaminated body fluids); or by perinatal transmission from infected mother to infant.[1]

After inoculation, infection may follow several alternative pathways.[2,3,47,48] Perhaps in some cases the infection is successfully aborted, although this has never been documented. Alternatively, the virus infects and begins to replicate in one or more types of susceptible cells. Circulating CD4 lymphocytes and macrophages are most commonly affected, although epithelial cells of the gastrointestinal tract, uterine cervical cells, and glial cells of the central nervous system (CNS) may also be targets.

At this point, HIV could conceivably enter a latent state with little replication and no antibody response,[9,48,49] although in the overwhelming majority of infections the virus probably replicates sufficiently to produce detectable levels of viral antigens and elicit host antibody production within a few weeks to months. During this period the patient often experiences a few days of clinical symptoms suggestive of a viral illness. In many cases these symptoms are probably ignored, although in some cases a mononucleosis-like syndrome or some other significant symptom complex appears.[4,5]

As the host's immune system mounts its initial antibody response to HIV, viral antigen is neutralized and disappears or is detectable only at low levels. The patient usually becomes asymptomatic and remains so for a period that may range from weeks to many years. HIV antibodies, but usually not HIV antigens, are detectable in the serum, and viral nucleic acid is detectable in infected cells. During this period, viral replication is held in check. The majority of infected individuals exist in this state and are identified by screening of serum for HIV antibody. A few individuals have become seronegative for HIV antibody during this period — a rare phenomenon of unknown clinical significance.[50] Even these individuals, however, continue to show presence of HIV genome in peripheral blood mononuclear cells.[49]

Major challenges for the immediate future are to understand why HIV disease is contained during this asymptomatic period and to conduct prospective studies to learn how to intervene with effective clinical management before symptoms and signs of disease emerge.

In most if not all cases, viral replication eventually resumes or accelerates. Activation of the cellular immune system by antigenic stimulation from other infectious agents may be one factor in promoting increased HIV replication. The time required for viral replication to resume, the subsequent rate of progression of disease, and the specific clinical syndromes that appear vary from person to person.

As viral replication proceeds, CD4 lymphocytes are destroyed by HIV infection and cell fusion, and monocyte-macrophages are rendered dysfunctional. Damage to these key cells probably leads to abnormal activation of other immune mechanisms and accounts for the observed dysfunction of B-cell and cytotoxic T-cell response. The clinical syndromes observed at any time depend partly on the degree of immunocompromise and partly on direct effects of HIV, particularly in the CNS. AIDS is diagnosed when a syndrome indicative of severe immunocompromise appears. Syndromes of less severity have been lumped under the term ARC (AIDS-related complex), and represent HIV disease that has not yet progressed to AIDS.

As the immune system deteriorates, the host becomes not only increasingly vulnerable to opportunistic infections and malignancies, but also is less able to slow the process of HIV replication. Antibodies to HIV p24 antigen decrease in titer and may become undetectable, while viral core antigens reappear. Eventually an untreatable complication results in death.[2,3,47,48]

■ NOMENCLATURE

An increasingly sophisticated understanding of the spectrum of HIV infection has evolved because of laboratory tests identifying the virus and epidemiologic studies delineating the natural history of infection. Terminology has undergone a parallel evolution. For clinical and research purposes, some terminology, such as "AIDS-related complex" or "ARC," is now of limited use in characterizing patients and monitoring progression along the disease spectrum.

What we now know to be HIV-related disease was at first identified only as a clinical syndrome of otherwise unexplained immune deficiency termed acquired immunodeficiency syndrome, or "AIDS." An infectious etiologic agent was suspected, but not yet identified, and there was no laboratory test for the suspected agent. For both clinical and case reporting purposes, a definition was needed so that epidemiologic studies could proceed. The term AIDS was deliberately defined to characterize only the most unequivocal examples of acquired immunodeficiency. As additional progressive, seriously disabling, and fatal syndromes have been identified and attributed to HIV, the definition has been modified to include them.[6]

Early in the epidemic, a number of other clinical syndromes were recognized as related to AIDS because they occurred among populations at risk for AIDS and because afflicted individuals often developed AIDS. These conditions were subsumed under the term AIDS-related complex, or ARC.

With the identification and isolation of HIV and the development of diagnostic tests specific for HIV infection, the virus was detected in asymptomatic individuals, and in persons with ARC and AIDS. It is now clear that the great majority of infected individuals do not have AIDS. Unfortunately, further studies suggest that progression to AIDS is common, and for all types of HIV infection, progression appears to be the rule rather than the exception. In the individual patient, the probability and rate of disease progression correlate with the activity of the virus in the host and the degree of destruction of the host's immune system. For both clinical prognostication and research purposes, characteristics that reflect these phenomena are being employed to classify patients within the disease spectrum.

The term ARC is vague with respect to prognosis and is not descriptive of the severity of immune system derangement or the level of activity of HIV in the infected host. As such, it is of limited use as a clinical diagnosis or as an identifying term for case reporting. Because of this, its use should be discouraged in favor of other classification schemes.

Similarly, the term AIDS is of limited value. It is not precise because there is a significant variation in prognosis within the subset of patients fulfilling the Centers for Disease Control (CDC) definition of AIDS. In addition, when used as a designation for the HIV epidemic, it focuses attention away from the remainder of the spectrum of HIV disease. The report of the Presidential Commission on the HIV Epidemic states:

> *The term AIDS is obsolete. HIV infection more correctly defines the problem. The medical, public health, political, and community leadership must focus on the full course of HIV infection rather than concentrating on the later stages of disease (ARC and AIDS). Continual focus on the later stages of disease rather than the entire spectrum of HIV infection has left our nation unable to deal adequately with the epidemic.*[51]

The term AIDS continues to have some use as a designation for the severe end of the spectrum of HIV disease characterized by severe immunologic derangement and morbidity-producing syndromes resulting from the direct effects of HIV and from opportunistic infections and malignancies.

■ THE POST-INOCULATION PERIOD

Much is still unknown about the events occurring in the period immediately after inoculation of the host with HIV.

A mononucleosis-like syndrome has been documented with acute HIV infection in many cases. Viral syndrome-like clinical signs may even occur in a majority of HIV infections, but may be attributed to benign viral illnesses and go unrecognized.[4,5]

Most often, HIV infection is detected in asymptomatic individuals, and observations indicate that a clinically latent stage ranging from months to years is the rule. Most infected persons are thought to manifest detectable HIV antigens and HIV antibodies within six months of infection. However, some do not and thus escape detection by the usual HIV-antibody screening tests.[9,48,49]

Small amounts of HIV nucleic acid provirus in a small number of infected host cells might be the only initial manifestation of HIV infection.

The polymerase chain reaction (PCR) technique for detecting HIV nucleic acid sequences among the relatively large amount of host nucleic acid[7,8] has begun to contribute to our understanding of this period of infection.[49] This technique is described in detail in another chapter.

Data have been published suggesting that some individuals will not produce detectable antibodies for as long as 35 months after infection.[9,49] Whether this is a rare occurrence or a common phenomenon with far-reaching implications remains to be determined.

■ CLINICAL PRESENTATIONS AND CLASSIFICATION OF HIV

HIV infection may present in any of the following ways: as an acute viral syndrome, often resembling infectious mononucleosis[4,5]; as an asymptomatic state characterized only by laboratory evidence of HIV infection; as a lymphadenopathy syndrome termed "persistent generalized lymphadenopathy" (PGL); as chronic constitutional symptoms, often systemic and nonspecific (weight loss, fever, night sweats); as a neurologic syndrome resulting from direct effects of HIV; as a chronic diarrheal illness; as a syndrome resulting from an opportunistic infection or malignancy; and as any combination of these. These presentations are discussed in detail in other chapters.

The CDC has presented a classification system emphasizing clinical presentation of the illness. This system is intended for "public health purposes, including disease reporting and surveillance, epidemiologic studies, prevention and control activities, and public health policy planning." The CDC classification is not intended for establishing prognosis: "Classification in a particular group is not explicitly intended to have prognostic significance, nor to designate severity of illness." Thus, this system is of limited use in predicting the course of an individual patient. The system is summarized below.[10]

TABLE 1. SUMMARY OF CLASSIFICATION SYSTEM FOR HUMAN T-LYMPHOTROPIC VIRUS TYPE III/ LYMPHADENOPATHY-ASSOCIATED VIRUS

Group I.   Acute infection
Group II.   Asymptomatic infection*
Group III.   Persistent generalized lymphadenopathy*
Group IV.   Other disease
  Subgroup A.   Constitutional disease
  Subgroup B.   Neurologic disease
  Subgroup C.   Secondary infectious diseases
    Category C-1.   Specified secondary infectious diseases listed in the CDC surveillance definition for AIDS**
    Category C-2.   Other specified secondary infectious diseases
  Subgroup D.   Secondary cancers**
  Subgroup E.   Other conditions

---

* *Patients in Groups II and III may be subclassified on the basis of a laboratory evaluation.*

** *Includes those patients whose clinical presentation fulfills the definition of AIDS used by the CDC for national reporting.*

■ PROGRESSION ALONG THE SPECTRUM — CLASSIFICATION

Classifying a patient within the clinical spectrum of HIV disease and following disease progression over time is done most effectively by using clinical symptoms and signs and laboratory measurements to classify disease state. Evolution and modification of classification schemes is a continuing process as more is learned about HIV-related disease and about which measures are most useful for predicting and monitoring a person's clinical course.[11,52]

One example of a classification system for the spectrum of HIV-related disease is the Walter Reed staging classification, which uses T4-helper-cell counts and clinical data.[12] Several studies have used this system (or modifications of it) in their study design.[12-15] The system has been criticized for using lymphadenopathy syndrome as a prognostic measure when several studies suggest that this syndrome alone does not correlate with prognosis,[11,16-20] and for failing to include thrombocytopenia as a clinical condition that may have prognostic value.[13,14]

The following table summarizes this classification. The classification system is based on the observation that T4 lymphocytes (CD4 lymphocytes, T-helper cells) are progressively lost as HIV infection progresses.

TABLE 2.   THE WALTER REED STAGING CLASSIFICATION FOR HIV INFECTION*

STAGE	HIV ANTI-BODY OR VIRUS ISOLA-TION	CHRONIC LYMPHADE-NOPATHY	T-HELPER CELLS/ CUBIC MM	DHS	THRUSH	O.I.
WR 0	—	—	>400	NL	—	—
WR 1	(+)	—	>400	NL	—	—
WR 2	(+)	(+)	>400	NL	—	—
WR 3	(+)	±	(<400)	NL	—	—
WR 4	(+)	±	(<400)	(P)	—	—
WR 5	(+)	±	(<400)	(C and/or +)	—	—
WR 6	(+)	±	(<400)	PC	±	(+)

* *The essential criteria for assignment to each stage are indicated by parentheses. DHS denotes delayed hypersensitivity; NL, normal; P, partial cutaneous anergy, which is defined as an intact cutaneous response to only one of the four test antigens; C, complete cutaneous anergy to the four test antigens; and O.I., opportunistic infection.*

To be clinically useful, a classification scheme must divide the clinical spectrum of disease into categories that correspond to available management strategies. In terms of presently available therapies, a division at CD4 lymphocyte counts of 200 and 500 cells/cubic mm offers a crude system which might be useful to clinicians as an interim classification scheme. The cut-offs at 200 and 500 reflect the design of clinical studies, rather than a discontinuity in the spectrum of HIV disease. Studies have demonstrated the benefits of AZT therapy for patients with CD4 counts below 500 cells/cubic mm and of prophylaxis against Pneumocystis pneumonia. Patients with higher cell counts benefit from education, baseline screening, periodic evaluation, and some management alterations because of HIV infection.

■ PROGRESSION ALONG THE SPECTRUM — USEFUL DIAGNOSTIC PARAMETERS

Laboratory values that have been reported to correlate with disease progression include elevation of erythrocyte sedimentation rate (ESR),[20] anemia,[20] thrombocytopenia,[18,21,22] T4 lymphocyte counts,[18,20,30,53-55] T-helper/suppressor ratios,[21] serum β_2-microglobulin,[20] serum and urine neopterin levels,[15,56,57] and serum levels of HIV p24 antigen.[14,20,23-27,53] The use of these measurements for clinical management is a major goal, but only preliminary recommendations can be made at present.

Erythrocyte Sedimentation Rate.   An ESR above 40 mm/hour carries a poorer prognosis, as a more rapid progression to AIDS is often observed in patients with this finding. A possible explanation for the elevated ESR in HIV-infected patients is that the mono- or polyclonal increases in immunoglobulins elevate the erythrocyte sedimentation rate,[28] and HIV infection causes a polyclonal B-cell activation with immunoglobulin production.[29] However, the ESR is elevated in many chronic illnesses, infections, and malignancies other than HIV infection.

Unexplained Anemia.   Unexplained anemia is associated with a poorer prognosis.[11,20] No specific mechanism has been discovered to relate anemia to HIV pathogenesis, and, like the elevated ESR, it is often found in other chronic diseases.

Thrombocytopenia.   Thrombocytopenia has been associated with progression to AIDS.[11,18,21,22] Two mechanisms have been proposed: (1) immune complex and complement deposits on platelets leading to clearance by the macrophage system; and (2) specific antiplatelet antibodies. Either of these mechanisms could be triggered by the non-specific B-cell activation and antibody production observed in HIV-infected patients.[29]

T Lymphocytes and Helper/Suppressor Ratios.   Currently, the T4 lymphocyte (helper lymphocyte) count is the variable most commonly monitored as a predictor of disease progression. Experience suggests a correlation between a low T4 count and poor prognosis, with no obvious breakpoint in the correlation. An absolute T4 count below 150/cubic mm or a falling T4 count correlates with progression, while T4 counts above 400 cells/cubic mm have a much lower probability of rapid progression in studies and clinical experience to date.[11,14,18-20,30,53-55] This correlation is not surprising, since the T4 lymphocyte is a major target cell of HIV. The T4 lymphocyte carries the CD4 receptor on its surface. This receptor is the attachment site for HIV when the virus initiates infection. The destruction of T4 lymphocytes in turn has profound effects on other components of the immune system.[2,3]

The ratio of T-helper lymphocytes to T-suppressor lymphocytes, the helper/suppressor or T4:T8 ratio, correlates with prognosis. Ratios in healthy individuals are generally above 1.5, whereas values below 0.8 carry a poorer prognosis.

Neopterin Levels.   Neopterin is a pterin compound arising during the metabolism of folic acid. It has been found in increased amounts in the serum and urine of patients with viral illnesses and malignancies. Neopterin is reported to be a marker of T-lymphocyte and cellular immune system activation.[31,32] It has been found in increased amounts in HIV-infected patients and reported to be of prognostic value.[15,33,56,57]

In vitro experiments suggest that antigenic stimulation of latently HIV-infected T lymphocytes may result not only in activation of the lymphocyte, but also in the reactivation of HIV from a latent state to active replication of the virus.[34,35,58] These observations have led some authors to conclude that T-cell activation, indicated by elevated neopterin levels, is a harbinger of progression and that therapies should avoid T-cell activation and consider immunosuppression instead.[36] The utility of neopterin levels for predicting progression must await additional evaluation in prospective studies. There is general agreement that, when possible, antigenic stimulation (e.g., by co-infection) should be avoided in HIV-infected individuals. However, the use of immunosuppressive therapy to prevent progression to AIDS, while an interesting concept, is not generally accepted at present. The precise use of neopterin levels in clinical management is yet to be determined.

β_2-Microglobulin Levels. β_2-microglobulin occurs on the surface of all nucleated cells, where it is noncovalently associated with the membrane glycoprotein class I HLA gene products. It is sometimes called the "light chain" of the HLA class I antigens. Structurally, it is a polypeptide consisting of 96 amino acid residues containing a single disulfide bridge; it also has considerable homology with the constant heavy-chain regions of the immunoglobulin molecule. It is released into serum during cell turnover.[37]

Although the precise function of β_2-microglobulin in vivo remains unclear, it is considered a nonspecific marker of infectious, inflammatory, malignant, and autoimmune disease activity.[37,38] It is noteworthy that during these disease processes, cellular immunity is often activated, and cell turnover, as well as β_2-microglobulin production, are increased. Elevated serum β_2-microglobulin levels have been observed in numerous malignancies. In lymphoproliferative disorders the serum level correlates with tumor load, and in multiple myeloma the levels are of prognostic value.[39] Elevated urinary levels of β_2-microglobulin have also been used as a marker for proximal renal tubule dysfunction, since it is synthesized in relatively constant amounts, passes through the glomerular filter, and is 99.9 percent reabsorbed by the proximal tubule of the kidney.[40] β_2-microglobulin can be assayed using commercially available enzyme-linked immunoassay kits. The assay is relatively inexpensive.

In several studies of HIV-infected individuals, serum levels of β_2-microglobulin have been reported to correlate with disease activity and with T-helper lymphocyte counts.[20,23-27,37,38] In one study, a β_2-microglobulin level above 3.0 micrograms/ml was the best single predictor of progression.[20] A hypothesis is that antigenic stimulation of the cellular immune system by HIV, cytomegalovirus, or other antigens, leads to increased cell turnover, which both increases production of β_2-microglobulin and stimulates renewed replication of latent HIV, resulting in disease progression. A role for β_2-microglobulin seems to exist in clinical management, but at present the details of how to use specific levels to make decisions about an individual patient are not clear.

HIV p24 Antigen.   The p24 antigen is the major HIV core protein. Serum levels of p24 antigen increase shortly after HIV infection and decline when p24 antibody appears. Both a low level or a subsequent decrease in anti-p24 antitibody and a high level or an increase in p24 antigen correlate with disease progression and a poor prognosis.[14,20,23-27,53] Levels of p24 antigen are increasingly used in studies to monitor efficacy of drug treatments. p24 antigen levels have been shown to decrease during therapy with AZT.[27,41] Commercial enzyme immunoassay kits for HIV p24 antigen are available. Some clinicians determine p24 antigen levels before starting AZT therapy and, after several months of treatment, look for a decrease in these levels as an indicator of successful inhibition of HIV. However, details of how to use p24 antigen levels for clinical management are not yet worked out.

■ USE OF MULTIPLE FACTORS FOR PROGNOSTICATION

One study examined the prognostic value of combinations of factors.[20] In a study of a cohort of homosexual men the following values were shown to have independent predictive value:

- serum β_2-microglobulin >3.0 micrograms/ml
- T4 lymphocyte count <200/cubic millimeter
- T4 lymphocyte percent of total lymphocytes <25 percent
- p24 antigen level present
- packed red-cell volume (hematocrit) <40 percent.

The three-year progression rate for subjects with two or more of these values was 57 percent, compared with 7 percent for subjects with normal values. The two-year progression rate for subjects with four or more abnormalities was 100 percent.

Additional guidelines for prognostication will certainly evolve as information emerges from natural-history studies now in progress.

■ FACTORS RELATED TO PROGRESSION

Several factors have been proposed as risks for more rapid progression of HIV infection.

Age.   A greater age at diagnosis has correlated with a poorer prognosis in several studies.[18,20]

Activation of Cellular Immunity.   Exposure to antigenic stimuli capable of activating the cellular immune system, such as sexually transmitted diseases, may increase risk for progression.[3] This phenomenon is suggested by in vitro data showing that when latently HIV-infected lymphocytes in cell culture are activated by infection with a second virus, the HIV begins to replicate.[34,35,58] Some studies suggest a relation between sexually transmitted diseases and progression of infection.[42,43]

Immunosuppression.   Although there is no proof, it has been assumed that drugs or other conditions leading to immunosuppression will adversely affect prognosis.

Malnutrition.   Whether malnutrition is an independent risk for progression is unclear. It is generally assumed that malnutrition predisposes to progression of infectious diseases.

■ THERAPEUTIC INTERVENTIONS TO LIMIT PROGRESSION

AZT therapy has been shown to inhibit HIV in vivo, to improve diagnostic variables reflecting the severity of HIV infection, and to prolong survival in patients with HIV infection and CD4 counts below 500 cells/cubic mm.[27,41,44-46] Questions still unanswered include whether the benefits of this drug outweigh the risks for individuals with less advanced disease, or if prophylaxis after accidental HIV exposure (such as a needlestick injury) is warranted.

Although no data exist to demonstrate their efficacy, the practices of minimizing exposure to infectious diseases and other potential antigenic stimuli (such as intravenous street drugs), avoiding immunosuppressive drugs, and maintaining good nutrition seem intuitively sensible and worth encouraging.

REFERENCES

1. Friedland GH, Klein RS. Transmission of the human immunodeficiency virus. N Engl J Med 1987; 317:1125-35.
2. Ho DD, Pomerantz RJ, Kaplan JC. Pathogenesis of infection with human immunodeficiency virus. N Engl J Med 1987; 317:278-86.
3. Fauci AS. The human immunodeficiency virus: infectivity and mechanisms of pathogenesis. Science 1988; 239:617-22.
4. Tindall B, Barker S, Donovan B, et al. Characterization of the acute clinical illness associated with human immunodeficiency virus infection. Arch Intern Med 1988; 148:945-9.
5. Fox R, Eldred LJ, Fuchs EJ, et al. Clinical manifestations of acute infection with human immunodeficiency virus in a cohort of gay men. AIDS 1987; 1:35-8.
6. Revision of the CDC surveillance case definition for acquired immunodeficiency syndrome. MMWR 1987; 36(suppl 1S).
7. Ou C, Kowk S, Mitchell SW, et al. DNA amplification for direct detection of HIV-1 in DNA of peripheral blood mononuclear cells. Science 1988; 239:295-7.
8. Mullis KB, Faloona FA. Specific synthesis of DNA in vitro via a polymerase-catalyzed chain reaction. Methods Enzymol 1987; 155:335-50.
9. Ranki A, Valle S, Krohn M, et al. Long latency precedes overt seroconversion in sexually transmitted human-immunodeficiency-virus infection. Lancet 1987; 2:589-93.
10. Classification system for human T-lymphotrophic virus type III/Lymphadenopathy virus infections. MMWR 1986; 35:336-8.
11. Kaslow RA, Phair JP, Friedman HB, et al. Infection with the human immunodeficiency virus: clinical manifestations and their relationship to immune deficiency. Ann Intern Med 1987; 107:474-80.
12. Redfield RR, Wright DC, Tramont EC. The Walter Reed staging classification for HTLV-III/LAV infection. N Engl J Med 1986; 314:131-2.
13. Terragna A, Dodi F, Anselmo M, et al. The Walter Reed staging classification in the follow-up of HIV infection. N Engl J Med 1986; 315:1355-6.
14. Allain J, Laurian Y, Paul DA, et al. Long-term evaluation of HIV antigen and antibodies to p24 and gp41 in patients with hemophilia. N Engl J Med 1987; 317:1114-21.
15. Fuchs D, Reibnegger G, Wachter H, et al. Neopterin levels correlating with the Walter Reed staging classification in human immunodeficiency virus (HIV) infection. Ann Intern Med 1987; 107:784-5.
16. Lang W, Anderson RE, Perkins H, et al. Clinical, immunologic, and serologic findings in men at risk for acquired immunodeficiency syndrome. JAMA 1987; 257:326-30.
17. Osmond D, Chaisson R, Moss A, Krampf W. Lymphadenopathy in asymptomatic patients seropositive for HIV. N Engl J Med 1987; 317:246.
18. Eyster ME, Gail MH, Ballard JO, et al. Natural history of human immunodeficiency virus infections in hemophiliacs: effect of T-cell subsets, platelet counts, and age. Ann Intern Med 1987; 107:1-6.
19. Goedert JJ, Biggar RJ, Melbye M, et al. Effect of T4 count and cofactors on the incidence of AIDS in homosexual men infected with the human immunodeficiency virus. JAMA 1987; 257:331-4.
20. Moss AR, Bacchetti P, Osmond D, et al. Seropositivity for HIV and the development of AIDS or AIDS related condition: three year follow up of the San Francisco General Hospital cohort. Br Med J 1988; 296:745-50.
21. Abrams DI, Kirpov DD, Goedert JJ, et al. Antibodies to human T-lymphocyte virus type III and development of the acquired immunodeficiency syndrome in homosexual men presenting with immune thrombocytopenia. Ann Intern Med 1986; 104:47-50.

22. Walsh C, Krigel R, Lennette E, Karpatkin S. Thrombocytopenia in homosexual patients: prognosis, response to therapy, and prevalence of antibody to the retrovirus associated with the acquired immuno-deficiency syndrome. Ann Intern Med 1985; 103:542-5.

23. Paul DA, Falk LA, Kessler HA, et al. Correlation of serum HIV antigen and antibody with clinical status in HIV-infected patients. J Med Virol 1987; 22:357-63.

24. Goudsmit J, Lange JM, Paul DA, Dawson GJ. Antigenemia and antibody titers to core and envelope antigens in AIDS, AIDS-related complex, and subclinical human immunodeficiency virus infection. J Infect Dis 1987; 155:558-60.

25. Goudsmit J, De Wolf F, Paul DA, et al. Expression of human immunodeficiency virus antigen (HIV-Ag) in serum and cerebrospinal fluid during acute and chronic infection. Lancet 1986; 2:177-80.

26. Lange JM, De Wolf F, Danner SA, et al. Persistent HIV antigenaemia and decline of HIV core antibodies associated with transition to AIDS. Br Med J 1986; 293:1459-1462.

27. Jackson GG, Paul DA, Falk LA, et al. Human immunodeficiency virus (HIV) antigenemia (p24) in the acquired immunodeficiency syndrome (AIDS) and the effect of treatment with zidovudine (AZT). Ann Intern Med 1988; 108:175-80.

28. Talstad I, Haugen HF. The relationship between the erythrocyte sedimentation rate (ESR) and plasma proteins in clinical materials and models. Scand J Clin Lab Invest 1979; 39:519-24.

29. Seligmann M, Pinching AJ, Rosen FS, et al. Immunology of human immunodeficiency virus infection and the acquired immunodeficiency syndrome. Ann Intern Med 1987; 107:234-42.

30. Polk BF, Fox R, Brookmeyer R, et al. Predictors of the acquired immunodeficiency syndrome developing in a cohort of seropositive homosexual men. N Engl J Med 1987; 316:61-6.

31. Kern P, Rokos H, Dietrich M. Raised serum neopterin levels and imbalances of T-lymphocyte subsets in viral diseases, acquired immune deficiency syndrome and related lymphadenopathy syndromes. Bio-medicine and Pharmacotherapy 1984; 38:407-11.

32. Huber C, Fuchs D, Niederwieser D, et al. Neopterin, a new biochemical marker for clinical assessment of cell-mediated immune response. Klin Wochenschr 1984; 62:103-13.

33. Hutterer J, Fuchs D, Eder G, et al. Neopterin as a discriminating and prognostic parameter in healthy homosexuals, ARC and AIDS patients . Wien Klin Wochenschr 1987; 99:531-5.

34. Gendelman HF, Leonard J, Weck K, et al. Herpesviral transactivation of the human immunodeficiency virus (HIV) by long terminal repeat sequence [Abstract]. III International Conference on AIDS. Washington, 1987; 13.

35. Luciw P, Tong-Sarksen SE, Matija Peterlin B. T-cell activation increases gene expression directed by the HIV LTR: implications for pathogenesis in AIDS [Abstract]. III International Conference on AIDS. Washington, 1987; 6.

36. Wachter H, Blecha HG, Fuchs D, et al. Activation of the macrophage/lymphocyte system in AIDS, ARC and AIDS risk groups. Wien Klin Wochenschr 1986; 98:449-54.

37. Karlsson FA, Wibell L, Evrin PE. β_2-microglobulin in clinical medicine. Scand J Clin Lab Invest 1980; 40(suppl 154):27-37.

38. Forman DT. β_2-microglobulin — an immunogenetic marker of inflammatory and malignant origin. Ann Clin Lab Sci 1982; 12:447-52.

39. Child JA, Kushwaha MR. Serum β_2-microglobulin in lymphoproliferative and myeloproliferative diseases. Hematological Oncology 1984; 2:391-401.

40. Statius van Eps LW, Schardijn GH. Value of determination of β_2-microglobulin in toxic nephropathy and interstitial nephritis. Wien Klin Wochenschr 1984; 96:673-8.

41. Chaisson RE, Allain JP, Leuther M, Volberding PA. Significant changes in HIV antigen level in the serum of patients treated with azidothymidine. N Engl J Med 1986; 315:1610-1.

42. Weber JN, Wadsworth J, Rogers LA, et al. Three-year prospective study of HTLV-III/LAV infection in homosexual men. Lancet 1986; 1:1170-82.

43. Weber JN, McCreaner A, Berrie E, et al. Factors affecting seropositivity to HTLV-III/LAV and progression of disease in sexual partners of patients with AIDS. Genitourin Med 1986; 62:177-80.

44. Hirsch MS. Azidothymidine. J Infect Dis 1988; 157:427-31.

45. Fischl MA, Richman DD, Grieco MH, et al. The efficacy of azidothymidine (AZT) in the treatment of patients with AIDS and AIDS-related complex. N Engl J Med 1987; 317:185-91.

46. Richman DD, Fischl MA, Grieco MH, et al. The toxicity of azidothymidine (AZT) in the treatment of patients with AIDS and AIDS-related complex. N Engl J Med 1987; 317:192-7.

47. Haseltine WA. Replication and pathogenesis of the AIDS virus [Review]. J Acquir Immune Defic Syndr 1988; 1:217-40.

48. Haseltine WA. Silent HIV infections. N Engl J Med 1989; 320:1487-9.

49. Imagawa DT, Lee MH, Wolinsky SM, et al. Human immunodeficiency virus type 1 infection in homosexual men who remain seronegative for prolonged periods. N Engl J Med 1989; 320:1458-62.

50. Farzadegan H, Polis MA, Wolinsky SM, et al. Loss of human immunodeficiency virus type 1 (HIV-1) antibodies with evidence of viral infection in asymptomatic homosexual men. A report from the Multi-center AIDS Cohort Study. Ann Intern Med 1988; 108:785-90.

51. Report of the Presidential Commission on the Human Immunodeficiency Virus Epidemic. Washington, D.C.: Presidential Commission on the Human Immunodeficiency Virus Epidemic, 1988:xvii.

52. Redfield RR, Tramont EC. Toward a better classification system for HIV infection. N Engl J Med 1989; 320:1414-6.

53. Eyster ME, Ballard JO, Gail MH, et al. Predictive markers for the acquired immunodeficiency syndrome (AIDS) in hemophiliacs: persistence of p24 antigen and low T4 cell count. Ann Intern Med 1989; 110:963-9.

54. Taylor JM, Fahey JL, Detels R, Giorgi JV. CD4 percentage, CD4 number, and CD4:CD8 ratio in HIV infection: which to choose and how to use. J Acquir Immune Defic Syndr 1989; 2:114-24.

55. Lang W, Perkins H, Anderson RE, et al. Patterns of T lymphocyte changes with human immuno-deficiency virus infection: from seroconversion to the development of AIDS. J Acquir Immune Defic Syndr 1989; 2:63-9.

56. Kramer A, Wiktor SZ, Fuchs D, et al. Neopterin: a predictive marker of acquired immune deficiency syndrome in human immunodeficiency virus infection. J Acquir Immune Defic Syndr 1989; 2:291-6.

57. Melmed RN, Taylor JM, Detels R, et al. Serum neopterin changes in HIV-infected subjects: indicator of significant pathology, CD4 T cell changes, and the development of AIDS. J Acquir Immune Defic Syndr 1989; 2:70-76.

58. Zagury D, Bernard J, Leonard R, et al. Long-term cultures of HTLV-III-infected T cells: a model of cytopathology of T-cell depletion in AIDS. Science 1986; 231:850-3.

4.1.2

Acute HIV Infection

Suzanne M. Crowe, M.B.B.S., F.R.A.C.P., and Michael S. McGrath, M.D., Ph.D.

Acute human immunodeficiency virus (HIV) infection may present as an infectious mononucleosis-like syndrome, or less commonly as an acute neurologic illness (meningitis, encephalitis, polyneuropathy, or myelopathy). Individuals infected with HIV may develop this acute illness before developing antibodies directed toward HIV components (seroconversion). The incidence of HIV mononucleosis is not accurately known. In an Australian study, eleven of 12 men who seroconverted were questioned retrospectively and reported an illness consistent with acute HIV syndrome.[1] Acute HIV infection has been described in homosexual men,[1] intravenous drug users,[2] in a hemophiliac,[3] a health care worker,[4] and in the female sexual partner of a bisexual man.[5] Thus, it is part of the clinical spectrum of disease associated with HIV infection and should be considered in the differential diagnosis of infectious mononucleosis-like syndromes and acute neurologic disorders.

■ INCUBATION PERIOD

The interval from infection to onset of illness in acute HIV infection is reported to vary from six days to six weeks.[2] In many instances the date of exposure is uncertain. The first report of this illness, the British needlestick case[4] (a nurse caring for a patient with AIDS sustained a needlestick injury while resheathing a hypodermic needle), revealed that the onset of illness occurred thirteen days after parenteral exposure. The incubation period may be longer in homosexual men because of the smaller dose of inoculum and the nonparenteral route of infection.[2] There have been infrequent instances in which the incubation period is much longer — up to 6 months.[13,14] However, documentation of exposure in these reports is less reliable.

■ CLINICAL PRESENTATION

The illness begins with the abrupt onset of nonspecific symptoms including fever, sweats, rigors, myalgia, neuralgia, headaches, and gastrointestinal disturbances (see Table 1).

Approximately three quarters of patients complain of a sore throat; this is invariably associated with pharyngeal erythema.[1] The presence of exudate and small ulcers involving the palate and buccal mucosa have been reported.[6,7]

A macular, erythematous rash develops during the course of illness in about fifty percent of patients.[7] The rash is initially more prominent on the chest and trunk and later involves the extremities.[4] The individual lesions are sparse, up to one centimeter in diameter, and fade within one week.[6] The rash may resemble roseola.[1] Other dermatologic manifestations include urticaria,[2] alopecia,[8] and desquamation of palms and soles.[1]

TABLE 1.   CLINICAL FEATURES IN 12 CASES OF ACUTE
HIV INFECTION*

	N	Percent
fever/sweats	11	92
myalgia/arthralgia	11	92
malaise/lethargy	10	83
lymphadenopathy	9	75
sore throat	9	75
anorexia/nausea/vomiting	8	67
headaches/photophobia	7	58
rash	6	50
diarrhea	4	33

*   *Modified with permission from Cooper DA, Gold J, Maclean P, et al.*[1] *Reprinted with permission of
The Lancet.*

Generalized lymphadenopathy has been observed in approximately three quarters of individuals acutely infected with HIV. Splenomegaly[1] and tender hepatomegaly with elevation of liver enzymes have also been frequent findings in these patients.[1,6,8]

The HIV is neurotropic[9] and neurologic disease may occur as a manifestation of acute infection. Photophobia occurs in over fifty percent of patients[1]; however, laboratory documented acute aseptic meningitis has been reported in only two patients.[2] HIV has been isolated from the cerebrospinal fluid (CSF) of patients who developed acute meningitis coincident with seroconversion.[10] Acute encephalopathy is also a rare consequence of acute HIV.[11] HIV-associated encephalopathy is characterized by a nonspecific prodromal period that lasts up to two weeks and the subsequent development of mood changes, confusion, incontinence, and seizures.[11] Neurologic examination may reveal altered mental status without localizing focal signs, including plantar responses, which may be extensor. Recently, acute facial palsy and sensori-motor peripheral neuropathy have been described, associated with seroconversion.[5] Depression, apparently unrelated to external conditions, is notable in some patients, and may persist for several months.[1,6]

Symptoms that appear acutely after infection with HIV generally resolve within two to three weeks. Lymphadenopathy, splenomegaly, lethargy, fever, and myalgia often continue for several months.[1,6]

■ DIAGNOSIS

The development of commercial antigen capture assays to detect HIV antigens (especially HIV p24) may allow earlier diagnosis of HIV infection. Whereas seroconversion occurs uncommonly during acute HIV illness, HIV antigenemia can be demonstrated as soon as two weeks after infection.[15] In a recent study, sequential samples of serum from 35 men who seroconverted showed HIV antigen in five subjects up to 16 weeks prior to seroconversion.[16] In a second study, nine of 14 individuals had detectable HIV antigen prior to seroconversion. Some of these subjects remain antigenemic. In general, there is less detectable HIV antigen within three to six months[15] and recurrence of antigenemia late in disease. Human immunodeficiency virus p24 antigen may be present in cerebrospinal fluid.[16] Persistence within cerebrospinal fluid is thought to reflect severe central nervous system disease.

■ SEROCONVERSION

Seroconversion, or the state at which antibodies to HIV viral components become detectable, has been reported to occur from eight days[11] to ten weeks[2] after the onset of acute illness. Antibodies directed against the various retroviral components do not develop simultaneously; antibodies to the envelope glycoproteins (gp160 and gp120) and to the major core protein (p24) may be detected up to four weeks before those directed against the transmembrane protein (p41) and phosphoprotein (p17).[2]

■ DIFFERENTIAL DIAGNOSIS

Acute HIV infection produces a constellation of symptoms that are similar to those induced by several other infectious agents. Care must be taken by the clinician to exclude infection with these other microorganisms before a diagnosis of acute HIV infection is made. Depending on the individual's presentation, infection with Epstein–Barr virus (EBV), cytomegalovirus (CMV), *Toxoplasma gondii*, *Treponema pallidum*, rubella, herpes simplex virus, and hepatitis B virus should be excluded before making a diagnosis of acute HIV infection.

■ LABORATORY FINDINGS

Lymphopenia with normal T4:T8 ratio (the comparison of leu 3/T4+ helper T cells with leu 2/T8+ suppressor T cells, a ratio usually greater than one) and thrombocytopenia are common laboratory abnormalities that occur with the onset of symptoms.[1] Following this, a marked proliferation of suppressor T cells occurs, and reaches a maximum rate approximately two weeks after the onset of illness. This leu 2/T8+ cell proliferation results in an inverted T-cell ratio.[6] Simultaneously, atypical lymphocytes appear in the peripheral blood. Recovery from the acute illness is associated with gradual and incomplete resolution of the leu2/T8+ T-cell lymphocytosis, with sustained inversion of T4:T8 ratio,[6] a phenomenon also seen with other viral infections including EBV and CMV.[12] Some patients develop a polymorphonuclear leukocytosis, rather than lymphopenia, during the acute illness.[2,5] Transient rises in hepatic transaminase occur commonly[1,6,7] and the lactate dehydrogenase may be markedly elevated.[8]

The CSF in two reported patients with acute meningitis[2] and in three patients with encephalopathy[1] may be entirely normal or have up to 30 lymphocytes per cubic millimeter with mildly increased protein (up to 1 g/l) and a normal glucose. HIV has been cultured from blood and CSF during the acute illness before seroconversion.[2,10]

■ SUMMARY AND CONCLUSIONS

Illness attributed to acute HIV infection generally occurs within two to three weeks of exposure to the virus. An infectious mononucleosis-like syndrome is the most common presentation; however, various acute neurologic conditions have been described. Development of antibodies is delayed when compared with other viral infections. Detectable HIV antigens in the serum may provide diagnosis during the acute illness.

The number of individuals in whom seroconversion occurs without the development of acute symptoms is not known. Whether these individuals have a prognosis different from the prognosis in those acquiring HIV infection with symptoms is also unknown.

HIV infection must be differentiated from other acute infectious mononucleosis-like syndromes. The delay before seroconversion is noteworthy because during this period the individual, negative by current AIDS antibody screening techniques, may, however, transmit HIV.

REFERENCES

1. Cooper D A, Gold J, Maclean P, et al. Acute AIDS retrovirus infection: Definition of a clinical illness associated with seroconversion. Lancet 1985; 1:537-40.

2. Ho DD, Sarngadharan MG, Resnick L, et al. Primary human T lymphotropic virus type III infection. Ann Intern Med 1985; 103:880-3.

3. Tucker J, Ludlam CA, Craig A, et al. HTLV-III infection associated with glandular-fever-like illness in a haemophiliac. Lancet 1985; 1:585.

4. Editorial. Needlestick transmission of HTLV-III from a patient infected in Africa. Lancet 1984; 11:1376-7.

5. Piette AM, Tussau F, Vignon D, et al. Acute neuropathy coincident with seroconversion for anti LAV/HTLV-III. Lancet 1986; 1:852.

6. Biggs B, Newton-John H. Acute HTLV-III infection: A case followed from onset to seroconversion. Med J Aust 1986; 144:545-6.

7. Lindskov R, Lindhardt BO, Weismann K, et al. Acute HTLV-III infection with roseola-like rash. Lancet 1986; 1:447.

8. Romeril KR. Acute HTLV-III infection. New Zealand Med J 1985; 98:401.

9. Shaw GM, Harper ME, Hahn BH, et al. HTLV-III infection in brains of children and adults with AIDS encephalopathy. Science 1985; 227:177-81.

10. Ho D, Rota T, Schooley R, et al. Isolation of HTLV-III from cerebrospinal fluid and neural tissues of patients with neurologic syndromes related to the acquired immunodeficiency syndrome. N Engl J Med 1985; 313:1493-7.

11. Carne CA, Tedder RS, Smith A, et al. Acute encephalopathy coincident with seroconversion for anti-HTLV-III. Lancet 1985; 11:1206-8.

12. Drew WL, Mills J, Levy JA, et al. Cytomegalovirus infection and abnormal T-lymphocyte subset ratios in homosexual men. Ann Intern Med 1985; 103:61-3.

13. Pristeria R, Seebacher C, Casini M, et al. Acute infection by HIV in drug addicts [Abstract]. Washington, DC: III International Conference on AIDS, 1987; 178.

14. Matheron S, Dormont D, Rey MA, et al. Kinetics of HIV infection after IV exposure to blood from an AIDS patient [Abstract]. Washington, DC: III International Conference on AIDS, 1987; 67.

15. Allain JP, Laurian Y, Paul DA, et al. Serological markers in early stages of human immunodeficiency virus infection in hemophiliacs. Lancet 1986; 2:1233-6.

16. Goudsmit J, de Wolf F, Paul DA, et al. Expression of human immunodeficiency virus antigen (HIV-Ag) in serum and cerebrospinal fluid during acute and chronic infection. Lancet 1986; 2:177-80.

Definition of ARC

Donald I. Abrams, M.D.

H IV infection is now understood as a continuum with a predictable natural history ending in the immune exhaustion now termed AIDS. AIDS-related complex (ARC) is being gradually abandoned as a clinical description. However, because ARC was an important concept in earlier descriptions of HIV disease, a brief note on its history is provided here as a reminder of medicine's evolving understanding of this pandemic.

The clinical conditions described as "AIDS related" were recognized up to two years before AIDS was formally described in 1981. As early as 1979, physicians caring for large numbers of homosexual men in San Francisco and New York had begun to note an increased incidence of generalized lymphadenopathy and constitutional symptoms in this population.[1,2] Lymph-node biopsies generally revealed benign reactive changes, and the condition was initially labeled "gay lymph-node syndrome (GLNS)."

In mid-1981, the first formal definitions of the syndrome of acquired immunodeficiency were published in the medical literature. Early reports of the physical findings in patients with the disorder revealed a high incidence of generalized lymphadenopathy along with the malignancies and opportunistic infections that defined AIDS at that time.[3] Attention was again turned to the members of the homosexual community who had been recognized as having the "gay lymph-node syndrome." Were these two phenomena connected in any way? Would patients with this benign lymphadenopathy go on to develop the more severe manifestations of acquired immunodeficiency?

In 1981, researchers from both coasts reported the lymphadenopathy syndrome to the Centers for Disease Control. Prospective natural-history study cohorts were assembled in medical centers in New York and California. After reviewing medical records from a number of New York City patients with lymphadenopathy, the Centers for Disease Control published the initial description of "persistent generalized lymphadenopathy (PGL)" in homosexual men in May 1982.[4]

In subsequent reports on PGL, however, slightly different criteria were used for including patients in each PGL cohort. Moreover, PGL was given a variety of different acronyms or names: chronic lymphadenopathy syndrome (CLS), extended lymphadenopathy syndrome (ELAS), idiopathic lymphadenopathy syndrome (ILS), lymphadenopathy syndrome (LAS, LAN, LNS), generalized persistent lymphadenopathy (GPL), chronic polyadenopathy, lymphadenomegaly syndrome, and chronic unexplained lymphadenopathy (CUL). Investigators who associated the lymphadenopathy syndrome with progression toward full-blown AIDS, even before HIV was identified as the common causal agent, designated the condition as acquired immunodeficiency-like syndrome and AIDS-related lymphadenopathy. "Lesser AIDS" was also proposed as a descriptive term to characterize patients with lymphadenopathy and other constitutional symptoms.

Early in the observation of natural history cohorts, some patients began to develop more life-threatening manifestations of AIDS,[5-9] so lymphadenopathy and other evidence of immune dysfunction were then described as "pre-AIDS" or as "AIDS prodrome." All of these terms described overlapping subsets of patients. The plethora of names served only to add to the general confusion about PGL's significance in patients in AIDS risk groups.

In an attempt to establish a more workable definition and to assure uniformity of the subset of patients being followed in prospective studies of natural history and therapeutic intervention trials, an extramural AIDS working group of the National Institutes of Health participated in a telephone conference call on June 10, 1983. Participants in this ad hoc working group included Donald Abrams (University of California, San Francisco), James Allen (Centers for Disease Control), Donald Armstrong (Memorial Sloan-Kettering Institute), Genrose Copley (National Cancer Institute), Robert Edelman (National Institutes of Allergy and Infectious Disease), Alvin Friedman-Kien (New York University), Michael Gottlieb (University of California, Los Angeles), Evan Hersh (M.D. Anderson), and Jack Killen (National Cancer Institute). The stated purpose of the conference call was "to attempt to develop a common definition accepted by all working group members for the variety of conditions variously referred to as lymphadenopathy syndrome, AIDS prodrome, etc." and "to develop a minimum common data set to be collected on all patients at their initial evaluation" (Killen JY: unpublished correspondence). The information developed was intended solely for use within the working group and was never meant to carry with it any official connotation. The members all agreed that "any title should not imply a prodromal condition to overt AIDS, given our current state of knowledge and a variety of psychosocial and medical/financial considerations." It was Dr. Killen from the National Cancer Institute who first suggested the name "AIDS-related complex" (ARC) during the course of this conference call. Ultimately, all members agreed upon ARC as an acceptable name.[9]

Although the term ARC was initially devised to describe a "complex," many clinicians and patients used it to pigeonhole various "conditions" that were not diagnostic of AIDS but that clearly distinguished patients infected with HIV as having "disease" above and beyond that seen in asymptomatic seropositive patients. Now that HIV has been identified as the cause of AIDS, and an inexorable progression has proved to be the natural history of HIV infection, it is more logical to think of these various manifestations as gradients of host response to infection with the agent, as opposed to static, separate, nonoverlapping syndromes.

Published classification systems for HIV infection stratified the retrovirus-related illness into various stages. The NIH schema categorized the population largely on the basis of clinical features,[11] whereas the Walter Reed staging classification relied heavily on T4 lymphocyte counts and immune phenotyping.[12] Both, however, assumed that the scope of viral infection ranged from well-appearing, asymptomatic seropositive persons to persons with severely deranged immune systems and life-threatening opportunistic infections. In 1986, the CDC reformulated a staging system for HIV infection; this was further impetus to eliminate the term ARC from the working vocabulary of AIDS investigators.[13] But it was long-term prospective studies of HIV-infected cohorts that finally made it clear that immune exhaustion and AIDS were the likely outcome of untreated HIV infection[10,14] and that the concept of "healthy" or "moderately affected" (ARC) HIV-infected persons was inaccurate.

In October 1988, the Committee for the Oversight of AIDS Activities of the Institute of Medicine, National Academy of Sciences, stated its belief that "the term ARC is no longer useful, either from a clinical or a public health perspective." Instead, "HIV infection itself should be considered a disease.[15]" With that recommendation, the term ARC will probably be retired to history.

REFERENCES

1. Metroka CE, Cunningham-Rundles S, Pollack MS, et al. Persistent generalized lymphadenopathy in homosexual men. Ann Intern Med 1983; 99:585-91.

2. Abrams DI, Lewis BJ, Beckstead JH, et al. Persistent diffuse lymphadenopathy in homosexual men: Endpoint or prodrome? Ann Intern Med 1984; 100:801-8.

3. Centers for Disease Control. Epidemiologic aspects of the current outbreak of Kaposi's sarcoma and opportunistic infections. N Engl J Med 1982; 306:248-52.

4. Centers for Disease Control. Persistent, generalized lymphadenopathy among homosexual males. MMWR 1982; 31:249-50.

5. Mathur-Wagh U, Enlow RW, Spigland I, et al. Longitudinal assessment of persistent generalized lymphadenopathy (PGL) in homosexual men: relation to the acquired immunodeficiency syndrome. Lancet 1984; 1:1033-8.

6. Mathur-Wagh U, Mildvan D, Senie RT. Follow-up at 4 1/2 years on homosexual men with generalized lymphadenopathy. N Engl J Med 1985; 313:1542-3.

7. Abrams DI, Mess T, Volberding PA. Lymphadenopathy: Endpoint or prodrome? Update of a 36 month prospective study. Adv Exp Med Biol 1985:187:73-84.

8. Fishbein DB, Kaplan JE, Spira TJ et al. Unexplained lymphadenopathy in homosexual men: A longitudinal study. JAMA 1985; 254:930-5.

9. Gottlieb MS, Wolfe P, Hardy D, et al. Persistent generalized lymphadenopathy: The UCLA experience. Adv Exp Med Biol 1985; 187:85-92.

10. Winkelstein W Jr. Epidemiological observations on the causal nature of the association between infection by the human immunodeficiency virus and the acquired immunodeficiency syndrome. Washington, D.C.: Scientific Forum on the Etiology of AIDS, American Foundation for AIDS Research, 1988.

11. Haverkos HW, Gottlieb MS, Killen JY, Edelman R. Classification of HTLV-III/LAV related diseases. J Infect Dis 1985:152:1095.

12. Redfield RR, Wright DC, Tramong EC. The Walter Reed staging classification for HTLV-III/LAV infection. N Engl J Med 1986; 314:131-2.

13. Centers for Disease Control. Classification system for human T lymphotropic virus type III/lymphadenopathy associated virus infection. MMWR 1986; 35:334-9.

14. Moss AR, Bacchetti P, Osmond D, et al. Seropositivity for HIV and the development of AIDS or AIDS related condition: three-year follow-up of the San Francisco General Hospital cohort. Br Med J 1988; 296:745-50.

15. Institute of Medicine/National Academy of Sciences. Confronting AIDS: Update 1988. Washington, DC: National Academy Press, 1988; 37.

Persistent Generalized Lymphadenopathy (PGL)

Donald I. Abrams, M.D.

The Centers for Disease Control (CDC) defines HIV-related persistent generalized lymphadenopathy (PGL) as palpable lymphadenopathy (lymph-node enlargement of 1 cm or greater) at two or more extrainguinal sites persisting for more than three months in the absence of other illness or conditions that could explain the findings.[1] PGL is currently staged as Group III HIV infection in the CDC system.

The PGL syndrome is a common manifestation of HIV infection, although HIV's role in the pathophysiology of the syndrome is still uncertain. Before HIV disease was recognized as a continuous and progressive process, PGL was regarded as related to AIDS but as possibly distinct from it. Clinicians hoped that PGL represented an alternative and more benign course of the disease process that caused AIDS. Subsequent studies have demonstrated that HIV-infected patients with PGL do progress to AIDS. Although the presence or absence of PGL has little prognostic value compared to other measures of HIV replication and immune system compromise, PGL remains important as a clinical manifestation of HIV infection. As a syndrome, however, it should be differentiated from other causes of lymphadenopathy.

■ HISTORY OF HIV-RELATED PGL

Before the HIV epidemic first appeared in 1979, most cases of diffuse lymphadenopathy in the gay male population were seen in patients with secondary syphilis or viral infection (e.g., cytomegalovirus, Epstein–Barr virus, or hepatitis). The syndrome was self-limited or responded to treatment of the underlying condition. After 1979, clinicians began to see increasing numbers of homosexual patients with persistent enlarged nodes, constitutional symptoms, and splenomegaly. Node biopsy usually showed benign, reactive changes. The first studies of AIDS cases in 1981 reported lymphadenopathy associated with *Pneumocystis carinii* pneumonia and Kaposi's sarcoma, as well as benign, reactive changes detected through node biopsy. Subsequently, lymphadenopathy was found to occur in all groups at risk for HIV infection.

Demographically and geographically, the PGL syndrome closely paralleled the distribution of HIV infection, appearing first in New York, San Francisco, and Los Angeles, and subsequently in London, Atlanta, and other cities.

■ CLINICAL FEATURES OF THE PGL SYNDROME

Lymphadenopathy may develop at the time of HIV infection, often in association with an acute viral-like syndrome,[2,3] often within a few months of seroconversion for HIV antibody. PGL is less likely to occur in late stages of HIV disease. In some patients, the disappearance of longstanding adenopathy has been followed by progression of HIV disease.[4]

Patients with PGL may be asymptomatic or have any of the systemic or localized signs and symptoms of HIV disease. The clinical features of the lymphadenopathy syndrome reported by different institutions have been remarkably uniform.[5-8]

In San Francisco, a prospective study of the syndrome in 200 patients was begun in 1981 and continued for 60 months.[9,10] One-third of patients reported having a viral-like syndrome within two months of developing lymphadenopathy. Two-thirds noted an enlarged lymph node without prior illness. All but six patients reported that the lymphadenopathy had developed since 1979, when the incidence of AIDS began to increase. Thirty percent of patients were asymptomatic. Seventy percent described symptoms similar to those in full-blown AIDS. Of the latter group, half experienced fatigue, low-grade intermittent fevers, and night sweats occurring more than five times a month. Some patients correlated episodes of fever, emotional stress, extreme fatigue, and drug use with enlarged nodes and pain. Some men reported that the tenderness and size of the nodes diminished when they stopped taking medications for interim infections. One-third of patients, usually those who had suffered the antecedent viral-like illness, reported a weight loss of more than five pounds. An equal number reported weight gain, which most attributed to physical inactivity caused by fatigue.

Examination of most patients revealed no remarkable changes except in the lymphoreticular system. The average number of enlarged node groups per patient was 10, counting right and left sides separately. Thus, it is not difficult to diagnose the lymphadenopathy syndrome during a physical examination. Axillary and inguinal adenopathy are almost universal. Occipital and posterior auricular nodes were occasionally associated with complaints of shooting pains in the scalp, most likely caused by nerve compression.

The distribution of affected node groups in the San Francisco General Hospital cohort suffering from HIV-related lymphadenopathy is shown in Table 1.

TABLE 1. NODE GROUPS INVOLVED IN 200 PATIENTS WITH HIV-RELATED LYMPHADENOPATHY AT SAN FRANCISCO GENERAL HOSPITAL

NODE GROUP	% OF PATIENTS	NODE GROUP	% OF PATIENTS
Axillary	98	Submandibular	37
Inguinal	98	Submental	36
Posterior cervical	86	Occipital	30
Preauricular	51	Supraclavicular	26
Epitrochlear	51	Anterior cervical	17
Postauricular	47	Popliteal	9
Femoral	43	Trapezial	7

Although nearly one-third of patients had palpable spleens, abdominal computed tomographic scans of a smaller group of lymphadenopathy patients showed splenic enlargement in three-quarters of the group.[11] Radiographic studies of patients have shown splenomegaly, retroperitoneal lymphadenopathy, and thickening of the rectal mucosa consistent with a chronic proctitis. Chest x-rays in patients with the benign reactive syndrome are generally negative for hilar or mediastinal adenopathy.[12] The presence of thoracic adenopathy may indicate that an opportunistic infection or occult malignancy is present.

■ PGL AND PROGNOSIS FOR HIV DISEASE PROGRESSION

Several studies have found that the presence of PGL does not predict HIV disease progression[4,13-17] in contrast to other markers such as low T4 lymphocyte counts,[4,14-20] p24 antigenemia,[14,17,21] and elevated β_2-microglobulin[14] and neopterin levels.[22,23] The presence of PGL can best be viewed as having played the role of a surrogate marker for HIV infection in the pre-HIV serology era. It allowed clinicians to identify an AIDS-associated condition even before HIV was discovered.

■ HISTOPATHOLOGY AND PATHOPHYSIOLOGY OF PGL

The pathophysiology of PGL and its relationship to HIV infection are unclear. PGL may represent a specific immune response mounted by only some patients to HIV infection or an unrecognized coinfection; alternatively, it may represent an unproductive process triggered by either.

Biopsies of lymph nodes in patients with PGL show nondiagnostic, benign reactive changes with follicular hyperplasia.[10,24,25] Increases in follicular dendritic cells, which are associated with HIV p24 antigen, have been reported.[26]

■ DIFFERENTIAL DIAGNOSIS

Diffuse lymphadenopathy in homosexual men may be caused by the disorders that cause adenopathy in non-HIV infected patients as well as by the opportunistic infections and malignancies associated with HIV disease. Table 2 lists some of the conditions reported in lymphadenopathy associated with HIV disease.

Kaposi's Sarcoma.   Kaposi's sarcoma (KS), alone or associated with mucocutaneous lesions, may be present in lymphadenopathy of neoplastic origin. Patients with KS may have peripheral nodes showing the same pattern of follicular hyperplasia as that in the lymphadenopathy syndrome.[27,28] The majority of patients also exhibit signs of peripheral lymphadenopathy, but KS's characteristic cutaneous or mucosal lesions should lead the physician to the correct diagnosis.[27-29] Early in the epidemic, up to 20 percent of patients with KS were diagnosed on the basis of lymph-node biopsies alone in the absence of cutaneous lesions. However, these patients usually had more marked constitutional symptoms, abnormal complete blood counts, or elevated erythrocyte sedimentation rates (ESR).

TABLE 2.   DIFFERENTIAL DIAGNOSIS OF AIDS RELATED LYMPHADENOPATHY*

NEOPLASMS

Kaposi's sarcoma, Hodgkin's disease
Non-Hodgkin's lymphoma (usually B-cell origin)

INFECTIONS

Pneumocystis carinii pneumonia, toxoplasmosis
Mycobacterium avium-intracellulare or *M. tuberculosis*
Cryptococcus neoformans, Coccidioides immitis

MISCELLANEOUS

Angioimmunoblastic lymphadenopathy, angiofollicular hyperplasia (Castleman's disease),
lymphadenopathy syndrome (reactive hyperplasia)

---

*   *Source: Abrams DI. Lymphadenopathy syndrome in male homosexuals. In: Gallin JI, Fauci AS, eds. Advances in host defense mechanisms, vol. 5. New York: Raven Press, 1985:75-97. (Reprinted with permission of Raven Press, New York.)*

Hodgkin's and Non-Hodgkin's Lymphomas.   Both Hodgkin's and non-Hodgkin's lymphomas, especially the aggressive B-cell variants, have been seen with increased frequency in homosexual patients.[30-32] These patients often appear with peripheral lymphadenopathy. They may show nongeneralized lymphadenopathy or disproportionate size and firmness in a particular group of nodes in the setting of generalized adenopathy. Similarly, patients with lymphoma may have more severe constitutional symptoms and abnormal complete blood counts or sedimentation rates, or both. Either hilar/mediastinal or bulky retroperitoneal lymphadenopathy should lead the clinician to suspect possible nonbenign adenopathy and particularly to pursue the possibility of diagnosing a lymphoma.

■ OPPORTUNISTIC INFECTIONS

Patients presenting with opportunistic infections may also have peripheral lymphadenopathy. The subset of patients whose first manifestation of AIDS is *Pneumocystis carinii* pneumonia, however, has a lower incidence of this physical finding when first examined.[33]

Mycobacterial Infection.   Patients with mycobacterial infection, both *Mycobacterium tuberculosis* and *M. avium intracellulare*, have been first diagnosed on the basis of lymph-node biopsy.[34-36] The majority of our patients, however, do not require surgical biopsy for diagnosis. Cytologic examination or culture of fine-needle aspiration from lymph nodes[35] or blood or bone-marrow specimens most often make the diagnosis. Bone-marrow biopsy is used to evaluate marked cytopenias, particularly anemia, in association with an elevated ESR. Although lymph nodes in patients with AIDS and mycobacterial infection often do not demonstrate typical caseating granulomata, acid-fast bacilli stains and cultures are valuable in making the final diagnosis. In our patient population, bulky intraabdominal adenopathy is also characteristic of mycobacterial infections.[37]

Histoplasmosis and Coccidioidomycosis.   Lymph-node biopsy has been reported as useful in a few cases of disseminated fungal infections, particularly histoplasmosis and coccidioidomycosis.[38] In these cases, physicians most frequently choose to do lymph-node biopsies because of the severity of the patient's constitutional symptoms and the presence of abnormal laboratory or x-ray findings.

Cryptococcus neoformans.   Cryptococcal infection in HIV disease has been diagnosed by fine-needle aspiration of a cervical lymph node,[39] an uncommon method of diagnosis. Adenopathy is not a common presentation.

Toxoplasmosis.   Rarely, nodes have also shown histologic changes suggestive of toxoplasmosis.[40] Disseminated toxoplasmosis is not a common diagnosis based on lymph-node biopsy in HIV-infected patients. Often pathologic material suggests a diagnosis of toxoplasma, but further evaluation fails to identify the organism.

Other Causes of HIV-associated Lymphadenopathy.   Other causes of PGL in HIV-infected patients include angioimmunoblastic lymphadenopathy and angiofollicular hyperplasia, or Castleman's disease.[41,42]

■ INDICATIONS FOR FINE-NEEDLE ASPIRATION OR BIOPSY OF LYMPH NODES

Since biopsies are nondiagnostic in patients with PGL, an important clinical decision is when to sample lymph-node tissue for cytologic analysis and culture. Experience suggests that an identifiable subset of stable asymptomatic patients with PGL are most likely to have nondiagnostic results and thus will not benefit from fine-needle aspiration or biopsy. Fine-needle aspiration or biopsy of lymph nodes in HIV-infected patients is indicated in the following situations[43]: (1) marked constitutional symptoms with an otherwise negative evaluation; (2) nongeneralized lymphadenopathy; (3) a single disproportionately enlarging node in a patient with generalized lymphadenopathy; (4) bulky mediastinal or abdominal adenopathy; and (5) any peripheral cytopenia, elevated ESR, or both, in conjunction with an otherwise negative evaluation.

Fine-needle aspiration is a first option when sampling of lymph-node tissue is indicated.[35,44] This procedure is preferable to surgical biopsy because of its lesser pain, inconvenience, cost, and potential for complications. Although a negative fine-needle aspirate does not exclude an underlying opportunistic infection or malignancy, a positive finding makes surgical excision of the node unnecessary. Adequate material for diagnosing mycobacterial infection, KS, non-Hodgkin's lymphoma, and Hodgkin's disease can be obtained when this procedure is carried out and the results are analyzed by experienced personnel.

Several publications support these recommendations.[45-47] Rashleigh-Belcher et al. from the Middlesex Hospital reported the results of lymph-node biopsies in 39 homosexual men with unexplained PGL.[45] Biopsies were performed under general anesthesia in hospital. Twenty-six patients underwent axillary, nine underwent cervical, and four underwent inguinal lymph-node biopsy. Thirty-eight of the biopsies demonstrated florid follicular hyperplasia. No patterns of follicular involution, lymphoma, or tumor were found. One patient's lymph node had caseating granulomata without acid-fast bacilli. This particular patient had a prior history of marked weight loss, night sweats, and an elevated ESR. The majority of the patients in this cohort were discharged from the hospital on the first postoperative day without complications. Four patients subsequently developed superficial wound infections, one developed a hematoma, and one developed a seroma. One patient had an unexplained episode of pyrexia. Thirty-seven of these patients had antibodies to HIV at the time of their lymph-node biopsy. Another patient became HIV antibody-positive after the biopsy. Twelve other Middlesex cohort patients with PGL were biopsied at outlying hospitals. The tissue specimens of all 12 demonstrated florid follicular hyperplasia.

Rashleigh-Belcher concluded that lymph-node biopsy of HIV-seropositive patients who were otherwise well is not indicated. They based their conclusion on the absence of pathologic diagnoses resulting from lymph-node biopsy and the fact that specific therapeutic intervention was needed in only one patient, who could probably have been diagnosed with mycobacterial disease by another manner. These investigators recommended lymph-node biopsy in HIV-seronegative or HIV-seropositive patients with severe constitutional symptoms, splenomegaly, increased erythrocyte sedimentation rate, cytopenias, oral candida, or hilar lymphadenopathy. Support for this policy was also offered by groups from St. Stephen's, Westminster, and Charing Cross Hospitals.[46,47]

Levine et al., in a University of Southern California natural history study of PGL, performed sequential node biopsy on 40 homosexual men under consideration as potential subjects.[48] In six patients, diagnoses other than florid follicular hyperplasia were found. The non-PGL diagnoses included small cleaved lymphoma in two patients, focal KS in two patients, disseminated tuberculosis in one, and *Histoplasma capsulatum* in one. The authors contend that clinical and laboratory data from these six patients were indistinguishable from those of the 34 PGL patients. Although the authors fail to include many parameters useful in separating the PGL subset from patients with other causes of HIV-related lymphadenopathy, their stress on the increased validity of data obtained from a fully biopsied cohort is well taken. The group warns that in prospective studies of PGL patients in whom lymph-node biopsy is not a requirement for entrance to the study, many patients may already be harboring an eventual AIDS diagnosis. Studies with the highest percentage of unbiopsied patients enrolled would, therefore, possibly be slanted toward a greater rate of evolution to full-blown AIDS. However, other investigators continue to maintain that lymph-node biopsy in typical cases of the reactive syndrome is not necessary.

REFERENCES

1. Classification system for human T-lymphotropic virus type III/lymphadenopathy-associated virus infections. MMWR 1986; 35:334-9.

2. Tindall B, Barker S, Donovan B, et al. Characterization of the acute clinical illness associated with human immunodeficiency virus infection. Arch Intern Med 1988; 148:945-9.

3. Cooper DA, Gold J, Maclean P, et al. Acute AIDS retrovirus infection. Definition of a clinical illness associated with seroconversion. Lancet 1985; 1:537-40.

4. El-Sadr W, Marmor M, Zolla-Pazner S, et al. Four-year prospective study of homosexual men: correlation of immunologic abnormalities, clinical status, and serology to human immunodeficiency virus. J Infect Dis 1987; 155:789-93.

5. Abrams DI. Lymphadenopathy: the San Francisco experience. In: Friedman-Kein AE, Laubenstein LJ, eds. The epidemic of Kaposi's sarcoma and opportunistic infections. New York: Masson, 1984:81-8.

6. Abrams DI, Lewis BJ, Beckstead JH, et al. Persistent diffuse lymphadenopathy in homosexual men: endpoint or prodrome? Ann Intern Med 1984; 100:801-8.

7. Persistent, generalized lymphadenopathy among homosexual males. MMWR 1982; 31:249-51.

8. Metroka CE, Cunningham-Rundles S, Pollack MS, et al. Generalized lymphadenopathy in homosexual men. Ann Intern Med 1983; 99:585-91.

9. Abrams DI. Lymphadenopathy syndrome in male homosexuals. In: Gallin JI, Fauci AS, eds. Advances in host defense mechanisms, vol. 5. New York: Raven Press, 1985:75-97.

10. Abrams DI, Kaplan LD, McGrath MS, Volberding PA. AIDS-related benign lymphadenopathy and malignant lymphoma: clinical aspects and virologic interactions. AIDS Res 1986; 2(Suppl 1):S131-S140.

11. Moon KL Jr, Federle MP, Abrams DI, et al. Kaposi's sarcoma and lymphadenopathy syndrome: limitations of abdominal CT in acquired immunodeficiency syndrome. Radiology 1984; 150:479-83.

12. Stern RG, Gamsu G, Golden JA, et al. Intrathoracic adenopathy: differential feature of AIDS and diffuse lymphadenopathy syndrome. AJR 1984; 142:689-92.

13. Daul CB, deShazo RD, Andes WA. Human immunodeficiency virus infection in hemophiliac patients. A three-year prospective evaluation. Am J Med 1988; 84:801-9.

14. Moss AR, Bacchetti P, Osmond D, et al. Seropositivity for HIV and the development of AIDS or AIDS related condition: three year follow up of the San Francisco General Hospital cohort. Br Med J 1988; 296:745-50.

15. Kaplan JE, Spira TJ, Fishbein DB, et al. A six-year follow-up of HIV-infected homosexual men with lymphadenopathy. Evidence for an increased risk for developing AIDS after the third year of lymphadenopathy. JAMA 1988; 260:2694-7.

16. Eyster ME, Gail MH, Ballard JO, et al. Natural history of human immunodeficiency virus infections in hemophiliacs: effects of T-cell subsets, platelet counts, and age. Ann Intern Med 1987; 107:1-6.

17. Polk BF, Fox R, Brookmeyer R, et al. Predictors of the acquired immunodeficiency syndrome developing in a cohort of seropositive homosexual men. N Engl J Med 1987; 316:61-6.

18. Eyster ME, Ballard JO, Gail MH, et al. Predictive markers for the acquired immunodeficiency syndrome (AIDS) in hemophiliacs: persistence of p24 antigen and low T4 cell count. Ann Intern Med 1989; 110:963-9.

19. Taylor JM, Fahey JL, Detels R, Giorgi JV. CD4 percentage, CD4 number, and CD4:CD8 ratio in HIV infection: which to choose and how to use. J Acquir Immune Defic Syndr 1989; 2:114-24.

20. Lang W, Perkins H, Anderson RE, et al. Patterns of T lymphocyte changes with human immunodeficiency virus infection: from seroconversion to the development of AIDS. J Acquir Immune Defic Syndr 1989; 2:63-9.

21. Allain J-P, Laurian Y, Paul DA, et al. Long-term evaluation of HIV antigen and antibodies to p24 and gp41 in patients with hemophilia. Potential clinical importance. N Engl J Med 1987; 317:1114-21.

22. Kramer A, Wiktor SZ, Fuchs D, et al. Neopterin: a predictive marker of acquired immune deficiency syndrome in human immunodeficiency virus infection. J Acquir Immune Defic Syndr 1989; 2:291-6.

23. Melmed RN, Taylor JM, Detels R, et al. Serum neopterin changes in HIV-infected subjects: indicator of significant pathology, CD4 T cell changes, and the development of AIDS. J Acquir Immune Defic Syndr 1989; 2:70-6.

24. O'Murchadha MT, Wolf BC, Neiman RS. The histologic features of hyperplastic lymphadenopathy in AIDS-related complex are nonspecific. Am J Surg Pathol 1987; 11:94-9.

25. Stanley MW, Frizzera G. Diagnostic specificity of histologic features in lymph node biopsy specimens from patients at risk for the acquired immunodeficiency syndrome. Hum Pathol 1986; 17:1231-9.

26. Porwit A, Bottiger B, Pallesen G, et al. Follicular involution in HIV lymphadenopathy. A morphometric study. APMIS 1989; 97:153-65.

27. Bhana D, Templeton AC, Master SP, Kyalwazi SK. Kaposi's sarcoma of lymph nodes. Br J Cancer 1970; 24:464-70.

28. Finkbeiner WE, Egbert BM, Groundwater JR, Sagebiel RW. Kaposi's sarcoma in young homosexual men: a histopathologic study with particular reference to lymph node involvement. Arch Pathol Lab Med 1982; 106:261-4.

29. Moskowitz LB, Hensley GT, Gould EW, Weiss SD. Frequency and anatomic distribution of lymphadenopathic Kaposi's sarcoma in the acquired immunodeficiency syndrome: an autopsy series. Hum Pathol 1985; 16:447-56.

30. Schoeppel SL, Hoppe RT, Dorfman RF, et al. Hodgkin's disease in homosexual men with generalized lymphadenopathy. Ann Intern Med 1985; 102:68-70.

31. Ziegler JL, Beckstead JA, Volberding PA, et al. Non-Hodgkin's lymphoma in 90 homosexual men. Relation to generalized lymphadenopathy and the acquired immunodeficiency syndrome. N Engl J Med 1984; 311:565-70.

32. Knowles DM, Chamulak GA, Subar M, et al. Lymphoid neoplasia associated with the acquired immunodeficiency syndrome (AIDS). The New York University Medical Center experience with 105 patients (1981-1986). Ann Intern Med 1988; 108:744-53.

33. Epidemiologic aspects of the current outbreak of Kaposi's sarcoma and opportunistic infections. N Engl J Med 1982; 306:248-52.

34. Freeman ML, Talbot GH. Nongranulomatous mycobacterial lymphadenitis in homosexual patients. Lab Invest 1983; 48:27a. abstract.

35. Bottles K, McPhaul LW, Volberding P. Fine-needle aspiration biopsy of patients with acquired immunodeficiency syndrome (AIDS): experience in an outpatient clinic. Ann Intern Med 1988; 108:42-5.

36. Hewlett D Jr, Duncanson FP, Jagadha V, et al. Lymphadenopathy in an inner-city population consisting principally of intravenous drug abusers with suspected acquired immunodeficiency syndrome. Am Rev Resp Dis 1988; 137:1275-9.

37. Nyberg DA, Federle MP, Jeffrey RB, et al. Abdominal CT findings of disseminated *Mycobacterium avium-intracellulare* in AIDS. AJR 1985; 145:297-9.

38. Abrams DI, Robia M, Blumenfeld W, et al. Disseminated coccidioidomycosis in AIDS. N Engl J Med 1984; 310:986-7.

39. Molina J-M, Oksenhendler E, Daniel M-T, Clauvel J-P. Fine-needle aspiration and cryptococcosis in the acquired immunodeficiency syndrome (AIDS). Ann Intern Med 1988; 108:772.

40. Ioachim HL. Toxoplasma lymphadenitis. In: Ioachim HL, ed. Lymph node biopsy. Philadelphia: JB Lippincott Co. 1985; 91.

41. Blumenfeld W, Beckstead JH. Angioimmunoblastic lymphadenopathy with dysproteinemia in homosexual men with acquired immune deficiency syndrome. Arch Pathol Lab Med 1983; 107:567-9.

42. Lachant NA, Sun NC, Leong LA, et al. Multicentric angiofollicular lymph node hyperplasia (Castleman's disease) followed by Kaposi's sarcoma in two homosexual males with the acquired immunodeficiency syndrome (AIDS). Am J Clin Pathol 1985; 83:27-33.

43. Abrams DI. AIDS-related lymphadenopathy: the role of biopsy. J Clin Oncol 1986; 4:126-7.

44. Bottles K, Cohen MB, Brodie H, et al. Fine-needle aspiration cytology of lymphadenopathy in homosexual males. Diagn Cytopathol 1986; 2:31-5.

45. Rashleigh-Belcher HJ, Carne CA, Weller IV, et al. Surgical biopsy for persistent generalized lymphadenopathy. Br J Surg 1986; 73:183-5.

46. Farthing CF, Henry K, Shanson DC, et al. Clinical investigations of lymphadenopathy, including lymph node biopsies, in 24 homosexual men with antibodies to the human T-cell lymphotropic virus type III (HTLV-III). Br J Surg 1986; 73:180-2.

47. Scott HJ, Glynn MJ, Lane IF, et al. Strategy for lymph node biopsy in homosexual men suspected of having LAV/HTLV-III related disease. Br J Surg 1986; 73:186-7.

48. Levine AM, Meyer PR, Gill PS, et al. Results of initial lymph node biopsy in homosexual men with generalized lymphadenopathy. J Clin Oncol 1986; 4:165-9.

4.2

Long-Term Management and Follow-up of HIV-Infected Patients

History and Physical Examination of HIV-Infected Patients

S.R. Hernandez, M.D.

This chapter offers primary-care providers some guidelines for managing HIV-infected patients.[1,2] Primary-care providers should be prepared to:

- collect a database of initial observations for comparison with future ones;
- manage troubling symptoms;
- diagnose and treat opportunistic infections and malignancies early in the course of HIV disease;
- educate the patient about unsafe sexual practices, needle sharing, and other modes of transmission to prevent further spread of HIV infection;
- minimize or avoid immune stimulation from infectious agents or other antigens;
- initiate appropriate antibiotic prophylaxis against selected infectious agents;
- initiate and manage appropriate anti-HIV therapies, including zidovudine (AZT) and investigational new drugs;
- closely observe patients' emotional and psychological condition as well as their psychosocial support and coping mechanisms;
- refer patients to appropriate subspecialists for evaluations.

The course of HIV infection is chronic and progressive, and is characterized by many acute and chronic problems. Some of these are caused directly by HIV and some by opportunistic infections and malignancies. While the course of disease is variable, the progression is predictable, so it is important to record initial observations for future comparison. The clinical spectrum of HIV infection and testing to detect HIV infection are described in other chapters.

■ TAKING THE HIV-INFECTED PATIENT'S HISTORY

Date and History of HIV Infection. Determining the approximate date of HIV infection is useful for predicting progression from asymptomatic to symptomatic HIV disease (or to full-blown AIDS). How long a patient has been infected may also influence clinical decisions, such as whether to initiate antiviral therapy or prophylactic regimens. Long-term prospective studies suggest that the majority of HIV-infected patients remain asymptomatic for 3 to 5 years after infection.

Establishing the approximate date of infection is easiest in individuals who were infected through blood transfusion or accidental needle stick and in patients whose histories disclose an acute viral or mononucleosis-like syndrome. Occasionally a patient may be seen with a history of either a single sexual exposure to an HIV-infected individual or a single instance of another high-risk behavior, such as one-time intravenous drug use involving shared needles. In these instances, the date of infection may be relatively easy to identify (if the patient reports no other risk behaviors).

Previous Medical Illness.   A detailed history of recent illnesses may clarify the present stage of the patient's HIV disease and the degree of immuno-compromise. Future management problems can be partially anticipated on the basis of sequelae or recurrences of previous illnesses, so all chronic medical conditions should be fully described. Particular attention should be paid to identifying any problems that may be exacerbated by concurrent HIV infection or treatment (e.g., bacterial pneumonias, parasitic infections, viral infections, and sexually-transmitted disease (STD)). Probing the patient's handling of previous illnesses may also indicate what psychological, financial, and logistical resources the patient has for coping with illness and therapy.

A history of complications from drug use should be ascertained. If the patient is an intravenous drug-user (IVDU), the physician should inquire about staphylococcal disease, endocarditis, abscesses, and hepatitis. A history of previous surgeries, complications of illnesses (such as multiple-lobe involvement or bacteremia associated with pneumonias), and details of potentially recurrent problems such as herpes simplex and syphilis (i.e., anatomic site, frequency, severity, and past therapy) should be obtained. HIV-infected intravenous drug users are at high risk for tuberculous infections and should receive an intradermal (Mantoux) test with 5 TU tuberculin PPD. If a positive induration equal to or greater than 5 mm occurs, the patient should receive appropriate therapy.[9]

Tuberculin Skin Test (PPD) History.   HIV-infected patients with a prior *M. tuberculosis* infection are at high risk for reactivation. Patients with histories of positive PPDs for which they never received therapy should receive anti-tuberculosis prophylaxis with isonicotine hydrazine (INH) for a minimum of 12 months unless liver disease or active alcohol abuse contraindicates this. Some experts believe that the isoniazid therapy should extend beyond the minimum 12 months.[9]

Geography of Present and Prior Residence.   Because infections endemic to geographic areas may escape consideration if the patient no longer resides there, the location of the patient's birth and both present and prior residence should be documented. In an HIV-infected patient, long-dormant infections may reactivate and cause life-threatening disease. For example, coccidioidomy-cosis may reactivate in individuals who acquired their primary infection while living in the Southwestern U.S., Sonoran desert, or California's San Joaquin Valley. Patients from the Central States, such as Indiana, Ohio, Mississippi, and Tennessee, are at risk for reactivation of histoplasmosis.

Allergies and Reactions.   When recording drug reactions and allergies, specific attention should be paid to antibiotic allergies. The type of allergic response should be made as clear as possible.

Current Therapeutic Drugs and Medications.   Many HIV-infected patients seek out black-market drugs, nontraditional therapies, and/or several different physicians in addition to the treatment they receive at the clinic or hospital. The provider should assume that patients may be seeking such outside therapies and inquire about the use of over-the-counter drugs, herbal remedies, and alternative therapies.

Use of Drugs.   Habitual or recreational use of drugs, alcohol, and tobacco may affect the patient's health. It is important to determine what drugs the patient is using, by what routes they are administered, how frequently they are used, and whether these drugs involve additional risk behaviors (e.g., unsafe sex, needle sharing).

Psychosocial History.   HIV infection is often a source of major emotional and psychological trauma. Many HIV-infected individuals lack traditional family support, so an assessment of emotional and logistical support systems is needed. The provider should try to identify the patient's major fears and primary mechanisms of coping, as well as potential gaps in the patient's support system.

Review of System.   It is very important to obtain a history of the most common symptoms associated with chronic HIV infection. These are: systemic symptoms (fever, weight loss, fatigue, night sweats, malaise), rash (skin changes), swollen lymph nodes, changes in vision, oral lesions, cough, abdominal pain, diarrhea, cervical and vaginal atypia, personality changes, difficulty in concentrating, short-term memory loss, headaches, myalgias, arthralgias, pain syndromes (e.g., postherpetic neuralgias), and abnormal bleeding.

For each of these symptoms, it is important to determine how long they lasted and whether the patient was treated for them (and how).

■ PHYSICAL EXAMINATION

HIV-related conditions can affect every anatomic structure and organ system. Particular emphasis should be placed on identifying the end-organ findings most commonly associated with HIV infection. Baseline observations early in the course of HIV infection facilitate early recognition of new problems as they emerge at later stages.

Vital Signs.   The patient's weight, temperature, respiratory and heart rates, and blood pressure provide objective evidence of changes in clinical status. These should be recorded at each clinic visit. Orthostatic measurements of blood pressure and heart rate should be recorded if hypovolemia or autonomic neuropathy is suspected.

Skin.   Skin lesions commonly encountered in HIV-infected patients are described in detail in other chapters. Some skin findings commonly associated with HIV infection are summarized in Table 1.

TABLE 1.   COMMON DERMATOLOGIC CONDITIONS ASSOCIATED WITH HIV*

I. **INFECTIOUS**
   Folliculitis
   APPEARANCE: Red papules at hair follicles, some with a central pustule
   LOCATION: Face, trunk
   CLINICAL CHARACTERISTICS: Tender or quite pruritic; furuncles may accompany

continued on next page

continued from previous page

TABLE 1. COMMON DERMATOLOGIC CONDITIONS ASSOCIATED WITH HIV*

Bullous Impetigo
>APPEARANCE: Flaccid superficial blisters
>
>LOCATION: Inguinal fold, axilla
>
>CLINICAL CHARACTERISTICS: Painless

Herpes Zoster: active
>APPEARANCE: Dermatomal painful blisters
>
>LOCATION: Unilateral, trunk, head and neck, most common
>
>CLINICAL CHARACTERISTICS: Pain often precedes lesions. Dissemination and secondary infection uncommon

Herpes Zoster: resolved
>APPEARANCE: Hypopigmented scars
>
>LOCATION: Trunk, head and neck, most common
>
>CLINICAL CHARACTERISTICS: Pain or dysesthesia may persist for months to years

Herpes Simplex
>APPEARANCE: Grouped blisters becoming ulcerations
>
>LOCATION: Genital, perianal, facial
>
>CLINICAL CHARACTERISTICS: Recurrent, often persistent. Suspect any persistent ulcer

Tinea Pedis: Unguium
>APPEARANCE: Thick, crumbly nails
>
>LOCATION: Toenails more often than fingernails
>
>CLINICAL CHARACTERISTICS: Does not cause paronychia

Tinea Pedis: Cruris
>APPEARANCE: Scaly patches with central clearing
>
>LOCATION: Upper thigh, inguinal crease
>
>CLINICAL CHARACTERISTICS: Spares scrotum. Positive KOH distinguishes from inguinal seborrheic dermatitis

Condyloma Acuminatum (Genital Warts)
>APPEARANCE: Tiny to large, flat to polypoid, skin-colored to hyperpigmented papules
>
>LOCATION: Penile shaft, perianal, vagina, cervix, oral mucosa
>
>CLINICAL CHARACTERISTICS: Asymptomatic, sexually transmitted.

Molluscum Contagiosum
>APPEARANCE: Pearly 1–5 mm dome-shaped papule with central umbilication
>
>LOCATION: Genitalia, face
>
>CLINICAL CHARACTERISTICS: Asymptomatic. Sexually transmitted

II. INFLAMMATORY
Seborrheic Dermatitis
>APPEARANCE: Erythematous, waxy (greasy) scales
>
>LOCATION: Nasolabial fold, retroauricular scalp, eyebrows, central trunk, and groin
>
>CLINICAL CHARACTERISTICS: Minimally symptomatic. Very, very common, almost universal

continued on next page

continued from previous page

TABLE 1.   COMMON DERMATOLOGIC CONDITIONS ASSOCIATED WITH HIV*

Psoriasis
 APPEARANCE: Thick, well marginated red plaques
 LOCATION: Elbows, knees, scalp, knuckles, gluteal cleft
 CLINICAL CHARACTERISTICS: Variably pruritic. Occurs at site of trauma.

Pruritic Rashes
 APPEARANCE: Urticarial papules, red scaly patches, plaques. Frequent excoriations
 LOCATION: Arms, legs, trunk
 CLINICAL CHARACTERISTICS: Intense pruritus. Etiologies largely unknown. Suspect drugs, insect bites, folliculitis

III. NEOPLASTIC
Kaposi's Sarcoma
 APPEARANCE: Oval; papule nodes, or plaques. Average 1–2 cm
 LOCATION: Trunk, retroauricular, legs. Oral mucosa, especially on hard palate
 CLINICAL CHARACTERISTICS: Appear at sites of injury. Edema may precede clinical lesions, especially on legs or around eyes

* *Compiled by Timothy Berger, M.D.*

Lymph Nodes.   Lymph nodes, including the cervical (anterior and posterior), pre- and postauricular, supraclavicular, epitrochlear, axillary, inguinal, and femoral, should be systematically examined at every visit. Overall size, asymmetry of right- and left-sided groups, disproportionate enlargement of a single group, texture, and tenderness should be noted. Compare with any previously recorded measurements to identify rapidly-enlarging individual nodes.

Eye.   Baseline visual acuity, pupillary size/reactivity, and visual-field examination should be recorded. Lids, conjunctiva, cornea, anterior chamber, lens, posterior chamber, and fundus should be examined with an ophthalmoscope. Abnormal findings should be noted.

Oral Cavity.   The oropharynx should be carefully evaluated for lesions associated with HIV infection. Oropharyngeal lesions may be ulcers (syphilis, herpes zoster or simplex), vesicles (herpes zoster or simplex), plaques (hairy leukoplakia), macules (Kaposi's sarcoma), exudates (candidiasis), nodules (lymphoma, Kaposi's sarcoma), and diffusely inflamed tissue (candidiasis, herpes simplex, periodontitis). The sides of the tongue should be routinely examined for hairy leukoplakia.

Chest.   The patient's respiratory rate and baseline auscultatory findings should be recorded. Pulmonary problems, often presenting with subtle physical exam findings, are common in HIV-infected patients.

Cardiovascular System.   Baseline cardiovascular findings, including jugular venous pressure, pulses, heart sounds, and any murmurs, should be recorded. Endocarditis is a common complication of intravenous drug use. Pericardial effusions (usually clinically silent) occasionally occur in HIV-infected patients.

Abdomen.   The patient should be checked for abdominal masses and the baseline size of the liver and spleen should be recorded.

Male Genitalia.   The testicles should be carefully examined for lumps that may be suggestive of a tumor. Induration, tenderness, and swelling in the epididymis can be a sign of an STD caused by gonococcus or chlamydia, or more rarely, a sign of tuberculosis. The penis and scrotum should be examined for other signs of STD (ulcerative or vesicular lesions, warts). The foreskin should be retracted, and the glans and urethral meatus should be inspected for evidence of lesions or discharge. Smears of any urethral discharge should be evaluated for chlamydia and gonococcus.

Female Genitalia.   External genitalia should be inspected for warts and ulcerative or vesicular lesions suggestive of STD. The cervix should be inspected for cervicitis (associated with chlamydia and herpes simplex infections) or other lesions. A Pap smear should be obtained regularly.[3,4] Yeast infection may be recurrent.

Anus and Rectum.   Rectal lesions and rectal pain are common among gay men. Both visual and digital exams should search for evidence of discharge, fissures, proctitis, abcesses, traumatic tears, and specific lesions associated with STD (condylomata accuminata, condylomata lata and other syphilitic lesions, lesions associated with HSV, chlamydia, and gonorrhea). Anorectal carcinomas have been reported in young, HIV-infected men, although an increased incidence has not been proven. Stool should be screened for occult blood.

Musculoskeletal System.   A baseline description of joints and bony structures should be taken. Any abnormal findings — presence of synovitis, limitation of motion, focal tenderness, overlying erythema, increased temperature — should be recorded. Reiter's-like arthritic syndromes have been reported in HIV-infected patients.[5,6] Musculoskeletal problems are associated with STD (gonococcal arthritis, chlamydia-associated Reiter's syndrome), IVDU-associated infections (abscesses, osteomyelitis, septic joints), and other infectious diseases (tuberculous arthritis and osteomyelitis) reported in HIV-infected patients. Muscle bulk and strength may be affected by neuropathic processes and by poorly-understood wasting syndromes, so baseline descriptions should be recorded. Diffuse tenderness may indicate myositis, which has been reported as an idiopathic effect of zidovudine therapy.[7,8]

Nervous System.   Because HIV is neurotropic, many HIV-associated opportunistic infections and malignancies affect the nervous system. Reports estimate that 40 percent to 80 percent of HIV-infected individuals eventually manifest neurologic and/or psychiatric symptoms. Because of this, complete and well-documented baseline neurologic and mental-status exams are critical.

There are many tools for evaluating mental status. An abbreviated mental status exam can be used. An alternative is a symptom check list on which the patient can report his or her symptoms.

REFERENCES

1. Northfelt DW, Hayward RA, Shapiro MF. The acquired immunodeficiency syndrome is a primary care disease. Ann Intern Med 1988; 109:773-5.

2. The acquired immunodeficiency syndrome (AIDS) and infection with the human immunodeficiency virus (HIV). Health and Public Policy Committee, American College of Physicians; and the Infectious Diseases Society of America. Ann Intern Med 1988; 108:460-9.

3. Pomerantz RJ, de la Monte SM, Donegan SP, et al. Human immunodeficiency virus (HIV) infection of the uterine cervix. Ann Intern Med 1988; 108:321-7.

4. Schrager L, Friedland G, Klein R, et al. Increased risk of cervical and/or vaginal squamous atypia in women infected with HIV [Abstract]. Proceedings of the Third International Conference on AIDS. Washington: U.S. Department of Health and Human Services and WHO, 1987.

5. Lin RY. Reiter's syndrome and human immunodeficiency virus infection. Dermatologica 1988; 176:39-42.

6. Duvic M, Johnson TM, Rapini RP, et al. Acquired immunodeficiency syndrome-associated psoriasis and Reiter's syndrome. Arch Dermatol 1987; 123:1622-32.

7. Bessen LJ, Greene JB, Louie E, et al. Severe polymyositis-like syndrome associated with zidovudine therapy of AIDS and ARC. N Engl J Med 1988; 318:708.

8. Gorard DA, Henry K, Guiloff RJ. Necrotizing myopathy and zidovudine. Lancet 1988; 1:1050-1.

9. Tuberculosis and human immunodeficiency virus infection: recommendations of the Advisory Committee for the Elimination of Tuberculosis (ACET). MMWR 1989; 38:236-8, 243-50.

Laboratory Testing and Management of HIV-Infected Patients

S.R. Hernandez, M.D.

T his chapter reviews long-term management considerations for HIV-infected patients, including baseline laboratory studies, indications for prophylaxis against *Pneumocystis carinii* pneumonia (PCP) and for anti-HIV therapy, prognostication, and psychosocial and behavioral issues.

■ SCREENING AND BASELINE LABORATORY TESTS

Baseline laboratory studies should include a complete blood count (CBC), differential blood count, erythrocyte sedimentation rate (ESR), platelet count, serum electrolytes, blood urea nitrogen (BUN) and creatinine, liver function tests, serum lactic dehydrogenase (LDH), serologic tests for syphilis, urinalysis, and a tuberculin skin test (PPD). Stool samples should also be examined if the patient is a sexually active gay man.

Early in the course of HIV infection, patients may have a normal CBC. In several studies, anemia (usually with features resembling the anemia of chronic disease) has been reported as a useful prognostic marker for progression of HIV disease.[1,2] The anemia may rarely be autoimmune-mediated.[3,4] If it is associated with other cytopenias, a fungal or mycobacterial infection or a malignancy infiltrating the bone marrow should be considered.

Varying degrees of thrombocytopenia may be found in HIV-infected patients. Antiplatelet antibodies have been well-described in HIV-related idiopathic thrombocytopenic purpura.[1,5-7]

The ESR usually becomes elevated during progression to AIDS.[2] When a precipitous rise from baseline occurs associated with a new symptom complex, the provider should consider a bacterial, fungal, or mycobacterial infection. If an opportunistic infection is diagnosed, the ESR can be a useful marker for response to therapy. At times, the ESR may exceed 100 mm/hr, in which case a lymphomal or a disseminated mycobacterial or fungal disease should be considered.

Serum electrolytes, BUN, and creatinine can indicate acid-base, renal function, and body-fluid abnormalities. The combination of low sodium and high potassium may be a clue to a hypoadrenal state. Urinalysis is an inexpensive test and can detect pyuria (bacterial, mycobacterial, chlamydial infections), hematuria (bleeding, glomerulonephritis, infections), and proteinuria (nephrotic syndrome). Ketonuria and a high urine specific gravity may reflect inadequate caloric intake or fluid intake, respectively.

Liver-function tests can rule out both cholestatic and hepatocellular processes caused by infections, malignancies, and drug toxicities. Elevated serum aminotransferase levels may be caused by viruses such as cytomegalovirus (CMV) or hepatitis B virus (HBV). Similarly, antibiotic, antiviral, and antifungal agents may be hepatotoxic. Elevated alkaline phosphatase may reflect neoplastic invasion, disseminated acid-fast bacteria (AFB), or fungal infection involving the liver. When it occurs, cholestasis is usually seen later in the course of HIV disease and may be associated with hepatobiliary obstruction caused by cryptosporidium or CMV.

In most asymptomatic HIV-infected patients, the LDH level is normal. Increased levels are reported in patients with pulmonary PCP and higher levels correlate with a poorer prognosis.[8] Thus, a new increase in the serum LDH level in a coughing patient should raise the suspicion of PCP. Elevated serum LDH has been occasionally observed in other pulmonary conditions associated with HIV infection[9] and in patients with non-Hodgkin's lymphomas.

HIV and syphilis often occur in persons in the same risk groups. Syphilis in HIV-infected patients may occur with subtle signs and follow a more rapid course than in the non-HIV-infected patients, so all HIV-infected patients should be screened for syphilis with a serum VDRL.

The PPD (together with candida or mumps control) should be used to detect previous *M. tuberculosis* infection so that prophylaxis with isoniazid (INH) can be considered. A negative PPD and negative control do not rule out prior tuberculosis exposure; rather, in the HIV-infected patient, they suggest anergy, a marker of depressed cellular immunity. Individuals with a PPD reaction greater than 5 mm should have a chest radiograph, the diagnosis of active TB should be excluded, and prophylaxis with INH should be started as discussed below.

Additional Studies.   Some clinicians recommend obtaining additional studies on a routine or selected basis. These include chest radiograph, serum uric acid and cholesterol, serum proteins, serologies for HBV surface antigen, serum cryptococcal antigen, and toxoplasma serology.

A chest radiograph is of limited value in an asymptomatic individual, although if no previous radiographs are on record, it may be useful to acquire one as a baseline for future comparison.

For unknown reasons, serum uric acid and serum cholesterol usually decrease to subnormal levels during progression to AIDS. However, this effect has not yet proved useful for prognostication and management.

Hypergammaglobulinemia is frequently observed in HIV-infected patients and reflects a polyclonal proliferation of B-cells. It is thought to be directly mediated by HIV infection and antigenic stimulation[10] and may be a direct effect of stimulated B cells that secrete immunoglobulins in 10-fold greater quantities than in non-HIV-infected persons. Most studies do not demonstrate a clinically useful association between hypergammaglobulinemia and HIV prognosis or disease progression.

Hepatitis B virus exposure is common among intravenous drug users (IVDUs) and other individuals exposed to HIV and other STDs. Most HIV-infected gay men and IVDUs have been exposed to HBV and have detectable antibodies to the virus. Screening for HBV antibody can identify individuals with chronic hepatitis, and may in turn influence decisions about using hepatotoxic medication. HBV-negative sexual partners of chronic HBV surface-antigen carriers can be offered vaccination against HBV. HBV-negative HIV-infected patients who are at risk for HBV because of high-risk behaviors (sexual or drug) can be vaccinated against HBV.

Cryptococcus is the most common life-threatening fungal infection in HIV-infected patients,[11,12] so some clinicians suggest assaying asymptomatic HIV-infected patients' serum for cryptococcal antigen and repeating the assay every three to six months if the result is negative. A rare patient may be asymptomatic for cryptococcal infection but have low titers of serum cryptococcal antigen. When this occurs, fungal blood cultures should be obtained. If these are negative, serial antigen measurements and close follow-up are indicated. If the patient's serum is positive, therapy with amphotericin B should be initiated. Many clinicians do not regard baseline and periodic screening for serum cryptococcal antigen as useful but do measure antigen levels when symptoms and signs of infection (such as unexplained fever or severe headache) occur.

Toxoplasma IgG (IFA) can be useful as a baseline test in HIV-infected patients. Most cases of toxoplasmosis in HIV-infected patients are thought to occur because of the reactivation of an old infection. CNS toxoplasmosis is often diagnosed presumptively (headache, fever, seizure, or focal neurologic signs coupled with abnormal CT scan) and treated empirically, using clinical and radiologic response rather than biopsy as confirmation. A positive toxoplasma serology at baseline can strengthen such an inferential diagnosis. Baseline serologic studies show evidence of past *Toxoplasma gondii* infection in over 50 percent of U.S. adults.[13]

Occasionally toxoplasmosis can be diagnosed inferentially when a patient's baseline-negative toxoplasma serology is coupled with seroconversion and findings suggestive of acute infection (e.g., CNS lesions). However, patients with advanced HIV disease are unlikely to mount a detectable acute serologic response (antitoxoplasma IgM or a four-fold rise in antitoxoplasma IgG) to an acute toxoplasma infection.

A single toxoplasma serology is useful only if it is negative, in which case toxoplasmosis is an unlikely cause for the patient's clinical condition. Most HIV-infected patients with toxoplasmosis as well as many with no evidence of toxoplasmosis have positive toxoplasma serologies, so positive serologies are not reliable as evidence of infection.[14] Thus, baseline toxoplasma serology is useful in a patient who is seronegative on baseline testing but who subsequently mounts a serologic response. It is also useful for identifying prior infection to support initiation of empiric therapy for CNS disease.

■ STUDIES FOR PROGNOSTICATING AND STAGING HIV INFECTION

The following are some tests reported as useful for staging and prognosis in HIV infection:

- Total T4 lymphocyte counts and T4:T8 (helper/suppressor) lymphocyte ratios[2,6,15-19]
- serum p24 HIV antigen[2,19-26]
- ESR[2]
- serum hemoglobin[1,2]
- serum β_2-microglobulin[2,21-24]
- neopterin levels[27]
- decline of antibody to p24 and p17 HIV *gag* proteins[24-27,29-32]
- anergy to subcutaneously-injected antigens[33]

T4 Lymphocyte Counts and T4:T8 Ratios.   T4 lymphocyte counts and T4:T8 ratios have generated the greatest volume of published data and clinical experience. They have also been used in establishing the criteria for initiating

zidovudine (AZT) therapy. Despite the relatively high cost and technical difficulty in performing these counts, they are the currently recommended studies
for staging and monitoring HIV infection.

β_2-Microglobulin.   Some cohort studies suggest that β_2-microglobulin correlates with HIV disease activity[2,21-24] and in one study it was the best predictor
of disease progression.[2] Serum levels can be inexpensively determined with
commercially available test kits that can be used in any clinical laboratory.
Unfortunately, published clinical data are insufficient for guiding the clinician
in using this test for patient management. Many clinicians do not use this test,
while others feel that its low cost justifies it as a baseline study along with T4
counts and that its clinical role will be clarified. It may eventually replace T4
counts as a prognostic tool.

Anergy.   Anergy is not a quantitative marker. However, it can be conve-
niently detected with commercial test kits or, less expensively, with a candida
skin test and other control antigens (such as trichophyton or CMI when a PPD
is placed). The Walter-Reed staging classification for HIV infection uses cutaneous anergy along with T4 cell counts <400/cubic mm to characterize advanced stages of HIV infection[33] (partial cutaneous anergy = reactivity to some
antigens; complete cutaneous anergy = no skin-test reactivity).

HIV p24 Antigen.   Clinicians use HIV p24 antigen (HIV core protein) serum levels as an index of ongoing HIV replication and thus of disease stage and
activity. A clinical role for this test has not been defined. p24 assays are expensive, sensitive to methodological variations, and undetectable at certain levels,
so they cannot be quantitated except in the later stages of HIV infection. For
all these reasons, the assay is useless for monitoring the early stages of HIV
disease. Some clinicians monitor p24 antigen assays periodically and use the
appearance of antigen as an indication for initiating AZT therapy, although
others argue that this strategy denies the patient the possible benefit of earlier
AZT therapy (e.g., whenever T4 count drops or is low). Some clinicians also
obtain assays to document a decrease in p24 antigen levels during AZT therapy
although they do not use the result to alter therapy.

Serum and Urine Neopterin Levels.   In a few preliminary studies, serum
and urine neopterin levels have correlated with T4 counts. However, there is
still insufficient evidence to recommend this test for routine clinical use.

■ FORMULATION OF MANAGEMENT STRATEGY

The following guidelines are useful, with the understanding that other formulations are possible. Time and additional clinical experience will bring more
changes in the way HIV infection is managed.

The stage and prognosis of an individual's HIV disease should be assessed so
that the patient and clinician can jointly decide upon follow-up intervals, monitoring, prophylaxis against PCP, antiviral therapy, and other aspects of management. One possible management strategy is to divide patients into three
groups based on T4 lymphocyte counts:

> **Group 1:** T4 count >500 cells/cubic mm;
>
> **Group 2:** T4 count 200–500 cells/cubic mm;
>
> **Group 3:** T4 count <200 cells/cubic mm.

Group 1 Patients.   Complete blood count, differential count, platelet, ESR, liver function tests, serum electrolytes/BUN/creatinine, and T4 lymphocyte count are obtained at each visit. If the T4 count is decreasing or is in the 500 to 800 cells/cubic mm range, a 3-month follow-up is scheduled. Otherwise, the patient is followed at 6-month intervals.

For Group 1 patients, the benefits of either AZT antiviral therapy or prophylaxis against PCP have not been demonstrated as of August 1989. For those Group 1 patients wishing to participate, enrollment in experimental clinical protocols may be recommended (if available) so that the patients' responses and drug toxicity can be objectively evaluated.

Group 2 Patients.   The patient is evaluated every 3 months with laboratory studies obtained at each visit (see Group 1). For patients on AZT, monthly monitoring is sufficient. For symptomatic and asymptomatic patients in this group, AZT therapy has been effective in limiting progression of HIV disease in clinical trials. Experimental antiviral protocols (if available) and/or AZT therapy are recommended.

Group 3 Patients.   The patient is evaluated at least every 3 months and the same laboratory studies used in Groups 1 and 2 are obtained. Experimental antiviral protocols (if available) and/or AZT therapy is recommended. Prophylaxis against PCP is recommended and supported by experimental data for all patients in Group 3 (symptomatic and asymptomatic).

AZT Treatment of Asymptomatic Patients.   Evidence is accumulating that early intervention slows progression to symptomatic HIV disease. Because of this, treatment of asymptomatic patients is less controversial than it once was. The currently available data on AZT therapy are from clinical trials conducted with symptomatic patients. Many clinicians feel that the benefit shown in these trials justifies treatment with AZT for asymptomatic patients with low T4 counts — e.g., in Groups 2 and 3. Others feel that until benefit is shown by clinical trials in asymptomatic patients (now in progress) the risk from toxicity is too great to justify treatment. An intermediate practice is to examine other indicators of HIV disease progression (e.g., p24 antigen) in patients in Groups 2 and 3 and offer AZT therapy to those at greater risk based on these additional tests.

■ AZT THERAPY

AZT therapy is discussed in detail in a separate chapter. To detect anemia or neutropenia, a CBC should be obtained when therapy begins and should be repeated every one to two weeks for two months and once per month thereafter. Side-effects of AZT include headaches, high fever, severe rashes, and nausea. Many clinicians withhold AZT during therapy for significant opportunistic infections (OIs) and resume it after recovery (e.g., three to four weeks after diagnosis of an OI) if there is no contraindication. Some clinicians fear that abrupt discontinuation of AZT may lead to a "rebound" of HIV disease and prefer to continue AZT at low doses during treatment of OIs. Asymptomatic HIV-infected patients are far less likely to require dose-reductions for anemia or neutropenia than more immunocompromised patients. They may also tolerate the drug for longer periods without interruption by acute opportunistic infections or bothersome side effects.

■ PROGNOSTICATION

As with many other chronic medical conditions, the prognosis for HIV disease can be determined only within broad and often unsatisfyingly vague ranges. These are defined by statistical data derived from long-term prospective studies of patient cohorts and from anecdotal reports of clinical experience. Evidence from these sources indicates that HIV disease progresses to full-blown AIDS and eventually to death. However, progression rates are variable and may be slowed by HIV antiviral therapy and perhaps by other medical interventions. There is reason to believe that therapeutic options will continue to improve. Modification of behaviors (such as smoking, drug use, and exposure to STDs) have not been proven to slow HIV disease progression, but they seem intuitively worthwhile and often cause subjective feelings of improved health. Any prognosis should be presented in a perspective that acknowledges both the severity of HIV disease and the cautious optimism that exists for altering its course. Patients should be encouraged to ask questions about transmission, natural history, and prognosis so that they can become active participants in understanding the clinical spectrum of their disease.

The majority of HIV-infected patients can expect to be asymptomatic for approximately 3 to 5 years after infection.[2] Laboratory values identified from cohort studies that suggest low risk for progression in the short term include T4 lymphocytes >400 cells/cubic mm, T4:T8 ratio >0.6, ESR <15 mm/hour, hemoglobin >13.5 g/deciliter, β_2-microglobulin <3.0 mg/liter.[2]

Some values derived from cohort studies suggest either significant risk for progression to AIDS over the next 3 years or HIV disease already at a more advanced stage. These include:

- T4 lymphocytes <200 cells/cubic mm
- T4:T8 ratio <0.4
- ESR >40 mm/hour
- hemoglobin <12 g/deciliter
- β_2-microglobulin >5.0 mg/liter
- detectable serum HIV p24 antigen.

The specific numbers cited above are arbitrarily selected cutoff values from cohort studies. Their use should not obscure the fact that HIV disease is a continuous spectrum. Their value in the clinical management of individual patients is unproven.

Profound abnormalities on the tests listed above, anergy, and opportunistic infections (CDC-defining AIDS infections as well as candidiasis, hairy leukoplakia, herpes zoster) indicate more advanced HIV disease, a worse short-term prognosis, and greater justification for initiating HIV antiviral therapy.

Although quantitative tests such as T4 lymphocyte counts and β_2-microglobulin correlate statistically with disease progression, isolated determinations may vary. Factors affecting such values include the random variation inherent in the assay, the patient's short-term state of health, improper sample handling, and laboratory errors. It is the ethical responsibility of clinicians to take the time to discuss the significance of T4 lymphocytes and other tests with the patient in a sensitive manner. Many patients interpret insignificant changes in T4 levels as evidence of profound changes in their condition, so it is important to clarify the limitations of prognostic tests.

■ PSYCHOSOCIAL, PHILOSOPHICAL, AND LEGAL ISSUES

A major role of the primary-care provider is to offer and arrange support during stressful and progressive illness. Considerations are discussed in other chapters.

Difficult management issues must eventually be confronted and these are best addressed with the patient's full participation. These often include prolongation of life through cardiac resuscitation and intubation, medical and financial issues, durable power of attorney, and social and logistical support if the patient can no longer live independently. Because HIV disease is progressive, fatal, and frequently involves sudden medical crises and a decline in mental ability, these issues should be raised and resolved as early as possible while the patient is still able to participate in making the decision.

The provider should ask the patient who else knows of his/her seropositivity and review issues of confidentiality related to landlords, employers, insurance, and healthcare agencies. Depending on the patient's needs, referrals may be made to social workers, legal assistance, ministers, healers, priests, psychologists, and community agencies.

■ PROPHYLAXIS/SUPPRESSION OF INFECTIOUS DISEASES

HIV-infected patients are at risk for activation and frequent recurrences of infections by organisms normally held in check by the immune system, such as candida, *Pneumocystis carinii*, *M. tuberculosis*, *Cryptococcus neoformans*, salmonella species, *Toxoplasma gondii*, and herpes simplex virus. Use of long-term antibiotic treatment to suppress these infectious agents may be necessary. Therapeutic and prophylactic treatment for each organism is discussed in detail in other chapters.

Prophylaxis against opportunistic infections has been best documented for PCP. More than 80 percent of all patients with AIDS develop PCP. In 65 percent of this population, PCP is the first opportunistic infection diagnosed. Data exist to support PCP prophylaxis for patients who have survived an episode of PCP. Many clinicians currently feel that PCP prophylaxis should be offered to patients who have T4-cell counts below 200/cubic mm, regardless of whether an AIDS-defining OI or malignancy has been diagnosed.

In February 1989, the Food and Drug Administration (FDA) approved a Treatment IND for aerosolized pentamidine as prophylaxis for PCP in individuals with a history of PCP or a T-cell count <200/cubic mm. The recommended dose is 300 mg of aerosolized pentamidine every four weeks using a RespirGard II (or equivalent) nebulizer. Full FDA licensing of aerosolized pentamidine is expected very shortly.

Active TB is a commonly diagnosed infection in HIV-infected people. Although data on the efficacy of INH preventive therapy in HIV-infected persons have not yet been published, INH reduces the incidence of active TB in a variety of TB risk groups. Thus any HIV-infected person, regardless of age, who has a positive tuberculin skin test reaction, has not been treated for active TB, and has no evidence of active TB, should be offered INH preventive therapy unless it is medically contraindicated. The Advisory Committee for the Elimination of Tuberculosis (ACET) recommends considering a tuberculin skin test positive in an HIV-infected person if there is greater than or equal to a 5 mm induration. The appropriate duration of INH prophylaxis for such patients has not been tested in clinical trials. ACET and the San Francisco General Hospital tuberculosis clinic recommend 12 months of prophylactic INH therapy. Other clinicians have offered therapy for 9 months. Some experts have suggested prolonging INH preventive therapy beyond 12 months and even for the lifetime of the patient.[34]

■ BEHAVIOR MODIFICATION

The Question of Immune Stimulation and Disease Progression.   In vitro studies describe increased HIV replication in HIV-infected cells after immunologic activation.[35-37] Although the clinical relevance of these data is unknown, they raise the question of whether stimulation of an HIV-infected person's immune system (by immunizations, STDs, other infections, intravenous drug injections, etc.) may cause more rapid progression of HIV disease by activating quiescent HIV in lymphocytes and macrophages. In the absence of definitive clinical data, it seems prudent to advise HIV-infected patients to take sensible precautions for avoiding infections (e.g., safer sex, good hygiene, avoid sharing dirty needles, etc.).

Unsafe Sexual Practices.   A newly acquired STD is a manifestation of recent unsafe sexual practices. Both self-interest and public-health concerns dictate that the HIV-infected patient change such high-risk behavior. Counseling should include a discussion of the danger of transmitting HIV to others, the possibility that the patient's own HIV infection may be accelerated by STD-related antigenic stimulation of the immune system, and the hypothetical possibility of becoming superinfected by more virulent HIV strains during unsafe sex with another HIV-infected person. Safer sex issues are discussed in detail elsewhere.

Substance Abuse.   Intravenous drug use involving shared needles creates two risks for the HIV-infected patient: transmission of HIV infection to others and the acquisition of other infectious agents. Even without needle sharing, the injection of antigens may activate the patient's immune system, thus promoting progression of HIV disease. The clinician's goal should be to involve the HIV-infected IVDU in a supportive and structured drug rehabilitation program. Short of this, the importance of clean needles and the use of bleach to clean his or her apparatus should be emphasized. Issues relating to intravenous drug use are discussed in detail in another chapter.

Other Behaviors.   Tobacco and alcohol have adverse and preventable health consequences and should be discouraged. Inadequately cooked or washed foods and unpasteurized milk can transmit bacterial or parasitic infections and should be avoided.

■ ROUTINE HEALTH MAINTENANCE CONSIDERATIONS

Cancer Screening.   Customary cancer screening should be provided for HIV-infected patients. Recent literature has reported HIV as a potential risk factor for cervical dysplasia.[38-41] Thus a Pap smear should be done yearly on all women whose previous smears have been normal. If there is a history of atypia, then a Pap should be done on initial visit and every three to six months thereafter. As would be done for any patient, HIV-infected men and women should be screened for all cancers expected in their age groups.

Immunizations.   Immunizations for HIV-infected persons are discussed in detail in another chapter. The CDC recommends that HIV-infected patients receive routine immunizations as outlined in Table 1.[42-46] However, these recommendations remain controversial. Some clinicians and researchers feel that stimulation of the immune system by immunizing antigens may activate latent HIV and promote disease progression.

Hepatitis B vaccine should be given to HIV-infected persons for the same reasons it is given to non-HIV-infected persons.[47,48]

TABLE 1. CDC RECOMMENDATIONS FOR ROUTINE IMMUNIZATION OF HIV-INFECTED CHILDREN, ADOLESCENTS, AND ADULTS

KNOWN HIV INFECTION

Vaccine	Asymptomatic	Symptomatic
DTP[1]	yes	yes
OPV[2]	no	no
IPV[3]	yes	yes
MMR[4]	yes	yes[8]
HbCV[5]	yes	yes
Pneumococcal[6]	yes	yes
Influenza virus[7]	no[9]	yes

Reprinted with permission of CDC, MMWR 1989; 38:205.
1. *DTP = diphtheria and tetanus toxoids and pertussis vaccine, adsorbed; DTP may be used up to the seventh birthday.*
2. *OPV = oral, live attenuated poliovirus vaccine; contains poliovirus types 1, 2, and 3.*
3. *IPV = inactivated poliovirus vaccine; contains poliovirus types 1, 2, and 3.*
4. *MMR = live measles, mumps, and rubella virus vaccine.*
5. *HbCV = Haemophilus influenzae type b conjugate vaccine.*
6. *Pneumococcal polysaccharide vaccine.*
7. *Inactivated influenza virus vaccine.*
8. *Should be considered.*
9. *Not contraindicated.*

■ HIV DISEASE AND PETS

Several infectious agents reported to afflict patients with HIV disease are sometimes contracted from animals. These include toxoplasma, cryptosporidium, campylobacter, salmonella, and cat-scratch bacillus. However, there are no studies to suggest that pets have been responsible for a significant number of infections in HIV-infected patients. Because pets are often a major source of support and comfort for patients with HIV disease, clinical recommendations focus instead on avoiding zoonoses. Advice has been variable, reflecting a lack of definitive data, and has included: the cleaning of litter boxes daily by a non-HIV infected person, or, if no alternative exists, using gloves and washing hands afterwards; not feeding pets uncooked meat or unpasteurized milk; not adopting stray pets; not adopting a new pet; and avoiding pet turtles.[49]

■ MANAGEMENT OF COMMON PROBLEMS

The patient should understand the need for reporting new symptoms as they develop. These include fever and other systemic symptoms, skin lesions, cough, dysphagia, diarrhea, thrush, headache, and lymphadenopathy. Evaluation of these symptoms is discussed in other chapters. He or she should understand where to go, what number to call in an emergency, and how and when to schedule follow-up visits with the clinician.

REFERENCES

1. Kaslow RA, Phair JP, Friedman HB, et al. Infection with the human immunodeficiency virus: clinical manifestations and their relationship to immune deficiency. A report from the Multicenter AIDS Cohort Study. Ann Intern Med 1987; 107:474-80.

2. Moss AR, Bacchetti P, Osmond D, et al. Seropositivity for HIV and the development of AIDS or AIDS related condition: three year follow up of the San Francisco General Hospital cohort. Br Med J 1988; 296:745-50.

3. Puppo F, Torresin A, Lotti G, et al. Autoimmune hemolytic anemia and human immunodeficiency virus (HIV) infection. Ann Intern Med 1988; 109:249-50.

4. Schreiber ZA, Loh SH, Charles M, Abeebe LS. Autoimmune hemolytic anemia in patients with the acquired immune deficiency syndrome (AIDS). Blood 1983; 62:117a.

5. Abrams DI, Kiprov DD, Goedert JJ, et al. Antibodies to human T-lymphotropic virus type III and development of the acquired immunodeficiency syndrome in homosexual men presenting with immune thrombocytopenia. Ann Intern Med 1986; 104:47-50.

6. Eyster ME, Gail MH, Ballard JO, et al. Natural history of human immunodeficiency virus infections in hemophiliacs: effects of T-cell subsets, platelet counts, and age. Ann Intern Med 1987; 107:1-6.

7. Walsh C, Krigel R, Lennette E, Karpatkin S. Thrombocytopenia in homosexual patients. Prognosis, response to therapy, and prevalence of antibody to the retrovirus associated with the acquired immuno-deficiency syndrome. Ann Intern Med 1985; 103:542-5.

8. Lipman ML, Goldstein E. Serum lactic dehydrogenase predicts mortality in patients with AIDS and pneumocystis pneumonia. West J Med 1988; 149:486-7.

9. Silverman BA, Rubinstein A. Serum lactate dehydrogenase levels in adults and children with acquired immune deficiency syndrome (AIDS) and AIDS-related complex: possible indicator of B cell lymphoproliferation and disease activity. Effect of intravenous gammaglobulin on enzyme levels. Am J Med 1985; 78:728-36.

10. Seligmann M, Pinching AJ, Rosen FS, et al. Immunology of human immunodeficiency virus infection and the acquired immunodeficiency syndrome. An update. Ann Intern Med 1987; 107:234-42.

11. Grant IH, Armstrong D. Management of infectious complications in acquired immunodeficiency syndrome. Am J Med 1986; 81:59-72.

12. Kovacs JA, Kovacs AA, Polis M, et al. Cryptococcosis in the acquired immunodeficiency syndrome. Ann Intern Med 1985; 103:533-8.

13. Krick JA, Remington JS. Toxoplasmosis in the adult — an overview. N Engl J Med 1978; 298:550-3.

14. Israelski DM, Remington JS. Toxoplasmic encephalitis in patients with AIDS. Infect Dis Clin North Am 1988; 2:429-45.

15. Kaplan JE, Spira TJ, Fishbein DB, et al. Lymphadenopathy syndrome in homosexual men. Evidence for continuing risk of developing the acquired immunodeficiency syndrome. JAMA 1987; 257:335-7.

16. Polk BF, Fox R, Brookmeyer R, et al. Predictors of the acquired immunodeficiency syndrome developing in a cohort of seropositive homosexual men. N Engl J Med 1987; 316:61-6.

17. Goedert JJ, Biggar RJ, Melbye M, et al. Effect of T4 count and cofactors on the incidence of AIDS in homosexual men infected with human immunodeficiency virus. JAMA 1987; 257:331-4.

18. El-Sadr W, Marmor M, Zolla-Pazner S, et al. Four-year prospective study of homosexual men: correlation of immunologic abnormalities, clinical status, and serology to human immunodeficiency virus. J Infect Dis 1987; 155:789-93.

19. Eyster ME, Gail MH, Ballard JO, et al. Natural history of human immunodeficiency virus infections in hemophiliacs: effects of T-cell subsets, platelet counts, and age. Ann Intern Med 1987; 107:1-6.

20. de Wolf F, Lange JM, Houweling JT, et al. Numbers of CD4+ cells and the levels of core antigens of and antibodies to the human immunodeficiency virus as predictors of AIDS among seropositive homosexual men. J Infect Dis 1988; 158:615-22.

21. Allain J, Laurian Y, Paul DA, et al. Long-term evaluation of HIV antigen and antibodies to p24 and gp41 in patients with hemophilia. N Engl J Med 1987; 317:1114-21.

22. Paul DA, Falk LA, Kessler HA, et al. Correlation of serum HIV antigen and antibody with clinical status in HIV-infected patients. J Med Virol 1987; 22:357-63.

23. Goudsmit J, Lange JM, Paul DA, Dawson GJ. Antigenemia and antibody titers to core and envelope antigens in AIDS, AIDS-related complex, and subclinical human immunodeficiency virus infection. J Infect Dis 1987; 155:558-60.

24. Goudsmit J, de Wolf F, Paul DA, et al. Expression of human immunodeficiency virus antigen (HIV-Ag) in serum and cerebrospinal fluid during acute and chronic infection. Lancet 1986; 2:177-80.

25. Lange JM, Paul DA, Huisman HG, et al. Persistent HIV antigenaemia and decline of HIV core antibodies associated with transition to AIDS. Br Med J 1986; 293:1459-62.

26. Jackson GG, Paul DA, Falk LA, et al. Human immunodeficiency virus (HIV) antigenemia (p24) in the acquired immunodeficiency syndrome (AIDS) and the effect of treatment with zidovudine (AZT). Ann Intern Med 1988; 108:175-80.

27. Pederson C, Nielsen CM, Vestergaard BF, et al. Temporal relation of antigenaemia and loss of antibodies to core antigens to development of clinical disease in HIV infection. Br Med J 1987; 295:567-9.

28. Hutterer J, Fuchs D, Eder G, et al. Neopterin as discriminating and prognostic parameter in healthy homosexuals, ARC and AIDS patients. Wien Klin Wochenschr 1987; 99:531-5.

29. McDougal JS, Kennedy MS, Nicholson JK, et al. Antibody response to human immunodeficiency virus in homosexual men. Relation of antibody specificity, titer, and isotype to clinical status, severity of immunodeficiency, and disease progression. J Clin Invest 1987; 80:316-24.

30. Schupbach J, Haller O, Vogt M, et al. Antibodies to HTLV-III in Swiss patients with AIDS and pre-AIDS and in groups at risk for AIDS. N Engl J Med 1985; 312:265-70.

31. Lange JM, Coutinho RA, Krone WJ, et al. Distinct IgG recognition patterns during progression of subclinical and clinical infection with lymphadenopathy associated virus/human T lymphotropic virus. Br Med J 1986; 292:228-30.

32. Weber JN, Clapham PR, Weiss RA, et al. Human immunodeficiency virus infection in two cohorts of homosexual men: neutralising sera and association of anti-*gag* antibody with prognosis. Lancet 1987; 1:119-22.

33. Lange JM, de Wolf F, Krone WJ, et al. Decline of antibody reactivity to outer viral core protein p17 is an earlier serological marker of disease progression in human immunodeficiency virus infection than anti-p24 decline. AIDS 1987; 1:155-9.

34. Redfield RR, Wright DC, Tramont EC. The Walter Reed staging classification for HTLV-III/LAV infection. N Engl J Med 1986; 314:131-2.

35. Tuberculosis and human immunodeficiency virus infection: Recommendations of the Advisory Committee for the Elimination of Tuberculosis (ACET). MMWR 1989; 38:236-50.

36. Folks TM, Justement J, Kinter A, et al. Cytokine-induced expression of HIV-1 in a chronically infected promonocyte cell line. Science 1987; 238:800-2.

37. Zagury D, Bernard J, Leonard R, et al. Long-term cultures of HTLV-III-infected T cells: a model of cytopathology of T-cell depletion in AIDS. Science 1986; 231:850-3.

38. Nabel G, Baltimore D. An inducible transcription factor activates expression of human immunodeficiency virus in T cells. Nature 1987; 326:711-3.

39. Pomerantz RJ, de la Monte SM, Donegan SP, et al. Human immunodeficiency virus (HIV) infection of the uterine cervix. Ann Intern Med 1988; 108:321-7.

40. Letters to the Editor: Is infection with HIV a risk factor for cervical intraepithelial neoplasia? Lancet 1987; 2:1277-8.

41. Cervical dysplasia and HIV infection. Lancet 1988; 1:237-9.

42. Henry MJ, Stanley MW, Cruikshank S, Carson L. Association of human immunodeficiency virus-induced immunosuppression with human papillomavirus infection and cervical intraepithelial neoplasia. Am J Obstet Gynecol 1989; 160:352-3.

43. Immunization of children infected with human immunodeficiency virus — supplementary ACIP statement. Immunization Practices Advisory Committee. MMWR 1988; 37:181-3.

44. Immunization of children infected with human T-lymphotropic virus type III/lymphadenopathy-associated virus. MMWR 1986; 35:595-8,603-6.

45. Recommendations of the Immunization Practices Advisory Committee (ACIP). General recommendations on immunization. MMWR 1989; 38:205-14, 219-27.

46. ACIP. Pneumococcal polysaccharide vaccine. MMWR 1989; 38:64-76.

47. Prevention and control of influenza. MMWR 1988; 37:361-4, 369-73.

48. Recommendations for protection against viral hepatitis. MMWR 1985; 34:313-24, 329-35.

49. Update on hepatitis B prevention. MMWR 1987; 36:353-60, 366.

50. Gorczyca K. Safe pet guidelines for people with AIDS/HIV. Third ed. San Francisco: Pets Are Wonderful Support (PAWS), 1989.

Immunization of HIV-Infected Persons

P.T. Cohen, M.D., Ph.D.

The recommendations of the United States Public Health Service Immunization Practices Advisory Committee (ACIP) for active and passive immunization of HIV-infected persons are similar to those for non-HIV-infected persons. Certain live virus vaccines, however, are not recommended for HIV-infected persons. This section reviews vaccine recommendations for HIV-infected persons, and discusses the following questions.

- Will live virus vaccines cause severe disease in HIV-infected persons?
- Will antigenic stimulation from the immunization activate latent HIV infection and promote progression of HIV disease?
- Will the HIV-infected patient's immune system respond to immunization?

Asymptomatic persons need not be screened for HIV infection solely for the purpose of receiving an immunization. As discussed below, there is no evidence that asymptomatic HIV-infected persons experience more adverse effects from routine immunizations than uninfected individuals. Except for the use of inactivated rather than live poliovirus vaccine, routine immunization recommendations are identical for HIV-infected and non-HIV-infected asymptomatic persons. Unresolved issues exist for BCG vaccine, which is administered routinely in some parts of the world. It is not recommended for use in the United States.

Table 1 lists routine immunizations recommended for HIV-infected persons.[1-3,41] Schedules for administration are found in standard references[3-5] and are discussed here only if recommendations differ from those for non-HIV-infected persons.

■ LIVE VACCINES IN HIV-INFECTED PATIENTS

Measles, Mumps, Rubella (MMR) Vaccine. ACIP recommends that administration of MMR vaccine be considered for all HIV-infected persons.[1] Previously, this vaccine combination was recommended only for asymptomatic HIV-infected persons.[2] The recommendation was changed because of reports of severe measles in nonvaccinated, symptomatic HIV-infected children[7] and because of the absence of significant adverse effects from measles, mumps, and rubella (MMR) vaccines in symptomatic HIV-infected patients.[2,8,9] Viruses in the MMR vaccine are not transmitted from the vaccinated individual to others.[2,10-12]

Symptomatic (immunocompromised) HIV-infected children should receive MMR vaccine at 15 months — the age currently recommended for other children. When there is an increased risk of exposure to measles, such as during an outbreak, these children should receive vaccine at even younger ages. At such times, infants 6 to 11 months old should receive monovalent measles vaccine and be revaccinated with MMR at 12 months or older. Children 12 to 14 months old should receive MMR and do not need revaccination.[2,8]

TABLE 1.   CDC RECOMMENDATIONS FOR ROUTINE IMMUNIZATION OF HIV-INFECTED CHILDREN, ADOLESCENTS, AND ADULTS.

KNOWN HIV INFECTION

Vaccine	Asymptomatic	Symptomatic
DTP[1]	yes	yes
OPV[2]	no	no
IPV[3]	yes	yes
MMR[4]	yes	yes[8]
HbCV[5]	yes	yes
Pneumococcal[6]	yes	yes
Influenza virus[7]	no[9]	yes

Reprinted with permission of CDC, MMWR 1989; 38:205.
1. *DTP = diphtheria and tetanus toxoids and pertussis vaccine, adsorbed. DTP may be used up to the seventh birthday.*
2. *OPV = oral, live attenuated poliovirus vaccine; contains poliovirus types 1, 2, and 3.*
3. *IPV = inactivated poliovirus vaccine; contains poliovirus types 1, 2, and 3.*
4. *MMR = live measles, mumps, and rubella virus vaccine.*
5. *HbCV = Haemophilus influenzae type b conjugate vaccine.*
6. *Pneumococcal polysaccharide vaccine.*
7. *Inactivated influenza virus vaccine.*
8. *Should be considered.*
9. *Not contraindicated.*

Poliomyelitis Vaccine.   ACIP recommends that HIV-infected persons be immunized against poliomyelitis if they have not been adequately immunized in the past. Inactivated poliovirus vaccine (IPV) should be used for immunization rather than live oral polio vaccine (OPV).[13] Immunosuppressed persons receiving OPV may be at increased risk for vaccine-associated paralytic disease, a complication observed in immunologically normal persons with a frequency of 1 in 5.5 million doses.[14] This is presently a theoretical concern, however, because studies have not revealed an increased incidence of OPV complications in HIV-infected persons.[9,15]

Because the attenuated virus in OPV is shed in bodily secretions, it may infect the recipients' household contacts. IPV is therefore recommended when immunizing any member of an HIV-infected person's household, whether they are immunosuppressed or not.[2]

BCG Vaccine.   BCG vaccine (for control of tuberculosis) contains a live attenuated strain of Mycobacterium bovis. BCG immunization is not recommended for persons with symptomatic HIV infection, and it is not recommended in areas of the world where the risk of exposure to tuberculosis is low, such as in the United States. The World Health Organization recommends that in populations with a high risk of tuberculosis, asymptomatic HIV-infected children should be immunized with BCG as soon after birth as possible.[16]

BCG vaccine has been associated with a case of disseminated Mycobacterium bovis in a 29-year-old AIDS patient[17] and with BCG adenitis in 3 infants with symptomatic HIV infection.[18]

BCG vaccination is a major weapon in tuberculosis control in many non-industrialized countries, including parts of Africa where there is a high prevalence of HIV infection. These are areas where resources for recognizing HIV infection are limited. Moreover, tuberculosis is a common infection in HIV-infected persons. Whether BCG immunization of HIV-infected persons poses risks that require modification of routine BCG immunization strategy remains unresolved.

Vaccinia Virus (Smallpox) Vaccine.   A case of disseminated vaccinia (smallpox) occurred after a military recruit with asymptomatic HIV infection received live vaccinia virus vaccine.[19] Smallpox vaccination is no longer medically indicated for anyone except laboratory workers occupationally exposed to the virus. Its use is justified in the military only as a defense against enemy use of the vaccinia virus as a biologic weapon.[20,21]

■ OTHER (NON-LIVE-VIRUS) VACCINES IN HIV-INFECTED PERSONS

DTP and *Haemophilus Influenzae* b.   Routine immunization for diphtheria, pertussis, tetanus (DTP), and *Haemophilus influenzae* type b is recommended for HIV-infected persons in accordance with ACIP's recommendations for all persons.[3,22,23]

Pneumococcal Vaccine.   Because of the high incidence of invasive pneumococcal infections seen in HIV-infected patients, symptomatic or asymptomatic HIV-infected persons over two years old should receive a single immunization with pneumococcal polysaccharide vaccine. The pneumococcal vaccine consists of purified, capsular polysaccharide vaccine. Pneumococcal vaccine is recommended for all adults and children over two years old with chronic illnesses or conditions associated with immunosuppression. The ACIP decision to recommend it for asymptomatic HIV-infected persons is a recent change.[41] Previously, it was not recommended for asymptomatic HIV-infected persons.[2,3,24]

Influenza Vaccine.   ACIP recommends that symptomatic HIV-infected persons over 6 months old be immunized annually with inactivated influenza virus vaccine.[1,6] For asymptomatic HIV-infected persons, ACIP does not recommend routine influenza vaccination[1] but suggests that "vaccination is a prudent precaution" in all HIV-infected persons over 6 months old.[6] Studies of HIV-infected persons have not shown unusual side effects or acceleration of HIV disease after influenza vaccination.[24,25] Yearly influenza vaccination is also indicated for household contacts of patients with symptomatic HIV infection and should be considered for health-care workers who have contact with HIV-infected patients.[3]

Hepatitis B Virus Vaccine.   ACIP recommends hepatitis B virus (HBV) vaccine for persons with high or moderate risk for HBV infection who lack evidence of protective anti-hepatitis B surface antibodies (anti-HBs).[27,28] These recommendations do not differ for HIV-infected persons except that plasma-derived vaccine (rather than recombinant vaccine) is recommended for immunocompromised persons.

Plasma-derived HBV vaccine should be administered in the deltoid muscle in adults and the anterolateral thigh muscle in infants and children. In adults, the vaccine's immunogenicity is significantly lower when the buttock is the injection site.[29] The vaccine may be given subcutaneously to persons at risk for hemorrhage.

Higher antigen doses of the vaccine are recommended for immunocompromised adults (40 micrograms) than for healthy adults (10 micrograms). These doses may also be advisable for asymptomatic HIV-seropositive adults.[30] The adult formulation of plasma-derived vaccine contains 20 micrograms of antigen/ml, while the recombinant vaccine contains only 10 micrograms/ml, and requires a 4.0 ml injection volume. This volume is too large for easy injection into the deltoid muscle and contains more aluminum hydroxide adjuvant (2.0 mg) than is currently recommended (1.25 mg per dose).[28]

Immunization consists of three injections over a six-month period. Some HIV-seropositive patients do not develop protective levels of anti-HBs after immunization.[30-32] Thus, clinicians should consider determining anti-HBs levels after completing the immunization schedule in HIV-infected persons. Nonresponding, non-HIV-infected persons may respond to an additional series of vaccinations, but HIV-seropositive patients may not.[33] Inadequately immunized HIV-infected patients will benefit from counseling about their greater risk of becoming HBV carriers,[33] precautions about sexual partners who are HBV carriers, and use of prophylactic immunoglobulin if HBV exposure occurs.

Many HIV-infected persons are at risk for HBV infection — homosexually active men, users of illicit injectable drugs, recipients of certain blood products, sexual contacts of HBV carriers, persons with multiple sexual partners, and infants born to HBV-positive mothers.

Health workers who risk contact with body fluids and secretions of HIV-infected persons and who do not have antibodies to HBV are also at risk and should be vaccinated with hepatitis B vaccine.

■ PASSIVE IMMUNIZATION IN HIV-INFECTED PATIENTS

In some circumstances, passive immunization with immune globulin (IG) can protect against selected infections, as discussed below.

Intravenous Immune Globulin.   High-dose (5 g protein/100 ml) intravenous immune globulin (IGIV) administered at regular intervals (monthly or biweekly) is under investigation as a way to prevent infections in HIV-infected children.[1,3] Use of intravenous immune globulin for this purpose is controversial. The dose range for treating immunodeficient persons is 100 to 300 mg/kg body weight, or based on package-insert instructions.[3]

Measles Prophylaxis.   IG (16.5 g protein/100 ml) can be used to modify or prevent measles infection in HIV-infected persons if it is administered within six days of exposure. For symptomatic HIV-infected persons exposed to measles, ACIP recommends IG prophylaxis regardless of whether the patient has been vaccinated for measles or has a past history of measles. The IG dose should be 0.5 ml/kg (82.5 mg/kg; maximum dose 15 ml or 2,475 mg) given intramuscularly. ACIP strongly recommends IG for exposed asymptomatic HIV-infected persons who are measles susceptible (unvaccinated, with no clear past history of measles), and particularly for infants less than one year old and pregnant women. The recommended dose is 0.25 ml/kg (maximum dose 15 ml) intramuscularly. Intramuscular IG may not be needed if the patient is already receiving high dose (100–400 mg/kg) intravenous immune globulin regularly and has received a dose within the past three weeks.[1,8]

Varicella Zoster.   For symptomatic HIV-infected persons with significant exposure to varicella-zoster virus (e.g., exposure through household contact, close indoor contact of more than one hour, sharing a hospital room, prolonged face-to-face contact), ACIP recommends treatment with varicella-zoster immune globulin (VZIG). The dose should be determined from the manufacturer's specifications. VZIG is available from some American Red Cross distribution centers.[2,4,34]

Viral Hepatitis.   ACIP has published detailed recommendations for prophylaxis with IG and hepatitis B hyperimmune globulin (HBIG) following exposure to viral hepatitis (hepatitis A, B, and non-A, non-B). These recommendations do not differ for HIV-infected persons.[27,28]

■ SEROLOGIC RESPONSE OF HIV-INFECTED PERSONS TO IMMUNIZATION

Published data suggest that many HIV-infected patients respond to immunization and many others do not. Although one study reports normal immunologic responses to influenza immunization in 55 HIV-infected patients (asymptomatic and symptomatic),[25] suboptimal responses were reported in studies of HIV-infected hemophiliacs receiving influenza, pneumococcal[34] and HBV[35] vaccination, and asymptomatic and symptomatic homosexual men receiving HBV[30,31] and influenza[26] vaccination.

These studies show that absence of symptoms is not equivalent to immunocompetence — a significant fact because several current ACIP recommendations use the presence or absence of symptoms as a management criterion. There are no established guidelines for followup and management of HIV-infected patients after attempted immunization has failed. Possible options include readministration of the vaccine regimen, booster doses added to the standard regimen, and counseling for nonresponders. More data are needed to evaluate these options.

■ RISK OF PROGRESSION OF HIV DISEASE AFTER IMMUNIZATION

HIV infection progresses from a quiescent "latent" state in an asymptomatic patient to increasing destruction of essential components of the immune system in the symptomatic patient. Published in vitro studies describe increased HIV replication in HIV-infected cells after immunologic activation.[36-38] These data raise the question of whether stimulation of an HIV-infected person's immune system by immunizations could cause progression of HIV disease by activating quiescent HIV in lymphocytes and macrophages.

Comprehensive studies are needed to definitively address this concern. To date, the sparse clinical data do not suggest worsening of HIV disease after immunization. Several hundred HIV-seropositive military recruits have received routine immunizations without adverse consequences.[20,39] Immunization of HIV-infected infants and children has not been associated with disease progression.[9,15] Pneumococcal and influenza vaccines have been administered to HIV-seropositive men without changes in their HIV p24 antigen levels,[20,40] which suggests that HIV replication did not increase after immunization.

REFERENCES

1. Immunization of children infected with human immunodeficiency virus — supplementary ACIP statement. MMWR 1988; 37:181-3.
2. Immunization of children infected with human T-lymphotropic virus type III/lymphadenopathy-associated virus. MMWR 1986; 35:595-8,603-66.
3. Committee on infectious diseases, American Academy of Pediatrics. Report of the committee on infectious diseases, Twenty-first edition 1988. American Academy of Pediatrics, Elk Grove Village, IL. 1988.
4. Adult immunization. Recommendations of the Immunization Practices Advisory Committee. MMWR 1984; 33(suppl 1):1S-68S.
5. General recommendations on immunization. MMWR 1983; 32:1-8, 13-7.
6. Prevention and control of influenza. MMWR 1988; 37:361-4, 369-73.
7. Measles in HIV-infected children, United States. MMWR 1988; 37:183-6.
8. Measles prevention. MMWR 1987; 36:409-18, 423-5.
9. von Reyn CF, Clements CJ, Mann JM. Human immunodeficiency virus infection and routine childhood immunisation. Lancet 1987; 2:669-72.
10. Recommendation of the Immunization Practices Advisory Committee (ACIP). Measles prevention. MMWR 1982; 31:217-24, 229-31.
11. Rubella prevention. MMWR 1984; 33:301-10, 315-8.
12. Recommendations of the immunization practices advisory committee (ACIP): mumps vaccine. MMWR 1982; 31:617-20, 625.
13. Poliomyelitis prevention: enhanced-potency inactivated poliomyelitis vaccine — supplementary statement. MMWR 1987; 36:795-8.
14. Nkowane BM, Wassilak SG, Orenstein WA, et al. Vaccine-associated paralytic poliomyelitis. United States: 1973 through 1984. JAMA 1987; 257:1335-40.
15. McLaughlin M, Thomas P, Onorato I, et al. Live virus vaccines in human immunodeficiency virus-infected children: a retrospective survey. Pediatrics 1988; 82:229-33.
16. Use of BCG vaccines in the control of tuberculosis: a joint statement by the ACIP and the advisory committee for elimination of tuberculosis. MMWR 1988; 37:663-75.
17. Disseminated *Mycobacterium bovis* infection from BCG vaccination of a patient with acquired immunodeficiency syndrome. MMWR 1985; 34:227-8.
18. Blanche S, Le Deist F, Fischer A, et al. Longitudinal study of 18 children with perinatal LAV/HTLV-III infection: attempt at prognostic evaluation. J Pediatr 1986; 109:965-70.
19. Redfield RR, Wright DC, James WD, et al. Disseminated vaccinia in a military recruit with human immunodeficiency virus (HIV) disease. N Engl J Med 1987; 316:673-6.
20. Halsey NA, Henderson DA. HIV infection and immunization against other agents. N Engl J Med 1987; 316:683-5.
21. Smallpox vaccine. MMWR 1985; 34:341-2.
22. Diphtheria, tetanus, and pertussis: guidelines for vaccine prophylaxis and other preventive measures. Immunization Practices Advisory Committee. MMWR 1985; 34:405-14, 419-26.
23. Polysaccharide vaccine for prevention of Haemophilus influenzae type b disease. MMWR 1985; 34:201-5.
24. Update: pneumococcal polysaccharide vaccine usage — United States. MMWR 1984; 33:273-6, 281.
25. Huang KL, Ruben FL, Rinaldo CR Jr, et al. Antibody responses after influenza and pneumococcal immunization in HIV-infected homosexual men. JAMA 1987; 257:2047-50.
26. Nelson KE, Clements ML, Miotti P, et al. The influence of human immunodeficiency virus (HIV) infection on antibody responses to influenza vaccines. Ann Intern Med 1988; 109:383-8.
27. Recommendations for protection against viral hepatitis. MMWR 1985; 34:313-24, 329-35.
28. Update on hepatitis B prevention. MMWR 1987; 36:353-60, 366.
29. Suboptimal response to hepatitis B vaccine given by injection into the buttock. MMWR 1985; 34:105-8, 113.
30. Collier AC, Corey L, Murphy VL, Handsfield HH. Antibody to human immunodeficiency virus (HIV) and suboptimal response to hepatitis B vaccination. Ann Intern Med 1988; 109:101-5.
31. Carne CA, Weller IV, Waite J, et al. Impaired responsiveness of homosexual men with HIV antibodies to plasma derived hepatitis B vaccine. Br Med J 1987; 294:866-8.
32. Drake JH, Parmley RT, Britton HA. Loss of hepatitis B antibody in human immunodeficiency virus-positive hemophilia patients. Pediatr Infect Dis J. 1987; 6:1051-4.

33. Hadler SC. Hepatitis B prevention and human immunodeficiency virus (HIV) infection. Ann Intern Med 1988; 109:92-4.

34. Varicella-zoster immune globulin for the prevention of chickenpox. MMWR 1984; 33:84-90, 95-100.

35. Ragni MV, Ruben FL, Winkelstein A, et al. Antibody responses to immunization of patients with hemophilia with and without evidence of human immunodeficiency virus (human T-lymphotropic virus type III) infection. J Lab Clin Med 1987; 109:545-9.

36. Folks TM, Justement J, Kinter A, et al. Cytokine-induced expression of HIV-1 in a chronically infected promonocyte cell line. Science 1987; 238:800-2.

37. Zagury D, Bernard J, Leonard R, et al. Long-term cultures of HTLV-III-infected T cells: a model of cytopathology of T-cell depletion in AIDS. Science 1986; 231:850-3.

38. Nabel G, Baltimore D. An inducible transcription factor activates expression of human immunodeficiency virus in T cells. Nature 1987; 326:711-3.

39. Human T-lymphotropic virus type III/lymphadenopathy-associated virus antibody prevalence in U.S. military recruit applicants. MMWR 1986; 35:421-4.

40. Nelson KE, Clements ML, Miotti P, et al. The influence of human immunodeficiency virus (HIV) infection on antibody responses to influenza vaccines. Ann Intern Med 1988; 109:383-8.

41. CDC. ACIP: General recommendations on immunization. MMWR 1989; 38:205-27.

Clinical Applications of Antiviral Therapy: Overview

Paul A. Volberding, M.D.

Because HIV (human immunodeficiency virus) infection results in immune depletion, which leads in the majority of cases to AIDS, there has been increased demand for effective antiretroviral agents. Contributing to this pressure has been the ongoing failure of attempts at immune restoration and the limitations of prophylaxis and therapy for AIDS-related infections and cancers. This chapter reviews current research and antiviral agents scheduled for further investigation in ongoing or upcoming clinical trials.

Optimism about developing successful anti-HIV agents arises from the rapid growth in basic information about the HIV's life cycle. Each of the major steps in this cycle offers a potential site for anti-HIV interventions:

1. viral attachment to cell surface receptors;
2. viral penetration into the host cell;
3. transcription of the viral genome;
4. integration of viral genome into host DNA;
5. translation of viral gene products; and
6. assembly and budding of intact viral progeny.

Drugs directed at the sites of viral transcription have already been found active in vitro and in vivo. Drugs directed at other sites are now being tested in humans. Below are discussions of agents in or approaching clinical testing, including the earlier experience with zidovudine (AZT). A separate chapter discusses the clinical use of AZT.

■ DRUGS TO INHIBIT HIV BINDING TO CELLS OR PENETRATION INTO CELLS

Peptide T. HIV binds to the surface of susceptible cells by attaching to the CD4 protein. The small polypeptide, peptide T, has been reported to block this binding, possibly because of structural similarities to HIV envelope glycoprotein.[1] Although controversial,[2] antiviral activity has been reported in vitro from at least one laboratory, and some clinical benefit has been reported in one small uncontrolled study in Sweden.[3] In this trial, patients were treated and their clinical symptoms remained stable. Other laboratories have not, to date, confirmed the in vitro antiviral activity of peptide T. Efforts to confirm the in vitro studies are in progress; an investigational new drug (IND) status has been granted for peptide T by the FDA for Phase I human trials.

AL721. AL721 is a combination of the neutral glycerides phosphatidyl choline and phosphatidyl ethanolamine in a molar ratio of 7:2:1, hence the compound's name. In an Israeli study, this mixture was reported to have antiviral activity[4]; similar results have been reported in this country. AL721 is postulated to act by altering the membrane composition of lymphocytes in a way that inhibits viral penetration of lymphocytes. In vivo evidence is limited to a small, uncontrolled Israeli study ; more careful, controlled trials are now underway in the United States.

Dextran Sulfate.   Dextran sulfate is a polysulfated polysaccharide, thus carrying a large anionic charge. Antiviral activity in vitro has been reported in several laboratories.[5-7] The drug is thought to attach itself to host cell surfaces, conferring a negative charge that limits viral binding to CD4. Phase I trials of oral dextran sulfate demonstrated acceptable toxicity (primarily mild hepatic enzyme changes), but no efficacy was shown. This may be due to the limited oral bioavailability of this compound.

■ SOLUBLE CD4

An interesting new approach to inhibiting HIV infection involves the use of truncated portions of the CD4 antigen, genetically constructed to be small enough to be soluble yet still contain the HIV binding site.[8-11] This has been shown to block HIV infection of lymphocytes in vitro. Phase I trials are completed and Phase II trials are beginning in order to compare CD4 to AZT as well as to combine these two agents. Modifications of the structure of soluble CD4 to enhance its serum half life are being made. These agents are also expected to enter clinical trials.

■ DRUGS TO BLOCK HIV TRANSCRIPTION

Many compounds have been developed to block HIV transcription, especially by inhibiting the enzyme reverse transcriptase, which catalyzes this event. Some of these have already been tested and found ineffective, such as suramin, HPA23, and ribavirin.

Foscarnet.   This drug, developed in Sweden for treating cytomegalovirus, has in vitro activity against HIV.[17] It requires parenteral administration, limiting its practicality, but small-scale clinical trials are in progress, using foscarnet alone or with AZT.

Zidovudine.   To date, the most successful drug in this category of blockers of HIV transcription is the nucleoside analog 3'-azido-3'deoxythymidine, also known as zidovudine, Retrovir, and most commonly, azidothymidine (AZT). AZT is demonstrably quite active in blocking HIV replication and infection of cells in vitro. In an initial Phase I trial, toxicity was acceptable and suspicions of clinical benefit led rapidly to a much larger Phase II trial.[18] This was conducted in 282 patients, approximately half of whom had severe ARC and half of whom had recently recovered from their first episode of *Pneumocystis carinii* pneumonia (PCP). Patients were randomized to receive either placebo or 250 mg of AZT 6 times daily. Patients were stratified by CD4 cell counts at entry to the trial. After approximately six months, all patients were offered treatment with AZT because of a statistically very significant decrease in mortality in patients receiving AZT therapy over patients in the placebo group.[19]

Since then (February 1987), ready access to this drug by prescription has produced a large body of clinical data. Controlled trials are now being conducted in a variety of other HIV-infected patient populations. To date, these trials show that AZT offers clinical benefit to patients with CD4 counts below 500 cells/cubic mm. While toxicity is common, especially hematologic toxicity such as severe anemia and neutropenia,[20] AZT is widely used to treat patients with AIDS and severe ARC. Suggestions for the clinical use of AZT are discussed in a separate chapter.

Zidovudine Analogs.   In addition to AZT, a variety of other nucleoside analogs have been developed. These include dideoxycytidine (ddC) and dideoxyinosine (ddI).[21,22] Newer agents in this group include D4T and CS87. All have demonstrated anti-HIV activity in vitro.

ddC has been tested in a Phase I trial that was interrupted because of the occurrence of painful distal axonal neuropathies in many patients. A follow-up Phase I trial reduced this toxicity by alternating lower doses of dideoxycytidine with AZT. Phase I clinical testing of ddI has also been promising: there is evidence of efficacy and less hematologic toxicity than AZT has at a total daily dose of 1200 mg. ddI has been made available under a broad treatment IND as Phase II trials are conducted.

■ DRUGS THAT BLOCK VIRAL ASSEMBLY

Alpha and Beta Interferon.   We understand much less about viral protein translation and assembly than about either attachment or transcription. Nevertheless, evidence suggests a role for alpha and beta interferon in interrupting this phase of the HIV life cycle.

Alpha interferon is demonstrably active in blocking HIV replication in vitro,[23] and in vivo studies using alpha interferon alone or in combination with AZT are currently in progress. A major limitation of alpha interferon as it has been generally used in Kaposi's sarcoma is the subjective toxicity of the compound. It is not known, however, if the large doses that seem to be required for anti-neoplastic activity will be required for antiviral activity. Beta interferon, also active in vitro against HIV, is also being studied in vivo.

Castanospermine and Deoxynojirimycin.   The plant alkaloids castanospermine and deoxynojirimycin have anti-HIV activity in vitro.[12,13] The antiviral mechanism appears to involve inhibition of glucosidase I, an enzyme that catalyzes glycosylation of the envelope proteins gp120 and gp41. Glycosylation may be necessary for viral binding to the CD4 receptor.[14,15] A clinical trial of deoxynojirimycin has begun.

■ GLQ-223 (TRICOSANTHIN, "Q")

GLQ-223 is a protein toxin from the root of a plant in the Chinese cucumber family, *Tricosanthes kirilowii*. It is the first drug found that has the ability to selectively kill HIV-infected cells in vitro.[16] Unlike most other antiviral drugs, which act primarily by preventing new infections in human cells, GLQ-223 selectively kills already HIV-infected macrophages. The specific mechanism by which the drug kills only HIV-infected cells is still under investigation, but tricosanthin is known to inactivate ribosomes in vitro. Adding an agent like GLQ-223 to the existing armamentarium of antiviral drugs could allow clinicians to attack the reservoir of HIV-infected cells while other drugs block the spread of virus to new cells. Tricosanthin has already been used clinically in China on a limited basis as an abortifacient and as a treatment for choriocarcinoma, suggesting that its toxicity may be acceptable. FDA approval for Phase I studies are scheduled for completion by late 1989; a non-FDA-approved clinical trial is also in progress. Early reports suggest a high rate of severe neurologic toxicity with limited evidence of efficacy.

■ PROSPECTS FOR FUTURE DRUG DEVELOPMENT

There remains a good deal of optimism about the development of potential anti-HIV agents. Drugs can be developed and tested to interfere at all points in the virus's life cycle. We hope that one or more of these drugs will be extremely active against HIV or that combinations of agents with non-overlapping toxicities may be able to inhibit HIV replication without impairing the ability of the cellular immune system to repopulate itself.

REFERENCES

1. Pert CB, Hill JM, Ruff MR, et al. Octapeptides deduced from the neuropeptide receptor-like pattern of antigen CD4+ in brain potently inhibit human immunodeficiency virus receptor binding and T-cell infectivity. Proc Nat Acad Sci 1986; 83:9254-8.
2. Dagani R. Controversy surrounds new AIDS drug called peptide T. Chemical and Engineering News July 20, 1987.
3. Wetterberg L, Alexius B, Saaf J, et al. Peptide T in treatment of AIDS. Lancet 1987; 1(8525):159.
4. Sarin PS, Gallo RC, Scheer DI, et al. Effects of a novel compound (AL721) on HTLV-III infectivity in vitro. N Engl J Med 1985; 313:1289-90.
5. Ueno R, Kuno S. Dextran sulfate, a potent anti-HIV agent in vitro having synergism with zidovudine. Lancet 1987; 1(8546):1379.
6. Berenbaum MC. Anti-HIV synergy between dextran sulfate and zidovudine. Lancet 1987; 2(8556):461.
7. Mitsuya H, Looney DJ, Kuno S, et al. Dextran sulfate suppression of viruses in the HIV family: inhibition of virion binding to CD4+ cells. Science 1988; 240:646-9.
8. Hussey RE, Richardson NE, Kowalski M, et al. A soluble CD4 protein selectively inhibits HIV replication and syncytium formation. Nature 1988; 331:78-81.
9. Deen KC, McDougal JS, Inacker R, et al. A soluble form of CD4 (T4) protein inhibits AIDS virus infection. Nature 1988; 331:82-4.
10. Traunecker A, Luke W, Karjalainen K. Soluble CD4 molecules neutralize human immunodeficiency virus type 1. Nature 1988; 331:84-6.
11. Smith DH, Byrn RA, Marsters SA, et al. Blocking of HIV-1 infectivity by a soluble, secreted form of CD4 antigen. Science 1987; 238:1704-7.
12. Pal R, Hoke GM, Sarngadharan MG. Role of oligosaccharides in the processing and maturation of envelope glycoproteins of human immunodeficiency virus type 1. Proc Natl Acad Sci USA 1989; 86:3384-8.
13. Gruters RA, Neefjes JJ, Tersmette M, et al. Interference with HIV-induced syncytium formation and viral infectivity by inhibitors of trimming glucosidase. Nature 1987; 330:74-7.
14. Fennie C, Lasky LA. Model for intracellular folding of the human immunodeficiency virus type 1 gp120. J Virol 1989; 63:639-46.
15. Montefiori DC, Robinson WE Jr, Mitchell WM. Role of protein N-glycosylation in pathogenesis of human immunodeficiency virus type 1. Proc Natl Acad Sci USA 1988; 85:9248-52.
16. McGrath MS, Hwang KM, Caldwell SE, et al. GLQ-223: an inhibitor of human immunodeficiency virus replication in acutely and chronically infected cells of lymphocyte and mononuclear phagocyte lineage. Proc Natl Acad Sci USA 1989; 86:2844-8.
17. Sandstrom EG, Kaplan JC, Byington RE, Hirsch MS. Inhibition of human T-cell lymphotropic virus type III in vitro by phosphonoformate. Lancet 1985; 1(8444):1480-2.
18. Yarchoan R, Klecker RW, Weinhold KJ, et al. Administration of 3'-azido-3'deoxythymidine, an inhibitor of HTLV-III/LAV replication, to patients with AIDS or AIDS-related complex. Lancet 1986; 1(8481):575-80.
19. Fischl MA, Richman DD, Grieco MH, et al. The efficacy of azidothymidine (AZT) in the treatment of patients with AIDS and AIDS-related complex. N Engl J Med 1987; 317:185-91.
20. Richman DD, Kornbluth RS, Carson DA. Failure of dideoxynucleosides to inhibit human immunodeficiency virus replication in cultured human macrophages. Journal of Experimental Medicine 1987; 166:1144-9.

21. Hamamoto Y, Nakashima H, Matsui T, et al. Inhibitory effect of 2′,3′-didehydro-2′,3′-dideoxy-nucleosides on infectivity of human immunodeficiency virus. Antimicrob Agents Chemother 1988; 31:907-10.

22. Yarchoan R, Broder S. Development of antiretroviral therapy for the acquired immunodeficiency syndrome and related disorders. N Engl J Med 1987; 316:557-63.

23. Ho DD, Hartshorn KL, Rota TR, et al. Recombinant human interferon ∝-A suppresses HTLV-III replication in vitro. Lancet 1985; 1(8429):602-4.

Clinical Applications of Antiviral Therapy: Use of Zidovudine

Paul A. Volberding, M.D.

I n controlled Phase II testing, zidovudine (azidothymidine, AZT, Retrovir) has been shown to have clinical benefit for patients with T4 (CD4+ lymphocyte) cell counts less than 500 per cubic mm. This chapter discusses the use of AZT in the clinical management of patients with HIV infections.

■ APPLICABILITY OF AZT

AZT is currently available for use in the United States by conventional prescription. Initially, AZT was FDA approved for AIDS patients with histories of *Pneumocystis carinii* pneumonia (PCP) and in patients with severe symptomatic HIV disease (ARC) (<200 T4 cells), because successful clinical trials were conducted in patients with these conditions.[1-3] These limited FDA indications posed problems for the clinician: the definition of ARC remained imprecise and limiting use to the specific indication of PCP made little intuitive sense, given our understanding that PCP is only one of many opportunistic infections occurring in the setting of HIV infection. More recent data provide justification for treating all patients who have T4 counts less than 500 cells/cubic mm with AZT.

One placebo-controlled clinical trial (ACTG 016, National Institute of Allergy and Infectious Diseases (NIAID)) showed that AZT (1200 mg/day in 6 doses) inhibits progression to AIDS in patients with T4 counts in the 200-to-500 cells/cubic mm range (patients were enrolled in the study if they had T4 counts in the range of 200 to 800 cells/cubic mm and one symptom of HIV disease, but there were so few patients in the 500-to-800 range that it is not possible to reach any conclusions about the benefits for this subgroup of the study). The study enrolled 713 patients. Half were treated with AZT and half with placebo. Thirty-six members of the placebo group progressed to more severe disease, compared to 14 subjects in the AZT-treated group. The study was discontinued when this difference between progression in the two groups became too great to justify continued administration of placebo to the control group. The incidence of severe side effects was relatively low (5 percent), a noteworthy difference from the high incidence of side effects (as much as 50 percent) in patients with more advanced HIV disease (Fauci A: personal communication).

Another double-blind placebo-controlled clinical trial (ACTG Protocol 019) demonstrated that AZT was beneficial in asymptomatic HIV-infected patients with CD4+ counts below 500 cells/cubic mm. This trial enrolled 3200 asymptomatic HIV-infected participants between July 1987 and July 1989. Subjects were stratified into three groups according to CD4+ counts (<200; 200 to 500; or >500 CD4+ lymphocytes/cubic mm). Each stratum was randomly assigned to either placebo, AZT 100 mg 5 times a day, or AZT 300 mg 5 times a day. The protocol was modified and portions terminated in August 1989 because monitors observed striking and statistically significant benefit from AZT therapy for individuals with <500 CD4+ cells/cubic mm at entry. Roughly 1300 subjects had <500 CD4+ cells/cubic mm at entry. Of these, 74 developed significant symptomatic HIV disease (AIDS or "advanced ARC") during follow-up, which ranged from four months to two years, with a mean of one year. Thirty-eight of these subjects were in the placebo group, compared to 19 in the 1500/mg/day AZT group and 17 in the 500 mg/day AZT group. p24 antigen levels and CD4+ cell counts also indicated benefit from AZT therapy for patients with <500 CD4+ cells/cubic mm. Because of the striking benefit shown for AZT treatment and the lack of a statistically significant difference between the two AZT doses, the study was terminated in patients with <500 CD4+ cells/cubic mm. All placebo-treated patients with <500 CD4+ cells/cubic mm at entry were switched to AZT (500 mg/day). For patients with more than 500 CD4+ cells/cubic mm at entry, there was no statistically significant difference between treatment arms as of August 1989. This segment of the study was continued with the modification that placebo-treated patients would receive AZT if their CD4+ counts fell below 500 cells/cubic mm.

For patients in the <500 CD4+ cells/cubic mm stratum, side effects from AZT were significantly fewer on the 500 mg/day regimen. Serious hematologic side effects occurred in 12 percent of patients taking 1500 mg/day, compared to 3 percent in patients taking 500 mg/day. Nausea was not significantly different between the two regimens, occurring in 3.3 to 5 percent of AZT-treated patients but only rarely in patients receiving placebo.

The possibility of arresting or slowing HIV replication before clinical illness develops creates great pressure and reasonable optimism for using AZT in less severely ill HIV-infected patients. Earlier data suggest[4] that HIV-infected patients will develop AIDS and that this progression is more rapid in patients with rapidly falling CD4 counts, detectable p24 HIV antigen, and elevated β_2-microglobulin.[4-7] Thus, AZT treatment or an equally effective antiviral therapy should be offered to patients with CD4 counts below 500 cells/cubic mm. However AZT treatment should be undertaken with an awareness of the risks and benefits in different subgroups of patients.

■ DOSAGE AND TOXICITY

The original recommended dose of AZT was 1000 to 1200 mg/day (given as 200 mg 5 or 6 times daily). The ACTG Protocols indicate that lower doses (500 to 600 mg/day) are as effective and the FDA agrees. The most common currently recommended regimens are 100 mg five times a day (sparing the patient from a nocturnal dose) or 200 mg three times a day. The subjective toxicity is usually quite acceptable. Many patients complain of mild nausea; occasionally a mild-to-moderate agitational or confused state occurs, but both of these side effects often decrease with continued drug administration. Patients very rarely require drug discontinuation or dosage reduction because of subjective toxicities.

In contrast to subjective toxicities, objective toxicities from AZT are common and often severe, frequently resulting in drug-dosage modification or discontinuation. In the first Phase II trial, the principal toxicity was hematologic.[8] In the past year, continued experience with AZT has confirmed this finding. As many as 50 percent of AIDS patients on continuous full-dose therapy experience severe hematologic toxicity that manifests as anemia or neutropenia.

Toxicity is much more common in patients with more advanced disease (as indicated by cytopenias prior to drug administration), low CD4 counts, or a previous diagnosis of AIDS. Adverse hematologic effects occur much more frequently in patients with <200 CD4 cells/cubic mm (and even more frequently in patients with fewer than 100 cells/cubic mm) than in patients whose CD4 counts are higher. Because AZT is the only currently available effective anti-HIV therapy, and because there is no available test to indicate that treatment can be stopped, treatment should continue indefinitely. Monitoring should be repeated more frequently at first and should focus on evidence of drug toxicity. A complete blood count (CBC) should be taken before initiating therapy, and should be repeated weekly or biweekly for patients with symptomatic HIV disease, AIDS, or hematologic abnormalities. Asymptomatic patients on 500 mg/day dosage without hematologic abnormalities require less frequent monitoring — e.g., a CBC before therapy, after 2 weeks of therapy, and monthly thereafter.

Anemia and Neutropenia.   The optimal modification of AZT therapy when toxicity occurs is still somewhat unclear. Alternative antiretroviral drugs are being developed and represent an option if available. Lacking this option, many clinicians will continue AZT therapy as long as the patient's clinical status permits. Even when patients develop transfusion-dependent anemia, these clinicians will continue full-dose AZT therapy. Others decrease the dosage or temporarily discontinue therapy if severe anemia develops.

In the setting of severe drug-induced neutropenia, management issues are much simpler. Most clinicians would continue AZT therapy at full dose until absolute neutrophil counts fall below 750 cells/cubic mm; many continue full-dose therapy until the absolute neutrophil count is <500. Most interrupt therapy or reduce the dose when these toxicity thresholds have been reached.

Recommendations.   Our current recommendation at San Francisco General Hospital is to continue full-dose AZT for isolated transfusion-dependent anemia but to decrease dosage or interrupt therapy when neutrophil counts fall below 500. Our experience is that many patients who require dosage adjustments will, after that point, be unable to tolerate full-dose regimens. Recent trials suggest that a reduced dose regimen (e.g., 100 mg, 5 times a day) may be as effective and have less toxicity, although this has not been proved for all subsets of patients.

■ AZT DURING ACTIVE OPPORTUNISTIC INFECTION

Questions often arise about continued use of AZT after a patient develops an acute AIDS-defining opportunistic infection such as pneumocystis pneumonia. Therapeutic regimens for AIDS-related opportunistic infections and malignancies are often associated with hematologic toxicity. For this reason, we prefer to interrupt AZT therapy while treating the acute opportunistic infection and reintroduce AZT after the patient recovers from that episode. Generally, it is possible to reinstitute AZT within three to four weeks after an opportunistic infection is diagnosed.

■ AZT IN AIDS-RELATED MALIGNANCIES

The situation is somewhat more difficult in the setting of AIDS-related malignancies because anti-neoplastic therapy is generally used on a much more chronic basis than treatment for AIDS-defining opportunistic infections. Clinical trials combining anti-neoplastic agents with AZT are in progress, but clinical experience to date suggests that in many cases, additive toxicity limits the use of one or both drugs. Deciding which drug to initiate first and which to continue in the face of hematologic toxicity can be difficult.

Patients with aggressive B-cell lymphomas related to HIV infection require immediate, aggressive chemotherapy to manage their life-threatening malignancy. At present, we recommend against continuing or initiating AZT therapy until such a malignancy is controlled.

Kaposi's sarcoma (KS), on the other hand, is often much more indolent. Our general practice with KS has been to stabilize the patient on either chemotherapy or AZT first and then to cautiously and carefully monitor the second agent as it is added to the patient's regimen. If the KS is relatively more aggressive or if it involves visceral structures such as the lungs, chemotherapy may be recommended without AZT. In patients with very indolent and limited cutaneous KS, we have in many cases interrupted chemotherapy to allow the patient to benefit from AZT.

■ HIV ENCEPHALOPATHY

The use of AZT in HIV encephalopathy is under investigation but is currently favored by most clinicians. Anecdotes have been published on the sometimes-rapid and striking neurologic improvement made possible by AZT therapy.[8,9] Ongoing clinical trials will establish whether these anecdotes are the exception or the rule. In the meantime, we would recommend a trial of AZT for HIV-related neurologic disorders, including encephalopathy.

■ AZT FOR POST-EXPOSURE PROPHYLAXIS OF HIV EXPOSURE

There is considerable interest in the use of AZT after occupational exposure to HIV-contaminated blood products. A clinical trial of AZT in the therapy of health-care workers accidentally injured by needles and other HIV-contaminated objects has been designed by Burroughs-Wellcome pharmaceutical company. There are some data from animal experiments with other retroviral infections to suggest that prompt initiation of a brief course of AZT may successfully abort retroviral infections.[10-12] If so, much of health workers' concern for their own risk of HIV infection may be eliminated. At this point, however, there are not sufficient data to prove that AZT therapy is beneficial in these circumstances. Questions on this application should be directed to clinical research centers. The Centers for Disease Control's study of health-care workers exposed to HIV suggests that the current risk of infection following exposure is less than 1 percent.[13]

■ FUTURE DEVELOPMENTS IN AZT THERAPY

One of the most interesting aspects of AZT therapy is the possibility that the drug may have increased activity when combined with other agents, especially those with immune-stimulating activities. Clinical trials of AZT and recombinant interleukin-2, for example, are being initiated. Another area of interest is the potential development of sustained-release forms of AZT to reduce the need for frequent and inconvenient oral administration. It is not known, however, if AZT's intracellular activity requires maintenance of a specific serum level of the compound. It may, for example, be possible to use a much higher and less frequent dosage without compromising drug activity intracellularly. Clinical trials exploring this and other questions are being initiated.

■ AZT RESISTANCE AND FAILURE

Recent reports have described the emergence of HIV strains with reduced sensitivity or resistance to AZT,[14] recurrence of HIV replication in the presence of AZT in vitro and in vivo,[15,16] and failure of AZT to maintain clinical remission of HIV disease.[17] In the most widely publicized study, viral isolates were obtained from 11 patients who had been treated with AZT for more than six months. Viral isolates from these patients showed progressively less sensitivity to AZT with longer duration of therapy; isolates from five patients showed markedly reduced sensitivity.[14]

These reports are of concern. However, AZT resistance has been described only in a small number of patients and has not been shown to be common. Furthermore, in the small numbers of patients from whom HIV-resistant isolates were obtained, the reduced sensitivity to AZT did not correlate with a reduced clinical response. These findings do not alter evidence that AZT prolongs life in patients with AIDS and symptomatic and asymptomatic HIV disease. Thus, at present, drug resistance is not a sufficient concern to justify modification of recommendations for AZT therapy.

REFERENCES

1. Hirsch MS. Azidothymidine. J Infect Dis 1988; 157:427-431.
2. Fischl MA, Richman DD, Grieco MH, et al. The efficacy of azidothymidine (AZT) in the treatment of patients with AIDS and AIDS-related complex. A double-blind, placebo-controlled trial. N Engl J Med 1987; 317:185-91.
3. Richman DD, Fischl MA, Grieco MH, et al. The toxicity of azidothymidine (AZT) in the treatment of patients with AIDS and AIDS-related complex. N Engl J Med 1987; 192-7.
4. Moss AR, Bacchetti P, Osmond D, et al. Seropositivity for HIV and the development of AIDS or AIDS related condition: Three year follow-up of the San Francisco General Hospital cohort. Br Med J 1988; 296:745-50.
5. Eyster ME, Gail MH, Ballard JO, et al. Natural history of human immunodeficiency virus infections in hemophiliacs: effects of T-cell subsets, platelet counts, and age. Ann Intern Med 1987; 107:1-6.
6. de Wolf F, Goudsmit J, Paul DA, et al. Risk of AIDS related complex and AIDS in homosexual men with persistent HIV antigenemia. Br Med J 1987; 295:569-72.
7. Allain JP, Laurian Y, Paul DA, et al. Long-term evaluation of HIV antigen and antibodies to p24 and gp41 in patients with hemophilia. N Engl J Med 1987; 317:1114-21.
8. Yarchoan R, Berg G, Brouwers P, et al. Response of human-immunodeficiency-virus-associated neurological disease to 3'-azido-3'deoxythymidine. Lancet 1987; 1:132-5.
9. Price RW, Brew B, Siditis J, et al. The brain in AIDS: central nervous system HIV-1 infection and AIDS dementia complex. Science 1988; 239:586-92.
10. Ruprecht RM, OBrien LG, Rossoni LD, et al. Suppression of mouse viraemia and retroviral disease by 3'-azido-3'deoxythymidine. Nature 1986; 323:467-9.
11. Sharpe AH, Jaenisch R, Ruprecht RM. Retroviruses and mouse embryos: a rapid model for neurovirulence and transplacental antiviral therapy. Science 1987; 236:1671-4.
12. Tavares L, Roneker C, Johnston K, et al. 3'-azido-3'deoxythymidine in feline leukemia virus-infected cats: a model for therapy and prophylaxis of AIDS. Cancer Res 1987; 47:3190-4.
13. Update: Acquired immunodeficiency syndrome and human immunodeficiency virus infection among health-care workers. MMWR 1988; 37:229-34, 239.
14. Larder BA, Darby G, Richman DD. HIV with reduced sensitivity to zidovudine (AZT) isolated during prolonged therapy. Science 1989; 243:1731-4.
15. Smith MS, Brian EL, Pagano JS. Resumption of virus production after human immunodeficiency virus infection of T lymphocytes in the presence of azidothymine. J Virol 1987; 61:3769-73.
16. Reiss P, Lange JMA, Boucher CA, Danner SA, Goudsmit J. Resumption of HIV antigen production during continuous zidovudine treatment. Lancet 1988; 1:421.
17. Bach MC. Failure of zidovudine to maintain remission in patients with AIDS. N Engl J Med 1989; 320:594-5.

HIV-Related Pharmacology

Roberta J. Wong, Pharm.D.

This chapter summarizes common side effects and interactions of medica-tions that are frequently used to treat HIV-related conditions. Patients with HIV infection may have more frequent, unusual, and severe side effects to medications than non-HIV-infected patients. For example, such reactions have been well documented in patients with *Pneumocystis carinii* pneumonia who are being treated with pentamidine and trimethoprim-sulfamethoxazole.[1-3]

Medication side effects should be considered whenever new symptoms appear in HIV-infected patients on multiple drug regimens. Patients should become active participants in observing and documenting side effects and should immediately notify their healthcare providers of any adverse reactions.

■ DRUGS COMMONLY USED IN TREATING HIV-INFECTED PATIENTS

Table 1 alphabetically lists those drugs commonly used for treating oppor-tunistic infections and neoplasms. The most common side effects are also noted. Table 2 lists medications commonly used, along with dosage regimens. Table 3 lists common side effects and the drugs likely to cause them; Table 4 suggests drugs of choice for treating infectious complications of HIV infection and describes typical side effects.

TABLE 1. MEDICATIONS FOR TREATMENT OF OPPORTUNISTIC INFECTIONS AND NEOPLASMS*

Abbreviations: GI = gastrointestinal
N/V = nausea/vomiting
SIADH = syndrome of inappropriate diuretic hormone

MEDICATION	TRADE NAME	SIDE EFFECTS
Para-amino-salicylic acid (PAS)	Reezipas, Teebacin	Sore throat, diarrhea, GI distress, myalgia, arthralgias[4,5]
Amphotericin	Fungizone	Acute: fever, chills, nausea, anorexia, headache, vomiting, thrombophlebitis[6,7]
		Chronic: anemia, hypokalemia, hypomagnesemia, renal failure
Bleomycin	Blenoxane	Acute: N/V, fever, alopecia, stomatitis, anaphylaxis[8]
		Chronic: pneumonitis
Clindamycin	Cleocin	Diarrhea, rash, pseudomembranous colitis, N/V[9,10]
Clofazimine	Lamprene	Red or purple skin, rash, GI distress[11]

continued on next page

continued from previous page

TABLE 1. MEDICATIONS FOR TREATMENT OF OPPORTUNISTIC INFECTIONS AND NEOPLASMS*

MEDICATION	TRADE NAME	SIDE EFFECTS
Dapsone	Dapsone	Methemoglobinemia, leukopenia, hepatotoxicity, rash, N/V[12]
Doxorubicin	Adriamycin	Acute: red urine, fever, myelosuppression, N/V, stomatitis, phlebitis[13]
		Chronic: alopecia, congestive heart failure
Ethambutol	Myambutol	Anorexia, vomiting, rash, retinitis[11,14]
Ganciclovir	Cytovene	Neutropenia, diarrhea, nausea, phlebitis[15]
Isoniazid	INH	N/V, acidosis, neuropathy, blood dyscrasias[11]
Pentamidine	Pentam	Acute: hypoglycemia, hypotension, rash, facial flushing, metallic taste[16]
		Chronic: hyperglycemia, leukopenia, anemia
Pyrimethamine	Daraprim	Neutropenia, rash, drug fever, thrombocytopenia[17]
Rifampin	Rifamate	Heartburn, gas, orange-red body fluids[11,14]
Sulfadiazine		Neutropenia, rash, drug fever, thrombocytopenia[17]
Sulfamethoxazole-Trimethoprim	Septra, Bactrim	Myelosuppression, crystalluria, rash, kernicterus, N/V[18,19]
Trimethoprim	Proloprim	Myelosuppression, increased serum creatinine, rash, N/V[12]
Vinblastine	Velban	N/V, leukopenia, alopecia, stomatitis[20]
Vincristine	Oncovin	Alopecia, paresthesias, uric acid nephropathy, SIADH, paralytic ileus[21]

*   *Compiled by the author.*

TABLE 2. MEDICATIONS AND DOSAGE REGIMENS COMMONLY USED IN HIV-INFECTED PATIENTS*

MEDICATION	TRADE NAME	DOSAGE
Acyclovir	Zovirax	200 mg 3–5 times po qd Tx 200 mg po tid maintenance[22]
Alprazolam	Xanax	1–2 mg po q 6–8 hrs[23]
Amitriptyline	Elavil, Endep	various (10–150 mg qd)[24]
Clotrimazole	Mycelex	dissolve 1–5 troches qd[25]
Diazepam	Valium	5–10 mg po q 6–8 hrs[26]
Diphenoxylate with atropine	Lomotil	1–2 po q 6 hrs[27]
Folinic Acid	Wellcovorin Leucovorin	5–10 mg po qd[28]
Haloperidol	Haldol	various[29]
Ibuprofen	Motrin, Rufen	400–600 mg po qid[30]

continued on next page

continued from previous page

TABLE 2.   MEDICATIONS AND DOSAGE REGIMENS COMMONLY USED IN HIV-INFECTED PATIENTS*

MEDICATION	TRADE NAME	DOSAGE
Ketoconazole	Nizoral	200–400 mg po qd[31]
Loperamide	Imodium	1–2 2 mg capsules po q 6 hrs[32]
Lorazepam	Ativan	1–2 mg po q 6–8 hrs[33]
Metoclopramide	Reglan	10–20 mg po q 6 hrs use for nausea, prn[34]
Metronidazole	Flagyl	250 mg tid[35]
Morphine sulfate	Roxanol MS Contin	various[36]
Prochlorperazine	Compazine	10–25 mg po q 6 hr[37]
Temazepam	Restoril	15–30 mg po qhs[38]
Triazolam	Halcion	0.25–0.5 mg po qhs[39]
Tylenol with codeine		325 mg Tylenol with 30–60 mg codeine po q 6 hrs, prn[36]
Zidovudine	Retrovir	100 mg 5x/day or 200 mg 3x/day

*   Compiled by the author.

TABLE 3.   SIDE EFFECTS AND POSSIBLE DRUGS PER SIDE EFFECT*

Abbreviations: supp = suppositories
susp = suspension
SIADH = syndrome of inappropriate diuretic hormone

SIDE EFFECT	POSSIBLE DRUGS
Abdominal cramps	Loperamide
Acidosis	Isoniazid
Adrenal insufficiency	Ketoconazole
Alopecia	Bleomycin, doxorubicin, vinblastine, vincristine
a.m. drowsiness	Temazepam, triazolam, lorazepam
Anaphylaxis	Bleomycin
Anemia	Amphotericin, pentamidine, dapsone, zidovudine (AZT)
Anorexia	Amphotericin, ethambutol
Arthralgias	Aminosalicylic acid, isoniazid
Ataxia	Temazepam
Blurred vision	Amitriptyline, diphenoxylate with atropine
Bronchospasm/coughing	Aerosolized pentamidine
Chills	Amphotericin
Constipation	Amitriptyline, diphenoxylate with atropine, morphine, prochlorperazine, tylenol with codeine
Crystalluria	Sulfamethoxazole-trimethoprim
Diarrhea	Acyclovir, aminosalicylic acid, clindamycin, clotrimazole, 5-flucytosine, ganciclovir, metoclopramide, nystatin susp/supp
Disulfiram reaction	Metronidazole

continued on next page

continued from previous page

TABLE 3. SIDE EFFECTS AND POSSIBLE DRUGS PER SIDE EFFECT*

SIDE EFFECT	POSSIBLE DRUGS
Dizziness	Acyclovir, diphenoxylate with atropine, lorazepam, loperamide, metoclopramide, morphine, temazepam
Drowsiness	Alprazolam, diazepam, lorazepam, morphine, tylenol with codeine
Dry mouth	Amitriptyline, diphenoxylate with atropine, prochlorperazine, tylenol with codeine
Dystonic reactions	Haloperidol
Facial flushing	Pentamidine
Fatigue	Metoclopramide
Fever	Amphotericin, bleomycin, doxorubicin, pyrimethamine, sulfadiazine, sulfamethoxazole-trimethoprim
GI distress	Aminosalicylic acid, clofazimine, folinic acid, ibuprofen, morphine, rifampin
Headache	Acyclovir, amphotericin
Hemolytic anemia	Dapsone
Hepatotoxicity	Dapsone, 5-flucytosine, isoniazid, ibuprofen, ketoconazole, sulfamethoxazole-trimethoprim
Hyperglycemia	Pentamidine
Hypoglycemia	Pentamidine
Hypokalemia	Amphotericin
Hypomagnesemia	Amphotericin
Hypotension	Alprazolam, diazepam, pentamidine
Kernicterus	Sulfamethoxazole-trimethoprim
Leukopenia/neutropenia	Dapsone, 5-flucytosine, ganciclovir, pentamidine, pyrimethamine, vinblastine
Methemoglobinemia	Dapsone
Myalgias	Aminosalicylic acid
Myelosuppression/blood dyscrasias	Dapsone, doxorubicin, ibuprofen, isoniazid, pentamidine, prochlorperazine, sulfamethoxazole-trimethoprim, clotrimazole, zidovudine
Nausea	Aminosalicylic acid, amphotericin, bleomycin, clindamycin, clotrimazole, dapsone, doxorubicin, 5-flucytosine, ganciclovir, isoniazid, ketoconazole, loperamide, metronidazole, nystatin supp/susp, pyrimethamine, sulfamethoxazole-trimethoprim, tylenol with codeine, vinblastine
Neutropenia	Pentamidine, pyrimethamine, sulfadiazine, sulfamethoxazole-trimethoprim
Paralytic ileus	Vincristine
Paresthesias/peripheral neuropathy	Vincristine, isoniazid
Pneumonitis	Bleomycin
Pruritis	Ketoconazole
Rash	Clindamycin, clofazimine, dapsone, ethambutol, folinic acid, ibuprofen, isoniazid, pentamidine, pyrimethamine, sulfadiazine, sulfamethoxazole-trimethoprim, trimethoprim
Red-purple skin	Clotrimazole, haloperidol, metoclopramide

continued on next page

continued from previous page

TABLE 3.   SIDE EFFECTS AND POSSIBLE DRUGS PER SIDE EFFECT*

SIDE EFFECT	POSSIBLE DRUGS
Red urine	Doxorubicin, rifampin
Renal dysfunction	Amphotericin, nonsteroidal anti-inflammatory agents, pentamidine, sulfamethoxazole-trimethoprim
Respiratory depression	Alprazolam, diazepam, tylenol with codeine
Retinitis	Ethambutol
Retrograde amnesia	Alprazolam, lorazepam, triazolam
Sedation	Amitriptyline, haloperidol, antihistamines, benzodiazepines, narcotics
SIADH	Vincristine
Sore throat	Aminosalicylic acid
Stomatitis	Bleomycin, doxorubicin, vinblastine
Taste alterations (metallic)	Clotrimazole, metronidazole, morphine, nystatin supp/susp, pentamidine
Thrombocytopenia	Pyrimethamine, sulfadiazine, sulfamethoxazole-trimethoprim
Thrombophlebitis	Amphotericin, doxorubicin, ganciclovir
Uric acid nephropathy	Vincristine
Vomiting	Aminosalicylic acid, amphotericin, bleomycin, clindamycin, dapsone, doxorubicin, ethambutol, 5-flucytosine, isoniazid, ketoconazole, metronidazole, sulfamethoxazole-trimethoprim, vinblastine
Weakness	Metoclopramide

*   *Compiled by the author.*

TABLE 4.   DRUGS OF CHOICE FOR TREATING INFECTIOUS COMPLICATIONS OF HIV INFECTION

Abbreviations: supp = suppositories
susp = suspension
N/V = nausea/vomiting

DRUG AND DOSAGE	SIDE EFFECTS	COMMENTS
***Pneumocystis carinii* pneumonia**		
1. TMP 15–20 mg/kg/d (4 divided doses) SMX 75–100 mg/kg/d (4 divided doses) IV or po for 14–21 days	Neutropenia, hepato-toxicity, fever, rash, N/V, azotemia, thrombocytopenia, kernicterus[18,19]	Switch to alternate drug in 50%–60% cases: if no response in 7–10 days or deterioration after 4–5 days of Tx; oral therapy can be used for mild cases
2. Pentamidine 4 mg/kg/d for 14–21 days IV (IM = causes sterile abscess)	Hypoglycemia, hyper-glycemia, rash, facial flushing, metallic taste, anemia, leukopenia, azotemia, orthostatic hypotension[16]	Switch to alternate drug in 50%–60% cases: if N/R 7–10 days or deterioration after 4–5 days of Tx

continued on next page

continued from previous page

TABLE 4.   DRUGS OF CHOICE FOR TREATING INFECTIOUS COMPLICATIONS OF HIV INFECTION

DRUG AND DOSAGE	SIDE EFFECTS	COMMENTS
***Pneumocystis carinii* pneumonia**		
3. Dapsone 100 mg/d po TMP 20 mg/kg/d (4 divided doses po) for 21 days	Hemolytic anemia, methemoglobinemia, hepatotoxicity, rash, N/V, leukopenia[12]	None
4. Aerosolized pentamidine: various doses under investigation	Bronchospasm, coughing[41,42]	Full inspiration and exhalation needed; use apparatus that produces 1.5- to 3-micron particles
***Cryptococcus neoformans* meningitis**		
1. Amphotericin 0.5–0.6 mg/ kg/d over 4 to 6 hours for 6 weeks, then maintenance	Acute: fever, chills, N/V, anorexia, headache, thrombophlebitis Chronic: hypokalemia, hypomagnesemia, azotemia, anemia[6,7]	Target 1.5–2 g over 6 weeks maintenance
2. 5-Flucytosine po 75–100 mg/kg/d (4 divided doses) for 6 weeks	Leukopenia (30%), nausea, vomiting, diarrhea, hepatotoxicity[43,44]	Not commonly used in patients with HIV infection or with bone marrow suppression; absorption delayed with antacid
3. Fluconazole 200–400 mg qd[45]		Investigational
***Toxoplasma gondii* meningitis**		
1. Pyrimethamine 100 mg LOAD, then 25–50 mg/d Sulfadiazine 4 g LOAD, then 1 g every 6 hours	Neutropenia, rash, drug fever, thrombocytopenia[17,18]	80%–85% response in 1–2 weeks (use with folinic acid), suppression with Tx indefinite; relapse common if Tx stopped
2. Folinic acid 10 mg every day	GI upset[28]	Use with sulfadiazine and pyrimethamine
3. Clindamycin 1200–3600 mg/d	Nausea/vomiting, diarrhea, rash[9,10]	Experimental dose and efficacy being studied
Cytomegalovirus retinitis/pneumonia		
1. Ganciclovir: experimental 5–7.5 mg/kg/d (2 doses) for 10 days, then 5/mg/ kg/d (5–7× per week)	Diarrhea, nausea, neutropenia, phlebitis[46]	Acyclovir ineffective in patients with HIV infection; may be useful in prevention of CMV infection in organ transplant patients

continued on next page

continued from previous page

TABLE 4.   DRUGS OF CHOICE FOR TREATING INFECTIOUS COMPLICATIONS OF HIV INFECTION

DRUG AND DOSAGE	SIDE EFFECTS	COMMENTS
Cytomegalovirus retinitis/pneumonia		
2. Foscarnet (phosphonoformate) experimental: 60 mg/kg qd × 2 weeks maintenance: 60–120 mg/kg/d	Anemia, increased serum creatinine[45]	
Candidiasis (Thrush)		
1. Clotrimazole troches (5 troches qd)	Nausea, diarrhea, altered taste[25]	Instruct patients to allow troches to dissolve slowly; DO NOT CHEW
2. Nystatin Vag Supp 100,000 U/tab tid	Nausea, diarrhea, altered taste[47]	Dissolve slowly
3. Nystatin Susp 100,000 U/ml 5–10 cc qid	Nausea, diarrhea, altered taste[48]	Rinse mouth with plain water after use
4. Ketoconazole 200 mg qd	N/V, hepatotoxicity, adrenal insufficiency[31]	Antacids delay absorption and prevent dissolution
Aspergillosis		
1. Amphotericin[49]		
Cryptosporidiosis		
1. No agent proven effective. Replace fluids; consider antimotility agents and/or hyperalimentation.[50]		
Coccidioidomycosis		
1. Meningitis: Amphotericin[51]		
2. Nonmeningitis: Ketoconazole[51]		
Histoplasmosis		
1. Amphotericin[52]		Maintenance with ketoconazole common
Mycobacterium avium intracellulare		
1. 3–4 drug therapies, none proven to be effective[11]		Recent work in San Francisco with Amikacin promising. Clofazimine may be used. Ansamycin available from CDC.

REFERENCES

1. Gordin FM, Simon GL, Wofsy CB, Mills J. Adverse reactions to trimethoprim-sulfamethoxazole in patients with acquired immunodeficiency syndrome. Ann Intern Med 1984; 100:495-9.

2. Jaffe HS, Abrams DI, Ammann AJ, et al. Complications of clotrimazole in treatment of AIDS-associated *Pneumocystis carinii* pneumonia in homosexual men. Lancet 1983; 2:1109-11.

3. Weinke TH, Sixt C, de Matos-Marques B, et al. Adverse reactions to trimethoprim-sulfamethoxazole (TMP-SMZ) in AIDS patients with *Pneumocystis carinii* pneumonia (PCP) [Abstract]. Stockholm: IV International Conference on AIDS 1988; 421.

4. Way EL. The absorption, distribution, excretion and fate of para-aminosalicylic acid. J Pharmacol Exp Ther 1948; 93:368.

5. Bobrowitz ID, Robins DE. Ethambutol-isoniazid versus PAS-isoniazid in original treatment of pulmonary tuberculosis. Am Rev Respir Dis 1967; 96:428-38.

6. Maddux MS, Barriere SL. A review of complications of amphotericin B therapy: recommendations for prevention and management. Drug Intell Clin Pharm 1980; 14:177-81.

7. Hoeprich PD. Chemotherapy of systemic fungal diseases. Annu Rev Pharmacol Toxicol 1978; 18:205-31.

8. Bennett JM, Reich SD. Bleomycin. Ann Intern Med 1979; 90:945-8.

9. Rolston KV, Hoy J. Role of clindamycin in the treatment of central nervous system toxoplasmosis. Am J Med 1987; 83:551-4.

10. Dannemann BR, Israelski DM, Remington JS. Intravenous clindamycin: An alternative treatment for AIDS patients with toxoplasmic encephalitis. Carmel: Western Society for Clinical Investigation, February 19, 1988. abstract.

11. Diagnosis and management of mycobacterial infection and disease in persons with human immunodeficiency virus infection. Centers for Disease Control, U.S. Department of Health and Human Services. Ann Intern Med 1987; 106:254-6.

12. Leoung GS, Mills J, Hopewell PC, et al. Dapsone-trimethoprim for *Pneumocystis carinii* pneumonia in the acquired immunodeficiency syndrome. Ann Intern Med 1986; 105:45-8.

13. Blum RH, Carter SK. Adriamycin. A new anticancer drug with significant clinical activity. Ann Intern Med 1974; 80:249-59.

14. Sunderam G, McDonald RJ, Maniatis T, et al. Tuberculosis as a manifestation of the acquired immunodeficiency syndrome (AIDS). JAMA 1986; 256:262-6.

15. Felsenstein D, D'Amico DJ, Hirsch MS, et al. Treatment of cytomegalovirus retinitis with 9-[1-hydroxy-1(hydroxymethyl) ethoxymethyl] guanine. Ann Intern Med 1985; 103:377-80.

16. Wharton JM, Coleman DL, Wofsy CB, et al. Trimethoprim-sulfamethoxazole or pentamidine for *Pneumocystis carinii* pneumonia in the acquired immunodeficiency syndrome. A prospective randomized trial. Ann Intern Med 1986; 105:37-44.

17. Haverkos HW. Assessment of therapy for toxoplasma encephalitis. The TE Study Group. Am J Med 1987; 82:907-14.

18. Rubin RH, Swartz MN. Trimethoprim-sulfamethoxazole. N Engl J Med 1980; 303:426-32.

19. Gleckman R, Alvarez S, Joubert DW. Drug therapy reviews: trimethoprim-sulfamethoxazole. Am J Hosp Pharm 1979; 36:893-906.

20. Volberding PA, Abrams DI, Conant M, et al. Vinblastine therapy for Kaposi's sarcoma in the acquired immunodeficiency syndrome. Ann Intern Med 1985; 103:335-8.

21. Mintzer DM, Real FX, Jovino L, Krown SE. Treatment of Kaposi's sarcoma and thrombocytopenia with vincristine in patients with acquired immunodeficiency syndrome. Ann Intern Med 1985; 102:200-2.

22. Strauss SE, Seidlin M, Takiff H, et al. Oral acyclovir to suppress recurring herpes simplex virus infections in immunodeficiency patients. Ann Intern Med 1984; 100:522-4.

23. Evans RL, Alprazolam (Xanax). Drug Intell Clin Pharm 1981; 15:633-8.

24. Pollack MH, Rosenbaum JF. Management of antidepressant-induced side effects: a practical guide for the clinician. J Clin Psychiatry 1987; 48:3-8.

25. Owens NJ, Nightingale CH, Schweizer RT, et al. Prophylaxis of oral candidiasis with clotrimazole troches. Arch Intern Med 1984; 144:290-3.

26. Davison K, Farquharson RG, Khan MC, Majid A. A double blind comparison of alprazolam, diazepam, and placebo in the treatment of anxious out-patients. Br J Clin Pharmacol 1985; (Suppl 1):37s-43s.

27. Barowsky H, Schwartz SA. Method for evaluating diphenoxylate hydrochloride. JAMA 1962; 180:1058-61.

28. Luft BJ, Brooks RG, Conley FK, et al. Toxoplasmic encephalitis in patients with acquired immune deficiency syndrome. JAMA 1984; 252:913-7.

29. Kessler KA, Waletzky JP, Clinical use of the antipsychotics. Am J Psychiatry 1981; 138:202-9.

30. Kantor T. Ibuprofen. Ann Intern Med 1979; 91:877-82.

31. Heel RC, Brogden RN, Carmine A, et al. Ketoconazole: a review of its therapeutic efficiency in superficial and systemic fungal infections. Drugs 1982; 23:1-36.

32. Heel RC, Brogden RN, Speight TM, Avery GS. Loperamide: a review of its pharmacological properties and therapeutic efficacy in diarrhoea. Drugs 1978; 15:33-52.

33. Ameer B, Greenblatt DJ. Lorazepam: a review of its clinical pharmacological properties and therapeutic uses. Drugs 1981; 21:162-200.

34. Albibi R, McCallum RW. Metoclopramide: pharmacology and clinical application. Ann Intern Med 1983; 98:86-95.

35. Koch-Weser J, Goldman P. Drug therapy: metronidazole. N Engl J Med 1980; 303:1212-8.

36. Levy MH. Pain management in advanced cancer. Semin Oncol 1985; 12:394-410.

37. Frytak S, Moertel CG. Management of nausea and vomiting in the cancer patient. JAMA 1981; 245:393-6.

38. Heel RC, Brogden RN, Speight TM, Avery GS. Temazepam: a review of its pharmacological properties and therapeutic efficacy as an hypnotic. Drugs 1981; 21:321-40.

39. Hirsch MS. AIDS Commentary. Azidothymidine. J Infect Dis 1988; 157:427-31.

40. Pakes GE, Brogden RN, Heel RC, et al. Triazolam: a review of its pharmacological properties and therapeutic efficacy in patients with insomnia. Drugs 1981; 22:81-110.

41. Conte JE Jr, Hollander H, Golden JA. Inhaled or reduced-dose intravenous pentamidine for *Pneumocystis carinii* pneumonia. A pilot study. Ann Intern Med 1987; 107:495-8.

42. Montgomery AB, Debs RJ, Luce JM, et al. Aerosolized pentamidine as sole therapy for *Pneumocystis carinii* pneumonia in patients with acquired immunodeficiency syndrome. Lancet 1987; 2:480-3.

43. Bennett JE, Dismukes WE, Duma RJ, et al. A comparison of amphotericin b alone and combined with flucytosine in the treatment of cryptococcal meningitis. N Engl J Med 1979; 301:126-31.

44. Medoff G. Controversial areas in antifungal chemotherapy: short-course and combination therapy with amphotericin b. Rev Infect Dis 1987; 9:403-7.

45. Jacobson MA, Crowe S, Levy J, et al. Effect of Foscarnet therapy on infection with human immunodeficiency virus in patients with AIDS. J Infect Dis 1988; 158:862-5.

46. Jacobson MA, Mills J. Serious cytomegalovirus disease in the acquired immunodeficiency syndrome (AIDS). Clinical findings, diagnosis, and treatment. Ann Intern Med 1988; 108:585-94.

47. Lawson RD, Bodey GP. Comparison of clotrimazole troche and nystatin vaginal tablet in the treatment of oropharyngeal candidiasis. Curr Ther Res Clin Exp 1980; 27:774-9.

48. Barrett AP. Evaluation of nystatin in prevention and elimination of oropharyngeal Candida in immunosuppressed patients. Oral Surg Oral Med Oral Pathol 1984; 58:148-51.

49. Medoff G, Kobayashi GS. Strategies in the treatment of systemic fungal infections. N Engl J Med 1980; 302:145-55.

50. Soave R, Armstrong D. Cryptosporidium and cryptosporidiosis. Rev Infect Dis 1986; 8:1012-23.

51. Whiteside ME, Barkin JS, May RG, et al. Enteric coccidiosis among patients with the acquired immunodeficiency syndrome. Am J Trop Med Hyg 1984; 33:1065-72.

52. Holmberg K, Meyer RD. Fungal infections in patients with AIDS and AIDS-related complex. Scan J Infect Dis 1986; 18:179-92.

Symptom Management Guidelines

Jeannee Parker Martin, R.N., M.P.H., and Jerome Schofferman, M.D.

A IDS manifests itself through a variety of symptoms related to unusual opportunistic infections and neoplasms. Often these symptoms can be easily associated with a specific opportunistic infection or neoplasm; sometimes they cannot. The following recommended interventions for alleviating or palliating the symptoms of AIDS have been tested in over 300 persons cared for by the AIDS Home Care and Hospice Program in San Francisco. Guidelines[1-3] for management are listed by the symptom, in alphabetical order. Physician's Desk Reference (1986) was used for all medications listed, unless otherwise noted.[4]

The medications ultimately identified for the management of various symptoms were arrived at after much trial and error. It is important to determine the characteristics of the individual patient, all symptoms this person is experiencing, and other factors which might enhance or impede utilization of these interventions. See also the documents related to treatment of each of the opportunistic infections or malignancies mentioned.

■ **SYMPTOM: DIARRHEA**

Etiology: cryptosporidiosis; cytomegalovirus (CMV); Kaposi's sarcoma (KS); *Mycobacterium avium intracellulare* (MAI); unknown etiology.

Comments: Diarrhea is common in most persons with AIDS. It is extremely irritating to the skin, especially when perianal lesions are present. A regular regime of skin care should be maintained, including cleansing of the area with warm soapy water, thorough drying of the area, and application of ointment (A and D) or other skin barrier cream or ointment.

Interventions: Discontinue foods that may aggravate diarrhea (e.g., Ensure can increase symptoms). *Mild diarrhea*: Kaopectate 60 ml to 120 ml after each bowel movement. Psyllium hydrophilic mucilloid (Metamucil) 1 tablespoon stirred into 8 oz glass of water taken orally 1 to 3 times per day. *Severe diarrhea*: Diphenoxylate hydrochloride with atropine (Lomotil, 2 tablets po qid or 10 ml Lomotil liquid qid; then adjust dose to individual response). Loperamide (Imodium) 4 mg po at onset of diarrhea; then decrease to 2 mg po after each unformed stool. Adjust dose to individual response. Incontinence pads, such as Attends, Depends, Chux; bedside commode chair.

■ **SYMPTOM: DYSPNEA, PRODUCTIVE COUGH; NONPRODUCTIVE COUGH WITH *PNEUMOCYSTIS CARINII* PNEUMONIA (PCP).**

Etiology: CMV, KS lesions in lungs, MAI, PCP.

Comments: Symptoms of PCP may recur on intermittent basis (dry cough, increased dyspnea, temperature elevations). Discussions should include decisions for hospitalization if acute symptoms develop or for palliative therapy that may be provided at home. Also, many patients will experience adverse reactions to trimethoprim-sulfamethoxazole (Septra) treatment (skin eruptions, pruritus, urticaria erythema) and will be maintained on pentamidine for acute episodes or for prophylaxis.

Interventions: Instruct patient in positioning techniques and techniques for energy conservation. Relaxation and controlled breathing exercises may also be helpful. Oxygen therapy continuously or as needed. Oxygen concentrator may be more cost effective for long term home care intervention. Oral morphine solution (10 to 20 mg/cc) for dyspnea and tachypnea to reduce respiratory rate and anxiety; begin with oral morphine solution 5 mg to 10 mg po q 4 hours around the clock. Adjust dose to individual response.[5] Scopolamine 1 patch (0.5 scopolamine) every 72 hours applied behind the ear to reduce pulmonary secretions. Cough expectorant/suppressant to help clear secretions. PCP prophylaxis: sulfamethoxazole 100 mg/kg and trimethoprim 20 mg/kg (Septra) given po in equally divided doses every 6 hours for 14 days. Or, pentamidine isethionate intramuscular injection or intravenously one time monthly.

■ SYMPTOM: EDEMA

Etiology: KS lesions

Comments: Edema associated with KS lesions will not usually be relieved by diuretics. Edema is related to local lymphatic blockage and not to systemic involvement.

Interventions: Elevate affected extremities. Use support stockings if possible. Apply cool moist towels for facial edema. Elevate head of bed. Low dose radiation therapy may relieve cause.

■ SYMPTOM: FEVER

Etiology: cryptosporidiosis, MAI, PCP; often fever of unknown origin.

Comments: Because fevers are one of the most persistent problems in most persons with AIDS, attention should be given to personal care and comfort measures. Because of copious perspiration, frequent linen changes may be necessary around the clock. A regime for cleansing and drying skin should be developed due to frequent diaphoresis and potential for skin breakdown.

Interventions: Acetaminophen 650 mg or aspirin 650 mg q 4 hrs around the clock to maintain temperature below 100°F. May need to alternate acetaminophen and aspirin q 2 hours around the clock. If fever unresponsive to above, ibuprofen (Motrin) 400 to 600 mg q 4 hours may relieve fevers. Motrin should be given with meals or milk. For temperature greater than 101.5°F, monitor for signs of acute infection. Give sponge bath for comfort. If appropriate, notify MD for antibiotic therapy. Encourage fluids, as tolerated.

■ SYMPTOM: MEMORY LOSS, CONFUSION, WEAKNESS

Etiology: lymphoma, meningitis, progressive multifocal leukoencephalopathy, toxoplasmosis.

Comments: There often will be no definitive diagnosis despite multiple neurologic complications. These symptoms are difficult to anticipate and may cause severe mental status changes necessitating 24-hour supervision by an attendant.

Interventions: Instruct caregivers in neurologic symptoms; help them understand and cope with these changes. Talk to patient in simple, short sentences. Keep calendar at bedside with appointments to help minimize confusion. Use large clock in room. Arrange for 24-hour care as mental status deteriorates to ensure safe environment: friends, family, attendants, and volunteers may be able to share coverage at different times of the day or night. Iorazepam (Ativan) 2 mg to 6 mg po q day.

■ SYMPTOM: NAUSEA, VOMITING

Etiology: CMV, KS, MAI, cryptosporidiosis; general deterioration; or medication induced, e.g., by morphine sulfate or chemotherapy.

Comments: Internal KS lesions may cause decreased peristalsis and symptoms of nausea and vomiting. These are not generally continuous symptoms in the person with AIDS. However, the interventions should be incorporated into the treatment plan so that prompt action can be taken should symptoms arise.

Interventions: Low residue diet. Intake in small amounts. Prochlorperazine (Compazine) 5 mg to 10 mg po qid or 25 mg rectally bid. Higher doses may be indicated to control nausea. Haloperidol (Haldol) 0.5 mg to 5.0 mg po bid or tid. Start at lowest dose and modify as needed. Dose may vary greatly between individuals. Promethazine hydrochloride (Phenergan) 25 mg po or rectally q 4 to 6 hours. Metoclopramide hydrochloride (Reglan) 10 mg tablets or syrup po tid (30 minutes after meals). Higher doses than in traditional settings and combinations of antiemetics also may be necessary to control nausea.

■ SYMPTOM: ORAL LESIONS

Etiology: *Candida albicans*, KS, herpes zoster.

Comments: Therapy usually will need to continue for the entire course of the illness because of underlying immunodeficiency. *C. albicans* will quickly recur when treatment is stopped even for short periods of time.

Interventions: Assess routinely for white, cottage cheese-like patches (*C. albicans*); dark blue or purple nodules or plaques (KS); localized vesicles (herpes). Rinse mouth frequently with dilute mouthwash. Brush teeth with soft toothbrush bid. For oral candidiasis: clotrimazole (Mycelex) troches 5 times daily for 14 consecutive days. Nystatin oral suspension 4 ml to 6 ml swish and swallow qid. For esophageal candidiasis: ketoconazole 200 mg one to two times daily.

■ SYMPTOM: PAIN

Etiology: edema due to KS, KS lesions in GI tract, herpes simplex type II, peripheral neuropathy, nonspecific complaints of discomfort.

Comments: Although pain management has not been a difficult problem in most AIDS patients, it is important to remember that pain is difficult to measure. Medication dosages should be modified to keep the person comfortable at home. Staff education may be necessary to ensure understanding of these higher doses.

Interventions: Acetaminophen 650 mg po or rectally q 4 hours. Codeine sulfate tablets 30 mg to 60 mg tablets every 4 hours. Oral morphine solution (10 to 20 mg/cc); begin with OMS 10 mg to 20 mg po q 4 hours around the clock. Adjust dose to individual response. Massage therapy and relaxation exercises can often reduce symptoms. Assign volunteer therapist as appropriate. Family/friends often have many suggestions for alternative therapies for pain control. If not harmful to the patient, these should be encouraged. Such interventions may greatly reduce anxiety related to pain or discomfort.

■ SYMPTOM: SKIN LESIONS

Etiology: KS, herpes simplex type II, perineal *C. albicans*.

Comments: KS lesions are distinctive dark blue or purple nodules or plaques which commonly are found on the feet or ankles, then progress proximally. Lesions are not open or ulcerated. KS is associated with widely disseminated lesions that may also affect pulmonary status, cause gastrointestinal complications, and urinary retention. Herpes simplex type II is a common venereal disease in homosexual or bisexual men. It appears as localized clusters of vesicles usually around the anus and is often a reactivation of a previous infection. Perianal *Candida albicans* therapy usually will need to continue for the entire course of the illness due to underlying immunodeficiency. Candida will quickly recur when treatment is stopped even for short periods of time.

Interventions: KS lesions: For ulcerated or draining lesions, cleanse with warm soapy water. Rinse and apply wet to dry dressing or Neosporin ointment bid. If lesions are not draining, may be left open to air. Herpes simplex lesions: Gloves should be worn during examination and/or application of medication to the vesicles to prevent transmission of herpes virus. Vesicles are highly contagious. Acyclovir (Zovirax) ointment 5 percent topically to adequately cover all lesions every 3 hours 6 times per day for 7 days. Acyclovir (Zovirax) tablets 200 mg 5 times per day for 14 days; then 3 times per day until healed. After each bowel movement, rectum should be cleansed gently with warm water and patted dry with soft towel. Toilet paper may abrade the vesicles and should not be used. Sitz bath and analgesics may relieve associated discomfort. Candida lesions: clotrimazole (Mycelex) cream to affected area bid. (morning and evening). After each bowel movement, rectum should be cleansed gently with warm water and patted dry with soft towel. Toilet paper may abrade the vesicles and should not be used. Sitz bath and analgesics may relieve associated discomfort.

■ SYMPTOM: VISION IMPAIRMENT, BLINDNESS

Etiology: cytomegalovirus (CMV), retinitis.

Comments: Vision impairment and loss are sometimes rapid and unexpected by the person with AIDS. Counseling and emotional support will be essential to help the person understand the implications of a diagnosis of CMV.

Interventions: Instruct patient and caregivers about symptoms related to CMV and help them cope with changes that may occur. Occupational therapy to help reorient person to house and to rearrange furnishings as necessary to allow increased level of independence. Contact local organizations for the blind for resources such as talking books, large print newspapers, and radios for the blind. Attendant for meal preparation or referral to home meals program, if patient is unable to safely manage stove or oven. Ganciclovir is an experimental drug being tested in the treatment of CMV. Check locally for availability.

REFERENCES

1. Durham J, Cohen F, eds. The person with AIDS: nursing perspectives. New York: Springer, 1987.
2. Martin J. Physical assessment guidelines for nurses. In: Durham JD, Cohen FL, eds. The person with AIDS: nursing perspectives. New York: Springer, 1987:161-77.
3. Lillard J, Lotspeich P, Gurich J, Hesse J. Acquired immunodeficiency syndrome in home care: maximizing helpfulness and minimizing hysteria. Home Healthc Nurs 1984; 2:11-4.
4. Physician's Desk Reference, 40th ed. Oradell: Medical Economics Company, 1986.
5. Twycross R, Lack S. Oral morphine in advanced cancer. Beaconsfield, England: Beaconsfield Publishers, Ltd., 1984.

Physical Assessment Guidelines for Case Management

Jeannee Parker Martin, R.N., M.P.H.

T he physical and neurologic changes in the person with AIDS are multiple and varied. It is rare that the person with AIDS has only one opportunistic infection or only one simple manifestation of this complicated illness. Rather, most individuals have three or more diagnosed infections and symptoms of several others. Early diagnosis and treatment of some opportunistic infections will prevent their exacerbation or recurrence in the future. Prompt recognition of undiagnosed symptoms and subsequent control of their manifestations will enhance patient comfort and quality of life as the illness progresses.

The following physical assessment guidelines for nurses have been developed to aid the entire home-care team in early identification of new infections or changing symptoms. The nurse instructs other members of the multidisciplinary team, the person with AIDS, and other family members or friends; and these guidelines can be used to assist them in the identification of new problems and to explore alternatives for care. They should be used in conjunction with the preceding document: "Symptom Management Guidelines."

TABLE 1. AIDS HOME CARE AND HOSPICE PROGRAM PHYSICAL ASSESSMENT GUIDELINES*

Document absence (0) or presence (+). If present, describe in detail (e.g., frequency, severity, etc.).

CONSTITUTIONAL SYMPTOMS

__ fevers
__ malaise
__ fatigue
__ night sweats
__ change in appetite
__ weight loss

PHYSICAL FINDINGS

T___ P___ RR___ BP___ (sitting)
P___ BP___ (standing)
weight ___

INTEGUMENT

__ pruritus (itching)
__ pain
__ usual skin care

__ lesions: describe location, size, drainage
__ rash: describe
__ decubitis ulcers: describe
__ color

continued on next page

continued from previous page

TABLE 1.   AIDS HOME CARE AND HOSPICE PROGRAM PHYSICAL ASSESSMENT GUIDELINES*

CONSTITUTIONAL SYMPTOMS	PHYSICAL FINDINGS

INTEGUMENT

__ temperature
__ integrity
__ tumor
__ petechiae
__ tenderness on palpation: identify location
__ vesicles

MUCOUS MEMBRANES

lips, mouth, throat

__ pain	__ cold sores
__ dysphagia	__ oral lesions (e.g., white plaques of candida; vesicles)
__ dryness	__ odor
__ usual oral care: describe	

NEUROLOGIC

__ memory loss per report of patient or family	__ orientation
__ confusion	__ judgment
__ insight	__ concentration
	__ thought content
	__ delusions
	__ hallucinations

HEAD/NECK

__ headache	__ nuchal rigidity (stiff neck)
__ syncope	__ gag reflex
__ dysphagia	__ speech: clear
__ dysphasia	

EYES

__ change in vision, blurring	check visual acuity (ability to read print or to recognize number of fingers held up)
__ pain	

EARS

__ change in hearing	note any hearing deficit
__ earache	

continued on next page

continued from previous page

TABLE 1. AIDS HOME CARE AND HOSPICE PROGRAM
PHYSICAL ASSESSMENT GUIDELINES*

CONSTITUTIONAL SYMPTOMS	PHYSICAL FINDINGS

NOSE

__ change in smell	
__ congestion	
__ frequent dribbling	

MOTOR

__ falls	observe gait, transfers, observe tremors, extrapyramidal signs if taking phenothiazines
__ seizures (if yes, describe)	
__ tremors	muscle strength testing as indicated
__ weakness	

SENSORY

__ numbness, tingling, burning of extremities	if indicated, check sensation to touch, temperature
__ bowel or bladder incontinence	

RESPIRATORY

__ cough	__ cyanosis
__ productive (if so, describe sputum color and amount)	__ depth and rhythm of respirations
__ SOB (at rest and/or with exertion required to participate)	__ lung exam
__ chest pain (associated with respiration), describe	__ auscultation
__ orthopnea	__ percussion
__ oxygen use	__ palpation; fremitus

CARDIOVASCULAR

__ chest pain	__ heart sounds
__ SOB	__ rhythm
__ leg pain	__ rate
__ cold hands or feet	__ presence of murmur or gallop (S3, S4)
	__ edema
	__ peripheral pulses
	__ skin color and perfusion

GASTROINTESTINAL

__ anorexia	abdominal exam:
__ nausea	__ presence of bowel tones in all four quadrants
__ vomiting	__ distention

continued on next page

continued from previous page

TABLE 1. AIDS HOME CARE AND HOSPICE PROGRAM PHYSICAL ASSESSMENT GUIDELINES*

CONSTITUTIONAL SYMPTOMS	PHYSICAL FINDINGS

GASTROINTESTINAL

__ change in taste	__ tenderness and/or guarding
__ diarrhea	**rectal exam:**
__ constipation	__ stool (home test for occult blood)
__ usual bowel regimen	__ hemorrhoids
__ fecal incontinence	

GENITOURINARY

__ hesitancy	__ urinary device
__ frequency	__ external catheter
__ dysuria	__ indwelling catheter (size, type, date of insertion)
__ burning	__ discharge
__ hematuria	__ inflammation
__ incontinence	__ lesions
	__ edema

ENDOCRINE

__ fatigue	__ facial edema (pitting or nonpitting)
__ palpitations with sweating	
__ easy bruising	

*   *Compiled by the author*

HIV Infection in Women

Lauren Poole, R.N., M.S.

Approximately 9 percent of adult AIDS cases in the United States occur in women; the number of women with HIV infection must be many orders greater. This chapter summarizes important facts about the epidemiology of HIV infection in women, including the role of intravenous drug use (IVDU) and the possibilities of perinatal transmission, for those involved in their health care. Clinical history, presentation, and counseling issues for women are also discussed.

■ EPIDEMIOLOGY OF HIV INFECTION IN WOMEN

According to surveillance data published by the Centers for Disease Control (CDC), as of January 1989, 52 percent of women diagnosed with AIDS in the U.S. are intravenous drug users, 30 percent were exposed to HIV through heterosexual contact, and 11 percent received HIV-infected blood or blood products. The transmission category for the remaining 7 percent is currently classified by the CDC as "undetermined" because the risk factors are unknown. A significant trend noted between 1982 and 1986, however, is the increase in percentage of female cases classified as heterosexually transmitted,[1] which has increased a hundredfold since the 15 percent of heterosexually transmitted cases reported in January 1986.[2]

About half of the women with AIDS in the U.S. are aged 30 to 39; 90 percent of adult female cases occur in women 20 to 50.[1] CDC surveillance data indicate that over 71 percent of all adult female AIDS cases are among black and Hispanic women — 51.6 percent black and 19.5 percent Hispanic.[3] This disproportionate number of black and Hispanic women with AIDS primarily reflects the prevalence of IVDU in some black and Hispanic communities, particularly those on the East Coast. Although most states have reported adult female AIDS cases to the CDC, over half of these cases have been reported from northeastern states — one-half of them in New York alone.

Fifty-nine percent of women with AIDS reported to the CDC have subsequently been reported as dead, compared to 50 percent of men (personal communication, Ann Hardy, CDC, 1988). AIDS has a significant impact on mortality patterns for women in areas where HIV infection is common — it is now the leading cause of death for women aged 30 to 34 years in New York City.[4]

■ PERINATAL TRANSMISSION

The vast majority of adults with HIV infection are in their reproductive years. The effect of this on childbearing is critical: according to CDC surveillance data, the risk factor for about 78 percent of the children with AIDS in the U.S. is a parent with AIDS or in an AIDS risk group.[3]

It is assumed that these children were born to infected mothers and that they acquired HIV infection during the perinatal period. While the exact mechanisms of perinatal transmission remain unknown, both transplacental and postpartum transmission have been suggested by several case reports:

1. An infant delivered by cesarean section had no postnatal contact with her infected mother's cervix but developed AIDS at six months of age.[5]

2. Evidence of HIV was found in tissues from a 20-week abortus of a seropositive, asymptomatic mother.[6]

3. Evidence of HIV was found in tissue from a 28-week baby born by cesarean section to a mother terminally ill with AIDS[7]; the infant had no contact with the mother's cervix.

4. Postnatal transmission of HIV has been suggested in a case in which the mother, who was infected by a postpartum blood transfusion, apparently transmitted HIV to her infant through breast milk[8]; the infant had no contact with the mother's cervix.

The risk of infection via cervical secretions is unclear, but HIV has been documented in cervical secretions.[9,10]

The relative risk of HIV infection to the fetus of an infected woman is not known. In an early study of infected mothers who had previously delivered infants who developed AIDS, 57 percent (6 of 14) babies born subsequently were also infected.[11] In contrast, no babies born to women infected by artificial insemination showed evidence of HIV infection after one year of follow-up.[12] Because these were small studies, it is important to emphasize that the risk estimates found in them are varied and uncertain. The largest most recently published study was done by a European collaborative group and demonstrated a 24 percent vertical transmission rate in 271 children born to HIV-infected mothers.[13]

At this time, outcomes for the newborn cannot be predicted by the clinical status of the mother during pregnancy. Infected babies have been born to women who are asymptomatic seropositives as well as to mothers with AIDS and ARC. A mother with AIDS can also deliver a baby with no evidence of disease.[14] Transmission from an infected woman to older children or to other household members who are not her sexual partners has never been documented.

▪ EVALUATION AND CLINICAL PRESENTATIONS

EVALUATION OF WOMEN IN HEALTH-CARE SETTINGS

Intravenous drug users in treatment programs and those who bear the physical stigmata of IV drug use are at risk for HIV infection. Other women at risk, however, are not easily identified. A comprehensive history that addresses possible risk factors for HIV infection will help identify some women at risk.

Appropriate questions should be incorporated into the social, sexual, and medical portions of the patient history. Documentation of patient responses to these questions must be done in a way that maximizes confidentiality.

1. "Have you ever been tested for antibodies to the AIDS virus? If so, what was the result of your test? When and why were you tested?"

2. "Since the late 1970s, have you ever injected drugs into your body with a needle? If yes, have you shared needles with other people?" If a woman is or has been an IVDU, a history of the type of drugs used and the extent of drug use and needle sharing should be obtained.

3. "Since 1979, have you ever had sexual relations with a person at risk for AIDS — someone who injects drugs, a gay or bisexual man, a hemophiliac, or a person from Haiti or central Africa?" If yes, further history should be taken on the clinical status of the person at risk, the type of sexual activity involved, the duration of the relationship, and the use and type of contraception.

4. "Have you had any anonymous sexual partners or partners that you did not know well who may possibly have been in AIDS risk groups?" Many women do not know the risk status of all their sexual partners. The question is most relevant if the patient lives where HIV infection is common.

5. "Have you tried to become pregnant through artificial insemination since the late 1970s? If yes, where?" Again, this question is most relevant if the patient has lived where HIV infection is common.

6. "Have you received a transfusion of blood or blood products since 1979?" If yes, ask when, where, and how much blood. The risk is higher if a woman received a transfusion before 1985 in an area where HIV was common.

7. When applicable, "Are you from Haiti or central Africa?"

8. "Is there any other reason why you think you might be at risk of exposure to HIV?" This question may lead to the patient's revealing an additional possible risk factor, such as providing health care to people with AIDS or HIV infection. The question also gives the woman a chance to express her fears about AIDS so that the health-care worker can evaluate her needs for information.

Even when such histories are taken, not all women at risk will be identified. Many women are unaware of their risk for HIV infection because they are unaware of the drug use or homosexual activities of their current or past sexual partners.

CLINICAL PRESENTATION

The signs and symptoms of HIV infection are the same for women as they are for men with one notable exception: women rarely present with Kaposi's sarcoma (KS), the most common AIDS-related malignancy. Women with AIDS most frequently present with *Pneumocystis carinii* pneumonia (PCP), the most common AIDS-related opportunistic infection in all risk groups defined by the CDC. Sixty-six percent of women diagnosed with AIDS as of October 1988 had PCP as their initial diagnosis; 3 percent had KS as their initial diagnosis.[1] The remaining 31 percent had other AIDS-related opportunistic infections without PCP or KS.

Gynecological Disorders

Few studies have been published on manifestations of HIV infection that may be unique to women. At the Fourth International AIDS Conference in

1988, investigators from Newark, New Jersey, presented clinical data on 169 women with HIV infection,[15] which revealed a high percentage of women with gynecological disorders as well as very high maternal morbidity and mortality. Whether these findings were related to HIV infection or to other patient characteristics (such as IVDU and poverty) was not adequately addressed. The study found that the average life expectancy of its subjects between diagnosis of AIDS and death was very short (mean, 14.5 weeks in 20 women). The meaning of this finding is unclear; it is as likely that the women entered the health-care system late in their HIV infection as that there is a sexual difference in the natural history of HIV infection.

An earlier study of 18 HIV-infected women at Walter Reed Army Institute of Research reported that six of eight women with CDC-defined AIDS had persistent vaginal candidiasis.[16] Since persistent oral candidiasis is a common AIDS-related disorder, this finding is probably related to HIV infection. The Walter Reed study also reported that 10 of the 18 women presented with clinical manifestations of HIV infection but had been inaccurately diagnosed, despite a history of numerous medical evaluations.[16]

Another possible clinical manifestation of HIV infection is cervical neoplasia; there appears to be an increased risk of this condition among HIV-infected women.[17-19] Human papillomavirus or immunosuppression (or both) may act as cofactors in the development of cervical neoplasia.

Role of Pregnancy in HIV Infection

The patient's pregnancy may affect both the natural history of HIV infection and the clinical presentation of her AIDS-related disease(s).

Pregnancy is associated with changes in cellular immunity — specifically, the ratio of T-helper to T-suppressor cells is decreased during both pregnancy and HIV infection.[20] Pregnancy in an HIV-infected woman may accelerate the progression of HIV infection. One study followed 15 women, asymptomatic at childbirth, for 30 months after their deliveries. During the follow-up period, five of these women developed AIDS, seven developed ARC, and only three remained asymptomatic.[21] Based on this study, the idea has become widely held that pregnancy exacerbates the progression of HIV infection.

Our study of progression among pregnant women for Project AWARE at San Francisco General Hospital shows no evidence that HIV disease progresses more rapidly in subjects who were pregnant or who were postpartum during their participation in AWARE. The number of women in our study is small, however. There remains a theoretical risk that pregnancy could accelerate progression of HIV disease, but there is no firm evidence for it. Case–control studies following both pregnant and nonpregnant HIV seropositive women are needed to answer the question.

AIDS-related opportunistic infections can be particularly fulminant during pregnancy. There are a number of published case reports of women who developed opportunistic infections while pregnant.[20,22,23] The women presented with rapidly progressive disease and died within weeks of their diagnoses, despite treatment. Diagnosis of clinical manifestations of HIV infection is complicated by pregnancy because some symptoms of HIV infection are similar to those commonly seen in pregnancy — for example, fatigue, anorexia, weight loss, and shortness of breath. Health-care workers caring for pregnant women in HIV risk groups must assess these women carefully for signs and symptoms of HIV infection.

TABLE 1.   MEDICAL PROBLEMS ASSOCIATED WITH WOMEN IVDUs AT HIGH RISK FOR HIV INFECTION

Abscesses	Pneumonia
Amenorrhea and erratic menses	Poor dental hygiene
Anemia	Poor nutritional status
Bacteremia	Septicemia
Cardiac disease, esp. endocarditis	Sleep disturbances
Cellulitis	Tetanus
Hepatitis (acute and chronic)	Tuberculosis
Phlebitis	Venereal diseases

TABLE 2.   OBSTETRICAL COMPLICATIONS ASSOCIATED WITH HEROIN ADDICTION

Abortion	Intrauterine death
Abruptio placenta	Intrauterine growth retardation
Amnionitis	Placental insufficiency
Breech presentation	Postpartum hemorrhage
Previous Cesarean section	Preeclampsia
Chorioamnionitis	Premature labor
Eclampsia	Premature rupture of membranes
Gestational diabetes	Septic thrombophlebitis

TABLE 3.   PHYSICAL EXAM FINDINGS ASSOCIATED WITH NARCOTIC ADDICTION IN WOMEN

Dermatologic:	Presence of infections, abscesses, thrombosed veins, herpes infections, pyodermas, icterus
Dental:	Status of dental hygiene; pyorrhea or abscessed cavities
Otolaryngeal:	Rhinitis; excoriation of nasal septum
Respiratory:	Presence of asthma, rales; signs of interstitial pulmonary disease
Cardiovascular:	Presence of increased pulmonary artery pressure; murmurs indicative of endocarditis or preexisting valvular disease
Breast:	Evidence of trauma: breast veins used for injection
Gastrointestinal:	Hepatomegaly
Genitourinary:	Evidence of venereal disease
Musculoskeletal:	Pitting edema; distortion of muscular landmarks due to subcutaneous abscesses or brawny edema

■ COUNSELING WOMEN WITH HIV INFECTION

Counseling issues differ for women depending on whether they are uninfected but at risk for HIV infection, seropositive but asymptomatic, or women with symptomatic HIV infection or AIDS. This section discusses appropriate prevention and transmission information for women in each group as well as prepregnancy and pregnancy counseling for both HIV-infected and high-risk women.

WOMEN AT RISK FOR HIV INFECTION: GENERAL CONSIDERATIONS

Antibody Testing

Women at risk should be counseled on how HIV is transmitted and how to avoid or minimize their exposures. Programs designed to meet the needs of women at risk who are or may become pregnant should make the HIV antibody test understandable and readily available. The CDC recommends antibody testing for women at high risk but emphasizes that many women are unaware of their risks for HIV infection.[21,26,27] The most important part of any such program is identifying women at risk and educating them to prevent exposure to (and transmission of) HIV. The best way to prevent perinatal transmission of HIV is to prevent its transmission to women.

TABLE 4.   INDICATIONS FOR HIV ANTIBODY TESTING IN WOMEN PRIOR TO OR DURING EARLY PREGNANCY

- Women with signs or symptoms of HIV infection and women who have delivered HIV-infected babies
- Women who have used intravenous drugs for nonmedical purposes since 1979
- Women who have been sex partners of men at risk for HIV infection (i.e., IV drug users, bisexuals, homosexuals, hemophiliacs, men from Haiti or central Africa)
- Women who have lived in HIV-endemic areas (e.g., Haiti, Burundi, Rwanda, Zaire, Congo, Tanzania, Kenya) since 1979
- Women who have been donor-inseminated since January 1979, unless donor was screened for HIV before insemination
- Women who received blood products between January 1, 1979 and June 1, 1985.

Guidelines for Preventing Transmission

Women at risk of sexual exposure to HIV should minimize their risks by following the guidelines below, which were developed by the Women's AIDS Network and other groups in San Francisco. They apply both to women at risk and to women who are already infected.

1. Know your sex partner. Ask questions about past sexual history, drug use, HIV antibody test results.

2. Unless you know that a sex partner is not infected, don't allow his or her blood (including menstrual blood), semen, urine, vaginal secretions, or feces to enter your vagina, anus, or mouth.

3. Have male partners use condoms for vaginal, oral, and anal sex.

4. Use contraceptive foams, jellies, or creams that contain the spermicide nonoxynol-9.

5. If you think you might be infected, never allow your blood, urine, vaginal secretions, or feces to enter another person's body. Always have male partners use a condom for sex.

The Women's AIDS Network guidelines do not advise women to avoid the exchange of saliva. Most authorities agree that kissing is not an effective means of transmitting HIV. However, because HIV has been isolated from saliva, women should be advised that transmission of HIV through saliva exchange (deep kissing) is theoretically possible but highly unlikely.

Adherence to these guidelines markedly reduces the sexual transmission of HIV to and from women. One laboratory study on the effectiveness of condoms, for instance, showed that HIV did not pass through latex or lambskin condoms.[24] Another study showed that nonoxynol-9 inactivated HIV in vitro.[25]

COUNSELING HIV-INFECTED, ASYMPTOMATIC WOMEN

Guidelines for HIV-infected people have been published by the CDC.[28] These guidelines should be made available to seropositive woman and to women who may be infected.

The concerns expressed most frequently by seropositive women are fear of becoming ill; fear of transmitting HIV to their sexual partners and children; difficulty in communicating with potential sexual partners and in remaining sexually active; and not being able to bear children for fear they will become infected.

The CDC recommends that seropositive women avoid pregnancy until more is known about perinatal transmission of HIV.[21] This recommendation is often difficult for seropositive women to accept. Childbearing is a life goal for many women; the potential loss of that option can be devastating. Even more difficult is the situation of a woman who is already pregnant and then learns that she is infected with HIV. Although perinatal transmission is neither inevitable nor predictable, its likelihood is quite high. Infected women in late pregnancy and those in early pregnancy who do not elect to have an abortion will need extensive counseling and support.

To help health-care workers in the task of counseling these women, the CDC has published "Recommendations for Assisting in the Prevention of Perinatal Transmission of HTLV-III/LAV and AIDS."[21] Of particular significance is the CDC's recommendation that women at risk be tested for exposure to HIV before conceiving (if possible) or as soon as pregnancy is diagnosed. The CDC recommends that all repeatedly reactive initial tests be confirmed using one of the standard confirmatory tests.

Table 5 is based partially on the CDC's recommendations. It summarizes steps to be taken and issues to be addressed for seropositive and seronegative high-risk women who are or may become pregnant.

TABLE 5. PREGNANCY COUNSELING RECOMMENDATIONS FOR PREGNANT AND NONPREGNANT SEROPOSITIVE AND HIGH-RISK WOMEN

PREGNANT WOMEN

Seropositive

1. counsel about the meaning of the test and possible risk of disease in mother and baby

2. discuss option of pregnancy termination if early in the pregnancy and woman wishes to consider this option

3. teach how to prevent further exposure to HIV and how to prevent transmission to others

4. teach signs and symptoms of HIV infection and advise to report those promptly if they occur

5. refer for high-risk prenatal care

6. refer to social worker, therapist, support group if indicated

7. enlist pediatrician to follow newborn

8. obtain appropriate informed consent before disclosing antibody results to parties listed in 5,6,7,

Seronegative

1. counsel about the meaning of the test and how to prevent exposure

2. retest at an appropriate time interval if recent or continued exposure

3. teach signs and symptoms of HIV infection and advise to report promptly if they occur

4. monitor closely during pregnancy for signs and symptoms of HIV infection

5. encourage breast feeding if antibody tests remain negative throughout pregnancy and if risk behavior has ceased

NONPREGNANT WOMEN

Seropositive

1. counsel about the meaning of the test and possible development of disease in the woman and risk of infection to newborn if pregnancy occurs

2. discuss postponing pregnancy until more is known about perinatal transmission and risk of disease progression in infected pregnant women

3. teach how to avoid further exposure to HIV and how to prevent transmission to others

4. refer for medical follow-up and obtain appropriate informed consent before disclosing antibody result

5. teach signs and symptoms of HIV infection and advise to report such symptoms promptly if they occur

6. enlist psychosocial help if indicated

7. discuss contraception

Seronegative

1. counsel about the meaning of the test and how to prevent exposure

2. retest at appropriate time if recent or continued exposure and pregnancy is desired or occurs

3. advise that, if antibody remains negative and risk behavior has ceased, woman is no longer at high risk

COUNSELING WOMEN WITH SYMPTOMATIC HIV INFECTION AND AIDS

The issues that women with symptomatic HIV infection and AIDS must deal with overlap those of asymptomatic seropositives and women at risk. Fear of transmitting HIV to others is a major concern to these women. Prevention guidelines for them are the same as for women who are asymptomatic. Unlike women at risk or women who are not clinically ill with HIV infection, those with symptomatic HIV infection and AIDS must deal with grief over the loss of their previous body image, sexual freedom, and potential for childbearing. They must also come to grips with the imminent loss of their own lives. Grief and many other emotions triggered by an ARC or AIDS diagnosis are discussed elsewhere. Several additional issues specific to women will be addressed here.

Women with symptomatic HIV infection and AIDS experience a unique social isolation. Although women were among the first persons diagnosed with AIDS, they are still not widely perceived as at risk for AIDS, which is still widely seen as a man's disease. Moreover, women with AIDS are a diverse group with no parallel community to look to for support, as gay men can. There are very few programs or services designed for women with AIDS.

Being diagnosed with symptomatic HIV disease or AIDS is some women's first indication that their sexual partners are infected and that these partners are therefore probably IV drug users or bisexuals. This revelation creates a profound sense of anger and betrayal that adds to the emotional crisis provoked by the ARC or AIDS diagnosis.

Because most women with severe HIV disease are in their childbearing years, many already have children. A major concern for such women is care for their children if or when they become disabled or die. Many women with ARC and AIDS are also poor and have had to deal with the problems associated with poverty — inadequate housing, poor nutrition, lack of health care and child care — long before their diagnosis. All of these problems are exacerbated by the diagnosis.

Women with symptomatic HIV disease and AIDS are often part of households already dealing with the disease: their children and sexual partners may also be infected. When AIDS affects a whole family, the psychosocial needs are extensive.

REFERENCES

1. Guinan ME, Hardy A. Epidemiology of AIDS in women in the United States. 1981 through 1986. JAMA 1987; 257:2039-42.
2. AIDS Weekly Surveillance Report, Centers for Disease Control, January 20, 1986.
3. Update: acquired immunodeficiency syndrome — United States, 1981–1988. MMWR 1989; 38:229-36.
4. Holmes VF, Fernandez F. HIV in women: current impact and future implications. Physician Assistant 1989; 13:53.
5. Cowan MJ, Hellmann D, Chudwin D, et al. Maternal transmission of acquired immune deficiency syndrome. Pediatrics 1984; 73:382-6.
6. Jovaisas E, Koch MA, Schafer A, et al. LAV/HTLV-III in 20-week fetus. Lancet 1985; 2:1129.
7. Lapointe N, Michaud J, Pekovic D, et al. Transplacental transmission of HTLV-III virus. N Engl J Med 1985; 312:1325-6.
8. Ziegler JB, Cooper DA, Johnson RO, Gold J. Postnatal transmission of AIDS-associated retrovirus from mother to infant. Lancet 1985; 1:896-8.
9. Wofsy CB, Cohen JB, Hauer LB, et al. Isolation of AIDS-associated retrovirus from genital secretions of women with antibodies to the virus. Lancet 1986; 1:527-9.
10. Pomerantz RJ, de la Monte SM, Donegan SP, et al. Human immunodeficiency virus (HIV) infection of the uterine cervix. Ann Intern Med 1988; 108:321-7.

11. Scott GB, Fischl M, Klimas N, et al. Mothers of infants with the acquired immunodeficiency syndrome (AIDS): outcome of subsequent pregnancies [Abstract]. International Conference on Acquired Immunodeficiency Syndrome (AIDS). Atlanta, 1985:21.

12. Stewart GJ, Tyler JP, Cunningham AL, et al. Transmission of human T-cell lymphotropic virus type III (HTLV-III) by artificial insemination by donor. Lancet 1985; 2:581-5.

13. Mother-to-child transmission of HIV infection. The European Collaborative Study. Lancet 1988; 2:1039-43.

14. Rogers MF, Ewing EP Jr, Warfield D, et al. Virologic studies of HTLV-III/LAV in pregnancy: case report of a woman with AIDS. Obstet Gynecol 1986; 68(suppl):2s-6s.

15. Kloser P, Grigoriu A, Kapila R. Women with AIDS: a continuing study 1987 [Abstract]. IV International Conference on AIDS. Stockholm, 1988; 1:4065.

16. Wright DC, Rhoades J, Redfield RR. HTLV-III/LAV disease in heterosexual women [Abstract]. II International Conference on AIDS. Paris, 1986:154.

17. Bradbeer C. Is infection with HIV a risk factor for cervical intraepithelial neoplasia? Lancet 1987; 2:1277-8.

18. Cervical dysplasia and HIV infection. Lancet 1988; 1:237-9.

19. Maiman M, Fruchter RG, Serur E, Boyce JG. Prevalence of human immunodeficiency virus in a colposcopy clinic. JAMA 1988; 260:2214-5.

20. Minkoff H, deRegt RH, Landesman S, Schwarz R. *Pneumocystis carinii* pneumonia associated with acquired immunodeficiency syndrome in pregnancy: a report of three maternal deaths. Obstet Gynecol 1986; 67:284-7.

21. Recommendations for assisting in the prevention of perinatal transmission of human T-lymphotropic virus type III/lymphadenopathy-associated virus and acquired immunodeficiency syndrome. MMWR 1985; 34:721-6, 731-2.

22. Jensen LP, OSullivan MJ, Gomez del Rio M, et al. Acquired immunodeficiency (AIDS) in pregnancy. Am J Obstet Gynecol 1984; 148:1145-6.

23. Wetli CV, Roldan EO, Fojaco RM. Listeriosis as a cause of maternal death: an obstetric complication of the acquired immunodeficiency syndrome (AIDS). Am J Obstet Gynecol 1983; 147:7-9.

24. Conant M, Hardy D, Sernatinger J, et al. Condoms prevent transmission of AIDS-associated retrovirus. JAMA 1986; 255:1706.

25. Hicks DR, Martin LS, Getchell JP, et al. Inactivation of HTLV-III/LAV-infected cultures of normal human lymphocytes by nonoxynol-9 in vitro. Lancet 1985; 2:1422-3.

26. Update: heterosexual transmission of acquired immunodeficiency syndrome and human immunodeficiency virus infection — United States. MMWR 1989; 38:423-4, 429-34.

27. AIDS and human immunodeficiency virus infection in the United States: 1988 update. MMWR 1989; 38(Suppl 4):1-38.

28. Provisional Public Health Service inter-agency recommendations for screening donated blood and plasma for antibody to the virus causing acquired immunodeficiency syndrome. MMWR 1985; 34:1-5.

5

CLINICAL MANIFESTATIONS OF HIV INFECTION

EDITORS

Donald I. Abrams, M.D., and P.T. Cohen, M.D., Ph.D.

5.1

Systemic Symptoms of HIV Infection

Systemic Symptoms of HIV Infection: Differential Diagnosis

P.T. Cohen, M.D., Ph.D.

S ystemic symptoms are frequently observed in patients infected with the human immunodeficiency virus (HIV), even in the absence of identifiable secondary diseases. For this discussion, systemic symptoms refer to symptoms often associated with disease, but that do not by themselves suggest any specific anatomic region, organ system, disease process, or etiologic agent as their cause. Thus, systemic symptoms are nonspecific and nonlocalizing. Examples include fever, night sweats, anorexia, weight loss, lethargy, and malaise. They may be caused by HIV itself or by occult secondary infections or malignancies.[1-3]

The same symptoms are frequently reported to primary care clinicians by patients who have no serious medical illness and may be caused by brief, self-limited illness, or by drugs or medications. Psychological factors may cause depression, lethargy, weight loss, and malaise. Patients preoccupied with bodily functions may incorrectly equate feeling warm or cold with fever, or may perceive temporary body fluid differences or weight measurements from different scales as weight loss. The threshold for seeking and reporting these symptoms may be especially low if patients consider themselves to be at risk for HIV disease.

In the absence of findings to specify their cause, systemic symptoms have a differential diagnosis that includes symptoms resulting from: any of the "traditional" causes of fever of unknown origin[4-6]; acute[7-11,20,21] or chronic[3,12-14,22] infection with HIV; or a secondary problem due to infection with HIV.[15-19]

It is important that conditions unrelated to AIDS be considered in the differential diagnosis of systemic symptoms. They include: infections, inflammatory bowel disease, neoplasms, necrotic tissue from trauma, vasculitidies, drug reactions, inflammatory arthritidies, occupational/environmental/hazardous material exposure, pulmonary emboli, thermoregulatory disorders, hemolytic states, Addisonian state, hyperthyroidism, granulomatous diseases, and functional or factitious conditions.

Some infectious agents that are possible causes of fever or other systemic symptoms in a patient infected with HIV are listed in Table 1.[15-18]

TABLE 1.

BACTERIA

Mycobacterium avium complex	*Haemophilus influenzae*	*Treponema pallidum*
Mycobacterium tuberculosis	Shigella species	Legionella species
Staphylococcus aureus	Salmonella species	Chlamydia species
Streptococcus pneumoniae	*Listeria monocytogenes*	*Nocardia asteroides*
Clostridium perfringens	Anaerobic species	

VIRUSES

HIV	Herpes simplex virus	Adenoviruses
Hepatitis viruses	Cytomegalovirus	Papova viruses
Epstein–Barr virus	Varicella virus	

FUNGI

Aspergillus species	*Cryptococcus neoformans*	Candida species
Histoplasma capsulatum	Coccidioides	

PROTOZOA

Cryptosporidium species	*Pneumocystis carinii*	Entamoeba species
Toxoplasma gondii	Isospora species	

The following are noninfectious conditions that are possible causes of fever or other systemic symptoms:

TABLE 2.

MALIGNANCIES	PSYCHOLOGICAL	MISCELLANEOUS
Kaposi's sarcoma	Depression	Drug reaction
Hodgkin's disease	Factitious	Adrenalitis
Non-Hodgkin's lymphoma	Functional	

REFERENCES

1. Fauci AS, Masur H, Gelmann EP, et al. The acquired immunodeficiency syndrome: an update. Ann Intern Med 1985; 102:800-11.
2. Francis DP, Jaffe HW, Fultz PN, et al. The natural history of infection with the lymphadenopathy associated virus human T lymphotrophic virus type III. Ann Intern Med 1985; 103:719-22.
3. Volberding PA. The clinical spectrum of the acquired immunodeficiency syndrome: implications for comprehensive care. Ann Intern Med 1985; 103:729-31.
4. Vickery DM, Quinnell RK. Fever of unknown origin: an algorithmic approach. JAMA 1977; 238:2183-8.
5. Jacoby GA, Swartz MN. Fever of undetermined origin. N Engl J Med 1973; 289:1407-10.
6. Petersdorf RG, Beeson PB. Fever of unexplained origin: report on 100 cases. Medicine 1961; 40:1-30.

7. Carne CA, Smith A, Elkington SG, et al. Acute encephalopathy coincident with seroconversion for anti HTLV-III. Lancet 1985; 2:1206-8.
8. Tucker J, Ludlam CA, Craig A, et al. HTLV-III infection associated with glandular fever like illness in a haemophiliac. Lancet 1985; 1:585.
9. Cooper DA, Gold J, Mackan P, et al. Acute AIDS retrovirus infection. Lancet 1985; 1:537-40.
10. Needlestick transmission of HTLV-III from a patient infected in Africa. Lancet 1984; 2:1376-7.
11. Ho DD, Sarngadharan MG, Resnick L, et al. Primary human T lymphocyte virus type III infection. Ann Intern Med 1985; 103:880-3.
12. Abrams DI. Lymphadenopathy syndrome in male homosexuals. In: Gallin JI, Fauci AS, eds. Acquired immunodeficiency syndrome. New York: Raven Press, 1985:75-97.
13. Quinn TC. Early symptoms and signs of AIDS and the AIDS related complex. In: Ebbeson P, Biggar RJ, Melbye M, eds. AIDS. Copenhagen: Munksgaard, 1984; 69-81.
14. Valle SL, Saxinger C, Ranki A, et al. Diversity of clinical spectrum of HTLV-III infection. Lancet 1985; 1:301-4.
15. Fauci AS, Macher AM, Longo DL, et al. Acquired immunodeficiency syndrome: epidemiologic, clinical, immunologic, and therapeutic considerations. Ann Intern Med 1984; 100:92-106.
16. Gold JWM. Clinical spectrum of infections in patients with HTLV-III associated diseases. Cancer Res 1985; 45(Suppl):4652S-4654S.
17. Armstrong D, Gold JWM, Dryjanski J, et al. Treatment of infections in patients with the acquired immunodeficiency syndrome. Ann Intern Med 1985; 103:738-43.
18. Wofsy CB. Opportunistic infections in AIDS. In: Focus on AIDS: a clinical appraisal. Symposium proceedings. Miami: Merieux Institute, Inc., 1984:6-10.
19. Greene JB, Slepian MJ. A clinical approach to opportunistic infections complicating the acquired immunodeficiency syndrome. In: Friedman-Kien AE, Laubenstein LJ, eds. AIDS: the epidemic of Kaposi's sarcoma and opportunistic infections. New York: Masson Publishing USA, 1984:89-95.
20. Fox R, Eldred LJ, Fuchs EJ, et al. Clinical manifestations of acute infection with human immunodeficiency virus in a cohort of gay men. AIDS 1987; 1:35-8.
21. Tindall B, Barker S, Donovan B, et al. Characterization of the acute clinical illness associated with human immunodeficiency virus infection. Arch Intern Med 1988; 148:945-9.
22. Kaslow RA, Phair JP, Friedman HB, et al. Infection with the human immunodeficiency virus: clinical manifestations and their relationship to immune deficiency, a report from the multicenter AIDS cohort study. Ann Intern Med 1987; 107:474-80.

Systemic Symptoms of HIV Infection: Evaluation

P.T. Cohen, M.D., Ph.D.

■ GENERAL CONSIDERATIONS

In evaluating a patient with systemic symptoms and signs who may be infected with the human immunodeficiency virus (HIV), the clinician's goal is to derive useful information for management, prognosis, and prevention of spread, while avoiding unjustified harm to the patient.

Causes of systemic symptoms range from serious illness to harmless or self-limited conditions. For patients with the latter conditions, much expense, anxiety, and inconvenience result from aggressive evaluation. On the other hand, for patients with serious illness, morbidity or death may occur if a "wait and watch" approach is adopted. This is particularly true in immunosuppressed patients in whom symptoms may be minimal even with life-threatening infections. Clearly, the clinician's keen judgment is required to select the proper pace and depth of evaluation.

Systemic symptoms may be the first recognized indicator of HIV infection. Identification of HIV infection at the earliest stage possible is an important goal. When initially recognized, many HIV-infected individuals are asymptomatic or minimally ill.[1,2] Unfortunately, evidence now indicates that progression, over months to years, to severe immunocompromise and death is the rule not the exception for HIV-infected persons.[13] Among the benefits of early identification of HIV infection are behavior modification to prevent spread to others; avoidance of potentially adverse factors such as malnutrition, drug abuse, exposure to antigenic stimuli (e.g., drugs, sexually transmitted diseases) that might activate HIV[12]; treatment with antiviral therapy (zidovudine or experimental protocol therapies) to slow progression of disease and destruction of the immune system; prophylaxis against some opportunistic infections; and vigilant clinical management to maintain health and recognize new problems.

The evaluation process should seek objective evidence to document that a disease process accounts for the observed symptoms. Inexpensive and harmless methods (history, physical examination, laboratory screening tests) should be used to search for clues that may suggest a more specific focus for further evaluation. Patients at risk obviously may have illnesses not specifically associated with HIV infection. Thus, all potential causes of systemic symptoms must be considered in all patients. Patients in certain risk groups may be at risk for other illnesses; for example, IV drug users may have endocarditis or occult abscesses, and patients with many different sexual partners may have sexually transmitted diseases other than HIV infection.

■ CLUES FROM THE PATIENT'S HISTORY

Information about the duration and frequency of symptoms, and whether the symptoms are "hard" (drenching night sweats, documented unintentional loss of more than 10 percent of body weight, documented persistent fever for four weeks, falling asleep often) or "soft" (feeling warm at night for three nights, loss of appetite, "low energy") is important for the evaluation process. Additionally, symptoms suggestive of HIV-related tumors or infections, risk factors for HIV infection, use of drugs or medications that may explain the symptoms, and other medical or psychosocial factors that may cause the symptoms should be noted.

Assessment of the risk for HIV infection should include queries about past history indicative of HIV infection (including results of HIV antibody testing if available) or illness suggesting immunosuppression. Information about intravenous drug use (particularly with needle sharing), number of sexual contacts since 1978 (when HIV probably appeared in the United States), sexual contact or needle sharing with persons infected with HIV, and receipt of blood products is also important.

■ CLUES FROM THE PHYSICAL EXAMINATION

Some symptoms and signs that are often found on physical examination, along with the AIDS-related conditions they suggest, are presented in Table 1.[3-7]

TABLE 1.   FINDINGS THAT SUGGEST CONDITIONS ASSOCIATED WITH HIV INFECTION

SYMPTOM/SIGN	SIGNIFICANCE/HIV-RELATED CONDITION
Fever, toxic appearance	Objective evidence of illness
Headache	Toxoplasmosis, cryptococcus, HIV encephalitis
Dementia	HIV dementia
Visual problems	
Cotton-wool exudates	*Pneumocystis carinii*, cytomegalovirus, toxoplasmosis
Chorioretinitis	Cytomegalovirus
Oral exudate	Oral candida
Oral lesions	Kaposi's sarcoma, herpetic ulcers, hairy leukoplakia
Odynophagia	Esophageal candida, esophageal herpes simplex
Adenopathy	Infectious diseases, lymphomas
Hepatomegaly	
Splenomegaly	
Diarrhea	Parasites, bacteria, protozoa
Skin conditions	Herpes zoster, herpes simplex, Kaposi's sarcoma, fungal infections, impetigo
Petechiae	Thrombocytopenia

■ LABORATORY AND DIAGNOSTIC TESTING

The extensiveness of testing depends upon the probability of finding significant illness. The following is not intended as a dogmatic formula, but it illustrates the spectrum of approaches and presentations.

Patients with "soft" symptoms, no objective abnormal findings on physical examination, and no apparent risk for HIV infection may be best served by reassurance, and reevaluation if symptoms persist. If doubt remains for the clinician or patient, basic laboratory and diagnostic screening tests may provide further reassurance or reveal additional clues. This level of testing might include the following tests:

- erythrocyte sedimentation rate
- complete blood, differential, and platelet counts
- serum electrolytes
- blood urea nitrogen and creatinine
- liver function
- serum calcium and phosphorus
- serologic test for syphilis
- stool analysis for occult blood
- urinalysis.

Suspicion of acute illness should be greater if the patient is known to have HIV infection on the basis of past illness or HIV antibody testing, or if the patient presents with measurable fever, an ill appearance, documented weight loss, or other compelling abnormalities. In this situation, more aggressive evaluation is indicated and might include:

- CD4 (T4, helper cell) lymphocyte count
- chest radiography
- sputum evaluation for pathogens
- blood cultures for bacteria, mycobacteria, and fungi
- stool cultures for leukocytes, bacterial pathogens, ova, and parasites
- serum for cryptococcal and hepatitis B antigens
- histoplasmosis, coccidioidomycosis, and toxoplasmosis serologies.

Serologies for Epstein–Barr virus and cytomegalovirus, as well as viral cultures, may be considered if results will alter management options.

If headache or other nonspecific central nervous system symptoms are prominent, a lumbar puncture should be done and cerebrospinal fluid examined for pyogenic bacteria and mycobacteria, fungi, syphilis, and biochemical and cellular abnormalities.

If no focal or specific findings are forthcoming, more invasive and expensive procedures, such as body imaging by gallium scanning, computer-assisted tomography, or magnetic resonance imaging, may be considered on a case-by-case basis to search for adenopathy, abscesses, tumors, organomegaly, or other pathologic findings.

Obviously, any abnormal findings should be the focus of additional diagnostic testing, imaging, and procedures, such as skin, liver, or lymph node biopsy; endoscopy; and bronchoscopy.

■ DIRECT TESTING FOR HIV INFECTION

For a patient not already known to be infected with HIV, if risk factors exist, or if the symptoms are not easily dismissed and are persistent, then testing for HIV infection is appropriate. Currently the most useful test for this purpose is the HIV antibody test.[14,15]

A positive HIV antibody test will emphasize HIV related conditions in the differential diagnosis and investigation, but it will not rule out other conditions as the cause of systemic symptoms. A negative HIV antibody test does not rule out early HIV infection since antibodies may not be produced for three to six months after HIV infection occurs. Thus, the antibody test result usually does not help to limit the scope of the evaluation in an acutely ill patient without localizing symptoms and signs. Its value lies in: (1) clarifying management considerations if a secondary cause for the systemic symptoms is found, (2) supporting HIV infection as a cause for the symptoms if a work-up excludes other potential etiologies, and (3) identifying the individual as needing long-term management for HIV infection.

The clinician or another knowledgeable person should inform the patient of the risks and benefits of testing for HIV and obtain the patient's consent. Confidentiality of the results should be guaranteed to the fullest extent possible. Both clinician and patient need to be aware of the potential for discrimination, emotional hardship, and rejection (by friends, lovers, and associates) that may result from disclosure of positive test results. The possibility of false-positive results must be recognized.[16] Regulations may require reporting of positive test results to government agencies, and subpoena of medical records in the event of legal proceedings is possible.

If the patient is clinically well and suspicion of serious illness is low, then to insure confidentiality, testing at an anonymous testing site might be considered. However, if the work-up must proceed at a rapid pace, and if the medical record must reflect the test result because subsequent management will be altered by it, then anonymous testing is not realistic.

■ INDICATIONS FOR HOSPITALIZATION

For most patients, all or a large part of the evaluation and management can be achieved in an outpatient setting. Hospital admission is indicated if the patient is toxic, has fever and is neutropenic, is actively bleeding and thrombocytopenic, or if the evaluation process must be accelerated because morbidity or suffering will occur if the outpatient pace is continued.

■ THE NONDIAGNOSTIC EVALUATION

If no cause for the systemic symptoms is found, and if the patient's HIV antibody test is negative, then antibody testing should be repeated in several months if HIV infection remains a consideration because of risk factors.

If HIV infection is documented, but no secondary cause for the systemic symptoms is found, further evaluation should be directed at determining where the patient is located on the spectrum of HIV infection. Most useful in terms of prognosis and evaluation of therapeutic options are measures of immune system compromise and of HIV activity. Measures that correlate with poor prognosis include anemia, presence of HIV p24 antigen, elevated serum β_2-microglobulin, low T4 lymphocyte count, and depressed T4/T8 helper/suppressor ratios.[13] These are discussed in other chapters.

If measurement of one or several of these variables suggests advanced disease or significant immunocompromise (e.g., T4 count <500 cells/cubic mm; presence of p24 antigen), then zidovudine therapy should be considered and discussed with the patient in terms of risks and benefits. For patients with less advanced disease, experimental protocols with zidovudine or other experimental treatments is an option.

When systemic symptoms persist and no specific cause is identified, the remaining diagnostic maneuver, by default, is observation over time — watching and waiting for the emergence of new clues. If necessary, fever can be managed with antipyretics as in other patients. Specific therapy is less defined for malaise, weight loss, and fatigue. Good nutrition and fluid intake, adequate rest, and abstinence from harmful drugs, including nicotine, alcohol, and caffeine, are straightforward measures worth trying. A search for modifiable psychological factors, such as fear, depression, and situational problems with family, work, and personal relationships may be productive.

Modification of high-risk behaviors will prevent HIV infection from spreading to others. This includes (1) abstaining from intravenous drug use, or at least from needle sharing[8]; and (2) practicing "safe sex," including limiting the number of sexual partners. Safer sexual practices will also ensure that the patient is not exposed to sexually transmitted diseases as sources of antigenic stimulation — a proposed mechanism of activation of latent HIV infection.[12]

The CDC surveillance definition for a case of AIDS is fulfilled if the HIV antibody test is positive in the presence of a greater than 10 percent unexplained weight loss of baseline body weight, and unexplained chronic weakness and documented fever for more than 30 days.[17] Patients with lymphadenopathy involving two or more extrainguinal sites (and persistent for at least three months) fulfill the criteria for persistent generalized lymphadenopathy syndrome.[1,9-11]

■ FOLLOW-UP INTERVAL

The interval for follow-up in the outpatient evaluation process must be determined on a case-by-case basis, but in the absence of specific infections or other morbidity-producing conditions, periodic follow-up evaluation every three to six months seems reasonable in patients with HIV disease. The patient should be instructed to contact the clinician by phone, or return for reevaluation on an emergent basis if new symptoms develop.

REFERENCES

1. Valle SL, Saxinger C, Ranki A, et al. Diversity of clinical spectrum of HTLV-III infection. Lancet 1985; 1:301-4.
2. Weiss SH, Goedert JJ, Sarngadharan MG, et al. Screening test for HTLV-III (AIDS agent) antibodies: specificity, sensitivity, and applications. JAMA 1985; 253:221-5.
3. Gold JWM. Clinical spectrum of infections in patients with HTLV-III associated diseases. Cancer Res 1985; 45(Suppl):4652S-4654S.
4. Armstrong D, Gold JWM, Dryjanski J, et al. Treatment of infections in patients with the acquired immunodeficiency syndrome. Ann Intern Med 1985; 103:739-43.
5. Greene JB, Slepian MJ. A clinical approach to opportunistic infections complicating the acquired immunodeficiency syndrome. In: Friedman-Kien AE, Laubenstein LJ, eds. AIDS: the epidemic of Kaposi's sarcoma and opportunistic infections. New York: Masson USA, 1984:89-95.
6. Wofsy CB. Acquired immunodeficiency syndrome (AIDS). In: Rakel RE, ed. Conn's current therapy. Philadelphia: W.B. Saunders, 1985:1-9.
7. McShane DJ. The spectrum of AIDS in clinical practice. In: Focus on AIDS: a clinical appraisal. Symposium proceedings. Miami: Merieux Institute, Inc., October 8, 1984:34-9.

8. Des Jarlais DC, Friedman SR, Hopkins W. Risk reduction for the acquired immunodeficiency syndrome among intravenous drug users. Ann Intern Med 1985; 103:755-9.

9. Fauci AS, Masur H, Gelmann EP, et al. The acquired immunodeficiency syndrome: an update. Ann Intern Med 1985; 102:800-11.

10. Quinn TC. Early symptoms and signs of AIDS and the AIDS related complex. In: Ebbesen P, Biggar RJ, Melbye M, eds. AIDS. Copenhagen: Munksgaard, 1984:69-81.

11. Abrams DI. Lymphadenopathy syndrome in male homosexuals. In: Gallin JI, Fauci AS, eds. Acquired immunodeficiency syndrome. New York: Raven Press, 1985:75-97.

12. Fauci AS. The human immunodeficiency virus: infectivity and mechanisms of pathogenesis. Science 1988; 239:617-22.

13. Moss AR, Bacchetti P, Osmond D, et al. Seropositivity for HIV and the development of AIDS or AIDS related condition: three year follow up of the San Francisco General Hospital cohort. Br Med J 1988; 296:745-50.

14. Centers for Disease Control. Update: Serologic testing for antibody to human immunodeficiency virus. MMWR 1988; 36:833-40.

15. Schwartz JS, Dans PE, Kinosian BP. Human immunodeficiency virus test evaluation, performance and use. JAMA 1988; 259:2574-9.

16. Meyer KB, Pauker SG. Screening for HIV: Can we afford the false positive rate? N Engl J Med 1987; 317:238-41.

17. Centers for Disease Control. Revision of the CDC surveillance case definition for acquired immunodeficiency syndrome. MMWR 1987; 36(Suppl 1S):3S-15S.

5.2

Oral Aspects

Opportunistic Infections of the Mouth

Deborah Greenspan, B.D.S.

Oral manifestations of human immunodeficiency virus (HIV) disease are common and include newly described oral lesions and novel presentations of previously known opportunistic diseases. Recognition requires careful history-taking and examination of the patient's oral cavity. Dentists are in a unique position to recognize early oral lesions during routine examinations. All oral lesions must be diagnosed by means of appropriate investigative techniques, including smears, cultures, and biopsies. Special stains should be used when necessary.[1-3]

■ CANDIDIASIS

Candidiasis is a fungal disease most frequently caused by the species *Candida albicans*. A number of factors can predispose patients to develop the disease: infancy, old age, antibiotic therapy, steroid and other immunosuppressive drugs, xerostomia, anemia, endocrine disorders, and primary and acquired immunodeficiency.[4]

CLINICAL FEATURES

The clinical features of oral candidiasis vary.[5] The oral lesions can be classified as pseudomembranous, atrophic, chronic hyperplastic, and as angular cheilitis.[6] They may be associated with a variety of symptoms, including complaints of a burning mouth, problems eating spicy food, and changes in taste. (See color plates 5.2.1.a and 5.2.1.b.)

Pseudomembranous Candidiasis. Pseudomembranous candidiasis is also known as thrush. It is characterized by the presence of creamy white plaques on the oral mucosa. The mucosa may appear red where the plaque is visible. The white plaques can be removed by scraping, which leaves a bleeding surface. This type of candidiasis may involve any part of the oral mucosa.

Atrophic Candidiasis. Atrophic candidiasis appears clinically as a red lesion. It is commonly seen on the palate and dorsum of the tongue. It may be acute or chronic but is more commonly chronic when associated with HIV infection.

Chronic Hyperplastic Candidiasis. Chronic hyperplastic candidiasis appears clinically as both red and white lesions. It may appear anywhere in the oral cavity. The white areas are due to hyperkeratosis. Unlike the plaques of pseudomembranous candidiasis, they cannot be removed by scraping. If these lesions are biopsied to establish a diagnosis, candida hyphae are revealed by a PAS (periodic acid-Schiff) stain.

Angular Cheilitis.   Angular cheilitis appears clinically as redness and fissuring, either unilaterally or bilaterally at the corners of the mouth; it can appear alone or in conjunction with another form of candidiasis.

DIFFERENTIAL DIAGNOSIS

Candida is a commensal organism in the oral cavity. Candidiasis is diagnosed by its clinical appearance and by detection of organisms on smears and culture. Smears taken from clinical lesions are examined using potassium hydroxide (KOH), PAS, or Gram's stain. Smears are taken by gently drawing a wooden tongue depressor across the lesion. The specimen is then transferred into a drop of KOH on a glass slide and protected by a cover slip. The smear is examined under the microscope and the presence of candida is detected by finding hyphae and blastospores. (Hyphae and spores are only seen in smears from lesions and do not occur in the healthy individual in the carrier state.) Cultures are grown on specific media, such as Sabouraud's; they may be positive and yet reveal very low colony counts. This probably represents a carrier state rather than active infection.

Atrophic candidiasis must sometimes be distinguished from erythroplakia by biopsy. Chronic hyperplastic candidiasis must sometimes be distinguished from hairy leukoplakia and other white lesions by biopsy.[5] If a biopsy is performed, tissue should be taken from a representative area. Histologically, oral candidiasis reveals candida hyphae in the superficial epithelium when viewed under a PAS stain. The inflammatory responses often associated with candida infection may be absent in immunocompromised patients.

TREATMENT OF ORAL CANDIDIASIS

The most common forms of oral candidiasis associated with HIV infection are the pseudomembranous and atrophic forms and angular cheilitis. Response to treatment is often good; oral lesions and symptoms may disappear in a fairly short period (ranging from 2 to 5 days), but relapses are common because of the underlying immunodeficiency. As with other causes of oral candidiasis, recurrences are common if the underlying problem persists. Oral candidiasis may be treated either topically or systemically.

Topical Treatment.   Topical treatments are preferred because they limit systemic absorption, but the effectiveness depends entirely on patient compliance. If formulations containing sweetening agents are used for long periods, daily fluoride rinses should be considered as concurrent treatment. The rinses, available as over-the-counter preparations, should be used for one minute once a day and then expectorated.

Several formulations are available for topical treatment. Mycelex (clotrimazole) troches can be used (10 mg, one tablet to be dissolved in the mouth 5 times a day). If used less frequently, this medication may not be as effective. Nystatin is available in a suspension, as a vaginal tablet, and as an oral pastille. Nystatin vaginal tablets (1 tablet, 100,000 units, dissolved in the mouth three times a day) can be used. Nystatin oral pastille is available as a 200,000-unit oral pastille (one or two pastilles dissolved slowly in the mouth 5 times a day). Nystatin suspension has a high sugar content and cannot be held in the mouth long enough to be effective. Topical creams and ointments containing nystatin (Mycolog) or clotrimazole may be useful in treating angular cheilitis.

Systemic Treatment. Systemic treatment may involve the use of ketoconazole (Nizoral). This is a 200 mg tablet that is taken with food once daily. Patient compliance is usually good. Very careful monitoring is necessary because of reported side effects, including hepatotoxicity.

PROGNOSTIC SIGNIFICANCE

Oral candidiasis may be of predictive value for the subsequent development of AIDS in persons in risk groups.[7-9] If oral candidiasis is diagnosed in a patient who lacks evidence of a predisposing factor, the patient should be referred for a work-up to determine if he or she has an HIV infection.

■ HISTOPLASMOSIS

Oral histoplasmosis has been reported in a female prostitute. The initial presentation of disease included a palatal perforation. Diagnosis was made from a histologic examination of a biopsy specimen from the hard palate.[13]

■ *MYCOBACTERIUM AVIUM-INTRACELLULARE*

A case of *Mycobacterium avium-intracellulare* has been reported that produced lesions in the oral cavity. Palatal and gingival granulomatous masses were seen on oral examination. A diagnosis of acid-fast bacilli (AFB) was made from a specially stained biopsy specimen. The AFB cultured from blood and sputum were identified as *Mycobacterium avium-intracellulare*.[12]

■ *CRYPTOCOCCUS NEOFORMANS*

Cryptococcus neoformans has been reported as causing an ulcerated mass in the hard palate of a patient with a previous history of *Pneumocystis carinii* pneumonia. Diagnosis was made from a biopsy of the palatal ulcer.[14]

■ HERPES SIMPLEX

Herpes simplex causes primary disease in the oral cavity. This may be followed by frequent recurrences. Primary herpetic gingivostomatitis is commonly seen in children and young adults. Following the primary episode, the virus becomes latent in the trigeminal ganglion. Recurrent oral herpes may be seen at any age and may occur extraorally or intraorally.

CLINICAL FEATURES

Recurrent herpes labialis occurs on the vermilion border of the lips. The patient may report a history of itching or pain, followed by the appearance of small vesicles. These rupture and form crusts. Recurrent intraoral herpes appears as clusters of painful small vesicles that rupture and ulcerate and usually heal within one week to 10 days. The lesions are found on the hard palate and gingiva.

DIFFERENTIAL DIAGNOSIS

Primary herpetic gingivostomatitis may be confirmed by rising antibody titers from initial and convalescent sera. Recurrent herpes may be confirmed by examining smears of lesions (treated with Papanicolaou stain) for multinucleated giant cells. Recently, it has become possible to demonstrate the presence of herpes simplex type 1 or type 2 by applying monoclonal antibodies to smears from the lesions.[15] The Syva kit (Syva Corporation, Palo Alto, Calif.) can easily be used for demonstrating HSV-1 and HSV-2. Cultures taken from fluid-filled vesicles may reveal the presence of herpes simplex (and its type) although vesicles present for several days may no longer reveal any virus. Recurrent intraoral herpes always occurs on keratinized mucosa (such as the hard palate and gingiva) and can therefore be distinguished from recurrent aphthous ulcers, which always appear on nonkeratinized mucosa. Recurrent intraoral herpes may appear more frequently in HIV-infected patients. The lesions may be painful and slow to heal.

TREATMENT

There is no effective cure for oral herpes simplex infections, but in some cases acyclovir may shorten the healing time for individual episodes. The optimum dosage of oral acyclovir has yet to be determined, but 1000 mg to 1200 mg (200 mg 5 or 6 times a day) may be useful in shortening the duration of oral lesions. Recurrent outbreaks of acyclovir-resistant herpes have been reported, including a case of an acyclovir-resistant oral HSV infection involving the facial skin, lips, nose, and mouth. After treatment with foscarnet, the lesions resolved.[16]

PROGNOSTIC SIGNIFICANCE

There is no known association between recurrent intraoral herpes and more rapid progression of HIV infection to AIDS. However, there is a clinical impression that recurrent HSV infections may be fairly common in patients with AIDS and other symptomatic HIV disease.[17]

■ HERPES ZOSTER

Herpes zoster (shingles) is caused by the varicella zoster virus (VZV). The disease is seen in the elderly and the immunosuppressed.

CLINICAL FEATURES

Oral herpes zoster is generally associated with skin lesions. There may be a prodrome of pain followed by multiple vesicles appearing on the facial skin, lips, and oral mucosa. Skin and oral lesions are frequently unilateral and follow the distribution of the maxillary and/or mandibular branches of the trigeminal nerve. The skin lesions form crusts and the oral lesions coalesce to form large ulcers. The ulcers frequently affect the gingiva, so tooth pain may be an early complaint.

DIFFERENTIAL DIAGNOSIS

The appearance of the lesions and their distribution are pathognomonic.

TREATMENT

Acyclovir may be useful in limiting the duration of the lesions.

■ HUMAN PAPILLOMAVIRUS LESIONS

Oral warts, papillomas, skin warts, and genital warts are associated with the human papillomavirus (HPV).[10] Anal warts have frequently been reported among homosexual men.[11]

CLINICAL FEATURES

Human papillomavirus lesions in the oral cavity may appear as solitary or multiple nodules. They may be sessile or pedunculated and appear as multiple, smooth-surfaced raised masses resembling focal epithelial hyperplasia or as multiple, small papilliferous or cauliflower-like projections (see color plate 5.2.1.c). Human papillomavirus types 7, 13, and 32 have been identified by this author in some of these oral warts.[18] Because the HPV types that have been found in HIV-infected individuals do not appear to be associated with anogenital warts, the term condyloma acuminata should probably not be used to describe them.

DIFFERENTIAL DIAGNOSIS

A biopsy is necessary for determining the histologic diagnosis. There is no known association between oral HPV lesions and more rapid progression of HIV disease to AIDS, but oral warts seem to be more common in HIV-infected individuals than in the general population.

TREATMENT

Oral HPV lesions can be treated surgically using local anesthetic. Carbon dioxide laser surgery is sometimes useful for multiple flat warts, but relapses occur and several repeat procedures may be necessary.

■ PERIODONTAL DISEASE

HIV-associated periodontal disease appears to be a fairly common problem in both asymptomatic and symptomatic patients. These conditions have been termed HIV-gingivitis (HIV-G) and HIV-periodontitis (HIV-P) because their presenting clinical features are often different from those in non-HIV-infected individuals.

CLINICAL FEATURES

HIV-G and HIV-P often occur in clean mouths where very little plaque or calculus is found to account for the gingivitis. The onset is often sudden and there is a rapid loss of bone and soft tissue. In HIV gingivitis, the gingiva may be reddened and edematous (see color plate 5.2.1.d). Patients sometimes complain of spontaneous bleeding. In acute-onset ulcerative gingivitis, ulcers occur at the tips of the interdental papilla and along the gingival margins. There are often complaints of severe pain. The ulcers heal, leaving the gingival papillae with a characteristic cratered appearance.

HIV-associated periodontitis may present as rapid loss of supporting bone and soft tissue. Typically, these losses occur simultaneously with no formation of gingival pockets. Sometimes only isolated areas of the mouth are involved.

Teeth may loosen and eventually fall out, but uninvolved sites can appear healthy. Necrotizing stomatitis may develop and areas of necrotic bone may appear along the gingival margin. The bone may eventually sequestrate. Patients with HIV-P and necrotizing stomatitis frequently complain of extreme pain and spontaneous bleeding.[18]

DIFFERENTIAL DIAGNOSIS

Diagnosis is made from the patient's history and clinical appearance. It is sometimes difficult to distinguish this type of periodontal disease from non-HIV-related disease. However, the complaints of severe pain, rapid onset, and rapid destruction in an often extremely clean mouth are unusual for non-HIV-related periodontal disease.[19,20]

TREATMENT

Patients may need to be referred to a periodontist. Penicillin is usually not helpful in controlling the disease. Reasonable success has been achieved using the following protocol: local debridement, irrigation with povidone-iodine, scaling and root planing, and maintenance with a chlorhexidine mouth rinse (Peridex-R). Recent studies show that the addition of chlorhexidine to this regimen produces significant improvement in periodontal condition. In some cases of necrotizing stomatitis, metronidazole (250 mg 4 times a day for 4 days) has proved helpful in managing the acute phase.[21-24]

DIFFERENT COURSE IN HIV INFECTION

The microbiology of periodontal disease in HIV-infected patients has not been fully described. Recurrences of acute episodes are common and response to conventional treatment may be poor. However, therapeutic strategies and frequent recall appointments can produce effective local treatment of patients' HIV-G and HIV-P.[23] There is as yet no known relationship between these conditions and the progression of HIV disease to AIDS.

■ ORAL ULCERATION

Oral ulcers resembling recurrent aphthous ulcers (RAU) are being reported with increasing frequency in HIV-infected persons. The cause of these ulcers is unknown, although many factors, including stress and infectious agents, have been suggested. In HIV-infected patients, the ulcers are well-circumscribed with erythematous margins. Minor, major, and herpetiform ulcers have been observed. The ulcers of the minor RAU type may appear as solitary lesions about 0.5 cm to 1 cm in size. The herpetiform type appear as clusters of small ulcers (1 mm to 2 mm), usually seen on the soft palate and oropharynx. The major RAU type appears as extremely large necrotic ulcers 2 cm to 4 cm in size. These are very painful and may persist for several weeks.[25]

DIAGNOSIS

The ulcers may present a diagnostic problem. Herpetiform RAU may resemble the lesions of Coxsackie virus infection, and major RAU may require biopsy to exclude malignancy, such as lymphoma. The ulcers usually occur on non-keratinized mucosa; this characteristic differentiates these ulcers from those caused by herpes simplex.

TREATMENT

The RAU-type ulcers usually respond well to topical steroids. Lidex ointment (0.05 percent) mixed with 50 percent Orabase should be applied five to six times per day. Decadron elixir used as a mouth rinse and then expectorated is helpful for multiple ulcers and for those where Lidex in Orabase is hard to apply. Cases have been reported of HIV-infected persons with oral and gastrointestinal aphthous-like ulcers. Systemic therapy (prednisone 40 to 60 mg/day for 7 to 10 days) has proven helpful in such cases.[26]

REFERENCES

1. Greenspan JS. Oral and dental diseases. In: Stites D, Stobo JD, Fudenberg HH, Wells JV, eds. Basic immunology. 6th ed. Los Altos, Calif.: Lange Medical Publishers, 1987:652-68.

2. Epstein JB, Truelove EL, Izutzu KT. Oral candidiasis: pathogenesis and host defense. Rev Infect Dis 1984; 6:96-106.

3. Greenspan D, Greenspan JS. Oral mucosal infection of AIDS? Dermatol Clin 1987; 5:733-7.

4. Pindborg JJ, Rindum J, Schiodt M, et al. Suggestion for a classification of oral candidiasis in patients with AIDS, ARC, and serum antibodies for LAV/HTLV III. J Dent Res 1986; 65:765. abstract.

5. Greenspan D, Pindborg JJ, Greenspan JS, Schiodt M. AIDS and the dental team. Copenhagen: Munksgaard, 1986:36-41.

6. Chandrasekar PH, Molinari JA. Oral candidiasis: forerunner of acquired immunodeficiency syndrome (AIDS)? Oral Surg Oral Med Oral Pathol 1985; 60:532-4.

7. Reichart PA, Gelderblom HR, Becker J, Kuntz A. AIDS and the oral cavity. The HIV infection: virology, etiology, origin, immunology, precautions and clinical observations in 110 patients. Int J Oral Maxillofac Surg 1987; 16:129-53.

8. Klein RS, Harris CA, Small CB, et al. Oral candidiasis in high-risk patients as the initial manifestation of the acquired immunodeficiency syndrome. N Engl J Med 1984; 311:354-8.

9. Tavitian A, Raufman JP, Rosenthal LE. Oral candidiasis as a marker for esophageal candidiasis in the acquired immunodeficiency syndrome. Ann Intern Med 1986; 104:54-5.

10. Scully C, Prime S, Maitland N. Papillomaviruses: their possible role in oral disease. Oral Surg Oral Med Oral Pathol 1985; 60:166-74.

11. Owen WF. Sexually transmitted diseases and traumatic problems in homosexual men. Ann Intern Med 1980; 92:805-8.

12. Volpe F, Schwimmer A, Barr C. Oral manifestations of disseminated *Mycobacterium avium intracellulare* in a patient with AIDS. Oral Surg Oral Med Oral Pathol 1985; 60:567-70.

13. Fowler CB, Nelson JR, Smith BR. A case of acquired immunodeficiency syndrome presented as a palatal perforation: report of a case and review of the literature. 40th Meeting of the American Association of Oral Pathologists. Toronto, 1986.

14. Glick M, Cohen SG, Cheney RT, et al. Oral manifestations of disseminated *Cryptococcus neoformans* in a patient with acquired immunodeficiency syndrome. Oral Surg Oral Med Oral Pathol 1987; 64:454-9.

15. Fung JC, Shanley J, Tilton RC. Comparison of the detection of herpes simplex virus in direct clinical specimens with herpes simplex virus-specific DNA probes and monoclonal antibodies. J Clin Microbiol 1985; 22:748-53.

16. MacPhail LA, Greenspan D, Schiodt M, et al. Acyclovir-resistant, foscarnet-sensitive oral herpes simplex type 2 lesion in a patient with AIDS. Oral Surg Oral Med Oral Pathol (in press).

17. Quinnan GV Jr, Masur H, Rook AH, et al. Herpes virus infections in the acquired immunodeficiency syndrome. JAMA 1984; 252:72-7.

18. Greenspan D, de Villiers EM, DeSouza Y, Greenspan JS. Unusual HPV types in oral warts in association with HIV infection. J Oral Path (in press).

19. Winkler JR, Murray PA. Periodontal disease. A potential intraoral expression of AIDS may be rapidly progressive periodontitis. CDA J 1987; 15:20-4.

20. Winkler JR, Grassi M, Murray PA. Periodontal disease in HIV-infected male homosexuals [Abstract]. III International Conference on AIDS. Washington, D.C., 1987:WP.144.

21. Murray PA, Grieve WG, Winkler JR. The humoral immune response in HIV-associated periodontitis [Abstract]. III International Conference on AIDS. Washington, D.C., 1987:THP.142.

22. Winkler JR, Grassi M, Murray PA. Clinical description and etiology of HIV-associated periodontal disease. In: Robertson PB, Greenspan JS, eds. Oral manifestations of AIDS. PSG Publishing Co., Inc., 1988.

23. Murray PA, Holt S. Microbiology of HIV-associated gingivitis and periodontitis. In: Robertson PB, Greenspan JS, eds. Oral manifestations of AIDS. PSG Publishing Co., Inc., 1988.

24. Grassi M, Williams CA, Winkler JR, Murray PA. Management of HIV-associated periodontal diseases. In: Robertson PB, Greenspan JS, eds. Oral manifestations of AIDS. PSG Publishing Co., Inc., 1988.

25. MacPhail LA, Greenspan D, Greenspan JS. Oral and pharyngeal ulcers in HIV-infected individuals. J Dent Res 1989; 68:415. abstract.

26. Bach MC, Howell DA, Valenti AJ, et al. Aphthous ulcerations of the gastrointestinal tract in patients with AIDS [Abstract]. V International Conference on AIDS. Montreal, 1989; M.B.P.247.

The Mouth:
Tumors, Idiopathic
Thrombocytopenic Purpura,
and Salivary Gland Disease

Deborah Greenspan, B.D.S.

■ KAPOSI'S SARCOMA

Kaposi's sarcoma (KS) may occur intraorally, either alone or in association with skin and disseminated lesions. Intraoral lesions have been reported in patients with lesions at other sites, but they may also be the first manifestation.[4]

Clinical Features. KS can appear as a red, blue, or purplish lesion. It may be flat or raised, solitary or multiple. The most common oral site is the hard palate, but lesions may be found on any part of the oral mucosa, including the gingiva, soft palate, and buccal mucosa (see color plate 5.2.2.a).

Differential Diagnosis. KS must be distinguished from hematomas, hemangiomas, vascular tumors, and pyogenic granulomas. Diagnosis is made by histologic examination. There are usually no bleeding problems associated with a biopsied oral KS lesion. However, it may be necessary to carefully distinguish the lesion from a vascular lesion such as a hematoma, hemangioma, other vascular neoplasm, or pigmented lesion. Prior aspiration may be helpful. Often the lesion appears suddenly. Early and late lesions can differ histologically, and early lesions may be difficult to diagnose because they resemble endothelial proliferation.[1] Once a patient has been diagnosed with KS, he or she should be referred for evaluation of HIV disease and appropriate treatment.[2]

Treatment. The prognostic significance of a KS diagnosis is discussed elsewhere. Localized therapy for oral KS lesions may be indicated if they become large and interfere with eating and talking.[2] Surgical management with the carbon dioxide laser may be indicated if the lesions are not overly vascular. Intralesion chemotherapy has been reported as effective in some cases. Radiation therapy may be indicated for large multiple lesions. However, a very severe and rapid onset of mucositis often occurs with radiation therapy.[3] The degree of mucositis is frequently out of proportion to the radiation dosage. However, severe mucositis can be minimized by using either a lower dosage over a longer period or doses of only 800 rads (Quivey J: personal communication).

■ LYMPHOMA

Clinical Features. Diffuse, undifferentiated non-Hodgkin's lymphoma (NHL) is a frequent HIV-associated malignancy. Lymphoma can occur anywhere in the oral cavity. There may be soft-tissue involvement with or without involvement of underlying bone. The lesion may present as a firm, painless swelling that may be ulcerated.

Differential Diagnosis.   Oral NHL lesions may be solitary and may some-times mimic dental infection. Diagnosis is made by histologic examination of biopsy specimens.

Treatment.   After diagnosis, the patient should be referred for evaluation of HIV disease and for treatment.

■ SQUAMOUS-CELL CARCINOMA

Several cases of squamous-cell carcinoma have been described in young homo-sexual men. These findings indicate an increased risk in this age group.[5,6] How-ever, there is no clear evidence to suggest that this increased incidence is directly related to HIV infection.

Clinical Features.   Squamous-cell carcinoma can appear as a red, white, or red-and-white area, or as an ulcer. The lesion can be raised or flat.

Differential Diagnosis.   Squamous-cell carcinoma must be differentiated from erythroplakia, leukoplakia, recurrent aphthous ulcer, and traumatic ul-cers. Diagnosis depends upon a histologic examination of biopsy specimens.

Treatment.   After diagnosis, the patient should be referred to an otorhino-laryngologist and radiation oncologist for treatment. There are no published data indicating whether the course of this tumor is different in HIV-infected patients than in non-HIV-infected patients.

■ IDIOPATHIC THROMBOCYTOPENIC PURPURA

Idiopathic thrombocytopenic purpura (ITP) has been described in relation to HIV infection. Oral lesions may be the first manifestation of this condition.

Clinical Features.   Petechiae, ecchymoses, and hematoma can occur any-where on the oral mucosa. Spontaneous bleeding from the gingiva can occur and patients may report finding blood in their mouths on waking.

Differential Diagnosis.   Idiopathic thrombocytopenic purpura must be dis-tinguished from other vascular lesions and KS. When ITP is suspected, blood and platelet counts should be obtained before other diagnostic procedures are performed. Treatment and prognostic significance are discussed elsewhere.

■ SALIVARY GLAND DISEASE

Salivary gland disease associated with HIV infection can present as xerostomia with or without salivary gland enlargement. Salivary gland enlargement has been reported in children and adults with HIV infection. The parotid gland is usually involved. Recently, Schiodt and others found that 9 of 12 patients (11 adults and 1 child) with HIV salivary gland disease had salivary gland enlarge-ment. Three had xerostomia. Biopsies from these patients' labial salivary glands showed histologic features similar to those seen in Sjögren's syndrome. No evidence of Epstein–Barr virus or cytomegalovirus was found.[7]

REFERENCES

1. Silverman S Jr, Migliorati CA, Lozada-Nur F, et al. Oral findings in people with or at high risk for AIDS: a study of 375 homosexual males. J Am Dent Assoc 1986; 112:187-92.

2. Ficarra G, Berson AM, Silverman S Jr, et al. Kaposi's sarcoma of the oral cavity: a study of 134 patients with a review of the pathogenesis, epidemiology, clinical aspects, and treatment. Oral Surg Oral Med Oral Pathol 1988; 66:543-50.

3. Watkins EB, Findlay P, Gelmann E, et al. Enhanced mucosal reactions in AIDS patients receiving oropharyngeal irradiation. Int J Radiat Oncol Biol Phys 1987; 13:1403-8.

4. Green TL, Beckstead JH, Lozada-Nur F, et al. Histopathologic spectrum of oral Kaposi's sarcoma. Oral Surg Oral Med Oral Pathol 1984; 58:306-14.

5. Marcusen DC, Sooy CD. Otolaryngologic and head and neck manifestations of acquired immunodeficiency syndrome (AIDS). Laryngoscope 1985; 95:401-5.

6. Greenspan JS, Silverman S Jr, Greenspan D. HIV infection and oral cancer [Abstract]. IV International Conference on AIDS. Stockholm, 1988; 2:2663.

7. Schiodt M, Greenspan D, Daniels TE, et al. Parotid gland enlargement and xerostomia associated with labial sialadenitis in HIV-infected patients. In: 2nd International Symposium on Sjögren's Syndrome. J Autoimmun (in press).

The Mouth: Hairy Leukoplakia and Epstein–Barr Virus

Deborah Greenspan, B.D.S.

■ ORAL HAIRY LEUKOPLAKIA

Oral hairy leukoplakia (HL) is a white lesion found predominantly on the lateral margins of the tongue. It was first seen in San Francisco in 1981 and reported in 1983.[1] Cases have now been reported from many parts of the world, including Africa.[2] Hairy leukoplakia has been seen in all the risk groups for HIV infection. Evidence for HIV infection has been found whenever it has been sought in patients with HL, and the condition thus appears to be a sign of HIV disease.[3,5] Rare cases have been reported in non-HIV-infected patients who are also immunosuppressed.[15]

CLINICAL APPEARANCE AND MANIFESTATIONS

The HL lesion can vary in size and appearance. It may be unilateral or bilateral. The lesions are white and can be small with fine corrugations. Some areas may be smooth and flat. The surface is irregular and may have prominent folds or projections, sometimes markedly resembling hairs. Lesions are found on the lateral margins of the tongue and may spread to cover the entire dorsal surface (see color plates 5.2.3.a and 5.2.3.b). They may also spread downwards onto the ventral surface of the tongue, where they usually have a flat appearance. Hairy leukoplakia lesions can also occur on the buccal mucosa, generally as flat lesions.[1] Patients are usually asymptomatic.

HAIRY LEUKOPLAKIA AND CANDIDIASIS

Candida albicans may be found in association with many HL lesions when cultured and smeared. Hyphae can be seen in PAS-stained sections. Administration of extensive antifungal therapy may change the appearance of the lesions but does not cause them to disappear.

Differential Diagnosis. Hairy leukoplakia lesions should be diagnosed by biopsy when possible to distinguish them from chronic candidiasis and other white lesions, such as lichen planus, squamous-cell carcinoma, and leukoplakia. In a known HIV-infected individual, biopsy is indicated if there is any doubt about the diagnosis.

Histopathology. The typical microscopic appearance of HL includes acanthosis, marked parakeratosis with the formation of ridges and keratin projections, areas of ballooning cells, and little or no inflammation in the connective tissue. The ballooning changes resemble koilocytosis. Cells are enlarged; some contain enlarged ballooning cells with pyknotic nuclei. Some contain peri-nuclear haloes.

HL is probably a viral-induced lesion. The authors have identified Epstein–Barr virus (EBV) in HL tissue.[8] An immunohistochemical investigation using peroxidase antiperoxidase and an antiserum to papillomavirus capsid antigen showed nuclear staining for papillomavirus antigen.[1]

Electron Microscopy.   In electronmicroscopic specimens, investigators have found structures consistent with a herpes group virus.[1] The structure consisted of 100 nm intranuclear virions and 240 nm encapsulated virus particles. Other structures are 48- to 52-nm particles visible in the suprabasal layer. Closer to specimen surfaces, where the nuclei are more condensed, arrays of these particles were seen and herpes group particles appeared in the same cell.[1] Several studies have described the appearance of these particles in HL biopsies.[6,7]

TREATMENT

Hairy leukoplakia is asymptomatic and does not require treatment. Patients with HL should be referred for evaluation of HIV disease and appropriate treatment. Occasionally, *Candida albicans* may be found in HL lesions. Treatment consists of antifungal medications. HL has disappeared in patients receiving high-dose acyclovir for herpes zoster.[10,11] Temporary elimination or almost complete clinical resolution of the lesion has occurred in patients treated with the experimental drug desciclovir in preliminary trials. Desciclovir is an analog of acyclovir. It is given orally and produces titers equivalent to intravenous acyclovir. However, HL lesions recurred one to four months after desciclovir treatment ended.[12] There are case reports of HL disappearing during treatment with ganciclovir, zidovudine, and aerosolized pentamidine. However, no case–control studies are available.

HAIRY LEUKOPLAKIA AND AIDS

Epidemiologically, HL appears to occur at the same time in the course of HIV infection as candidiasis.[13] A study showed that 48 percent of patients with hairy leukoplakia developed AIDS within 16 months of HL diagnosis.[4] More recently, a study reported that approximately 57 percent of patients with HL developed AIDS within 48 months of HL diagnosis.[14] Diagnosis of hairy leukoplakia, then, is an indication of both HIV infection and immunodeficiency. Its presence is an indication for a workup to evaluate and treat HIV disease.

■ EPSTEIN–BARR VIRUS

No evidence has been found of herpes simplex, varicella zoster, or cytomegalovirus in specimens investigated with a number of immunohistochemical techniques. However, strong evidence was found for the presence of EBV.[8] Anticomplement immunofluorescence with human reference sera containing antibodies to Epstein–Barr viral capsid antigen produced distinctive nuclear staining in 19 of 21 specimens. Control specimens included non-lesional mucosa from the same patients as well as biopsy specimens of other oral diseases. Southern blot hybridization with probes for EBV revealed the typical EBV-specific pattern. Reconstruction hybridization studies indicated that more than

200 viral molecules per cellular genome were present in many cases. Non-lesional biopsies from the same patient were negative.

The entire EBV genome is apparently present in the lesions. This was determined by isolating DNA from specimens and hybridizing it to Southern blots containing many different fragments of EBV DNA. They revealed hybridization at many positions on the blot, indicating many genomic components. Finally, hybridization of HL-lesion DNA, using a probe that recognized both ends of the EBV genome, revealed the pattern of linear EBV DNA. Antibody to EBV antigens was of a specificity and titer similar to antibody found in male homosexuals in San Francisco. Intraepithelial Langerhans' cells are reduced or absent in the HL lesion, and this decrease correlates with the presence of viral antigens.[9]

REFERENCES

1. Greenspan D, Greenspan JS, Conant M, et al. Oral "hairy" leukoplakia in male homosexuals: evidence of association with papillomavirus and a herpes group virus. Lancet 1984; 2:831-6.
2. Schiodt M, Pindborg JJ. AIDS and the oral cavity. Epidemiology and clinical oral manifestations of human immune deficiency virus infection: a review. Int J Oral Maxillofac Surg 1987; 16:1.
3. Greenspan JS, Mastrucci MT, Leggott PJ, et al. Hairy leukoplakia in a child. AIDS 1988; 2:143.
4. Greenspan D, Greenspan JS, Hearst NG, et al. Relation of hairy leukoplakia to infection with the human immunodeficiency virus and the risk of developing AIDS. J Infect Dis 1987; 155:475-81.
5. Greenspan D, Hollander H, Friedman-Kien A, et al. Oral hairy leukoplakia in two women, a haemophiliac and a transfusion recipient. Lancet 1986; 2:978-9.
6. Belton CM, Eversole LR. Oral "hairy" leukoplakia: ultrastructural features. J Oral Pathol 1986; 15:493-9.
7. Kansas RJ, Abrams AM, Jensen JL, et al. Oral hairy leukoplakia: ultrastructural observations. Oral Surg Oral Med Oral Pathol 1988; 65:333-8.
8. Greenspan JS, Greenspan D, Lennette ET, et al. Replication of Epstein–Barr virus within the epithelial cells of oral "hairy" leukoplakia, an AIDS-associated lesion. N Engl J Med 1985; 313:1564-71.
9. Daniels TE, Greenspan D, Greenspan JS, et al. Absence of Langerhans' cells in oral hairy leukoplakia, an AIDS-associated lesion. J Invest Dermatol 1987; 89:178.
10. Friedman-Kien AE. Viral origin of hairy leukoplakia. Lancet 1986; 2:694.
11. Resnick L, Herbst JS, Ablashi DV, et al. Regression of oral hairy leukoplakia after orally administered acyclovir therapy. JAMA 1988; 259:384-8.
12. Greenspan D, Greenspan JS, Chapman S, et al. Efficacy of BWA515U in treatment of EBV infection in hairy leukoplakia [Abstract]. III International Conference on AIDS. Washington, D.C., 1987; MP.223,47.
13. Feigal DW, Overby GL, Greenspan D, et al. Early oral lesions found in community cohorts: Is hairy leukoplakia more common than candidiasis? [Abstract]. IV International Conference on AIDS. Stockholm, 1988; 2:7582.
14. Greenspan D, Feigal DW, Greenspan JS, et al. Hairy leukoplakia and AIDS [Abstract]. IV International Conference on AIDS. Stockholm, 1988; 2:7795.
15. Greenspan D, Greenspan JS, de Souza Y, et al. Oral hairy leukoplakia in an HIV-negative renal transplant recipient. J Oral Pathol Med 1989; 18:32-4.

5.3

Dermatologic Aspects

5.3.1   Dermatologic Manifestations of HIV Infection — *Berger*

Dermatologic Manifestations of HIV Infection

Timothy G. Berger, M.D.

H IV-infected persons commonly have cutaneous abnormalities.[1,2] When observed for several months, almost 100 percent of such patients manifest skin disease.[3]

Some of the conditions seen are unique and pathognomonic for this disease — for example, Kaposi's sarcoma. More commonly, the conditions are nonspecific, looking similar in HIV-infected and non-HIV-infected individuals. However, HIV-infected individuals often have several simultaneous or sequential cutaneous conditions that are the key to suspecting underlying HIV infection.

In general, these cutaneous abnormalities are not prognostic of the level of immunosuppression. They may identify those at risk for the more rapid appearance of symptomatic HIV infection or AIDS (e.g., herpes zoster).[4] Cutaneous abnormalities may worsen as the disease progresses (i.e., seborrheic dermatitis, xerosis) or they may arise as fulminant infections following immunization. In at least one case, an asymptomatic U.S. Army recruit given vaccinia immunization developed widespread infection with the virus.[5] In general, however, live-virus immunization is tolerated by HIV-infected individuals.[6]

Cutaneous abnormalities are divided into two large groups: infectious and noninfectious. When appropriate, a more complete discussion of the differential diagnosis is included below.

■ DERMATOLOGIC MANIFESTATIONS OF *STAPHYLOCOCCUS AUREUS*

Staphylococcus aureus is the most common cause of cutaneous bacterial infection in HIV-infected individuals. Infection may occur before any other signs or symptoms of HIV infection. The following morphologic patterns may be present: bullous impetigo, ecthyma, folliculitis, hidradenitis-like plaques, abscesses, and cellulitis.

DIAGNOSIS

Bullous Impetigo. Bullous impetigo is most common in hot humid weather, presenting as very superficial blisters or erosions, most commonly seen in the groin or axilla. Since the blisters are so flaccid, they are very short-lived; often only erosions or yellow crusts are present. These lesions closely mimic cutaneous candidiasis.[7]

Ecthyma. Ecthyma is an eroded or superficially ulcerated lesion with a very adherent crust. If this crust is removed, a plane of purulent material teeming with staphylococci can often be found. Removal of this crust is necessary to treat the lesion topically.

Folliculitis.   Folliculitis due to *S. aureus* occurs most commonly in the hairy areas of the groin, axilla, or face (especially in men who shave). Follicular pustules are the primary lesion. Gram's stain and culture should be obtained to confirm the diagnosis and to allow selection of appropriate antibiotic therapy, such as dicloxacillin (500 mg 4 times a day). Often the follicular lesions are intensely pruritic, so other pruritic dermatoses like scabies may be suspected.[7] Occasionally follicular lesions will extend more deeply, forming abscesses. Rarely, all follicles across several square centimeters are infected, forming a large, violaceous, hidradenitis-like plaque. The plaque may be studded with pustules and have deep tracts connecting infected follicles. Their appearance may mimic Kaposi's sarcoma, but in KS overlying pustules are quite unusual (see color plates 5.3.1.a and 5.3.1.b).

TREATMENT

The treatment of cutaneous staphylococcal infections is determined by the depth of the infection. Very superficial lesions, like bullous impetigo, often respond to 7 to 10 days of an appropriate antistaphylococcal antibiotic, such as dicloxacillin (500 mg 4 times daily). Deeper lesions often require courses of treatment lasting for months. In addition, combinations of antibiotics, especially a penicillinase-resistant penicillin or cephalosporin plus rifampin (600 mg once daily), are often necessary to clear the infection. Adjunctive topical therapy is helpful in beginning treatment and reducing recurrences. Washing the infected area with an antibacterial agent (Hibiclens, Betadine, or benzoyl peroxide wash) helps remove crusts, dries lesions, and decreases surface bacterial concentration, thus reducing infectiousness. Topical antibiotics (clindamycin 1 percent or erythromycin 2 percent solutions) may be used regularly in chronically infected areas. Loculated abscesses must be incised and drained when fluctuant in order for antibiotics to be effective. When cellulitis of any significance or symptoms of bacteremia are present, hospital admission for treatment with intravenous antibiotics is appropriate. Since relapses and recurrences are common, regular washing with antibacterial soaps is often indicated.

Not all folliculitides in HIV-infected individuals are caused by bacteria. Culture-negative folliculitis is common and may demonstrate either polymorphonuclear leukocytes or eosinophils[8] on biopsy. These lesions are quite pruritic and are often very resistant to treatment.

■ CAT-SCRATCH DISEASE

Recently, a small gram-negative bacterium was identified in the primary skin lesions and involved lymph nodes of individuals with cat-scratch disease. Although usually restricted to these two sites in immunocompetent individuals, widespread infection can occur, if rarely. In San Francisco over the past three years, we have identified 15 individuals with HIV infection and cutaneous lesions containing a similar bacterium.[9,10] At least three of these patients also had osseous lesions. The condition was initially reported as atypical subcutaneous infection in AIDS patients[11] and as epithelioid angiomatosis.[12] Additional reports support the conclusion that this is not a rare condition.[13]

DIAGNOSIS

Clinically, the most characteristic lesions resemble pyogenic granulomas — fleshy, friable, protuberant papules-to-nodules that tend to bleed very easily (see color plate 5.3.1.c). In addition, deep cellulitic plaques, nodules, and lesions resembling folliculitis may occur. Lesions number from a few to hundreds. In addition to the skin, mucosal surfaces and bone may be involved. Angritt at the Armed Forces Institute of Pathology has demonstrated similar organisms in the lymph node, liver, and spleen.[14] Clinically, the lesions are frequently misdiagnosed as vascular tumors, especially Kaposi's sarcoma. Histologically, the lesions are characterized by a prominent vascular proliferation that forms an elevated papule (see color plate 5.3.1.d). Neutrophilic leukocytes are prominent in the interstitium. Basophilic aggregates are found adjacent to the vascular lumina, representing collections of the bacterium. The diagnosis is confirmed by identifying the causative organism in affected tissue using silver stains and electron microscopy. A reproducible method of culturing the organism is not yet available.

TREATMENT

Treating affected patients with erythromycin in full doses (500 mg 4 times daily for weeks to months) will lead to resolution of the lesions, as may rifampin. If the patient has only a few lesions, surgical removal may be curative. Unlike Kaposi's sarcoma, the cat-scratch lesions have not responded to radiation therapy. Two patients gave a history of cat exposure prior to the onset of their disease.

■ DERMATOLOGIC MANIFESTATIONS OF *PSEUDOMONAS AERUGINOSA*

Information on *Pseudomonas aeruginosa* infections in HIV-infected individuals is limited to anecdotal evidence. No studies have been conducted on this infection in AIDS patients, but we have diagnosed and treated several cases at San Francisco General Hospital.

Chronic ulcerations and macerated skin are susceptible to colonization by gram-negative bacteria, especially *P. aeruginosa*. We have seen one AIDS patient with chronic leg ulcers due to excoriation and folliculitis who developed pseudomonas overgrowth. He responded very slowly to intravenous antibiotics and local acetic-acid soaks. Two other patients developed macerated toe webs that became colonized with *P. aeruginosa*.[15] One died of pseudomonas sepsis, underscoring the potential danger of this usually benign condition for AIDS patients. A third patient developed pseudomonas sepsis while on zidovudine (AZT), including multiple subcutaneous nodules. These became fluctuant and required surgical drainage.[16] A fourth patient on ganciclovir (DHPG) developed buttocks lesions resembling ecthyma gangrenosum on two occasions; both required wide surgical excision.

■ HERPES SIMPLEX VIRUS

Early in the AIDS epidemic, chronic persistent herpes simplex infection (HSV) was recognized in AIDS patients.[17] Today, this finding is an index infection in establishing an AIDS diagnosis.[18]

DIAGNOSIS

As long as HIV-infected individuals' immune systems are still reasonably intact, the course of genital and oral-facial HSV recurrences may be similar to those in non-HIV-infected individuals. Herpes simplex virus should be considered in evaluating all ulcerative lesions. Perirectal ulcers in particular should be examined for HSV.

Lesions appear as grouped blisters that rupture, crust, and heal in 7 to 10 days. Once HIV-infected individuals have become severely immunosuppressed, they experience chronic lesions that continue to expand and form large, crusted erosions 2 to 10 cm or larger in diameter (see color plate 5.3.1.e). Lesions may be quite painful, especially if located perianally or periorally. A Tzanck smear dried, taken from the edge of the ulcer and stained with Giemsa or methylene blue, may be positive for multinucleated giant cells, giving a rapid diagnosis. Alternatively, fluorescent antibody testing or viral culture should be performed. If these are negative and clinical suspicion of HSV is high, a biopsy of skin from the edge of the ulcer should be performed. A portion of the tissue should also be cultured for virus, which may be positive even when swab cultures are negative. In addition to routine histologic examination, special stains and cultures should be performed for other possible infecting organisms, including spirochetes.

TREATMENT

Oral acyclovir has been extremely useful in managing HSV infections in HIV-infected patients. In the immunocompetent HIV-infected patient, either intermittent or chronic suppressive therapy may be used. In the immunosuppressed patient with chronic ulcerative lesions, acyclovir (200 mg to 400 mg by mouth 5 times daily) is given. This is continued until the ulcers heal. This may take several weeks. Chronic suppressive therapy with acyclovir (400 mg by mouth 2 to 3 times daily) is then instituted to reduce recurrences.

SPREADING, NECROTIZING, AND DISSEMINATED HSV INFECTIONS

Untreated lesions tend to enlarge slowly. New lesions at distant sites may appear, probably by cross-contamination rather than by hematogenous spread. It is unusual for herpes infections to disseminate even in immunosuppressed individuals.

Herpes simplex virus may rarely cause a necrotizing folliculitis that appears as 0.2 cm to 1 cm papules with firm central crusts. A biopsy is usually required to establish the diagnosis, since the site of infection is the epithelium along the hair shaft in the dermis.

ACYCLOVIR-RESISTANT HSV INFECTION

We have seen several individuals with large chronic perianal ulcers due to thymidine kinase-negative, acyclovir-resistant herpes simplex virus type 2.[19,20] This situation should be suspected when even high-dose intravenous acyclovir fails to improve the ulcers. The significance of acyclovir resistance in HIV-infected individuals is unknown.

■ HERPES ZOSTER INFECTION

DIAGNOSIS

Herpes zoster virus (HZV) infection is commonly seen during the course of HIV infection and is particularly common in healthy-appearing individuals before the onset of other symptoms.[4] Unlike zoster in non-HIV-infected individuals, in HIV-infected persons this dermatomal eruption may be particularly bullous, hemorrhagic, necrotic, and painful.

In individuals with normal immune systems, the duration of blisters and crusts is usually two or three weeks. This is also the approximate duration for significant pain, although intermittent paroxysms of pain may continue for a few more weeks. Scarring is minimal to mild. In severe cases, and occasionally in HIV-infected persons, excruciating and disabling pain may last for many months. In addition, necrotic lesions may last for up to six weeks and heal with severe scarring. This dermatomal scarring is characteristically seen in HIV-infected patients and should be looked for when evaluating at-risk individuals.

TREATMENT

Acyclovir. Treating HZV infection in HIV-infected patients is somewhat uncertain. Elderly individuals without HIV infection are often given relatively high-dose oral corticosteroids for several weeks to prevent post-zoster neuralgia, although the efficacy of this treatment is controversial. Younger individuals, which AIDS patients usually are, are not usually given systemic steroids, because the likelihood of post-zoster neuralgia is low. In addition, corticosteroids may cause immunosuppression in HIV-infected patients who are already immunosuppressed or at risk for immunosuppression.

High levels of acyclovir (achieved by intravenous administration) shorten the course of herpes zoster in immunocompromised patients. It is uncertain whether these serum levels can be achieved with an oral regimen, thus avoiding hospitalization for intravenous treatment.

Oral acyclovir may be effective in treating HZV infection, but indications and dosage are uncertain. If acyclovir is given, it should be initiated as soon as possible. Recommended doses are much higher than those for herpes simplex because of the relative insensitivity of the zoster virus to this medication. At San Francisco General Hospital, we recommend doses of 800 mg orally four to six times daily for five days. If new blisters are still appearing after this time, five more days of treatment are prescribed. Some authors believe that intravenous administration is more effective than oral.[21] Fortunately, side effects from this drug are rare, even at these high doses.

Since acyclovir reduces the initial pain, speeds healing, and reduces the risk of HZV dissemination, patients with symptomatic HIV disease or AIDS should be treated with acyclovir as soon as HZV infection occurs. The method of administration is determined by the patient's immune status and the pattern of zoster. If the patient has a reasonably intact immune system and does not have clinical features of disseminated or visceral infection, and if lesions are not near the eye (trigeminal nerve), then oral acyclovir (in the doses mentioned above) is probably adequate and beneficial.

In cases of significant immunosuppression, disseminated or visceral lesions, and perhaps when zoster affects the ophthalmic branch of the trigeminal nerve (eyelid or tip of the nose especially), intravenous acyclovir (10 to 12 mg/kg 3 times daily) is indicated. The possible increased risk for herpetic keratitis, retinal vasculitis, and uveitis supports intravenous treatment of persons with such zoster infections.[24] Only intravenous acyclovir can be guaranteed to reach adequate plasma levels to inhibit all HZV strains. Treatment is continued until the lesions are well crusted (usually about seven days) after which the drug may be discontinued or oral acyclovir may be given in full doses to complete the therapy. Treatment should probably be continued for two weeks. Early and vigorous treatment prevents the severe necrotic forms of zoster and helps relieve the terrible pain that can occur. Acyclovir treatment probably does not reduce the risk of post-herpetic neuralgia.

We have seen two patients with chronic verrucous lesions due to HZV.[23] Others have also reported similar patients. These lesions occurred during acyclovir therapy and isolates have been acyclovir-resistant. The significance of this finding is unknown.

Other Treatment.   Other treatments for zoster consist mostly of analgesics and topical care of skin lesions. In mild cases, soap and water are adequate for bathing skin lesions, but in severe cases, compresses (two or three times a day) are recommended to help remove necrotic debris. These should probably be followed by the use of an antibiotic ointment such as Silvadene (silver sulfadiazine) or bacitracin, which keeps the scabs soft and helps prevent them from sticking to dressings. Antibiotic ointments may also prevent secondary infection. Capsaicin cream (Zostrix), a substance-P depletor,[22] may reduce both acute and chronic zoster pain.

■ DERMATOLOGIC MANIFESTATIONS OF MOLLUSCUM CONTAGIOSUM

CLINICAL PRESENTATION

Molluscum contagiosum is a superficial cutaneous viral infection manifested as small (2 to 3 mm) flesh-colored hemispherical papules. Characteristically, there is a faint whitish core in the center of each papule, some of which may be slightly umbilicated. This eruption is seen commonly in young children (ages 3 to 8 years), whose lesions are scattered widely over face, arms, and trunk. In adults, this mild infection is usually sexually transmitted and occurs in the pubic area. In the nonimmunosuppressed individual, lesions tend to last for 6 to 12 months and then spontaneously resolve when the host develops resistance to the virus.

At San Francisco General Hospital, we have found that 10 percent to 20 percent of patients with AIDS and symptomatic HIV disease develop lesions of molluscum contagiosum, often quite widespread and over 100 in number. The forehead, beard area, and upper trunk are commonly involved. This is usually a sign of significant immunosuppression, since asymptomatic HIV-infected individuals have a much lower incidence of infection than those with AIDS or symptomatic HIV.[25-27]

Medical personnel, such as nurses and physicians, do not need to take precautions other than handwashing, however, because casual contact does not result in infection.

TREATMENT

There are no known medical complications of molluscum contagiosum. It does not affect internal organs or even cause significant symptoms on the skin. The objective of treatment is therefore primarily cosmetic and preventive.

Individual lesions can easily be treated by light cryotherapy using liquid nitrogen. If that is not available, pricking the lesion with a large-gauge needle and removing the white core (molluscum body) is also effective. Topical application of a tiny drop of cantharidin to each lesion for three to six hours will often induce sufficient inflammation to eradicate the lesions. Complete cure is difficult to achieve, and treatment is usually restricted to bothersome or distressing lesions.

■ HUMAN PAPILLOMAVIRUS (WARTS)

Superficial cutaneous infection with papillomavirus — warts — occurs with increased frequency in immunosuppressed patients. Lesions may be extensive and resistant to therapy.

CLINICAL PRESENTATION

In HIV-infected patients, the lesions may look like those seen in nonimmunosuppressed patients. Very extensive infections mimicking epidermodysplasia verruciformis have also been seen, although rarely, in HIV-infected individuals. Symptoms seldom result from these infections, except that warts on the soles of the feet may occasionally cause the feeling of having a "rock in the shoe" when walking, and warts around the fingernails may sometimes cause pain when the patient grasps something.

TREATMENT

Treatment is primarily cosmetic. In patients with AIDS and symptomatic HIV disease, the results may be disappointing. Even in persons with normal immunity, relapse of warts after treatment is common. In immunosuppressed persons, this is even more the case; relapse is almost to be expected. Standard treatment includes liquid nitrogen cryotherapy, the use of which is restricted primarily because of discomfort. Topical "anti-wart" medications containing salicylic and lactic acids dissolve keratin, and help primarily by debulking the callous-like cap over the wart. They may lead to complete disappearance of the lesions, however. In general, the treatment outlook for warts is poor in immunosuppressed patients. Referral to a dermatologist may be appropriate to help with these annoying lesions.

HUMAN PAPILLOMAVIRUS AND SEXUALLY TRANSMITTED CANCERS

Condyloma accuminata are of special significance in HIV-infected individuals. Cervical dysplasia and carcinoma are now clearly associated with human papillomavirus (HPV) infection.[28] Like the cervix, the anorectal area has a "transformation zone." HPV infection is very common in the genital and perianal area of homosexual men, especially those practicing receptive anal intercourse. In these men, even when visible warts are not present, cytological dysplasia can be seen on smears.[29] Cervical dysplasia is also extremely common in HIV-infected women.[30] In addition, bowenoid dysplasia is seen in biopsy material of wart-like lesions (bowenoid papulosis) from the genital area of homosexual men.[31] This pattern correlates closely with the presence of potentially carcinogenic HPV type 16. Papillomavirus is also found in the anorectal carcinomas of homosexual men.[32] These data strongly support the concept that anorectal cancer, like cervical carcinoma, is a consequence of sexually transmitted disease. HPV may be the inducing agent and by itself may be sufficient to produce cancer. HIV infection may be a cofactor enhancing this effect.

Unfortunately, anorectal warts in HIV-infected men are difficult to eradicate.[33] Nonetheless, an attempt should be made to eliminate all warts, especially those that are potentially premalignant lesions. The degree of cytologic atypia seen on biopsied condylomata may identify at least a portion of those harboring HPV with malignant potential.[34] The future availability of HPV typing may guide us in therapy. Until that time, complete eradication of all anogenital warts in male and female HIV-infected individuals should be the goal. If this is impossible, then careful evaluation and close follow-up are clearly necessary to identify any genital neoplasms at the earliest and most treatable stage.

■ VIRAL INFECTIONS OF THE SKIN: ACUTE HIV EXANTHEM

In acute primary HIV infection, a rash may develop in addition to a mononucleosis-like illness. The frequency of the rash in acute HIV infection may be as high as 50 percent.[35-38]

The rash is described as macular, maculopapular, or roseola-like. It usually does not itch. The rash is widely distributed over the trunk and limbs and may involve palms and soles. A collarette of scale may be present at the periphery of the rash area. An associated enanthem of oral erythema or superficial erosions may be present. The exanthem and enanthem spontaneously resolve within one to two weeks.

These features are similar to other viral exanthems and are not specific for HIV infection. This syndrome should be considered when diagnosing at-risk individuals exhibiting symptoms of acute viral syndrome. Detection of HIV antigen by enzyme immunoassay (EIA) may confirm the diagnosis of acute HIV infection in HIV antibody-negative persons.[39]

■ CUTANEOUS MYCOBACTERIAL INFECTION

Infections with *Mycobacterium avium-intracellulare* and *Mycobacterium tuberculosis* are seen with increased frequency in AIDS patients. These infections may be disseminated, unusual, and severe.[40,41] Despite this, cutaneous lesions caused by these organisms are unusual. They commonly present as chronic sinuses over involved lymph nodes (scrofula), chronic ulcerations, or hemorrhagic macules.[2,42] All biopsies from AIDS patients should be examined with appropriate stains to rule out the presence of mycobacteria in the tissue. When present, organisms are usually abundant. There has been one patient reported with *M. marinum* infection presenting as ecthyma.[43]

■ FUNGAL AND YEAST INFECTIONS

SUPERFICIAL FUNGAL AND YEAST INFECTIONS

The most common form of yeast infection in HIV-infected persons is thrush. This may be accompanied by angular cheilitis fissuring, maceration, and erythema of the corners of the mouth. Treatment includes clotrimazole troches for oral thrush and an anticandidal agent, such as nystatin (e.g., Mycolog ointment) or an imidazole cream, for the affected lateral lips.

Other superficial yeast and fungal infections can be broken down into two sections: intertriginous infections and nail, paronychial, and foot infections.

INTERTRIGINOUS INFECTIONS

Intertriginous infection may be caused by either candida or tinea and involve the groin, axillary vault, or inframammary areas. In these areas, candida presents as a vivid red, slightly eroded eruption in the depths of the folds. The surface is wrinkled and a white membrane may coat the eroded surface. A hallmark of this rash is satellite pustules extending out centrifugally from the eroded areas. In males, the scrotum is involved. A mildly burning pain may cause as much complaint as the pruritus does.

Tinea in the groin is usually pruritic. The scrotum is spared. The depth of the folds may be clear, and a well-demarcated, annular patch expands down the upper thigh. In more extensive cases, the lesions may extend through the pubic hair onto the lower abdomen and buttocks.

Both candida and tinea are diagnosed by potassium hydroxide examination of scales taken from the active border or a satellite pustule. Topical treatment is usually adequate and involves the application twice daily of an imidazole cream (clotrimazole, miconazole, or ketoconazole). Candidal lesions may be moister, so drying soaks may initially be helpful. Eroded lesions in intertriginous areas are very tender, so topical solutions may burn. Treatment is continued for 10 to 14 days. Since relapses are common, intermittent prophylactic treatment may be required.

In my experience, most HIV-infected individuals referred for a refractory intertriginous eruption have seborrheic dermatitis or psoriasis of the groin. This presents as variable pruritic erythematous patches with a fine scale. There are no central clearing and no satellite pustules. Scrotal involvement occurs, but it is not erosive or tender.

Rarely, persistent groin rashes are due to tinea. Persistence is usually caused by prescribing the wrong medication (i.e., nystatin), using a strong steroid with the antifungal agent (i.e., Lotrisone), or trying to treat with oral ketoconazole alone. With oral ketoconazole, due to poor gastric acidity, tissue levels are insufficient.[51] Addition of a topical imidazole is dramatically beneficial.

Candida Infection of the Nails.   Nails may be affected by both candida and tinea. Candida almost always affects the fingernails, frequently presenting as a paronychia (inflammation of the tissues surrounding the nail). There is tenderness, erythema, and bogginess of the proximal nail fold. Purulent material may be expressible. Infection tends to be chronic, in which case the cuticle is lost and the nail plate may become ridged or dystrophic. Onycholysis (separation of the nail plate from the nail bed) may also be present. The nail plate itself is usually not invaded, so nail-thickening, opacity, and crumbling are unusual.

Exposure to water is a significant predisposing factor in candidal nail infection. Dishwashers, bartenders, and housewives are at increased risk. Topical imidazole in solution form or 2 percent to 4 percent thymol in chloroform twice daily is the initial therapy. The onycholytic nail must also be trimmed away so that the medication can be applied at the most proximal area of onycholysis. In refractory cases, ketoconazole (given orally in doses of 200 mg to 400 mg daily) is helpful. Regular monitoring of liver functions is necessary because of the rare possibility of hepatotoxicity.

Tinea Infection of the Nails, Feet, and Hands.   Tinea infection of the nails, feet, and hands is common in HIV-infected persons, but it is also common in the non-HIV-infected, so it is not a specific marker of HIV infection. Tinea of the nail, in contrast to candida, involves primarily the nail plate, favors the toenails over the fingernails, and does not cause acute paronychia. Nails become opaque, thickened, and may split or crumble. There is often an associated tinea infection of the soles or toe-webs, manifested by chronic maceration, scaling, blistering, and/or thickening of the skin. Occasionally the palms will be involved in a similar manner. Tinea is especially likely as a diagnosis if two feet and one hand are affected. Occasionally tinea will spread to hairy areas, especially the face and lower legs, causing chronic plaque-like folliculitis. This may easily be mistaken for a chronic bacterial infection. Previous use of topical steroids may induce this pattern and mask the correct diagnosis.

Tinea of the palms and soles is improved with topical imidazole therapy twice daily. Cure, even with oral antifungals (griseofulvin or ketoconazole), is unlikely for the toenails but possible for the fingernails if therapy is continued for several months. Since relapse is common, constant use of topical antifungals is often necessary.

DEEP (SYSTEMIC) FUNGAL INFECTIONS

The following systemic infections have been reported in patients with symptomatic HIV disease and AIDS: candidiasis, cryptococcosis, histoplasmosis, coccidioidomycosis, sporotrichosis, actinomycosis, and phaehyphomycosis.[44-53] Only the first three present significant dermatologic problems.

Cryptococcosis.   Cryptococcosis is common in AIDS patients, usually causing meningitis. Cutaneous lesions may precede or occur simultaneously with the central nervous system (CNS) disease. In non-AIDS HIV-infected patients, 10 percent to 20 percent of patients with disseminated cryptococcosis have skin lesions. Lesions appear anywhere on the body but are most common on the head and neck. They begin as painless erythematous or hyperpigmented papules that may progress to nodules or ulcers. Lesions may present as a cellulitis or resemble herpes simplex or molluscum contagiosum.[45,46,52] Diagnosis is established by skin biopsy, cultured and appropriately stained. Finding cryptococcosis in the skin is almost certainly an indication of disseminated infection, so appropriate workup, especially of the CNS, is mandatory.

Histoplasmosis.   Disseminated histoplasmosis is becoming an increasingly common problem in AIDS patients living in histoplasma-endemic areas — it occurred in over 5 percent of AIDS patients in one series from Houston, Texas.[53] Most cases probably represent reactivation of old histoplasmosis rather than dissemination of newly acquired infections. This explains cases now being seen in New York City, Los Angeles, and San Francisco among individuals who previously lived in areas endemic for the disease. Skin involvement is present in about 10 percent of AIDS patients with disseminated histoplasmosis.[53] The cutaneous lesions are not specific and present as erythematous macules, papules, maculopapular dermatitic lesions, pustules, acneiform lesions, ulcerations, and plaques. Histology of the skin demonstrates granulomas; organisms are easily seen with special stains (e.g., methenamine silver). Therefore, skin biopsy is a good way to diagnose disseminated histoplasmosis. Bone-marrow biopsy and culture are positive in 69 percent of cases and blood culture is positive in 27 percent of cases. About 10 percent of patients with disseminated histoplasmosis present with sepsis, disseminated intravascular coagulopathy, and pulmonary, CNS, and renal failure. Patients with this presentation have all died from it.

Sporotrichosis.   Sporotrichosis most commonly presents as a disease of the skin and draining lymphatics. It is usually treated quite effectively with SSKI (supersaturated solution of potassium iodide). Rarely, sporotrichosis may disseminate. Disseminated sporotrichosis associated with HIV infection apparently begins as an asymptomatic pulmonary infection that spreads hematogenously to the skin and joints. Multiple widespread cutaneous ulcers and subcutaneous nodules are present.[47,48] Amphotericin-B is the treatment of choice.

■ CUTANEOUS MANIFESTATIONS OF SYPHILIS

Cutaneous presentations of primary and secondary syphilis in HIV-infected individuals are usually similar to those in non-HIV-infected persons. Unusual features of syphilitic infection have been reported in patients with HIV infection, however. One patient with AIDS had true negative treponemal (FTA-ABS) and nontreponemal (VDRL) serologies although he had cutaneous lesions of secondary syphilis.[54] Skin biopsy of a cutaneous lesion demonstrated the spirochete and established the diagnosis. The patient's HIV infection apparently delayed development of reactive antibody to *Treponema pallidum*, resulting in negative tests. Thus, in the HIV-infected person, a negative serologic test may not be adequate to rule out secondary syphilis. Another recent report documents palmoplantar keratoderma in an HIV-infected person's secondary syphilis.[55] His immune response to *T. pallidum* was atypical. All HIV-infected persons with confirmed neurosyphilis, seronegative secondary syphilis, and CNS relapse despite recommended therapy should be reported to the Centers for Disease Control (CDC) or local health department.

■ CNS MANIFESTATIONS OF SYPHILIS

Among both non-HIV-infected and HIV-infected persons, central nervous system (CNS) syphilitic infection may occur early, even in the primary or early secondary stage. Clinical CNS disease may be manifest as early as a few months after infection.[56] Recommended therapies may not be adequate to treat or prevent this complication in non-HIV-infected persons. Publications have suggested that early CNS involvement (even after standard treatment regimens) may be more common in HIV-infected individuals.[56,57] This may be due to a combination of HIV-related impaired cell-mediated immunity and suboptimal CNS levels of medication. HIV-infected individuals who have been treated with standard therapies for early syphilis should be followed carefully. If CNS signs or symptoms develop, appropriate evaluation for early CNS relapse should be performed, including lumbar puncture and VDRL on the cerebrospinal fluid. The CDC recommends that a CSF examination precede and guide therapy in all HIV-infected patients with latent syphilis present for longer than one year or for unknown duration.[58]

TREATMENT OF SYPHILIS IN THE HIV-INFECTED INDIVIDUAL

Because of reports of early CNS relapse, the CDC has issued guidelines for the treatment of syphilis in persons with HIV infection.[58] Patients with early syphilis are treated with 2.4 million units of benzathine penicillin given intramuscularly at a single session. There is disagreement on this issue. However, even patients with early syphilis require cerebrospinal fluid (CSF) examination if there are any clinical findings suggesting possible CNS involvement. Tetracycline (500 mg orally 4 times daily for 15 days) is used for penicillin-allergic patients. If compliance cannot be assured, hospitalization, desensitization to penicillin, and treatment with penicillin are recommended. Erythromycin is not recommended.[59] Quantitative nontreponemal tests are repeated at one, two, and three months and thereafter at three-month intervals until a satisfactory serologic response occurs. If an appropriate fall in titer does not occur (two dilutions by three months in primary or by six months in secondary), reevaluation and CSF examination should be performed.

For latent syphilis of longer than one year or of unknown duration, CSF examination is recommended for all HIV-infected patients. Benzathine penicillin should not be used to treat asymptomatic or symptomatic neurosyphilis in HIV-infected individuals.

Patients with neurosyphilis should be treated for at least 10 days with either aqueous crystalline penicillin G (2 to 4 million units IV every 4 hours/12 to 24 million units daily) or with procaine penicillin G (2.4 million units intramuscularly daily) plus probenecid (500 mg orally four times daily). The correct therapy for HIV-infected persons with late latent syphilis and a normal CSF examination is not known. Weekly injections of benzathine penicillin (2.4 million units for three consecutive weeks) is suggested. Frequent serologic reevaluation is recommended to document the adequacy of therapy. Serologic response may be slower than in patients with early syphilis.

■ PNEUMOCYSTIS

Two reports have documented *Pneumocystis carinii* cutaneous infection of the external auditory canal.[60,61] In these cases, polypoid lesions obstructed and protruded from the ear canals. Histology showed a dermal nodule composed of angiocentric perivascular amphophilic foamy material identical to that seen in pneumocystis lung infection. Organisms were identified by the Grocott stain. Neither patient had clinical pneumonia at the time of presentation, but one later developed pneumocystis pneumonia. Both cases were treated with trimethoprim—sulfamethoxazole and their cutaneous lesions healed.

■ PAPULOSQUAMOUS DISEASES: XEROSIS/ICHTHYOSIS

HIV-infected patients commonly complain of increasing dryness of the skin (xerosis).[43,62] Typically, the xerosis is most prominent on the anterior lower legs, but it may be quite widespread. In the winter, the xerosis is more severe and may be associated with dermatitis. The dermatitis presents as itching and dryness with areas of erythematous papules and fine scale on the posterior arms and lower legs. Those with an atopic diathesis (hay fever, asthma, or previous atopic dermatitis) are predisposed to this type of xerotic eczema. Excessive or frequent bathing with deodorant soaps is a frequent precipitating factor and should be discontinued. Mild topical steroid ointments (1 percent to 2.5 percent hydrocortisone or 0.025 percent triamcinolone) are applied to the dermatitic areas three times a day. All dry areas of the body are covered with a moisturizing lotion or cream (Eucerin, Lubriderm, Moisturel) after bathing and at bedtime. In HIV-infected patients, xerosis remains active to some degree, especially in the winter months.

Dry and thickened skin, as is seen in acquired ichthyosis, is an uncommon condition in AIDS patients. Thickening of the palms and soles may be present as well.[1,2] One reported patient (and two patients that we have seen) had acquired ichthyosis associated with a wasting syndrome.

■ SEBORRHEIC DERMATITIS

Seborrheic dermatitis is a common mild eruption, usually affecting the scalp and central areas of the face. It occurs in up to 5 percent of the non-HIV-infected population. The etiology of common seborrheic dermatitis is not understood, but it may be related to the presence of pityrosporon yeasts. It is usually a mild eruption that waxes and wanes. It may be mildly itchy, but it responds quickly to mild topical corticosteroid therapy. Flare-ups of this condition often occur when the afflicted individual is recovering from a severe illness or surgery. Increased severity of seborrheic dermatitis is seen in certain neurologic conditions, particularly Parkinson's disease.

INCIDENCE

Early in the AIDS epidemic, many patients with symptomatic HIV disease and AIDS had particularly severe seborrheic dermatitis. One study found an 83 percent incidence of seborrheic dermatitis associated with AIDS and a 42 percent incidence with symptomatic non-AIDS HIV disease.[63] Other studies have reported incidences in AIDS patients ranging from 25 percent to 45 percent.[25,64] These percentages are far above those to be expected in a population on the basis of flare-ups from severe illness alone. This author and colleagues have seen and managed many cases of this dermatosis in AIDS patients. It has become evident that seborrheic dermatitis in HIV-infected individuals has a broad clinical spectrum, ranging from typical seborrheic dermatitis to a widespread form more like inverse psoriasis or sebopsoriasis.

CLINICAL MANIFESTATIONS

Clinically, typical HIV-related seborrheic dermatitis occurs predominantly on the scalp, usually with mild involvement on the face (particularly in the brows, around the eyelashes, down the nasolabial folds, and in and around the ears). Occasionally, seborrheic dermatitis will also occur on the center of the chest, particularly in individuals with a lot of chest hair. It is less common in the axillae and groin. The dermatitis usually manifests itself as poorly defined, faint pink patches, with mild-to-profuse fine, loose, waxy scales. In a small percentage of patients, the seborrheic dermatitis is more extensive and is present on the scalp and large areas of the face. Involvement of the chest, axillae, and groin is not rare. The intertriginous lesions are clinically identical to those seen in Reiter's syndrome and psoriasis concurrent with HIV infection.

The most severe form of seborrheic dermatitis is seen in a small percentage of patients and consists of typical severe seborrheic dermatitis of the face and scalp, plus extensive involvement of the intertriginous areas. The axillae and groin are bright red and covered by a fine scale. The eruption moves out from the intertriginous areas onto the trunk and neck and may involve large areas of the body. Like classic seborrheic dermatitis, pruritus is generally mild. This severe form of seborrheic dermatitis may also be seen in non-HIV-infected persons, where it is quite unusual. This form may be called sebo-psoriasis or inverse psoriasis — a cross between seborrheic dermatitis and psoriasis. This severe form of seborrheic dermatitis is the presenting manifestation of HIV infection in cases we have observed (see color plate 5.3.1.f).

Several features of seborrheic dermatitis in HIV-infected patients may help to explain its increased incidence and severity in this group. First, we and other authors have noted that seborrheic dermatitis in AIDS patients may be disproportionately associated with central nervous system involvement.[43] Careful studies are needed to confirm these anecdotal observations. Second, the histology, like the clinical presentation in HIV-associated seborrheic dermatitis, is different from classic seborrheic dermatitis.[65] These histologic differences have not been useful in understanding the pathogenesis, however. Third, AIDS patients on ketoconazole have a decreased incidence of seborrheic dermatitis. This may support the role of yeast in seborrheic dermatitis.[25]

TREATMENT

Mild seborrheic dermatitis in HIV-infected patients is managed in the same manner as in non-HIV-infected patients. Mild topical steroids (e.g., 1 percent hydrocortisone), tar shampoos, and often, a topical imidazole (clotrimazole or ketoconazole) should be applied twice daily. Patients are very slow to respond to treatment with topical imidazoles alone. In my experience, topical imidazoles do improve the efficacy of steroid therapy; most importantly, they reduce the frequency with which medication must be applied. Since the seborrheic dermatitis is a chronic condition, maintenance therapy is required. Often if the patient uses 1 percent hydrocortisone cream plus an imidazole, maintenance therapy need be applied only twice weekly and rarely more than once daily.

In healthy individuals, the hallmark of widespread seborrheic dermatitis is a rapid response to mild treatment. In HIV-infected persons with extensive seborrheic dermatitis, therapy is often quite difficult. Lesions are often refractory to all but the most potent topical steroids, even when used in combination with topical imidazoles. Potent topical steroids are relatively contraindicated on the face and intertriginous areas, making therapy even more problematic. Some of these patients improve with tar and occasionally with ultraviolet light therapy (as used for treatment of psoriasis). Oral ketoconazole (200 mg to 400 mg daily) may benefit severely affected patients.

■ PSORIASIS

Psoriasis may coexist with HIV infection and AIDS. Pruritus and secondary infection are difficult management problems and are probably exacerbating factors. Side effects may limit the usefulness of available treatments, and certain therapies (e.g., methotrexate) are relatively contraindicated. Difficult cases are best managed by a dermatologist who is skilled in the treatment of both HIV infection and psoriasis.

Psoriasis is a chronic scaling skin disorder with a genetic basis in 50 percent of cases. The typical age at onset of psoriasis is the twenties to thirties. Sharply marginated red plaques with a thick silvery scale are typically present over the elbows, knees, and lumbosacral areas. Nail pitting and dystrophy and arthritis are features that may coexist with psoriasis. The psoriatic lesions may occasionally itch. The severity of the skin disease is extremely variable from one patient to another and for each patient over time.

PSORIASIS AND HIV INFECTION

Cases of psoriasis associated with HIV infection have been noted since early in the AIDS epidemic, and the incidence of psoriasis in HIV-infected persons may be higher (5 percent) than in the general population (1 percent to 2 percent).[66] Psoriasis has been reported in HIV-infected persons of both sexes and in patients with AIDS acquired by sexual transmission, intravenous drug use, and transfusion.

Psoriasis may first appear early in the course of HIV infection. Persons with no previous personal or family history of psoriasis may develop it even when the HIV infection is acquired late in life, as opposed to psoriasis in otherwise healthy individuals, in whom it usually appears before the age of 30. We have seen a homosexual male in his early sixties who was very sexually active for one year in his late fifties and then became celibate. Psoriasis first appeared soon after this period of sexual activity. Other findings associated with HIV infection appeared three years later. It may be, then, that HIV infection induces or permits the appearance of new psoriasis in a person with no personal or family history of the condition.

Not only is HIV infection associated with new cases of psoriasis, but it may also be associated with an exacerbation of longstanding stable psoriasis, which may advance as a patient's HIV infection progresses.[66] This is not universally true, however; some HIV-infected persons may have psoriasis that remains stable even as immunodeficiency progresses. Why some patients have advancing skin disease and others have stable skin disease (although both have similar immunosuppression) is unknown. Potential exacerbating factors include coexistent infections with bacteria and yeast, the physiological stress of repeated illnesses, or the psychological stress and anxiety induced by a progressively fatal disease. The elevated levels of alpha-interferon in HIV infection may be a precipitating factor.[67]

CLINICAL MANIFESTATIONS

The clinical appearance of psoriasis is similar in HIV-infected and non-infected individuals. However, the incidence of severe involvement of the axillae and groin (sebopsoriasis) is increased in HIV-infected patients. In addition, psoriatic erythroderma is not rare in these patients.[66] In my experience, the most common cause of an erythroderma in an AIDS patient (second to drug reactions) is psoriasis. As in routine psoriasis, pruritus may be a serious problem for the HIV-infected patient with psoriasis. Secondary infection of excoriated psoriatic plaques with *Staphylococcus aureus* is common. Repeated episodes of pyoderma and cellulitis are the rule; even sepsis is seen in rare cases in HIV-infected patients.

At least one series reported a poor prognosis for psoriatic HIV-infected patients. Many of them developed AIDS soon after diagnosis of psoriasis. Their average lifespan was 12 months.[68] In two patients I have treated until their deaths and in others I know about by report, the psoriasis cleared immediately before death.

TREATMENT

Therapy for psoriasis in otherwise healthy persons is imperfect, owing in part to our limited understanding of the condition's pathogenesis. Topical steroids, anthralin, ultraviolet light (UVB) with or without tar, PUVA (psoralens plus ultraviolet A), the retinoids, and immunosuppressives (especially methotrexate) are all useful. HIV-infected patients present additional challenges to an already inadequate armamentarium.

In general, psoriasis responds poorly to less than medium- or high-potency topical steroids. Use of potent topical steroids over large areas of the body leads, however, to systemic absorption, adrenal suppression, and possibly immunosuppression — obviously undesirable effects in patients with HIV infection. Topical steroids may also reduce local immunity, increasing the likelihood of cutaneous infections.

We have used tar plus UVB (Goeckermann therapy) with marginal success. One patient did develop Kaposi's sarcoma (KS) while on this therapy, and other authors have reported the appearance of KS or worsening of AIDS with UVB therapy.[66,68] KS, like psoriasis, is known to develop in areas of inflamed or traumatized skin (Koebner phenomenon); whether this is a cause-and-effect relationship is unknown. PUVA reduces T-cell numbers in atypical infiltrates in the skin and may even eliminate circulating atypical T lymphocytes. PUVA is also a cutaneous carcinogen. The safety of PUVA in HIV-infected patients has yet to be established, but two of four patients treated in one series developed KS on this therapy.[66] Methotrexate therapy has been associated with progressive immunosuppression or rapid demise (or both) when used in many HIV-infected persons and is probably contraindicated for skin or joint disease.[66,67] HIV testing for all psoriatic patients at risk should be considered before methotrexate therapy is started.

Some HIV-infected patients with severe psoriasis have responded favorably to etretinate, a retinoid.[66] The frequency of past or current liver disease due to hepatitis B infection in AIDS patients has limited etretinate's usefulness, but two erythrodermic patients we treated did respond to therapy with this agent. Others have found side-effects limiting.[68] Seven patients reported to date have had significant improvement of their psoriasis associated with zidovudine (AZT) therapy.[68-70] The response appears to be related to an adequate dose and to be correlated with macrocytosis.[70] Most of our patients with psoriasis who have taken AZT have had a significant initial improvement followed by a mild relapse after several weeks to months. Although the psoriasis has not returned to the pretreatment levels of severity, the response is not universal and does not appear to be related to the severity of the psoriasis.

■ REITER'S SYNDROME

Reiter's syndrome consists of the classic triad of arthritis, conjunctivitis, and urethritis. Incomplete forms (e.g., arthritis and other findings) have been recognized. Reiter's occurs predominantly in genetically predisposed (HLA-B27 positive) males, commonly following genitourinary or gastrointestinal infections. Like psoriasis, Reiter's may appear in HIV-infected patients.[66,71] Usually symptoms of HIV infection and Reiter's appear simultaneously or the HIV infection is symptomatic before the onset of Reiter's. We have seen one patient, however, who initially presented with classic cutaneous lesions of Reiter's before manifesting clinical symptoms of HIV infection.

INCIDENCE

Whether the incidence of Reiter's syndrome increases in HIV infection or merely coincides with it, and whether HIV infection permits the expression or exacerbates the features of Reiter's are unknown. Certainly the postulated precipitating events for Reiter's — genitourinary sexually transmitted diseases and gastrointestinal infectious illnesses — are common in HIV-infected individuals. In addition, many HIV-infected persons are young males — the population at risk for Reiter's.

CLINICAL MANIFESTATIONS

The classic cutaneous lesions of Reiter's syndrome occur in HIV-associated Reiter's as well and may help to establish the diagnosis. The palms and especially the soles develop superficial pustules that dry, forming keratotic papules. These coalesce until the soles are diffusely thickened and scaled. This is called keratoderma blennorrhagicum (see color plate 5.3.1.g). The nails are commonly affected; extensive subungual debris may appear, the nails may be horizontally ridged, and during severe flares, the nail plate may be so dystrophic as to appear absent. These nail findings may also be seen in psoriasis.

In the groin and axillae, red plaques identical to those seen in seborrheic dermatitis and psoriasis can be present. They rarely reach the extent seen in the latter two diseases, however. Histologically, skin biopsies from lesions of Reiter's syndrome and psoriasis show identical features. Biopsies are therefore not useful in distinguishing between these two conditions.

Oral and genital mucosa can also be involved. The glans penis may be covered by a dry, sharply marginated eruption called circinate balanitis. In the uncircumcised patient, lesions are more moist and may mimic candidiasis. On gross examination the arcuate nature and sharp border of the lesions, and a negative test for yeast (potassium hydroxide preparation), help to establish the diagnosis of circinate balanitis. Evanescent and often asymptomatic oral erosions may be present. A geographic tongue (i.e., showing migratory white patches) may also be found in patients with Reiter's syndrome.

TREATMENT

Therapy for the cutaneous lesions of HIV-associated Reiter's syndrome is identical to that for psoriasis. Methotrexate is contraindicated, but etretinate may be useful in severely affected patients. One of our patients with Reiter's syndrome and HIV infection has responded dramatically to zidovudine (AZT);

his skin lesions have almost entirely cleared and his joint symptoms have improved.

ATOPIC DERMATITIS

Atopic dermatitis may appear in both children and adults infected with HIV. In one series, 50 percent of infants with AIDS had atopic dermatitis.[72] Hemophilic children infected by transfusion may have flare-ups of previously quiescent atopic dermatitis.[73] Adults with a previous history of atopic disease may also note recurrence of atopy after diagnosis with AIDS.[74] They may develop atopic dermatitis when previously they had only respiratory atopic symptoms.

HYPERSENSITIVITY REACTIONS IN HIV-INFECTED PATIENTS

Since helper T cells and antigen-presenting cells are both targets of HIV and crucial in the development of many hypersensitivity reactions, these reactions should theoretically be infrequent in HIV-infected persons whose T cells are depleted. However, hypersensitivity reactions occur frequently, suggesting that normal numbers of T cells are not necessary for many hypersensitivity reactions to take place.

DRUG REACTIONS

Trimethoprim/sulfamethoxazole (TMP/SMX) is used frequently in managing pneumocystis pneumonia. The incidence of adverse reactions to the drug is very high; in one study, 62 percent of patients could not complete their course of therapy because of adverse reactions.[75] The most common reaction was cutaneous eruption, almost always maculopapular, occurring in 48 percent of treated patients and 78 percent of those suffering an adverse reaction. In 33 percent, the skin rash resolved during therapy, but in 66 percent progressive toxicity necessitated discontinuation of the drug. The rash did not always recur when the patient was rechallenged with the same therapy. Thus, in persons with HIV infection and pneumocystis pneumonia, the overall incidence of skin eruptions from TMP/SMX is about 10 times that in a non-HIV-infected population. The reasons for this difference are unknown. The high incidence of similar eruptions in patients with Epstein–Barr infection given ampicillin may be due to similar causes.

Other hypersensitivity reactions seen in HIV-infected patients are urticarial drug reactions, exfoliative erythroderma, fixed drug eruption, erythema multiforme, and toxic epidermal necrolysis. These reactions are most often due to antibiotics, especially TMP/SMX and the penicillins. Eruptions due to dapsone, ketoconazole, pyrimethamine, amphotericin-B, pentamidine, and zidovudine (AZT) are less common. The incidence of these reactions does not appear to be increased in HIV-infected patients, even though they receive multiple medications at frequent intervals, which increases their risk of developing adverse reactions.

INSECT BITE REACTIONS

Urticarial pruritic papules are a common morphologic lesion in HIV-infected patients. This form of lesion is clinically specific but etiologically nonspecific. In occasional patients, this lesion is associated with insect bites and is called papular urticaria. In HIV-infected patients in San Francisco, except for scabies mites, fleas are the insect most commonly causing papular urticaria. In Miami, mosquitoes may be the primary offender. A skin biopsy of the lesion can be useful in confirming the diagnosis of insect-bite reaction. Oral antihistamines combined with protection from biting insects leads to improvement in the lesions.

PHOTOSENSITIVITY

Photosensitivity in HIV-infected persons has been rarely reported.[77] Such reactions are not unusual, however; I have seen many cases here at San Francisco General Hospital and Dr. Penneys in Miami has had a similar experience. Erythematous patches and plaques appear during periods of increased sun exposure on exposed body parts, primarily the dorsa of the hands, extensor forearms, the side of the neck, and the face. The photosensitivity is due to the ultraviolet spectrum (UVB). Hypersensitive patients benefit from sun protection and sun screens. One patient from Miami responded to PUVA therapy.

Porphyria cutanea tarda (PCT) has been reported in six male patients with HIV infection, suggesting an association between the two.[76,82,83] Three patients had the familial form of the disease and three were sporadic cases. Many patients who are genetically susceptible to PCT develop the disease only after exposure to hepatotoxic agents (ethanol) or drugs that interfere with uroporphyrinogen decarboxylase (iron or estrogens, for example). Hepatitis may also precipitate clinical PCT. Why patients capable of developing PCT do so after HIV infection is unknown, but in many cases patients have been exposed to one or more of the precipitating factors noted above.

PRURITIC PAPULAR ERUPTIONS

Pruritic papules are common in HIV infection[78] and are due to various causes. *Staphylococcus aureus* folliculitis, eosinophilic folliculitis, demodicidosis,[84] insect-bite reactions, granulomas with no identifiable infectious agent (e.g., granuloma annulare[85]), papular eruption of HIV infection,[79] and other excoriated papular eruptions with no known etiology may all present as pruritic papules. Evaluation requires a skin biopsy and culture of the tissue. Unless a specific cause is found, therapy is extremely difficult. Our approach is to search for staphylococcal infection by culturing an unruptured pustule (if present). We then treat empirically for staphylococcus. About 50 percent of patients improve with this regimen, particularly those with positive cultures from the pustules. Topical steroids also help. Ultraviolet B therapy, like that given to patients with pruritus and renal failure,[81] has been useful in some patients when other topical measures have failed. Rarely, pruritus with no primary skin lesions may be the presenting sign of AIDS.[80]

■ DERMATOLOGIC MANIFESTATIONS OF NEOPLASTIC DISORDERS

Kaposi's sarcoma (KS) is a neoplasm of endothelial cells involving the skin and, at times, other internal organs. KS is common among the HIV-infected, but there is not an equal incidence in all risk groups. In one series, 46 percent of homosexual men with AIDS had KS at the time of their initial diagnosis. The incidence in heterosexual intravenous drug users is only 3.8 percent.[86]

CLINICAL PRESENTATION

KS may affect any portion of the cutaneous surface. Initially, it appears as red-to-brown flat macules (see color plates 5.3.1.h through l). Papules, nodules, and tumors may also be present or develop later. Lesions tend to orient themselves along the lines of cleavage, forming oval papules. They range in size from several millimeters to over 10 centimeters and may be widespread, grouped, or zosteriform, numbering from one to hundreds.

KS may affect mucosal surfaces and internal organs with or without involving the skin. Visceral involvement occurs in 72 percent of AIDS patients with KS, most often affecting the gastrointestinal tract (50 percent), lymph nodes (50 percent), and lungs (37 percent).[87]

NATURAL HISTORY AND PROGNOSIS

The natural history of AIDS-associated KS is not uniform, but the prognosis is poor. The average survival of patients is 18 months.[87] Most have generalized, slowly progressive disease; others have stable KS. Even more rarely, the disease may spontaneously resolve.[88] Generalized disease and coexistent opportunistic infections are poor prognostic findings; the latter are the most common cause of death.[87]

DIAGNOSIS

Diagnosis is established by biopsy of an affected organ (the skin being the most accessible, if it is involved). A palpable lesion, preferably one that has been present for at least several weeks, should be selected. Sites of prior trauma should be avoided. A 3.5- to 4-mm punch biopsy should be taken from the center of the lesion. Despite their vascular nature, lesions usually do not bleed excessively if the following precautions are followed: avoid foot and lower-leg lesions if possible; use xylocaine with epinephrine 1:100,000 and inject it at least 5 minutes before taking the biopsy; biopsy into the subcutaneous fat; and suture all wounds.

Except on the lower extremity, biopsy sites in KS lesions heal at the normal rate and the incidence of infection for this type of surgical wound is not increased. The most common errors in biopsying tissue that is not diagnostic are the following: choosing the wrong lesion; biopsying the edge of a lesion; crushing the tissue; and taking too small a punch biopsy (3 mm).

The pathological interpretation of tissue biopsies should be performed by someone skilled in evaluating HIV-associated KS lesions. Early lesions may be subtle and difficult to distinguish from the vascular reactivity associated with prior inflammation or stasis dermatitis. Changes may be focal, and so multiple sections are often required before a diagnostic area is found. Diagnostic pathologic findings must always be present to make the diagnosis of KS, especially in persons who exhibit no other evidence of HIV infection or who are HIV-seropositive but not immunosuppressed. Consultation should be sought if there is any question. It is best to avoid pathologic diagnoses that are equivocal — i.e., "possible KS." Clinical diagnoses should be made only rarely, since skin lesions are so accessible and biopsies so easy.

TREATMENT

Therapy aims at controlling symptoms, reducing edema, eliminating pain, and clearing lesions, but it is not thought to be curative. If treatment is necessary or elected, radiation and systemic alpha-interferon or chemotherapy are commonly used. Cutaneous lesions may be improved with local cryo-therapy or intralesional injections with vincristine or vinblastine.[89]

Other cutaneous carcinomas are unusual in HIV-infected patients. Basal-cell carcinoma is occasionally seen, but except for one report, aggressive cases have not been reported. In this patient, the cancer had been present eight years prior to transfusion-associated HIV infection, had not been surgically controlled on several occasions, and had metastasized.[90] Rarely, AIDS-associated lymphoma will present in the skin.[42]

■ SCABIES

Scabies in HIV-infected persons often takes the typical pattern of pruritic papules with accentuation in the intertriginous areas, genitalia, and finger-webs. With advancing immunosuppression, the infestation may be exaggerated, becoming more widespread and refractory to treatment, and sparing the characteristic areas.[91] Gamma benzene hexachloride applied from the neck down for 8 to 24 hours is usually curative.

In rare cases, true crusted or Norwegian scabies may occur in patients with AIDS.[92-94] Norwegian (crusted) scabies is nonpruritic and appears as thick crusts over large areas of the body. These crusts teem with mites and are highly contagious. Multiple courses of gamma benzene hexachloride may be required to cure the patient. As a portal of entry for bacterial pathogens, this form of scabies can lead to sepsis and death.[93]

■ MUCOCUTANEOUS PIGMENTATION DUE TO ZIDOVUDINE

In dark-skinned persons (Hispanics and blacks) treated with zidovudine (AZT), hyperpigmentation of the nails, oral mucosa, and skin may occur.[95-97] The hyperpigmentation appears to be related to increased melanogenesis in the areas of hyperpigmentation and not to drug deposition. Tests for adrenal insufficiency are normal in these patients.

HYPERPIGMENTATION IN NAILS

The initial manifestation is usually a bluish discoloration of the lunulae (proximal white portions) of the nails, most prominent on the thumbnails. This appears about one month after AZT therapy begins. In addition, hyper-pigmented longitudinal nail bands may appear. In very dark-skinned black persons, the whole nail-plate may turn black, beginning proximally and grow-ing distally, and eventually involving the whole nail. Usually all nails are af-fected, but changes are more marked on the fingernails. The pigment in the nail-plate stains like melanin when it is examined histologically.

HYPERPIGMENTATION IN ORAL MUCOSA

In three patients on AZT, we have observed bilateral black pigmentation of the lateral mid-tongue. The pigmentation occurs in the same location as hairy leukoplakia, but the relationship (if any) between the two is unclear —

only one of the three patients had leukoplakia when the pigmentation appeared.

HYPERPIGMENTATION OF THE SKIN

Cutaneous hyperpigmentation may also be noted, especially in areas exposed to the sun or rubbed by clothing (e.g., the belt line). An enhanced ability to tan may also be noted. In one biopsied patient, increased epidermal melanin and melanin-containing macrophages (melanophages) were found in the dermis. Electron microscopy demonstrated heavily melanized melanosomes in the dermal macrophages.

FACTORS AFFECTING HYPERPIGMENTATION

The degree of hyperpigmentation of the nails and skin is partly related to dosage of AZT: patients note a decrease in hyperpigmentation when the dose is decreased because of its toxicity. The pigmentation clears if the drug is discontinued. Cutaneous hyperpigmentation on the face may be improved by avoiding sun exposure and by using a high sun-protection factor sunscreen (SPF 15 or higher). Bleaching the skin with 2 percent to 4 percent hydroquinone cream is also useful when combined with a sunscreen.

REFERENCES

1. Kaplan MH, Sadick N, McNutt NS, et al. Dermatologic findings and manifestations of acquired immunodeficiency syndrome (AIDS). J Am Acad Dermatol 1987; 16:485-506.
2. Fisher BK, Warner LC. Cutaneous manifestations of the acquired immunodeficiency syndrome. Update 1987. Int J Dermatol 1987; 26:615-30.
3. Valle SL. Dermatologic findings related to human immunodeficiency virus infection in high-risk individuals. J Am Acad Dermatol 1987; 17:951-61.
4. Friedman-Kien AE, Lafleur FL, Gendler E, et al. Herpes zoster: a possible early clinical sign for development of acquired immunodeficiency syndrome in high-risk individuals. J Am Acad Dermatol 1986; 14:1023-8.
5. Redfield RR, Wright DC, James WD, et al. Disseminated vaccinia in a military recruit with human immunodeficiency virus (HIV) disease. N Engl J Med 1987; 316:673-6.
6. Halsey NA, Henderson DA. HIV infection and immunization against other agents. N Engl J Med 1987; 316:683-5.
7. Duvic M. Staphylococcal infections and the pruritus of AIDS-related complex. Arch Dermatol 1987; 123:1599.
8. Soeprono FF, Schinella RA. Eosinophilic pustular folliculitis in patients with acquired immunodeficiency syndrome. J Am Acad Dermatol 1986; 14:1020-2.
9. LeBoit PE, Berger TG, Egbert BM, et al. Epithelioid haemangioma-like vascular proliferations in AIDS: Manifestation of cat-scratch disease bacillus infection? Lancet 1988; 30:960-3.
10. Koehler JE, LeBoit PE, Egbert BM, Berger TG. Cutaneous vascular lesions and disseminated cat-scratch disease in patients with the acquired immunodeficiency syndrome (AIDS) and AIDS-related complex. Ann Intern Med 1988; 109:449-55.
11. Stoler MH, Bonfiglio TA, Steigbigel RT, Pereira M. An atypical subcutaneous infection associated with acquired immune deficiency syndrome. Am J Clin Pathol 1983; 80:714-8.
12. Cockerell CJ, Friedman-Kien AE. Epithelioid angiomatosis and cat scratch disease bacillus. Lancet 1988; 1:1334-5.
13. Knobler EH, Silvers DN, Fine KC, et al. Unique vascular skin lesions associated with human immunodeficiency virus. JAMA 1988; 260:524-7.
14. Angritt P. Case for diagnosis. Military Med 1988; 153:M26-7, 32.
15. Amonette RA, Rosenberg EW. Infection of toe webs by gram-negative bacteria. Arch Dermatol 1973; 107:71-3.
16. Schlossberg D. Multiple erythematous nodules as a manifestation of *Pseudomonas aeruginosa* septicemia. Arch Dermatol 1980; 116:446-7.
17. Seigal FP, Lopez C, Hammer GS, et al. Severe acquired immunodeficiency in male homosexuals manifested by chronic perianal ulcerative herpes simplex lesions. N Engl J Med 1981; 305:1439-44.

18. Centers for Disease Control. Revision of the CDC surveillance definition for acquired immunodeficiency syndrome. MMWR 1987; 36(Suppl 1):1S-15S.

19. Erlich KS, Jacobson MA, Koehler JE, et al. Foscarnet therapy for severe acyclovir-resistant herpes simplex virus type-2 infections with the acquired immunodeficiency syndrome (AIDS). An uncontrolled trial. Ann Intern Med 1989; 110:710-3.

20. Erlich KS, Mills J, Chatis P, et al. Acyclovir-resistant herpes simplex virus infections in patients with the acquired immunodeficiency syndrome. N Engl J Med 1989; 320:293-6.

21. Balfour HH. Acyclovir therapy for herpes zoster: advantages and adverse effects. JAMA 1986; 225:387-8.

22. Bernstein JE, Bickers DR, Dahl MV, Roshal JY. Treatment of chronic postherpetic neuralgia with topical capsaicin. J Am Acad Dermatol 1987; 17:93-6.

23. Pahwa S, Biron K, Lim W, et al. Continuous varicella-zoster infection associated with acyclovir resistance in a child with AIDS. JAMA 1988; 260:2879-82.

24. Seiff SR, Margolis T, Graham SH, O'Donnell JJ. Use of intravenous acyclovir for treatment of herpes zoster ophthalmicus in patients at risk for AIDS. Ann Ophthalmol 1988; 20:480-2.

25. Goodman DS, Teplitz ED, Wishner A, et al. Prevalence of cutaneous disease in patients with acquired immunodeficiency syndrome (AIDS) or AIDS-related complex. J Am Acad Dermatol 1987; 17:210-20.

26. Matis WL, Triana A, Shapiro R, et al. Dermatologic findings associated with human immunodeficiency virus infection. J Am Acad Dermatol 1987; 17:746-51.

27. Redfield RR, Burke DS. HIV infection: the clinical picture. Sci Am 1988; 259:90-8.

28. Kaufman RH, Adams E. Herpes simplex virus and human papilloma virus in the development of cervical carcinoma. Clin Obstet Gynec 1986; 29:678-92.

29. Frazer IH, Crapper RM, Medley G, Brown TC. Association between anorectal dysplasia, human papilloma virus, and human immunodeficiency virus infection in homosexual men. Lancet 1986; 2:657-60.

30. Bradbeer C. Is infection with HIV a risk factor for cervical intraepithelial neoplasia? Lancet 1987; 1:277-8.

31. Nash G, Allen W, Nash S. Atypical lesions of the anal mucosa in homosexual men. JAMA 1986; 256:873-6.

32. Gal AA, Meyer PR, Taylor CR. Papillomavirus antigens in anorectal condyloma and carcinoma in homosexual men. JAMA 1987; 257:337-43.

33. Douglas JM Jr, Rogers M, Judson FN. The effect of asymptomatic infection with HTLV-III on the response of anogenital warts to intralesional treatment with recombinant ∝-interferon. J Infect Dis 1986; 154:331-4.

34. von Krogh G, Syrjanen SM, Syrjanen KJ. Advantage of human papilloma virus typing in the clinical evaluation of genitoanal warts. J Am Acad Dermatol 1988; 18:495-503.

35. Cooper DA, Maclean P, Finlayson R, et al. Acute AIDS retrovirus infection. Lancet 1985; 1:537-40.

36. Wantzin GRL, Lindhardt BO, Weismann K, Ulrich K. Acute HTLV III infection associated with exanthema, diagnosed by seroconversion. Br J Derm 1986; 115:601-6.

37. Ho DD, Sarngadharan MG, Resnick L, et al. Primary human T-lymphotropic virus type III infection. Ann Intern Med 1985; 103:880-3.

38. Rustin MHA, Ridley CM, Smith MD, et al. The acute exanthem associated with seroconversion to human T-cell lymphotropic virus III in a homosexual man. J Infect Dis 1986; 12:161-3.

39. Kessler HA, Blaauw B, Spear J, et al. Diagnosing human immunodeficiency virus infection in seronegative homosexuals presenting with an acute viral syndrome. JAMA 1987; 258:1196-9.

40. Zakoski P, Fligiel S, Berlin OGW, Johnson BL Jr. Disseminated *Mycobacterium avium-intracellulare* infection in homosexual men dying of acquired immunodeficiency. JAMA 1982; 248:2980-2.

41. Sunderam G, McDonald RJ, Maniatis T, et al. Tuberculosis presenting as a manifestation of the acquired immunodeficiency syndrome (AIDS). JAMA 1986; 256:362-6.

42. Penneys NS, Hicks B. Unusual cutaneous lesions associated with acquired immunodeficiency syndrome. J Am Acad Dermatol 1985; 13:845-52.

43. Kaplan MH, Sadick N, McNutt NS, et al. Dermatologic findings and manifestations of acquired immunodeficiency syndrome (AIDS). J Am Acad Dermatol 1987; 16:485-506.

44. Holmberg K, Meyer RD. Fungal infections in patients with AIDS and AIDS-related complex. Scand J Infect Dis 1986; 18:179-92.

45. Borton LK, Wintroub BU. Disseminated cryptococcosis presenting as herpetiform lesions in a homosexual man with acquired immunodeficiency syndrome. J Am Acad Dermatol 1984; 387-90.

46. Rico MJ, Penneys NS. Cutaneous cryptococcosis resembling molluscum contagiosum in a patient with AIDS. Arch Dermatol 1985; 121:901-2.

47. Bibler MR, Luber HJ, Glueck HI, Estes SA. Disseminated sporotrichosis in a patient with HIV infection after treatment for acquired factor VIII inhibitor. JAMA 1986; 256:3125-6.

48. Lipstein-Kresch E, Isenberg HD, Singer C, et al. Disseminated *Sporothrix schenckii* infection with arthritis in a patient with acquired immunodeficiency syndrome. J Rheumatol 1985; 12:805-8.

49. Yeager BA, Hoxie J, Weisman RA, et al. Actinomycosis in the acquired immunodeficiency syndrome-related complex. Arch Otolaryngol Head Neck Surg 1986; 112:1293-5.

50. Duvic M, Lowe L, Rios A, et al. Superficial phaeohyphomycosis of the scrotum in a patient with the acquired immunodeficiency syndrome. Arch Dermatol 1987; 123:1597-8.

51. Lake-Bakaar G, Tom W, Lake-Bakaar D, et al. Gastropathy and ketoconazole malabsorption in the acquired immunodeficiency syndrome (AIDS). Ann Intern Med 1988; 109:471-3.

52. Concus AP, Helfand RF, Imber MJ, et al. Cutaneous cryptococcosis mimicking molluscum contagiosum in a patient with AIDS. J Infect Dis 1988; 158:897-8.

53. Johnson PC, Khardori N, Najjar AF, et al. Progressive disseminated histoplasmosis in patients with acquired immunodeficiency syndrome. Am J Med 1988; 85:152-8.

54. Hicks CB, Benson PM, Lupton GP, Tramont EC. Seronegative secondary syphilis in a patient infected with the human immunodeficiency virus (HIV) with Kaposi's sarcoma. Ann Intern Med 1987; 107:492-5.

55. Radolf JD, Kaplan RP. Unusual manifestations of secondary syphilis and abnormal humoral immune response to *Treponema pallidum* antigens in a homosexual man with asymptomatic human immuno-deficiency virus infection. J Am Acad Dermatol 1988; 18:423-8.

56. Berry CD, Hooton TM, Collier AC, Lukehart SA. Neurologic relapse after benzathine penicillin therapy for secondary syphilis in a patient with HIV infection. N Engl J Med 1987; 316:1587-9.

57. Johns DR, Tierney M, Felsenstein D. Alteration in the natural history of neurosyphilis by concurrent infection with the human immunodeficiency virus. N Engl J Med 1987; 316:1569-72.

58. Recommendations for diagnosing and treating syphilis in HIV-infected patients. MMWR 1988; 37:600-2, 607-9.

59. Duncan WC. Failure of erythromycin to cure secondary syphilis in a patient infected with the human immunodeficiency virus. Arch Dermatol 1989; 125:82-4.

60. Coulman CU, Greene I, Archibald RWR. Cutaneous pneumocystosis. Ann Intern Med 1987; 106:396-8.

61. Schinella RA, Breda SD, Hammerschlag PE. Otic infection due to *Pneumocystis carinii* in an apparently healthy man with antibody to the human immunodeficiency virus. Ann Int Med 1987; 106:399-400.

62. Farthing CF, Staughton RCD, Payne CM. Skin disease in homosexual patients with acquired immune deficiency syndrome (AIDS) and lesser forms of human T cell leukaemia virus (HTLV III) disease. Clin Exp Dermatol 1985; 10:3-12.

63. Mathes BM, Douglass MC. Seborrheic dermatitis in patients with acquired immunodeficiency syn-drome. J Am Acad Dermatol 1985; 13:947-51.

64. Eisenstat BA, Wormser GP. Seborrheic dermatitis and butterfly rash in AIDS. N Engl J Med 1984; 311:189.

65. Soeprono FF, Schinella RA, Cockerell CJ, Comite SL. Seborrheic-like dermatitis of acquired immuno-deficiency syndrome. J Am Acad Dermatol 1986; 14:242.

66. Duvic M, Johnson TM, Rapini RP, et al. Acquired immunodeficiency syndrome-associated psoriasis and Reiter's syndrome. Arch Dermatol 1987; 123:1622-32.

67. Quesada JR, Gutterman JU. Psoriasis and ∝-interferon. Lancet 1986; 1:1466-8.

68. Duvic M, Rios A, Brewton GW. Remission of AIDS-associated psoriasis with zidovudine. Lancet 1987; 2:627.

69. Ruzicka T, Froschl M, Hohenleutner U, et al. Treatment of HIV-induced retinoid-resistant psoriasis with zidovudine. Lancet 1987; 2:1469-70.

70. Kaplan MH, Sadick NS, Wieder J, et al. Antipsoriatic effects of zidovudine in human immunodeficiency virus-associated psoriasis. J Am Acad Dermatol 1989; 20:76-82.

71. Winchester R, Bernstein DH, Fischer HD, et al. The co-occurrence of Reiter's syndrome and acquired immunodeficiency. Ann Intern Med 1987; 106:19-26.

72. Scott GB, Buck BE, Leterman JG, et al. Acquired immunodeficiency syndrome in infants. N Engl J Med 1984; 310:76-81.

73. Ball LM, Harper JI. Atopic eczema in HIV-seropositive haemophiliacs. Lancet 1987; 1:627-8.

74. Parkin JM, Eales LJ, Galazka AR, Pinching AJ. Atopic manifestations in the acquired immune deficiency syndrome: response to recombinant interferon gamma. Br Med J 1987; 294:1185-6.

75. Gordin FM, Simon GL, Wofsy CB, Mills J. Adverse reactions to trimethoprim-sulfamethoxazole in patients with the acquired immunodeficiency syndrome. Ann Intern Med 1984; 100:495-9.

76. Lobato MN, Berger TG. Porphyria cutanea tarda associated with the acquired immunodeficiency syn-drome. Arch Dermatol 1988; 124:1009-10.

77. Toback AC, Longley J, Cardullo AC, et al. Severe chronic photosensitivity in association with acquired immunodeficiency syndrome. J Am Acad Dermatol 1986; 15:1056-7.

78. Colebunders R, Mann JM, Francis H, et al. Generalized papular pruritic eruption in African patients with human immunodeficiency virus infection. AIDS 1987; 1:117-21.

79. James WD, Redfield RR, Lupton GP, et al. A papular eruption associated with human T cell lym-photropic virus type III disease. J Am Acad Dermatol 1985; 13:563-6.

80. Shapiro RS, Samorodin C, Hood AF. Pruritus as a presenting sign of acquired immunodeficiency syndrome. J Am Acad Dermatol 1987; 16:1115-7.

81. Buchness MR, Lim HW, Hutchens VA, et al. Eosinophilic pustular folliculitis in the acquired immuno-deficiency syndrome. N Engl J Med 1988; 318:1183-6.

82. Wissel PS, Sordillo P, Anderson KE, et al. Porphyria cutanea tarda associated with the acquired immune deficiency syndrome. Am J Hematol 1987; 25:107-13.

83. Hogan D, Card RT, Ghadially R, et al. Human immunodeficiency virus infection and porphyria cutanea tarda. J Am Acad Dermatol 1989; 20:17-20.

84. Dominey A, Rosen T, Tschen J. Papulonodular demodicidosis associated with acquired immunodeficiency syndrome. J Am Acad Dermatol 1989; 20:197-201.

85. Ghadially R, Sibbald RG, Water JB, Haberman HF. Granuloma annulare in patients with human immunodeficiency virus infections. J Am Acad Dermatol 1989; 20:232-5.

86. DeJarlais DC, Marmor M, Thomas P, et al. Kaposi's sarcoma among four different AIDS risk groups. N Engl J Med 1984; 310:1119.

87. Lemlich G, Schwam L, Lebwohl M. Kaposi's sarcoma and acquired immunodeficiency syndrome. Post-mortem findings in 24 cases. J Am Acad Dermatol 1987; 16:319-25.

88. Janier M, Vignon MD, Cottenot F. Spontaneously healing Kaposi's sarcoma in AIDS. N Engl J Med 1985; 312:1638-9.

89. Odom RB, Goette DK. Treatment of cutaneous Kaposi's sarcoma with intralesional vincristine. Arch Dermatol 1978; 114:1693-4.

90. Sitz KV, Keppen M, Johnson DF. Metastatic basal cell carcinoma in acquired immunodeficiency syndrome-related complex. JAMA 1987; 257:340-3.

91. Sadick N, Kaplan MH, Pahwa SG, Sarngadharan MG. Unusual features of scabies complicating human T-lymphotropic virus type III infection. J Am Acad Dermatol 1986; 15:482-6.

92. Rau RC, Baird IM. Crusted scabies in a patient with acquired immunodeficiency syndrome. J Am Acad Dermatol 1986; 15:1058-9.

93. Glover R, Young L, Goltz RW. Norwegian scabies in acquired immunodeficiency syndrome: report of a case resulting in death from associated sepsis. J Am Acad Dermatol 1987; 16:396-8.

94. Drabick JJ, Lupton GP, Tompkins K. Crusted scabies in human immunodeficiency virus infection. J Am Acad Dermatol 1987; 17:142.

95. Furth PA, Kazakis AM. Nail pigmentation changes associated with azidothymidine (zidovudine). Ann Intern Med 1987; 107:350.

96. Panwalker AP. Nail pigmentation in the acquired immunodeficiency syndrome (AIDS). Ann Intern Med 1987; 107:943-4.

97. Greenberg RG, Berger TG. Nail and mucocutaneous hyperpigmentation of azidothymidine therapy. J Am Acad Dermatol (in press).

5.4

Neurologic Aspects

Neurologic Dysfunction: Overview

Yuen T. So, M.D., Ph.D.

Neurologic complications are frequent in patients infected with HIV. Autopsy studies of patients who died of AIDS or symptomatic HIV infection revealed pathologic abnormalities in the nervous system in 75 percent to 90 percent of patients.[2-4] Symptoms and signs of neurologic dysfunction were seen in 30 percent to 40 percent of AIDS patients in several large clinical series.[1,2,5] Moreover, 10 percent of AIDS patients presented with neurologic symptoms and signs before the recognition of other AIDS-related diseases.[2]

A very high incidence of cognitive dysfunction, in the range of 50 percent to 87 percent, was found in one study administering detailed neuropsychologic testing to HIV-infected patients.[8] Another study, however, found considerably lower incidence using more conservative criteria in a nonreferral population.[6] It is important to point out that all these prevalence and incidence figures are approximate; the estimates depend on patient selection and diagnostic criteria, as well as on the pattern of patient referral to academic centers.

All HIV-infected patients are at risk for developing an extraordinarily wide range of neurologic disorders. Cerebral symptoms and signs are the most common: headache, encephalopathy, dementia, seizures, and focal neurologic deficits such as hemiparesis, ataxia, hemisensory loss, or hemianopsia. Peripheral neuropathy is seen in approximately 35 percent of hospitalized AIDS patients.[7] Myelopathies include both spinal cord compression by epidural tumor or abscess and intrinsic spinal cord diseases due to viral infections or other causes. Myopathy, though relatively uncommon, is also well recognized.

A high index of suspicion is necessary in the clinical management of HIV-infected patients because relatively trivial neurologic symptoms may be the first indicator of a serious underlying disorder. Since any portion of the neuraxis may be involved, it is worthwhile to attempt an anatomic localization of the lesion during the initial evaluation of patients. This helps to narrow the differential diagnosis before proceeding with further imaging and laboratory studies. Since multiple neurologic diseases often coexist in this patient population, close surveillance is needed even if a presumptive diagnosis has been made. A change in clinical condition often necessitates a thorough reevaluation.

REFERENCES

1. Snider WD, Simpson DM, Nielsen S. Neurological complications of the acquired immune deficiency syndrome: analysis of 50 patients. Ann Neurol 1983; 14:403-18.

2. Levy RM, Bredesen DE, Rosenblum ML. Neurological manifestations of the acquired immunodeficiency syndrome (AIDS): experience at UCSF and review of the literature. J Neurosurg 1985; 62:475-95.

3. Rosenblum ML, Levy RM, Bredesen DE. AIDS and the nervous system. New York: Raven Press, 1988.

4. de la Monte SM, Schooley RT, Hirsch MS, Richardson EP. Subacute encephalomyelitis of AIDS and its relation to HTLV-III infection. Neurology 1987; 37:562-9.

5. Koppel BS, Wormser GP, Tuchman AJ, et al. Central nervous system involvement in patients with acquired immune deficiency syndrome (AIDS). Acta Neurol Scand 1985; 71:337-53.

6. Goethe KE, Mitchell JE, Marshall DW, et al. Neuropsychological and neurological function of human immunodeficiency virus seropositive asymptomatic individuals. Arch Neurol 1989; 46:129-33.

7. So YT, Holtzman DM, Abrams D, Olney R. Peripheral neuropathy associated with AIDS: prevalence and clinical features from a population-based survey. Arch Neurology 1988; 45:945-8.

8. Grant I, Atkinson JH, Hesselink JR, et al. Evidence for early central nervous system involvement in acquired immunodeficiency syndrome and other human immunodeficiency virus infections: studies with neuropsychologic testing and magnetic resonance imaging. Ann Intern Med 1987; 107:828-36.

Neurologic Dysfunction: Intracranial Disorders

Yuen T. So, M.D., Ph.D.

The central nervous system disorders seen in AIDS patients can be divided into four general categories: (1) primary infection of the brain by HIV; (2) opportunistic infections by parasitic, fungal, viral, and bacterial organisms; (3) central nervous system (CNS) neoplasms; and (4) complications of systemic disorders.

■ PRIMARY HIV INFECTION OF THE BRAIN

AIDS Dementia Complex. The syndrome has been variously called subacute encephalitis, AIDS dementia complex (ADC), HIV encephalopathy or encephalitis, and multifocal giant-cell encephalitis. Although the pathogenesis of this disorder is still unclear, accumulating evidence suggests that direct HIV infection may play an important role.[11] The exact prevalence of this dementia is debated, but its frequency clearly increases with advancing stages of HIV infection. It is probably uncommon in HIV-seropositive individuals in early stages of HIV disease,[5] but it is frequently encountered in AIDS patients with systemic symptoms.[6]

Poor concentration, forgetfulness, psychomotor slowing, and social withdrawal are typical presenting symptoms; these are often difficult to distinguish from symptoms of depression. Symptoms generally evolve over months, although acute presentation may be precipitated by metabolic derangements or an infectious illness. Seizures or myoclonus sometimes occur. Aside from the findings of dementia on clinical examination, hyperreflexia, Babinski's sign, and frontal-release signs such as snout and grasp reflexes are often present. The neurologic deficits seen in AIDS dementia are usually diffuse; hence, severe or asymmetrical focal deficit would suggest an alternate diagnosis such as cerebral mass lesions or progressive multifocal leukoencephalopathy (PML). Computed tomographic (CT) or magnetic resonance imaging (MRI) scans of the brain may be normal, or may show nonspecific cerebral atrophy. In addition, MRI often shows patchy or diffuse white matter abnormalities.

■ OPPORTUNISTIC INFECTIONS OF THE CNS

Toxoplasma gondii. CNS toxoplasmosis is the most common cause of intracerebral mass lesions in AIDS patients. Frequencies of 3 percent to 40 percent have been reported, reflecting the considerable regional variation in exposure to the organism.[1,2,7] Most of the cases in the United States are probably a result of reactivation of a latent infection. Common initial symptoms are headache, personality change, seizures, hemiparesis, hemisensory loss, and other focal neurologic deficits. CT scan of the brain usually shows single or multiple lesions in the supratentorial fossa, and less commonly in the posterior fossa. Ring or nodular contrast-enhancement of the CT lesions is usually present. MRI is more sensitive in detecting lesions, and consistently shows more than one cerebral lesion.

Cryptococcus neoformans.   This is the most common fungal infection of the CNS, presenting usually as a subacute meningitis.[8] Headache and fever are the most common symptoms. Some patients also present with acute encephalopathy or cranial-nerve palsies. Nuchal rigidity suggests meningeal inflammation but is frequently absent in AIDS patients. In fact, some patients may have a completely normal neurologic examination. Hence, a new headache that does not remit should be investigated with lumbar puncture unless contraindicated by cerebral mass lesions. CT or MRI is usually normal, although rarely CNS cryptococcoma may be seen. Cerebrospinal fluid (CSF) examination should include a determination of the cryptococcal antigen titer, since an elevated titer may occasionally be the only CSF abnormality.

Aseptic Meningitis.   Like other patients with meningitis, patients with aseptic meningitis often present initially with a headache. Focal neurologic signs are uncommon. Many patients with this syndrome probably have a primary HIV meningoencephalitis.[4,13] The meningitis often first manifests at the time of seroconversion and tends to recur spontaneously.[2]

Progressive Multifocal Leukoencephalopathy (PML).   PML is a subacute or chronic progressive illness with dementia, hemiparesis, hemianopsia, ataxia, and other focal deficits.[9] If the focal deficits are mild, it may be difficult to distinguish PML from AIDS dementia complex. CT or MRI reveals focal or diffuse lesions in the white matter, usually without contrast enhancement or mass effect. The brainstem or cerebellum may be solely involved in about 10 percent of cases. The natural history is that of progressive decline until death.

Viral Encephalitis.   The herpesviruses are the most important. Both herpes simplex (HSV-1) and herpes zoster have been associated with encephalitis.[2] The etiologic role of another herpesvirus, cytomegalovirus (CMV), is unclear, although CMV is occasionally isolated from the CSF and histologic evidence of infection is frequently seen in the brain at autopsy.

Fungal Encephalitis.   Reported cases include candidiasis, aspergillosis, coccidioidomycosis, and mucormycosis.[3] Diagnosis is usually made by demonstration of the fungus from biopsy tissues.

Neurosyphilis.   Although neurosyphilis is not an opportunistic infection, a recent report suggests that neurosyphilis in HIV-infected patients may be more refractory to therapy and may progress more rapidly than it does in the non-HIV-infected population.[14] More extensive experience is needed to clarify these observations.

■ CNS NEOPLASMS

Although Kaposi's sarcoma is the most common systemic neoplasm in AIDS, it rarely spreads to the CNS. Non-Hodgkin's lymphoma is a more important cause of neurologic dysfunctions. Primary CNS lymphoma, without evidence of systemic lymphoma, is second only to CNS toxoplasmosis as a cause of cerebral mass lesions in AIDS patients.[12] The symptoms and signs as well as the radiologic appearance are often indistinguishable from those of toxoplasmosis, and a confident diagnosis is possible only with brain biopsy. Systemic lymphomas invade the CNS by spreading along the leptomeninges, causing cranial nerve palsy, polyradiculopathy, and spinal cord compression. Intraparenchymal mass lesions are uncommon. Cytologic examination of the CSF is essential for the diagnosis.

■ COMPLICATIONS OF SYSTEMIC DISEASES

Metabolic Encephalopathy.   Common causes in AIDS patients include adverse reaction to therapeutic drugs, drug overdose, hypoxia, hyponatremia, hypoglycemia (e.g., secondary to pentamidine treatment), and organ failures. Rarely, Wernicke's encephalopathy has been reported.[15]

Strokes.   Cerebral infarction and transient ischemic attacks are seen infrequently in HIV-infected patients.[10] They may be a result of marantic endocarditis, vasculitis, meningovascular syphilis, and systemic hypotension.

■ SYMPTOMS, NEUROLOGIC SIGNS, AND DIFFERENTIAL DIAGNOSIS

Headache.   Headache is a difficult clinical problem in patients with HIV disease. While many patients undoubtedly have benign headaches, headaches may also herald a wide range of intracranial disorders. Meningitis, encephalitis, cerebral mass lesions, and progressive multifocal leukoencephalopathy can all present with headache. Any new headache that persists should be investigated with CT or MRI, followed by a lumbar puncture unless contraindicated by the presence of mass lesions.

Seizures.   All the CNS disorders discussed earlier in this chapter can manifest as generalized or focal seizures. Status epilepticus may also occur. The common causes in descending order of frequency are cerebral mass lesions, encephalitis (including AIDS dementia complex), and meningitis.[17] In about 20 percent of patients, no definite cause can be found despite thorough evaluation. Treatment with phenobarbital or phenytoin (Dilantin) provides excellent symptomatic control, although patients with mass lesions tend to be more refractory to therapy.

Dementia.   Most cases of dementia are due to AIDS dementia complex. Mass lesions and PML can present with personality change and cognitive decline, but they are usually associated with more prominent focal deficits.

Altered Mental Status.   Acute encephalopathy is distinguished from dementia by the more rapid progression of symptoms and the frequent association with an altered level of consciousness. Differential diagnosis includes metabolic encephalopathy from systemic diseases, opportunistic infections, neoplasms, strokes, and a postictal confusional state. Moreover, patients with underlying dementia are extremely susceptible to metabolic and infectious derangements and frequently present with altered mental state.

Posterior Fossa Symptoms and Signs.   Isolated involvement of the posterior fossa is uncommon. Symptoms and signs include vertigo, diplopia, headache, cerebellar ataxia, and cranial nerve deficits. If the brainstem parenchyma is involved, long-tract signs such as hemiparesis and hemisensory loss are common. Differential diagnosis includes the following.

TABLE 1.   POSTERIOR FOSSA SYMPTOMS AND SIGNS —
DIFFERENTIAL DIAGNOSIS

EXTRAAXIAL (i.e., cranial neuropathies)	INTRAAXIAL (i.e., brainstem and cerebellum involvement)
Cryptococcal meningitis	Cryptococcal meningitis
Leptomeningeal lymphoma	CNS toxoplasmosis
Aseptic meningitis	Primary CNS lymphoma
Herpes zoster	Progressive multifocal leukoencephalopathy (PML)
Mononeuropathy multiplex	Tuberculoma
Tuberculous meningitis	

■ DIAGNOSTIC STUDIES

Brain CT Scan and MRI.   Although MRI is more sensitive than CT in detecting CNS abnormalities,[16] CT with double-dose contrast is an excellent alternative.[18] There is no pathognomonic radiologic appearance for any of the CNS disorders seen in AIDS patients. However, several patterns are clinically helpful. Widespread white matter abnormalities without contrast enhancement or mass suggest either PML or AIDS dementia complex. The lesions of AIDS dementia complex tend to be more diffuse, less well demarcated, and more prominent in the frontal regions. Cerebral mass lesions suggest either abscesses or primary CNS lymphoma. Ring or nodular enhancement with contrast may be seen in either, and there is no reliable way to distinguish the two types of lesions. However, multiple lesions probably favor toxoplasmosis, and a solitary lesion seen on MRI would favor a diagnosis of lymphoma. Hydrocephalus may occur with mass lesions that obstruct CSF outflow. When it occurs in isolation, it is usually associated with one of the meningitides, such as cryptococcal meningitis or basilar meningitis in neurosyphilis.

Lumbar Puncture.   Routine CSF studies are frequently abnormal in patients in all stages of HIV infection. Elevated protein, hypoglycorrhachia, pleocytosis, or some combination of the three are seen in meningitis, encephalitis, and CNS neoplasms. More specific tests like CSF VDRL, cryptococcal antigen titer, and microbiological studies (including viral and mycobacterial cultures) should be routinely carried out. Cytologic examination is useful in the diagnosis of lymphoma, especially in patients with leptomeningeal metastasis of systemic non-Hodgkin's lymphoma.

Brain Biopsy.   Biopsy is probably the only reliable method for making a confirmatory diagnosis of intracranial disorders such as toxoplasmosis, lymphoma, and PML. In view of the considerable morbidity of open-brain biopsy, we favor an empiric treatment approach to patients who are clinically stable and have multiple radiologically verifiable lesions. We use an antitoxoplasmosis regimen of pyrimethamine and sulfadiazine, and follow these patients with daily neurologic examinations and weekly imaging studies. Brain biopsy is considered if there is clinical deterioration or no radiologic response at the end of a 10-day course of antibiotic treatment. Brain biopsy is also considered for those patients who are either neurologically unstable or have only a solitary lesion on brain MRI. Obviously, there cannot be any simple rule; other clinical factors and, above all, the patient's wishes, should be taken into consideration.

TABLE 2. TREATMENT AND PROGNOSIS

DIAGNOSIS	TREATMENT	PROGNOSIS
AIDS dementia complex	Zidovudine (AZT)	Partial clinical improvement in some patients[19]
Toxoplasmosis	Sulfadiazine and pyrimethamine; clindamycin in combination with pyrimethamine may be an alternative	Good initial response but recurrence common[7]
Cryptococcal meningitis	Amphotericin B and 5-fluorocytosine	High recurrence rate without maintenance therapy[8]
CNS lymphoma	Radiation therapy	Tumor is radiosensitive, but recurrence rate is high and patients often die of other opportunistic infections[20]
Aseptic meningitis	None	Spontaneous remission, but recurrent meningitis is common[2]
Progressive multifocal encephalopathy	None	Progression until death[9]
Herpes simplex encephalitis	Acyclovir	Variable; paradoxically, more immunocompromised patients may have less fulminant courses[2]

REFERENCES

1. Snider WD, Simpson DM, Nielsen S. Neurological complications of the acquired immune deficiency syndrome: analysis of 50 patients. Ann Neurol 1983; 14:403-18.

2. Levy RM, Bredesen DE, Rosenblum ML. Neurological manifestations of the acquired immunodeficiency syndrome (AIDS): experience at UCSF and review of the literature. J Neurosurg 1985; 62:475-95.

3. Rosenblum ML, Levy RM, Bredesen DE. AIDS and the nervous system. New York: Raven Press, 1988.

4. Ho DD, Rota TR, Schooley RT, et al. Isolation of HTLV-III from cerebrospinal fluid and neural tissues of patients with neurologic syndromes related to the acquired immune deficiency syndrome. N Engl J Med 1985; 313:1493-7.

5. Goethe KE, Mitchell JE, Marshall DW, et al. Neuropsychological and neurological function of human immunodeficiency virus seropositive asymptomatic individuals. Arch Neurol 1989; 46:129-33.

6. Grant I, Atkinson JH, Hesselink JR, et al. Evidence for early central nervous system involvement in the acquired immunodeficiency syndrome (AIDS) and other human immunodeficiency virus (HIV) infections. Studies with neuropsychologic testing and magnetic resonance imaging. Ann Intern Med 1987; 107:828-36.

7. Luft BJ, Remington JS. AIDS commentary. Toxoplasmic encephalitis. J Infect Dis 1988; 157:1-6.

8. Zuger A, Louie E, Holzman RS, et al. Cryptococcal disease in patients with the acquired immunodeficiency syndrome. Diagnostic features and outcome of treatment. Ann Intern Med 1986; 104:234-40.

9. Berger JR, Kaszovitz B, Post MJ, Dickinson G. Progressive multifocal leukoencephalopathy associated with human immunodeficiency virus infection. A review of the literature with a report of sixteen cases. Ann Intern Med 1987; 107:78-87.

10. Engstrom JW, Lowenstein DH, Bredesen DE. Cerebral infarctions and transient neurologic deficits associated with acquired immunodeficiency syndrome. Am J Med 1989; 86:528-32.

11. Navia BA, Price RW. The acquired immunodeficiency syndrome dementia complex as the presenting or sole manifestation of human immunodeficiency virus infection. Arch Neurol 1987; 44:65-9.

12. So YT, Couchais A, Davis RL, et al. Neoplasms of the central nervous system in acquired immuno-deficiency syndrome. In: Rosenblum ML, Levy RM, Bredesen DE, eds. AIDS and the nervous system. New York: Raven Press, 1988.

13. Carne CA, Tedder RS, Smith A, Sutherland S, et al. Acute encephalopathy coincident with seroconver-sion for anti-HTLV-III. Lancet 1985; 2:1206-8.

14. Johns DR, Tierney M, Felsenstein D. Alteration in the natural history of neurosyphilis by concurrent infection with the human immunodeficiency virus. N Engl J Med 1987; 316:1569-72.

15. Foresti V, Confalonieri E. Wernicke's encephalopathy in AIDS. Lancet 1987; 1:1499.

16. Levy RM, Mills CM, Posin JP, et al. The superiority of cranial magnetic imaging (MRI) to computed tomographic (CT) brain scans for the diagnosis of cerebral lesions in patients with AIDS [Abstract]. II International Conference on AIDS. Paris, 1986; 37.

17. Holtzman DM, Kaku DA, So YT. New onset seizures associated with human immunodeficiency virus infection. Etiology and clinical features in 100 cases. Am J Med 1989 (in press).

18. Post MJ, Kursunoglu SJ, Hensley GT, et al. Cranial CT in acquired immunodeficiency syndrome: spectrum of diseases and optimal contrast enhancement technique. AJR 1985; 145:929-40.

19. Yarchoan R, Klecker RW, Weinhold KJ, et al. Administration of 3'-azido-3'-deoxythymidine, an in-hibitor of HTLV-III/LAV replication, to patients with AIDS or AIDS-related complex. Lancet 1986; 1:575-80.

20. Formenti SC, Gill PS, Lean E, et al. Primary central nervous system lymphoma in AIDS. Results of radiation therapy. Cancer 1989; 63:1101-7.

Spinal Cord Disorders

Yuen T. So, M.D., Ph.D.

S pinal cord disorders are less common than intracranial and peripheral nervous system diseases. Sensory disturbance or gait instability is the usual clinical presentation. Early clinical signs are spasticity, hyperreflexia, and loss of superficial abdominal reflexes. Paraparesis or quadriparesis, Babinski's sign, loss of sphincter control, and a spinal level of sensory loss are seen in the more severe cases. Back pain or spine tenderness (or both) often accompany the acute myelopathies and, if present, should suggest a potential neurologic emergency.

■ VACUOLAR MYELOPATHY

Vacuolar myelopathy, a pathologic entity that resembles subacute combined degeneration of pernicious anemia, is the most common spinal cord disorder in HIV infection; it is seen in the postmortem examination in up to 30 percent of patients.[2,3] However, the clinical correlate of vacuolar myelopathy is recognized less frequently. Symptoms of myelopathy are usually subacute or chronic. If paresthesias are prominent, myelopathy may be confused with peripheral neuropathy. However, brisk tendon reflexes (with preservation of ankle jerks) and posterior column signs (such as impaired joint-position sense) should suggest a spinal cord involvement. Vacuolar myelopathy often coexists with AIDS dementia complex, and both conditions cause spasticity and paraparesis. Thus, it may be difficult to separate the spinal cord involvement in AIDS patients with dementia.

■ ACUTE MYELOPATHIES

Though less common than vacuolar myelopathy, acute spinal cord dysfunction is important to recognize in AIDS patients. Symptoms and signs of cord dysfunction may progress rapidly, often accompanied by back pain or spine tenderness. The causes include spinal-cord compression from lymphomatous metastasis,[1,6] tuberculous spinal abscess,[10] and infections by cytomegalovirus or herpesvirus.[1,4,8] In addition, a rare acute myelopathy at the time of HIV seroconversion has been described.[9]

■ DIAGNOSIS AND TREATMENT

In emergency-room settings, spinal cord compression should be looked for in patients with acute back pain and deteriorating neurologic deficits. Magnetic resonance imaging (MRI) scans of the appropriate spinal cord segments or myelography with follow-up computed tomographic (CT) scan is the diagnostic test of choice. If radiologic studies are negative, the cerebrospinal fluid (CSF) should be evaluated for evidence of infection or meningeal lymphomatosis. Prognosis depends on the residual neurologic function at the time treatment is initiated. If the CSF findings support an infectious etiology, empiric antimicrobial therapy should be considered in patients who are neurologically unstable.

In patients with vacuolar myelopathy, radiologic studies are usually normal, although MRI rarely shows areas of increased signal within the spinal cord. CSF studies may be normal or may show nonspecific abnormalities. Somatosensory-evoked potential is a useful adjunct to document a conduction defect in the sensory pathways of the spinal cord. The etiology of vacuolar myelopathy is unknown, and no treatment is available at present.[3,11]

REFERENCES

1. Levy RM, Bredesen DE, Rosenblum ML. Neurological manifestations of the acquired immunodeficiency syndrome: experience at UCSF and review of the literature. J Neurosurg 1985; 62:475-95.
2. Petito CK, Navia BA, Cho ES, et al. Vacuolar myelopathy pathologically resembling subacute combined degeneration in patients with the acquired immunodeficiency syndrome. N Engl J Med 1985; 312:874-9.
3. Rosenblum M, Scheck AC, Cronin K, et al. Dissociation of AIDS-related vacuolar myelopathy and productive HIV-1 infection of the spinal cord. Neurology 1989; 39:892-6.
4. Tucker T, Dix RD, Katzen C, et al. Cytomegalovirus and herpes simplex virus ascending myelitis in a patient with acquired immune deficiency syndrome. Ann Neurol 1985; 18:74-9.
6. Ziegler JL, Drew WL, Miner RC, et al. Outbreak of Burkitt's like lymphoma in homosexual men. Lancet 1982; 2:631-3.
8. Dix RD, Bredesen DE, Erlich KS, Mills J. Recovery of herpesviruses from cerebrospinal fluid of immunodeficient homosexual men. Ann Neurol 1985; 18:611-4.
9. Denning DW, Anderson J, Rudge P, Smith H. Acute myelopathy associated with primary infection with human immunodeficiency virus. Br Med J 1987; 294:143-4.
10. Doll DC, Yarbro JW, Phillips K, Klatt C. Mycobacterial spinal cord abscess with an ascending polyneuropathy. Ann Intern Med 1987; 106:333-4.
11. Yarchoan R, Berg G, Brouwers P, et al. Response of human-immunodeficiency-virus-associated neurological disease to 3'-azido-3'-deoxythymidine. Lancet 1987; 1:132-5.

Disorders of the
Peripheral Nerves

Yuen T. So, M.D., Ph.D.

■ DISTAL SYMMETRIC POLYNEUROPATHY

Several distinct neuropathy syndromes have been described in patients infected with HIV.[1] The most common is a distal symmetric polyneuropathy (DSPN) that affects approximately 35 percent of hospitalized AIDS patients with systemic symptoms.[3,5] This neuropathy manifests as subacute onset of numbness and tingling in a stocking or glove distribution. Burning dysesthesias over the soles and the distal portion of the digits are frequent presenting complaints that bring the patients to medical attention. Early and consistent clinical signs are bilaterally depressed ankle reflex and impaired vibration sensation in the toes. The etiology of DSPN is probably multifactorial. Some patients undoubtedly have neuropathy from well-recognized toxins such as alcohol, vincristine, and isoniazid. However, no etiology can be ascertained in the majority of the remaining patients; both autoimmune mechanisms and viral infection have been suggested as possible etiologies.

Electromyography (EMG) and nerve-conduction studies are useful in differentiating DSPN from the less common neuropathy syndromes described below. There is no treatment that has been convincingly shown to alter the clinical course of DSPN; an initial report of success with zidovudine (AZT) has been challenged by subsequent studies.

■ INFLAMMATORY NEUROPATHIES

Mononeuropathy multiplex and inflammatory demyelinating neuropathy have also been recognized in HIV-infected patients.[2,6] They differ from DSPN because they tend to occur in otherwise asymptomatic seropositive individuals and in symptomatic patients who have relatively intact immune systems. These neuropathies usually produce patchy motor and sensory deficits, whereas DSPN is a symmetrical and predominantly sensory neuropathy. Symptoms of the inflammatory neuropathies may appear suddenly or may evolve over several days or weeks. Cranial nerve palsy is occasionally seen. The pathogenesis is probably immune-mediated, although the exact mechanism is unknown. Some patients with mononeuropathy multiplex or demyelinating neuropathy have improved after plasmapheresis.[6]

■ LUMBOSACRAL POLYRADICULOPATHY

This disorder is seen primarily in AIDS patients with systemic symptoms.[4] Patients present with rapidly progressive weakness and areflexia of the lower extremities, often with patchy sensory loss and sphincter disturbances. It is an uncommon disorder, although it is important to recognize because of its poor prognosis.

There are probably several different causes for the lumbosacral polyradiculopathy syndrome, although the common site of pathology appears to be in the cauda equina or lumbosacral roots. Imaging studies of the lumbosacral spine should be performed to rule out any compressive lesions. In about half of the patients, an intensely inflammatory cerebrospinal fluid (CSF) (>400 white cells/cubic millimeter, >40 percent polymorphonuclear cells) is seen.[8] Cytomegalovirus (CMV) is often recovered from the CSF of these patients, and autopsy studies have revealed the characteristic intraneuronal inclusion bodies of CMV. Although occasional patients have improved after treatment with ganciclovir, weakness usually progresses rapidly to complete paralysis, and most patients succumb within two to three months. In another group of the patients, a moderate or low-grade pleocytosis (<100 white cells/cubic millimeter, mostly mononuclear) is seen instead. Some cases are due to leptomeningeal lymphoma, but some have no definable cause. These patients' disease tends to have a more indolent clinical course, and partial recovery has been seen.

■ RARE NEUROPATHIES

Although some degree of autonomic involvement is often detectable in AIDS patients with peripheral neuropathy, severe autonomic dysfunction is rare.[7] Sensory ataxia is also rare despite the almost universal presence of sensory symptoms in AIDS-related neuropathies. The only report to date described a patient with ataxia, Romberg sign, and no motor finding initially; inflammatory changes were seen in the dorsal root ganglia at autopsy.[9]

REFERENCES

1. Parry GJ. Peripheral neuropathies associated with human immunodeficiency virus infection. Ann Neurol 1988; 23(Suppl):S49-S53.
2. Lipkin WI, Parry GJ, Kiprov D, Abrams D. Inflammatory neuropathy in homosexual men with lymphadenopathy. Neurology 1985; 10:1479-83.
3. So YT, Holtzman DM, Abrams DI, Olney RK. Peripheral neuropathy associated with acquired immunodeficiency syndrome. Prevalence and clinical features from a population-based survey. Arch Neurol 1988; 45:945-8.
4. Eidelberg D, Sotrel A, Vogel H, et al. Progressive polyradiculopathy in acquired immune deficiency syndrome. Neurology 1986; 36:912-6.
5. Cornblath DR, McArthur JC. Predominantly sensory neuropathy in patients with AIDS and AIDS-related complex. Neurology 1988; 38:794-6.
6. Cornblath DR, McArthur JC, Kennedy PG, et al. Inflammatory demyelinating peripheral neuropathies associated with human T-cell lymphotropic virus type III infection. Ann Neurol 1987; 21:32-40.
7. Craddock C, Pasvol G, Bull R, et al. Cardiorespiratory arrest and autonomic neuropathy in AIDS. Lancet 1987; 2:16-8.
8. So YT, Holtzman DM, Olney RK. The spectrum of progressive lumbosacral polyradiculopathy seen in acquired immune deficiency syndrome. Neurology (Suppl) 1989:382.
9. Elder G, Dalakas M, Pezeshkpour G, Sever J. Ataxic neuropathy due to ganglioneuronitis after probable acute human immunodeficiency virus infection. Lancet 1986; 2:1275-6.

5.5

Pulmonary Aspects

Respiratory System:
A General Approach

Peter M. Small, M.D., and Philip C. Hopewell, M.D.

There is a high incidence of pulmonary disease in patients with AIDS and presumably in patients at earlier stages of HIV infection as well. The majority of these diseases are infectious, but neoplastic and idiopathic inflammatory conditions also occur.

The most common pulmonary infection in AIDS patients is *Pneumocystis carinii* pneumonia (PCP), occurring alone in 58 percent and with Kaposi's sarcoma in an additional 5 percent of patients who meet CDC criteria for AIDS.[1,2] In addition to *P. carinii*, AIDS patients are predisposed to a variety of other fungal, mycobacterial, bacterial, and viral pulmonary opportunistic infections. AIDS patients also appear to have a high incidence of pulmonary infections that are not defined by the CDC as HIV-related opportunistic infections.[4]

Both Kaposi's sarcoma (KS) and lymphoma may involve the lungs of AIDS patients. Pulmonary KS is usually seen in patients with extensive extrapulmonary disease.[5] Non-Hodgkin's lymphoma in patients with HIV infection may involve pleura, intrathoracic lymph nodes, and lung parenchyma.

Idiopathic inflammatory pulmonary disease is clearly associated with HIV disease. Infiltration of the lungs with lymphocytes (in a pattern consistent with lymphocytic interstitial pneumonitis) is common in children with AIDS,[6] and is increasingly being diagnosed in adults.[7] Nonspecific interstitial pneumonitis was reported as the causative factor in 32 percent of all cases of pneumonitis in AIDS patients at the NIH over a four-year period.[8] Alveolar proteinosis has also been identified as a cause of respiratory failure and death[9] in patients with pulmonary disease. One study showed that 72 percent (88 out of 122) of HIV-infected individuals without evidence of infectious or neoplastic disease had lymphocytic alveolitis on bronchoscopic lavage, suggesting that the lungs may be involved early in the course of HIV infection.[10]

■ DIFFERENTIAL DIAGNOSIS

It is important to remember that not all lung disease in patients with HIV infection or AIDS is necessarily related to HIV infection. Patients may also have pulmonary diseases (such as asthma, pneumococcal pneumonia, or other disorders) that are common in the general population.

In addition to these usual pulmonary diseases, AIDS patients are prone to a unique spectrum of pulmonary disease. Table 1 lists the pulmonary disorders found in 441 patients with AIDS cared for in New York and California institutions.[3] These disorders make up the majority of the differential diagnosis of lung disease in patients with AIDS.

TABLE 1.   PULMONARY INVOLVEMENT IN 441 PATIENTS
WITH AIDS

Infections*	No. of Patients (%)
P. carinii	373 (85)
M. avium-intracellulare	79 (17)
Cytomegalovirus	74 (17)
M. tuberculosis	19 (4)
Legionella	19 (4)
Pyogenic bacteria	11 (2)
Cryptococcus neoformans	9 (2)
Other fungi	6 (1)
Herpes simplex	2 (<1)
Toxoplasma gondii	1 (<1)
Kaposi's sarcoma	36 (8)

* *More than one organism may be present in a single patient (from Murray et al.[3]). Adapted from the*
New England Journal of Medicine, *1984; 310:1682-8.*

Although there are no recent compilations of data similar to those in Table
1, important changes regarding pulmonary involvement include: (1) increased
incidence of serious pyogenic infections; (2) recognition that *M. tuberculosis* is
of increasing importance; (3) decline in diagnosis of legionella; and (4) increased frequency of lymphocytic and nonspecific interstitial pneumonitis.[11]

■ GENERAL APPROACH

Given the array of diagnoses possible for pulmonary disease in patients with
HIV infection, respiratory complaints must be taken seriously and evaluated
promptly. Patients with AIDS should be taught to recognize and report respiratory symptoms. The first step in the diagnostic evaluation of such symptoms
should be to exclude "routine" pulmonary diseases rather than to automatically
assume that the symptom is HIV-related. Having excluded possible common
diseases, the clinician should direct the diagnostic approach toward identifying
the disorders listed in Table 1.[12,13] The sequence of diagnostic studies should be
determined logically and progress from noninvasive to more invasive studies.[14]
Diagnosis requires coordination among clinical services and among clinicians,
radiologists, pathologists, and microbiologists. A system should be developed
to ensure that all appropriate studies are done expeditiously and accurately.
The specific diagnostic approach is described in detail in subsequent chapters.

■ HISTORY AND PHYSICAL EXAMINATION

Like most respiratory disorders, pulmonary involvement in patients with HIV
infection produces nonspecific signs and symptoms. Commonly, patients have
had systemic symptoms such as fever, malaise, and weight loss for several weeks
to months before developing pulmonary symptoms. Occasionally, however,
the initial subjective manifestations of AIDS may be respiratory symptoms. In a
group of patients with AIDS and pulmonary involvement studied by Stover
and coworkers,[15] 89 percent reported cough and 64 percent dyspnea. The

cough was productive in 39 percent. Pleuritic pain (20 percent) and hemoptysis (3 percent) were also reported. Acute symptoms were much more common among patients with pyogenic bacterial pneumonias, and often included shaking chills. Symptoms in patients with opportunistic infections, especially *P. carinii* pneumonia, tended to be more indolent, although they were rapidly progressive in a few instances.

Physical findings may be very useful in establishing or suggesting a diagnosis of AIDS or AIDS-related complex (ARC), but they are not particularly helpful in defining a specific pulmonary process. Pulmonary findings are more useful in suggesting that respiratory symptoms in a high-risk patient are not caused by an AIDS-related disorder. For example, the finding of diffuse wheezing would suggest the diagnosis of asthma. Findings that are consistent with localized consolidation of the lung, if confirmed radiographically, would be most indicative of an acute pyogenic bacterial pneumonia (these occur with greater frequency in patients with HIV infection, but are not necessarily related[4]). Findings associated with an AIDS-related pulmonary process include diffuse rales, indicating a widespread infiltrative process. A large pleural effusion, such as might be associated with Kaposi's sarcoma (KS), would cause limited expansion of the affected hemithorax, dullness to percussion, and decreased breath sounds.

Ancillary or extrapulmonary findings that may provide circumstantial evidence for an AIDS-related pulmonary process include the following: retinitis or endophthalmitis due to cytomegalovirus[16] or disseminated candidiasis[17]; mouth lesions such as thrush[18] or hairy leukoplakia[19]; neurologic findings that may indicate cryptococcal disease[20] or toxoplasmosis[21] (either of which can involve the lungs); diffuse lymphadenopathy caused by HIV[22]; and cutaneous lesions of Kaposi's sarcoma, which are nearly always present (and usually extensive) in patients who also have pulmonary KS.[5]

REFERENCES

1. Update: acquired immunodeficiency syndrome — United States. MMWR 1986; 35:17-21.

2. Peterman TA, Drotman DP, Curran JW. Epidemiology of the acquired immunodeficiency syndrome (AIDS). Epidemiol Rev 1985; 7:1-21.

3. Murray JF, Felton CP, Garay SM, et al. Pulmonary complications of the acquired immunodeficiency syndrome: report of a National Heart, Lung, and Blood Institute workshop. N Engl J Med 1984; 310:1682-8.

4. Chaisson RE. Infections due to encapsulated bacteria, salmonella, shigella, and campylobacter. In: Sande MA, Volberding PA, eds. Medical management of AIDS. Philadelphia: W.B. Saunders, 1988:249-51.

5. Kaplan LD, Hopewell PC, Jaffe H, et al. Kaposi's sarcoma involving the lung in patients with the acquired immunodeficiency syndrome. Jour AIDS 1988; 1:23-30.

6. Rubinstein A, Morecki R, Silverman B, et al. Pulmonary disease in children with acquired immune deficiency syndrome and AIDS-related complex. J Pediatr 1986; 108:498-503.

7. Morris JC, Rosen MJ, Marchevsky A, Teirstein AS. Lymphocytic interstitial pneumonia in patients at risk for the acquired immune deficiency syndrome. Chest 1987; 91:63-7.

8. Suffredini AF, Ognibene FP, Lack EE, et al. Nonspecific interstitial pneumonitis: a common cause of pulmonary disease in the acquired immunodeficiency syndrome. Ann Intern Med 1987; 107:7-13.

9. Ruben FL, Talamo TS. Secondary pulmonary alveolar proteinosis occurring in two patients with acquired immune deficiency syndrome. Am J Med 1986; 80:1187-90.

10. Guillon JM, Denis M, Mayaud C, et al. HIV-related alveolitis. Chest 1988; 94:1264-70.

11. Murray JF, Garay SM, Hopewell PC, et al. Pulmonary complications of the acquired immunodeficiency syndrome: an update. Am Rev Resp Dis 1987; 135:504-9.

12. Chaisson RE, Theuer CP, Elias D, et al. HIV seroprevalence in patients with tuberculosis [Abstract]. Program and Abstracts of the Twenty-eighth Interscience Conference on Antimicrobial Agents and Chemotherapy. Los Angeles: American Society for Microbiology, 1988:571.

13. Bronnimann DA, Adam RD, Galgiani JN, et al. Coccidioidomycosis in the acquired immunodeficiency syndrome. Ann Intern Med 1987; 106:372-9.

14. Hopewell PC. Diagnosis of *Pneumocystis carinii* pneumonia. Inf Dis Clin N Am 1988; 2:409-18.

15. Stover DE, White DA, Romano PA, et al. Spectrum of pulmonary diseases associated with the acquired immune deficiency syndrome. Am J Med 1985; 78:429-37.

16. Egbert PR, Pollard RB, Gallagher JG, Merigan TC. Cytomegalovirus retinitis in immunosuppressed hosts. II. Ocular manifestations. Ann Intern Med 1980; 93:664-70.

17. Edwards JE, Foos RY, Montgomerie JZ, Guze LB. Ocular manifestations of candida septicemia: review of 76 cases of hematogenous candida endophthalmitis. Medicine 1974; 53:47-75.

18. Klein RS, Harris CA, Small CB, et al. Oral candidiasis in high-risk patients as the initial manifestation of the acquired immunodeficiency syndrome. N Engl J Med 1984; 311:354-8.

19. Greenspan JS, Greenspan D, Lenette ET, et al. Replication of Epstein–Barr virus within the epithelial cells of oral "hairy" leukoplakia, an AIDS associated lesion. N Engl J Med 1985; 313:1564-71.

20. Zuger A, Louie E, Holzman RS, et al. Cryptococcal disease in patients with the acquired immunodeficiency syndrome, diagnostic features and outcome of treatment. Ann Intern Med 1986; 104; 234-40.

21. Pons VG, Jacobs RA, Hollander H. Nonviral infections of the central nervous system in patients with acquired immunodeficiency syndrome. In: Rosenblum ML, Levy RM, Bredesen DE, eds. AIDS and the nervous system. New York: Raven Press, 1988:263-9.

22. Metroka CE, Cunningham-Rundles S, Pollack MS, et al. Generalized lymphadenopathy in homosexual men. Ann Intern Med 1983; 99:585-91.

Respiratory System: Radiographic Findings

Peter M. Small, M.D., and Philip C. Hopewell, M.D.

T he chest radiograph is almost always the first diagnostic study undertaken to determine the cause of respiratory symptoms or physical findings related to the lungs. Only rarely does the chest film yield a definitive diagnosis; however, findings point toward the next steps in the evaluation. Patients from HIV risk groups or with known AIDS may have "standard" pulmonary disorders that are not related to the immunosuppression per se, such as asthma or viral or bacterial pneumonias. The chest film, together with the history and physical examination, helps to sort out these processes and to indicate who should undergo further diagnostic testing for an HIV-related pulmonary process.

A wide variety of abnormalities found on the chest radiograph may indicate an HIV-related disorder. However, there is considerable overlap among the diagnoses that can produce a given finding. Thus, none of the findings should be viewed as specific for a particular disease.[1]

■ DIFFERENTIAL DIAGNOSIS

The differential diagnosis associated with radiographic abnormalities can identify the following respiratory symptoms or findings in a patient with AIDS or HIV infection.

Diffuse Interstitial Infiltration. This radiographic pattern, generally involving all portions of the lungs in an even pattern, is most commonly caused by *P. carinii*.[1,3] Several variations on the basic pattern may be seen. The infiltration may be somewhat heterogeneously distributed throughout the lung or it may be more miliary in appearance. Interstitial infiltrates may be limited to the upper lung fields in those patients who develop *P. carinii* pneumonia (PCP) while receiving aerosolized pentamidine.[2] A diffuse interstitial pattern also may occur with cytomegalovirus (CMV),[1] *Mycobacterium tuberculosis*,[4] *M. avium* complex, histoplasmosis,[5] and coccidioidomycosis.[6] In some instances, particularly in patients with disseminated *Mycobacterium avium* complex infections, it is difficult to determine if the detected organism is the cause of the radiographic abnormality or if it is secondary to bacteremia or fungemia. More than one organism may be present (e.g., *P. carinii* commonly coexists with CMV or *M. avium* complex).

Malignancies are much less common than infections as a cause of diffuse interstitial infiltration of the lungs. Pulmonary Kaposi's sarcoma has been reported as a cause of this radiographic pattern, although it is usually associated with other radiographic findings.[7,8] Both Hodgkin's and non-Hodgkin's lymphomas may cause parenchymal infiltrates on the chest films of patients with AIDS, although they more commonly present as mediastinal mass, adenopathy, or pleural effusions.

Diffuse interstitial infiltrates are seen in several idiopathic disorders. Lymphoid interstitial pneumonitis, although not exclusively an HIV-related diagnosis, has been reported in patients with ARC and may be a response to an undefined lung infection.[9] Chest films have shown fine bilateral interstitial reticular and reticulonodular infiltration. Nonspecific interstitial pneumonitis without identifiable infection and alveolar proteinosis also present with diffuse infiltrates in patients with AIDS.[10,15]

Diffuse Airspace Consolidation.   Essentially any of the infectious and non-infectious processes described above as causing diffuse interstitial infiltration may also cause widespread airspace consolidation. Such consolidation, particularly when due to pneumocystis pneumonia, increases as the disorder becomes more severe. Infectious organisms other than *P. carinii* are much less likely to cause diffuse consolidation.

Focal Airspace Consolidation.   Focal consolidation is probably caused by bacterial pneumonia[16] but may also be caused by *Mycoplasma pneumoniae* or viruses other than CMV, such as adenovirus or influenza.[1,3] *P. carinii* may also cause localized abnormalities (especially in patients who have received aerosolized pentamidine), as may *M. tuberculosis* and *Mycobacterium avium* complex.[1,11]

Nodular Lesions.   Pulmonary Kaposi's sarcoma is the most likely cause of nodular lesions scattered throughout the lungs.[8] Nodular infiltrations may also occur in patients with mycobacterial and fungal infections or toxoplasmosis.

Cavitary Lesions.   True cavitation on a chest roentgenogram is unusual in patients with AIDS. However, pneumatoceles are fairly common in patients with PCP. Organisms such as *M. tuberculosis* and *M. avium* complex, which commonly cause cavitary lesions in nonimmunosuppressed hosts, rarely do so in patients with AIDS. However, tuberculosis may cause cavitation in HIV-infected patients who do not yet have an AIDS-defining diagnosis. Cavitation may be seen in bacterial pneumonias (such as those caused by *S. aureus*, anaerobic infections, or klebsiella species) and in fungal processes. Pneumocystis pneumonia causes cystic changes in the lungs, particularly during the healing process, and has been reported to present as a cavitary nodule.[17]

Pleural Effusion.   Pleural effusions, particularly if they are large, are most likely to be caused by Kaposi's sarcoma. Smaller effusions are seen in association with nearly all of the infectious processes; thus, the finding of a small effusion is of little diagnostic value.

Intrathoracic Adenopathy.   Intrathoracic adenopathy may occur in patients with Kaposi's sarcoma, lymphoma, and infectious processes — particularly tuberculosis and cryptococcus. Adenopathy is very uncommon with PCP; when present, it is probably due to another process. The differential diagnosis of lymphadenopathy also includes Castleman's disease[12] and should include metastatic malignancies other than KS. Surprisingly, the diffuse lymphadenopathy syndrome, an HIV-related disorder, is not associated with intrathoracic adenopathy.[13]

Pneumothorax.   Spontaneous pneumothorax has been noted in association with pneumocystis pneumonia.[14] Pneumothorax may also occur after a pulmonary diagnostic procedure, such as a transbronchial biopsy.

Normal Chest Film. A normal chest film may indicate that the respiratory symptoms reported by the patient are not caused by lung disease or that the disease is not sufficiently advanced to cause radiographic findings. Approximately 5 percent to 10 percent of patients with proven PCP have normal chest films. Other pathogens, such as CMV and *M. avium* complex, may also be present without causing abnormal chest films. For these reasons, if the patient's symptoms are judged to be significant, further evaluation is warranted.

■ RADIOGRAPHIC ABNORMALITIES IN HIV-ASSOCIATED DISORDERS

Although radiographic findings are not specific for particular diagnosis in patients with HIV infection, certain patterns of abnormalities are highly suggestive. This section complements the chapter on pulmonary radiographic findings, in which the differential diagnosis of various radiographic abnormalities is described.

Pneumocystis carinii **Pneumonia.** The radiographic pattern most commonly seen with pneumocystis pneumonia is a diffuse interstitial infiltration.[1] Usually the infiltration is linear, but on occasion may be finely nodular. It tends to be distributed homogeneously throughout the lungs but may be uneven, involving one lung or even one lobe more heavily than another.[3] Patients receiving aerosolized pentamidine prophylaxis who develop PCP may have infiltrates that are limited to the upper lung fields.[2] More severe disease may cause diffuse airspace consolidation; at times, this consolidation may be extremely dense throughout all parts of the lungs. Air bronchograms may show such consolidation. Much less commonly, PCP may cause localized infiltrations and solitary nodules.[17] Spontaneous pneumothorax has also been reported in these patients.[14] Bullae are occasionally seen in patients who have recovered from PCP. Although intrathoracic lymphadenopathy and small pleural effusions may be seen in patients with PCP, these findings suggest the presence of another process.

Mycobacterium tuberculosis. The radiographic manifestations of *M. tuberculosis* in otherwise asymptomatic HIV-seropositive persons are no different from those seen in seronegative persons with this infection.[19] In contrast, pulmonary disease caused by *M. tuberculosis* in patients with AIDS is characterized by an atypical radiographic presentation. In reactivation disease, the radiograph frequently resembles the pattern classically associated with primary tuberculosis in immunocompetent hosts: prominent hilar and mediastinal adenopathy, noncavitating infiltrates, and no upper-lobe predominance. Diffuse or miliary infiltrates are also common. AIDS patients with sputum cultures positive for *M. tuberculosis* may also have normal chest radiographs.[4]

Cytomegalovirus. Because CMV occurs so commonly in association with other organisms, the radiographic pattern produced by CMV alone is not well defined. However, the organism has been associated with diffuse reticular interstitial infiltration.[1]

Mycobacterium avium **Complex.** Like CMV, the pulmonary abnormalities caused by *M. avium* complex have not been clearly defined, in part because it is often found in association with other organisms. In a retrospective review of patients with apparent pulmonary disease caused by *M. avium* complex, the radiographic findings included mediastinal adenopathy, localized and diffuse alveolar infiltrates, interstitial infiltrates, and normal chest films.[20]

Fungal Infections.   HIV infection predisposes the patient to a variety of pulmonary fungal infections, including histoplasmosis, cryptococcus, and coccidioidomycosis. Other fungi (such as aspergillus and candida) rarely cause pulmonary disease in these patients. Fungal pneumonias produce a wide range of radiographic findings,[6,20,21] including intrathoracic adenopathy, focal nodules, diffuse interstitial and nodular infiltrations, focal airspace consolidation, and cavitary lesions.

Bacterial Pneumonia.   Bacterial pneumonias in patients with AIDS tend to produce lobar or segmental consolidation. However, diffuse patchy infiltration can also be seen.

Kaposi's Sarcoma.   Kaposi's sarcoma may cause a wide variety of radiographic manifestations. Diffuse coarse interstitial infiltrates, alveolar consolidation, or scattered nodular lesions may be seen. Pleural effusion and intrathoracic lymphadenopathy are common.[8,22]

Lymphoma.   There does not appear to be any specific radiographic manifestation of HIV-related lymphoma. Solitary pulmonary lesions, pleural effusions, and infiltration of the pulmonary parenchyma — both with and without intrathoracic adenopathy — have all been seen.

Lymphoid Interstitial Pneumonitis.   In the few adult patients reported with lymphoid interstitial pneumonitis, the chest films have shown diffuse interstitial and alveolar infiltrates, with occasional nodular densities.[23]

Nonspecific Interstitial Pneumonitis.   In a review of 152 episodes of clinical pneumonia seen during a four-year period at the National Institutes of Health, 32 percent were idiopathic, nonspecific pneumonitis. Thus, pulmonary symptoms that generally present with an interstitial infiltrate on chest x-ray may not have an identifiable cause.[10]

Alveolar Proteinosis.   Histologic examination of the lungs of two patients who died from respiratory failure showed secondary alveolar proteinosis with interstitial infiltrates. Although both patients had prior opportunistic infections, one had no evidence of an AIDS-defining infection when he died of respiratory failure. This suggests that secondary alveolar proteinosis itself may play a pathologic role in respiratory failure.[15]

REFERENCES

1. Suster B, Akerman M, Orenstein M, Wax MR. Pulmonary manifestations of AIDS: review of 106 episodes. Radiology 1986; 161:87-93.

2. Abd AG, Nierman DM, Ilowite JS, et al. Bilateral upper lobe *Pneumocystis carinii* pneumonia in a patient receiving inhaled pentamidine prophylaxis. Chest 1988; 94:329-31.

3. Cohen BA, Pomeranz S, Rabinowitz JG, et al. Pulmonary complications of AIDS: radiologic features. AJR 1984; 143:115-22.

4. Pitchenik AE, Rubinson HA. The radiographic appearance of tuberculosis in patients with the acquired immune deficiency syndrome (AIDS) and pre-AIDS. Am Rev Respir Dis 1985; 131:393-6.

5. Mandell W, Goldberg DM, Neu HC. Histoplasmosis in patients with the acquired immune deficiency syndrome. Am J Med 1986; 81:974-8.

6. Bronnimann DA, Adam RD, Galgiani JN, et al. Coccidioidomycosis in the acquired immunodeficiency syndrome. Ann Intern Med 1987; 106:372-9.

7. Ognibene FP, Steis RG, Macher AM, et al. Kaposi's sarcoma causing pulmonary infiltrates and respiratory failure in the acquired immunodeficiency syndrome. Ann Intern Med 1985; 102:471-5.

8. Kaplan LD, Hopewell PC, Jaffe H, et al. Kaposi's sarcoma involving the lung in patients with the acquired immunodeficiency syndrome. Jour AIDS 1988; 1:23-30.

9. Morris JC, Rosen MJ, Marchevsky A, Teirstein AS. Lymphocytic interstitial pneumonia in patients at risk for the acquired immune deficiency syndrome. Chest 1987; 91:63-7.

10. Suffredini AF, Ognibene FP, Lack EE, et al. Nonspecific interstitial pneumonitis: a common cause of pulmonary disease in the acquired immunodeficiency syndrome. Ann Intern Med 1987; 107:7-13.

11. Milligan SA, Stulbarg MS, Gamsu G, Golden JA. *Pneumocystis carinii* pneumonia radiographically simulating tuberculosis. Am Rev Respir Dis 1985; 132:1124-6.

12. Lachant MA, Sun MCJ, Leong LA, et al. Multicentric angiofollicular lymph node hyperplasia, Castleman's disease, followed by Kaposi's sarcoma in two homosexual males with the acquired immunodeficiency syndrome (AIDS). Am J Clin Pathol 1985; 83:27-33.

13. Stern RG, Gamsu G, Golden JA, et al. Intrathoracic adenopathy: differential features of AIDS and diffuse lymphadenopathy syndrome. Am J Radiol 1984; 142:689-92.

14. Goodman PC, Daily C, Munagi H. Spontaneous pneumothorax in *P. carinii* pneumonia in the acquired immunodeficiency syndrome. Am J Radiol 1986; 147:29-31.

15. Ruben FL, Talamo TS. Secondary pulmonary alveolar proteinosis occurring in two patients with acquired immune deficiency syndrome. Am J Med 1986; 80:1187-90.

16. Chaisson RE. Infections due to encapsulated bacteria, salmonella, shigella, and campylobacter. In: Sande MA, Volberding PA, eds. Medical management of AIDS. Philadelphia: W.B. Saunders, 1988:249-51.

17. Barrio JL, Suarez M, Rodriguez JL, et al. *Pneumocystis carinii* pneumonia presenting as cavitating and noncavitating solitary pulmonary nodules in patients with the acquired immunodeficiency syndrome. Am Rev Respir Dis 1986; 134:1094-6.

18. Wheat LJ, Slama TG, Zeckel ML. Histoplasmosis in the acquired immune deficiency syndrome. Am J Med 1985; 78:203-10.

19. Chaisson RE, Theuer CP, Elias D, et al. HIV seroprevalence in patients with tuberculosis [Abstract]. Program and Abstracts of the Twenty-eighth Interscience Conference on Antimicrobial Agents and Chemotherapy. Los Angeles: American Society for Microbiology, 1988:571.

20. Marinelli DL, Albelda SM, Williams TM, et al. Nontuberculous mycobacterial infection in AIDS: clinical, pathologic, and radiographic features. Radiology 1986; 160:77-82.

21. Wasser L, Talavera W. Pulmonary cryptococcosis in AIDS. Chest 1987; 92:692-5.

22. Garay SM, Belenko M, Fazzini E, Schinella R. Pulmonary manifestations of Kaposi's sarcoma. Chest 1987; 91:39-43.

23. Teirstein AS, Rosen MJ. Lymphocytic interstitial pneumonia. Clin Chest Med 1988; 9:467-71.

Pulmonary Function Tests and Gallium Citrate Lung Scans

Peter M. Small, M.D., and Philip C. Hopewell, M.D.

Patients with respiratory symptoms who are at risk for HIV infection should be initially evaluated with a chest roentgenogram. If the film is normal, further screening studies should be performed to determine if even more rigorous diagnostic efforts are needed. Tests of pulmonary function — especially the single breath diffusing capacity for carbon monoxide (DLCO) and measurement of the alveolar to arterial oxygen tension difference $P(A - a)O_2$ with exercise — have proven to be particularly helpful.

Curtis and coworkers[1] reported the results of pulmonary function tests in 125 patients with AIDS or suspected AIDS. The results of bronchoscopy were compared for those who had *Pneumocystis carinii* pneumonia (PCP) and those who did not. Patients with PCP had statistically significant reductions in vital capacity (VC), total lung capacity (TLC), and DLCO. Abnormalities in these measurements were sensitive to the presence of *P. carinii*. Specifically, the sensitivity of the TLC was 71.4 percent; VC, 85.2 percent; and DLCO, 89.35 percent. This indicates that although not perfect, these tests are highly likely to reveal abnormalities in pulmonary function among patients with *P. carinii*. However, all tests were very nonspecific and had relatively low negative predictive values, indicating that an abnormal test could not be definitively associated with *P. carinii* and that a negative result did not exclude *P. carinii* as a possible diagnosis.

Gagliardi and coworkers[2] have reported using a combination form of spirometry that measures the forced expiratory volume in 1 second (FEV_1), forced vital capacity (FVC), TLC, and the $P(A - a)O_2$ with rest and exercise to provide both a sensitive and specific indicator of the presence of *P. carinii*. Using these measurements, these investigators constructed two formulas.

Formula 1.

$$\frac{FEV_1 / FVC \times [P(A - a)O_2\ exercise - P(A - a)O_2\ rest]}{\%\ predicted\ TLC} = {>}10$$

Formula 2.

$$\frac{FEV_1 / FVC \times [P(A - a)O_2\ exercise - P(A - a)O_2\ rest]}{\%\ predicted\ VC} = {>}12$$

If the number derived from formula 1 was greater than 10, or the number derived from formula 2 was greater than 12, the specificity for *P. carinii* was 100 percent, although the sensitivity was only 77 percent and 76 percent, respectively. A reduction in the minimum score should increase sensitivity but decrease specificity.

Pulmonary function tests have also been used to follow the course of *P. carinii* pneumonia (PCP) in patients with AIDS.[3,4] In general, there was little improvement in VC, TLC, or DLCO during the first 30 days after treatment was begun. However, longer-term follow-up demonstrated improvement in the DLCO in the small number of patients studied.[3] These changes did not correlate with the presence or absence of *P. carinii* in bronchoscopic specimens.

Increased uptake of gallium citrate by the lung has been noted in a number of inflammatory and neoplastic disorders.[5] After intravenous administration of this isotope to patients with PCP, the pulmonary concentration of this isotope is enhanced, presumably due to changes in blood flow and leukocyte influx. Such enhancement can be detected even before there are any radiographic abnormalities.[6] Like pulmonary function tests, the gallium lung scan is quite sensitive but nonspecific for diagnosing PCP. In a study by Curtis et al.,[1] gallium scanning had a 90.7 percent sensitivity in patients with proven PCP, but was only 40.9 percent specific and had a negative predictive value of 69.2 percent. Thus, gallium scanning cannot be used for definitive diagnosis of PCP, but a negative study cannot completely exclude the possibility of this pneumonia.

Along with chest radiography as a screening test for persons with or suspected of having AIDS, pulmonary function measurements and gallium lung scans each incrementally add evidence to the detection of pulmonary processes requiring more definitive diagnostic evaluations. The chest film should be the first study performed. If an abnormality suggests an HIV-related process, more definitive diagnostic studies should be undertaken. If the chest film is normal, further screening using pulmonary function studies should be employed. These should include measurement of DLCO, $P(A - a)O_2$, or both. Abnormalities identified by either of these studies indicate the need for further evaluation.

If pulmonary function tests are normal, a gallium lung scan should be performed. Increased uptake (if present) should be evaluated. Such a sequence of diagnostic studies represents a cost-effective and efficient strategy for diagnostic evaluations in HIV-infected patients.[7,8]

REFERENCES

1. Curtis J, Goodman P, Hopewell P. Noninvasive tests in the diagnostic evaluation for *P. carinii* pneumonia in patients with or suspected of having AIDS. Am Rev Respir Dis 1986; 133:A182. abstract.

2. Gagliardi AT, White DA, Stover DE, Zaman MK. A noninvasive index for the diagnosis of *Pneumocystis carinii* pneumonia (PCP) in patients with the acquired immunodeficiency syndrome (AIDS). Am Rev Respir Dis 1986; 133:A183. abstract.

3. Coleman DL, Dodek PM, Golden JA, et al. Correlation between serial pulmonary function tests and fiberoptic bronchoscopy in patients with *Pneumocystis carinii* pneumonia and the acquired immunodeficiency syndrome. Am Rev Respir Dis 1984; 129:491-3.

4. Wharton JM, Coleman DL, Wofsy CB, et al. Trimethoprim sulfamethoxazole or pentamidine for *Pneumocystis carinii* pneumonia in the acquired immunodeficiency syndrome. Ann Intern Med 1986; 105:37-44.

5. Siemsen JK, Grebe SF, Waxman AD. The use of gallium-67 in pulmonary disorders. Sem in Nucl Med 1978; 8:235-49.

6. Bitran J, Bekerman C, Weinstein R, et al. Patterns of gallium-67 scintigraphy in patients with acquired immunodeficiency syndrome and the AIDS-related complex. J Nucl Med 1987; 28:1103-6.

7. Coleman DL, Hattner RS, Luce JM, et al. Correlation between gallium lung scans and fiberoptic bronchoscopy in patients with suspected *Pneumocystis carinii* pneumonia and the acquired immune deficiency syndrome. Am Rev Respir Dis 1984; 130:1166-9.

8. Hopewell PC. Diagnosis of *Pneumocystis carinii* pneumonia. Infect Dis Clin N Am 1988; 2:409-18.

Respiratory System: Techniques for Definitive Diagnosis

Peter M. Small, M.D., and Philip C. Hopewell, M.D.

The screening studies described in the previous chapter serve to identify patients needing further evaluation. These studies do not provide specific diagnosis. Definitive diagnoses can be established only by identifying specific pathogens in lung-derived specimens or by specific histopathologic changes in lung cells or tissue samples.

■ SPUTUM EXAMINATION

Microscopic examination and culture of sputum specimens are the most expeditious and least invasive means of obtaining diagnostic material from the lungs. Conventional techniques (e.g., sputum Gram's stain and examination for acid-fast bacilli) are usually the most appropriate first step in evaluating HIV-infected patients with pulmonary disease.

Because the most frequent pulmonary pathogen encountered in patients with AIDS is *Pneumocystis carinii*, techniques for detecting this organism have been extensively investigated. Two early studies using examination of expectorated sputum demonstrated that the procedure had a sensitivity of approximately 55 percent in patients with AIDS.[1,2] Ng and colleagues[9] have increased the sensitivity to approximately 75 percent by digestion and concentration of the sputum. To reduce contamination of the sputum with oral debris, patients are instructed not to eat for 8 hours prior to sputum induction. They then brush their teeth and oral cavity vigorously and gargle several times with water before inhaling a mist of 3 percent to 5 percent saline generated by an ultrasonic nebulizer. The sputum produced is generally clear and resembles saliva but consists of material from the lower respiratory tract.

The specimens are then partially liquefied, concentrated by centrifugation, and then stained. Any stain for *P. carinii* may be used. However, because there tends to be more trophozoites and fewer cysts in sputum, Giemsa-like stains may show more organisms than stains for cyst walls. The use of a fluorescent monoclonal antibody stain may further improve the sensitivity.[12] (Induced sputum can also be examined for other organisms. However, without clinical evidence of tuberculosis or a fungal infection, the yield on routine examination for these organisms is very low.)

The negative predictive value of sputum examination is approximately 60 percent,[2,9] which is not sufficiently high to exclude *P. carinii* as a possible diagnosis even when the sputum examination is negative. Thus, in a patient with abnormalities on the screening studies described previously, a negative sputum examination cannot terminate the evaluation.

■ BRONCHOALVEOLAR LAVAGE AND BRONCHOSCOPY

Early in the AIDS epidemic, clinicians recognized that lung biopsy and bronchoalveolar lavage specimens obtained with the fiberoptic bronchoscope were highly sensitive for diagnosing pulmonary disorders, especially PCP.[3-5] Broaddus et al.[6] reported that bronchoalveolar lavage had a sensitivity for *P. carinii* of 85 percent and for all other organisms combined, a sensitivity of 76 percent. Transbronchial biopsy was 97 percent sensitive for *P. carinii* and 54 percent for all other organisms combined. Used together, the two procedures were determined to be 100 percent sensitive for *P. carinii* and 94 percent for other organisms combined. The predictive value of a bronchoscopic examination (including bronchoalveolar lavage) that did not show *P. carinii* ranged from 92 to 100 percent; true negativity was established by examining subsequent (within 32 days) biopsies, an autopsy, or by following the clinical course of the patient for 30 days. The lower predictive value was calculated by assuming that patients had false-negative results, while the higher value was obtained by assuming that they were true negatives.

More recently, several investigators have reported a higher sensitivity for bronchoalveolar lavage.[7,8] It has therefore been suggested that lavage alone should be performed and that transbronchial biopsy not be used unless the lavage is nondiagnostic. This approach avoids the complications of transbronchial biopsy — pneumothorax and hemorrhage. Broaddus et al.[6] reported that pneumothorax occurred in 9 percent of patients in whom biopsy was performed; approximately 50 percent required tube thoracostomy for reexpansion of the lung, but serious hemorrhage did not occur. The same institution reported that the use of fluoroscopy for guiding the transbronchial biopsy did not influence the frequency of pneumothorax.[13]

Bronchoscopy is nearly always performed on an awake, lightly sedated patient. Topical anesthesia is used for both upper and lower airways. Careful inspection of the airways should be performed to detect any intraluminal abnormalities, particularly endobronchial Kaposi's sarcoma. These lesions are generally seen in patients who also have extensive cutaneous lesions. Their appearance is sufficiently distinctive to allow a definitive diagnosis to be made simply by visualization: they are cherry-red and resemble the submucosal hemorrhages that may be produced by trauma from the bronchoscope.[14] Thus, it is important to inspect the airways carefully while advancing the bronchoscope rather than while withdrawing it. Endobronchial Kaposi's sarcoma lesions tend to occur at bronchial bifurcations. Biopsy is generally difficult; moreover, because of the highly vascular nature of the tumor, serious bleeding may occur.

After inspection of the airways, bronchoalveolar lavage is performed. The bronchoscope is advanced until it is wedged, usually in the right middle or lower lobe. If the process is focal rather than diffuse (as judged from the chest film), lavage should be performed in the abnormal area. Sterile, nonbacteriologic saline is then instilled (usually in 20 ml aliquots, for a total volume of 100 ml to 120 ml). Suction is applied after each bolus of fluid. Often there is little return until after 40 ml to 60 ml has been instilled. The total volume returned should be 50 ml to 60 ml.

Institutions differ in how they process bronchoalveolar lavage fluid. Analysis should, however, include appropriate stains for *P. carinii*, acid-fast organisms, and fungi. In addition, the material should be cultured for mycobacteria and fungi. Staining and culturing for legionella species and viruses should be considered, depending on epidemiologic circumstances and available facilities.

■ TRANSBRONCHIAL BIOPSY

If transbronchial biopsy is performed, it should take place after the lavage is completed. Contraindications include the presence of an uncorrectable coagulopathy (absolute contraindication) and mechanical ventilation (relative contraindication). The procedure is hazardous in an uncooperative patient.

If the pulmonary process is diffuse, the biopsy is usually taken from the right lower lobe. Fluoroscopic guidance is not essential in patients with diffuse abnormalities, but it is required if the process is focal. The number of biopsies taken varies considerably among institutions, but sufficient material should be obtained for both microbiologic and histologic examinations. An appropriately stained touch imprint of the tissue is a very accurate means of identifying *P. carinii*.[8] Fixed tissue sections should also be stained for *P. carinii*. As described for lavage fluid, tissue should be stained and cultured for mycobacteria, fungi, and perhaps Legionella species and viruses. Standard hematoxylin and eosin staining should also be done.

After the biopsies are obtained, the airway should be observed for significant bleeding. After the procedure, a frontal view chest film should be taken with the patient exhaling fully to determine if a pneumothorax has occurred.

Other diagnostic techniques (such as brush biopsies and transthoracic needle aspiration of the lung) have been evaluated for diagnosing opportunistic pulmonary disease.[4,11] The sensitivity of brush biopsy is unacceptably low compared with bronchoalveolar lavage and transbronchial biopsy. Transthoracic needle aspiration has an unacceptable rate of complications when used in patients with diffuse infiltrative disease, although it is valuable in evaluating focal lesions.

■ OPEN-LUNG BIOPSY

In patients without AIDS, open-lung biopsy produces a high diagnostic yield. However, the appropriate role of this procedure in patients with known or suspected AIDS-related pulmonary disease is debatable.[4,15] It is clearly indicated for patients who, despite bronchoalveolar lavage, have progressive, undiagnosed pulmonary disease and cannot tolerate transbronchial biopsy because of uncorrectable coagulopathy or high-pressure mechanical ventilation. It can yield important information in patients who have no diagnosis despite full bronchoscopic evaluation, including bronchoalveolar lavage and transbronchial biopsy.[16] Open-lung biopsy has also been useful in diagnosing lymphocytic interstitial pneumonia and nonspecific interstitial pneumonia, both of which may resemble opportunistic infections.[17]

Tissue obtained by open-lung biopsy should be processed and examined as described for tissue obtained by transbronchial biopsy. It is essential that not all tissue be put in formalin but that a sufficient amount be kept unpreserved for microbiologic examinations.

In view of the potential complexity, discomfort, and expense of the diagnostic evaluation of HIV-related pulmonary problems, it is essential that clinicians and hospitals develop a systematic approach that is applicable in most instances. It is equally important that each institution evaluate the cumulative results of local practices to determine which elements of the diagnostic scheme are valuable and which are not. Periodic review of such information can be crucial to shaping an expeditious and cost-efficient approach.

REFERENCES

1. Pitchenik AE, Ganjei P, Torres A, et al. Sputum examination for the diagnosis of *Pneumocystis carinii* pneumonia in the acquired immunodeficiency syndrome. Am Rev Respir Dis 1986; 133:226-9.
2. Bigby TD, Margolskee D, Curtis JL, et al. The usefulness of induced sputum in the diagnosis of *Pneumocystis carinii* pneumonia in patients with the acquired immunodeficiency syndrome. Am Rev Respir Dis 1986; 133:515-8.
3. Coleman DL, Dodek PM, Luce JM, et al. Diagnostic utility of fiberoptic bronchoscopy in patients with *Pneumocystis carinii* pneumonia and the acquired immune deficiency syndrome. Am Rev Respir Dis 1983; 128:795-9.
4. Murray JF, Felton CP, Garay SM, et al. Pulmonary complications of the acquired immunodeficiency syndrome: report of a National Heart, Lung, and Blood Institute workshop. N Engl J Med 1984; 310:1682-8.
5. Stover DE, White DA, Romano PA, Gellene RA. Diagnosis of pulmonary disease in acquired immunodeficiency syndrome (AIDS): role of bronchoscopy and bronchoalveolar lavage. Am Rev Respir Dis 1984; 130:659-62.
6. Broaddus C, Dake MD, Stulbarg MS, et al. Bronchoalveolar lavage and transbronchial biopsy for the diagnosis of pulmonary infections in the acquired immunodeficiency syndrome. Ann Intern Med 1985; 102:747-52.
7. Murray T, Grossman G, Bruade J, Staton G. Is transbronchial biopsy necessary for diagnosis of pulmonary infections with AIDS? Am Rev Respir Dis 1986; 133:A182. abstract.
8. Golden JA, Hollander H, Stulbarg MS, Gamsu G. Bronchoalveolar lavage as the exclusive diagnostic modality for *Pneumocystis carinii* pneumonia. Chest 1986; 90:18-22.
9. Ng VL, Gartner I, Weymouth LA, et al. The use of mucolysed induced sputum for the identification of pulmonary pathogens associated with human immunodeficiency virus infection. Arch Pathol Lab Med 1989; 113:488-93.
10. Blumenfeld W, Wagar E, Hadley WK. Use of the transbronchial biopsy for diagnosis of opportunistic pulmonary infection in acquired immunodeficiency syndrome (AIDS). Am J Clin Pathol 1984; 81:1-5.
11. Wallace JM, Batra P, Gong H Jr, Overfors C-O. Percutaneous needle lung aspiration for diagnosing pneumonitis in the patient with acquired immunodeficiency syndrome. Am Rev Respir Dis 1985; 131:389-92.
12. Kovacs JA, Ng VL, Masur H, et al. Diagnosis of *Pneumocystis carinii* pneumonia: improved detection in sputum with use of monoclonal antibodies. N Engl J Med 1988; 318:589-93.
13. Milligan SA, Luce JM, Golden J, et al. Transbronchial biopsy without fluoroscopy in patients with diffuse roentgenographic infiltrates and the acquired immunodeficiency syndrome. Am Rev Respir Dis 1988; 137:486-8.
14. Kaplan LD, Hopewell PC, Jaffe H, et al. Kaposi's sarcoma involving the lung in patients with the acquired immunodeficiency syndrome. Jour AIDS 1988; 1:23-30.
15. Stulbarg MS, Golden JA. Open lung biopsy in the acquired immunodeficiency syndrome (AIDS). Chest 1987; 91:639-40.
16. Fitzgerald W, Bevelaqua FA, Garay SM, Aranda CP. The role of open-lung biopsy in patients with the acquired immunodeficiency syndrome. Chest 1987; 91:659-61.
17. Morris JC, Rosen MJ, Marchevsky A, Teirstein AS. Lymphocytic interstitial pneumonia in patients at risk for the acquired immune deficiency syndrome. Chest 1987; 91:63-7.

Physiologic Consequences and Management of Respiratory System Involvement

Peter M. Small, M.D., and Philip C. Hopewell, M.D.

In general, patients with pulmonary disorders associated with AIDS have no significant pre-existing lung disease. Thus, most symptoms and physical and laboratory findings are the result of an acute or subacute process. *P. carinii* pneumonia (PCP), the most commonly occurring condition, is exclusively an intraalveolar process with little or no direct involvement of the interstitium of the affected lung.[1] Alveoli are incapable of participating in gas exchange with capillary blood, thus causing hypoxia because of intrapulmonary shunting of blood.

Typically, patients with PCP are hypoxemic and, at least in part to compensate for the hypoxemia, have below normal values of arterial CO_2 tension with a respiratory alkalosis. As discussed in a previous chapter, the hypoxemia tends to worsen with exercise, resulting in an increase in the $P(A - a)O_2$. As the alveolar-filling defect becomes more severe, hypoxemia increases, causing respiratory failure and death if the process is not checked. Besides hypoxemia, alveolar filling causes the lung to become less compliant; this makes breathing harder work.

Management of patients requires treating the underlying process (if possible) and supplying supplemental oxygen. In patients with marked shunting, endotracheal intubation and mechanical ventilation may be necessary both to deliver high concentrations of oxygen and to take over the work of breathing.

Other pulmonary processes tend not to be restricted to alveolar spaces, and may predominantly involve the interstitium.[1] The physiologic consequences are, however, quite similar to those produced by *P. carinii*. Kaposi's sarcoma may cause both parenchymal infiltration and large pleural effusions, which then cause hypoxemia.[2]

REFERENCES

1. Marchevsky A, Rosen MJ, Chrystal G, Kleinerman J. Pulmonary complications of the acquired immunodeficiency syndrome: a clinicopathologic study of 70 cases. Hum Pathol 1985; 16:659-70.
2. Ognibene FP, Stein RG, Macher AM, et al. Kaposi's sarcoma causing pulmonary infiltrates and respiratory failure in the acquired immunodeficiency syndrome. Ann Intern Med 1985; 102:471-5.

COLOR
PLATES

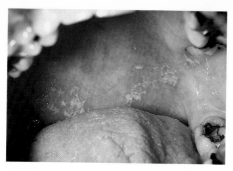

5.2.1.a Pseudomembranous candidiasis. Creamy white patches on erythematous mucosa.

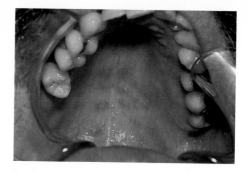

5.2.1.b Atrophic candidiasis appearing as palatal erythema.

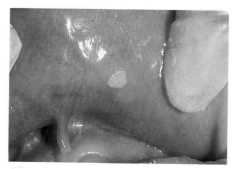

5.2.1.c Wart on labial mucosa.

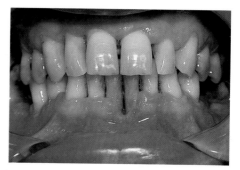

5.2.1.d HIV-associated periodontal disease showing localized destruction of the gingival tissue.

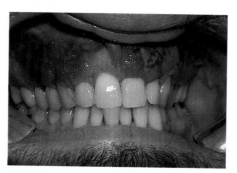

5.2.2.a Kaposi's sarcoma occurring on the gingiva.

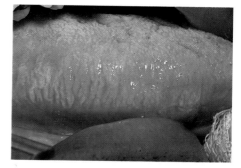

5.2.3.a Hairy leukoplakia appearing as corrugations on the lateral margin of the tongue.

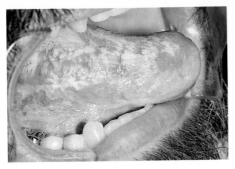

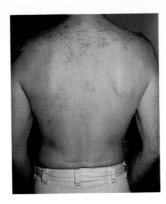

5.3.1.a
Staphylo-
coccal
folliculitis.

5.2.3.b   More extensive hairy leukoplakia
appearing as corrugations and plaques on the
lateral margin of the tongue.

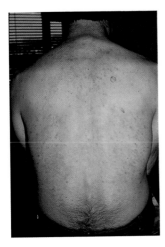

5.3.1.b
Folliculitis
that on biop-
sy showed
acute fol-
licular inflam-
mation with
a significant
component
of eosinophils.

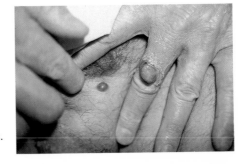

5.3.1.c   Friable angiomatous nodules of the
finger and scrotum in a patient with bacillary
angiomatosis or disseminated cat-scratch disease and AIDS. Reproduced with kind permission from *Annals of Internal Medicine*
1988; 109:451.

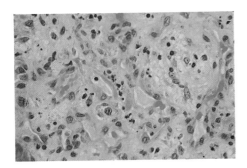

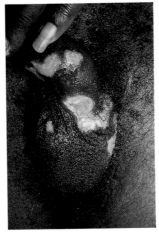

5.3.1.e
Extensive
genital her-
pes simplex
virus infec-
tion as the
presenting
manifesta-
tion of HIV
infection.

5.3.1.d   Biopsy specimen of a patient with
bacillary angiomatosis or disseminated cat-
scratch disease and AIDS. There is a proliferation of plump vessels in an edematous
stroma with significant numbers of polymorphonuclear leukocytes. The granular basophilic material adjacent to the vessels in the
center represents aggregates of the bacilli
(hematoxylin and eosin stain x177).

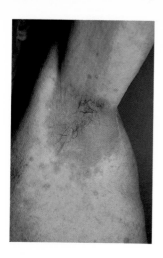

5.3.1.f Seborrheic dermatitis with axillary involvement. This cleared with oral ketoconazole plus topical steroids.

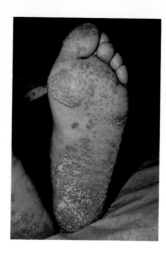

5.3.1.g Classic keratoderma blennorrhagicum in an AIDS patient with Reiter's syndrome.

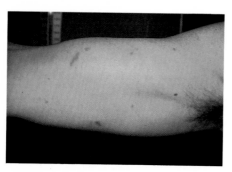

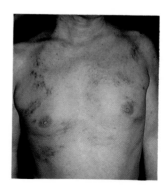

5.3.1.i Epidemic Kaposi's sarcoma (KS) in AIDS. Extensive plaques of the trunk.

5.3.1.h Epidemic Kaposi's sarcoma (KS) in AIDS. Typical oblong papules and plaques of the arm.

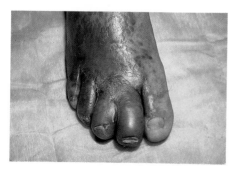

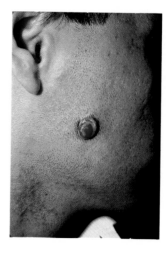

5.3.1.k Epidemic Kaposi's sarcoma (KS) in AIDS. KS presenting as friable angiomatous nodules. This solitary lesion had erupted over several weeks. No other lesions were found on a total skin examination.

5.3.1.j Epidemic Kaposi's sarcoma (KS) in AIDS. Pedal edema and plaques of KS.

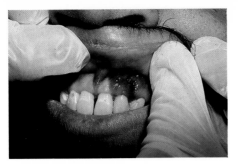

5.3.1.l   Epidemic Kaposi's sarcoma (KS) in AIDS. Oral plaque as the only lesion at presentation.

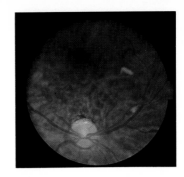

5.11.1.a Cotton-wool spots.

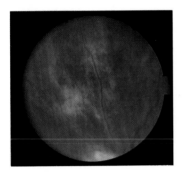

5.11.1.b CMV retinitis. Note perivascular distribution.

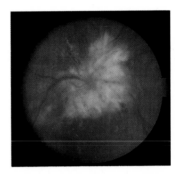

5.11.1.c CMV optic neuritis and retinitis.

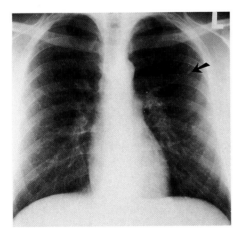

5.15.1.a   Non-Hodgkin's lymphoma. Initial chest radiograph shows small peripheral lung nodule (arrow).

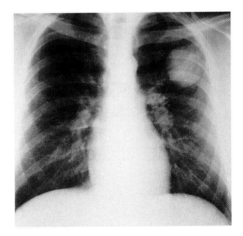

5.15.1.b   Non-Hodgkin's lymphoma. Chest film six weeks later shows dramatic increase in size.

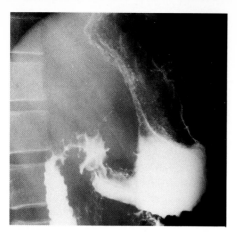

5.15.1.c   Cytomegalovirus gastritis. Barium GI shows diffuse ulceration and thickened folds throughout stomach and duodenum.

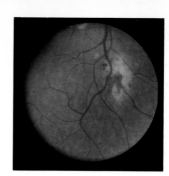

6.4.6.a Typical appearance of CMV retinitis in a patient with AIDS.

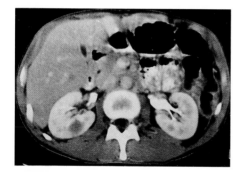

5.15.1.d   Non-Hodgkin's lymphoma. Bilateral renal masses were biopsied and proved to be lymphoma.

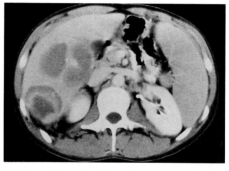

5.15.1.e   Non-Hodgkin's lymphoma. Multiple hepatic masses.

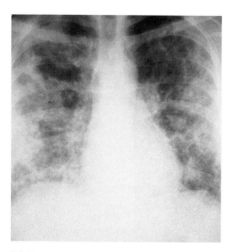

6.5.2.a   PCP with nodular infiltrates.

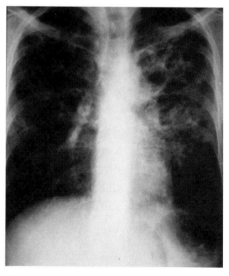

6.5.2.b   Cystic lesions after an episode of PCP.

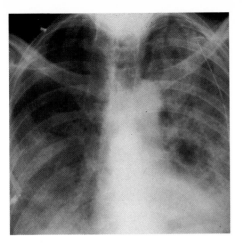

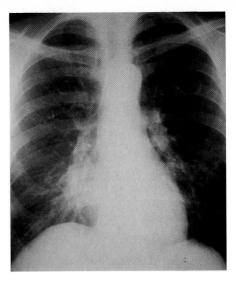

6.5.2.c   Predominant left-sided disease with pneumothorax with chest tube and PCP.

6.5.2.d   Unilateral alveolar infiltrate in PCP.

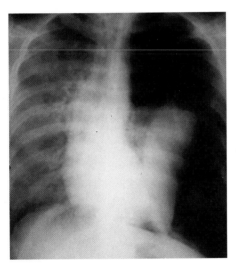

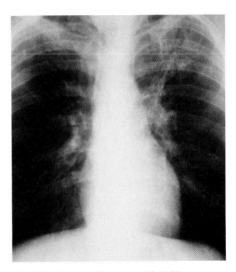

6.5.2.e   Left tension pneumothorax with PCP.

6.5.2.f   Apical infiltrates with PCP.

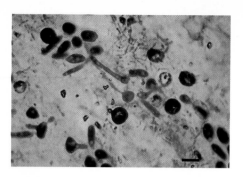

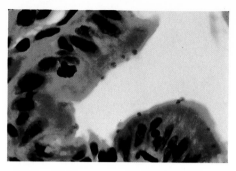

6.5.5.a Cryptosporidia oocysts seen in a modified Kinyoun acid-fast stain of a direct fecal smear from an infected patient (examined under oil immersion). Reproduced with kind permission from the *Journal of Infectious Diseases* 1983; 147:824-8.

6.5.5.b Cryptosporidia lined up along the villi of the small bowel (hematoxylin and eosin stain x177).

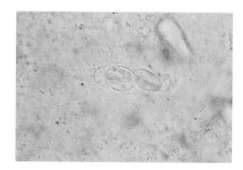

6.5.7.a *Isospora belli* oocyst seen in an iodine wet-mount of unconcentrated stool from an infected patient.

5.6

Cardiovascular Aspects

5.6.1   Cardiac Involvement in AIDS — *Cheitlin*

Cardiac Involvement in AIDS

Melvin D. Cheitlin, M.D.

C linically significant cardiac problems in AIDS patients are unusual; however, cardiac abnormalities are not uncommon, especially when they are sought using echocardiography. Cardiomyopathy, cardiac tamponade, and congestive heart failure have been reported, but the vast majority of incidentally discovered cardiac abnormalities are clinically silent. The significance of these findings is not yet apparent.

Cardiac involvement, especially by focal myocarditis (but usually without clinical signs of cardiac or pericardial involvement) or cardiac tamponade, is not unusual among AIDS patients. Some of these pericardial and myocardial abnormalities are caused by organisms known to cause myocarditis, but there are many instances where the etiology is unknown. The possibility that HIV infection is responsible cannot be ruled out; in fact, HIV was identified in a myocardial biopsy from one patient with unexplained right-ventricular dysfunction.[1]

In the vast majority of patients there is no need for specialized studies like echocardiography. If a patient has an increase in cardiac size on the chest x-ray or if clinical signs of left or right heart-failure occur, an echocardiogram is helpful in identifying pericardial effusion or right- or left-ventricular dilatation. If the venous pressure rises, echocardiography is definitely indicated to detect impending tamponade. This should be followed by pericardiocentesis. If left-ventricular dilatation and hypocontractility occur (especially if the patient develops congestive heart failure and pulmonary congestion), then endomyocardial biopsy is recommended in order to identify a treatable organism.

■ BACKGROUND AND SIGNIFICANCE OF CARDIAC INVOLVEMENT IN AIDS

Cardiovascular abnormalities have been reported in AIDS patients clinically, echocardiographically, and at autopsy. Pericardial involvement with effusion and even cardiac tamponade, echocardiographic abnormalities, and clinical cardiomyopathy with right- and left-sided congestive heart failure have all been reported, either as isolated cases or as a small series of retrospective echocardiograms done on patients with AIDS. The frequency of abnormalities specifically related to AIDS in consecutively studied patients is not known. The etiology of these abnormalities is also unclear. Since HIV infection in AIDS patients results in profound suppression of T-cell macrophage-mediated immunity, and since there are significant abnormalities in B-cell lymphocyte function resulting in abnormalities of humoral immunity, patients frequently face life-threatening superinfections by bacterial, fungal, parasitic, and viral organisms. Some of these — herpes simplex,[2] cytomegalovirus, cryptococcosis,[3] toxoplasmosis, and histoplasmosis — are known to cause pericarditis and myocarditis in the absence of AIDS, so the presence of definite myocardial disease in an AIDS patient does not necessarily mean that the disease is due to HIV.

Echocardiography has identified abnormalities in 25 percent to 75 percent of patients with AIDS.[4-6] Most abnormalities that can be recognized by echocardiography have been reported, including the presence of pericardial fluid, mitral valve prolapse, chamber-size abnormalities, and wall-motion abnormalities. Although these abnormalities could be due to infection with HIV, there are many other possible reasons for the echocardiographic irregularities. Among AIDS patients in whom cardiac abnormalities are common, the incidence of alcohol and intravenous drug abuse is high. Abnormal wall motion and ejection fraction can be due to direct myocardial involvement because of HIV infection, but these functional parameters are also load-dependent and can be due to abnormalities of preload and afterload (possibly caused by hypovolemia, sepsis, or pulmonary hypertension from pulmonary disease).

■ POSSIBLE MECHANISMS OF CARDIAC INJURY IN HIV-INFECTED PATIENTS

Severe pulmonary disease is frequent in AIDS patients with cardiac abnormalities; right-ventricular dilatation and failure are not unusual. At San Francisco General Hospital, we evaluated two patients with AIDS and *Pneumocystis carinii* pneumonia (PCP) who had pulmonary hypertension with increased pulmonary vascular resistance (proven by catheterization) leading to early right-ventricular hypertrophy. The patients had normal chest x-rays. With right-ventricular dilatation, especially if a pericardial abnormality is present, left-ventricular-filling characteristics can be altered and result in echocardiographic abnormalities. For instance, secundum atrial septal defects are a common congenital cardiac abnormality and may be associated with mitral valve prolapse because of diastolic distortion of the left ventricle caused by diastolic distension of the right ventricle.

Drugs used in the treatment of AIDS may at times result in cardiac abnormalities; it has been reported that intravenous pentamidine, for example, causes the arrhythmia Torsad des Pointes.[7] Myocardial dysfunction can also occur in chronically ill patients with significant emotional stress, marked elevations in sympathetic tone and catecholamines, or in those patients with nutritional abnormalities. It is not known whether the reported high incidence of echocardiographic abnormalities in AIDS patients is specifically related to HIV infection, to superinfection with other organisms, or to factors unrelated to HIV infection — no echocardiographic studies comparing HIV antibody-positive groups of patients to appropriate controls have yet been done.

Since AIDS was first recognized in 1981, individual case reports describing both clinical and autopsy evidence of cardiac abnormalities have appeared. The most obvious of these abnormalities has been pericarditis — at times seen with cardiac tamponade. Frequently the etiology of pericarditis was not identified, although in some cases known pathogens such as *Mycobacterium tuberculosis*,[8] staphylococcus,[9] cryptococcosis, and herpes simplex were found, presumably functioning as opportunistic infections permitted by the patients' immunodeficient state. In addition, Kaposi's sarcoma[10] and non-Hodgkin's lymphomas[11-14] involving the heart and pericardium have been reported. In many of the autopsy series, this involvement has been clinically silent. Also, nonbacterial thrombotic endocarditis[15] has been described, as has infective endocarditis — at times with unusual organisms.[16]

■ REPORTS OF CARDIAC FINDINGS AT AUTOPSY

1. In 1984, Welch et al.[17] reviewed medical records, biopsy specimens, and autopsy material from 36 patients with AIDS. Metastatic Kaposi's sarcoma was seen in eight patients, and four had high-grade lymphomas. Thirty-five of the 36 patients had at least one opportunistic infection, and 83 percent of the patients had multiple fatal infections. The heart was normal in 25 of the 36 cases. In six cases, a focal interstitial fibrosis was seen; acute microscopic foci of myocardial necrosis were identified in two patients with otherwise normal hearts. Kaposi's sarcoma involved the epicardium in three subjects, and one case had extensive involvement of the myocardium.

2. Also in 1984, Guarda et al.[18] reported a retrospective review of autopsies on 13 men with AIDS. One had a cytomegalovirus infection involving multiple organ systems, including the heart. Two patients had nonbacterial thrombotic endocarditis, and one had a microscopic focus of recent myocardial infarction. Two had Kaposi's sarcoma involving the pericardium and epicardium. In all 13 patients, the cardiac involvement was incidental to HIV infection.

3. Silver et al.[10] reported 1984 autopsy findings on 18 National Institutes of Health patients without cardiac symptoms during life. Five (28 percent) had deposits of Kaposi's sarcoma in the heart — the only abnormality found. As an addendum, two additional patients were reported, one with acute myocarditis of unknown etiology.

4. In 1985, Cammarosano and Lewis[19] reported autopsy findings on 41 patients with AIDS, 10 of whom had major pathologic cardiac findings: 4 had Kaposi's sarcoma, 3 had nonbacterial thrombotic endocarditis, 2 had fibrinous pericarditis of unknown etiology, and 1 had *Cryptococcus neoformans* myocarditis as part of a generalized infection.

5. At the IV International AIDS Conference in Stockholm, several autopsy studies were abstracted. La Font et al. reported 50 cases of "myocarditis" selected at autopsy from 137 consecutively autopsied AIDS patients.[20] They divided the patients into 3 groups, depending on whether clinical evidence of cardiac disease was absent (29 patients), mild (13 patients), or severe (14 patients). Cardiac involvement led to death in 10 of 14 severely affected patients. A known pathogen was identified in 5 of 10 patients dying with heart failure. LaFont et al. concluded that severe myocarditis can lead to heart failure and that many AIDS patients studied had myocardial involvement with no demonstrable pathogen.[20] In another abstract from this same group,[21] selenium deficiency was suspected as a cause of cardiomyopathy in some patients since their serum selenium was low compared to that in a control population. There was improvement of the left-ventricular shortening fraction upon selenium repletion.

6. Finally, Anderson et al. from the Armed Forces Institute of Pathology compared the frequency of "myocarditis" at necropsy in patients dying from AIDS in the United States to AIDS patients in Puerto Rico.[22]

Forty percent of 91 U.S. patients had myocarditis compared to 26 percent of 46 Puerto Rican patients. Most of the U.S. patients had no known pathogens, whereas 75 percent of the Puerto Rican patients had myocardial involvement by known pathogens. The investigators believed that the incidence of myocarditis of unknown etiology was higher in the U.S. population.

■ REPORTS OF ECHOCARDIOGRAPHIC ABNORMALITIES IN AIDS

All studies of echocardiographic abnormalities in AIDS patients reported to date are retrospective and without controls.

1. In 1984, Fink et al. reported a study of 15 AIDS patients, 13 of whom were studied by echocardiography.[23] None of the patients exhibited clinical evidence of myocardial disease. In three patients, cardiac tamponade had developed, and three patients had echocardiographic left-ventricular hypokinesia. Two patients had dilated right ventricles, one with right-sided marantic endocarditis and one with mitral regurgitation. Three were asymptomatic patients with left-ventricular dysfunction of unknown etiology. Thus in this study, 73 percent of the 15 AIDS patients had cardiac abnormalities.

2. In 1985, Issenberg[4] reported a study of 12 children with AIDS and 10 with ARC (6 months to 6 years of age). Echocardiographic abnormalities were found in 64 percent of both groups, with pericardial effusion in 18 percent and left-ventricular dilatation and decreased contractility in 45 percent.

3. In 1985, Sherron[5] reported 23 patients, aged 4 to 48 months, with AIDS or ARC. Ten (44 percent) had cardiac symptomology. Follow-up studies were done in 9 patients at 3-month intervals. Seventeen patients (74 percent) had signs of left-ventricular dysfunction, with fractional shortening less than 28 percent in 15 patients. Five patients had a moderate pericardial effusion, all with left-ventricular dysfunction.

4. Himelman et al. from the University of California, San Francisco (UCSF) conducted quantitative echocardiography on 20 hospitalized patients with AIDS and 44 ambulatory patients with AIDS, ARC, or asymptomatic HIV infection and compared the echocardiographic findings to those 20 control patients with leukemia whose echocardiograms had been measured in Himelman's laboratory.[24] They found 7 patients with "dilated cardiomyopathy" among the hospitalized AIDS patients and none in the ambulatory, asymptomatic HIV-infected patients or leukemia controls ($p < 0.05$). There were 7 pericardial effusions among the hospitalized AIDS patients and 6 among the controls — not a significant difference.

5. Several abstracts on echocardiographic abnormalities were reported at the IV International Conference on AIDS in Stockholm. Levy et al. observed 60 HIV-seropositive patients with 2-D echocardiography, 50 with ECG, and 44 with 24-hour ambulatory ECGs.[25] None of the patients was suspected of having cardiac disease; however, 50 percent had cardiac abnormalities. Nine patients had left-ventricular dilatation, 9 had pericardial effusion, and 9 had left-ventricular hypokinesia.

6. Lipschultz et al. from Children's Hospital in Boston studied 33 pediatric AIDS patients with echocardiography and found a similarly high incidence of cardiac abnormalities, including 3 patients with sympathetic dilated cardiomyopathy.[26]

■ REPORTS OF MYOCARDIAL INVOLVEMENT IN AIDS

1. In 1986, Cohen et al.[27] reported three fatal cases of AIDS with striking clinical, echocardiographic, and morphologic findings of dilated cardiomyopathy. At autopsy, dilatation of all the chambers was seen, along with focal inflammatory infiltrates with lymphocytes and histiocytes, and myocyte necrosis. No viral pathogens were found. All these patients had abnormal echocardiograms consistent with left-ventricular dilated cardiomyopathy. The study population consisted of 24 AIDS patients from two hospitals, yielding a 12.5 percent (3 of 24) incidence of cardiomyopathy among AIDS patients with clinical signs of cardiac disease.

2. In 1987, Roldan et al.[28] published the largest retrospectively reviewed series, which included 54 autopsies of AIDS patients; 5 of those studied were IV drug users. Cardiac pathologic changes were seen in 30 of the 54 patients (55 percent); cardiac abnormalities were seen in 25 of these 30 patients (83 percent), myocardial abnormalities in 25 (83 percent), and myocarditis as defined by lymphocyte infiltration in 17 (56 percent). Of these 17 patients, *Toxoplasma gondii* was seen in 6 patients, 1 of whom died with overwhelming myocarditis. Myocarditis with myocardial necrosis of unknown origin was seen in 11 of the 54 patients (20 percent). Pericardial disease was found in five patients with accompanying myocardial disease. In this series, the only patient who had symptomatic myocardial disease was the patient who died with toxoplasmic myocarditis.

3. In 1987, Corboy et al.[29] reported the autopsies of 3 male homosexual AIDS patients (aged 29, 42, and 45) with dilated cardiomyopathy. In each case, the heart had four-chamber dilatation; upon histologic examination, areas of myocytolysis and mild interstitial fibrosis were found, but no etiologic agents or cellular infiltrates were seen.

4. In 1987, Calabrese et al.[1] reported a 32-year-old man with a four-year history of AIDS who developed congestive heart failure and whose echocardiogram revealed a markedly dilated right ventricle. The left-ventricular ejection fraction was 61 percent. It was determined by catheterization that there was no pulmonary hypertension present, so a right-ventricular endomyocardial biopsy was done. No inflammatory cells were seen; the only pathogen evident was HIV. Extensive degenerative changes in numerous myocytes were seen. For virologic study, a co-culture of myocytes from a single specimen and HIV-sensitive phytohemagglutinin-stimulated lymphoblasts showed syncytial cells by day 7. By day 14, the supernate had detectable reverse transcriptase activity. HIV antigen was detectable by antigen capture assay on day 21. The authors mention the possibility that HIV was in the blood and not in the myocardial tissue.

5. At San Francisco General Hospital, 96 consecutive autopsies performed on AIDS patients between 1981 and 1986 were reviewed for gross and microscopic evidence of cardiac involvement. Eighty-eight cases had histologic sections of the heart, all of which were reviewed. Eighteen patients of these 88 patients (20.5 percent) had myocardial involvement, and 9 (10.2 percent) had myocardial inflammatory infiltration. None had clinical or autopsy evidence of left-ventricular dilated cardiomyopathy. Six patients had Kaposi's sarcoma involving the heart, four had pericardial effusion, four had pericardial inflammatory changes without effusion, and nine had one or more small foci of inflammatory myocardial infiltration. No organisms were identified in four of these patients. Two had a cryptococcal abscess; in three, a specific fungus was found as part of a diffuse multi-organ involvement. We concluded that although cardiac microscopic foci of cellular infiltration are not unusual in AIDS, they are most often incidental to the widespread fungemia and do not cause clinically significant cardiac disease.

REFERENCES

1. Calabrese LH, Proffitt MR, Yen-Liebermann B. Congestive cardiomyopathy and illness related to the acquired immunodeficiency syndrome (AIDS) associated with isolation of retrovirus from myocardium. Ann Intern Med 1987; 107:691-2.

2. Freedberg RS, Gindea AJ, Dieterich DT, Greene JB. Herpes simplex pericarditis in AIDS. NY State J Med 1987; 87:304-6.

3. Schuster M, Valentine F, Holzman R. Cryptococcal pericarditis in an intravenous drug abuser. J Infect Dis 1985; 152:842.

4. Issenberg HJ, Charytan M, Rubinstein A. Cardiac involvement in children with acquired immune deficiency syndrome. Am Heart J 1985; 110:710. abstract.

5. Sherron P, Pickoff AS, Ferrer PL, et al. Echocardiographic evaluation of myocardial function in pediatric AIDS patients. Am Heart J 1985; 110:710. abstract.

6. Reitano J, King M, Cohen H, et al. Cardiac function in patients with acquired immune deficiency syndrome (AIDS) or AIDS prodrome. J Am Coll Cardiol 1984; 3:525. abstract.

7. Wharton JM, Demopulos PA, Goldschlager N. Torsad de pointes during administration of pentamidine isethionate. Am J Med 1987; 83:571-6.

8. D'Cruz IA, Sengupta EE, Abrahams C, et al. Cardiac involvement, including tuberculous pericardial effusion, complicating acquired immune deficiency syndrome. Am Heart J 1986; 112:1100-2.

9. Stechel RO, Cooper DJ, Greenspan J, et al. Staphylococcal pericarditis in a homosexual patient with AIDS-related complex. New York State J Med 1986; 86:592-3.

10. Silver MA, Macher AM, Reichert CM, et al. Cardiac involvement by Kaposi's sarcoma in acquired immune deficiency syndrome (AIDS). Am J Cardiol 1984; 53:983-5.

11. Guarner J, Brynes RK, Chan WC, et al. Primary non-Hodgkin's lymphoma of the heart in two patients with acquired immunodeficiency syndrome. Arch Pathol Lab Med 1987; 111:254-6.

12. Balasubramanyam A, Waxman M, Kazal HL, Lee MH. Malignant lymphoma of the heart in acquired immune deficiency syndrome. Chest 1986; 90:243-6.

13. Gill PS, Chandraratna PA, Meyer PR, Levine AM. Malignant lymphoma: cardiac involvement at initial presentation. J Clin Oncol 1987; 5:216-24.

14. Ioachim HL, Cooper MC, Hellman GC. Lymphomas in men at high risk for acquired immune deficiency syndrome (AIDS). A study of 21 cases. Cancer 1985; 56:2831-42.

15. Garcia I, Fainstein V, Rios A, et al. Nonbacterial thrombotic endocarditis in a male homosexual with Kaposi's sarcoma. Arch Intern Med 1983; 143:1243-4.

16. Trepeta RW, Edberg SC. *Corynebacterium diphtheriae* endocarditis: sustained potential of a classical pathogen. Am J Clin Pathol 1984; 81:679-83.

17. Welch K, Finkbeiner W, Alpers CE, et al. Autopsy findings in the acquired immune deficiency syndrome. JAMA 1984; 252:1152-9.

18. Guarda LA, Luna MA, Smith JL Jr, et al. Acquired immune deficiency syndrome: postmortem findings. Am J Clin Pathol 1984; 81:549-57.

19. Cammarosano C, Lewis W. Cardiac lesions in acquired immune deficiency syndrome (AIDS). J Am Coll Cardiol 1985; 5:703-6.

20. LaFont A, March C, Wolff M, et al. Myocarditis in AIDS: etiology and prognosis [Abstract]. Stockholm: IV International Conference on AIDS 1988; 1:404.

21. Zazzo JF, LaFont A, Chappuis PL, et al. Nonobstructive cardiomyopathy (NOCM) and selenium deficiency in AIDS [Abstract]. Stockholm: IV International Conference on AIDS 1988; 1:400.

22. Anderson D, deVinatea M, Marches A, et al. Myocarditis at necropsy in patients with AIDS from the United States and Puerto Rico [Abstract]. Stockholm: IV International Conference on AIDS 1988; 1:403.

23. Fink L, Reicheck N, Sutton MG. Cardiac abnormalities in acquired immune deficiency syndrome. Am J Cardiol 1984; 54:1161-3.

24. Himelman RB, Chung WS, Chernoff D, et al. Cardiac manifestations of HIV infection: a prospective echocardiographic study [Abstract]. Stockholm: IV International Conference on AIDS 1988; 1:400.

25. Levy WS, Simon GL, Ron AM, et al. Clinically silent cardiac abnormalities in patients with HIV infection [Abstract]. Stockholm: IV International Conference on AIDS 1988; 1:401.

26. Lipschultz SE, Chanock S, Sanders SP, et al. Cardiac manifestation of positive HIV infection [Abstract]. Stockholm: IV International Conference on AIDS 1988; 1:400.

27. Cohen IS, Anderson DW, Virmani R, et al. Congestive cardiomyopathy in association with acquired immunodeficiency syndrome. N Engl J Med 1986; 315:628-30.

28. Roldan EO, Moskovitz L, Hensley GT. Pathology of the heart in acquired immunodeficiency syndrome. Arch Pathol Lab Med 1987; 111:943-6.

29. Corboy JR, Fink L, Miller WT. Congestive cardiomyopathy in association with AIDS. Radiology 1987; 165:139-41.

5.7

Endocrinologic Aspects

5.7.1   Endocrine Abnormalities — *Hellerstein*

Endocrine Abnormalities

Marc Hellerstein, M.D., Ph.D.

A number of endocrinologic abnormalities have been reported in patients with HIV infection,[1,2,10] but their clinical importance remains largely uncertain. Many are likely to be non-specific responses to infection, stress, and malnutrition. Many others are due to infiltration of endocrine glands by tumor or infection. In this chapter, we review adrenal, testicular, pituitary, pancreatic, and thyroidal abnormalities in HIV infection.

■ ADRENAL FUNCTION

Of all endocrine deficiencies in AIDS patients, adrenal insufficiency has received the most attention. At autopsy, the incidence of adrenal involvement has been very high in several series.[2-4] Bricaire et al. found abnormal adrenal glands in 64 of 83 AIDS patients at postmortem examination.[2] Of these, 37 showed inflammation and 22 showed necrosis. Cytomegalovirus (CMV) was present in the adrenals in 44 cases, Kaposi's sarcoma (KS) in 3, and cryptococcosis, toxoplasmosis, and tuberculosis in 1 each. The extremely high incidence of adrenal CMV has been confirmed by others.[3,4] CMV was present in 81 of 164 AIDS patients at autopsy, and 75 percent of patients with CMV infection had involvement of the adrenals.[3] The adrenal was the third most common site for CMV in another series of AIDS patients, following the lungs and gastrointestinal tract.[4] In an animal model of T-cell deficiency (the nude mouse), murine CMV replicates in high titer in the adrenal gland, resulting in destructive adrenalitis.[5] However, the clinical significance of these adrenal lesions in AIDS patients has been questioned,[6] since maximal necrosis in one large series was always less than 70 percent and generally less than 55 percent. This is far less than the percentage of adrenal destruction usually required for adrenal insufficiency.

The incidence of clinical or biochemical adrenal insufficiency in patients with AIDS is in fact much lower, despite a number of case reports reporting the association.[7-9] Of the 32 cases analyzed in Glasgow et al.'s series,[6] only two had been suspected premortem of having adrenal insufficiency. In a careful study of endocrine abnormalities in ambulatory AIDS patients by Dobs et al.,[10] 36 of 39 tested had a normal response to ACTH (serum cortisol >20 micrograms/dl), with a mean baseline value of 14 ($\pm$1) rising to 30 ($\pm$2) at 60 minutes. On the other hand, the incidences of hyponatremia, hyperkalemia, and hypotension are high in AIDS patients.[11,12] When new patients with hyponatremia (serum sodium, <133) and hypovolemia (urine sodium, <20) were tested, four of seven had inadequate cortisol response to ACTH.[11] AIDS patients treated with suramin had a 20 percent to 30 percent incidence of clinical or biochemical adrenal insufficiency.[13] This is unlikely to have clinical importance because suramin has not been found to be an effective treatment and has no current indications.[13]

Ketoconazole, which is used to treat certain fungal infections, inhibits adrenal corticosteroid synthesis and blunts the cortisol response to ACTH.[14]

This may be an underrecognized cause of impaired adrenal reserve and even frank adrenal insufficiency with Addisonian crisis.[37] Rifampin also alters the metabolism of glucocorticoids, thereby increasing hormone excretion values or necessitating higher exogenous steroid doses to maintain therapeutic effect.

The most extensive and sophisticated study of adrenal function in AIDS patients is that of Membreno et al.[15] at San Francisco General Hospital. They reported that the basal serum cortisol level is increased in hospitalized AIDS patients (432 ±28 vs. 298 ±22 nmol/L in controls), presumably due to stress. The mean ACTH response was normal in the AIDS group. However, the serum cortisol at 60 minutes post-ACTH was within one standard deviation (SD) of normal in only 48 percent of AIDS patients and within two SD in 86 percent. Moreover, steroids of the 17-deoxy series (corticosterone and 18-hydroxy-DOC) were significantly lower in AIDS patients, although aldosterone and 18-hydroxycortisone were in the normal range. Prolonged ACTH administration (three days) resulted in exaggeration of the differences, with lower 18-hydroxy-DOC, corticosterone, DOC, and cortisol in the AIDS group compared to non-HIV-infected patients. Of the adrenal insufficient patients, all had low ACTH (<20 pmol/L), low aldosterone, hyperkalemia, and hypotension. None had hyperpigmentation. Finally, two of two patients tested had an inadequate 18-DOC response to corticotropin-releasing hormone (CRH).

Membreno et al. concluded from this careful investigation that there is an abnormal response of 17-deoxy corticosteroids to acute or prolonged ACTH administration in patients with AIDS and less so in patients with symptomatic HIV infection. Moreover, a role for the pituitary is suggested by the normal aldosterone (i.e., zona glomerulosa function) and by the decreased response to CRH. The authors proposed a pathogenesis for progressive adrenal dysfunction in AIDS patients, beginning with a putative 17-deoxy regulator from the pituitary that selectively decreases during HIV infection, progresses to inadequate ACTH, and finally culminates in clinical adrenal insufficiency if primary adrenal involvement occurs. This proposed pathogenesis remains to be tested, and the clinical implications of these intriguing findings remain uncertain (i.e., Can an impaired 17-deoxy steroid response to ACTH be used prospectively to predict impending adrenal insufficiency?). Whether these abnormalities are specific to HIV infection or reflect non-specific stress also remains to be established.

Diagnosing adrenal insufficiency in AIDS patients can be difficult. If classical biochemical criteria are met (e.g., basal cortisol levels less than 5 micrograms/dl and ACTH-stimulated increase of less than 7 micrograms/dl), the diagnosis of frank adrenal insufficiency is clear. The absolute cortisol level after ACTH stimulation has also been used as a simple diagnostic criterion in other settings (a peak value of 20 micrograms/dl or more purportedly indicates normal adrenal reserve).[16] Based on AIDS patients studied at San Francisco General Hospital, Biglieri has proposed, however, that the normal response be defined as peak levels of 22 micrograms/dl or greater.[17,18]

If unexplained hyperkalemia persists despite normal cortisol response to ACTH, this may represent hyporeninemic hypoaldosteronism, which has been reported in hospitalized AIDS patients.[12] Serum potassium normalized with mineralocorticoid therapy alone (fludrocortisone 0.1 to 0.2 mg/day) in this syndrome. It is therefore important to make the diagnosis, since glucocorticoid treatment can be avoided. The etiology of hyporeninemic hypoaldosteronism in both AIDS patients and non-HIV-infected patients is not known.

Treating proven adrenal insufficiency in AIDS patients is essentially the same as in other clinical settings. Stress doses (180 to 200 mg of hydrocortisone in divided doses) should be given during acute illnesses. Chronic overtreatment should be avoided to prevent worsening an already immunosuppressed condition. However, it should be emphasized that AIDS is not a contraindication to pharmacologic glucocorticoid therapy (e.g., in central nervous system (CNS) toxoplasmosis). Ketoconazole should be used with caution and adrenal function should be monitored.[14] Clinicians should also be aware of the effects of rifampin on steroid metabolism.[37]

■ TESTICULAR FUNCTION

The most common endocrine abnormality in HIV infection found in Dobs et al.'s study[10] was a low serum testosterone level. Patients with symptomatic HIV infection had serum testosterones of 292 ± 70 ng/dl; AIDS patients had serum testosterones of 401 ± 30 ng/dl. Both these levels were significantly lower than in patients with asymptomatic HIV infection (567 ± 49) or in non-HIV-infected controls (608 ± 121). The testosterone value was low in 42 percent of symptomatic HIV-infected patients (3 of 7) and 50 percent of AIDS patients (20 of 40). Clinically, 67 percent (28 of 42) of AIDS patients complained of loss of libido and 33 percent complained of impotence.

Hypogonadism was hypogonadotropic in 75 percent of cases studied (18 of 24). However, seven of eight patients given gonadotropin-releasing hormone (GnRH) had a normal gonadotropin response. This suggests but does not prove that pituitary function was normal and the lesion was central. The finding that low serum testosterone correlated with weight loss and a low lymphocyte count was consistent with CNS etiology since stress or a catabolic state (or both) are known to cause central hypogonadotropic hypogonadism in other settings.[19-21] The fact that 55 percent of hypogonadal versus 26 percent of eugonadal men died within twelve months was also consistent with a nonspecific causality. Thus, central hypogonadism is common among patients with AIDS and advanced HIV infection but is not due to HIV infection per se. It does, however, appear to correlate with degree of illness. Since there have been no studies on the effects of testosterone replacement in patients with chronic illnesses, the net benefits and risks remain unknown. Subjective or performance benefits to sex-steroid replacement remain untested. Accordingly, the management implications of hypogonadism in HIV infection remain completely unknown. In addition, some clinicians have expressed concerns about possible legal liabilities that they may incur if sexual function is restored to HIV-infected patients who may then possibly infect their partners.

■ PITUITARY FUNCTION

Pituitary infiltration (e.g., *Toxoplasma gondii*) has been reported to cause hypopituitarism in AIDS patients.[22] The evidence for pituitary dysfunction in the absence of a mass lesion is only indirect (i.e., inadequate ACTH response to adrenal insufficiency[15] or hypogonadotropic hypogonadism,[10] though the latter may well not be due to pituitary dysfunction). Elevated serum prolactin levels correlating with progression of disease have been reported in men with AIDS,[23] though the clinical significance of this is unknown.

■ PANCREATIC FUNCTION

The pancreatic disturbance of most clinical importance in HIV infection is secondary to pentamidine treatment for *Pneumocystis carinii* pneumonia (PCP). Pentamidine-induced hypoglycemia is extremely common in AIDS patients treated for PCP — 14 percent to 28 percent.[24,25] For unknown reasons, this incidence is much higher than in non-AIDS patients who are also treated for PCP — i.e., a range of 6.2 percent to 9.1 percent.[26,27] Moreover, symptomatic hypoglycemia is more common among AIDS patients (25 percent)[25] than it is among non-HIV-infected patients (1.2 percent).[26]

The basis of pentamidine hypoglycemia is well understood. Pentamidine is a potent B-cell toxin,[26] so much so that it has been used experimentally for treating malignant insulinomas.[27] Destruction of B cells may result in an unphysiologic release of stored insulin with resulting hypoglycemia. Patients experiencing pentamidine hypoglycemia can therefore progress later to diabetes mellitus, with or without ketoacidosis.[26,28] It is important to recognize that the long tissue half-life of pentamidine can result in hypoglycemia days or weeks after discontinuing a therapeutic course.[24,25] The true incidence of pentamidine hypoglycemia is therefore likely to be even greater than estimated from in-hospital studies.

It is possible to predict patients at greatest risk for pentamidine hypoglycemia.[24,25] The most important predictors are azotemia (40 percent of hypoglycemic patients in one study[24] and 100 percent in another[25] developed azotemia during pentamidine therapy), total dose and duration of pentamidine therapy, and a history of previous pentamidine therapy.[24] In such patients, extreme vigilance must be maintained to prevent this potentially life-threatening complication. Conversely, these patients should be tested for diabetes with blood or urine tests after recovering from PCP.

The reason for this increased sensitivity of AIDS patients to pentamidine hypoglycemia is unknown. There are reports of CMV[29] or CMV DNA[30] in the pancreas of AIDS patients at autopsy. Another possibility is that interleukin-1 (IL-1), which is known to be a B-cell toxin,[31] may be elevated in AIDS patients with chronic fevers and infections. However, this has yet to be demonstrated.

■ THYROID FUNCTION

Any chronic illness associated with malnutrition or inflammation can cause abnormalities in thyroid function tests. This has been called the "euthyroid sick" syndrome, to indicate that the thyroid gland is normal but that systemic illness is present and alters thyroid hormone physiology. It would therefore not be surprising if thyroid function abnormalities were common in AIDS patients. However, thyroid function tests (TFTs) have been reported to be normal (e.g., normal TFTs and response to thyrotropin-releasing hormone[10]). Reports of abnormalities in TFTs in HIV infection have appeared.[32,33] Patients hospitalized with PCP, especially non-survivors, had the low T_3 levels expected in severe non-thyroidal illness. However, these patients did not have elevated reverse T_3 values, in contrast to medical intensive-care-unit patients and ambulatory HIV-infected patients (those with asymptomatic and symptomatic infections and those with AIDS), all of whom had normal T_3 and reverse T_3 levels. Thus, the classic "euthyroid sick" syndrome does not appear to be common in HIV infection, for unclear reasons. There have been reports of pneumocystosis of the thyroid gland,[34] CMV involvement of the thyroid,[35] and KS in the thyroid.[36]

The clinical effect of most HIV-related endocrine abnormalities is uncertain, except for the wasting syndrome cachexia. It is likely that many if not most of these abnormalities are due to non-specific stress. Even so, various infectious and neoplastic complications or treatments of AIDS can involve the endocrine glands, so patients should be monitored for adrenal insufficiency and pentamidine-induced hypoglycemia in particular.

REFERENCES

1. Aron DC. Endocrine complications of the acquired immunodeficiency syndrome. Arch Intern Med 1989; 149:330-3.

2. Bricaire F, Marche C, Zoubi D, et al. [Adrenal lesions in AIDS: anatomopathological study]. Ann Med Interne (Paris) 1987; 138:607-9.

3. Klatt EC, Shibata D. Cytomegalovirus infection in the acquired immunodeficiency syndrome. Clinical and autopsy findings. Arch Pathol Lab Med 1988; 112:540-4.

4. Guarda LA, Luna MA, Smith JL Jr, et al. Acquired immune deficiency syndrome: postmortem findings. Am J Clin Pathol 1984; 81:549-57.

5. Shanley JD, Pesanti EL. Murine cytomegalovirus adrenalitis in athymic nude mice. Arch Virol 1986; 88:27-35.

6. Glasgow BJ, Steinsapir KD, Anders K, Layfield LJ. Adrenal pathology in the acquired immune deficiency syndrome. Am J Clin Pathol 1985; 84:594-7.

7. Greene LW, Cole W, Greene JB, et al. Adrenal insufficiency as a complication of the acquired immunodeficiency syndrome. Ann Intern Med 1984; 101:497-8.

8. Guenthner EE, Rabinowe SL, Van Niel A, et al. Primary Addison's disease in a patient with the acquired immunodeficiency syndrome. Ann Intern Med 1984; 100:847-8.

9. Tapper ML, Rotterdam HZ, Lerner CW, et al. Adrenal necrosis in the acquired immunodeficiency syndrome. Ann Intern Med 1984; 100:239-41.

10. Dobs AS, Dempsey MA, Ladenson PW, Polk BF. Endocrine disorders in men infected with human immunodeficiency virus. Am J Med 1988; 84:611-6.

11. Vitting KE, Gardenswartz MH, Zabetakis PM, et al. Frequency of hyponatremia (HN), hypoadrenalism and non-osmolar vasopressin release in the acquired immunodeficiency syndrome (AIDS). Fed Proc 1988; 47:221. abstract.

12. Kalin MF, Poretsky L, Seres DS, Zumoff B. Hyporeninemic hypoaldosteronism associated with acquired immune deficiency syndrome. Am J Med 1987; 82:1035-8.

13. Kaplan LD, Wolfe PR, Volberding PA, et al. Lack of response to suramin in patients with AIDS and AIDS-related complex. Am J Med 1987; 82:615-20.

14. Pont A, Williams PL, Loose DS, et al. Ketoconazole blocks adrenal steroid synthesis. Ann Intern Med 1982; 97:370-2.

15. Membreno L, Irony I, Dere W, et al. Adrenocortical function in acquired immunodeficiency syndrome. J Clin Endocrinol Metab 1987; 65:482-7.

16. May ME, Carey RM. Rapid adrenocorticotropic hormone test in practice. Retrospective review. Am J Med 1985; 79:679-84.

17. Membreno L, Cobb E, Biglieri EG, Brodie H. Reduced ACTH stimulation of 17-deoxysteroids, deoxycorticosterone (DOC), corticosterone (B), 18-hydroxy-DOC of the adrenocortical zona fasciculata (ZF) in acquired immunodeficiency syndrome (AIDS). Clin Res 1986; 35:428A. abstract.

18. Dere W, Klein R, Biglieri EG. Focal adrenocortical steroid defects acquired in AIDS. Program of the Endocrine Society, 67th Annual Meeting, 1985; 136. abstract.

19. Woolf PD, Hamill RW, McDonald JV, et al. Transient hypogonadotropic hypogonadism caused by critical illness. J Clin Endocrinol Metab 1985; 60:444-50.

20. Nakashima A, Koshiyama K, Uozumi T, et al. Effects of general anesthesia and severity of surgical stress on serum LH and testosterone in males. Acta Endocrinol (Copenh) 1975; 78:258-69.

21. Rudman D, Fleischer AS, Kutner MH, Raggio JF. Suprahypophyseal hypogonadism and hypothyroidism during prolonged coma after head trauma. J Clin Encocrinol Metab 1977; 45:747-54.

22. Milligan SA, Katz MS, Craven PC, et al. Toxoplasmosis presenting as panhypopituitarism in a patient with the acquired immunodeficiency syndrome. Am J Med 1984; 77:760-4.

23. Croxson TS, Chapman WE, Miller LK, et al. Prolactin levels in men with AIDS [Abstract]. II International Conference on Acquired Immunodeficiency Syndrome. Paris, 1986.

24. Waskin H, Stehr-Green JK, Helmick CG, Sattler FR. Risk factors for hypoglycemia associated with pentamidine therapy for pneumocystis pneumonia. JAMA 1988; 260:345-7.

25. Stahl-Bayliss CM, Kalman CM, Laskin OL. Pentamidine-induced hypoglycemia in patients with the acquired immune deficiency syndrome. Clin Pharmacol Ther 1986; 39:271-5.

26. Bouchard P, Sai P, Reach G, et al. Diabetes mellitus following pentamidine-induced hypoglycemia in humans. Diabetes 1982; 31:40-5.

27. Osei K, Falko JM, Nelson KP, Stephens R. Diabetogenic effect of pentamidine. In vitro and in vivo studies in a patient with malignant insulinoma. Am J Med 1984; 77:41-6.

28. Bryceson A, Woodstock L. The cumulative effect of pentamidine dimethanesulphonate on the blood sugar. East Afr Med J 1969; 46:170-3.

29. Agha FP, Nostrant TT, Abrams GD, et al. Cytomegalovirus cholangitis in a homosexual man with acquired immune deficiency syndrome. Am J Gastroenterol 1986; 81:1068-72.

30. Keh WC, Gerber MA. In situ hybridization for cytomegalovirus DNA in AIDS patients. Am J Pathol 1988; 131:490-6.

31. Mandrup-Poulsen T, Bendtzen K, Nerup J, et al. Affinity-purified human interleukin I is cytotoxic to isolated islets of Langerhans. Diabetologia 1986; 29:63-7.

32. LoPresti J, Fried J, Nicoloff J. Unique alternations in thyroid function tests in AIDS. Clin Res 1988; 36:386A. abstract.

33. LoPresti JS, Fried JC, Spencer CA, Nicoloff JT. Unique alterations of thyroid hormone indices in the acquired immunodeficiency syndrome (AIDS). Ann Intern Med 1989; 110:970-5.

34. Gallant JE, Enriquez RE, Cohen KL, Hammers LW. *Pneumocystis carinii* thyroiditis. Am J Med 1988; 84:303-6.

35. Frank TS, LiVolsi VA, Connor AM. Cytomegalovirus infection of the thyroid in immunocompromised adults. Yale J Biol Med 1987; 60:1-8.

36. Krauth PH, Katz JF. Kaposi's sarcoma involving the thyroid in a patient with AIDS. Clin Nucl Med 1987; 12:848-9.

37. Kyriazopoulou V, Parparousi O, Vagenakis AG. Rifampicin-induced adrenal crisis in Addisonian patients receiving corticosteroid replacement therapy. J Clin Endocrinol Metab 1984; 59:1204-6.

5.8

Hematologic Aspects

5.8.1   HIV-Related Immune Thrombocytopenic Purpura — *Abrams*

HIV-Related Immune Thrombocytopenic Purpura

Donald I. Abrams, M.D.

Immune thrombocytopenic purpura (ITP) is perhaps one of the most clinically challenging of the AIDS-related conditions. ITP, a diagnosis most frequently encountered in its acute form in children after viral infections and in its chronic presentation in middle-aged women, was first recognized as potentially related to AIDS by Morris et al. in 1982.[1] They described a cluster of 11 cases of autoimmune thrombocytopenic purpura in homosexual men in New York City. Demographic backgrounds and immunologic changes were very similar to those being described in patients with the newly recognized acquired immunodeficiency syndrome. Subsequently, the problem has also been recognized in narcotics addicts and hemophiliacs without other manifestations of AIDS.[2,3]

Thrombocytopenia is a recognized complication in many patients with confirmed AIDS diagnoses. A percentage of patients with Kaposi's sarcoma (KS) has been noted to develop low platelet counts either at the time of their diagnosis or during therapy.[4] A similar phenomenon has been recognized in patients diagnosed with AIDS-related lymphomas. Patients with pneumocystis pneumonia may initially have mild thrombocytopenia or, more commonly, develop impressive drops in platelet count during treatment. The rapid fall in platelets occurring during therapy for AIDS-related pneumocystis pneumonia is generally assumed to be drug-induced.[5] Many of our patients, however, have platelet-associated immunoglobulin before therapy, and it remains present at the time of thrombocytopenia.[6] Lowering of the platelet count could, in fact, be secondary to clearance of a previously blocked reticuloendothelial system that now recognizes and removes antibody-coated platelets.[7,8]

Platelet count depression (100,000 to 150,000/cubic mm) has been observed in approximately 58 percent of patients in our cohort undergoing evaluation for the syndrome of persistent generalized lymphadenopathy (PGL). In our study of the natural history of ITP, thrombocytopenia in connection with the lymphadenopathy syndrome appears to be associated with an increased risk of progression from lymphadenopathy syndrome to bona fide AIDS.[9] Thrombocytopenia, then, has been observed with all of the major clinical manifestations of HIV infection. Like peripheral lymphadenopathy, it may be a nonspecific response to the viral infection.

In addition to occurring with other manifestations of AIDS, thrombocytopenia as an isolated complication has emerged in a group of patients. The two largest studies of this patient population have come from New York University and San Francisco General Hospital.[10,11] The experiences at these two centers are striking in their similarities.

Thirty-five homosexual males with isolated thrombocytopenia have been studied at SFGH.[6,11,12] The mean age of the cohort is 33.6 years (range: 23 to 47 years). Thirty-two patients are white, three are Hispanic. One patient was diagnosed with immune thrombocytopenia in April of 1980. Four patients were diagnosed in 1982. An apparent seasonal clustering of cases was observed in 1983; 14 of 18 patients appeared between April and July. Similarly, 7 of 12 cases in 1984 were diagnosed in May and June.

■ CLINICAL FEATURES

The clinical presentation of patients with isolated thrombocytopenia has been generally benign. No patient has suffered from major gastrointestinal or central nervous system bleeding during the course of follow-up observation. The mean duration of follow-up care is currently greater than 50 months. Six patients denied any antecedent bleeding before their diagnosis of ITP. These patients were generally found to be thrombocytopenic on routine blood testing done for other reasons, generally AIDS anxiety. Easy bruisability and petechiae were the most common manifestations in presenting complaints reported in over 50 percent of the patients. Five patients reported epistaxis; five, gingival bleeding; and five, rectal bleeding. Two patients sought medical attention because of blood in their ejaculate. The mean duration from onset of symptoms to the diagnosis of ITP in the cohort was one month.

Physical examination revealed evidence of mucosal bleeding. Cutaneous or palatal petechiae, or ecchymoses, were noted in the majority of patients. Twenty of our 35 evaluated patients had varying degrees of peripheral lymphadenopathy. Because of the marked severity of the thrombocytopenia, these patients were included in our ITP cohort rather than in the subset of patients with generalized lymphadenopathy. However, there is clinical overlap in these two groups. Six patients had minimal splenomegaly on palpation. Splenic enlargement is not a usual feature of non-AIDS-related immune thrombocytopenia. Oral candida was present in two patients at the time of their initial evaluation.

■ LABORATORY FEATURES

Initial laboratory findings in the cohort of 35 thrombocytopenic patients revealed a mean platelet count of 21,000/cubic mm (range: 3,000 to 69,000/cubic mm). Platelet-associated immunoglobulin was detected by a fluorescence-activated flow cytometric assay in all 30 patients tested. Bone marrow aspirates and biopsies performed on 25 patients were consistent with peripheral destruction showing adequate to increased megakaryocytes. Mild anemia (hematocrits: 37 percent to 39.9 percent) was present in four patients. White blood cell counts averaged 6600/cubic mm. The general absence of anemia or leukopenia, or both, was used to define these patients as having isolated thrombocytopenia.

Numerous patients with AIDS or related conditions have initially appeared at our clinic with pancytopenia. Although these patients may also show platelet-associated immunoglobulin on testing and evidence of immune platelet destruction, patients with pancytopenia are not included in this discussion of the ITP cohort.

■ LYMPHOCYTE STUDIES

Analysis of lymphocyte subsets in patients with non-AIDS-related autoimmune thrombocytopenia might be expected to show an increase in the helper-cell population, with a resultant elevated T lymphocyte helper/suppressor ratio. As reported in the original New York City cohort, patients with AIDS-related thrombocytopenia show the same inversion of the helper/suppressor ratio seen in AIDS and its related conditions. The total lymphocyte count in our cohort of 35 patients averaged 1700/cubic mm (range: 800 to 3100/cubic mm). Monoclonal antibody phenotyping of the T lymphocytes revealed a mean OKT3 number of 1378/cubic mm (range: 1700 to 2600/cubic mm). The absolute number of helper T cells, as determined by OKT4 monoclonal antibody, was decreased to 390/cubic mm (range: 70 to 750/cubic mm). OKT8 suppressor cytotoxic T lymphocytes averaged 1200/cubic mm (range: 600 to 2800/cubic mm). The resultant helper/suppressor T-lymphocyte ratio in our cohort was 0.45 (range: 0.1 to 0.8). This, again, was an unexpected phenotype in patients with an autoimmune phenomenon and supported the contention that ITP in homosexual men was related to infection with HIV.

Subsequent evaluation of HIV antibody status in our cohort revealed 100 percent seropositivity. Of 25 patients evaluated by the ELISA, 21 were positive and 4 were borderline. All four borderline cases were confirmed as positive via Western blot. In the New York series, antibodies to HIV were detected in sera from 13 of 14 thrombocytopenic patients evaluated by an indirect immuno-fluorescence assay.[10] These investigators compared the geometric mean titer of HIV antibody in their patients with titers in healthy homosexual seropositive controls and 12 seropositive homosexual patients with AIDS and secondary thrombocytopenia. Patients with isolated thrombocytopenia had levels of antibody equivalent to those of healthy controls. Patients with AIDS and secondary thrombocytopenia had lower titers at levels that approached statistical significance.

■ THE MECHANISM OF ITP

The mechanism of AIDS-related immune thrombocytopenic purpura (ITP) remains a matter of some controversy. Two alternative hypotheses that have been investigated are reviewed here. Clinical case studies supporting a relationship between reticuloendothelial system function and status of thrombocytopenia in individual patients are also described.

Walsh et al. of New York University presented findings indicating that in their cohort of homosexual men with AIDS-related ITP, the mechanism of thrombocytopenia was different from that in classic autoimmune thrombocytopenia.[13] Their patients had higher levels of platelet-associated immunoglobulin and platelet complement than patients with classic autoimmune thrombocytopenic purpura. Platelet eluates from the majority of patients with classic ITP were capable of binding to platelets from other patients. Such binding only occurred in 1 of 10 eluates from the homosexual population.

Twenty-one of 24 patients with AIDS-related thrombocytopenia had elevated levels of circulating immune complexes; none of five patients with classic ITP tested showed immune complexes. Of the circulating immune complexes detected in the homosexual ITP population, 79 percent were capable of binding to normal platelets, whereas homosexuals with thrombocytopenic purpura had neither serum IgG nor platelet IgG capable of binding to normal platelets. The homosexual patients, however, did have immune complexes that were capable of binding to platelets.

Walsh and colleagues thus contend that, in contrast to classic autoimmune thrombocytopenic purpura, in which an antiplatelet IgG is directed against platelet antigenic determinants, AIDS-related ITP appears to result from the deposition of immune complexes and complement on platelets. They further hypothesize that the immune-complex deposition occurs on platelet Fc receptors. Monocytes or macrophages would then bind to free Fc domains of exposed IgG molecules or to platelet-bound complement by their C3B receptors. The authors suggest that ITP in homosexual men may thus be viewed as an epiphenomenon related to the presence of circulating immune complexes rather than a true autoimmune disorder.

Data to support a contrary mechanism were reported by Stricker et al. in their evaluation of the San Francisco thrombocytopenia cohort.[6] Twenty-nine of 30 homosexual men with ITP were found to have a serum antibody that bound to a target platelet antigen of 25,000 daltons. This antibody activity was not detectable in patients with classic ITP or in patients with thrombocytopenia secondary to nonimmune mechanisms. The antibody was shown to bind via the $F(ab')_2$ portion of the molecule, indicating that it was, in fact, a true autoantibody and not an immune complex as postulated by Walsh et al. The 25,000-dalton antigen was found to be an integral part of the platelet membrane rather than an adsorbed antigen, since it resisted trypsin hydrolysis and thrombin stimulation of platelets.

No cross-reactivity could be demonstrated between the platelet-associated antigen and components of the HIV core protein. The serum antibody did react, however, with the 25,000-dalton antigen associated with cultured herpes simplex virus, types I and II. It appeared that the antigen was derived from the green monkey kidney cells in which the herpes simplex viruses were grown, rather than from the actual herpes species themselves. The significance of this observation is being investigated further. The presence of elevated circulating immune complexes in only 7 to 11 of the patients with AIDS-related ITP tested in the San Francisco cohort reduces the likelihood of an immune complex mediated mechanism even further.

In a control group of 16 patients with AIDS-related lymphadenopathy or bona fide AIDS, platelet-associated IgG was detected in all five patients studied. The unique antibody to the 25,000-dalton antigen was detected in 15 of 16 patients studied. This control group had no thrombocytopenia at the time these determinations were made. The question of why some patients with AIDS and ARC have normal platelet counts in the presence of platelet-associated IgG and the 25,000-dalton antibody remains unanswered. An attractive hypothesis is that Fc-receptor-mediated clearance is defective in patients with AIDS, as it is in other patients with chronic infectious diseases and hypergammaglobulinemia.[8,14] Defective reticuloendothelial system clearance in the face of antibody-coated platelets results in a normal platelet count.[7] The spleen, preoccupied with other responsibilities, relegates removal of antibody-coated platelets to a low priority. In patients whose reticuloendothelial function is relatively "unblocked," thrombocytopenia could then develop in the face of immunoglobulin coating of the platelets.

Our clinical observations support the contention that patients presenting with isolated thrombocytopenia as their only manifestation of infection with HIV generally are clinically "healthy" compared with the majority of patients with AIDS and other AIDS-related conditions.[11,12] Further support of this hypothesis involves a patient in our cohort whose thrombocytopenia was not corrected by splenectomy; he maintained a stable low platelet count in the 30,000/cubic mm range. He developed an illness characterized by low-grade fever, malaise, and minimal right-upper-quadrant tenderness. Mild transaminase elevations occurred. During the acute hepatitis-like illness, his platelet count rose to normal. With resolution of symptoms, the thrombocytopenia recurred.

Perhaps even more dramatic and suggestive evidence that effective reticuloendothelial clearance is a prerequisite for thrombocytopenia in AIDS is provided by findings in two of our patients who remained untreated for their AIDS-related thrombocytopenia. Both patients maintained average platelet counts in the 10,000 to 30,000/cubic mm range over a two-year period. No therapeutic interventions occurred. Both patients ultimately progressed to develop pneumocystis pneumonia. One patient presented with some prodromal symptoms, mild anemia, and elevation of the sedimentation rate, one month before the diagnosis of pneumonia. At the time of diagnosis and hospitalization, one month later, the platelet count was 400,000/cubic mm. The second patient, who had maintained 30,000 platelets for two years, developed pneumocystis pneumonia and presented with a normal platelet count. Similarly, a third patient who had been treated with a short course of steroids stopped therapy because of the development of an intolerable peripheral neuropathy. Eight months later, he developed fevers and a rising platelet count. At the time of hospitalization for commencement of therapy for cryptococcal meningitis, the patient had 150,000 platelets. During therapy with amphotericin-B and 5-FC, the patient's platelet count plummeted rapidly to his previous 20,000 range. The mechanism was felt to be drug induced. However, the recurrent thrombocytopenia could, in fact, have reflected "unblocking" of the reticuloendothelial system in response to clearance of cryptococcal disease.

A final example in support of this hypothesis is shown by a patient in whom splenectomy was unsuccessful. After a prolonged hospitalization with multiple surgical and infectious complications, the patient was discharged with a platelet count of 40,000/cubic mm. Over the following weeks, he developed progressive malaise, low-grade fevers, and left shoulder pain. A staphylococcal osteomyelitis was ultimately diagnosed. The platelet count at that time was normal. After three weeks of antibiotic therapy, the platelet count had again dropped to the 40,000 to 50,000/cubic mm range.

■ RESPONSE TO THERAPIES

One of the more challenging aspects of the clinical management of patients with AIDS-related ITP has been investigating therapeutic approaches. Even in the earliest cases, the possibility that thrombocytopenia might somehow be associated with immunosuppression seen in AIDS made the use of steroids problematic. Similarly, the effect of second-line therapy, splenectomy, on an already impaired immune system, made the clinician think twice before recommending this intervention. At this time, however, data have been collected on each of these therapies that suggest no real evidence of further clinically significant immune suppression.

The following traces the experience at San Francisco General Hospital that has led to our present recommendations for treatment of patients with AIDS-related ITP. The initial reflex was to employ the above standard modalities of therapy, steroids and splenectomy; however, we also evaluated other interventions. In view of an apparent lack of significant bleeding complications in our cohort of patients and their desire to avoid further potentially immunocompromising therapies, a current alternative practice of careful observation without therapy in the nonbleeding patient has become standard.

Response to Prednisone.   One difficulty in assessing the response to steroid therapy has been the lack of a standard measure of response. In reporting on prednisone treatment in 17 patients with AIDS and thrombocytopenia, Walsh et al. described an "excellent" response as a return of platelet count to greater than 100,000/cubic mm while on prednisone, and a "moderate" response as a rise in platelet count to over 50,000/cubic mm.[10] The response did not need to be persistent on steroid tapering to be considered excellent or moderate. In their cohort treated with initial doses of 60 to 100 mg/day followed by tapering, eight patients achieved an excellent response, and eight others a moderate response. Only one patient did not respond to prednisone therapy. However, upon tapering the steroids, the platelet counts were noted to fall to previous or lower levels in 13 patients. Only two patients maintained normal platelet counts after cessation of steroid therapy. The sustained remissions persisted for 17 and 36 months at the time of publication of these results. Two other patients in their series maintained moderate responses.

By the same response criteria, 19 of 24 patients in the San Francisco series initially begun on prednisone (1 mg/kg by mouth every day) achieved an initial response,[11,12] translating to a 79 percent response rate. However, again, only two of our patients maintained normal platelet counts after tapering of steroid therapy. Although a rise in platelet count is often associated with cessation of clinical bleeding in patients with bleeding problems due to thrombocytopenia, the lack of major clinical bleeding in patients with AIDS-related ITP makes the significance and clinical utility of such subnormal platelet-count rises questionable. If one then evaluates responses to prednisone on the basis of whether they were sustained or transient, only 4 of the total of 41 patients in both series achieved sustained complete responses from steroid therapy (see Table 1).

TABLE 1.   RESPONSE TO THERAPY IN PATIENTS WITH AIDS-RELATED IMMUNE THROMBOCYTOPENIA*

TREATMENT	NUMBER OF PATIENTS		
	SF (%)	NY (%)	TOTAL (%)
PREDNISONE (1 mg/kg/day, minimum: 21 days)	24	17	41
Sustained complete response on therapy	2 (8)	2 (12)	4 (10)
Partial response	17 (71)	14 (82)	31 (76)
Platelet count normalized, then fell	8	6	14
Platelet count rose to subnormal, then fell	9	8	17
Complete response, 12 months off therapy	2	—	2
No response	5 (21)	1 (6)	6 (15)
SPLENECTOMY	15	10	25
Sustained complete response	10 (66)	10 (100)	20 (80)

continued on next page

continued from previous page

TABLE 1. RESPONSE TO THERAPY IN PATIENTS WITH
AIDS-RELATED IMMUNE THROMBOCYTOPENIA*

TREATMENT	NUMBER OF PATIENTS		
	SF (%)	NY (%)	TOTAL (%)
Splenectomy failures	5 (33)	0	5 (20)
OTHER THERAPIES DURING STEROID TREATMENT			
Vincristine, 2.0 mg IV weekly (1 to 6 weeks)	5		
Partial response	1		
No response	4		
Danazol, 200 mg qid for three months	5		
No response	5		

* Compiled by the authors.

None of the patients treated in either series developed an episode of opportunistic infection or malignant transformation while on prednisone therapy. However, the transient rise in platelet count in 31 of 41 patients did not occur without some adverse side effects. The complications of treatment were similar to those described in patients without AIDS on prolonged steroid courses. Weight gain and moon faces developed in 15 of the 24 patients treated in our series. Fourteen patients developed oral candidiasis while on therapy. Marked dysphoric reactions described as an almost amphetamine-like reaction were described by 10 patients during the course of their prednisone therapy. Steroid acne and activation of herpes labialis were also seen in 50 percent of our cohort. One patient developed a severe proximal myopathy of the lower extremities that was felt to be consistent with a steroid myopathy. A severe distal sensory neuropathy caused cessation of steroid treatment in another patient, after which the symptom resolved. A third patient with a past history of treatment for pulmonary tuberculosis 20 years before developing ITP experienced an episode of headache and fever after six months of steroid therapy. Cerebrospinal fluid examination revealed a monocytosis and negative cultures. In three weeks the patient's symptomatology had abated and a repeat lumbar puncture was negative. The etiology of this episode remains unclear. The patient ultimately developed the AIDS dementia complex and died.

Serial measurements of lymphocyte subsets were performed on seven of our patients during the initiation of prednisone treatment.[11] The pre-therapy helper/suppressor ratio averaged 0.45. With the institution of prednisone therapy, a decrease in total lymphocyte count occurred in patients treated. An equivalent depression was noted in both the OKT4- and OKT8-positive populations during steroid therapy, resulting in no significant change from the baseline helper/suppressor ratio. Post-treatment ratios drawn up to three months after the initiation of therapy averaged 0.37 in this subset. The mean duration of steroid therapy in the 24 patients treated was 10 months. The median duration was five months. This reflects the tendency for a more protracted trial of steroid therapy in patients diagnosed more recently. The range of total duration of steroid therapy is from 3 weeks to 36 months in our patient population.

Of note is that lymph nodes of ITP patients who initially had associated peripheral lymphadenopathy on physical examination became impalpable during prednisone treatment. As these patients were tapered off steroids, the generalized lymphadenopathy was again appreciable.

Response to Splenectomy.   The overall response rate to splenectomy in the combined New York and San Francisco series is 80 percent. This compared favorably with the success of surgery in non-AIDS-related ITP.[15] All 10 patients reported by Walsh et al. had excellent responses; their platelet counts became normal after splenectomy, and no postoperative complications were reported. Previous steroid treatment had failed in these 10 New York patients undergoing surgery. Surgery was performed at a mean time of 3.6 months (± 0.7 months) after diagnosis except in one patient who underwent splenectomy 33 months after initial diagnosis.

In our cohort, splenectomy has been performed on 15 patients with AIDS-related ITP. In two patients, this procedure was the initial therapy; the remaining patients underwent splenectomy after failure of a steroid trial. Ten of the 15 splenectomized patients achieved sustained complete remissions and normal platelet counts postoperatively. Four of the five surgical failures occurred within the first month postoperatively. One patient suffered a relapse four months after the surgery. Most of these splenectomized patients underwent surgery within the first six months of ITP diagnosis. One of the responders, however, only agreed to surgery after 19 months of steroid therapy. Three patients had serial T-cell subset analysis before and after splenectomy. A post-splenectomy lymphocytosis was observed; a twofold to threefold increase in both helper and suppressor cell subsets yielded no change in the actual helper/suppressor lymphocyte ratio.

Postoperative complications after splenectomy have been minimal in our patients with isolated AIDS-related thrombocytopenia. Two patients developed postoperative episodes of pneumonitis. One patient suffered a draining pancreatic fistula after accidental resection of a portion of the pancreas. This patient ultimately developed a string of infectious complications including pleural-based Legionnaire's disease, staphylococcal sepsis, disseminated varicella, and ultimately, staphylococcal osteomyelitis. No postoperative mortality has occurred. In general, patients experienced a normal postoperative convalescence. This contrasts somewhat with the SFGH experience with splenectomy in patients with full-blown AIDS. In this subset of patients, the procedure has been associated with substantially increased morbidity and occasional mortality.

Intravenous Gamma Globulin.   High-dose intravenous gamma globulin has been reported to reverse immune thrombocytopenic purpura in some patients, even though the effect may be transient.[16] The exact mechanism is unclear, but it has been suggested that the rise in platelet count may be due to competitive inhibition of macrophage binding of platelets by increased reticuloendothelial system blockade.[17] Reports of the efficacy of intravenous gamma globulin in AIDS-related ITP have appeared. Tertian reported on 12 patients with AIDS-related thrombocytopenia treated with high-dose intravenous gamma globulin.[18] All patients had platelet counts less than 50,000/cubic mm at the initiation of therapy. Seven patients were severe hemophiliacs, three were intravenous drug users, and two were homosexual men. The dose schedule ranged from 0.5 g/kg/day in 1 day to 0.4 g/kg/day in 5 days. A total of one to nine treatments per patient was given. Indications for high-dose intravenous gamma globulin therapy were bleeding episodes and preoperative splenectomy or other surgery. A response was noted in 11 of 12 patients. A rapid rise in platelet count to normal and lasting for an average of 6 to 21 days was reported. The single nonresponder was a hemophiliac. The transient platelet elevation was felt to be beneficial for preoperative elimination of thrombocytopenia before splenectomy.

Other Therapies.   Other therapies have been evaluated in combination with an initial course of steroids in some members of the San Francisco cohort. Five patients received from one to six weekly intravenous injections of vincristine (2.0 mg). In four patients, no response was observed. One patient receiving a full six weeks of vincristine therapy achieved a normal platelet count at week 4. However, platelets fell again to subnormal levels at week 6 despite continued prednisone and vincristine.

Danazol has been reported to have some efficacy in non-AIDS-related immune thrombocytopenic purpura.[19] It also reportedly may invert abnormal helper/suppressor lymphocyte ratios. Fischl et al. reported the use of danazol (800 mg by mouth every day for at least 3 months) in six cases of AIDS-related thrombocytopenia.[20] Three of their thrombocytopenic patients had previous AIDS opportunistic infections without KS. The remaining three had chronic lymphadenopathy, weight loss, and oral thrush. All had the classic defect in cellular immunity. Initial platelet counts ranged from 9,000 to 34,000/cubic mm. Four of six patients achieved platelet-count elevation ranging from 65,000 to 125,000/cubic mm, and the response typically occurred after three months of therapy. Two patients achieved normal T-lymphocyte ratios; three others experienced a progressive increase in the subset of T helper/inducers without normal T-lymphocyte ratios.

Five patients in the San Francisco cohort were treated with danazol (200 mg by mouth 4 times/day for at least 3 months) together with their initial course of prednisone therapy. In none of these five patients was any substantial response noted in either platelet count or T-lymphocyte helper/suppressor ratio.

Three patients in our cohort have undergone plasma exchange in an attempt to alleviate their thrombocytopenia.[21] This was done in the hope of removing either circulating immune complexes or an autoantibody aimed at specific target platelet membrane antigens. One patient underwent treatment with the staphylococcal protein A column. Although transient platelet elevations were noted immediately after procedure, no sustained responses were obtained with this treatment.

No Therapy.   Sixteen patients in the New York series were reported as receiving no treatment for their thrombocytopenia.[10] The mean platelet count of this group was 79,000/cubic mm (range: 32,000 to 135,000/cubic mm). Four of these patients had normal platelet counts without any therapeutic intervention 5 to 10 months after the diagnosis. One of the four developed AIDS 22 months after initial ITP diagnosis.

Sustained complete remissions in response to prednisone therapy occur infrequently. Many of our patients are reluctant to undergo splenectomy. In view of the fact that no serious bleeding complications have been observed in our series of markedly thrombocytopenic patients, no therapy has been recommended to most of our recently diagnosed patients with AIDS-related ITP.

Patients with platelet counts initially as low as 8000/cubic mm at presentation have elected to receive no treatment and have done well, with observation, over the past 4.5 years. Two of our untreated patients who had maintained platelet counts in the 20,000 to 30,000/cubic mm range for up to two years developed AIDS. Both these patients achieved normal platelet counts at the time of diagnosis of their opportunistic infection.

■ NATURAL HISTORY OF ITP

ITP, now well recognized as an AIDS-related condition, is similar to persistent generalized lymphadenopathy, as it has been presumed that thrombocytopenia is an alternative phenotypic response to infection with HIV. The natural history to date of patients who initially have had isolated thrombocytopenia as their only manifestation of HIV infection is discussed below. A percentage of the ITP cohort has progressed to develop the more severe manifestations of AIDS. Case histories of some of our patients from the San Francisco General Hospital cohort with ITP evolving to AIDS are presented to stress an unusual fluctuation of platelet count in relation to overall health status.

Thrombocytopenia, similar to lymphadenopathy, clearly appears to be a frequent secondary response to infection with HIV. Studies on a group of hemophilia patients in France clearly delineate the temporal sequence between infection with HIV and the development of thrombocytopenia.[18] In this subset, serial serum samples allowed investigators to date the time of seroconversion. The interval between the first seropositive serum specimen and the development of thrombocytopenia in six hemophilic patients was 12, 15, 21, 24, 33, and 36 months, respectively.

Because some patients with thrombocytopenia seemed otherwise well, it was initially hoped that thrombocytopenia would perhaps be their only manifestation of infection with HIV. Unfortunately, however, serial follow-up of San Francisco patients with ITP[11,12] and of the New York University cohort[10] has shown progression to AIDS. Evolution of a bona fide AIDS diagnosis has occurred in patients who have received specific therapy for their ITP with steroids, splenectomy, or both, as well as in patients who have chosen no therapeutic interventions. Case histories of five patients in the SFGH cohort whose ITP progressed to AIDS are presented below.

The San Francisco Experience.   Patient 1 was initially diagnosed with ITP in January 1982. He was treated intermittently with steroid therapy for 19 months until he consented to undergo splenectomy. The surgery was uncomplicated, and the patient achieved a complete sustained response and a normal platelet count. However, he subsequently developed fevers, weight loss, and diarrhea. In November 1984, a diagnosis of small-bowel lymphoma was made. The patient died after cytotoxic chemotherapy.

Patient 2 was noted to have thrombocytopenia in February 1982. After two months of steroid therapy, his platelet count had only reached a maximum of 50,000/cubic mm. Because in our earlier experience attempts were made in all patients to achieve "safe" levels of platelets, this patient was referred for splenectomy. He achieved a complete sustained response with a normal platelet count after splenectomy. Coincident with splenectomy, the patient's sexual partner of 21 years was diagnosed with pneumocystis pneumonia. The ITP patient did well until he developed cough, fever, diarrhea, and weight loss. He was diagnosed with pneumocystis pneumonia in November 1984, and the condition was successfully treated. In March 1985, evaluation of the patient's confusion yielded the diagnosis of cerebral toxoplasmosis. Despite an initial resolution of the CNS lesions to appropriate antibiotic therapy, the patient died.

Patient 3 was diagnosed with ITP in October 1983. Biopsy of an enlarged lymph node at the time of diagnosis revealed a necrotizing granuloma, and a coincident diagnosis of cat-scratch disease was entertained. The patient had a three-month trial of oral steroids. He complained of CNS dysphoria as well as development of a painful sensory distal neuropathy. Steroids were discontinued in January 1984. The patient subsequently continued to have a stable depressed platelet count in the 20,000/cubic mm range. In late January 1985, one year after discontinuing steroids, his platelet count began to rise spontaneously. At that time he also began to develop increased constitutional symptoms with fevers, night sweats, and weight loss. Blood cultures ultimately grew *Cryptococcus neoformans*. Cerebrospinal fluid confirmed the diagnosis of cryptococcal meningitis with sepsis. At the time of admission to the hospital to initiate amphotericin B therapy, the patient's platelet count had risen to 150,000/cubic mm. Three weeks after the institution of amphotericin B and 5-flucytosine (5-FC), the patient developed severe thrombocytopenia and had a platelet count of 20,000/cubic mm. The mechanism of thrombocytopenia was felt to be drug induced. He ultimately died from uncontrolled gastrointestinal hemorrhage.

Patient 4 was diagnosed with ITP in February 1984. The patient chose, in conjunction with a health-care provider, to be followed with close observation and no therapeutic intervention. He continued to have a stable platelet count in the 5,000 to 10,000/cubic mm range for the ensuing 22 months. In December 1985, he complained of general malaise and low-grade fevers. His hematocrit had fallen to 37 percent. Erythrocyte sedimentation rate was elevated for the first time in his two years of follow-up. His platelet count had risen to 90,000/cubic mm. The patient returned to the clinic one month later acutely short of breath and was diagnosed with pneumocystis pneumonia. At the time of his admission for commencement of antibiotic therapy, his platelet count was 450,000/cubic mm. The patient died during the second week of his hospitalization for pneumocystis pneumonia.

Patient 5 was diagnosed with ITP in May 1984. His only therapy for ITP was plasma exchange for five courses; the staphylococcal protein A column was used on one occasion. In November 1985, his platelet count, which had been stable at approximately 30,000 to 40,000/cubic mm, rose to 139,000/cubic mm during an episode that was diagnosed as a bacterial pneumonia. However, the patient continued to have a positive gallium scan. This prompted sputum induction in February 1986, resulting in a positive diagnosis of pneumocystis pneumonia. The patient's platelet count at the initiation of therapy was 204,000/cubic mm. He successfully recovered from the episode of pneumocystis, and two months later his platelet count was 89,000/cubic mm.

The mean time from initial diagnosis of ITP to the development of AIDS in these five patients was 26 months.

The New York Experience.   The experience with progression to AIDS in the New York cohort is similar to that seen in our patient population. Walsh et al. reported that 6 of their 33 patients followed for a mean of 20 months (±2 months) developed bona fide AIDS.[10] Thus, the overall rate of progression in the 68 patients reported in the literature from the New York and San Francisco series after approximately 2 years of follow-up is 11 of 68 patients or 16 percent.

Patients in the New York University cohort developing AIDS were diagnosed 16.6 months (mean) after their ITP diagnosis (range: 1 to 37 months). No association between the severity of thrombocytopenia and the ultimate development of AIDS was observed by Walsh and colleagues. Four of these patients had a history of previous prednisone therapy; four had undergone splenectomy. One patient who developed AIDS had no intervening therapy. These investigators also reported that this patient's platelet count became normal before the development of AIDS.

Lymphadenopathy as an associated AIDS-related condition was reported in seven members of the New York series. Five patients presented with significant lymphadenopathy at the time of diagnosis of thrombocytopenia. One of these patients developed Kaposi's sarcoma. Two other patients reportedly developed lymphadenopathy 12 and 23 months after the diagnosis of thrombocytopenia, and one of these also developed Kaposi's sarcoma two years later. The investigators conclude that if the seven patients with lymphadenopathy are excluded from analysis of the ITP cohort evolving to AIDS, 4 of 26 patients with thrombocytopenia alone could be described as having developed AIDS over the 20 months of follow-up. Whether it is necessary to analyze the presence of lymphadenopathy and thrombocytopenia as independent prognostic variables in this manner will require further observation of these cohorts.

■ HIV INFECTION AND COAGULATION STUDIES

Hematologic abnormalities are a common finding in patients with AIDS. Cytopenias involving all of the cellular elements of blood have been well described. The association of immune thrombocytopenia with AIDS and related conditions is established. The findings of coagulation abnormalities in a subset of patients with AIDS-related opportunistic infections and the clinical observations that led to the recognition of the presence of a lupus anticoagulant in patients with pneumocystis pneumonia are reviewed below. Recommendations for screening AIDS patients with prolonged bleeding times are made and the clinical relevance of the lupus anticoagulants in the setting of AIDS is also discussed.

Lupus Anticoagulants.   The observation of a lupus anticoagulant in patients with AIDS, particularly those with opportunistic infections, has been recently confirmed in two separate studies and represents the first coagulation disorder reported in association with AIDS.[22-24] Our awareness of this abnormality stemmed from observations on patients admitted to San Francisco General Hospital for bronchoscopic confirmation of a suspected diagnosis of pneumocystis pneumonia. Before the procedure, these patients routinely underwent coagulation panel screening, including prothrombin time, partial thromboplastin time, and platelet count. Patients were frequently noted to have prolongation of their partial thromboplastin time. Hematology consultation was often requested to evaluate this laboratory abnormality.

A typical patient profile is represented by a 32-year-old male who was admitted with a history of two months of fatigue, a 20-pound weight loss, and two weeks of fever and nonproductive cough. He denied any history of bleeding or bruising. Physical examination showed a patient in moderate respiratory distress, febrile to 40.1°C, with a respiratory rate of 32. The patient appeared chronically ill and had oral candida and shoddy peripheral lymphadenopathy. His chest was clear. Initial laboratory examination showed a hemoglobin of 9.8 g/dl and a leukocyte count of 12,500/cubic mm, with 78 percent polymorphonuclear leukocytes, 4 percent bands, 13 percent lymphocytes, and 5 percent monocytes. The platelet count was normal at 310,000/cubic mm. Results of liver function tests were normal. Coagulation studies showed a normal prothrombin time and a partial thromboplastin time of 54.3 seconds (normal, 24 to 34 seconds).

When the prolongation of the partial thromboplastin time was investigated, an inhibitor screen involving 50:50 mixing showed no correction of the PTT with 50 percent normal plasma. This finding indicated the presence of an inhibitor to coagulation. Partial thromboplastin time with kaolin incubation remained prolonged at 54.2 seconds. The lack of correction with incubation excludes the possibility of a pre-kallikrein deficiency. Assays for particular coagulation factors, including Factors II, VIII, IX, XI, and XII, revealed no deficiency that could explain prolongation of the partial thromboplastin time. The Russell viper venom time was prolonged in this patient at 68.8 seconds (normal: 24 to 37 seconds) and failed to correct with the addition of 50 percent normal plasma. This confirmed the inhibitor as a lupus anticoagulant. Results of platelet aggregation studies were normal.

In order to further assess the frequency of the finding of the lupus anticoagulant in hospitalized patients with AIDS, 34 consecutive patients were evaluated at San Francisco General Hospital during the month of August 1984.[22,23] None of the patients had a known history of systemic lupus erythematosus, autoimmune disorders, use of chlorpromazine, or a history of malignancy other than KS. Twenty-four of the 34 patients had prolonged partial thromboplastin times. Nine patients had PTTs from 35 to 40 seconds, seven from 40 to 45 seconds, and eight showed prolongation greater than 45 seconds. Only 1 of the 34 patients had a prolonged prothrombin time.

Confirmation of the presence of a lupus anticoagulant by Russell viper venom time was only performed if clinically indicated to differentiate a lupus anticoagulant from a true coagulopathy before performing an invasive procedure. Six patients from the group of 34 had Russell viper venom times performed and all were prolonged. In addition, in five other patients, results of mixing studies showed immediate prolongation, again confirming the presence of an inhibitor. Virtually all of the 34 patients had been admitted for evaluation and treatment of an AIDS-related opportunistic infection.

The lupus anticoagulant is an acquired coagulation inhibitor first described in patients with systemic lupus erythematosus.[25] Since that time, it has also been noted in association with other immune disorders, myeloproliferative disorders, neoplastic disease, pregnancy, and secondary to certain drugs.[26-31] The anticoagulant is an immunoglobulin, either IgG or IgM, that interferes with all phospholipid-dependent coagulation assays. Lupus anticoagulants inhibit coagulation at the level of the prothrombin activator complex consisting of calcium, Factors Va, Xa, and phospholipid.[32] They do not, however, interfere with the action of specific coagulation factors and are generally felt to be an in vitro phenomenon. No clinical bleeding diathesis is associated with the presence of a lupus anticoagulant except in the presence of thrombocytopenia, hypoprothrombinemia, functional platelet abnormality, or an underlying coagulopathy. Thrombotic episodes, however, have been reported in 20 percent to 50 percent of patients with the lupus anticoagulant.[33] One patient in our series of 34 developed a massive deep venous thrombosis of the lower extremity requiring heparin anticoagulation. It was felt that this episode was a manifestation of the concomitant presence of a circulating lupus anticoagulant. However, full evaluation to rule out the possibility of disseminated intravascular coagulation was equivocal.

Cohen et al. of George Washington University Medical Center report the presence of circulating coagulation inhibitors in 10 of 50 homosexual patients with AIDS evaluated over a two-year period.[24] All but one of their patients had proven opportunistic infection. The single exception was a patient who had Kaposi's sarcoma alone. None of their 10 patients demonstrated a biologic false positive test for lues. None of the 10 had positive antinuclear antibody or rheumatoid factors. All had a polyclonal gammopathy.

The coagulation profiles of the 10 patients showed moderately prolonged activated partial thromboplastin times ranging from 40 to 53 seconds. Three patients had concomitant elevations in the prothrombin time that correlated with mild deficiencies of factor II activity. None of the prolongations of activated partial thromboplastin time was corrected with the addition of normal platelet-poor plasma. The circulating anticoagulants were thought to be lupus anticoagulants in seven patients.

Immunoelectropheresis studies were performed on the isolated immunoglobulins and showed inhibitory activity to coagulation. These studies showed the coagulation inhibitors to be either monoclonal IgG lambda or polyclonal IgM. This finding is in keeping with previously published evaluations of the lupus anticoagulant.[34] In six of those seven patients, lupus anticoagulant immunoglobulin characterization revealed an IgM. The authors speculate that the overwhelming predominance of IgM type anticoagulants in patients with AIDS may, in fact, reflect acuteness of the infections in these clinical situations. They further observed that the lupus anticoagulant activity tended to disappear in those patients whose acute opportunistic infections subsequently responded to therapy. In one patient, the circulating inhibitor of coagulation developed only after longstanding KS was complicated by additional *Mycobacterium avium-intracellulare* infection. This further strengthened the observation that the lupus anticoagulant is associated with AIDS-related opportunistic infection.

The clinical significance of the lupusagulant in patients with AIDS-related opportunistic infections is noteworthy. The finding of aned prolongation of the activated partial thromboplastin time in initial evaluation of a patient scheduled to undergo an invasive procedure should not preclude the intervention. If no clinical history of bleeding is noted, the lupus anticoagulant should be suspected. Added complications would not be expected to occur in the setting of a lupus anticoagulant except in situations associated with marked hypoprothrombinemia, thrombocytopenia, or platelet dysfunction.[26,27,31,35] Such patients with associated abnormalities could be adequately protected by prophylactic administration of platelet transfusions or fresh frozen plasma before undergoing invasive procedures.[3] Patients with a prolonged activated partial thromboplastin time secondary to a lupus anticoagulant may safely undergo invasive procedures for diagnosis and therapy.

REFERENCES

1. Morris L, Distenfeld A, Amorosi E, Karpatkin S. Autoimmune thrombocytopenic purpura in homosexual men. Ann Intern Med 1982; 96:714-7.

2. Savona S, Nardi MA, Lennette ET, Karpatkin S. Thrombocytopenic purpura in narcotics addicts. Ann Intern Med 1985; 102:737-41.

3. Ratnoff OD, Menitove JE, Aster RH, Lederman MM. Coincident classic hemophilia and "idiopathic" thrombocytopenic purpura in patients under treatment with concentrates of antihemophilic factor (factor VIII). N Engl J Med 1983; 308:439-42.

4. Abrams DI, Chinn EK, Lewis BJ, et al. Hematologic manifestations in homosexual men with Kaposi's sarcoma. Am J Clin Pathol 1984; 81:13-8.

5. Jaffe HS, Abrams DI, Ammann AJ, et al. Complications of co-trimoxazole in treatment of AIDS-associated *Pneumocystis carinii* pneumonia in homosexual men. Lancet 1983; 2:1109-11.

6. Stricker RB, Abrams DI, Corash L, Shuman MA. Target platelet antigen in homosexual men with immune thrombocytopenia. N Engl J Med 1985; 313:1375-80.

7. Kelton JG, Carter CJ, Rodger C, et al. The relationship among platelet-associated IgG, platelet lifespan and reticuloendothelial cell function. Blood 1984; 63:1434-8.

8. Bender BS, Frank MM, Lawley TJ, et al. Defective reticuloendothelial system Fc-receptor function in patients with acquired immunodeficiency syndrome. J Infect Dis 1985; 152:409-12.

9. Abrams DI. Lymphadenopathy related to the acquired immunodeficiency syndrome in homosexual men. Med Clin North Am 1986; 70:693-706.

10. Walsh C, Krigel R, Lennette E, Karpatkin S. Thrombocytopenia in homosexual patients: prognosis, response to therapy, and prevalence of antibody to the retrovirus associated with the acquired immunodeficiency syndrome. Ann Intern Med 1985; 103:542-5.

11. Abrams DI, Kiprov DD, Goedert JJ, et al. Antibodies to human T-lymphotropic virus type III and development of the acquired immunodeficiency syndrome in homosexual men presenting with immune thrombocytopenia. Ann Intern Med 1986; 104:47-50.

12. Abrams DI, Kiprov DD, Volberding PA. Isolated thrombocytopenia in homosexual men: longitudinal follow-up. Adv Exp Med Biol 1985; 187:117-22.

13. Walsh CM, Nardi MA, Karpatkin S. On the mechanism of thrombocytopenic purpura in sexually active homosexual men. N Engl J Med 1984; 311:635-6.

14. Frank MM, Hamburger MI, Lawley TJ, et al. Defective reticuloendothelial system Fc-receptor function in systemic lupus erythematosus. N Engl J Med 1979; 300:518-23.

15. Pizzuto J, Ambriz R. Therapeutic experience on 934 adults with idiopathic thrombocytopenic purpura: multicentric trial of the cooperative Latin American group on hemostasis and thrombosis. Blood 1984; 64:1179-83.

16. Fehr J, Hofmann V, Kappeler U. Transient reversal of thrombocytopenia in idiopathic thrombocytopenic purpura by high-dose intravenous gamma globulin. N Engl J Med 1982; 306:1254-8.

17. Salama A, Mueller-Eckhardt C, Kiefel V. Effect of intravenous immunoglobulin in immune thrombocytopenia. Competitive inhibition of reticuloendothelial system function by sequestration of autologous red blood cells? Lancet 1983; 2:1935.

18. Tertian G, Boue F, Lebras P, et al. Thrombocytopenia in ARC: management with high dose IV IgG. Vox Sang 1987; 52:9. abstract.

19. Ahn YS, Harrington WJ, Simon SR, et al. Danazol for the treatment of idiopathic thrombocytopenic purpura. N Engl J Med 1983; 308:1396-9.

20. Fischl MA, Ahn YS, Klimas N, et al. Use of danazol in autoimmune thrombocytopenic purpura associated with the acquired immunodeficiency syndrome. Blood 1984; 64(Suppl 1):2362. abstract.

21. Kiprov DD, Lippert R, Sandstrom G, et al. Acquired immunodeficiency syndrome (AIDS). Apheresis and operative risks. J Clin Apheresis 1985; 2:427-40.

22. Bloom EJ, Abrams DI, Rodgers GM. Lupus anticoagulant in the acquired immunodeficiency syndrome. Blood 1984; 64:241a. abstract.

23. Bloom EJ, Abrams DI, Rodgers GM. Lupus anticoagulant in the acquired immunodeficiency syndrome. JAMA 1986; 256:491-3.

24. Cohen AJ, Philips TM, Kessler CM. Circulating coagulation inhibitors in the acquired immunodeficiency syndrome. Ann Intern Med 1986; 104:175-80.

25. Conley CL, Hartman RC. A haemorrhagic disorder caused by circulating anticoagulant in patients with disseminated lupus erythematosus. J Clin Invest 1952; 31:621-2.

26. Margolius A Jr, Jackson DP, Ratnoff OD. Circulating anticoagulants: a study of 40 cases and a review of the literature. Medicine 1961; 40:145-202.

27. Feinstein DI, Rapaport SI. Acquired inhibitors of blood coagulation. Prog Hemost Thromb 1972; 1:75-95.

28. Shapiro SS, Thiagarajan P. Lupus anticoagulants. Prog Hemost Thromb 1982; 6:263-85.

29. Schleider MA, Nachman RL, Jaffee EA, et al. A clinical study of the lupus anticoagulant. Blood 1976; 48:499-509.

30. Lubbe WF, Butler WS, Palmer SJ, et al. Lupus anticoagulant in pregnancy. Br J Obstet Gynaecol 1984; 91:357-63.

31. Boxer M, Ellman L, Carvalho A. The lupus anticoagulant. Arthritis Rheum 1976; 19:1244-8.
32. Shapiro SS, Thiagarajan P, DeMarco L. Mechanism of action of the lupus anticoagulant. Ann NY Acad Sci 1981; 370:359-65.
33. Mueh HR, Herbst KP, Rapaport SI, et al. Thrombosis in patients with lupus anticoagulant. Ann Intern Med 1980; 92:156-9.
34. Thiagarajan P, Shapiro SS, DeMarco L. Monoclonal immunoglobulin M coagulation inhibitor with phospholipid specificity. J Clin Invest 1980; 66:397.
35. Regan MG, Lackner H, Karpatkin S. Platelet function and coagulation profile in lupus erythematosus: studies in 50 patients. Ann Intern Med 1974; 81:462-8.

5.9

Renal Aspects

Azotemia and Proteinuria

Michael H. Humphreys, M.D., and Patricia Schoenfeld, M.D.

This chapter describes the three major processes producing azotemia in patients with HIV infection[1,2]: (1) prerenal azotemia due to renal hypoperfusion, often resulting from hypovolemia due to poor fluid intake; (2) acute renal failure caused by ischemic tubular necrosis and drug nephrotoxicity; and (3) chronic or progressive renal insufficiency resulting from structural renal disease, most commonly associated with focal and segmental glomerulosclerosis (FSGS) and the nephrotic syndrome, although other forms of glomerular disease are also seen.

Diagnosis of azotemia and acute renal failure are described. A table of potentially nephrotoxic drugs used in treating HIV-related opportunistic infections is also provided.

■ PRERENAL AZOTEMIA

Prerenal azotemia in HIV-infected patients is no different than in non-HIV-infected patients. Symptomatic hypovolemia can usually be detected by increased thirst, orthostatic hypotension, and diminished urinary output. Chemical indices of the urine indicate sodium conservation (urine sodium concentration <20 meq/liter or a low fractional sodium excretion). This form of azotemia usually reverses itself quickly with adequate rehydration.

■ ACUTE RENAL FAILURE

Acute renal failure in the HIV-infected patient is often a manifestation of drug-induced nephrotoxicity. A number of agents with proven or possible nephrotoxicity are used in treating the opportunistic infections associated with HIV; a partial list of these is given in Table 1.

TABLE 1. SOME DRUGS USED IN THE TREATMENT OF HIV-RELATED COMPLICATIONS*

PROVEN NEPHROTOXICITY	NO PROVEN NEPHROTOXICITY	UNKNOWN
Pentamidine	Trimethoprim/sulfamethoxazole	Interferon
Rifampin	Spiramycin	Interleukin
Dapsone	Ketoconazole	Zidovudine (AZT)
Amphotericin B		

* *Compiled by the authors.*

When drug-induced azotemia develops, it usually is interpreted as an indication to discontinue the drug. This poses difficult therapeutic dilemmas if no adequate alternative therapy exists. When renal insufficiency develops, the clinician must remember to adjust doses of any concurrent medications that are renally metabolized or excreted.

Patients with HIV infection may also develop acute renal failure from other causes (e.g., acute tubular necrosis, acute glomerulonephritis, or acute interstitial nephritis).[1,2] Usually, the clinical presentation and findings in the urinary sediment provide sufficient data to identify the azotemia's underlying cause. When acute renal failure becomes severe, hemodialysis should be offered, since experience both at San Francisco General Hospital and other centers indicates that many of these patients can recover renal function.[3,4]

■ CHRONIC RENAL FAILURE

Progressive renal insufficiency in the patient with HIV infection is frequently accompanied by nephrotic-range proteinuria (>3.5 g/24 hr). It can be caused by a variety of glomerular abnormalities; lesser degrees of proteinuria may also occur. Interest has centered on the possibility that this combination of azotemia and nephrotic-range proteinuria reflects a specific renal syndrome in HIV-infected patients. Centers in New York, Miami, and Los Angeles have reported specific histologic and ultrastructural abnormalities that are believed to indicate HIV-associated renal involvement.[1]

■ LESIONS

Histologic examination of the kidneys, either by renal biopsy or at autopsy, reveals a very high incidence of FSGS. This lesion can be found as a variable percentage of the idiopathic nephrotic syndrome in non-HIV-infected adults, but it is also associated with intravenous drug use as so-called heroin nephropathy. However, not all HIV-infected patients with this form of nephrotic syndrome have intravenous drug use as an associated risk factor; the lesion has also been observed in young children[5] and patients who were later diagnosed with AIDS.[4] Moreover, the clinical course of the disease appears to differ from that of FSGS in non-HIV-infected intravenous drug users.[6]

Characteristics of the renal lesion include glomerular changes of FSGS with variable staining for immunoglobulins on immunofluorescent study, and a marked degree of tubular dilatation and interstitial fibrosis. The electron microscope reveals a high incidence of tubuloreticular structures in endothelial cell cytoplasm. Nuclear inclusions are also common.[7-9] Clinical correlates of this condition include rare hypertension associated with the renal disease,[4] relatively large kidneys as determined by renal ultrasound,[4,10] and rapid progression of renal failure to end-stage renal disease within weeks to months.[3-6]

The true incidence of this lesion in HIV-infected patients remains controversial. An autopsy series from San Francisco failed to disclose any such glomerular lesions in 35 patients with AIDS,[11] and a larger series from the National Institutes of Health did not identify any AIDS patients with nephrotic syndrome. The same series found a very low incidence of sclerotic glomerular lesions.[12] Both clinical and autopsy experience at San Francisco General Hospital have failed to reveal a high incidence of FSGS in patients with AIDS seen by the Division of Nephrology for renal and electrolyte problems or when patients were examined postmortem.[13]

OTHER RENAL PATHOLOGIES

Autopsy series have demonstrated other, relatively minor, pathologic changes in the kidneys of patients with AIDS. These include cytomegalovirus inclusions, granulomas from fungal infections, Kaposi's sarcoma, lymphoma, and other mild abnormalities.[11-13] In addition, clinical series have documented a variety of other glomerular lesions, including post-infectious glomerulonephritis, minimal change and membranous nephropathies, and membranoproliferative glomerulonephritis.[1,2,13,14] We have seen few cases of HIV-associated FSGS at San Francisco General Hospital but a much wider variety of renal lesions than reported from Downstate Medical Center in Brooklyn[3] and the University of Miami.[5]

The widely varying incidence of HIV-associated nephropathy reported from different centers is largely dependent on the patient populations seen at those centers. Most of the cases of HIV-associated nephropathy identified to date have been among blacks and intravenous drug users,[3-5,13,15] and centers with large concentrations of these patients report far higher rates of renal pathologies than centers treating largely gay white males. In San Francisco, where the vast majority of AIDS cases are among gay white men, relatively few cases of glomerular lesions have been seen. It is possible that risk factors and race determine the likelihood that HIV-infected patients will develop renal abnormalities. For example, unrecognized infectious agents transmitted by inoculation of blood but not by sexual contact could be a transmission mechanism. In addition, blacks in general have a greater risk of contracting renal disease.[16] They are particularly susceptible to FSGS.[17,18] Further experience will be needed before the true incidence of this lesion in various HIV-infected populations can be determined.

DIAGNOSIS

Diagnostic evaluation of azotemia and proteinuria in a patient with HIV infection or AIDS should include quantitation of 24-hour urinary protein excretion and creatinine clearance and a search for other systemic illnesses that could lead to a glomerular abnormality and nephrotic syndrome. If the patient's clinical condition permits, renal biopsy may be recommended to establish the histopathology. This is particularly useful because of multiple possible causes of nephrotic syndrome in these patients, including membranous nephropathy related to hepatitis B infection, membranoproliferative disease, and other forms of immune-complex-mediated glomerular damage.[13,14] Since there is no effective therapy for the underlying lesion, the treatment of FSGS is limited to supportive care. The benefits of renal biopsy for diagnostic purposes in patients with HIV infection must be determined on an individual basis.

SUPPORTIVE TREATMENT

Efforts should be made to maintain the nutritional support of these patients with protein and caloric intakes greater than 1.0 g/kg and 35 kcal/kg per day, respectively. If renal insufficiency occurs, appropriate attention must be paid to adjusting the dosage of potentially toxic drugs used in treating associated conditions. Hypertension must also be treated when it occurs.

■ PROGNOSIS

The prognosis for AIDS patients with FSGS-related nephrotic syndrome appears to be very poor. Experience at centers in New York and Miami suggests that patients with FSGS progress in a period of months to end-stage renal disease requiring dialysis. Once on dialysis, patients die within a 3- to 11-month period, presumably due to their underlying HIV-associated problems.[3-5] The patient's poor prognosis, together with negligible rehabilitation while on dialysis, must lead clinicians to seriously consider withholding routine recommendation for dialysis treatment to such patients.

REFERENCES

1. Humphreys MH, Schoenfeld PY. Renal complications in patients with the acquired immunodeficiency syndrome (AIDS). Am J Nephrol 1987; 7:107.
2. Humphreys MH, Schoenfeld PY. AIDS and renal disease. Kidney 1987; 20:7-12.
3. Rao TK, Friedman EA, Nicastri AD. The types of renal disease in the acquired immunodeficiency syndrome. N Engl J Med 1987; 316:1062-8.
4. Bourgoignie JJ, Meneses R, Ortiz C, et al. The clinical spectrum of renal disease associated with human immunodeficiency virus. Am J Kidney Dis 1988; 12:131-7.
5. Pardo V, Meneses R, Ossa L, et al. AIDS-related glomerulopathy: occurrence in specific risk groups. Kidney Int 1987; 31:1167-73.
6. Rao TK, Filippone EJ, Nicastri AD, et al. Associated focal and segmental glomerulonephritis in the acquired immunodeficiency syndrome. N Engl J Med 1984; 310:669-73.
7. Chander P, Soni A, Suri A, et al. Renal ultrastructural markers in AIDS-associated nephropathy. Am J Pathol 1987; 126:513-26.
8. Cohen AH, Nast CC. HIV-associated nephropathy: a unique combined glomerular, tubular, and interstitial lesion. Mod Pathol 1988; 1:87-97.
9. D'Agati V, Suk J-I, Carbone L, et al. The pathology of HIV-associated nephropathy: a detailed morphologic and comparative study. Kidney Int (in press).
10. Schaffer RM, Schwartz GE, Becker JA, et al. Renal ultrasound in acquired immune deficiency syndrome. Radiology 1984; 153:511-3.
11. Welch K, Finkbeiner W, Alpers CE, et al. Autopsy findings in the acquired immune deficiency syndrome. JAMA 1984; 252:1152-9.
12. Balow JE, Mackner AM, Rook AH. Paucity of glomerular disease in acquired immunodeficiency syndrome (AIDS). Abstracts Am Soc Nephrol 1989; 18:29A. abstract.
13. Mazbar S, Humphreys MH. AIDS-associated nephropathy is not seen at San Francisco General. Am Soc Nephrol 1987; 20:55A. abstract.
14. Gardenswartz MH, Lerner CW, Selingson GR, et al. Renal disease in patients with AIDS: a clinico-pathologic study. Clin Nephrol 1984; 21:197-204.
15. Pardo V, Aldana M, Colton RM, et al. Glomerular lesions in the acquired immunodeficiency syndrome. Ann Intern Med 1984; 104:429-34.
16. Rostand SG, Kirk KA, Rutsky BA, et al. Racial differences in the incidence of treatment for end-stage renal disease. N Engl J Med 1982; 306:1276-9.
17. Cunningham EE, Zielenzy MA, Venuto RC. Heroin-associated nephropathy. A nationwide problem. JAMA 1983; 250:2935-6.
18. Korbet SM, Schwartz MM, Lewis EJ. The prognosis of focal segmental glomerular sclerosis of adulthood. Medicine 1986; 65:304-11.

Fluid and Electrolyte Abnormalities

Michael H. Humphreys, M.D., and Patricia Schoenfeld, M.D.

S erum electrolyte abnormalities are common in patients with AIDS. These include hyponatremia, hyperkalemia, hypokalemia, and acid–base disturbances. This chapter describes the clinical manifestations, diagnosis, and treatment of these conditions.

■ HYPONATREMIA

Hyponatremia in the AIDS patient can usually be related to one of three possible causes: fluid loss, inappropriate secretion of antidiuretic hormone, or adrenal insufficiency. Hyponatremia with hypovolemia results from loss of sodium-containing fluids, most commonly through diarrhea, accompanied by replacement consisting primarily of water to produce dilutional hyponatremia. Hyponatremic patients are often symptomatically hypovolemic with urine retention and urine sodium concentrations <20 meq/liter; the hyponatremia is corrected through restoration of adequate sodium and extracellular fluid volume.

Hyponatremia may also result from the syndrome of inappropriate secretion of antidiuretic hormone (SIADH) in the setting of central nervous system (CNS) or pulmonary infections caused by cytomegalovirus, tuberculosis, fungal, and *Pneumocystis carinii* infections.[2,5] The hyponatremia in these patients is accompanied by plasma and extracellular fluid volumes that are normal to slightly expanded, normal renal function, and urine electrolytes that reveal a concentrated urine with a sodium concentration usually greater than 20 meq/liter. Managing this form of hyponatremia consists of restricting water to an amount equivalent to the daily urine output so that insensible water loss progressively leads to a negative water balance and a rise in serum sodium concentration. Of course, the underlying opportunistic infections must also be treated if possible.

A third cause of hyponatremia in AIDS patients is related to abnormalities in adrenal steroid synthesis and secretion. Many patients will, on specific testing such as cosyntropin stimulation, exhibit subtle-to-florid abnormalities of adrenal function.[1,3] These range from slight impairments in glucocorticoid production to frank adrenal insufficiency; isolated mineralocorticoid deficiency is only rarely seen.[3] Despite this spectrum of abnormalities, clinical symptoms are rare. It is possible that in some of these patients, hyponatremia may result from glucocorticoid deficiency, although further experience will be needed to determine both the frequency with which this occurs and the necessity for glucocorticoid replacement therapy. Ketoconazole, prescribed for fungal infections, has been shown to block adrenal steroid biosynthesis.[4]

Diagnosis of hyponatremia depends on evidence from the patient's clinical history, physical examination of alterations in body fluid homeostasis, and laboratory studies of renal function. Hypouricemia is frequently seen in patients with inappropriate secretion of antidiuretic hormone. Urinary electrolytes are also helpful in assessing the hyponatremic patient. Management is based on the underlying pathophysiology.

■ HYPOKALEMIA

Hypokalemia may reflect excessive renal and extrarenal potassium losses through protracted vomiting and diarrhea. It may also result from acquired tubular dysfunction caused by nephrotoxic drugs such as rifampin, amphotericin B, and pentamidine. Hyperkalemia may reflect mineralocorticoid hormone deficiency, due either to frank adrenal insufficiency or to a more selective defect in aldosterone biosynthesis.[6]

■ ACID–BASE DISTURBANCES

The most common acid–base disturbances in AIDS patients are respiratory in origin and are caused by pulmonary involvement with opportunistic infections. Respiratory alkalosis is usually the initial disturbance. As lung involvement worsens and gas exchange deteriorates, hypercapnia and respiratory acidosis occur. Metabolic acidosis with a normal anion gap develops in patients with protracted diarrhea and in those patients who develop impaired renal acidification as a manifestation of drug-induced nephrotoxicity. A few patients with isolated mineralocorticoid deficiency and metabolic acidosis have been reported.[6] Patients with renal insufficiency develop progressive metabolic acidosis with an increased anion gap. Metabolic alkalosis results from severe vomiting; however, this does not seem to be a common disturbance in AIDS patients.

REFERENCES

1. Greene LW, Cole W, Greene JB, et al. Adrenal insufficiency as a complication of the acquired immunodeficiency syndrome. Ann Intern Med 1984; 101:497-8.
2. Vitting KE, Gardenswartz MH, Zabetakis PM, et al. Frequency of hyponatremia (HN), hypoadrenalin, and nonosmolar vasopressin release in the acquired immunodeficiency syndrome (AIDS). Abstracts Am Soc Nephrology 1986; 19:64A. abstract.
3. Membreno L, Irony I, Dere W, et al. Adrenocortical function in acquired immunodeficiency syndrome. J Clin Endocrinol Metab 1987; 65:482-7.
4. Pont A, Williams PL, Loose DS, et al. Ketoconazole blocks adrenal steroid synthesis. Ann Intern Med 1982; 97:370-2.
5. Tang WW, Feinstein EI, Massey SG. Hyponatremia (HN) in patients with acquired immune deficiency syndrome (AIDS) and the AIDS-related complex (ARC). Abstracts Am Soc Nephrology 1987; 20:64A. abstract.
6. Kalin MF, Poretsky L, Seres DS, Zumoff B. Hyporeninemic hypoaldosteronism associated with acquired immunodeficiency syndrome. Am J Med 1987; 82:1035-8.

HIV-Associated Nephropathy and ESRD in Patients with AIDS

Patricia Schoenfeld, M.D., and Michael H. Humphreys, M.D.

■ INCIDENCE OF HIV-ASSOCIATED NEPHROPATHY

The incidence of HIV-associated renal disease varies from 10 percent at Downstate Medical Center in Brooklyn,[1] to 8 percent at the University of Miami/Jackson Memorial Hospital,[2] to 2 percent at San Francisco General Hospital.[3] This variation may be a reflection of different risk factors for HIV infection in those cities as well as of other factors in the epidemiology of HIV-associated nephropathy. In New York, 50 percent of patients with HIV-associated nephropathy are IV drug users,[1] while in Miami, the HIV-infected population is more diverse — about 30 percent are intravenous drug users, 25 percent are Haitian, and the remainder are homosexual or heterosexual partners of infected persons and those with unknown risk factors.[2] In contrast, in San Francisco, where the incidence of renal disease is lowest, 84 percent of HIV-infected persons are gay or bisexual men, 1.7 percent are intravenous drug users, and 11.6 percent are both gay or bisexual and use intravenous drugs.[3] The incidence of HIV-associated nephropathy in other parts of the country varies with the numbers of HIV-infected patients with these risk factors.

The national incidence of HIV-related renal involvement may be inferred from data collected by the Department of Defense during its screening of new military recruits. The overall seroprevalence is 1.3/1000 (2,232 HIV-seropositive individuals among 1,752,191 tested), and varies widely according to geographic region. The incidence of seropositivity in this group is 0.74/1000/yr. Among seropositives, about 1 percent had renal abnormalities, but specific information regarding the nature and severity of their renal disease is not available. Based on these crude figures and the estimates from the Centers for Disease Control (CDC) that 1 to 1.5 million persons are infected with HIV in the U.S., it might be expected that 10,000 to 15,000 persons may develop renal disease in association with HIV infection.[4]

■ HIV DISEASE AND PATIENTS WITH ESRD

True incidence and prevalence data are not available for patients with end-stage renal disease (ESRD). Estimates of the number of HIV-infected patients being treated with dialysis have been obtained from a number of sources, including several surveys conducted by the CDC. The first of these was a study of 520 patients reported by Peterman et al. that showed a Western-blot–confirmed positive rate of 0.8 percent.[5] Subsequently, the CDC established a voluntary HIV disease dialysis registry that collected data from 1291 patients on hemodialysis between June 1986 and June 1988 from 27 facilities. This survey unfortunately does not include data from the country as a whole and therefore is not a fair sample of the U.S. dialysis population. The results, however, are very similar to the Peterman data in that there were 10 HIV-seropositive patients reported, for a prevalence of 0.8 percent.[6]

Additional data provided by the CDC are from the annual HCFA facility surveys required of all dialysis facilities in the U.S. participating in the Medicare dialysis program. For three years (1985–1987), this survey included two questions: "Does your facility treat patients known to be HIV-positive?" and "What is the number of patients treated with HIV disease?" Table 1 summarizes these surveys.[7]

TABLE 1. U.S. DIALYSIS UNITS TREATING HIV-INFECTED PATIENTS

YEAR	TOTAL CENTERS	NO. CENTERS WITH HIV+ PATIENTS	TOTAL NO. PATIENTS	PATIENTS WITH HIV INFECTION	PERCENT HIV+ PATIENTS
1985	1254	134	80,151	244	0.3
1986	1350	238	87,760	546	0.6
1987	1486	351	97,225	924	1.0

These data undoubtedly underestimate the true numbers of patients with ESRD and HIV disease, since only about 30 percent to 40 percent of facilities routinely screen all or high-risk patients for HIV infection. These results do, however, indicate a steady rise in the numbers of patients undergoing dialysis who have HIV disease, and they are consistent with the rough estimate of the total number of HIV-infected patients with renal abnormalities determined from the military recruit figures.

■ HIV TESTING IN PATIENTS WITH ESRD

It is common practice to give ESRD patients blood transfusions for anemia or during kidney transplantation. The presence of transfusion recipients and other high-risk groups in the dialysis population creates concern about the need for routine serologic testing of dialysis patients and transplant recipients. This issue is further complicated by the passage of laws in several states requiring informed consent for HIV testing, a move that makes uniform testing of patients more difficult. Informal surveys indicate that about 30 percent of facilities test all patients for HIV disease and 40 percent screen high-risk patients. An increasing number of facilities require HIV testing for transient dialysis; many now refuse to accept HIV-seropositive patients for transient or permanent dialysis.

The rationale for routine testing of patients on dialysis is concern about possible transmission of HIV during dialysis treatment. Such a fear is unfounded: all experience to date indicates that the process of chronic hemodialysis is not associated with the transmission of HIV except for the risk from blood transfusion for anemic patients.[8,9] Furthermore, all patients with ESRD found to be HIV-seropositive have had other known risk factors for HIV infection.[9]

The American Association of Kidney Patients sponsored a conference in November 1987 that re-affirmed its 1986 position that routine testing of all dialysis patients is not necessary for infection control.[10] HIV testing is not necessary or recommended for admission to hemodialysis or peritoneal dialysis programs.

Patients should not be discriminated against in the provision of dialysis care. Specifically, patients requiring acute, chronic, or transient dialysis should not be denied treatment or admission to dialysis units on the basis of their HIV test result or the lack thereof.

However, because of rapid increases in knowledge of HIV disease and the development of effective therapy for HIV-infected patients, the rationale for testing patients with ESRD has changed over the past year. It may now be appropriate and clinically indicated to test patients in the following situations:

1. *When there is potential clinical benefit to the individual:*

    a. a positive HIV test may affect the choice of dialysis modality;

    b. knowledge of HIV status may be useful for medical management, including anti-HIV therapy, prophylaxis against certain infections, new treatment protocols, etc.; and

    c. knowledge of HIV status may be an incentive to control behavior that may contribute to progression of disease.

2. *Where public health and infection control may be affected:*

    a. knowledge of serostatus may be an incentive for behavior modification to prevent spread to others; and

    b. such knowledge may be of benefit to another individual (e.g., person with an accidental needlestick injury).

Whenever performed, HIV antibody testing should be accompanied by the following: (1) informed patient consent; (2) appropriate pre- and post-test professional counseling; (3) assurance of the confidentiality of the test results; and (4) use of appropriate confirmatory testing for all positive screening results, with confirmation by a second sample if possible.

Dialysis units may not always be able to ensure confidentiality of test results or provide appropriate counseling. While developing their own educational programs, they should become familiar with community AIDS educational and social services useful to their patients and encourage clients to use them.[8]

■ DIALYSIS OF THE PATIENT WITH AIDS

Modality Selection. Selection of dialysis method in patients with AIDS should be based primarily on the patient's clinical needs. Other considerations such as infection control precautions, economic concerns, and staffing may play a role in this decision, but they should be secondary to the medical and psychosocial needs of the patient. Access to dialysis treatment should not be limited by restriction to a single method (i.e., either hemodialysis or peritoneal dialysis), and patients with HIV disease should not be discriminated against in the provision of care.

Clinical AIDS.   Patients with advanced HIV disease and ESRD are very ill and often require prolonged or repeated hospitalizations. Such patients have most often been treated with chronic hemodialysis as inpatients. Survival times are commonly short and rehabilitation is minimal. In patients who are well enough to receive treatment as outpatients, it may be possible to consider chronic ambulatory peritoneal dialysis (CAPD) or home hemodialysis if social support is adequate. We have had one patient with Kaposi's sarcoma who has performed CAPD therapy successfully in conjunction with several courses of chemotherapy.

The generally dismal outcome in dialysis patients with advanced HIV disease raises the possibility that starting dialysis at all in such patients may be inappropriate. The presence of progressive neurological disease and dementia in HIV-infected patients makes the benefits of dialysis even more difficult to justify and may result in the need to stop dialysis therapy in some patients. At present, most nephrologists individualize treatment options for each patient, taking into consideration the wishes of the patient, family, companions, and the motivation of the patient to prolong life, even if for a very short period.

Earlier Stages of HIV Disease.   Patients with earlier stages of HIV infection are often asymptomatic or have milder chronic symptoms, such as lymphadenopathy or intermittent diarrheal illness. Such patients do well at a dialysis center, but they may also be good candidates for CAPD or home hemodialysis if they meet the usual selection criteria for self-care and home dialysis. Home dialysis and, in particular, CAPD, offer several advantages over center-based hemodialysis: lack of blood exposure, fewer equipment concerns, and reduced risk of virus transmission to staff and others.

CAPD therapy may offer other potential advantages over hemodialysis treatment. These can be summarized as follows:

1. CAPD may theoretically result in less stimulation of the HIV-infected T cell than hemodialysis. Conventional cellulosic membranes can result in membrane-induced stimulation of cytokines, which may increase viral replication in the stimulated lymphocyte. While evidence exists that standard hemodialysis membranes produce chronic stimulation of the immune system, there is no evidence that such stimulation is deleterious to HIV-infected patients.

2. Patients on CAPD have been reported to have better humoral immune function than those on hemodialysis.[11]

3. Nutritional benefit may result from peritoneal absorption of glucose. However, protein loss into the dialysate, especially during peritonitis, may cancel this benefit.

4. Use of CAPD obviates the leukopenia induced by standard dialysis membranes in patients who are often chronically leukopenic as a result of HIV disease.

5. Higher hematocrits in patients on CAPD may allow the use of AZT and other specific HIV/AIDS therapies.

A potential disadvantage of CAPD is an increased risk of peritonitis. However, data on the frequency of peritonitis in HIV-infected patients are not currently available. Experience at San Francisco General Hospital indicates that the rates of peritonitis in AIDS patients are similar to those of other patients with comparable lifestyles and adherence to good technique. Since many patients who develop HIV-associated nephropathy and ESRD are intravenous drug users, they may not be ideal candidates for self-care, especially those patients who continue to abuse drugs. Finally, patients with AIDS have more frequent illness and infectious complications than other patients on CAPD, thus placing greater care demands on staff and physicians.

Specific HIV Disease Treatment. With the advent of effective treatment for some complications of HIV infection and evidence that AZT prolongs survival, the use of these therapies in the AIDS patient on dialysis must be considered. AZT has been shown to double the survival time in patients who survive their first infection with pneumocystis pneumonia. It is now being used in other situations to prevent the occurrence of serious infections. Information on the use of AZT in patients with reduced renal function is limited; the drug is excreted by the kidney, so decreased clearance occurs during renal failure. Burroughs Wellcome has recommended that dosages be reduced by about 20 percent in patients with renal insufficiency. Of greater concern, however, is the hematologic toxicity of the drug, which results in the need for blood transfusion in many patients. It is unclear whether patients with ESRD can tolerate this toxicity if anemia is already present. The anticipated availability of erythropoietin may obviate this concern, provided the hormone is effective in patients with profound immunosuppression and drug-induced marrow toxicity.

Other therapies that should be considered in dialysis patients with HIV disease are the various prophylactic regimens used for pneumocystis pneumonia. These include the use of trimethoprim/sulfamethoxazole and aerosolized pentamidine. Further data need to be collected on the effectiveness and safety of such treatment in patients with ESRD.

REFERENCES

1. Rao TK, Friedman EA, Nicastri AD. The types of renal disease in the acquired immunodeficiency syndrome. N Engl J Med 1987; 316:1062-8.
2. Pardo V, Meneses R, Ossa L, et al. AIDS-related glomerulopathy: occurrence in specific risk groups. Kidney Int 1987; 31:1167-73.
3. Mazbar S, Humphreys MH. AIDS-associated nephropathy is not seen at San Francisco General. Am Soc Nephrol 1987; 20:55A. abstract.
4. Baker J, Wright C. Presentation to NKF-NIH AIDS Task Force. Bethesda, Md.: National Institutes of Health, 1988. Unpublished.
5. Peterman TA, Lang GR, Mikos NJ, et al. HTLV-III/LAV infection in hemodialysis patients. JAMA 1986; 255:2324-6.
6. Marcus R, Solomon SL, Favero MS, et al. Abst Kidney Int 1989; 35:256.
7. Panlilo A. Presentation to NKF-NIH AIDS Task Force, Bethesda, Md.: National Institutes of Health, 1988. Unpublished.
8. Perez GO, Ortiz C, De Medina M, et al. Lack of transmission of human immunodeficiency virus in chronic hemodialysis patients. Am J Nephrol 1988; 8:123-6.
9. Rao TK, Landesman SH, Friedman EA. Seroprevalence of antibody to human immunodeficiency virus (HIV) in patients treated by maintenance hemodialysis. Abs Kidney Int 1989; 35:242.
10. American Association of Kidney Patients. Consensus Conference on AIDS and Renal Disease. Washington, D.C.: National Association of Patients on Hemodialysis and Transplantation, 1978.
11. Giacchino F, Pozzato M, Piccoli G. Evaluation of the influences of peritoneal dialysis on cellular immunity by the E-rosette inhibition test. Artif Organs 1984; 8:156-60.

5.10

Gastrointestinal and Hepatobiliary Aspects

Approach to AIDS Patients with Gastrointestinal Symptoms: Overview

Scott L. Friedman, M.D.

■ FREQUENCY OF GASTROINTESTINAL SYMPTOMS

Gastrointestinal and hepatobiliary symptoms are among the most frequent complaints in AIDS, and a methodical effort is required to identify symptoms that are treatable. Best estimates suggest that 50 percent to 93 percent of all AIDS patients will have marked gastrointestinal symptoms during the course of their illness.[1,2] The most frequent symptom is diarrhea, which is usually chronic and associated with weight loss and malnutrition. Odynophagia and dysphagia, abdominal pain, and jaundice are less frequently seen but they present equally difficult diagnostic and management challenges. Gastrointestinal bleeding is rare and is as likely to be due to non-HIV-related pathology as to specific opportunistic infections or neoplasms.

■ EVALUATION OF GASTROINTESTINAL SYMPTOMS

Three general points must be considered when evaluating gastrointestinal symptoms in HIV-infected patients:

1. The clinical signs and symptoms alone rarely suggest a specific etiology, so that all notable gastrointestinal complaints should be investigated by sufficiently objective studies to identify specific infections or neoplasms associated with advanced HIV infection or AIDS.

2. Multiple gastrointestinal infections are the rule, making it important to distinguish between true pathogens and secondary colonization. Evidence of tissue invasion by an infectious agent is the hallmark of true pathogenicity.

3. The overriding goal of evaluation is to promptly identify those infections susceptible to specific therapy. Examples of treatable infections include salmonella, shigella, campylobacter, herpesvirus, and cytomegalovirus infections, as well as others not unique to AIDS. In particular, homosexual men with AIDS who have had multiple sexual partners are more likely than other AIDS patients to have gastrointestinal complications from protozoal and bacterial infections, including amebiasis, giardiasis, and chlamydial and treponemal infections.[3] With changing sexual habits within the gay community in response to the AIDS epidemic, transmission of "gay bowel" pathogens appears to be declining.[11]

Among the more difficult management issues in the HIV-infected patient is deciding how extensively to investigate gastrointestinal symptoms. The clinician must always weigh the discomfort and invasiveness of a procedure against the severity of the patient's complaints and the likelihood of identifying a treatable condition. Thus, for example, patients who are incapacitated by abdominal pain or diarrhea should be more extensively evaluated with endoscopic or imaging studies than patients whose symptoms do not interfere with daily activities. On the other hand, the physician should not hesitate to use procedures when the discomfort to the patient is minimal, such as collecting stool samples for examination or culture.

■ PRECAUTIONS FOR GASTROINTESTINAL PROCEDURES

Recent studies underscore the low transmissibility of HIV by casual contact.[4] Furthermore, no cases have been reported in which HIV infection has been transmitted to health-care personnel or patients via contaminated endoscopic instruments. Nonetheless, high standards of instrument care and protection must be maintained to insure the safety of patients and health professionals.

The following guidelines have been used by San Francisco General Hospital. Universal body substance precautions should be applied to all patients regardless of HIV status. Personnel performing or observing any gastrointestinal procedures should wear gowns, gloves, masks, and protective eyewear to avoid contact with body fluids.[5,8,9] Needles must be disposed of carefully. Lensed instruments must be thoroughly washed and disassembled to remove any secretions or debris and then disinfected or sterilized after each use. The use of immersible instruments and automated washing stations is recommended. A variety of disinfectants is suitable for this purpose, including 1 percent glutaraldehyde sporicidin, 6 percent hydrogen peroxide, or 25 percent ethanol, for 10 to 30 minutes. Both glutaraldehyde and 25 percent ethanol have been shown to inactivate the reverse transcriptase activity of HIV.[6,12] Iodophors should be avoided because of their inability to kill mycobacteria.[7]

Among gastrointestinal endoscopists and assistants, there is a broad spectrum of perceived risk and precautions.[13] In one recent survey,[10] one-third of respondents cited their reluctance to participate in endoscopic procedures in patients with AIDS. They also reported that almost one-half of their institutions utilize a separate instrument for patients with AIDS. While it is appropriate to demonstrate concern regarding the safety of endoscopic procedures, such an approach may create a false sense of security on the part of endoscopy personnel while performing procedures in non-AIDS patients. In fact, a greater risk may be present in dealing with asymptomatic HIV-infected patients undergoing endoscopy for other reasons. Thus, stringent infection control precautions must be applied to all patients.

REFERENCES

1. Gazzard BG. HIV disease and the gastroenterologist. Gut 1988; 29:1497-505.
2. Malenbranche R, Guerin JM, Laroche AC, et al. Acquired immunodeficiency syndrome with severe gastrointestinal manifestations in Haiti. Lancet 1983; 2:873-7.
3. Quinn TC, Stamm WE, Goodell SE, et al. The polymicrobial origin of intestinal infections in homosexual men. N Engl J Med 1983; 309:576-82.
4. Friedland GH, Saltzman BR, Rogers MF, et al. Lack of transmission of HTLV-III/LAV infection to household contacts of patients with AIDS or AIDS-related complex with oral candidiasis. N Engl J Med 1986; 314:344-8.
5. Conte JE, Hadley WK, Sande M, et al. Infection control guidelines for patients with the acquired immunodeficiency syndrome (AIDS). N Engl J Med 1983; 309:740-4.

6. Spire B, Barre-Sinoussi F, Montagnier L, Chermann JC. Inactivation of lymphadenopathy associated virus by chemical disinfectants. Lancet 1984; 2:899-901.

7. Nelson KE, Larson PA, Schraufnagel DE, Jackson J. Transmission of tuberculosis by flexible fiber-bronchoscopes. Am Rev Respir Dis 1983; 127:97-100.

8. Gerberding JL. Recommended infection-control policies for patients with human immunodeficiency virus infection. An update. N Engl J Med 1986; 315:1562-4.

9. Centers for Disease Control. Recommendations for preventing transmission of infection with human T-lymphotropic virus type III/lymphadenopathy-associated virus in the workplace. MMWR 1985; 34:682-6, 691-5.

10. Raufman JP, Strauss EW. Gastrointestinal endoscopy in patients with acquired immune deficiency syndrome: an evaluation of current practices. Gastrointest Endosc 1987; 33:76-9.

11. Self-reported behavioral change among gay and bisexual men — San Francisco. MMWR 1985; 34:613-5.

12. Cleaning and disinfection of equipment for gastrointestinal flexible endoscopy: interim recommendations of a Working Party of the British Society of Gastroenterology. Gut 1988; 29:1134-51.

13. Raufmann J-P, Straus EW. Endoscopic procedures in the AIDS patient: risks, precautions, indications, and obligations. Gastroenterol Clin North Am 1988; 17:495-506.

Diarrhea

Scott L. Friedman, M.D.

Diarrhea is the most common gastrointestinal symptom in AIDS, reported in 50 percent[1] to 90 percent[2] of all AIDS patients. There is considerable geographic variation in the frequency of diarrhea and the spectrum of enteric pathogens. Diarrhea is extremely common in Africa and Haiti, where the term "slim disease" has been applied to the wasting syndrome associated with chronic diarrhea.[46,52] In the U.S., diarrhea is also frequent among persons with AIDS. In a study of AIDS patients from New York, 80 percent of homosexuals had diarrhea, whereas diarrhea was present in only 58 percent of those whose risk factor was parenteral drug use.[53] The frequency of protozoal, viral, and bacterial pathogens also varies. *Isospora belli* is a frequent pathogen in Haiti, for example, but is less commonly observed in the U.S. and Western Europe.[54] Excretion of enteric viruses, in particular adenovirus and rotavirus, has been identified in a large percentage of homosexuals from Australia,[55] whereas none was observed in a smaller cohort from the eastern United States.[56] Enteric infection with *Mycobacterium avium-intracellulare* is more common among Eastern U.S. intravenous drug users than among homosexuals.[53]

■ DIFFERENTIAL DIAGNOSIS

A wide variety of protozoal, viral, and bacterial organisms have been implicated as diarrheal pathogens in patients with HIV infection and AIDS (see Table 1). Some, like *Mycobacterium avium-intracellulare*, are unique to AIDS; others, like cryptosporidium, cause self-limited diarrheal illness in healthy hosts and chronic diarrhea in immunosuppressed patients.[60]

TABLE 1. DIARRHEA IN HIV-INFECTED PATIENTS AND PATIENTS WITH AIDS: DIFFERENTIAL DIAGNOSIS

INFECTIONS

Protozoan	Bacterial
Cryptosporidium*	*Mycobacterium avium-intracellulare**
Isospora belli	Salmonella*
Microsporidium	Shigella*
	Campylobacter*
	Clostridium difficile
	Small bowel overgrowth
	Vibrio parahemolyticus

continued on next page

continued from previous page

TABLE 1. DIARRHEA IN HIV-INFECTED PATIENTS AND PATIENTS WITH AIDS: DIFFERENTIAL DIAGNOSIS

INFECTIONS

Viral	Fungal	Non AIDS-Specific Pathogens
Cytomegalovirus*	Candida	Giardia
Herpes simplex	*Histoplasma capsulatum*	*Entamoeba histolytica*
Enteroviruses(?)		"Non-pathogenic" Entamoeba *Strongyloides stercoralis*
Adenovirus(?)		

Neoplasms	Idiopathic
Lymphoma	"AIDS enteropathy"
Kaposi's sarcoma	

*   *More frequent.*

The majority of HIV-infected patients with diarrhea have one or more identifiable pathogens. Gastrointestinal infection has been identified in over half of AIDS patients with diarrhea in recent studies.[3,57] Simultaneous infections with more than one organism were common, emphasizing the need to exclude all pathogens thoroughly when evaluating diarrheal symptoms.

Protozoans are the most frequent type of gastrointestinal pathogen identified in persons with AIDS. Cryptosporidium in particular is a major source of morbidity because it causes intractable diarrhea that results in profound weight loss and malnutrition. In a large series from Baltimore, the most common pathogen associated with diarrhea was cryptosporidium. In another series, cryptosporidium was identified in one-third of all patients with diarrhea associated with AIDS.[4] The small bowel is the most common site of luminal involvement,[5] but cryptosporidial organisms have also been identified in the appendix,[6] rectal mucosa, and stomach, as well as the biliary tree[5] and respiratory tract.[7] The site of involvement within the gastrointestinal tract does not appear to affect the clinical presentation, except in rare cases of cryptosporidial cholecystitis,[8] when right upper-quadrant pain is the predominant symptom.

Patients with cryptosporidiosis are almost always symptomatic, although rare asymptomatic carriage of the organism has been seen in immunocompetent hosts.[9] Prominent clinical features include diarrhea (up to 17 liters per day) associated with frank malabsorption[4] and evidence of intestinal secretion.[10] Abdominal pain is seen in one-half to two-thirds of all patients and is usually dull, crampy, and predominantly epigastric or upper abdominal.[4,5] The mechanism of diarrhea in cryptosporidiosis is unknown; it has been suggested that the organisms rest on the villous surface of the enterocyte and impair cell function by releasing cellular toxins. Careful morphologic evaluation of cryptosporidial infection in experimental animals using electron microscopy has demonstrated that the organism enters the host cell by internalization within a sac of host membrane.[30] This study has further demonstrated that cryptosporidia can be identified within the cytoplasm of M cells (immunologic cells found in the large intestine) within Peyer's patches, allowing for sampling by intestinal lymphoid cells. Recently, a culture system facilitating complete growth of cryptosporidia in vitro has been developed; this may enable investigators to clarify the pathogenic features of this infection.[11]

Isospora belli is a protozoal organism related to cryptosporidium and is occasionally identified in AIDS patients with diarrhea. The infection is clinically indistinguishable from that due to cryptosporidium, with watery diarrhea and weight loss being prominent symptoms.[32] Unlike cryptosporidium, however, isospora oocysts enter, rather than rest upon, the enterocyte. The pathogenic significance of this mode of infection is unclear.[4] Extraintestinal isosporiasis within mesenteric lymph nodes has been reported in a single patient with AIDS.[19]

Microsporidia are small (1 to 5 micron) protozoal organisms that have been seen in the intestinal mucosa of AIDS patients. It is uncertain whether they actually cause diarrheal illness.[12] When infected tissue is examined using electron microscopy, they can be recognized best by their characteristic ultrastructure,[13,31] although the organisms may also be visible in Giemsa-stained smears of specimens from small-bowel biopsies.[36]

Diarrhea due to non-opportunistic protozoa such as *Entamoeba histolytica* is surprisingly uncommon in AIDS. A recent study suggests that *E. histolytica* is not necessarily a pathogen in homosexual men even when isolated from the stool.[37] Pathogenic zymodemes of this organism can be identified by their isoenzyme pattern.[58] The significance of finding "non-pathogenic" protozoa such as *Entamoeba coli*, *Entamoeba hartmanni*, *Endolimax nana*, *Iodamoeba buetschlii*, and *Dientamoeba fragilis* in AIDS patients is unknown. No direct association between these organisms and diarrhea has been described in AIDS patients, but finding one or more of these is likely to signify that more pathogenic organisms are also present.

Diarrhea due to bacterial infection is seen with moderate frequency in AIDS patients. *Mycobacterium avium-intracellulare* (MAI) and salmonella are the most commonly observed bacterial pathogens. The hallmark of MAI infection in the intestines, as in other tissues, is the relative paucity of tissue response. Intestinal involvement with MAI is common but often asymptomatic. Up to 60 percent of patients with MAI identified at autopsy have gastrointestinal involvement,[14] yet few clinical series recognize MAI as an intestinal pathogen antemortem. The small bowel is the most common site of infection; organisms have been identified in the colon as well.[14,15] Antemortem identification of MAI is usually only possible through bowel biopsy. A small subset of patients with intestinal MAI develop a clinical syndrome strikingly similar to Whipple's disease. As in Whipple's disease, patients with pseudo-Whipple's disease caused by MAI develop severe malabsorption and small-bowel atrophy associated with submucosal macrophages laden with organisms. In these cases, however, the organisms are acid-fast *M. avium* bacilli instead of the Whipple's bacillus.[16] Pseudo-Whipple's due to MAI can also be distinguished by the absence of two common features of true Whipple's disease — arthralgias and biopsy evidence of dilated small-bowel villous lacteals.[17] More recently, a patient has been described who developed terminal ileitis with stricture formation and obstruction due to infiltration with atypical mycobacteria.[32]

Recurrent salmonella bacteremia, with or without clinical enteritis, has a twenty-fold higher incidence in patients with AIDS than in healthy populations.[18] AIDS patients with salmonellosis have watery, non-bloody diarrhea and stool cultures positive for salmonella. Subtypes most commonly seen include *Salmonella typhimurium* and *S. choleraesuis*.[34,38-40] No clear explanation has been established for the increased incidence of this bacterial infection in patients with AIDS. Other bacterial infections include shigella and campylobacter. There have been recent reports of multiply antibiotic-resistant *Campylobacter jejuni* and campylobacter bacteremia in AIDS.[41,42] This organism may be a cause of chronic diarrhea. Similarly, recurrent shigella infection associated with bacteremia may be more common in AIDS. The cases reported thus far have been due to *Shigella flexneri*.[43] Some patients with AIDS may have achlorhydria, which predisposes them to bacterial overgrowth within the proximal small bowel, although the exact incidence of this is unknown. *Chlamydia trachomatis* may also be more common in AIDS patients with diarrhea.[3]

Candida species have not been clearly established as diarrheal pathogens in AIDS. The presence of yeast in areas of intestinal pathology is not uncommon; this finding most likely represents secondary colonization rather than primary fungus-induced disease. Isolated cases of colitis or colonic masses due to histoplasmosis have also been reported.[44,45]

Viral infection of the gastrointestinal tract by cytomegalovirus (CMV) occurs commonly in AIDS patients. Cytomegalovirus is the most common pathogen identified in autopsy series.[20] Of patients with CMV, virtually all will have gastrointestinal involvement.[21] The colon is the most common enteric site of CMV infection, which can manifest itself as patchy or diffuse colitis associated with watery diarrhea.[22] Diarrhea results from mucosal vasculitis via invasion of vascular endothelium. The sequence may ultimately lead to perforation or infarction, or both, associated with hematochezia.[23]

Herpes simplex virus does not cause diarrhea via enteric infection, but AIDS patients may develop chronic perianal ulcerations with mucopurulent discharges that may be interpreted as diarrhea.[24] In a study cited earlier, 26 percent of all AIDS patients with diarrhea had herpes simplex.[3] Distal herpes proctitis, associated with proctalgia and bladder or bowel dysfunction, is seen in AIDS patients but does not by itself represent an opportunistic infection, since herpetic proctitis is commonly seen among otherwise healthy gay men.[25] However, severe mucocutaneous herpes infection persisting for one month without healing is considered an opportunistic infection, thereby establishing an AIDS diagnosis in an HIV-seropositive individual.[26] Herpes virus is often cultured from enteric ulcerations in association with other pathogens in AIDS patients. Such findings, however, do not exclude herpes as a secondary infection within these ulcers.[27] Other enteric viruses are less frequently observed and are not clearly established as significant pathogens. As noted previously, rotavirus and adenovirus are frequently isolated from homosexuals in Australia, but not the U.S. However, the presence of these viruses does not correlate closely with gastrointestinal symptoms.

In rare instances, neoplasms in AIDS patients can cause diarrhea. Gastrointestinal involvement by non-Hodgkin's lymphoma occurred in 15 of 88 patients with AIDS and extranodal lymphoma.[28] Such tumors may lead to lymphatic obstruction and enteropathy with protein loss. Kaposi's sarcoma (KS) involves the gastrointestinal tract in up to 40 percent of AIDS patients with skin or lymph-node KS (or both), but it is rarely identified as a cause of diarrhea in this population.[29] A single case of diarrhea due to protein-losing enteropathy in a patient with enteric Kaposi's sarcoma has been described.[35] Patients with no identifiable diarrheal pathogen have been characterized as having "AIDS enteropathy," although it seems likely that as diagnostic methods improve, many of them will be shown to have pathogens as well. Patients with idiopathic diarrhea are particularly common in Africa, where severe wasting is referred to as "slim disease."[46] It is uncertain yet whether this represents a truly different disease from that observed in the United States and Europe.

■ IS HIV AN ENTERIC PATHOGEN?

The recent identification of HIV in rectal and small-bowel biopsies of AIDS patients[47] has raised two possibilities: (1) the gastrointestinal tract is a portal of entry for primary HIV infection; and (2) local HIV infection of gastrointestinal tissue contributes to gastrointestinal symptoms.

The clearest evidence thus far that HIV may directly enter the body via the gastrointestinal tract has been in patients with a mononucleosis-like illness associated with oral and esophageal ulcerations and acute HIV illness following seroconversion.[48,49,59] Retroviral-like particles have been identified within the esophageal ulcers, although their presence does not establish the esophagus as the initial site of viral invasion. This syndrome is often associated with transient nausea, vomiting, and diarrhea.[59]

It is uncertain that HIV can directly cause diarrhea, since in the original report by Nelson et al.,[47] the virus could only be identified in cells within the lamina propria and not within epithelial cells. The only evidence of HIV tropism for intestinal cells has been in cell-culture studies, in which colon carcinoma cell lines could be transfected with HIV.[50,51] Thus, infection of non-epithelial cells within intestinal tissue could arise via systemic infection with HIV. It remains to be determined whether the mucosal immunologic abnormalities observed thus far in AIDS are due to HIV in the intestinal wall.

■ EVALUATION

HISTORY AND PHYSICAL EXAMINATION

The clinical history is not highly useful for establishing a specific diagnosis in AIDS patients with diarrhea, since co-infection by more than one enteric pathogen is the rule.[1] A careful history can, however, help in localizing the segment of luminal gastrointestinal tract that is most severely involved. For example, symptoms of cramps, bloating, and nausea suggest gastric or small-bowel involvement or both, raising the possibility of infection with cryptosporidium, *Isospora belli*, or giardia. Hematochezia usually implies large-bowel inflammation; most commonly this results from colonic infection by cytomegalovirus, shigella, chlamydia, or campylobacter. Tenesmus, or a sense of rectal urgency, indicates inflammation of the rectal mucosa or proctitis. It occurs most often as a result of herpes, shigella, or campylobacter infections. Symptoms describing the character, frequency, color, or odor of the stool are nonspecific in AIDS and are therefore of little value in diagnosing specific infections.

A history of sexual promiscuity, especially when it includes multiple anonymous homosexual contacts, broadens the differential diagnosis of diarrhea, since one must consider not only enteric infections unique to AIDS, but also the spectrum of infections commonly seen in many healthy homosexual men.[61,62] These include infections by giardia, amoeba, gonococcus, chlamydia and treponema.

The physical exam also provides few diagnostic clues in the evaluation of diarrhea in HIV-infected patients. Peripheral lymphadenopathy, hepatospleno-megaly, and abdominal tenderness are commonly seen in association with diarrhea, yet these findings have little diagnostic value.

LABORATORY EVALUATION

The overriding goal in the evaluation of diarrhea is to identify treatable infections while avoiding diagnostic invasiveness. Careful evaluation of diarrhea is likely to reveal an infectious cause in the majority of patients.[65,71] The following outline provides a procedure for evaluating diarrhea in patients with HIV infection:

Identify treatable infections:

1. If patient has diarrhea, obtain stool specimen.

    Culture for:

    Salmonella
    Shigella
    Campylobacter
    Clostridium difficile

    Examine for:

    Ova and parasites
    Acid-fast bacilli smear for:
    Cryptosporidium
    Isospora belli

2. If patient has rectal bleeding, tenesmus, or both, perform flexible sig-moidoscopy with mucosal biopsy.

    Pathology exam for:

    Cytomegalovirus
    Herpesviruses
    Neoplasm

    Culture for:

    Gonococci
    Campylobacter
    Chlamydia
    Mycobacterium avium-intracellulare
    Herpesviruses

3. If diarrhea and weight loss persist in an otherwise active patient, perform upper endoscopy.

    Aspirate secretions:

    Examine for ova and parasites
    Culture for bacteria and colony count

    Biopsy small-bowel mucosa:

    Specimen pathology and culture as for #2 above

As can be seen above, all patients with symptomatic diarrhea (defined here in functional terms as a significant increase in the frequency of and decrease in the consistency of the patient's stools) should have multiple stool specimens cultured for routine enteric pathogens and examined for ova and parasites. Specific organisms identified in this way should be treated. Stool should also be examined with Ziehl–Neelsen stain in order to identify cryptosporidia.[63] Up to six specimens for ova and parasites may be required in order to exclude cryptosporidium and *Isospora belli*.[54,65] In practical terms, there is no urgency in finding cryptosporidia or *M. avium*, since at present no effective means exist for eradicating these organisms. In contrast, *Isospora belli* is responsive to antibiotics.

If stool exams are negative or identify untreatable infections, the decision to undertake more extensive evaluation should be based on the degree to which diarrhea alone contributes to the patient's overall debility. For example, it would be reasonable to further evaluate the HIV-infected patient who has severe diarrhea and weight loss but who otherwise feels well and remains active. Here, one might consider upper endoscopy or small-bowel capsule biopsy to obtain specimens of small-bowel mucosa for pathologic exam and intestinal fluid for ova and parasite exam and bacterial and fungal culture. Tests used to identify fat malabsorption, such as fecal-fat quantitation and the D-xylose test are not specific, since they are abnormal in almost all AIDS patients with diarrhea, regardless of etiology.[1,12] Similarly, hypokalemia and true intestinal-fluid secretion have been commonly observed but are not associated with any single infection.[12]

A second circumstance justifying an invasive work-up is symptoms suggesting colitis, proctitis, or both. Here a flexible sigmoidoscopy with mucosal biopsy may reveal a treatable infection. All tissue should be examined for microscopic hallmarks of cytomegalovirus or herpesvirus infection, since these may be treatable. In addition, tissue should be cultured for bacterial enteric pathogens, chlamydia, and viruses. Sigmoidoscopy may also reveal evidence of infections or non-infectious colitis not unique to AIDS. These include pseudomembranous colitis due to *C. difficile*, amebiasis, lymphogranuloma venereum, gonorrheal proctitis, Crohn's disease, or idiopathic ulcerative colitis. Barium contrast studies of the gastrointestinal tract are not helpful in the evaluation of diarrhea, since non-specific multifocal abnormalities are almost always present.[64]

■ TREATMENT

When evaluation of diarrhea identifies an enteric pathogen, specific therapy should be administered if available. Chronic administration of alternating antibiotics may be necessary for recurrent salmonella, shigella, campylobacter, or isospora.[54,66] Patients whose work-up fails to identify a treatable infection should be treated symptomatically with antidiarrheals such as Lomotil, Imodium, or opiates. On occasion, we use an empiric trial of oral antibiotics or antiparasite therapy for the possibility of small-bowel overgrowth, undetected campylobacter, isospora enteritis, or undetected protozoa. Sulfonamides, quinolones, tetracyclines, or metronidazole may be appropriate in this setting. A somatostatin analogue has been useful in controlling watery diarrhea in individual cases; larger trials are underway to evaluate the value of this treatment.[69,70] Some patients treated with AZT may show resolution of cryptosporidial-associated diarrhea.[65] If clinical signs of dehydration are present, intravenous fluid repletion is indicated. Nutritional support may be important for these patients.

■ **DEFINITION AND CLINICAL FINDINGS OF AIDS ENTEROPATHY**

A substantial number of AIDS patients have diarrhea and wasting without evidence of enteric infections; such patients are described as having "AIDS enteropathy." No standard definition of this entity exists, and in our experience patients with idiopathic diarrhea are clinically indistinguishable from those in whom an enteric pathogen is identified.

Unexplained diarrhea is more commonly seen in patients with symptomatic HIV infection not diagnosed as AIDS than among patients with AIDS.[57] Often the idiopathic diarrhea occurs before or at the time of initial AIDS diagnosis.[57,72]

Identifying HIV and HIV mRNA in bowel tissue of patients with AIDS raises the possibility (as yet unproven) that HIV directly causes diarrhea.

Some have suggested that idiopathic diarrhea in AIDS is due to immunologic injury.[72] Other investigators have used electron microscopy to demonstrate "tubuloreticular particles" in the intestinal mucosa of AIDS patients and "activation" of rectal epithelial lymphocytes.[57,73,76] The particles are thought to be condensations of endoplasmic reticulum and are often associated with immunologically mediated tissue injury.

Evidence continues to amass, however, that most patients with "idiopathic" diarrhea have an enteric infection. My bias is that the severely impaired cellular immune response associated with AIDS is not likely to induce autoimmune intestinal injury. Furthermore, there are many viral — and possibly protozoal — pathogens that are undetectable by the diagnostic methods currently used. As the sensitivity of our diagnostic methods improves and the full spectrum of infections seen in AIDS is appreciated, it is likely that fewer patients will be considered to have "idiopathic" diarrhea. This position is underscored by a recent study from the National Institutes of Health demonstrating a high likelihood of identifying enteric pathogens in AIDS patients with "idiopathic" diarrhea when a truly comprehensive evaluation is undertaken (17 of 20 patients with diarrhea).[56] Thus, the failure to identify enteric infections in patients with unexplained diarrhea is more likely to reflect insensitive diagnostic methods than autoimmune enteric injury.

MANAGEMENT

AIDS patients with idiopathic diarrhea should be treated symptomatically. Empiric trials of antibiotics may be appropriate (see above). Anti-diarrheals, such as Imodium (2 capsules after each unformed stool, up to 8 capsules per day) or Lomotil (1 to 2 tablets 4 times per day), are often required. Health-care providers should provide opiates to control diarrheal symptoms as necessary, although these medications may induce drowsiness or impaired mental functioning. Bulk-forming agents, including Metamucil or bran, may be helpful in some cases. Nutritional repletion will increase the patient's sense of well-being, although it has not demonstrably prolonged survival. In severe cases, short- or long-term intravenous fluid repletion may be indicated.

■ **ENTERIC IMMUNE DEFECTS IN ARC AND AIDS**

The systemic immunologic defects characteristic of symptomatic HIV infection and AIDS are paralleled by similar abnormalities of the gastrointestinal immune system. Total intestinal submucosal lymphocyte counts in small bowel[77] and rectum[78] are reduced, with almost a complete absence of T4 helper cells[78] and reduction of the T4/T8 lymphocyte ratio. In addition, there are decreased numbers of enteric IgA plasma cells compared to those in controls. The extent of IgA depletion in this study did not correlate with circulating levels of IgA or nutritional status.[79] Finally, a deficiency of tryptase-positive chymase-negative mast cells has been reported, suggesting an absence of T-cell growth factors, which stimulate mast-cell development.[80]

The practical consequences of impaired gastrointestinal immune function have not been assessed directly. It is likely, however, that these humoral and cellular abnormalities contribute to the persistence of a wide array of gastro-intestinal infections in AIDS. This is supported by the fact that clearance of cryptosporidiosis may occur in patients treated with AZT.[65]

For unknown reasons, some AIDS patients have impaired gastric-acid secretion[74] with high serum gastrin values. In two small series, approximately half of 23 patients had little or no gastric-acid secretion.[74,75] This may account for the observed incidence of small-bowel overgrowth, which in 75 percent of cases was due to organisms normally present as mouth flora. An absence of gastric acid allows colonization of the upper small bowel by organisms normally killed within the acidic milieu of the stomach.

REFERENCES

1. Dworkin B, Wormser GP, Rosenthal WS, et al. Gastrointestinal manifestations of the acquired immunodeficiency syndrome: a review of 22 cases. Am J Gastroenterol 1985; 80:774-8.
2. Malebranche R, Guerin JM, Laroche AC, et al. Acquired immunodeficiency syndrome with severe gastrointestinal manifestations in Haiti. Lancet 1983; 2:873-7.
3. Laughon BE, Druckman DA, Vernon A, et al. Prevalence of enteric pathogens in homosexual men with and without acquired immunodeficiency syndrome. Gastroenterology 1988; 94:984-93.
4. Whiteside ME, Barkin JS, May RG, et al. Enteric coccidiosis among patients with the acquired immunodeficiency syndrome. Am J Trop Med Hyg 1984; 33:1065-72.
5. Pitlik SD, Fainstein V, Garza D, et al. Human cryptosporidioses: spectrum of disease. Arch Intern Med 1983; 143:2269-75.
6. Guarda LA, Stein SA, Cleary KA, Ordonez NG. Human cryptosporidiosis in AIDS. Arch Pathol Lab Med 1983; 107:562-6.
7. Forgacs P, Tarshis A, Ma P, et al. Intestinal and bronchial cryptosporidiosis in an immunodeficient homosexual man. Ann Intern Med 1983; 99:793-4.
8. Pitlik SD, Fainstein V, Rios A, et al. Cryptosporidial cholecystitis. N Engl J Med 1983; 308:967.
9. Current WL, Reese NC, Ernst JV, et al. Human cryptosporidiosis in immunocompetent and immunodeficient persons: studies of an outbreak and experimental transmission. N Engl J Med 1983; 308:1252-7.
10. Andreani T, LeCharpentier Y, Brovet J-C, et al. Acquired immunodeficiency with intestinal cryptosporidiosis: possible transmission by Haitian whole blood. Lancet 1983; 1:1187-90.
11. Current WL, Haynes TB. Complete development of Cryptosporidium in cell culture. Science 1984; 224:603-5.
12. Modigliani R, Bories C, Le Charpentier Y, et al. Diarrhea and malabsorption in acquired immune deficiency syndrome: a study of four cases with special emphasis on opportunistic protozoan infestations. Gut 1985; 26:179-87.
13. Dobbins WO, Weinstein WM. Electron microscopy of the intestine and rectum in acquired immunodeficiency syndrome. Gastroenterology 1985; 88:738-49.
14. Sohn CS, Schroff RW, Kliewer KE, et al. Disseminated *Mycobacterium avium-intracellulare* infection in homosexual men with acquired cell-mediated immunodeficiency: a histologic and immunologic study of two cases. Am J Clin Pathol 1983; 79:247-52.
15. Wolke A, Meyers S, Adelsberg BR, et al. *Mycobacterium avium intracellulare* associated colitis in a patient with acquired immunodeficiency syndrome. J Clin Gastroenterol 1984; 6:225-9.
16. Gillin JS, Urmacher C, West R, Shike M. Disseminated *Mycobacterium avium-intracellulare* infection in acquired immunodeficiency syndrome mimicking Whipple's disease. Gastroenterology 1983; 85:1187-91.
17. Roth RI, Owen RL, Keren DF, Volberding PA. Intestinal infection with *Mycobacterium avium* in acquired immune deficiency syndrome (AIDS). Dig Dis Sci 1985; 30:497-504.
18. Smith PD, Macher AM, Bookman MA, et al. *Salmonella typhimurium* enteritis and bacteremia in the acquired immunodeficiency syndrome. Ann Intern Med 1985; 102:207-9.

19. Restrepo C, Macher AM, Radany EH. Disseminated extraintestinal isosporiasis in a patient with acquired immune deficiency syndrome. Am J Clin Pathol 1987; 87:536-42.

20. Welch K, Finkbeiner W, Alpers CE, et al. Autopsy findings in the acquired immunodeficiency syndrome. JAMA 1984; 252:1152-9.

21. Reichert CM, O'Leary TJ, Levens DL, et al. Autopsy pathology in the acquired immunodeficiency syndrome. Am J Pathol 1983; 112:357-82.

22. Meiselman MS, Cello JP, Margaretten W. Cytomegalovirus colitis. Report of the clinical, endoscopic and pathologic findings in two patients with acquired immune deficiency syndrome. Gastroenterology 1985; 88:171-5.

23. Foucar E, Mukai K, Foucar K, et al. Colon ulceration in lethal cytomegalovirus infection. Am J Clin Pathol 1981; 76:788-801.

24. Siegel FP, Lopez C, Hammer GS, et al. Severe acquired immunodeficiency in male homosexuals manifested by chronic perianal ulcerative herpes simplex lesions. N Engl J Med 1981; 305:1439-44.

25. Goodell SE, Quinn TC, Mkrtichian PA-C, et al. Herpes simplex proctitis in homosexual men: clinical, sigmoidoscopic, and histopathological features. N Engl J Med 1983; 308:868-71.

26. Centers for Disease Control. Update on acquired immunodeficiency syndrome (AIDS) in the United States. MMWR 1982; 24:507-14.

27. Gertler SL, Pressman J, Price P, et al. Gastrointestinal cytomegalovirus infection in a homosexual man with severe acquired immunodeficiency syndrome. Gastroenterology 1983; 85:1403-6.

28. Ziegler JL, Beckstead JA, Volberding PA, et al. Non-Hodgkin's lymphoma in 90 homosexual men: relation to generalized lymphadenopathy and the acquired immunodeficiency syndrome. N Engl J Med 1984; 311:565-70.

29. Friedman S, Wright T, Altman D. Gastrointestinal manifestations of Kaposi's sarcoma in acquired immunodeficiency syndrome. Endoscopic and autopsy findings. Gastroenterology 1985; 89:102-8.

30. Marcial MA, Madara JL. Cryptosporidium: Cellular localization, structural analysis of absorptive cell-parasite membrane-membrane interactions in guinea pigs, and suggestion of protozoan transport by M cells. Gastroenterology 1986; 90:583-94.

31. Desportes I, Le Charpentier Y, Galian A, et al. Occurrence of a new microsporidian: *Enterocytozoon bieneusi* n.g., n.sp., in the enterocytes of a human patient with AIDS. J Protozool 1985; 32:250-54.

32. Dehovitz JA, Pape JW, Boncy M, Johnson WD Jr. Clinical manifestations and therapy of *Isospora belli* infection in patients with the acquired immunodeficiency syndrome. N Engl J Med 1986; 315:87-90.

33. Schneebaum CW, Novick DM, Chabon AB, et al. Terminal ileitis associated with *Mycobacterium avium intracellulare* infection in a homosexual man with acquired immune deficiency syndrome. Gastroenterology 1987; 92:1127-32.

34. Fischl MA, Dickinson GM, Sinave C, et al. Salmonella bacteremia as manifestation of acquired immunodeficiency syndrome. Arch Intern Med 1986; 146:113-5.

35. Laine L, Politoske EJ, Gill P. Protein-losing enteropathy in acquired immunodeficiency syndrome due to intestinal Kaposi's sarcoma. Arch Intern Med 1987; 147:1174-5.

36. Rijpstra AC, Canning EU, Van Ketel RJ, et al. Use of light microscopy to diagnose small-intestinal microsporidiosis in patients with AIDS. J Infect Dis 1988; 157:827-31.

37. Goldmeier D, Sargeaunt PG, Price AB, et al. Is *Entamoeba histolytica* in homosexual men a pathogen? Lancet 1986; 1:641-4.

38. Jacobs JL, Gold JW, Murray HW, et al. Salmonella infections in patients with the acquired immunodeficiency syndrome. Ann Intern Med 1985; 102:186-8.

39. Glaser JB, Morton-Kute L, Berger SR, et al. Recurrent *Salmonella typhimurium* bacteremia associated with the acquired immunodeficiency syndrome. Ann Intern Med 1985; 102:189-93.

40. Celum CL, Chaisson RE, Rutherford GW, et al. Incidence of salmonellosis in patients with AIDS. J Infect Dis 1987; 156:998-1002.

41. Perlman DM, Ampel NM, Schifman RB, et al. Persistent *Campylobacter jejuni* infections in patients with human immunodeficiency virus (HIV). Ann Intern Med 1988; 108:540-6.

42. Dworkin B, Wormser GP, Abdoo RA, et al. Persistence of multiply antibiotic-resistant *Campylobacter jejuni* in a patient with the acquired immune deficiency syndrome. Am J Med 1986; 80:965-70.

43. Mandell W, Neu HC. Shigella bacteremia in adults. JAMA 1986; 255:3116-7.

44. Naveau S, Roulot D, Cartier I, et al. Colite ulcereuse à *Histoplasma capsulatum* chez un patient atteint d'un syndrome d'immunodepressin acquire (SIDA). Gastroenterol Clin Biol 1986; 10:760-3.

45. Haggerty CM, Britton MC, Dorman JM, Marzoni FA Jr. Gastrointestinal histoplasmosis in suspected acquired immunodeficiency syndrome. West J Med 1985; 143:244-6.

46. Colebunders R, Francis H, Mann JM, et al. Persistent diarrhea, strongly associated with HIV infection in Kinshasa, Zaire. Am J Gastroenterol 1987; 82:859-64.

47. Nelson JA, Wiley CA, Reynolds-Kohler C, et al. Human immunodeficiency virus detected in bowel epithelium from patients with gastrointestinal symptoms. Lancet 1988; 1:259-61.

48. Cooper DA, Gold J, MacLean P, et al. Acute AIDS retrovirus infection. Definition of a clinical illness associated with seroconversion. Lancet 1985; 1:537-40.

49. Rabeneck L, Boyko WJ, McLean DM, et al. Unusual esophageal ulcers containing enveloped viruslike particles in homosexual men. Gastroenterology 1986; 90:1882-9.

50. Adachi A, Gendelman HE, Koenig S, et al. Production of acquired immunodeficiency syndrome-associated retrovirus in human and nonhuman cells transfected with an infectious molecular clone. J Virol 1986; 59:284-91.

51. Adachi A, Koenig S, Gendelman HE, et al. Productive, persistent infection of human colorectal cell lines with human immunodeficiency virus. J Virol 1987; 61:209-13.

52. Serwadda D, Mugerwa RD, Sewankambo NK, et al. Slim disease: a new disease in Uganda and its association with HTLV-III infection. Lancet 1985; 2:849-52.

53. Antony MA, Brandt LJ, Klein RS, Bernstein LH. Infectious diarrhea in patients with AIDS. Dig Dis Sci 1988; 33:1141-6.

54. Pape JW, Verdier R-I, Johnson WD Jr. Treatment and prophylaxis of *Isospora belli* infection in patients with the acquired immunodeficiency syndrome. N Engl J Med 1989; 320:1044-6.

55. Cunningham AL, Grohman JH, Harkness J, et al. Gastrointestinal viral infections in homosexual men who were symptomatic and seropositive for human immunodeficiency virus. J Infect Dis 1988; 158:386-91.

56. Smith PD, Lane HC, Gill VJ, et al. Intestinal infections in patients with the acquired immunodeficiency syndrome (AIDS). Etiology and response to therapy. Ann Intern Med 1988; 108:328-33.

57. Connolly GM, Shanson D, Hawkins DA, et al. Non-cryptosporidial diarrhoea in human immunodeficiency virus (HIV) infected patients. Gut 1989; 30:195-200.

58. Strachan WD, Chiodini PL, Spice WM, et al. Immunological differentiation of pathogenic and non-pathogenic isolates of *Entamoeba histolytica*. Lancet 1988; 1:561-3.

59. Gaines H, von Sydow M, Pehrson PO, Lundbegh P. Clinical picture of primary HIV infection presenting as a glandular-fever-like illness. Br Med J 1988; 297:1363-8.

60. Janoff EN, Smith PD. Perspectives on gastrointestinal infections in AIDS. Gastroenterol Clin North Am 1988; 17:451-63.

61. Baker RW, Peppercorn MA. Gastrointestinal ailments of homosexual men. Medicine 1982; 61:390-405.

62. Quinn TC, Stamm WE, Goodell SE, et al. The polymicrobial origin of intestinal infections in homosexual men. N Engl J Med 1983; 309:576-82.

63. Garcia LS, Bruckner DA, Brewer TC, Shimizu RY. Techniques for the recovery and identification of Cryptosporidium oocysts from stool specimens. J Clin Microbiol 1983; 18:185-90.

64. Wall SD, Ominsky S, Altman DF, et al. Multifocal abnormalities of the gastrointestinal tract in AIDS. AJR 1986; 146:1-5.

65. Connolly GM, Dryden MS, Shanson DC, Gazzard BG. Cryptosporidial diarrhoea in AIDS and its treatment. Gut 1988; 29:593-7.

66. Armstrong D. Opportunistic infections in the acquired immune deficiency syndrome. Semin Oncol 1987; 14(Suppl 3):40-7.

67. Culpepper-Morgan JA, Kotler DP, Scholes JV, Tierney AR. Evaluation of diagnostic criteria for mucosal cytomegalic inclusion disease in the acquired immune deficiency syndrome. Am J Gastroenterol 1987; 82:1264-70.

68. Rene E, Marche C, Chevalier T, et al. Cytomegalovirus colitis in patients with acquired immunodeficiency syndrome. Dig Dis Sci 1988; 33:741-50.

69. Cook DJ, Kelton JG, Stanisz AM, Collins SM. Somatostatin treatment for cryptosporidial diarrhea in a patient with the acquired immunodeficiency syndrome (AIDS). Ann Intern Med 1988; 108:708-9.

70. Robinson EN Jr, Fogel R. SMS 201-995, a somatostatin analogue, and diarrhea in the acquired immunodeficiency syndrome (AIDS). Ann Intern Med 1988; 109:680-1.

71. Smith PD, Janoff EN. Infectious diarrhea in human immunodeficiency virus infection. Gastroenterol Clin North Am 1988; 17:587-98.

72. Kotler DP, Gaetz HP, Lange M, et al. Enteropathy associated with the acquired immunodeficiency syndrome. Ann Intern Med 1984; 101:421-8.

73. Ozick L, Chander P, Agarwal A, Soni A. Tubuloreticular inclusions in colonic mucosa as diagnostic markers of AIDS. Am J Gastroenterol 1989; 84:195-7.

74. Lake-Bakaar G, Beidas S, El-Sakir R, et al. Impaired gastric acid secretion in AIDS. Gastroenterology 1987; 92:1488.

75. Budhraja M, Levendoglu H, Kocka F, et al. Duodenal mucosal T cell subpopulation and bacterial cultures in acquired immune deficiency syndrome. Am J Gastroenterol 1987; 82:427-31.

76. Weber JR, Dobbins WO. The intestinal and rectal epithelial lymphocyte in AIDS. An electron microscopic study. Am J Surg Pathol 1986; 10:627-39.

77. Rodgers VD, Fassett R, Kagnoff M. Abnormalities in intestinal mucosal T cells including those with the lymphadenopathy syndrome and acquired immunodeficiency syndrome. Gastroenterology 1986; 90:552-8.

78. Ellakany S, Whiteside TL, Schade RR, van Thiel DH. Analysis of intestinal lymphocyte subpopulations in patients with acquired immunodeficiency syndrome (AIDS) and AIDS-related complex. Am J Clin Pathol 1987; 87:356-64.

79. Kotler DP, Scholes JV, Tierney A. Intestinal plasma cell alterations in acquired immunodeficiency syndrome. Dig Dis Sci 1987; 32:129-38.

80. Irani AM, Craig SS, DeBlois G, et al. Deficiency of the tryptase-positive, chymase-negative mast cell type in gastrointestinal mucosa of patients with deficiency t-lymphocyte function. J Immunol 1987; 138:4381-6.

Weight Loss

Scott L. Friedman, M.D.

Weight loss is the most common and often most disturbing general symptom associated with AIDS. It is reported in 95 percent to 100 percent of AIDS patients.[1,2] Striking weight loss was observed even in the early clinical reports, occasionally preceding the actual diagnosis of AIDS.[3] The mean weight loss varies in clinical series from 25 to 35 pounds, but it may be more severe if associated with watery diarrhea.[1,3,4] Associated anorexia is the rule, although weight loss may be profound even with adequate caloric intake.[5]

■ DIFFERENTIAL DIAGNOSIS

Weight loss in AIDS is so common and the variety of illnesses so great that it is difficult to ascribe this symptom to a single opportunistic infection or neoplasm. It may be due to impaired caloric intake, excess caloric loss, or increased caloric utilization.[25] A systematic, careful approach to distinguish these possibilities is essential.[25] The few clinical studies specifically investigating weight loss have noted that it tends to be greater when diarrhea is present.[6,7] Thus, the differential diagnosis of weight loss in the AIDS patient is similar to that of diarrhea if patients have diarrheal symptoms. In addition, profound weight loss may indicate steatorrhea due to fat malabsorption, which is most often associated with infiltrative or infectious small-bowel disease caused by *Mycobacterium avium-intracellulare* (MAI), cryptosporidium, or cytomegalovirus (CMV). A more treatable, although less common, cause of fat malabsorption is pancreatic insufficiency, resulting from either chronic pancreatitis unrelated to HIV infection, opportunistic infection of the pancreas by cytomegalovirus, or pancreatitis induced by pentamidine treatment of *Pneumocystis carinii* infection.[13,24]

Adrenal insufficiency is a rare but treatable cause of wasting in the AIDS patient. In most cases, this condition has been ascribed to CMV infection of the adrenals.[8] In one case, adrenal insufficiency occurred before the diagnosis of AIDS.[9] A case of rifampicin-induced adrenal insufficiency has been reported.[14] All patients reported thus far have had weight loss, fever, hypotension, hyperkalemia, and hyponatremia. Hypoglycemia, eosinophilia, and hyperpigmentation have not always been present.[10] All patients also have abnormal ACTH (cosyntropyn) stimulation test results and have responded well to steroid replacement.

It must be remembered that weight loss and generalized wasting are common consequences of any overwhelming illness, including AIDS, and that such weight loss will often progress without evidence of malabsorption or anorexia.

■ EVALUATION

Specific investigation of weight loss is rarely indicated in AIDS patients, since an extensive evaluation is unlikely to identify a single cause. There are three notable exceptions:

1. patients whose laboratory and clinical features suggest adrenal insufficiency (see DIFFERENTIAL DIAGNOSIS, above);

2. patients with clinical and laboratory evidence of pancreatitis (increased amylase, abdominal pain, history of chronic alcohol abuse, pancreatic calcifications), in whom fat malabsorption may indicate pancreatic insufficiency; and

3. patients who otherwise feel relatively well and are ambulatory but have profound weight loss and diarrhea out of proportion to their general state of health. Although evaluation of this latter group may often yield non-specific findings, it is reasonable to evaluate these patients more aggressively to exclude treatable infections before considering nutritional supplements.

Patients with weight loss who have hypotension, hyperkalemia, and hyponatremia should have an ACTH stimulation test to exclude adrenal insufficiency.

Patients with increased amylase and abdominal pain in association with fat malabsorption should be treated empirically with pancreatic enzyme replacement as a diagnostic and therapeutic maneuver for pancreatic insufficiency. Such insufficiency is rare and can be caused by CMV pancreatitis, pancreatic KS, or pentamidine-induced pancreatitis. Non-invasive imaging of the pancreas (CT scan or ultrasonography) is also appropriate.

A reasonable workup in the mildly symptomatic HIV-infected patient who has disproportionate weight loss is similar to that outlined for the patient who has diarrhea. Emphasis should be placed on identifying treatable infections by using non-invasive means where possible, including careful stool exams and culture. Tests of small-bowel absorptive function, such as D-xylose absorption, fecal-fat quantitation, and serum B12, are not specific because results are abnormal in over half of all AIDS patients with diarrhea and weight loss regardless of which pathogens are present.[1,6,11]

Nutritional Abnormalities Associated with Weight Loss in AIDS. Evidence of malnutrition in AIDS patients is common and tends to be worse when diarrhea is present. In Kotler's study of 25 AIDS patients, all had depressed serum albumin, although values were significantly lower in patients with diarrhea.[7] Marked depletion of body fat, total-body potassium, and increase in extracellular fluid volume commonly occur.[19] Hypoalbuminemia has also been observed in Haitians[5] and children with AIDS.[12] Few other parameters of nutritional status have been studied. Pitchenick reported that of 11 Haitians with AIDS, 6 weighed less than 80 percent of ideal body weight and 9 had triceps skin-fold thicknesses below the 30th percentile.[5] No studies have examined nitrogen balance in AIDS patients.

Attention has been focused on the possibility that zinc deficiency in AIDS patients may contribute to impaired immune function; however, little evidence exists that zinc deficiency in AIDS contributes substantially to immunosuppression. Some clinical surveys of AIDS patients report significantly depressed zinc levels,[6] although others report normal levels.[5] Deficiencies of vitamin B12 and selenium[21] have also been seen; their frequency and relative contributions to the immunosuppression are unknown.

Protein-calorie malabsorption may itself induce intestinal mucosal atrophy, further exacerbating malnutrition. This has been clearly demonstrated in children with marasmus,[17] critically ill patients,[22] and those with AIDS.[18] In each instance, nutritional repletion may result in reversal of small-bowel mucosal abnormalities.[23]

■ TREATMENT

The primary therapeutic goal in the HIV-infected patient with weight loss is to identify all treatable infections contributing to diarrhea or general debility. When possible, specific antimicrobial therapy should be instituted for enteric protozoal or bacterial pathogens, such as *Entamoeba histolytica*, giardia, salmonella, campylobacter, or shigella.

Megestrol Acetate.   A preliminary report has suggested that a synthetic progesterone, megestrol acetate, may promote weight gain in patients with AIDS who do not have significant diarrhea.[15] Thirteen patients with AIDS were treated for a mean of 10 weeks, with all patients reporting some weight gain during the study, although four died of opportunistic infection. Only two of these patients were concurrently treated with zidovudine (AZT). Larger trials are reportedly planned to examine the efficacy of this promising treatment. In addition, AZT alone may contribute to weight gain, most likely by improving immunocompetence and reducing the frequency of opportunistic infection.[26]

Invasive Nutritional Supplements.   Few studies address the role of invasive nutritional supplementation; however, in our experience its indication is limited either to HIV-infected patients who appear relatively well but whose weight loss and diarrhea are disproportionately severe or to young children with HIV infection who fail to thrive. In either case, no clear evidence supports the notion that alimentation prolongs survival, although it may increase the patient's sense of well-being.

Enteral supplementation should be attempted initially, since intravenous hyperalimentation imposes the additional risk of catheter infections, bleeding, or thrombosis. No published studies are available comparing different enteral formulas, but at San Francisco General Hospital, elemental enteral formulas in which at least 30 percent of the total calories are provided as fat, usually in medium-chain triglycerides, are preferred. Formulas should be lactose-free to prevent diarrhea and should contain trace metals, including zinc and selenium. The optimal end point for enteral supplementation is uncertain. In general, supplementation should be maintained until either a reasonable improvement is documented or the patient develops a contraindication to its use (e.g., intractable diarrhea not responsive to anti-diarrheal medications).[16]

At present, intravenous hyperalimentation for AIDS patients is rarely indicated. Children or adult patients who have disproportionately severe diarrhea may require short-term alimention if enteral formulas are contraindicated or not tolerated. In addition, perioperative intravenous hyperalimentation may be appropriate to enhance wound healing and to speed recovery in the AIDS patient requiring surgery. The most effective hyperalimentation formulas for these patients have not been established; however, any formula employed should contain adequate trace metals.[16]

Ultimately the decision to offer parenteral nutritional supplements is highly subjective. The needs or desires of the debilitated patient must be weighed against the additional morbidity produced by nasogastric or intravenous catheters. The patient should be made aware of the lack of evidence that such supplementation substantially alters the overall course of the disease.

REFERENCES

1. Dworkin B, Wormser GP, Rosenthal WS, et al. Gastrointestinal manifestations of the acquired immunodeficiency syndrome: a review of 22 cases. Am J Gastroenterol 1985; 80:774-8.

2. Rene E, Marche C, Regnier B, et al. Manifestations digestives du syndrome d'immunodeficience acquise (SIDA); étude chez 26 patients. Gastroenterol Clin Biol 1985; 9:327-35.

3. Gottlieb MS, Groopman JE, Weinstein WE, et al. The acquired immunodeficiency syndrome. Ann Intern Med 1983; 99:208-20.

4. Portnoy D, Whiteside ME, Buckley E, MacLeod CL. Treatment of intestinal cryptosporidiosis with spiramycin. Ann Intern Med 1984; 101:202-4.

5. Pitchenick AE, Fischl MA, Dickinson GM, et al. Opportunistic infection and Kaposi's sarcoma among Haitians: Evidence of a new acquired immunodeficiency state. Ann Intern Med 1983; 98:277-84.

6. Gillin JS, Shike M, Alcode N, et al. Malabsorption and mucosal abnormalities of the small intestine in the acquired immunodeficiency syndrome. Ann Intern Med 1985; 102:619-22.

7. Kotler DP, Gaetz HP, Lange M, et al. Enteropathy associated with the acquired immunodeficiency syndrome. Ann Intern Med 1984; 101:421-8.

8. Tapper ML, Rotterdam HZ, Lerner CW, et al. Adrenal necrosis in the acquired immunodeficiency syndrome. Ann Intern Med 1984; 100:239-41.

9. Guenthner EE, Rabinowe SL, Van Niel A, et al. Primary Addison's disease in a patient with the acquired immunodeficiency syndrome. Ann Intern Med 1984; 100:847-8.

10. Green LW, Cole W, Greene JB, et al. Adrenal insufficiency as a complication of the acquired immunodeficiency syndrome. Ann Intern Med 1984; 101:497-8.

11. Modigliani R, Bones C, Le Charpentier Y, et al. Diarrhea and malabsorption in acquired immune deficiency syndrome: a study of four cases with special emphasis on opportunistic protozoan infestations. Gut 1985; 26:179-87.

12. Scott GB, Buck BE, Leterman JG, et al. Acquired immunodeficiency syndrome in infants. N Engl J Med 1984; 310:76-81.

13. Lambertus MW, Murthy AR, Nagami P, Goetz MB. Diabetic ketoacidosis following pentamidine therapy in a patient with the acquired immunodeficiency syndrome. West J Med 1988; 149:602-4.

14. Ediger SK, Isley WL. Rifampicin-induced adrenal insufficiency in the acquired immunodeficiency syndrome: difficulties in diagnosis and treatment. Postgrad Med J 1988; 64:405-6.

15. von Roenn JH, Murphy RL, Weber KM, et al. Megestrol acetate for treatment of cachexia associated with human immunodeficiency virus (HIV) infection. Ann Intern Med 1988; 109:840-1.

16. Hickey MS, Weaver KE. Nutritional management of patients with ARC or AIDS. Gastroenterol Clin North Am 1988; 17:545-61.

17. Brunser O, Castillo C, Araya M. Fine structure of the small intestine mucosa in infantile marasmic malnutrition. Gastroenterology 1976; 70:495-507.

18. Benkov KJ, Stawski C, Sirlin SM, et al. Atypical presentation of childhood acquired immune deficiency syndrome mimicking Crohn's disease: nutritional considerations and management. Am J Gastroenterol 1985; 80:260-5.

19. Kotler DP, Wang J, Pierson RN. Body composition studies in patients with the acquired immunodeficiency syndrome. Am J Clin Nutri 1985; 42:1255-65.

20. Harriman GR, Smith PD, Horne MK, et al. Vitamin B12 malabsorption in patients with acquired immunodeficiency syndrome. Clin Res 1987; 35:409A. abstract.

21. Dworkin BM, Rosenthal WS, Wormser GP, Weiss L. Selenium deficiency in the acquired immunodeficiency syndrome. J Parent Ent Nutrition 1986; 10:405-7.

22. Brinson RR, Anderson WM, Singh M. Hypoalbuminemia-associated diarrhea in critically ill patients. J Crit Illness 1987; 2:72-8.

23. Bentler M, Stanish M. Nutrition support of the pediatric patient with AIDS. J Am Dietetic Assn 1987; 87:488-91.

24. Vendrell J, Torre D, Zazz JF, et al. HIV and the pancreas. Lancet 1987; 2:1212.

25. Greene JB. Clinical approach to weight loss in the patient with HIV infection. Gastroenterol Clin North Am 1988; 17:573-86.

26. Yarchoan R, Klecker RW, Weinhold KJ, et al. Administration of 3'-azido-3'-deoxythymidine, an inhibitor of HTLV-III/LAV replication, to patients with AIDS or AIDS-related complex. Lancet 1986:1:575-80.

Dysphagia and Odynophagia Due to Esophagitis

Scott L. Friedman, M.D.

■ DIFFERENTIAL DIAGNOSIS

Dysphagia or odynophagia (or both) due to esophagitis is very common among AIDS patients. Both were recognized as prominent symptoms in early reports of the disease.[1] Their exact frequency has not been established, and not all patients with esophagitis are symptomatic. Instances of esophageal infection, unrecognized antemortem but revealed at autopsy, have been reported.[2]

The majority of patients with dysphagia/odynophagia have candidal esophagitis alone or in association with other infectious pathogens,[27] including cytomegalovirus (CMV), herpes simplex, and *Mycobacterium avium-intracellulare*. Kaposi's sarcoma, lymphoma, and other non-AIDS-specific disorders can also be present.

Cytomegalovirus and herpesvirus are the only other pathogens in HIV infection that commonly cause esophagitis. *M. avium* has been associated with esophageal disease by culture on rare occasion but is not clearly pathogenic in the esophagus. Cryptosporidiosis of the esophagus has been reported in a child.[21] It should be remembered that AIDS patients may have esophageal symptoms due to diseases not unique to HIV infection. These include esophagitis due to reflux or medications.

Candida. The specific incidence of candidal esophagitis depends on the risk group to which the HIV-infected population under study belongs. Ninety-three percent of Haitians with AIDS have oral thrush or candidal esophagitis,[3] whereas in one series of homosexual men, the incidence of candidal esophagitis was only 40 percent.[4] The association of oral thrush with candidal esophagitis approaches 100 percent, according to a recent study by Tavitian, who reported that in 10 patients with oral lesions consistent with thrush, all had endoscopic evidence of candidal involvement of the esophagus.[5] Although their study group was small, the authors suggest that all AIDS patients with oral candida should be assumed to have esophageal candida. While oral thrush often predicts concurrent esophagitis, the absence of thrush does not exclude the possibility of esophageal candidiasis.[6] Many studies, including Tavitian's, fail to distinguish between colonization and true infection by candida, making comparisons of data between patient series difficult. In addition, oral candida may be overdiagnosed, since these reports do not distinguish between thrush and hairy leukoplakia, a tongue lesion whose appearance is similar to that of candida.[7]

Cytomegalovirus. There is growing recognition that CMV may cause severe odynophagia. CMV may appear either as diffuse distal esophagitis or occasionally as large linear mucosal ulcerations.[8]

Herpesvirus. Herpesvirus has occasionally caused esophagitis in patients with AIDS and has also been reported as a rare cause of esophagitis in immunocompetent patients.[9] In healthy patients, herpes esophagitis is usually due to herpes simplex type 1 (HSV-1)[9]; however, we have seen AIDS patients with either HSV-1- or HSV-2-induced esophagitis (Friedman S: personal observation). The disease is similar to herpetic infections of other mucous membranes. The pathogenic features follow a predictable sequence: discrete vesicles appear first, followed by formation of shallow ulcers, and finally, coalescing into regions of diffuse inflammation indistinguishable from those resulting from other causes of esophagitis. It is during this late stage of diffuse esophagitis that most patients with herpes are usually evaluated. Herpes esophagitis is more commonly associated with severe odynophagia than is candida esophagitis.

Non-Specific Esophageal Ulceration.   A syndrome of oral and esophageal aphthous ulcerations, often coinciding with primary HIV infection, has been reported from several centers.[20,23-25] All but one patient were homosexual. The syndrome also may include a maculopapular rash, conjunctivitis, headache, night sweats, and lymphadenopathy. Dysphagia and odynophagia are prominent features. Biopsies of the esophageal ulcers typically reveal a chronic polymorphonuclear inflammatory infiltrate without fungal organisms or prominent endothelial- or epithelial-cell inclusions suggestive of CMV or herpes, respectively.[25] In situ hybridization of the ulcers in one study demonstrated HIV mRNA within mononuclear cells of the lamina propria.[25] Treatment with ganciclovir or ketoconazole is not effective. Corticosteroids may have promoted resolution of the ulcerations in three patients.[24,25] These findings suggest that acute HIV infection may be directly responsible for esophageal ulcerations in some patients. It is not clear if areas of ulcerations represent sites of HIV entry, since there is no evidence that HIV directly infects esophageal epithelium.

■ EVALUATION

There is no way to identify the specific cause of odynophagia in the HIV- infected patient based on symptoms or physical examination alone. Like other gastrointestinal symptoms, odynophagia in the presence of multiple co-infecting organisms makes it impossible to ascribe a symptom or sign to a single pathogen.

As seen in Table 1, endoscopy, with biopsy and specific culture, is the only method of establishing a specific etiology for the cause of dysphagia/odynophagia.

TABLE 1. EVALUATION OF DYSPHAGIA/ODYNOPHAGIA IN AIDS

1. **Barium Swallow (Double-Contrast)**
   Findings may be suggestive of infection or neoplasm, but not diagnostic
2. **Endoscopy**
   Gross:
       Candida: white plaques, friability
       CMV: single ulcer or diffuse esophagitis
       HSV: vesicles or shallow ulcers
   Micro: Look for tissue invasion by specific organism
       Candida: yeast forms
       CMV: inclusions in endothelial cells
       HSV: inclusions in epithelial cells
   Brush: May reveal specific organism
   Culture: Supportive evidence, but doesn't exclude superinfection
3. **Serology:** Not diagnostic

Evidence of tissue invasion is required to establish the pathogenicity of an infectious agent.

On gross examination, candida appears as a thick, cheesy, white exudate, often associated with marked mucosal friability and hemorrhage.[10] Brushings (though not diagnostic) display evidence of pseudomycelia, whereas diagnostic biopsies show true mucosal invasion by fungi.[10] Candida serology is not useful in the AIDS patient, even though it may have utility in the immunocompetent host.[11]

Cytomegalovirus usually produces single deep ulcerations or very large superficial ulcerations of the esophagus. Microscopically, CMV esophagitis displays evidence of vascular endothelial-cell invasion, often in association with a true vasculitis.[12]

Early herpes esophagitis appears as characteristically discrete vesicles that gradually resolve, leaving shallow ulcers. Biopsies and brushings for cytology from the margin of the ulcers (where active viral replication occurs) are most likely to show epithelial cell invasion and nuclear changes typical of herpes infections.

In general, cultures of esophageal biopsy specimens for fungi and viruses are less useful than biopsies, since cultures alone do not distinguish between true pathogens and secondary colonizers.

Barium-swallow radiography in the patient with odynophagia may reveal fungal plaques or mycelia of candida,[13] cytomegalovirus,[14] or herpes,[15] but the technique has a lower sensitivity than endoscopy. Studies of non-AIDS patients with candidal esophagitis suggest a false-negative rate of between 20 percent and 80 percent.[16,17]

■ TREATMENT

An empiric approach to managing esophageal symptoms is most reasonable in the HIV-infected patient. Given the preponderance of candidal infection, patients with odynophagia who have oral thrush should be treated empirically with ketoconazole, 200 mg/day (antifungal lozenges alone are rarely efficacious in this setting). If symptoms persist, endoscopy with biopsy and brushings should be performed to exclude CMV or herpes. Tavitian has found that in many patients, esophageal symptoms due to candida improve with treatment even though endoscopic evidence of infection persists.[18] In agreement with our experience, he points out that eradication of invasive candidiasis does not necessarily prolong survival. Furthermore, symptomatic improvement of esophageal symptoms is probably the most important goal, since it leads to increased oral intake and better nutritional status.

Patients with documented candidal esophagitis not responsive to ketoconazole have been reported.[18] The resistance may possibly be due to a lack of the gastric acid necessary for bio-availability of the drug.[26] Persistent symptoms in these patients may respond to miconazole (50 mg 4 times per day as a gel).[22] Truly refractory candida esophagitis may require treatment with amphotericin B. Herpes esophagitis responds to acyclovir (200 mg capsules every 4 hours), and, in our experience, resolution is not often followed by relapse. Recently an acyclovir derivative, ganciclovir, has been used for the treatment of cytomegalovirus infections.[19] Its role in treating esophageal CMV infection is not yet clear.

Endoscopy rarely fails to establish a definitive cause for esophagitis. The main difficulty arises in deciding which infection is causing symptoms when two or more are found in association. As stated earlier, the clinician should look for evidence of tissue invasion by either candida, CMV, or herpes. If more than one appears invasive, initial treatment for the more likely pathogen should be chosen. If symptoms persist, a trial of therapy for the remaining organism should be undertaken.

REFERENCES

1. Masur H, Michelis M, Greene JB, et al. An outbreak of community acquired *Pneumocystis carinii* pneumonia. Initial manifestations of a cellular immune dysfunction. N Engl J Med 1981; 305:1431-8.

2. Welch K, Finkbeiner W, Alpers CE, et al. Autopsy findings in the acquired immunodeficiency syndrome. JAMA 1984; 252:1152-9.

3. Malebranche R, Gueren JM, Laroche AC, et al. Acquired immunodeficiency syndrome with severe gastrointestinal manifestations in Haiti. Lancet 1983; 2:873-7.

4. Gottlieb MS, Groopman JE, Weinstein WE, et al. The acquired immunodeficiency syndrome. Ann Intern Med 1983; 99:208-20.

5. Tavitian A, Rauffman J, Rosenthal LE. Oral candidiasis as a marker for esophageal candidiasis in the acquired immunodeficiency syndrome. Ann Intern Med 1986; 104:54-5.

6. Scherl E, Siegel F, Geller S, Waye J. Gastrointestinal manifestations of acquired immunodeficiency syndrome. Gastroenterology 1984; 86:1235. abstract.

7. Greenspan D, Conant M, Silverman S, et al. Oral "hairy leucoplakia" in male homosexuals: evidence of association with both papillomavirus and a herpes group virus. Lancet 1984; 2:831-4.

8. St. Onge G, Bezahler GH. Giant esophageal ulcer associated with cytomegalovirus. Gastroenterology 1982; 83:127-30.

9. Solammedevi SV, Patwardhan R. Herpes esophagitis. Am J Gastroenterol 1982; 77:48-50.

10. Trier JS, Bjorkman DJ. Esophageal gastric and intestinal candidiases. Am J Med 1984; 77:39-48.

11. Kodsi BE, Wickremesinghe PC, Kozinn PJ, et al. Candida esophagitis: a prospective study of 27 cases. Gastroenterology 1976; 71:715-9.

12. Meiselman MS, Cello JP, Margaretten W. Cytomegalovirus colitis. Report of the clinical, endoscopic and pathologic findings in two patients with acquired immune deficiency syndrome. Gastroenterology 1985; 88:171-5.

13. Wall SD, Ominsky S, Altman DF, et al. Multifocal abnormalities of the gastrointestinal tract in AIDS. Am J Roentgenol 1986; 146:1-5.

14. Balthazar EJ, Megibow AJ, Hulnick DH. Cytomegalovirus esophagitis and gastritis in AIDS. AJR 1985; 144:1201-4.

15. Lerner CW, Tapper ML. Opportunistic infection complicating acquired immune deficiency syndrome. Medicine 1984; 63:155-64.

16. Eras P, Goldstein MJ, Sherlock PJ. Candida infection of the gastrointestinal tract. Medicine 1972; 51:367-79.

17. Holt H. Candida infection of the esophagus. Gut 1968; 9:227-31.

18. Tavitian A, Kaufman J, Rosenthal LE, et al. Ketoconazole resistant candida esophagitis in patients with acquired immunodeficiency syndrome. Gastroenterology 1986; 90:443-5.

19. Masur H, Lane HC, Palestine A, et al. Effect of 9-(1,3-dihydroxy-2-propoxymethyl)guanine on serious cytomegalovirus disease in eight immunosuppressed homosexual men. Ann Intern Med 1986; 104:41-4.

20. Rabeneck L, Boyko WJ, McLean DM, et al. Unusual esophageal ulcers containing enveloped virus-like particles in homosexual men. Gastroenterology 1986; 90:1882-9.

21. Kazlow PG, Shah K, Benkov KJ, et al. Esophageal cryptosporidiosis in a child with acquired immune deficiency syndrome. Gastroenterology 1986; 91:1301-3.

22. Deschamps MM, Pape JW, Verdier RI, et al. Treatment of candida esophagitis in AIDS patients. Am J Gastroenterol 1988; 83:20-1.

23. Gaines H, von Sydow M, Pehrson PO, Lundbegh P. Clinical picture of primary HIV infection presenting as a glandular-fever-like illness. Br Med J 1988; 297:1363-8.

24. Bach MC, Valenti AJ, Howell DA, Smith TJ. Odynophagia from aphthous ulcers of the pharynx and esophagus in the acquired immunodeficiency syndrome (AIDS). Ann Intern Med 1988; 109:338-9.

25. Kotler DP, Wilson CS, Haroutiounian G, Fox CH. Detection of human immunodeficiency virus-1 by 35S-RNA in situ hybridization in solitary esophageal ulcers in two patients with the acquired immune deficiency syndrome. Am J Gastroenterol 1989; 84:313-7.

26. Lake-Bakaar G, Tom W, Lake-Bakaar D, et al. Gastropathy and ketoconazole malabsorption in the acquired immunodeficiency syndrome (AIDS). Ann Intern Med 1988; 109:471-3.

27. Raufman J-P. Odynophagia/dysphagia in AIDS. Gastroenterol Clin North Am 1988; 17:599-614.

Abdominal Pain

Scott L. Friedman, M.D.

A bdominal pain in patients with HIV infection is uncommon. However, when it is acute and severe, it may portend a catastrophic complication. No data exist on the exact frequency of this symptom.[31,32]

■ DIFFERENTIAL DIAGNOSIS

When making a differential diagnosis for an HIV-infected patient with abdominal pain, the physician must consider not only the manifestations of opportunistic infections and neoplasms but also the more common causes of abdominal pain that occur in otherwise healthy persons.

The differential diagnosis for abdominal pain in HIV-infected patients, presented in Table 1, is organized by the pain's site of origin. For each organ system, a list of potential complications and their likely causes is noted. This information is based primarily on case reports, which are noted in the third column. The table excludes non-HIV-related diagnoses, which are more common causes of abdominal pain, even in patients with AIDS. Only one study has been published specifically addressing the evaluation of abdominal pain in patients with AIDS, and it underscores the wide spectrum of potential causes for abdominal pain in this patient population.[1] Overall, cytomegalovirus (CMV) infection of the bowel or biliary tract is the most common cause of abdominal pain in AIDS patients.

TABLE 1. ABDOMINAL PAIN: DIFFERENTIAL DIAGNOSIS

ORGAN	CAUSES
Stomach	
Gastritis or tumor	CMV,* cryptosporidium[2,3,26,27]
Focal ulcer	CMV,* candida[4,5,20]
Outlet obstruction	Cryptosporidium,* CMV, lymphoma[3,6,7]
Small Bowel	
Enteritis	Cryptosporidium,* CMV, MAI[3,8,21]
Obstruction	Lymphoma,* KS[9,10]
Perforation	CMV,* lymphoma[9,11]
Colon	
Colitis	CMV,* HSV, shigella,[11,12] salmonella, campylobacter, C. difficile[13,14]
Obstruction	Lymphoma,* KS[9]
Perforation	CMV,* lymphoma, HSV[11,15,22]
Appendicitis	KS,* cryptosporidium[16,28]
Liver and/or Spleen	
Infiltration	Lymphoma,* CMV, MAI[1,7]

continued on next page

continued from previous page

TABLE 1.   ABDOMINAL PAIN: DIFFERENTIAL DIAGNOSIS

ORGAN	CAUSES
Biliary Tract	
Cholecystitis	CMV,* cryptosporidium,* candida, enterobacter[3,4,23,24]
Papillary stenosis	CMV,* cryptosporidium,* KS[3,4,25]
Cholangitis	CMV*
Pancreas	
Inflammation	CMV,* KS, drug-induced (pentamidine)[17,29]
Mesentery	
Infiltration	MAI,* cryptococcus, KS,[1,18] lymphoma
Peritoneum	*Vibrio vulnificus,*[26] *M. tuberculosis*[30]

*   *More frequent.*

■ EVALUATION

The patient's history is important in identifying the origin of abdominal pain. In general, the associated symptoms and signs should help identify the particular organ involved. A specific work-up similar to that for a patient without HIV infection should be undertaken. The one exception is that abdominal sonography and computed tomography (CT) scanning are useful early in the assessment of abdominal pain and may highlight regions of disease not suspected clinically.[19] These unsuspected findings often include gallbladder wall–thickening, focal hepatic lesions, biliary ductal dilatation, adenopathy, or peritoneal thickening.

Table 2 defines abdominal pain in terms of the four most common pain syndromes, likely causes, and diagnostic methods. The duration and severity of symptoms dictate the urgency of evaluation. For example, patients with dull, insidious abdominal pain can be evaluated with less urgency than patients who develop acute, severe abdominal pain with evidence of peritonitis.

TABLE 2.   EVALUATION OF ABDOMINAL PAIN: PAIN "SYNDROMES"

SYMPTOMS	SUSPECT	DIAGNOSTIC METHOD
1. Dull pain, diarrhea, mild nausea, vomiting	Infectious enteritis	Stool cultures, stool stain for ova and parasites, sigmoidoscopy
2. Acute, severe pain, peritonitis	Perforation	Abdominal flat plate, abdominal x-ray, surgical consultation
3. Right upper quadrant pain, abnormal liver function tests	Cholecystitis, cholangitis, hepatic infiltrates	Liver function tests, CT/Sono, possibly ERCP, liver biopsy
4. Subacute pain, severe nausea/vomiting	Obstruction	Contrast study

■ TREATMENT

Managing abdominal pain begins with deciding if the patient requires surgical intervention.[36] In general, the indications for surgical intervention in HIV-infected patients are similar to those in patients without HIV infection. Specifically, intestinal perforation, obstruction, life-threatening inflammation, or cholecystitis must be managed surgically, despite the fact that the general debility of most AIDS patients increases their perioperative and postoperative risks. In two recent series, perioperative mortality (i.e., within 30 days) was 50 percent and 71 percent.[23,33] Postoperative complications may include wound infection, disseminated intravascular coagulation, gastrointestinal bleeding, and pneumonia.[34,35] Once surgery is undertaken, the surgeon should submit all specimens for viral and fungal culture as well as for routine pathologic examination. The main goal of surgery in the patient with abdominal pain should be palliation of symptoms; prolonged anesthesia time and extensive tissue resection should be avoided whenever possible.

The non-surgical management of abdominal pain is determined by the results of clinical evaluation. Any treatable infection contributing to the symptoms should be appropriately managed. Symptoms due to lymphoma or Kaposi's sarcoma may respond to chemotherapy or radiation therapy. Symptomatic treatment with analgesics may be indicated in addition to specific antibiotic or antineoplastic regimens.

REFERENCES

1. Potter DA, Danforth DN, Macker AM, et al. Evaluation of abdominal pain in the AIDS patient. Ann Surg 1984; 199:332-9.
2. Caya JG, Cohen EB, Allendorph MM, et al. Atypical mycobacterial and cytomegalovirus infection of the duodenum in a patient with acquired immunodeficiency syndrome: endoscopic and histopathologic appearance. Wis Med J 1984; 83:33-6.
3. Pitlik SD, Fainstein V, Garza D, et al. Human cryptosporidiosis: spectrum of disease. Arch Intern Med 1983; 143:2269-75.
4. Kavin H, Jonas RB, Chowdury L, Kabins S. Acalculous cholecystitis and cytomegalovirus infection in the acquired immunodeficiency syndrome. Ann Intern Med 1986; 104:53-4.
5. Scott BB, Jenkins D. Gastro-oesophageal candidiases. Gut 1982; 23:137-9.
6. Balthazar EJ, Magibow AJ, Hulnick DH. Cytomegalovirus esophagitis and gastritis in AIDS. AJR 1985; 144:1201-4.
7. Ziegler JL, Beckstead JA, Volberding PA, et al. Non-Hodgkin's lymphoma in 90 homosexual men: relation to generalized lymphadenopathy and the acquired immunodeficiency syndrome. N Engl J Med 1984; 311:565-70.
8. Urmacher C, Nielsen S. The histopathology of the acquired immune deficiency syndrome. Pathology 1985; 20:197-220.
9. Steinberg JJ, Bridges N, Feiner HD, Valensi Q. Small intestinal lymphoma in three patients with acquired immune deficiency syndrome. Am J Gastroenterol 1985; 80:21-6.
10. White JAM, King MH. Kaposi's sarcoma presenting with abdominal symptoms. Radiology 1964; 46:197-201.
11. Foucar E, Mukai K, Foucar K, et al. Colon ulceration in lethal cytomegalovirus infection. Am J Clin Pathol 1981; 76:788-801.
12. Goodell SE, Quinn TC, Mkrtichian PA-C, et al. Herpes simplex proctitis in homosexual men: clinical, sigmoidoscopic, and histopathological features. N Engl J Med 1983; 308:868-71.
13. Budhraja M, Levendoglu H, Sherer R. Spectrum of sigmoidoscopic findings in AIDS patients with diarrhea. Am J Gastroenterol 1985; 80:828. abstract.
14. Smith PD, Macker AM, Bookman MA, et al. *Salmonella typhimurium* enteritis and bacteremia in the acquired immunodeficiency syndrome. Ann Intern Med 1985; 102:207-9.
15. Frank D, Raicht RF. Intestinal perforation associated with cytomegalovirus infection in patients with acquired immune deficiency syndrome. Am J Gastroenterol 1984; 79:201-5.
16. Benkov KJ, Stawski C, Sirlin SM, et al. Atypical presentation of childhood acquired immune deficiency syndrome mimicking Crohn's disease: nutritional considerations and management. Am J Gastroenterol 1985; 80:260-5.

17. Mobley K, Rotterdam HZ, Lerner CW, Tapper ML. Autopsy findings in the acquired immune deficiency syndrome. Pathology 1985; 20:45-65.

18. Friedman S, Wright T, Altman D. Gastrointestinal manifestations of Kaposi's sarcoma in acquired immunodeficiency syndrome. Endoscopic and autopsy findings. Gastroenterology 1985; 89:102-8.

19. Jeffrey RB, Nyberg DA, Bottles K, et al. Abdominal CT in acquired immunodeficiency syndrome. AJR 1986; 146:7-13.

20. Campbell DA, Piercey JRA, Shnitka TK, et al. Cytomegalovirus-associated gastric ulcer. Gastroenterology 1977; 72:533-5.

21. Barone JE, Gingold BS, Arvanitis ML, Nealon TF. Abdominal pain in patients with acquired immune deficiency syndrome. Ann Surg 1986; 204:619-23.

22. Kram HB, Hino ST, Cohen RE, et al. Spontaneous colonic perforation secondary to cytomegalovirus in a patient with acquired immune deficiency syndrome. Crit Care Med 1984; 12:469-71.

23. Robinson G, Wilson SE, Williams RA. Surgery in patients with acquired immunodeficiency syndrome. Arch Surg 1987; 122:170-5.

24. Kahn DG, Garfinkle JM, Klonoff DC, et al. Cryptosporidial and cytomegaloviral hepatitis and cholecystitis. Arch Pathol Lab Med 1987; 11:879-81.

25. Schneiderman DJ, Cello JP, Laing FC. Papillary stenosis and sclerosing cholangitis in the acquired immunodeficiency syndrome. Ann Intern Med 1987; 106:546-9.

26. Chin KP, Lowe MA, Tong MJ, Koehler AL. *Vibrio vulnificus* infection after raw oyster ingestion in a patient with liver disease and acquired immune deficiency syndrome-related complex. Gastroenterology 1987; 92:796-9.

27. Elta G, Turnage R, Eckhauser FE, et al. A submucosal antral mass caused by cytomegalovirus infection in a patient with acquired immunodeficiency syndrome. Am J Gastroenterol 1986; 81:714-7.

28. Baker MS, Wille M, Goldman H, Kim HK. Metastatic Kaposi's sarcoma presenting as acute appendicitis. Milit Med 1986; 1:45-7.

29. Zuger A, Wolf BZ, El-Sadr W, et al. Pentamidine-associated fatal acute pancreatitis. JAMA 1986; 256:2383-5.

30. Barnes P, Leedom JM, Radin DR, Chandrasoma P. An unusual case of tuberculous peritonitis in a man with AIDS. West J Med 1986; 144:467-9.

31. Sievert W, Merrell RC. Gastrointestinal emergencies in the acquired immunodeficiency syndrome. Gastroenterol Clin North Am 1988; 17:409-18.

32. Macho JR. Gastrointestinal surgery in the AIDS patient. Gastroenterol Clin North Am 1988; 17:563-71.

33. Wexner SD, Smithy WB, Trillo C, et al. Emergency colectomy for cytomegalovirus ileocolitis in patients with the acquired immune deficiency syndrome. Dis Colon Rectum 1988; 31:755-61.

34. Ferguson CM. Surgical complications of human immunodeficiency virus infection. Am Surg 1988; 54:4-9.

35. Nugent P, O'Connell TX. The surgeon's role in treating acquired immunodeficiency syndrome. Arch Surg 1986; 121:1117-20.

36. Barone JE, Wolkomir AF, Muakkassa FF, Fares LG 2d. Abdominal pain and anorectal disease in AIDS. Gastroenterol Clin North Am 1988; 17:631-8.

Jaundice and Hepatomegaly

Scott L. Friedman, M.D.

Hepatomegaly, with or without jaundice, is a frequent finding in AIDS patients. In one retrospective study, hepatomegaly was detected clinically in over half of all patients.[1] The clinical examination probably underestimates the true incidence of hepatomegaly, since in the same series it was noted in 84 percent of patients postmortem. Hepatomegaly is usually associated with one or more liver-function test abnormalities, although in our experience significant jaundice due to parenchymal disease is uncommon.

■ DIFFERENTIAL DIAGNOSIS

Conditions associated with HIV infection account for the majority of cases of hepatomegaly (see Table 1). The hepatic histology is usually specific for the infection or neoplasm present; no features are common to all AIDS patients with hepatic disease.[2,25] Most studies have reviewed liver abnormalities in populations of homosexuals with AIDS, but the spectrum of hepatic disease is similar in another group, intravenous drug users with AIDS.[24]

TABLE 1. DIFFERENTIAL DIAGNOSIS OF JAUNDICE/HEPATOMEGALY IN AIDS

HEPATIC PARENCHYMAL DISEASE

More common
- *M. avium-intracellulare*
- Drug-induced, especially sulfa
- Cryptococcus
- Lymphoma
- Kaposi's sarcoma
- Cytomegalovirus
- Histoplasmosis
- Coccidioidomycosis
- Hepatitis B
- Microsporidiosis

Less common
- Chronic active hepatitis (in children)
- Peliosis hepatis

BILIARY DISEASE
- Cholangitis (cytomegalovirus, cryptosporidium)
- Lymphoma
- Kaposi's sarcoma

Mycobacterium avium-intracellulare is the most frequent hepatic pathogen in AIDS, occurring in from 19 percent to 70 percent of patients.[3] The pathologic hallmark of the infection is poorly formed granulomas containing acid-fast bacilli.[4] The organisms are rarely seen outside of granulomas.

Cryptococcus commonly infects the liver and always occurs in the setting of disseminated infection.[1] The organism is typically found in the sinusoid and is associated with a poor inflammatory response.

Kaposi's sarcoma (KS) has a predilection for periportal regions of the liver and is seen in 10 percent to 15 percent of liver biopsies.[1,5] On gross examination, tumor nodules appear as violaceous or hemorrhagic masses within hepatic parenchyma. Microscopically, the characteristic spindle cells and vascular slits of KS usually directly abut normal-appearing liver tissue.[6]

Cytomegalovirus (CMV) is overall the most frequent infectious pathogen in AIDS patients, with involvement reported in 5 percent to 25 percent of liver biopsies.[1,5] Typical viral inclusions are usually identified in Kupffer cells but can sometimes be seen in hepatocytes or sinusoidal endothelial cells.[1,7]

Noncryptococcal fungal infection may also occur. Histoplasma has recently been recognized as an opportunistic pathogen in AIDS patients and liver involvement is occasionally seen in patients with disseminated fungal disease.[8] Reported cases have shown caseating granulomas containing fungal organisms subsequently identified by culture. Disseminated coccidioidomycosis involving the liver has been reported, occurring coincident with acute pulmonary infection.[17]

Primary hepatic involvement by non-Hodgkin's lymphoma has been reported in 9 percent of 88 homosexual men with extranodal lymphoma and AIDS,[9] a higher rate than that found in non-HIV-infected patients with lymphoma. The lesions are usually focal and may be large.[10,26] Hodgkin's disease in the AIDS patient tends to display rapid extranodal spread and more aggressive cellular invasion, making liver involvement more likely.[11]

Drug-induced liver dysfunction in AIDS patients is most commonly due to sulfonamides used to treat pneumocystis infections.[2] The increased frequency of adverse reactions to these medications is now well-recognized in AIDS patients.[12] Liver involvement typically yields evidence of granulomas that often contain eosinophils.[2]

Acute or chronic liver disease attributable to hepatitis B infection is surprisingly rare among AIDS patients, given the high prevalence of serologic markers for this infection in the homosexual community.[13] In a large series reviewing liver biopsy and autopsy findings in 85 homosexual men with AIDS, only 5 percent of patients had evidence of chronic liver disease due to hepatitis B, despite a 76 percent prevalence of hepatitis B markers in serum.[14] A single case of microsporidian hepatitis has been reported.[18] Electron microscopy is necessary to definitively identify the organism.

Children with HIV infection may have an unusual form of chronic active hepatitis not yet seen in adults. Duffy recently reported four children who showed piecemeal necrosis (the hallmark of chronic active hepatitis) in the absence of serologic markers for past hepatitis B infection.[15] Inflammation was prominent and consisted primarily of T-suppressor lymphocytes. The pathologic features were distinctly different from those seen in patients with non-A, non-B hepatitis. It is unclear whether these findings reflect an infection not previously associated with HIV, a noninfectious consequence of HIV infection, or a direct result of HIV infection.

Peliosis hepatis, characterized by sinusoidal ectasia and blood-filled cystic spaces, has been described in patients with AIDS.[19] The lesions may contribute to intrahepatic cholestasis and may represent precursor lesions to Kaposi's sarcoma.

Biliary tract involvement in AIDS patients may at times be difficult to distinguish from hepatic parenchymal disease. Cholecystitis, cholangitis, and papillary stenosis due to CMV have been reported; affected patients usually complain of abdominal pain.[16,20,21] Patients with CMV viremia often have evidence of cholestasis even in the absence of symptoms, supporting a role for CMV in the papillary stenosis/cholangitis syndrome associated with AIDS.[23] Neoplastic biliary obstruction due to lymphomatous nodes or KS has been reported.[22] For suspected biliary-tract disease, ultrasonography is a useful diagnostic technique.

■ EVALUATION

The initial decision after evaluating the HIV-infected patient with jaundice, hepatomegaly, or both, is to determine if the findings are due to intrahepatic or extrahepatic disease. Simultaneous disease in both sites must also be considered. A history of mild jaundice, often associated with fevers and constitutional symptoms, is more consistent with intrahepatic disease. Symptoms of deep jaundice associated with pain of relatively acute onset instead suggest extrahepatic disease.

Because both patient history and hepatomegaly are nonspecific for establishing these conditions, further evaluation is always necessary. Laboratory tests are useful to help distinguish intrahepatic from extrahepatic disease in the AIDS patient. Elevations of alanine aminotransferase (ALT) and aspartate transaminase (AST) in the presence of normal bilirubin and alkaline phosphatase levels suggest intrahepatic pathology. Marked elevation of alkaline phosphatase is common in AIDS,[1,27,28] so an imaging procedure of the liver and biliary ducts is almost always indicated when jaundice or hepatomegaly is present. Abdominal computed tomography (CT) scan and sonogram are especially useful in identifying ductal dilatation, gallbladder pathology, and focal hepatic lesions. They should be employed early in the evaluation of jaundice and hepatomegaly.[10]

In intrahepatic disease, abnormalities of liver function tests do not usually suggest a specific etiology except when there is marked elevation of alkaline phosphatase. This finding correlates statistically with the presence of *Mycobacterium avium-intracellulare* infection in the liver in AIDS patients.[27] Elevations of ALT, AST, or both, are seen in 35 percent to 40 percent of patients, but neither the pattern nor the extent of elevation of these tests correlates with specific findings in the liver.[2,27]

The indications for liver biopsy in the patient in whom intrahepatic disease is suspected are not well-defined; however, in general, biopsy is appropriate only when symptomatic, treatable disease of the liver is suspected or when a specific diagnosis of hepatic disease is needed. Liver biopsies are abnormal in 90 percent to 100 percent of patients with AIDS,[2,27] yet in Schneiderman's careful retrospective review, liver biopsy identified a previously undiagnosed infection or neoplasm in only 2 of 26 patients. This suggests that the liver is rarely the sole site of disease. Specific infections or neoplasms are usually evident on tissue sections of appropriately stained biopsy material. When present, *M. avium* is almost always seen within hepatic granulomas, although occasionally it may be detectable only after culture of biopsy material for acid-fast bacilli.[4,27] Cryptococcus and histoplasma may also be associated with granulomas.[1,8]

Cytomegalovirus (CMV) is recognizable by its typical nuclear inclusions within Kupffer cells or hepatocytes.[1] Kaposi's sarcoma and lymphomas are easily identified by their homogeneous neoplastic appearance.[1,9] When lymphoma is suspected, the liver biopsy material should be fixed in paraformaldehyde to allow for thin plastic sections, which can better define histologic type. Drug-induced hepatitis may be recognized on occasion by the presence of eosinophils within granulomas.[2]

An extrahepatic cause for jaundice is suggested on CT by the presence of dilated ducts or other biliary abnormalities. Further evaluation, when indicated, may include endoscopic retrograde cholangiopancreatography (ERCP) if CT or ultrasound demonstrates dilation of extrahepatic ducts extending to the duodenum. In cases of papillary stenosis, endoscopic papillotomy can safely be performed provided that the patient's coagulation profile is normal. Ampullary and biopsy specimens collected during ERCP should be examined for the presence of viruses, protozoa, or neoplastic cells, and cultured for viruses, particularly CMV.

■ NONDIAGNOSTIC WORK-UP

An appreciable number of nonspecific findings are often present in liver biopsies of AIDS patients, in the absence of obvious infection or neoplasm. Welch reported sinusoidal dilation along with hepatic plate atrophy in a pattern similar to that of peliosis hepatis in 31 of 36 autopsies.[5] Granulomas are occasionally seen in the absence of fungal or bacterial organisms.[3,27] Microvesicular and macrovesicular steatosis were often seen in two clinical series and may have been due to malnutrition, since the findings were similar to those seen in patients with kwashiorkor.[2,27]

The significance of most of the nonspecific liver biopsy findings in AIDS patients is unclear. It is unknown whether they represent as-yet unidentified infections or noninfectious immunologic sequelae of HIV infection. Treatment is indicated only in those patients who have pain due to infiltration; small amounts of analgesia may be required.

Patients with jaundice due to extrahepatic disease often require intervention even when a specific infection is not diagnosed. In particular, surgery is indicated in patients with clinical evidence of cholecystitis and occasionally in those with severe cholangitis. Biliary obstruction may respond to endoscopic papillotomy if papillary stenosis or tumor is present at the ampulla of Vater. On rare occasion, neoplastic extrahepatic obstruction that is not amenable to papillotomy can be treated by transhepatic percutaneous drainage or endoscopic stent placement. However, the high risk of bacterial infection created by an indwelling catheter may make this a highly morbid procedure in the AIDS patient.

REFERENCES

1. Glasgow BJ, Anders K, Layfield LJ, et al. Clinical and pathologic findings of the liver in the acquired immune deficiency syndrome (AIDS). Am J Clin Pathol 1985; 83:582-8.
2. Lebovics E, Thung SN, Schaffner F, Radensky PW. The liver in the acquired immunodeficiency syndrome: a clinical and histologic study. Hepatology 1985; 5:293-8.
3. Orenstein MS, Tavitian A, Yonk B, et al. Granulomatous involvement of the liver in patients with AIDS. Gut 1985; 26:1220-5.
4. Greene JB, Sidhu GS, Lewin S, et al. *Mycobacterium avium intracellulare*: a cause of disseminated life threatening infection in homosexuals and drug abusers. Ann Intern Med 1982; 97:539-46.
5. Welch K, Finkbeiner WE, Alpers CE, et al. Autopsy findings in the acquired immunodeficiency syndrome. JAMA 1984; 252:1152-9.
6. Friedman S, Wright T, Altman D. Gastrointestinal manifestations of Kaposi's sarcoma in acquired immunodeficiency syndrome. Endoscopic and autopsy findings. Gastroenterology 1985; 89:102-8.

7. Mobley K, Rotterdam HZ, Lerner CW, Tapper ML. Autopsy findings in the acquired immune deficiency syndrome. Pathology 1985; 20:45-65.

8. Wheat LJ, Slama TG, Zeckel ML. Histoplasmosis in the acquired immune deficiency syndrome. Am J Med 1985; 78:203-10.

9. Ziegler JL, Beckstead JA, Volberding PA, et al. Non-Hodgkin's lymphoma in 90 homosexual men: relation to generalized lymphadenopathy and the acquired immunodeficiency syndrome. N Engl J Med 1984; 311:565-70.

10. Jeffrey RB, Nyberg DA, Bottles K, et al. Abdominal CT in acquired immunodeficiency syndrome. AJR 1986; 146:7-13.

11. Jaffe ES, Clark J, Steis R, et al. Lymph node pathology of HTLV and HTLV-associated neoplasms. Cancer Res 1985; 45:4662S-4664S.

12. Gordin FM, Simon GL, Wofsy CB, et al. Adverse reactions to trimethoprim-sulfamethoxazole in patients with the acquired immunodeficiency syndrome. Ann Intern Med 1984; 100:494-9.

13. Schreeder MT, Thompson SE, Hadler SC, et al. Hepatitis B in homosexual men: prevalence of infection and factors related to transmission. J Infect Dis 1982; 146:7-15.

14. Schneiderman DJ, Arenson DM, Cello JP. Hepatic disease in patients with the acquired immune deficiency syndrome. Gastroenterology 1986; 90:1620. abstract.

15. Duffy LF, Daum F, Kahn E, et al. Hepatitis in children with acquired immune deficiency syndrome. Histopathologic and immunocytologic features. Gastroenterology 1986; 90:173-81.

16. Pitlik SD, Fainstein V, Rios A, et al. Cryptosporidial cholecystitis. N Engl J Med 1983; 308:1967.

17. Bronnimann DA, Adam RD, Galgiani JN, et al. Coccidioidomycosis in the acquired immunodeficiency syndrome. Ann Intern Med 1987; 106:372-9.

18. Terada S, Reddy R, Jeffers LJ, et al. Microsporidian hepatitis in the acquired immunodeficiency syndrome. Ann Intern Med 1987; 107:61-2.

19. Czapar CA, Weldon-Linne M, Moore DM, Rhone DP. Peliosis hepatis in the acquired immunodeficiency syndrome. Arch Pathol Lab Med 1986; 110:611-3.

20. Schneiderman DJ, Cello JP, Laing FC. Papillary stenosis and sclerosing cholangitis in the acquired immunodeficiency syndrome. Ann Intern Med 1987; 106:546-9.

21. Viteri AL, Greene JF Jr. Bile duct abnormalities in the acquired immune deficiency syndrome. Gastroenterology 1987; 92:2014-8.

22. Robinson G, Wilson SE, Williams RA. Surgery in patients with acquired immunodeficiency syndrome. Arch Surg 1987; 122:170-5.

23. Jacobson MA, Cello JP, Sande MS. Cholestasis and disseminated cytomegalovirus disease in patients with the acquired immunodeficiency syndrome. Am J Med 1988; 84:218-24.

24. Dworkin BM, Stahl RE, Giardina MA, et al. The liver in acquired immune deficiency syndrome: emphasis on patients with intravenous drug abuse. Am J Gastroenterol 1987; 82:231-6.

25. Schneiderman DJ. Hepatobiliary abnormalities of AIDS. Gastroenterol Clin North Am 1988; 17:615-30.

26. Friedman SL. Gastrointestinal and hepatobiliary neoplasms in AIDS. Gastroenterol Clin North Am 1988; 17:465-86.

27. Schneiderman DJ, Arenson DM, Cello JP, et al. Hepatic disease in patients with the acquired immune deficiency syndrome (AIDS). Hepatology 1987; 7:925-30.

28. Kahn SA, Saltzman BR, Klein RS, et al. Hepatic disorders in the acquired immune deficiency syndrome: a clinical and pathological study. Am J Gastroenterol 1986; 81:1145-8.

Gastrointestinal Bleeding

Scott L. Friedman, M.D.

Gastrointestinal bleeding in AIDS patients is rare. Several clinical and autopsy series do not cite a single case of serious gastrointestinal hemorrhage in a combined total of 118 patients, suggesting that the frequency is less than 1 percent.[1-4]

■ DIFFERENTIAL DIAGNOSIS

Gastrointestinal bleeding in AIDS patients is as likely to arise from lesions not unique to HIV infection as from AIDS-defining opportunistic infections or neoplasms. Lesions not unique to HIV infection include peptic or stress-related ulcer disease, variceal hemorrhage due to portal hypertension, inflammatory bowel disease, diverticular disease or colonic polyps and neoplasia. None of these diseases occurs more commonly in HIV-infected and AIDS patients than in healthy persons. This section addresses only those infectious processes and neoplasms associated exclusively with HIV infection that may on rare occasion cause gastrointestinal bleeding.

TABLE 1. DIFFERENTIAL DIAGNOSIS OF GASTROINTESTINAL BLEEDING IN AIDS (EXCLUDING NON-AIDS-SPECIFIC DIAGNOSES)

UPPER GASTROINTESTINAL TRACT

Esophagitis	**Gastritis**
Herpes	Cryptosporidiosis
Cytomegalovirus	Cytomegalovirus
Candida	
Enteritis	**Neoplasms**
Salmonella	Kaposi's sarcoma
Campylobacter	Lymphoma

LOWER GASTROINTESTINAL TRACT

Colitis	**Neoplasms**
Cytomegalovirus	Kaposi's sarcoma
Shigella	Lymphoma
Amebiasis	

Cytomegalovirus (CMV) involvement of the gastrointestinal tract may cause bleeding by inducing vasculitis in affected tissue. The vasculitis results in ischemia, infarction, or both, all of which occur most commonly in the colon or distal small bowel.[5,6] A similar mechanism probably accounts for the bleeding associated with CMV infection of the esophagus and stomach.[7] Hemorrhage from colonic or esophageal infection may be due to either focal or diffuse inflammation.[5,7] Occasionally, patients can develop a pancolitis that is clinically similar to the colitis seen in patients with inflammatory bowel disease or mesenteric ischemia.[7]

Candida albicans infection may sometimes induce esophageal hemorrhage via direct fungal invasion, causing a severe erosive esophagitis.[8] In a large autopsy series of cancer patients from Memorial Sloan–Kettering Hospital, 20 of 70 patients (29 percent) had esophageal bleeding with established candidal esophagitis.[8] No reports of similar bleeding have been made in AIDS patients with this infection.

Herpes esophagitis has also (although rarely) been associated with esophageal hemorrhage in non-AIDS patients.[9] The later stages of herpes infection of the esophagus are associated with mucosal ulcerations that may coalesce into a diffuse hemorrhagic esophagitis.

Cryptosporidiosis may rarely cause enteritis associated with hematochezia,[10] although the majority of patients with cryptosporidiosis have severe diarrhea with little or no hemorrhage.[11]

Salmonella-, shigella-, or campylobacter-associated enteritis occurs with increased frequency in AIDS patients compared with non-AIDS patients.[12] These infections are associated with watery diarrhea that may be grossly or microscopically bloody.

Several enteric infections associated with hemorrhage occur with increased frequency in sexually active homosexual men, regardless of whether they have AIDS. These organisms include campylobacter, shigella, *Entamoeba histolytica*, and chlamydia.[13] The clinical features of such infections in AIDS patients are similar to those seen in otherwise healthy homosexual men.

Neoplasms associated with AIDS may occasionally cause intestinal bleeding. In a small series from San Francisco, Kaposi's sarcoma (KS) was the most common cancer found in patients with AIDS-related gastrointestinal bleeding.[17] Isolated cases have been reported in which ulcerated gastrointestinal KS lesions have bled spontaneously.[14,18] In general, however, KS lesions are asymptomatic. In a series of 20 patients with intestinal KS and AIDS from San Francisco General Hospital, no episodes of gastrointestinal bleeding occurred either spontaneously or after endoscopic biopsy.[15]

Primary intestinal lymphoma occurs more often in AIDS patients than in non-AIDS patients.[16] Bleeding from these tumors may occur.[17]

■ EVALUATION

Gastrointestinal bleeding in a patient with HIV infection should be evaluated with the same approach used in assessing a healthy patient. First determine how brisk the bleeding is and whether it arises from an upper- or lower-tract lesion. Coagulation parameters should be checked to insure that a coagulopathy is not contributing to blood loss. The color of rectal blood is an initial clue to its source. Bright red blood suggests lower-tract bleeding while melena suggests an upper-tract source. Orthostatic vital signs and placement of a nasogastric tube are initial diagnostic maneuvers appropriate for assessing the source and severity of hemorrhage. Upper endoscopy is usually necessary to define the source of any severe upper-tract bleeding. Colonoscopy is less practical for evaluating acute lower-tract hemorrhage than endoscopy is in upper-tract bleeding. We prefer to perform flexible sigmoidoscopy if lower gastrointestinal bleeding is present. If no source is evident and if bleeding is severe, we evaluate the patient with a nuclear red-blood-cell scan to define the approximate site of bleeding.

Endoscopic mucosal biopsy of briskly bleeding lesions is generally not appropriate because of the risk of more severe hemorrhage. Once a lesion is identified, we prefer to treat the patient on the basis of the gross findings and to repeat the examination, including mucosal biopsy, after the bleeding subsides. It is usually impossible to make a specific diagnosis at the time of acute bleeding, but endoscopy or sigmoidoscopy is important in identifying whether the bleeding arises from a focal lesion or from diffuse inflammation.

Less invasive diagnostic methods, including stool examination and culture, are indicated if blood loss is not severe enough to require endoscopy or sigmoidoscopy. However, mucosal biopsy demonstrating tissue invasion by infection or neoplasm is the most specific way of establishing a cause for gastrointestinal bleeding. The role of barium contrast studies in evaluating gastrointestinal bleeding is limited. Upper GI series or barium enema can be useful in localizing potential sites of bleeding if endoscopic procedures are not available.

■ TREATMENT

Appropriate management of severe gastrointestinal bleeding due to HIV-related diseases does not require a specific diagnosis. Treatment consists of blood-product support, and, if necessary, surgery. Attempts should be made to use endoscopic hemostatic techniques (e.g., heater probe or multipolar electrocautery) whenever possible.

The patients with chronic gastrointestinal blood loss in whom no treatable infection or neoplasm is found must be managed symptomatically. Intermittent blood-product replacement may be necessary to prevent severely symptomatic anemia. Surgery should be avoided, if possible, because of the considerable perioperative and postoperative risk to these severely debilitated patients.

REFERENCES

1. Rene E, March C, Regnier B, et al. Manifestations digestives du syndrome d'immunodeficience acquise (SIDA): étude chez 26 patients. Gastroenterol Clin Biol 1985; 9:327-35.
2. Malebranche R, Guerin JM, Laroche AC, et al. Acquired immunodeficiency syndrome with severe gastrointestinal manifestations in Haiti. Lancet 1983; 2:873-7.
3. Urmacher C, Nielsen S. The histopathology of the acquired immune deficiency syndrome. Pathology 1985; 20:197-220.
4. Welch K, Finkbeiner W, Alpers CE, et al. Autopsy findings in the acquired immune deficiency syndrome. JAMA 1984; 252:1152-9.
5. Meiselman MS, Cello JP, Margaretten W. Cytomegalovirus colitis. Report of the clinical, endoscopic and pathologic findings in two patients with acquired immune deficiency syndrome. Gastroenterology 1985; 88:171-5.
6. Foucar E, Mukai K, Foucar K, et al. Colon ulceration in lethal cytomegalovirus infection. Am J Clin Pathol 1981; 76:788-801.
7. Balthazar EJ, Megibow AJ, Hulnick DH. Cytomegalovirus esophagitis and gastritis in AIDS. AJR 1985; 144:1201-4.

8. Eras P, Goldstein MJ, Sherlock PJ. Candida infection of the gastrointestinal tract. Medicine 1972; 51:367-79.

9. Fishbein PG, Tuthill R, Kressel H, et al. Herpes simplex esophagitis: a cause of upper gastrointestinal bleeding. Am J Dig Dis 1979; 24:540-4.

10. Babb RR, Differding JL, Trollope ML. Cryptosporidia enteritis in a healthy professional athlete. Am J Gastroenterol 1982; 77:833-4.

11. Whiteside ME, Barkin JS, May RG, et al. Enteric coccidiosis among patients with the acquired immunodeficiency syndrome. Am J Trop Med Hyg 1984; 33:1065-72.

12. Glaser JB, Morton-Kute L, Bergeo SR, et al. Recurrent *salmonella typhimurium* bacteremia associated with the acquired immunodeficiency syndrome. Ann Intern Med 1985; 102:189-93.

13. Baker RW, Peppercorn MA. Gastrointestinal ailments of homosexual men. Medicine 1982; 61:390-405.

14. Potter DA, Danforth DN, Macher AM, et al. Evaluation of abdominal pain in the AIDS patient. Ann Surg 1984; 199:332-9.

15. Friedman S, Wright T, Altman D. Gastrointestinal manifestations of Kaposi's sarcoma in acquired immunodeficiency syndrome. Endoscopic and autopsy findings. Gastroenterology 1985; 89:102-8.

16. Ziegler JL, Beckstead JA, Volberding PA, et al. Non Hodgkin's lymphoma in 90 homosexual men: Relation to generalized lymphadenopathy and the acquired immunodeficiency syndrome. Gastroenterology 1983; 85:1403-6.

17. Cello JP, Wilcox CM. Evaluation and treatment of gastrointestinal tract hemorrhage in patients with AIDS. Gastroenterol Clin North Am 1988; 17:639-48.

18. Friedman SL. Gastrointestinal and hepatobiliary neoplasms in AIDS. Gastroenterol Clin North Am 1988; 17:465-86.

Hepatitis B Virus in AIDS

Scott L. Friedman, M.D.

■ PREVALENCE

The prevalence of seropositivity from past or present infection with hepatitis B virus (HBV) is high in AIDS patients, but no higher than in control patients belonging to the same high-risk groups for HIV infection. In a national case–control study of homosexual men with Kaposi's sarcoma or *Pneumocystis carinii* pneumonia, 94 percent of 46 patients were either HBsAg, anti-HBs- and/or anti-HBc-positive compared with 88 percent of 114 homosexual controls.[1] The majority of patients had evidence of past hepatitis B infection, as suggested by anti-HBs positivity in the absence of hepatitis B surface antigen.

The prevalence of past or present HBV infection in the male homosexual population was well recognized before the HIV epidemic. It has been related to the duration of homosexual activity, the number of non-steady sexual partners, and the frequency of anal–genital or oral–anal contact.[2] Subsequent clinical and autopsy studies in AIDS patients have confirmed a prevalence of positive hepatitis B serology approaching 90 percent.[3,4] One smaller study has suggested an unusually high prevalence of positive anti-HBc in serum, suggesting that ongoing HBV replication may be more common in persons with AIDS.[5]

In a recent multicenter survey, virtually all homosexual men who were seropositive for hepatitis delta virus (HDV) were also seropositive for HIV.[15] Among intravenous drug users (IVDUs) in New York, the prevalence of antibody to HDV and HIV were 67 percent and 58 percent, respectively, although the risk was independent — no relationship was observed between HDV and HIV positivity.[14]

■ CLINICAL FEATURES OF TYPE B VIRAL HEPATITIS IN AIDS

HBV-related symptomatic liver disease is rare in persons with AIDS, despite the high prevalence of serum markers reflecting past or present HBV infection. Rustgi reported that 27 of 30 patients with AIDS were seropositive for HBV, yet only 3 patients had chronic surface antigenemia and no patients had antibodies to the delta agent.[4] One of the 3 anti-HBs-positive patients in this study subsequently died, and postmortem examination showed no evidence of chronic hepatitis even though HBcAg was identified within hepatocytes. There appears to be no relationship between serum aspartate aminotransferase (AST) levels and indices of immune function or HBV replication.[16] In IVDUs who are both HDV- and HIV-antibody-positive, the severity of liver disease correlates with anti-HDV but not with anti-HIV.[14]

In a large combined clinical and autopsy series at San Francisco General Hospital, only 5 of 85 patients with positive HBV serology had pathologic evidence of chronic active hepatitis or cirrhosis — a prevalence rate no different from that reported in immunocompetent persons infected with HBV.[6] Based on the surprisingly low incidence of chronic liver disease in AIDS patients with type B viral hepatitis, Rustgi suggested that the lack of adequate immune response in AIDS patients may result in less T-cell-mediated liver injury than in immunocompetent hosts.[4] This may also mean a higher prevalence of patients with incubating HBV who are asymptomatic, which theoretically increases the risk of transmitting their unrecognized infection.[17]

■ HEPATITIS B — A COFACTOR IN THE ETIOLOGY OF AIDS?

Before HIV was identified in 1983–84, several authors had suggested that HBV might be etiologic in AIDS.[5,7,8] This suggestion was based on the parallel epidemiology of HIV infection and hepatitis B and on the identification of hepatitis B viral DNA in Kaposi's sarcoma tissue of two patients with AIDS.[9] McDonald in 1983 suggested that the AIDS agent might be similar to the delta agent — a small piece of nucleic acid requiring the presence of HBsAg to initiate infectivity.[8]

A study by Laure et al. has provided more direct evidence for the importance of HBV in HIV infection by demonstrating that HBV DNA is integrated into the host genome of lymphoid cells from patients with AIDS or symptomatic HIV infection.[10] This raises the possibility that HBV DNA may be required for HIV to exert its pathogenic effect in the target lymphocyte. Integration of viral DNA in this study was seen even in patients with no serologic markers of HBV. This additional important finding suggests that HBV may be present in more patients than serologic studies indicate. It also rekindles interest in HBV as a cofactor in the development of AIDS.

Many questions about the role of HBV in HIV infection and AIDS remain unanswered. Future studies will undoubtedly address the molecular mechanisms responsible for hepatitis virus infection of lymphoid cells and the pathogenic significance of this phenomenon. The findings may have implications for understanding HIV infection, AIDS, and hepatitis B.

■ THE HEPATITIS B VACCINE AND AIDS

There is no evidence that the hepatitis B vaccine (Heptavax B) can transmit HIV infection. This concern was initially raised because the hepatitis vaccine was produced largely from the serum of homosexual men, a known risk-group for HIV infection.[11,12] Stevens clearly established the lack of association between HIV infection and the hepatitis B vaccine by demonstrating that of 642 patients in New York who received the vaccine, only 2 developed AIDS, or an incidence of 2.4 cases per 1000, compared with an incidence of 4.4 cases per 1000 in an unvaccinated homosexual control population.[13] Furthermore, the purely theoretical concern about HIV contamination can be eliminated by preparing antigen for hepatitis B vaccine using recombinant DNA technology. In fact, if the theories implicating hepatitis B as a co-factor in HIV infection are correct, then use of the vaccine in seronegative high-risk patients might reduce the risk of HIV infection.

At present, the indications for using hepatitis B vaccine are the same as they were before the HIV epidemic: all patients who are or who will be at increased risk for hepatitis B should be vaccinated. This includes health-care personnel, hemodialysis and hemophilia patients, intimate contacts of hepatitis B carriers, and populations at high risk for the disease, such as IVDUs, homosexuals, and prostitutes.

It appears, however, that HIV-antibody-positive individuals have a suboptimal antibody response to hepatitis B vaccination.[18] Thus, these individuals should have HBV-antibody levels determined following vaccination.

REFERENCES

1. Rogers MF, Morens DM, Stewart JA, et al. National case control study of Kaposi's sarcoma and *Pneumocystis carinii* pneumonia in homosexual men. Part 2. Laboratory results. Ann Intern Med 1983; 99:151-8.

2. Schreeder MT, Thompson SE, Hadler SC, et al. Hepatitis B in homosexual men: prevalence of infection and factors related to transmission. J Infect Dis 1983; 146:7-15.

3. Glasgow BJ, Anders K, Layfield LJ, et al. Clinical and pathologic findings of the liver in the acquired immunodeficiency syndrome (AIDS). Am J Clin Pathol 1985; 83:582-8.

4. Rustgi VK, Hoofnagle JH, Gerin JL, et al. Hepatitis B virus infection in the acquired immunodeficiency syndrome. Ann Intern Med 1984; 101:795-7.

5. Wright T, Friedman S, Altman D. Hepatitis B virus infection is implicated in the pathogenesis of Kaposi's sarcoma in homosexual men. Gastroenterology 1983; 84:1402. abstract.

6. Schneiderman DJ, Arenson DM, Cello JP. Hepatic disease in patients with the acquired immune deficiency syndrome. Gastroenterology 1986; 90:1620. abstract.

7. Ravenholt RT. Role of hepatitis B virus in acquired immunodeficiency syndrome. Lancet 1983; 2:885-6.

8. McDonald MI, Hamilton JD, Durack DT. Hepatitis B surface antigen could harbor the infective agent of AIDS. Lancet 1983; 2:882-4.

9. Siddiqui A. Hepatitis B virus DNA in Kaposi's sarcoma. Proc Natl Acad Sci USA 1983; 80:4681-4.

10. Laure F, Zagury D, Saimot AG, et al. Hepatitis B virus DNA sequence in lymphoid cells from patients with AIDS and AIDS-related complex. Science 1985; 229:561-3.

11. Golden JA. No increased incidence of AIDS in recipients of hepatitis B vaccine. N Engl J Med 1983; 308:1163.

12. Szmuness W, Stevens CE, Harley EJ, et al. Hepatitis B vaccine: demonstration of efficacy in a controlled clinical trial on a high-risk population in the United States. N Engl J Med 1980; 303:833-41.

13. Golden JA. No increased incidence of AIDS in recipients of hepatitis B vaccine. N Engl J Med 1983; 308:1163-4.

14. Novick DM, Farci P, Croxson TS, et al. Hepatitis D virus and human immunodeficiency virus antibodies in parenteral drug abusers who are hepatitis B surface antigen positive. J Infect Dis 1988; 158:795-803.

15. Solomon RE, Kaslow RA, Phair JP, et al. Human immunodeficiency virus and hepatitis delta virus in homosexual men. A study of four cohorts. Ann Intern Med 1988; 108:51-4.

16. Rector WG Jr, Govindarajan S, Horsburgh CR Jr, et al. Hepatic inflammation, hepatitis B replication, and cellular immune function in homosexual males with chronic hepatitis B and antibody to human immunodeficiency virus. Am J Gastroenterol 1988; 83:262-6.

17. Hadler SC. Hepatitis B prevention and human immunodeficiency virus (HIV) infection. Ann Intern Med 1988; 109:92-4.

18. Collier AC, Corey L, Murphy VL, Handsfield HH. Antibody to human immunodeficiency virus (HIV) and suboptimal response to hepatitis B vaccination. Ann Intern Med 1988; 109:101-5.

Gastrointestinal Kaposi's Sarcoma and Non-Hodgkin's Lymphoma

Scott L. Friedman, M.D.

■ INCIDENCE OF GASTROINTESTINAL KAPOSI'S SARCOMA

Gastrointestinal involvement by Kaposi's sarcoma (KS) is frequent in patients with AIDS.[35] In two autopsy series, gastrointestinal KS was seen in 56 percent to 70 percent of all patients who had KS.[1,2] Most clinical series probably underestimate the overall incidence of luminal gastrointestinal involvement with KS, since intestinal lesions rarely lead to symptoms. In a prospective endoscopic evaluation of 50 homosexual men with AIDS and skin or lymph-node KS, 20 patients (40 percent) had evidence of gastrointestinal KS within the range of the flexible sigmoidoscope or upper endoscope.[3] The clinical pattern of gastrointestinal KS in U.S. AIDS patients resembles that in Africans with AIDS.[4] In contrast, the indolent variant of KS previously recognized in elderly men of European origin is only rarely associated with gastrointestinal involvement.[5]

The location of nonvisceral sites of KS (skin, lymph nodes) does not predict the likelihood of gastrointestinal KS, although in general, patients with extensive cutaneous lesions are more likely to have gastrointestinal involvement.[3,6] The absence of skin or lymph-node KS, however, does not exclude the possibility of gastrointestinal involvement, since patients have been seen with gastrointestinal disease in the absence of skin findings.[7] Patients with oral KS lesions are no more likely to have gastrointestinal KS than patients without oral lesions.[3]

Clinical Features of Gastrointestinal KS. Gastrointestinal KS, although often widely disseminated, rarely leads to symptoms. KS lesions are usually small and multiple, but may occasionally be bulky masses.[3] Several autopsy series have failed to demonstrate a single instance of death due primarily to a gastrointestinal KS lesion.[2,8] Similarly, in the author's prospective study, there were no proven clinical sequelae of gastrointestinal lesions in 20 patients with endoscopic evidence of KS.[3]

Rare clinical consequences of gastrointestinal KS lesions have been reported both before and since the HIV epidemic began. Gastrointestinal bleeding from ulcerated KS lesions has been reported,[9,36] as well as from renal allograft-associated,[10] African,[11] and European[12] variants of KS. Bowel involvement in non-HIV-infected patients has on rare occasion led to obstruction,[13] perforation with peritonitis,[14] or mesenteric cyst formation.[15] Intestinal KS has also been described in association with celiac disease,[16] protein-losing enteropathy,[17,18] and malabsorption.[19]

Gastrointestinal KS in AIDS patients has not been reported to cause many of these complications, but with the continued spread of HIV infection, it is likely that many of these clinical sequelae will eventually be seen. Hepatobiliary KS has also been reported. In fact, KS has been found in every solid organ except kidneys, heart, and brain.[20] Lesions in the liver are predominantly periportal and are usually asymptomatic,[20] but conceivably they could cause biliary obstruction if located in the distal common bile duct or lymph nodes near the hepatic hilus. Pancreatic KS lesions have also been seen[3] but have not been shown to cause pancreatitis.

Evaluation of Gastrointestinal KS.   Most gastrointestinal KS lesions are discovered incidentally during endoscopic procedures. Three morphologically distinct luminal KS lesions have been reported: maculopapular (often hemorrhagic) lesions, polypoid lesions, and umbilicated nodular lesions.[21] Each has a characteristic appearance, although occasionally cytomegalovirus infection (especially in the colon) may resemble hemorrhagic KS lesions.[22]

Endoscopic biopsy of KS lesions is safe; no complications (including perforation or bleeding) have been reported since KS was recognized as a manifestation of AIDS. The yield of endoscopic biopsy is relatively low. Overall, the likelihood of a positive biopsy of a characteristic lesion is only 23 percent.[3] The low yield is probably due to the submucosal location of the tumor, which makes it inaccessible to the standard biopsy instrument. This possibility is underscored by the findings in sigmoidoscopic biopsies, where larger biopsy instruments are used, in which 36 percent of patients with visible lesions are positive for KS. The smaller endoscopic biopsies are positive in only 13 percent of patients with visible KS.[3] Radiologic contrast studies often show KS lesions.[23] However, the low specificity and sensitivity of this technique compared with endoscopy make it a less desirable means of evaluating gastrointestinal KS.

Prognosis of Gastrointestinal KS.   Although visceral KS lesions rarely cause symptoms, AIDS patients with gastrointestinal involvement by KS have a poorer prognosis than those AIDS patients without gastrointestinal KS. In the author's study (see Table 1),[3] the 24-month survival in patients without gastrointestinal KS was significantly greater than in those who had gastrointestinal KS at the time of first evaluation.

TABLE 1.   SURVIVAL OF PATIENTS WITH AND WITHOUT GASTROINTESTINAL KAPOSI'S SARCOMA AT SIX-MONTH INTERVALS*

MONTHS AFTER DIAGNOSIS	NUMBER OF PATIENTS ALIVE		P VALUE†
	WITH GI KS	WITHOUT GI KS	
6	15/16 (94%)	21/21 (100%)	<0.10
12	11/16 (69%)	20/21 (95%)	<0.005
18	4/13 (31%)	15/16 (94%)	<0.001
24	1/9 (11%)	7/8 (88%)	<0.005

*   Friedman SL, Wright TL, Altman DF. *Gastrointestinal Kaposi's sarcoma in patients with acquired immune deficiency syndrome: endoscopic and autopsy findings. Reprinted with permission from* Gastroenterology 1985; 89:102-8.

†   *P values using one-sided Fisher's exact test.*

Why the prognosis is poorer in patients with gastrointestinal KS is unclear. It is possible that the extent of visceral KS involvement parallels the severity of immunosuppression and thus the patients' susceptibility to life-threatening infections.

Treatment of Gastrointestinal KS.   There is little reason to treat most gastrointestinal KS lesions because complete eradication of the tumor is not always possible and because so few lesions are symptomatic. In those patients who develop biliary or luminal obstruction or perforation due to KS lesions, surgery is the indicated treatment.

■ GASTROINTESTINAL OR HEPATOBILIARY LYMPHOMA

General Aspects.   A striking increase in non-Hodgkin's lymphoma (NHL), often accompanied by gastrointestinal involvement, has been recognized in persons with AIDS. Many of these patients have serologic evidence of Epstein–Barr virus (EBV) and/or human T-cell leukemia virus 1 (HTLV-1) infection, suggesting that one or both of these agents may contribute to the development of neoplasia.[24,25] Lymphoma may develop as the first manifestation of AIDS or as a later complication in a patient with an established diagnosis.[26] The tumors are almost all of B-cell origin.[26]

Clinical Features.   Almost all patients present with extranodal disease; approximately one-third have primary lymphoma of the gastrointestinal tract or hepatobiliary tree.[26] Any region may be involved; hepatic parenchymal lesions or rectal tumors are particularly common. Lymphoma has been seen in the oral mucosa,[26] esophagus,[27] stomach,[28-30] duodenum,[30] small bowel,[31] mesentery,[29] and colon.[31] Tumors may be single or multiple fungatory masses, often with associated hemorrhage. Rectal tumors may be insidious and can be mistaken for benign tissues or fistulae.[32]

Clinical sequelae of gastrointestinal NHL depend on the tumor's location. Because these tumors are very aggressive, it is unlikely that they remain asymptomatic for very long. Bleeding, intestinal obstruction, intussusception, and perforation have all been reported.[27,30,31] Hepatobiliary tumors may cause pain due to hepatic enlargement or biliary obstruction. They are often associated with jaundice and marked elevation of alkaline phosphatase.

Diagnosis of Gastrointestinal NHL.   Non-invasive imaging studies can be useful in identifying suspected NHL, although tissue evaluation is always required to establish the diagnosis. Computerized tomographic (CT) scanning or ultrasound are particularly useful for hepatobiliary lesions, whereas barium contrast studies or endoscopy are more appropriate for luminal tumors. Endoscopic biopsies are often positive when tumor is present. Tissue should be submitted for plastic embedding and staining with leukocyte common antigen.[33] Brushing for cytologic studies may have additional diagnostic value. Fine-needle aspiration of masses or enlarged lymph nodes has proven to be an extremely useful technique at San Francisco General Hospital.[34] An experienced cytologist and close interdisciplinary cooperation are essential for the method to succeed.

Treatment of Gastrointestinal NHL.   Treatment of NHL gastrointestinal lesions is almost always necessary because tumors are rarely asymptomatic. Either chemotherapy or radiation can produce significant tumor reduction, but early recurrences are quite common.[37] Surgical resection may be necessary for perforation, life-threatening obstruction, or occasionally for prophylaxis in anticipation of massive tumor lysis following chemotherapy.

REFERENCES

1. Welch K, Finkbeiner W, Alpers CE, et al. Autopsy findings in the acquired immune deficiency syndrome. JAMA 1984; 252:1152-9.
2. Guarda LA, Luna MA, Smith JL, et al. Acquired immune deficiency syndrome: postmortem findings. Am J Clin Pathol 1984; 81:549-57.
3. Friedman S, Wright T, Altman D. Gastrointestinal manifestations of Kaposi's sarcoma in acquired immunodeficiency syndrome: endoscopic and autopsy findings. Gastroenterology 1985; 89:102-8.
4. Lothe F, Murray JF. Kaposi's sarcoma: autopsy findings in the African. Acta Un Int Cancrum 1962; 18:429-51.
5. Rothman S. Some clinical aspects of Kaposi's sarcoma in the European and North American population. Acta Un Int Cancrum 1962; 18:364-71.
6. Saltz RK, Kurtz RC, Lightdale CJ, et al. Kaposi's sarcoma: gastrointestinal involvement and correlation with skin findings and immunologic function. Dig Dis Sci 1984; 29:817-23.
7. Gottlieb MS, Groopman JE, Weinstein WE, et al. The acquired immunodeficiency syndrome. Ann Intern Med 1983; 99:208-20.
8. Mobley K, Rotterdam HZ, Lerner CW, Tapper ML. Autopsy findings in the acquired immune deficiency syndrome. Pathology 1985; 20:45-65.
9. Potter DA, Danforth DN, Macher AM, et al. Evaluation of abdominal pain in the AIDS patient. Ann Surg 1984; 199:332-9.
10. Stribling J, Weitzner S, Smith GV. Kaposi's sarcoma in renal allograft recipients. Cancer 1978; 42:442-6.
11. Templeton AC. Studies in Kaposi's sarcoma, post mortem findings and disease patterns in women. Cancer 1972; 30:854-67.
12. Nesbitt S, Mark PF, Zimmerman HM. Disseminated visceral idiopathic hemorrhagic sarcoma (Kaposi's disease): report of a case with necropsy findings. Ann Intern Med 1945; 22:601-5.
13. White JAM, King MH. Kaposi's sarcoma presenting with abdominal symptoms. Radiology 1964; 46:197-201.
14. Mitchell N, Feder I. Kaposi's sarcoma with secondary involvement of the jejunum, with perforation and peritonitis. Ann Intern Med 1949; 31:324-9.
15. Sherwin B, Gordimer H. Kaposi's sarcoma. Case report with unique visceral manifestations. Ann Surg 1952; 135:118-23.
16. Sunter JP. Visceral Kaposi's sarcoma. Occurrence in a patient suffering from celiac disease. Arch Pathol Lab Med 1978; 102:543-5.
17. Novis BH, King H, Bank S. Kaposi's sarcoma presenting with diarrhea and protein losing enteropathy. Gastroenterology 1974; 67:996-1000.
18. Perrone V, Pergola M, Abate G, et al. Protein-losing enteropathy in a patient with generalized Kaposi's sarcoma. Cancer 1981; 47:588-91.
19. Bryk D, Farman J, Dalleman S, et al. Kaposi's sarcoma of the intestinal tract: roentgen manifestations. Gastrointest Radiol 1978; 3:425-30.
20. Urmacher C, Nielsen S. The histopathology of the acquired immune deficiency syndrome. Pathology 1985; 20:197-220.
21. Ahmed N, Nelson RS, Goldstein HM, Sinkovics JG. Kaposi's sarcoma of the stomach and duodenum. Endoscopic and roentgenologic correlations. Gastrointest Endosc 1975; 21:149-52.
22. Meiselman MS, Cello JP, Margaretten W. Cytomegalovirus colitis. Report of the clinical, endoscopic and pathologic findings in two patients with acquired immune deficiency syndrome. Gastroenterology 1985; 88:171-5.
23. Rose HS, Balthazar EJ, Megibow AJ, et al. Alimentary tract involvement in Kaposi's sarcoma: radiographic and endoscopic findings in 25 homosexual men. Am J Roentgenol 1982; 139:661-6.
24. Kaplan LD, Volberding PA, Abrams DI. Update on AIDS-associated non-Hodgkin's lymphoma in San Francisco. Washington, D.C.: III International Conference on AIDS, 1987; 9.
25. Levine AM, Gill PS, Muggia F. Malignancies in the acquired immunodeficiency syndrome. Curr Probl Cancer 1987; 11:209-55.
26. Ziegler JL, Beckstead JA, Volberding PA, et al. Non-Hodgkin's lymphoma in 90 homosexual men: relation to generalized lymphadenopathy and the acquired immunodeficiency syndrome. N Engl J Med 1984; 311:565-70.
27. Bernal A, del Junco GW. Endoscopic and pathologic features of esophageal lymphoma: a report of four cases in patients with acquired immune deficiency syndrome. Gastrointest Endosc 1986; 32:96-9.

28. Di Carlo EF, Amberson JB, Metroka CE, et al. Malignant lymphomas and the acquired immuno-deficiency syndrome. Evaluation of 30 cases using a working formulation. Arch Pathol Lab Med 1986; 110:1012-6.

29. Lind SE, Gross PL, Andiman WA, et al. Malignant lymphoma presenting as Kaposi's sarcoma in a homosexual man with the acquired immunodeficiency syndrome. Ann Intern Med 1985; 102:338-40.

30. Petersen JM, Tubbs RR, Savage RA, et al. Small noncleaved B-cell Burkitt-like lymphoma with chromo-some t(8; 14) translocation and Epstein-Barr virus nuclear-associated antigen in a homosexual man with acquired immune deficiency syndrome. Am J Med 1985; 78:141-8.

31. Steinberg JJ, Bridges N, Feiner HD, Valensi Q. Small intestinal lymphoma in three patients with acquired immune deficiency syndrome. Am J Gastroenterol 1985; 80:21-6.

32. Boylston AW, Cook HT, Francis ND, Goldin RD. Biopsy pathology of acquired immune deficiency syndrome (AIDS). J Clin Pathol 1987; 40:1-8.

33. Kurtin PJ, Pinkus GS. Leukocyte common antigen —diagnostic discriminant between hematopoietic and nonhematopoietic neoplasms in paraffin sections using monoclonal antibodies: correlation with immunologic studies and ultrastructural localization. Hum Pathol 1985; 16:353-65.

34. Bottles K, McPhaul LW, Volberding P. Fine-needle aspiration biopsy of patients with acquired immu-nodeficiency syndrome (AIDS): experience in an outpatient clinic. Ann Intern Med 1988; 108:42-5.

35. Friedman SL. Gastrointestinal and hepatobiliary neoplasms in AIDS. Gastroenterol Clin North Am 1988; 17:465-86.

36. Cello JP, Wilcox CM. Evaluation and treatment of gastrointestinal tract hemorrhage in patients with AIDS. Gastroenterol Clin North Am 1988; 17:639-48.

37. Kaplan LD, Abrams DI, Feigal E, et al. AIDS-associated non-Hodgkin's lymphoma in San Francisco. JAMA 1989; 261:719-24.

Anorectal Disease

Scott L. Friedman, M.D.

■ SPECTRUM OF ANORECTAL DISEASE IN HIV-INFECTED PATIENTS

Anorectal problems may occur in any HIV-infected patient, but they are particularly common among homosexual men. A broad array of anorectal problems are prevalent in the healthy homosexual population, partly because of the prevalence of anal intercourse and anilingus.[22,23] Anal warts and fissures, infections with lymphogranuloma venereum, gonorrhea, syphilis, and herpes viruses are well-recognized pathogens, although they do not necessarily imply immunodeficiency in their hosts. They have been the subject of numerous reports antedating the HIV epidemic.[1-3]

TABLE 1. ANORECTAL DISEASE IN HIV-INFECTED PATIENTS

INFECTIONS

Bacteria	Viruses	Fungi
Chlamydia trachomatis	Herpes simplex	*Candida albicans*
Lymphogranuloma venereum	Cytomegalovirus	
Neisseria gonorrhoeae		
Spirochetes	**Neoplasms**	
Shigella flexneri	Lymphoma	
Campylobacter jejuni	Kaposi's sarcoma	
Mycobacterium tuberculosis[20]	Squamous-cell carcinoma	
Leishmania[21]	Cloacogenic carcinoma	
Clostridium difficile	Condyloma acuminatum	

The frequency of anorectal disease among homosexual AIDS patients is quite high. In a large New York City series of 340 patients, the incidence of anorectal disease was 34 percent.[4] Perirectal abscesses, anal fistulae, and infectious proctitis were the most common findings, but lymphoma, ulcerations due to tuberculosis, and histoplasmosis were also seen. The overall healing rate following surgery or biopsy was extremely poor — only 12 percent of patients demonstrated prompt healing. Rectal perforation, incontinence, and persistent drainage complicated 90 percent of all diagnostic or therapeutic efforts in this series.

While a patient's recurrent anorectal disease associated with systemic symptoms may raise the possibility of AIDS, any anorectal infection alone does not qualify as an AIDS-defining opportunistic infection. Only cytomegalovirus, fungal infection, chronic perianal herpes infection lasting more than one month, or anorectal lymphoma or Kaposi's sarcoma in the presence of HIV antibody seropositivity establishes a diagnosis of AIDS.[5,6]

Anorectal carcinomas are more common in homosexual men than in other members of the population. Epidemiologic studies demonstrate an increased incidence of anal carcinomas in young unmarried males compared to married males.[7,8] Several recent reports have described this tumor specifically in homosexual men,[9-13] some of whom had AIDS. Furthermore, anorectal dysplasia in homosexual men is associated with presence of serum antibodies to HIV and a depressed T4/T8 lymphocyte ratio.[14] Expression of these tumors may not depend on immune deficiency, however. It is not clear whether the dysplasia results from immune suppression or if both these findings reflect a high frequency of anal-receptive intercourse. These neoplasms appear to result from chronic perianal herpes or papillomavirus infections acquired through sexual contact.[15] Morphologic studies have documented histologic progression, often in the same lesion, from benign condyloma acuminatum to marked dysplasia or squamous carcinoma.[16,17] Immune deficiency may enhance this progression: immunocompromised renal transplant patients display a 100-fold increase in incidence of carcinoma of the vulva and anus when compared to the immunocompetent population.[18] No increased incidence of anorectal carcinoma has been recognized in HIV-infected subgroups other than homosexual men.

■ APPROACH TO ANORECTAL SYMPTOMS IN HIV-INFECTED PATIENTS

A careful history of the HIV-infected homosexual patient who does not have AIDS may uncover symptoms of advancing HIV disease. Weight loss, fever, fatigue, and night sweats all raise the possibility of neoplasm or anorectal opportunistic infection.

Insidious presentation of rectal lymphoma is not uncommon. In HIV-infected patients and patients with AIDS, physical examination should include careful inspection of the skin and mucous membranes as well as palpation of the lymph nodes. Careful visual inspection of the anus for fissures and masses should precede digital examination. Palpation of the anal canal may reveal masses or fissures not otherwise evident. All patients with anorectal symptoms should have anoscopy and sigmoidoscopy (rigid or flexible) with mucosal biopsy, even if the mucosa appear unremarkable on gross examination.

Specimens should be evaluated for evidence of neoplasm or infection; when appropriate, they should be examined for bacterial (including gonococcal and chlamydial), viral, and fungal cultures. Laboratory evidence of leukopenia in patients not diagnosed with AIDS may further raise the index of suspicion for neoplasm or opportunistic infection. Computed tomographic scan may define the extent of disease if a neoplasm is identified.[19]

Based on clinical experience with anorectal disease in HIV-infected patients thus far, a conservative approach to surgical management seems warranted. All efforts should be directed toward identifying infections and providing symptomatic relief, reserving more aggressive measures for those in whom less invasive efforts fail.

REFERENCES

1. Quinn TC, Stamm WE, Goodell SE, et al. The polymicrobial origin of intestinal infections in homosexual men. N Engl J Med 1983; 309:576-82.
2. Baker RW, Peppercorn MA. Gastrointestinal ailments of homosexual men. Medicine 1982; 61:390-405.
3. Rompalo AM, Stamm WE. Anorectal and enteric infection in homosexual men. West J Med 1985; 142:647-52.
4. Wexner SD, Smithy WB, Milsom JW, Dailey TH. The surgical management of anorectal diseases in AIDS and pre-AIDS patients. Dis Colon Rectum 1986; 29:719-23.
5. Siegal FP, Lopez C, Hammer GS, et al. Severe acquired immunodeficiency in male homosexuals, manifested by chronic perianal ulcerative herpes simplex lesions. N Engl J Med 1981; 305:1439-44.
6. Lee MH, Waxman M, Gillooley JF. Primary malignant lymphoma of the anorectum in homosexual men. Dis Colon Rectum 1986; 29:413-6.
7. Daling JR, Weiss NS, Klopfenstein LL, et al. Correlates of homosexual behavior and the incidence of anal cancer. JAMA 1982; 247:1988-90.
8. Peters RK, Mack TM. Patterns of anal carcinoma by gender and marital status in Los Angeles County. Br J Cancer 1983; 48:629-36.
9. Li FP, Osborn D, Cronin CM. Anorectal squamous carcinoma in two homosexual men. Lancet 1982; 2:391.
10. Croxon T, Chabon AB, Rorat E, Barash IM. Intraepithelial carcinoma of the anus in homosexual men. Dis Colon Rectum 1984; 27:325-30.
11. Longo WE, Ballantyne GH, Gerald WL, Modlin IM. Squamous cell carcinoma in situ in condyloma acuminatum. Dis Colon Rectum 1986; 29:503-6.
12. Conant MA, Volberding P, Fletcher V, et al. Squamous cell carcinoma in sexual partner of Kaposi sarcoma patient. Lancet 1982; 1:286.
13. Read EJ, Orenstein JM, Chorba TL, et al. Listeria sepsis and small cell carcinoma of the rectum: an unusual presentation of the acquired immunodeficiency syndrome. Am J Clin Pathol 1985; 83:385-9.
14. Frazer IH, Medley G, Crapper RM, et al. Association between anorectal dysplasia, human papilloma virus, and human immunodeficiency virus in homosexual men. Lancet 1986; 2:657-60.
15. Daling JR, Weiss NS, Hislop G, et al. Sexual practices, sexually transmitted diseases, and the incidence of anal cancer. N Engl J Med 1987; 317:973-7.
16. Kovi J, Tillman RL, Lee SM. Malignant transformation of condyloma acuminatum. A light microscopic and ultrastructural study. Am J Clin Pathol 1974; 61:702-10.
17. Bogomoletz WV, Potet F, Molas G. Condyloma acuminata, giant condyloma acuminatum (Buschke-Lowenstein tumour) and verrucous squamous carcinoma of the perianal and anorectal region: a continuous precancerous spectrum? Histopathol 1985; 9:155-69.
18. Penn I. Cancers of the anogenital region in renal transplant patients. Analysis of 65 cases. Cancer 1986; 58:611- 6.
19. Albin J, Lewis E, Eftekhasi F, Shirkhoda A. Computed tomography of rectal and perirectal disease in AIDS patients. Gastrointest Radiol 1987; 12:67-70.
20. Lax JD, Haroutiounian G, Attia G, et al. Tuberculosis of the rectum in a patient with acquired immune deficiency syndrome. Report of a case. Dis Colon Rectum 1988; 31:394-7.
21. Rosenthal PJ, Chaisson RE, Hadley WK, Leech JH. Rectal leishmaniasis in a patient with acquired immunodeficiency syndrome. Am J Med 1988; 84:307-9.
22. Hyder JW, MacKeigan JM. Anorectal and colonic disease and the immunocompromised host. Dis Colon Rectum 1988; 31:971-6.
23. Barone JE, Wolkomir AF, Muakkassa FF, Fares LG 2d. Abdominal pain and anorectal disease in AIDS. Gastroenterol Clin North Am 1988; 17:631-8.

5.11

Ophthalmologic Aspects

Manifestations of HIV Infection in the Eye

James J. O'Donnell, M.D.

Ophthalmologists have a role and a responsibility in caring for AIDS patients. The majority of patients with severe HIV infection have eye problems, the most common of which are retinal cotton-wool spots, Kaposi's sarcoma (KS), and cytomegalovirus (CMV) retinitis. These problems can be accurately diagnosed and effectively managed in most cases. All AIDS patients should consult with an ophthalmologist.

Cotton-wool spots are white, superficial retinal lesions with feathered edges, distributed near the optic nerve along the major retinal vessels. KS lesions on the conjunctiva are red, painless elevations; on the eyelid they are purple, firm, nontender nodules of varying size. CMV appears as fluffy, white, superficial retinal lesions, often perivascular, with associated retinal hemorrhages. The ophthalmologist should also be alert to the possibility of other opportunistic infections of the eye.[1-7]

■ RETINAL COTTON-WOOL SPOTS

Cotton-wool spots in the retina are the most common ocular finding in severe HIV infection.[1-7,13-16] The lesions resemble cotton wool because of their white, feather-edged appearance (see color plate 5.11.1.a).

Pathogenesis of Cotton-Wool Spots. The cotton-wool spot is produced by an ischemic infarct in the superficial layer of the retina. This layer is composed of axons leading from the ganglion cells into the optic nerve. The infarct causes axonal swelling, and axoplasm and mitochondria accumulate. On light microscopy, the lesion appears as a cytoid body on the superficial retina, resembling a very large cell filled with cytoplasm.

The etiology of cotton-wool spots in HIV infection is uncertain. In autopsied cases, *Pneumocystis carinii* has been seen (by transmission electron microscopy) in the retina adjacent to the cotton wool-spots.[8,9] However, not all investigators have been able to find pneumocystis in the retina.[10] Whether this represents differences in microscopy technique, chance occurrence, or earlier treatment of *Pneumocystis carinii* remains to be determined. Also, HIV itself can infect the retina.[16]

Clinical Manifestations of Cotton-Wool Spots. In AIDS patients, cotton-wool spots are distributed near the optic nerve along the major retinal vessels. The lesions are usually less than one-quarter disc (optic nerve) diameter in size. Occasionally, small flame-shaped hemorrhages and small white-centered retinal hemorrhages are associated with these lesions. They should be distinguished from retinal exudates, which are yellow, smooth, marginated lesions found deeper in the retina.

In a few patients, the diagnosis of AIDS has been suspected because of the appearance of cotton-wool spots. A complete history, physical examination, and laboratory tests are, of course, necessary to confirm such a suspicion.

Patient Management Considerations.   There is no treatment for asymptomatic cotton-wool spots. As previously mentioned, *Pneumocystis carinii* should be suspected if other symptoms and signs of pneumocystis infection, such as dyspnea, are present.

Cotton-wool spots almost never produce symptomatic vision loss. Only rarely, when the lesion is due to an infarct in axons from the foveal area, is there loss of vision. Individual cotton-wool spots spontaneously disappear in about two months, but new spots may appear.

Research Prospects.   The relationship between *Pneumocystis carinii* and cotton-wool spots, the precise etiology of these lesions in HIV infection, and the significance of cotton-wool spots in relation to the stage of HIV disease should be explored.

■ KAPOSI'S SARCOMA OF THE CONJUNCTIVA AND EYELIDS

KS lesions of the conjunctiva or eyelids, or both, are the second most common ocular lesions seen in AIDS patients.[1-7,14]

Pathogenesis.   The pathogenesis of ocular KS lesions is the same as that of the systemic KS lesions seen in some patients with AIDS.

Clinical Manifestations   Lesions on the conjunctiva appear as bright red, painless spots of varying sizes and elevation. They are often hidden in the superior or inferior fornix. The patient's lids should be manually retracted and he or she should be instructed to look upward and downward on examination. Occasionally, associated subconjunctival hemorrhage is present. Lesions on the lid appear as purple, firm, nontender nodules of varying sizes and shapes.

Diagnostic Considerations for Ocular KS.   A KS diagnosis is almost always established by biopsy of lesions elsewhere in the patient. A conjunctival or lid-lesion biopsy is indicated only for the rare patient with HIV infection and a possible KS lesion present only in the periocular area.

Patient Management Considerations for Ocular KS.   Ocular KS rarely requires treatment. If lesions produce symptoms or unacceptable cosmetic problems (e.g., occasionally a large KS lesion on the eyelid will obscure the patient's vision), they may require treatment. Low-dosage radiation works well for shrinking ocular lesions. Kaposi's sarcoma lesions of the conjunctiva and eyelids rarely threaten vision.

■ CYTOMEGALOVIRUS RETINITIS

Cytomegalovirus retinitis is the most serious ocular complication of AIDS, occurring in about 10 to 15 percent of patients.[1-7,13,14,17-25]

Pathogenesis.   Opportunistic infection of the retina by CMV causes a severe, acute, progressive necrotic vasculitis and retinitis. Atrophy and pigment clumping follow necrosis.

Clinical Manifestations of Ocular CMV Infections. Cytomegalovirus retinitis is asymptomatic in some patients. When it is symptomatic, the patient may complain of decreased visual acuity, scotoma, photophobia, perception of flashes of light, sudden onset of the sensation of floating spots, redness, or pain. Slit-lamp examination may reveal anterior segment uveitis with detectable cells and flare in the anterior chamber and small keratic precipitates on the corneal endothelium. Cells may be seen in the vitreous. Cytomegalovirus retinitis lesions are fluffy, white, and superficial, with associated retinal hemorrhages. The lesions are often perivascular. The optic nerve is frequently involved and may be the site of initial inflammation (see color plates 5.11.1.b and 5.11.1.c).

Diagnostic Considerations. The ophthalmoscopic appearance of CMV retinitis in patients with AIDS or HIV infection is usually characteristic. The retina should be examined with an indirect ophthalmoscope through well-dilated pupils. Occasionally, a very small, early CMV lesion may be confused with a cotton-wool spot, but the rapid progression of CMV retinitis quickly resolves this confusion. Cytomegalovirus cultures of blood, urine, semen, or all of these should be performed to confirm the diagnosis.

Patient Management Considerations. Cytomegalovirus retinitis usually progresses quickly and involves the entire retina in a matter of weeks, so patients should be examined approximately every two weeks. Retinal drawings and fundus photography should be used in monitoring these patients. Fluorescein angiography is rarely necessary.

Dihydroxy propoxymethyl guanine (DHPG, ganciclovir) is an experimental drug that has shown promise as a treatment for CMV retinitis. This drug probably stops or slows the progression of CMV retinitis in most patients.[11,12,17-22] A large-scale randomized controlled trial of this new drug has not been performed. After initial treatment, patients probably have to be maintained on the drug to prevent recurrence. This is a considerable burden for the patient, since the drug is only available in IV form. A randomized controlled trial is being planned by Syntex.

The dosage regimen for treating CMV retinitis with ganciclovir is:
induction phase: 5 mg/kg every 12 hours for two weeks.
maintenance phase: 6 mg/kg per day, indefinitely.

An indication for treatment is sight-threatening CMV retinitis (retinitis involving — or near — the macula or fovea). Most clinicians discontinue zidovudine (AZT) if ganciclovir treatment is undertaken. A few patients have tolerated very low doses of AZT (e.g., 200 to 400 mg/day) during ganciclovir therapy; however, the risk of marrow suppression is very high. Patients to be treated with ganciclovir should have absolute neutrophil counts above 1000 cells/cubic mm. Side effects of ganciclovir include neutropenia (30 percent of patients), thrombocytopenia (occasional patients), rash and neurologic symptoms (rarely).

AZT therapy may complicate treatment of CMV retinitis. This anti-HIV drug is similar to ganciclovir in terms of toxicity, and their additive toxicities are unacceptable. This leads to a difficult dilemma when an AIDS patient on AZT develops CMV retinitis: the AZT must be stopped when ganciclovir is started. This is a difficult decision for patients and physicians faced with deciding between abandoning useful AZT therapy and treating progressive CMV retinitis, which often leads to blindness.

Untreated CMV retinitis usually progresses to complete blindness. Both eyes usually become involved. Treatment with ganciclovir or foscarnet is probably effective in altering this prognosis.

Research Prospects.   A controlled, randomized trial could establish the effectiveness of ganciclovir and foscarnet and any need for maintenance therapy. Oral rather than intravenous delivery of these drugs would greatly facilitate therapy. Eventually, a prospective, randomized treatment trial comparing ganciclovir to foscarnet needs to be performed.

Cytomegalovirus retinitis has also been treated with foscarnet.[23,24] This is also an intravenous drug. The main toxicity is renal. Clinical evidence suggests that foscarnet slows CMV retinitis much as ganciclovir does. Foscarnet is still being evaluated in Phase I studies and the optimal dose is not yet known. Foscarnet does not cause neutropenia and is compatible with AZT. It is also possible that AZT restores immune function, thus stabilizing CMV retinitis. The few reported cases of spontaneously stabilized retinitis may be instances of this effect.[25]

REFERENCES

1. Holland GN, Pepose JS, Pettit TH, et al. Acquired immune deficiency syndrome. Ocular manifestations. Ophthalmology 1983; 90:859-73.

2. Freeman WR, Lerner CW, Mines JA, et al. A prospective study of the ophthalmologic findings in the acquired immune deficiency syndrome. Am J Ophthalmol 1984; 97:133-42.

3. Holland GN. Ocular manifestations of the acquired immune deficiency syndrome. Int Ophthalmol Clin 1985; 25:179-87.

4. Schuman JS, Friedman AH. Retinal manifestations of the acquired immune deficiency syndrome (AIDS): cytomegalovirus, *Candida albicans*, cryptococcus, toxoplasmosis, and *Pneumocystis carinii*. Trans Ophthalmol Soc UK 1983; 103:177-90.

5. Pepose JS, Holland GN, Nestor MS, et al. Acquired immune deficiency syndrome: pathogenic mechanisms of ocular disease. Ophthalmology 1985; 92:472-84.

6. Newsome DA, Green WR, Miller ED, et al. Microvascular aspects of acquired immune deficiency syndrome retinopathy. Am J Ophthalmol 1984; 98:590-601.

7. Palestine AG, Rodrigues MM, Macher AM, et al. Ophthalmic involvement in acquired immune deficiency. Ophthalmology 1984; 91:1092-9.

8. Kwok S, O'Donnell JJ, Wood IS. Retinal cotton-wool spots in a patient with *Pneumocystis carinii* infection. N Engl J Med 1982; 307:184-5.

9. O'Donnell JJ, Kwok S, Wood IS. Retinal cotton-wool spots in acquired immunodeficiency syndrome. N Engl J Med 1982; 307:1705.

10. Holland GN, Gottlieb MS, Foos RY. Retinal cotton-wool patches in acquired immunodeficiency syndrome. N Engl J Med 1982; 307:1704.

11. Palestine AG, Stevens G, Lane HC, et al. Treatment of cytomegalovirus retinitis with dihydroxy propoxymethyl guanine. Am J Ophthalmol 1985; 101:95-101.

12. Felenstein D, D'Amico DJ, Hirsch MS, et al. Treatment of cytomegalovirus retinitis with 9-[2-dihydroxy-1 (hydroxymethyl) ethoxymethyl] guanine. Ann Intern Med 1985; 103:377-80.

13. Pepose JS, Nestor MS, Holland GN, et al. An analysis of retinal cotton-wool spots and cytomegalovirus retinitis in the acquired immune deficiency syndrome. Am J Ophthalmol 1983; 95:118-20.

14. O'Donnell JJ, Goodner EK, Shiba AH. A prospective study of eye disease in AIDS. Invest Ophthalmol Vis Sci 1986; 27:Suppl:122.

15. Mansour AM, Jampol LM, Logani S, et al. Cotton-wool spots in acquired immunodeficiency syndrome compared with diabetes mellitus, systemic hypertension, and central retinal vein occlusion. Arch Ophthalmol 1988; 106:1074-7.

16. Pomerantz RJ, Kuritzkes DR, de la Monte SM, et al. Infection of the retina by human immunodeficiency virus type I. N Engl J Med 1987; 317:1643-7.

17. Mills J, Jacobson MA, O'Donnell JJ, et al. Treatment of cytomegalovirus retinitis in patients with AIDS. Rev Inf Dis 1988; 10:Suppl 3:5522-31.

18. Jacobson MA, O'Donnell JJ, Brodie HR, et al. Randomized prospective trial of ganciclovir maintenance therapy for cytomegalovirus retinitis. J Med Virol 1988; 25:339-49.

19. Holland GN, Sidikaro Y, Kreiger AE, et al. Treatment of cytomegalovirus retinopathy with ganciclovir. Ophthalmology 1987; 94:815-23.

20. Henderly DE, Freeman WR, Causey DM, Rao NA. Cytomegalovirus retinitis and response to therapy with ganciclovir. Ophthalmology 1987; 94:425-34.

21. Treatment of serious cytomegalovirus infections with 9-(1,3-dihydroxy-2-propoxymethyl) guanine in patients with AIDS and other immunodeficiencies. Collaborative DHPG Treatment Study Group. N Engl J Med 1986; 314:801-5.

22. Jabs DA, Newman C, De Bustros S, Polk BF. Treatment of cytomegalovirus retinitis with ganciclovir. Ophthalmology 1987; 94:824-30.

23. Jacobson MA, O'Donnell JJ, Mills J. Foscarnet treatment of cytomegalovirus in patients with the acquired immunodeficiency syndrome. Antimicrob Agents Chemother 1989; 33:736-41.

24. Walmsley SL, Chew E, Read SE, et al. Treatment of cytomegalovirus retinitis with trisodium phosphonoformate hexahydrate (foscarnet). J Infect Dis 1988; 157:569-72.

25. Fay MT, Freeman WR, Wiley CA, et al. Atypical retinitis in patients with the acquired immunodeficiency syndrome. Am J Ophthalmol 1988; 105:483-90.

5.12

Otolaryngologic Aspects

5.12.1 Otolaryngologic Manifestations — *Sooy*

Otolaryngologic Manifestations

C. Daniel Sooy, M.D.

A IDS can manifest itself 41 percent to 71 percent of the time in the oto-laryngologic (ENT) head and neck area,[1-8] and as clinical experience increases, this approaches 100 percent during the course of HIV infection. Because of the nature and frequency of otolaryngologic presentations, an overview of the problems encountered is valuable to both the otolaryngologist and the primary care physician. Not only individuals with AIDS but also those with ARC and a lesser degree of HIV infection can be similarly affected. Common disease entities, when seen in these patients, can be due to unusual organisms and may require different therapeutic approaches. Certainly the most common complaints that patients with AIDS and ARC have in the order of decreasing frequency are dysphagia or odynophagia, sinusitis and postnasal drip, neck masses, nasal obstruction, and otologic problems, including infection and hearing loss.

Because the literature in many of these areas is just evolving, approaches to treatment are often determined by basic precepts or the clinical experience of physicians in large medical centers such as San Francisco General Hospital.

Additional considerations are HIV infection control precautions concerning secretions found in the head and neck.[9]

■ THE EAR

ACUTE OTITIS MEDIA

In the nonimmunosuppressed population, acute otitis media, or infection in the middle ear, is one of the most common diseases of childhood and usually manifests itself as ear pain and hearing loss. It is thought to be primarily due to eustachian tube dysfunction caused by upper respiratory infection and allergy in the pediatric population, and by upper respiratory infection, allergy, and nasopharyngeal tumors in the adult population. The usual etiologic agents are pneumococcus, β-hemolytic streptococcus, *Haemophilus influenzae*, *Branhamella catarrhalis*, and staphylococcus. Gram-negative bacteria are found more frequently in the neonate and the immunosuppressed.

Acute otitis media has been reported in pediatric AIDS patients[8,10-13] and can be the presenting manifestation.[5,8] The infection may be more common in this population, reflecting B-cell abnormalities,[14] or it may simply be the initial event prompting medical evaluation. Acute otitis media has been reported in the HIV-infected adult population,[4,15] but without apparent increase in incidence. Eustachian tube dysfunction appears common in both pediatric and adult AIDS populations, possibly due to HIV or recurrent upper respiratory tract viral infection. The extensive benign reactive lymphoid hyperplasia commonly seen as adenopathy can also involve the adenoidal tissue and lead to extensive adenoidal hypertrophy, obstruction, and eustachian tube dysfunction. Finally, nasopharyngeal tumors, which are almost exclusively Kaposi's sarcoma (KS), can contribute to eustachian dysfunction.

The actual role of allergy in HIV-associated acute otitis media is unclear, but AIDS patients do have increased eosinophilia and viral infections. Viral infections have been suggested by some authors to precipitate allergies.[10,15] More recent information suggests that allergy is almost twice as common in HIV-infected patients (Goetzl E: personal communication).

The bacteriology of acute otitis media in AIDS is not well defined; however, *Haemophilus influenzae* has been cultured in children and *Streptococcus pneumoniae* in adults with AIDS.[10,15] Thus, it would seem likely that the bacteriology of acute otitis media in AIDS patients may be similar to that in the non-AIDS population, with the exception that there may be more viral, fungal, and mycobacterial infections in patients with AIDS.

Because of the high likelihood of uncommon or resistant pathogens in AIDS patients, tympanocentesis to obtain material for bacterial culture should be considered before initiating therapy.

SEROUS OTITIS MEDIA

Serous otitis media is the most common cause of hearing loss in the non-AIDS pediatric population and is due to eustachian tube dysfunction, resolving acute otitis media, or both. It typically appears as hearing loss and aural fullness. There is no prospective evidence to date to suggest that this disease is more prevalent in children with AIDS than in other children. However, it does appear to be more common in adults with AIDS than in nonimmunosuppressed adults (author's personal experience). Serous otitis media and decreased eustachian tube function are presumably caused by viral infections (including HIV infection, which results in benign reactive hyperplasia of the adenoids), adenoidal hypertrophy, nasopharyngeal tumors, and possibly allergy.[16]

Treatment should be a trial of broad-spectrum antibiotics (e.g., Augmentin ([amoxicillin/clavulanate potassium] 500 mg tid for 10 days) and decongestants, followed by early myringotomy and ventilation-tube placement. Precautions to guard against HIV should be observed, since this virus has been cultured from samples of middle-ear fluid (Sooy, Evans, Levy: unpublished data). Finally, the patient should also have a careful nasopharyngeal exam to rule out tumor.

EXTERNAL OTITIS AND MALIGNANT EXTERNAL OTITIS

External otitis is an inflammation, usually bacterial or fungal in origin, of the external ear canal causing pain, drainage, and, occasionally, hearing loss. Bacterial external otitis occurs secondary to maceration from water or abrasion from trauma. It has been reported in AIDS patients[17] but, in our experience, has not been as common as one would expect. Fungal external otitis in AIDS patients is clearly more aggressive in this setting. We have seen complete bilateral erosion of the entire eardrum due to aspergillus external otitis. Malignant external otitis, a *Pseudomonas aeruginosa* osteitis of the skull base that is most commonly seen in diabetics, has been reported in a pediatric AIDS patient.[18]

Treatment should consist of local debridement of fungus, followed by application of topical antifungal agents on a daily basis until control is obtained. Should this fail, oral agents (ketoconazole 200 mg bid) and antifungal cultures and sensitivities may be necessary.

Dermatologic conditions that affect the rest of the body may also affect the skin of the ear canal. In our experience, seborrheic dermatitis is probably the most common dermatologic problem affecting the external auditory canal in AIDS patients. A conventional approach using a steroid cream (0.1 percent triamcinolone cream alone, applied twice daily) or otic drops (Tridesilon otic drops) is effective.

MASTOIDITIS

Mastoiditis has been seen in the AIDS population.[4,51] It can occur as an extension of acute otitis media that has been untreated or inadequately treated. It does not appear to be more common in AIDS patients than in the nonimmunosuppressed population.

Hospital admission and empiric treatment with antibiotics effective against *H. influenzae*, *S. pneumoniae*, and streptococcal strains of bacteria (e.g., cefuroxime) should be initiated after material for bacterial culture is obtained by tympanocentesis.

Radiographs of the involved mastoid should be obtained and if coalescence of the mastoid airspaces is found, then surgical drainage is indicated.

TUMORS OF THE EAR

In our experience, tumors of the ear almost exclusively consist of KS in AIDS patients. Non-Hodgkin's lymphoma of the earlobe has also been reported.[19] KS occurs more often in the auricle, less commonly in the external auditory canal, and least commonly in the tympanic membrane and middle ear. When KS involves the external canal, tympanic membranes, or middle ear, it can be accompanied by hearing loss.

Laser therapy is usually ideal for localized palliation. Obstructive disease of the external auditory canal secondary to tumor can be well managed by carbon dioxide or argon laser therapy. We find argon laser treatment most effective in cases in which the tumor extends onto the tympanic membrane, where it can be ablated without perforation. Radiation therapy is excellent for regional disease and probably is the treatment of choice for middle-ear involvement. Systemic treatment with chemotherapy can give excellent partial and complete responses for middle-ear involvement or when there are other areas of involvement.

HEARING LOSS

Some hearing loss of 25 db or better across the range of 250 to 8000 Hz occurred in 49 percent of 35 AIDS and ARC patients over the course of their disease.[20] This was confirmed in a study of seropositive active duty military recruits, suggesting some relationship to the stage of HIV infection.[52] The loss was mostly high-frequency sensory neural hearing loss (moderate to severe in 14 percent). Auditory brain-stem response was abnormal in 78 percent of 9 patients demonstrating latency greater than 2 standard deviations and having a highly degraded wave form.[20] This condition is not unlike demyelinating disease and is probably due to vascular myelopathy similar to that described by Petito et al.,[21] possibly secondary to HIV. Auditory brain-stem response suggests some hearing loss could be central in etiology and may provide a noninvasive marker for CNS disease and treatment.[53] Conductive hearing loss as a complication of AIDS is usually due to serous effusion of the middle ear or KS involving the external canal, drum, or middle ear. *Pneumocystis carinii* granulomas have been reported obstructing the canal.[54] This has responded to local excision and treatment with Septra. It has been suggested that this should be an index opportunistic disease for AIDS.

Sensorineural hearing loss in AIDS patients can easily be multifactorial. Certainly viral infection can be the cause; cytomegalovirus (CMV) has been well documented to cause hearing loss. CMV can be cultured in almost 100 percent of AIDS patients and is a major cause of organ dysfunction. Other viral infections may well include HIV, which has been shown to also be neurotrophic.[22,23] Fungal and mycobacterial infections of the ear have been observed to cause hearing loss in the non-AIDS population. Meningitis, which is relatively common in AIDS patients, is a well-recognized cause of hearing loss in non-AIDS patients.[24] Iatrogenic hearing loss could occur secondary to drug administration from antitumor agents (e.g., vincristine), antifungal agents (e.g., amphotericin), and antiviral agents and immune modulators (e.g., isoprinosine). All are used in treating AIDS patients. These drugs have all been documented to cause sensorineural hearing loss in the non-AIDS population. Another agent used for viral infections (2'-fluoro-5-iodo-aracytosine) has been documented to be neurotoxic in the AIDS patient and consequently is a possible source of hearing loss.[25]

Evaluation for hearing loss should proceed along conventional lines, using audiogram, auditory brain-stem response, and computed tomography (CT) or magnetic resonance imaging (MRI) scanning. It must be kept in mind that auditory brain-stem response can be abnormal in the AIDS or ARC patient even if hearing is normal (Sooy and Gardi: unpublished data). Blood work, cultures, and evaluation of cerebrospinal fluid should be done on an individual basis to rule out infectious etiologies. Syphilis has been responsible for hearing loss in AIDS but whether it is more common in this group is unclear.[55] Aggressive aural rehabilitation with hearing aids and assistive devices should be instituted whenever a significant loss is detected. Vertigo is not commonly reported in patients with HIV disease.[56] While it may be uncommon, it is more likely to be submerged in the multitude of symptoms seen in these patients.

■ FACIAL NERVE PARALYSIS

Paralysis of the seventh cranial nerve can occur in association with inflammatory neuropathies in AIDS and ARC patients,[26] and with other causes.[2,27] Cranial neuropathies secondary to central nervous system infections and tumors have been well documented in AIDS patients and should be considered. We have noted Ramsey–Hunt syndrome or herpes oticus with facial paralysis in both primary herpes zoster and recurrent zoster. Treatment for zoster is the administration of acyclovir (2 to 3 g per day divided into 5 doses), and following the paralysis with electrical testing. The use of steroids is controversial, particularly in this clinical setting.

■ NOSE AND PARANASAL SINUSES

We have observed large herpetic crusting nasal ulcers (up to 4 cm across) in five AIDS patients. The ulcers involved the nasal alae, vestibule, and perinasal skin. Four of the five patients responded to oral or intravenous acyclovir (2 g by mouth in 5 divided doses or 5 mg/kg every 8 hours); one patient whose virus was acyclovir-resistant in vitro did not respond to this treatment.

KS of the nasal mucosa occurs, but is rarely an isolated clinical problem. It usually can be treated symptomatically by laser or electrocauterization.

Epistaxis occurs primarily in individuals who have idiopathic thrombocytopenic purpura (ITP) or nasal–nasopharyngeal KS and it is managed in the same fashion as epistaxis in other coagulopathies or tumors. If a single bleeding point can be identified, it should be cauterized instead of packed. When packing is necessary, it is best done with salt pork carved to the size of the nasal vault and placed there with firm pressure. Over the next two days, the fat will render and the pack will loosen and come out easily. If salt pork is not available, gelfoam pledgets soaked with thrombin should be placed on the area of bleeding. Packing should be inserted as a backing if necessary.

Nasal obstruction can be due to KS, allergy, viral infection, or nasopharyngeal blockage by tumor.

Postnasal drip is frequently secondary to sinusitis but may have an allergic basis or be due to viral infection. When an allergic basis is suspected, topical therapy with Nasalcrom ([cromolyn sodium nasal solution, USP] 1 puff each nostril 3 times a day) should be the first treatment tried. Although steroid inhalers have not been shown to cause significant systemic suppression, the concern that they may increase immunosuppression makes them a theoretical second-choice treatment. However, we have used them frequently with much success and no complications (beclomethasone nasal spray, qd or tid).

Sinusitis is frequently a finding in AIDS or ARC patients. A number of lymphadenopathy patients seen by Dr. Donald Abrams at our institution have had this condition. Although there is only a small amount of data upon which to base empiric therapy,[10,15,28] a wide range of etiologic agents was found, including the bacterial agents *Haemophilus influenzae*, *Streptococcus pneumoniae*, *Trichomonas vaginalis*, *Staphylococcus aureus*, and *Legionella pneumophila*. Influenza virus was only recovered once. The most frequently cultured bacterial organisms were *H. influenzae* and *S. pneumoniae*. The most frequently cultured fungal organism was *Pseudoallescheria boydii*, and it was found to be as common as either of the bacterial pathogens in one series of 12 patients.[28]

Because of the diagnostic and therapeutic value of sinus irrigation, this treatment should be initiated early, particularly in the patient who is febrile, lethargic, or otherwise toxic in appearance. Culture should be analyzed for anaerobes, aerobes, legionella, viral, mycobacterial, and fungal organisms. Initial coverage should be based upon a smear of the sinus aspirate, when possible. If the intranasal exam reveals areas that are white, necrotic, or do not blanch, aggressive fungal infection is possible and a surgical drainage of the maxillary sinus by a Caldwell-Luc procedure and local debridement may be necessary. Consultation with an otolaryngologist is also helpful when the ethmoid, frontal, and sphenoid sinuses are involved. It is also important to recognize that both KS[28] and lymphoma have been reported to occur in the maxillary sinus of AIDS patients (Ziegler JL: personal communication).

■ NASOPHARYNX

The nasopharyngeal complications of AIDS are primarily related to obstruction, which can be caused by benign reactive hypertrophy of the adenoid pad secondary to HIV infection. The pad may completely fill the nasopharynx to the point of obstruction and cause recurrent nasopharyngitis. This has a distinct radiographic appearance that is homogeneous with symmetrical borders.[57] In this situation, conventional adenoidectomy is valuable; at surgery, a fresh specimen should be examined by a pathologist to rule out lymphoma. Obstruction can be secondary to tumor, which is most commonly KS. However, lymphoma of the nasopharynx should be suspected, since 89 percent of lymphomas in AIDS patients are extranodal.[19] Involvement in the nasopharynx accounts for 15 percent of the extranodal lymphomas occurring in the head and neck area of non-AIDS patients.[29]

Removal of localized tumor for symptomatic relief is best done by laser or suction cautery. For diffuse KS of the nasopharynx, radiation therapy is the treatment of choice unless there are plans to use systemic chemotherapy because of tumor in other locations.

■ ORAL AND OROPHARYNGEAL COMPLICATIONS

The oral cavity is probably the most common site of involvement in the head and neck for tumor and opportunistic infections in AIDS patients. Complaints of dysphagia and odynophagia usually bring patients to the otolaryngologist.

The oral lesions that cause dysphagia and odynophagia in AIDS can be divided into lesions of opportunistic infections (oral candidiasis, herpetic stomatitis, hairy leukoplakia, aphthous stomatitis, and other less common infections, such as *Mycobacterium avium-intracellulare*),[30] and tumors (KS, lymphoma, and squamous-cell carcinoma).[58]

Thrush or oral candidiasis, with its white pseudomembrane, is the most common oral opportunistic infection in AIDS. However, it may also assume an erythematous atrophic form. Oral candidiasis was found to be a harbinger of AIDS in 59 percent of high-risk patients studied by Klein.[31] If the patient has substernal pain, esophageal candidiasis should be suspected, since AIDS and ARC patients who have oral candidiasis may have concomitant esophageal candidiasis that requires treatment with ketoconazole.[32]

Mycelex troches ([clotrimazole] five times a day for two weeks) are effective treatment for acute oral candidiasis, but maintenance therapy is often necessary because this infection is frequently a chronic problem. Chelosis is common and also responds to anticandidal therapy.

Viral lesions are most commonly herpetic in etiology,[6] but we have cultured CMV. These lesions are often larger than would normally be expected and are characterized by a small rim of erythema around a necrotic center.

Giant intraoral ulcers commonly occur and may possibly be major aphthous ulcers. They may be quite large (up to 2 or 3 cm) and characteristically have a long, protracted clinical course. Large oral ulcers that are culture- and pathology-negative for an infectious process sometimes respond to Diprolene mixed with Orabase or dexamethasone elixir (given qid) without resorting to systemic steroid treatment. It is important to biopsy and culture those lesions that do not show improvement in 10 days, as erosive lymphomas can look similar.[58]

Hairy leukoplakia is a slightly raised, "hairy"-appearing white lesion most commonly found on the lateral border of the tongue.[33] The etiology is most likely the Epstein–Barr virus, which has been identified within the epithelial cells. Although this lesion is usually asymptomatic, treatment with acyclovir will give temporary resolution should it become a symptomatic problem. In a study of 110 high-risk patients who did not have AIDS at the time that hairy leukoplakia was diagnosed, 25 percent went on to develop AIDS.[34] Numerous other unusual infectious agents (e.g., MAI) less commonly occur.

HIV-associated salivary gland disease with parotid enlargement and xerostomia is a hallmark of pediatric AIDS. Whether it is directly associated with HIV or a Sjögren's-like phenomenon is unclear.

Squamous-cell carcinoma has been reported in AIDS patients,[35] who are appreciably younger than most patients who contract this tumor. It is noteworthy that these patients tend to fare poorly compared with older, nonimmunosuppressed patients who have tumors of a comparable stage (Sooy CD, Marinsen DC: unpublished data).

Treatment should be the same as for other epidermoid carcinomas of the head and neck of similar Tumor, Node, Metastasis (TNM) classification, keeping in mind the underlying disease.

Mucocutaneous KS of the oral cavity is common in AIDS. The hard palate is involved most frequently,[4] but occurrence anywhere in the oral cavity is not unusual. Additionally, occurrence in Waldeyer's ring, particularly the tonsils, is common.

Tonsillar enlargement occurs in both pediatric[36] and adult AIDS patients. Most commonly, it represents benign reactive lymphoid hyperplasia. The second most common cause is tonsillar involvement with KS, which can resemble acute infectious tonsillitis. Other portions of Waldeyer's ring can be similarly involved with KS.

Tonsillitis does occur, but as of yet does not appear to be more common. However, *Streptococcus pneumoniae* and *Haemophilus influenzae* take advantage of B-cell defects, and *Staphylococcus aureus* tends to persist in AIDS patients for reasons that are unclear.[37] Because of these considerations, one might expect tonsillitis to be more common.

There have been cases of tonsillar involvement with extranodal lymphoma (Ziegler J: personal communication). One should always watch for unilateral tonsillar enlargement or asymmetry. However, tonsillar lymphoma may also occur as an erosive, unilateral, or bilateral lesion. Tonsillectomy has a diagnostic role as a biopsy. It has been suggested as a cofactor predisposing to the development of severe infection in HIV-positive patients,[38] but it is probably a demographic coincidence.

Isolated exophytic oral lesions of KS are best treated with laser therapy, whereas the treatment for more extensive disease is radiation therapy or systemic chemotherapy. Intralesional chemotherapy with vinblastine sulfate (Velban) can be an effective alternative treatment with reduced systemic dosage. After a test dose of 0.01 mg to determine a response, a dose between 0.01 mg and 0.04 mg is used per square centimeter of lesion. The dose is administered with an allergist syringe (Conant MA: personal communication). It is important to remember that AIDS patients are susceptible to severe radiation mucositis, which requires a reduction in dose and prophylaxis for candida. Prophylaxis for herpetic infection should also be carried out if a strong history of this infection exists.

Lymphoma in the AIDS patient tends to be diagnosed at a later stage, and frequently involves the central nervous system. It tends to be extranodal and has a poor prognosis.[19] Most of the reports of lymphomas in the upper aerodigestive tract have noted their presence in the jaw, mandible, gingiva,[19,35,39] or tonsils. This suggests that extranodal lymphomas of the head and neck in AIDS patients may involve Waldeyer's ring less frequently than in non-AIDS patients. In non-AIDS patients there is a 66 percent incidence of extranodal lymphomas of the head and neck involving Waldeyer's ring.[29] Perhaps lymphoma is being underdiagnosed at this site. Tonsillar asymmetry should be considered as a possible first indication of lymphoma.

■ HYPOPHARYNX AND LARYNX

Lesions of the hypopharynx and larynx are common and often occur as dysphagia, odynophagia, or hoarseness. Candidal hypopharyngitis and laryngitis are less common than oral candida. Their presence does not necessarily correlate with that of candidal esophagitis; in fact, the hypopharynx can be relatively clear in the presence of significant candidal esophagitis. Treatment for candidal esophagitis or hypopharyngitis with ketoconazole should be initiated if symptoms are minimal. This treatment is also worthwhile for sore throat of unknown etiology.

Therapy for candida should be initiated with ketoconazole if the patient is not responding to Mycelex. For the patient who has extensive hypopharyngeal disease or significant substernal pain, esophagoscopy should be performed to rule out esophageal candidiasis, CMV, or herpetic infections. Viral infections of the hypopharynx and larynx are usually herpetic and can often be seen on indirect laryngoscopy. Should these infections fail to respond to a trial of acyclovir, direct laryngoscopy with biopsy and viral cultures may be necessary. CMV infection of the larynx has been reported.[40]

KS of the hypopharynx,[41,42] in our experience, is more common than KS of the larynx.[41,43] The most common site is the base of the tongue, but lesions may be located anywhere in the hypopharynx. They may be single, multiple, sessile, pedunculated, or massive enough to cause airway obstruction necessitating tracheotomy. Isolated or obstructing lesions are best palliated by laser alone or suction electrocautery before removal. Radiation therapy works well for more extensive local or regional disease. Chemotherapy is effective for regional or systemic disease.

We have not yet seen extranodal lymphomas in the hypopharynx (lingual tonsils) in AIDS patients. However, because it is the site of 12 percent of extranodal lymphomas in non-AIDS patients,[29] the base of the tongue should be carefully examined for asymmetry. Persistent hoarseness in AIDS patients is usually due to edema from lymphatic obstruction from tumor, chronic cough, or candidiasis of the larynx. Hoarseness may also be due to vocal cord involvement with KS. Management can require emergency airway control and laser resection followed by radiation if the patient is not going to receive chemotherapy. Vocal cord paralysis has been noted in two patients due to CMV involvement of the recurrent nerve. Vocal cord paralysis due to vincristine or vinblastine therapy for KS resolved after discontinuation of the vinca alkaloids. Vocal cord paralysis from vincristine or vinblastine has only been previously documented in non-AIDS patients.[44] This paralysis must be evaluated locally and as a cranial neuropathy in AIDS patients.

■ NECK MASSES

Neck masses are ubiquitous in HIV infection and are most frequently the result of adenopathy. Cervical adenopathy secondary to the benign reactive hyperplasia[45] caused by HIV is most commonly located in the posterior triangle.[46] Stable adenopathy should be monitored every 3 to 6 months and the same biopsy criteria should be used as for other neck masses. When patients move from ARC to full-blown clinical AIDS, their adenopathy may decrease. Of particular concern is the neck mass that is rapidly enlarging, tender, or predominant in size, since it can indicate tumor or opportunistic infection. The most common tumor is KS, which occurs in the lymph nodes; it can be easily identified on fine-needle aspiration. Second in frequency is non-Hodgkin's lymphoma, which may require open biopsy for definitive diagnosis.

Clinical guidelines for biopsy include (1) a rapidly enlarging mass, (2) a tender mass, (3) a mass that is larger than adjacent nodes, and (4) a node in a patient who has a change in his systemic symptoms. If FNA shows granulomas without organisms, or is nondiagnostic, open biopsy should be performed after adequate head and neck evaluation including nasopharyngoscopy and laryngoscopy.

Parotid enlargement is seen in both adults[4,47] and children.[11,12,48,49] In adults, parotid enlargement is usually discrete with a mass. Parotid enlargement is relatively unique to pediatric AIDS patients and is often diffuse. The etiology is unclear, but diffuse parotid enlargement could result from a Sjögren's-like syndrome, cytomegalovirus infection,[4] or could be due to HIV infection.[50]

Management of parotid enlargement should start with a decision as to whether the mass is diffuse or discrete. A discrete mass should be fine needle biopsied and treated on that basis. The diffusely enlarged parotid should be scanned by MRI. Should the mass become hard or increase rapidly in size, lymphoma or infection must be considered. If the mass is not hard or rapidly enlarging, the likelihood of lymphoma is lessened and the mass can be followed until more is known about this lesion. However, the risk of lymphoma does exist and the patient may elect to have the lesion removed.[59]

REFERENCES

1. Lanser MJ, Klein HZ, Marvin A. Pathologic quiz. Arch Otolaryngol 1985; 111:486.

2. Rosenberg RA, Schneider KL, Cohen NL. Head and neck presentations of acquired immunodeficiency syndrome. Laryngoscope 1984; 94:642-6.

3. Rosenberg RA, Schneider KL, Cohen NL. Head and neck presentations of acquired immunodeficiency syndrome. Otolaryngol Head Neck Surg 1985; 93:700-5.

4. Marcusen DC, Sooy CD. Otolaryngologic and head and neck manifestations of acquired immunodeficiency syndrome (AIDS). Laryngoscope 1985; 95:401-5.

5. Abemyor E, Calcaterra TC. Kaposi's sarcoma and acquired immunodeficiency syndrome: an update with emphasis on head and neck manifestations. Arch Otolaryngol 1983; 109:536-42.

6. Patow CA, Lewis DM, Macher AM. Infections and neoplastic manifestations in acquired immunodeficiency syndrome. New dimensions in otolaryngology. Vol. 2. Head and neck surgery. New York: Elsevier Science Publishers, 1985; 805-6.

7. Napier BL, McTighe AH, Snow TF, et al. Acquired immune deficiency syndrome presenting as oral pharyngeal and cutaneous sarcoma. Laryngoscope 1983; 93:1466-9.

8. Cooke D, Jahn A, Oleske J. Ear, nose and throat manifestations in acquired immune deficiency syndrome in children. Otolaryngol Head Neck Surg 1985; 94:68.

9. Sooy CD, Gerberding JL, Kaplan MJ. The risk for otolaryngologists who treat patients with AIDS and AIDS virus infection: report of an in-process study. Laryngoscope 1987; 97:430-4.

10. Church J, Durrani FK. Otitis media and sinusitis as a presentation of AIDS. Ann Allergy 1987. abstract.

11. Rubinstein A, Sicklick M, Gupta A, et al. Acquired immunodeficiency with reversed T4/T8 ratios in infants born to promiscuous and drug addicted mothers. JAMA 1983; 249:2350-6.

12. Ammann AJ. Is there an acquired immune deficiency syndrome in infants and children? Pediatrics 1983; 72:430-2.

13. Hellmann D, Cowan MJ, Ammann AJ, et al. Chronic active Epstein Barr virus infections in two immunodeficient patients. Clin Lab Observations 1983; 103:585-8.

14. Ammann AJ, Schiffman G, Abrams D, et al. B-cell immunodeficiency in acquired immune deficiency syndrome. JAMA 1984; 251:1447-54.

15. Poole MD, Postma D, Cohen MS. Pyogenic otorhinologic infections in acquired immune deficiency syndrome. Arch Otolaryngol 1984; 110:130-1.

16. Frick OL. Role of viral infections in asthma and allergy. Clin Rev Allergy 1983; 1:5-17.

17. Cooke D, Jahn A, Oleske J. Ear, nose, and throat manifestations in acquired immune deficiency syndrome in children. Program, Am Acad Otolaryngology — Head and Neck Surgery, Atlanta, October 1985.

18. Scott GB, Buck BE, Leterman JG, et al. Acquired immunodeficiency syndrome in infants. N Engl J Med 1984; 310:76-81.

19. Ziegler JL, Beckstead JA, Volberding PA, et al. Non-Hodgkin's lymphadenopathy and the acquired immunodeficiency syndrome. N Engl J Med 1984; 311:565-70.

20. Sooy D, Gardi J. Hearing loss in AIDS and ARC [Abstract]. Western Section Meeting, American Trilogic Society, Los Angeles, January 3, 1987.

21. Petito CK, Bradford AN, Cho E-S, et al. Vacuolar myelopathy pathologically resembling subacute combined degeneration in patients with the acquired immunodeficiency syndrome. N Engl J Med 1985; 312:874-9.

22. Ho DD, Rota TR, Schooley RT, et al. Isolation of HTLV-III from cerebrospinal fluid and neural tissues of patients with neurological syndromes related to the acquired immunodeficiency syndrome. N Engl J Med 1985; 313:1493-7.

23. Black PH. HTLV-III, AIDS, and the brain. N Engl J Med 1985; 313:1538-9.

24. Dodge PR, Davis H, Feigin RD, et al. Prospective evaluation of hearing impairment as a sequela of acute bacterial meningitis. N Engl J Med 1984; 311:869-74.

25. Gold JWM, Leyland-Jones B, Urmacher C, Armstrong D. Pulmonary and neurologic complications of treatment with *FIAC* (2'-fluoro-5-iodo-aracytosine) in patients with acquired immune deficiency syndrome (AIDS). AIDS Res 1984; 1:243-52.

26. Lipkin WI, Parry G, Kiprov D, Abrams D. Inflammatory neuropathy in homosexual men with lymphadenopathy. Neurology 1985; 35:1479-83.

27. Levy RM, Bredesen DE, Rosenblum ML. Neurological manifestations of the acquired immunodeficiency syndrome (AIDS): experience at UCSF and review of the literature. J Neurosurg 1985; 62:475-95.

28. Marcusen DC, Sooy CD. Bacteriology and treatment of sinusitis in the acquired immunodeficiency syndrome (unpublished).

29. Jacobs C, Weiss L, Hoppe RT. The management of extranodal head and neck lymphomas. Arch Otolaryngol Head Neck Surg 1986; 112:654-8.

30. Volpe F, Schwinmer A, Barr C. Oral manifestation of disseminated *Mycobacterium avium-intracellulare* in a patient with AIDS. Oral Surg Oral Med Oral Pathol 1985; 60:567-70.

31. Klein RS, Harris CA, Small CB, et al. Oral candidiasis in high-risk patients as the initial manifestation of the acquired immunodeficiency syndrome. N Engl J Med 1984; 311:354-8.

32. Tavitian A, Raufman JP, Rosenthal LE. Oral candidiasis as a marker for esophageal candidiasis in the acquired immunodeficiency syndrome. Ann Intern Med 1986; 104:54-5.

33. Greenspan JS, Greenspan D, Lennette ET, et al. Replication of Epstein—Barr virus within the epithelial cells of oral "hairy" leukoplakia, an AIDS-associated lesion. N Engl J Med 1985; 313:1564-71.

34. Epidemiologic notes and reports. Oral viral lesions (hairy leukoplakia) associated with the acquired immunodeficiency syndrome. MMWR 1985; 34:549-50.

35. Lozada F, Silverman S Jr, Conant M. New outbreak of oral tumors, malignancies and infectious diseases strikes young male homosexuals. J Calif Dent Assoc 1982; 10:39-42.

36. Hellman D, Cowan MJ, Ammann AJ, et al. Chronic active Epstein Barr virus infections in two immunodeficient patients. J Pediatr 1983; 103:585-8.

37. Armstrong D, Gold JWM, Dryjanski J, et al. Treatment of infections in patients with the acquired immunodeficiency syndrome. Ann Intern Med 1985; 103:738-43.

38. McCombie SC. Tonsillectomy as a co-factor in the development of AIDS. Med Hypotheses 1986; 19:291-3.

39. Figlin RA, Mariguchi JD, Coffey RA, Seijo O. Kaposi's sarcoma and immunoblastic sarcoma in the acquired immune deficiency syndrome. JAMA 1984; 251:342-3.

40. Jensen OA, Gerstoft J, Thomsen HK, Morner K. Cytomegalovirus retinitis in the acquired immunodeficiency syndrome (AIDS). Light-microscopical, ultrastructural and immunohistochemical examination of a case. Acta Ophthalmol 1984; 62:1-9.

41. Sooy CD, Ho COM, Wall SD. Spectrum of Kaposi's sarcoma of the hypopharynx in AIDS: its diagnosis, evaluation and management. In: Myers E, ed. New dimensions in otorhinolaryngology — head and neck surgery. Vol. 2. New York: Elsevier Science Publishers, 1985; 602-3.

42. Patow CA, Stark TW, Findlay PA, et al. Pharyngeal obstruction by Kaposi's sarcoma in a homosexual male with acquired immune deficiency syndrome. Otolaryngol Head Neck Surg 1984; 92:713-6.

43. Pitcock JK, Parey SE, Schwartz MR, Smith R. Kaposi's sarcoma of the larynx. Program, Am Acad Otolaryngology — Head and Neck Surgery, Atlanta, 1985; 81-2.

44. Delaney P. Vincristine induced laryngeal nerve paralysis. Neurology 1982; 32:1285-8.

45. Finkbeiner WE, Egbert BM, Groundwater TR, Sagebiel RW. Kaposi's sarcoma in young homosexual men. Arch Pathol Lab Med 1982; 106:261-4.

46. Abrams DI. Lymphadenopathy syndrome in male homosexuals. In: Gallin JI, Fauci AS, eds. Advances in host defense mechanisms. Vol. 5. New York: Raven Press, 1985; 75-97.

47. Ryan JR, Ioachim HL, Marmer J, Loubea JM. Acquired immune deficiency syndrome — related lymphadenopathies presenting in the salivary gland lymph nodes. Arch Otolaryngol 1985; 111:554-6.

48. Ammann A. AIDS in children. West J Med 1986; 145:230-1.

49. Ammann AJ. The acquired immunodeficiency syndrome in infants and children. Ann Intern Med 1985; 103:734-7.

50. Lecatsas G, Houff S, Macher A. Retrovirus-like particles in salivary glands, prostate and testes of AIDS patients. Proc Soc Exp Biol Med 1985; 178:653-5.

51. Kohan D, Rothstein SG, Cohen NL. Otologic disease in patients with acquired immunodeficiency syndrome. Ann Otol Rhinol Laryngol 1988; 97:636-40.

52. Bell AF, Atkins JS, Zajac R, et al. HIV and sensorineural hearing loss [Abstract]. IV International Conference on AIDS, Stockholm, 1988:7009.

53. Comi G, Medaglini T, Localtelli V, et al. Multimodality evoked potentials in acquired immunodeficiency syndrome. In: Berber C, Blum T, eds. Evoked Potentials III, 1987.

54. Breda SD, Gigliotti F, Hammerschlag PE, et al. *Pneumocystis carinii* in the temporal bone as a primary manifestation of the acquired immunodeficiency syndrome. American Otological Society Program, 1987:26. abstract.

55. Berry CD, Hooton TM, Collier AC, et al. Neurologic relapse after benzathine penicillin therapy for secondary syphilis in a patient with HIV infection. N Engl J Med 1987; 316:1587-9.

56. Geltma CL, Schupbach JE. Neuro-audiologic findings of a patient with acquired immune deficiency syndrome. ASHA 1986; 26:76.

57. Olsen WL, Jeffrey RB Jr, Sooy CD, et al. Lesions of the head and neck in patients with AIDS: CT and MR findings. AJR 1988; 151:785-90.

58. Greenspan JS, Greenspan D, Winkler JR. Diagnosis and management of the oral manifestations of HIV infection and AIDS. Infect Dis Clin North Am 1988; 2:373-85.

59. Shugar JM, Som PM, Jacobson AL, et al. Multicentric parotid cysts and cervical adenopathy in AIDS patients. A newly recognized entity: CT and MR manifestations. Laryngoscope 1988; 98:772-5.

5.13

Psychiatric Aspects

Psychosocial Impact of AIDS: Overview

James Dilley, M.D.

T his chapter provides an overview of the social and psychological problems facing people with AIDS. It describes coping mechanisms for patients and addresses the psychological issues faced by patients at different stages of their illness.

The social and psychological problems confronting an individual with AIDS can be enormous. These psychosocial problems and the unique medical uncertainty surrounding the disease combine to make AIDS different from virtually any other medical problem facing contemporary health-care providers. Certain psychosocial issues set AIDS patients apart from patients with other life-threatening illnesses.

It is well known that patients with AIDS are often stigmatized and subsequently experience social and emotional isolation. The stigma is multifaceted, and is partly due to attributes of the disease and partly to the social standing of the groups most commonly afflicted.

- AIDS is a new and complicated disease that is not well understood by the general population. Well-intentioned but uninformed individuals can have unfounded fears of contagion and be restrained toward people with AIDS.
- AIDS is most frequently a venereal disease. In addition, it is commonly found among intravenous drug users, who spread it through sharing "dirty needles." Both of these issues, sexuality and illicit drug use, can raise moral issues, thereby making it easy for patients and non-patients alike to develop an attitude of "blaming the victim" for the illness.
- Gay people have historically been stigmatized solely on the basis of their homosexuality.[1] Similarly, individuals who use intravenous drugs share, at best, a public image of being troubled, difficult, or frightening.
- At this time, AIDS is an incurable disease that in the U.S. predominantly strikes men in their early adult years.

■ COPING WITH AIDS

In addition to being stigmatized, AIDS patients must cope with the inexorable physical decline associated with the disease. Considerable psychological stamina is required after the diagnosis, since each new symptom, infection, or indication of weight loss is regarded as a sign of potential progression of disease.[2] Some patients become overwhelmed by hypochondria. Others may refuse to acknowledge their physical disabilities and minimize their need for care.

The probable duration of life after diagnosis can be estimated statistically from the opportunistic infection or neoplasm that produces the initial diagnosis of AIDS. Patients whose AIDS diagnosis is first based on the appearance of cryptococcal meningitis, for example, face a life expectancy of less than six months.[3] Patients first diagnosed with Kaposi's sarcoma, on the other hand, may remain feeling well for several years.

Nonetheless, AIDS patients generally find that their quality of life is compromised after diagnosis and that their health progressively deteriorates. In New York City, 86 percent of the first 1065 AIDS patients survived their initial hospitalization, but 46 percent of those survivors spent at least 30 percent of their remaining weeks or months in a hospital and 32 percent required hospitalization for at least half of their remaining lifetime.[3]

In addition to the weakness, persistent fevers, myalgias, and fatigue often suffered by patients with AIDS, the high incidence of neurologic disease further complicates coping with the diagnosis. Recent studies show that 30 percent to 40 percent of all AIDS patients will develop some neurologic dysfunction.[4-7] Of 180 patients evaluated neurologically over a three-year period, more than 50 percent eventually developed cognitive dysfunction. Thus, neurologic complications, including forgetfulness, poor concentration, lack of interest and difficulty with complex tasks are common. The complications of these central nervous system deficits may further impair the patient's ability to adapt to the stresses of their illness.

The major psychological issues for a person with AIDS change at different stages of the illness. The following psychological issues arise as the disease progresses[8]:

New Diagnosis

- Affective numbing vs. affective discharge; "denial"
- Need for emotional, financial, social support; self-esteem
- Fear of contaminating family, friends
- Fear of rejection: family, friends
- Pressure to make complicated treatment decisions
- Feelings of guilt and self-blame; illness as retribution
- Is there sex after diagnosis? Life-style changes

Mid-stage

- Loss of hope; emotional exhaustion
- More detailed grief work: anticipating and mourning loss of important people and objects
- Extent of treatment; pain control
- Unfinished business: life review; putting one's affairs in order

Terminal Care

- Adequate pain control; personal contact
- Work with family, friends
- Death and dying: honoring the patient's wishes

A patient's immediate reaction to a new AIDS diagnosis may be characterized as a normal stress response — anger, betrayal, and shock coexist with numbness and disbelief.[8] Some patients, however, most notably those with longstanding AIDS-related conditions (ARC), may experience relief.

After an initial adaptation, the implications of the diagnosis gradually become clearer. The patient must cope with the losses associated with a progressive illness, including the loss of employment, social role, and financial security. These losses, in turn, may diminish the patient's previous sense of social and professional worth. Similarly, feelings of depression and anxiety are common.

Guilt, low self-esteem, worthlessness, and the belief that the diagnosis is "retribution for past sins" have been reported.[9]

Anticipatory grieving occurs as thoughts of death and the possibility of pain-filled suffering predominate. The idea of suicide is a common finding, although in our experience in San Francisco, the actual number of people diagnosed with AIDS who harm themselves appears to be low. In a recent study of AIDS-related suicides in New York City, on the other hand, the incidence of suicide was significantly higher.[11] This points to the necessity of specifying and localizing psychosocial issues surrounding AIDS and HIV infection rather than assuming that there are general patterns.

As patients face the frustration of an encroaching illness, diffuse anger is often directed at medical institutions and personnel. The diagnosis may mean disclosure of the patient's membership in a high-risk group. Families and friends may then learn that the patient practices a life-style with which they disagree. Because of this, patients with AIDS are especially vulnerable to emotional rejection. Discrimination occurs frequently. Housing, employment, and health care are all areas in which AIDS patients are subjected to unfounded fears of contagion and prejudice. These experiences can increase the patient's own sense of unworthiness.

The ability of an individual to adapt successfully to life after diagnosis of a life-threatening disease depends on the following: (1) central nervous system compromise by the disease, (2) personality traits and coping mechanisms, (3) external support, and (4) social stigma.[10]

The AIDS patient is confronted with severe challenges on each of these fronts. Persons with ARC face similar problems; these are discussed elsewhere in this text.

REFERENCES

1. Larsen KS, Reed M, Hoffman S. Attitudes of heterosexuals toward homosexuality. J Sex Res 1980; 16:245-51.
2. Morin SF, Charles KA, Malyon AK. The psychological impact of AIDS on gay men. Am Psychol 1984; 39:1288-93.
3. Rivin BE, Monroe JM, Hubschman BP, et al. AIDS outcome: a first follow-up. N Engl J Med 1984; 311:857.
4. Snider WD, Simpson DM, Neilson S, et al. Neurological complications of acquired immune deficiency syndrome: analysis of 50 patients. Ann Neurol 1983; 14:403-18.
5. Levy RM, Bredesen DE, Rosenblum ML. Neurological manifestations of the acquired immune deficiency syndrome (AIDS): experience at UCSF and review of the literature. J Neurosurg 1985; 62:475-95.
6. Britton CB, Miller JR. Neurological complications in acquired immune deficiency syndrome (AIDS). Neurol Clin 1984; 2:315-39.
7. Petito CK, Navia BA, Cho ES, et al. Vascular myelopathy pathologically resembling subacute combined degeneration in patients with acquired immune deficiency syndrome. N Engl J Med 1985; 312:874-9.
8. Dilley J. Treatment issues and approaches in the psychological care of AIDS patients. In: Nichols S, Ostrow D, eds. Psychiatric aspects of AIDS. Washington D.C.: American Psychiatric Press, 1984; 62-76.
9. Dilley JW, Ochitill HN, Perl M, Volberding P. Findings in psychiatric consultations with patients with AIDS. Am J Psychiatry 1985; 142:82-5.
10. Holland JC. Psychological aspects of cancer. In: Holland JF, Frei E, eds. Cancer medicine, 2nd ed. Philadelphia: Lea and Febiger, 1982; 1175-1203.
11. Marzuk PM, Tierney H, Tardiff K, et al. Increased risk of suicide in persons with AIDS. JAMA 1988; 259:1333-7.

Altered Mental States: Clinical Syndromes and Diagnosis

James Dilley, M.D., Jay Baer, M.D., Alicia Boccellari, Ph.D., and Herbert Ochitill, M.D.

This chapter surveys the altered mental states associated with HIV infection. It summarizes common central nervous system (CNS) disease, describes clinical syndromes, including delirium, dementia, and depression, and provides detailed summaries of the elements used for diagnostic evaluations of an AIDS/HIV patient's altered mental states.

It is well recognized that at some point during the course of their disease, approximately 30 percent to 40 percent of all patients with AIDS will develop clinically obvious neurologic symptoms.[1,2] Many of the rest may have neuropsychiatric abnormalities that either go undetected, unreported, or are attributed to psychological factors.

This view is supported by data from direct observation of brain tissue, which reveal structural, pathologic abnormalities in over 75 percent of cases,[3-6] as well as data from neuropsychological testing of random samples of patients with AIDS.[7-9] Furthermore, the concept that HIV infection of neurologic tissues occurs in the majority of AIDS patients is suggested by recent research demonstrating: (1) HIV in the brain tissue of 10 of 16 patients with clinical features of encephalopathy; (2) isolation of the virus from the cerebrospinal fluid and neural tissues in some AIDS patients[10]; and (3) the discovery that virus-specific antibody to HIV is produced within the blood–brain barrier.[11] Table 1 lists other central nervous system diseases found in patients with AIDS or AIDS-related illness, together with their treatment.

The consequences of these neurologic complications can have profound effects on the behavior, mood, or cognitive status of AIDS patients. The physician should suspect an organic cause in all HIV-infected patients who show significant mental status changes. There is an abundance of anecdotal evidence, for example, that certain opportunistic infections — i.e., toxoplasmosis and cryptococcosis — cause depressions.

These patients, however, are also subject to the full range of mental illnesses that trouble the general population. Thus it is frequently difficult to discern if the causes of their psychiatric disturbance are organic or functional. The most severe clinical syndromes and mental disorders observed are reviewed briefly below; more exhaustive reviews are available.[12-14]

TABLE 1. COMMON CENTRAL NERVOUS SYSTEM DISEASE
STATES IN 315 PATIENTS WITH AIDS OR AIDS-RELATED
ILLNESS AND CNS DISEASE*

CNS DISEASE STATE	PERCENT	KNOWN MEDICAL TREATMENT
VIRAL SYNDROMES	30	
Subacute encephalitis	17	None
Atypical aseptic meningitis	7	None
Herpes simplex encephalitis	3	ARA-A or acyclovir
Progressive multifocal leukoencephalopathy	2	Possibly ARA-A
Other	1	
NONVIRAL SYNDROMES	51	
Toxoplasma gondii	32	Pyrimethamine + sulfadiazine
Cryptococcus neoformans	13	Amphotericin B & 5-fluorocytosine
Candida albicans	2	Amphotericin B & 5-fluorocytosine
Atypical mycobacteria	2	INH, ethambutol, & rifampin
Other	2	
NEOPLASMS	10	
Primary CNS lymphoma	5	Radiation therapy
CNS + systemic lymphoma	4	Radiation therapy + specific chemotherapy
Kaposi's sarcoma	1	Radiation therapy + chemotherapy
CEREBROVASCULAR ACCIDENT	3	Treat etiology
UNKNOWN	8	

* *Adapted, with permission, from Levy RM, Bredesen DE, Rosenblum ML. Neurological manifestations of the acquired immunodeficiency syndrome (AIDS): experience at UCSF and review of the literature. J Neurosurg 1985; 62:475-95.*

■ CLINICAL SYNDROMES

DELIRIUM

Delirium is one of the most common organic mental disorders seen in AIDS patients. Clinical features include a fluctuating level of consciousness, reversal of sleep—wake cycle, abnormal vital signs (often indicating autonomic hyperarousal) and, in many cases, psychotic phenomena (e.g., hallucinations).

The presence of psychotic symptoms may result in misdiagnosing a delirious state as a functional psychosis. Factors contributing to the development of delirium are summarized below.[13]

Primary Disease States

- Infectious, neoplastic, and cerebrovascular disease states (as in the chronic organic mental disorders)
- Meningitis and meningoencephalitis
    Acute HIV infection
    B-cell lymphoma

Kaposi's sarcoma
Fungal infections
Atypical mycobacterial infections
Other viral infections

- Other

Seizure disorders and postictal states
Treatment side effects (e.g., chemotherapy, interferon)

CNS Abnormalities Secondary to Systemic Processes

Sepsis
Hypoxemia from respiratory compromise (e.g., *Pneumocystis carinii*
   pneumonia)
Electrolyte imbalance
Acute renal failure

Environmental and Psychologic Factors

Visual loss (e.g., CMV retinitis)
Sensory understimulation
Inactivity
Disrupted circadian rhythms
Psychologic distress
Social isolation
Sleep loss

Delirium in medically ill patients is frequently acute in onset and resolves fully in four to seven days. In AIDS patients, however, it is frequently superimposed on, or evolves into, dementia.

DEMENTIA

Although it waxes and wanes, the dementia apparently caused by HIV brain infection is progressive and may appear anywhere in the course of the illness. The loss of cognitive capacities can be rapid or insidious, and may severely compromise a patient's ability to live independently. Cognitive functions that appear to be affected earlier in the course of this disorder include delayed memory, mental flexibility, visual–spatial memory, and overall speed of mental operations. In more advanced cases, there is often a marked impairment in judgment that necessitates a patient's hospitalization. At San Francisco General Hospital, an affective syndrome has appeared de novo in several patients who within weeks of diagnosis begin to manifest obvious signs of dementia. The syndrome is characterized by expansiveness, lability, and grandiosity that can reach delusional proportions. Irritability, hyperactivity, and insomnia are also observed.

DEPRESSION

Depression is often accompanied by suicidal thoughts, gestures, or attempts. For many patients, the acute mood-worsening is related to recent stress (e.g., receiving an AIDS diagnosis or perceiving rejection by loved ones). Patients with such an acute exacerbation of depression will usually respond to brief hospitalization and psychosocial interventions.

Suicidal thoughts are common, and perhaps ubiquitous, in patients with AIDS. The overwhelming majority of patients referred for psychiatric consultation at San Francisco General Hospital, regardless of the reason for consultation, experience these thoughts at some point(s) during their illness. It can be difficult to distinguish endogenous depression from either an advanced state of debility or from dementia; depression may coexist with either condition. Although the presence of HIV-related illness (e.g., toxoplasmosis or cryptococcosis) should always alert the clinician to the possibility of disease-related depression, de novo or recurrent depressive episodes can occur in this population. Patients with past histories of depression are at greater risk for repeated episodes.

Antidepressant drugs are helpful in depressed HIV patients and should be considered when patients manifest symptoms of major depression for more than two weeks, as well as after reversible organic causes for these symptoms have been addressed.

OTHER CLINICAL SYNDROMES

Patients with HIV-related illness may exhibit a number of psychotic symptoms (e.g., hallucinations) in conjunction with or independent of delirium, dementia, depression, and substance abuse. There is no single definition of "AIDS psychosis." In some patients, psychotic symptoms are simply the re-emergence of a pre-existing major psychiatric illness (e.g., schizophrenia). In other patients, the relationship between these symptoms and HIV infection remains unclear; serial observation of these patients may indicate whether these psychotic symptoms are the first evidence of HIV brain infection.

■ DIAGNOSIS

Diagnosis of altered mental states can be a complicated process, since AIDS patients are subject to many organic disturbances that can yield such a result. Important elements in the evaluation include:

1. **History of Present Illness.** The relationship between the onset of symptoms and physical/psychological insults should be explored. All evaluations should include questions about medication and recreational drug use.

2. **Mental Status Examination.** Special attention should be given to cognitive testing. The clinician's skills need to be perfected for assessment of attention, memory, orientation, language use, constructional ability, calculation, abstraction, and judgment. It is important to realize, however, that brief screening exams in common use (e.g., Mini Mental State Exam) often fail to detect the early deficits seen in HIV encephalopathy. The clinician should also pay attention to how a patient has been coping with life-threatening disease.

3. **Past Psychiatric History.** The patient with a pre-existing psychiatric disorder may or may not be experiencing a relapse. Relapse is likely if the current episode is symptomatically similar to past episodes. In our clinical experience at San Francisco General Hospital, the majority of patients requiring psychiatric hospitalization have no history of major psychiatric

illness, and do not have evidence of central nervous system insult. In some patients, the problem is clearly HIV encephalopathy; in other patients, it is not clear that the psychological disturbance is caused by HIV brain infection.

4. **Physical Examination.** This includes careful neurologic evaluation. Immune deficiency may blunt some signs or symptoms of illness and make them more difficult to detect.

5. **Consultation.** Other medical specialists should be consulted.

6. **Laboratory Evaluation.** Standard studies should be carried out. These include CBC, serum chemistry, urinalysis, thyroid panel, syphilis serology, serum cryptococcal antigen, and B12 level.

7. **Additional Studies.** When an organic cause is suspected, evaluation should include a computed tomographic scan of the head (or magnetic resonance imaging if available), lumbar puncture for cerebrospinal fluid examination (including cryptococcal antigen and titers for toxoplasmosis), and neuropsychological testing.

The results of these laboratory studies for central nervous system HIV infection can vary, and negative studies do not absolutely rule out infection.[15]

REFERENCES

1. Levy RM, Bredesen DE, Rosenblum ML. Neurological manifestations of AIDS: experience at UCSF and review of the literature. J Neurosurg 1985; 62:475-95.
2. Snider WD, Simpson DM, Nielson S, et al. Neurological complications of AIDS syndrome: analysis of 50 patients. Ann Neurol 1983; 14:403.
3. Britton CB, Miller JR. Neurological complications of AIDS. Neurol Clin 1984; 2:315.
4. Jordan BD, Navia BA, Cho ES, et al. Neurological complications of AIDS: an overview based on 110 autopsied patients [Abstract]. Atlanta: International Conference on AIDS, 1985:49.
5. Reichert CM, O'Leary TM, Levens DL, et al. Autopsy pathology in the acquired immune deficiency syndrome. Am J Pathol 1983; 112:357-82.
6. Welch K, Finkbeiner W, Alpers CE, et al. Autopsy findings in the acquired immune deficiency syndrome. JAMA 1984; 252:1152-9.
7. Tross S, Price R, Sidtis J, et al. Neuropsychological complications of AIDS [Abstract]. American College of Neuropsychopharmacology Meeting Abstracts, 1985:28.
8. Silberstein C, McKegney P, O'Dowd NA, et al. Neuropsychologic dysfunction in HTLV seropositives [Abstract]. Washington, D.C.: 139th Meeting of the American Psychiatric Association, Washington, D.C., 1986:128.
9. Loewenstein RJ, Rubinon DR. Psychiatric aspects of AIDS: the organic mental syndromes. In: Kurstak MT, Lipowski ZJ, eds. Viruses, immunity, and mental diseases. New York: Plenum Press (in press).
10. Ho DD, Rota TR, Schooley RT, et al. Isolation of HTLV-III from cerebrospinal fluid and neural tissues of patients with neurologic syndromes related to the acquired immunodeficiency syndrome. N Engl J Med 1985; 313:1493.
11. Resnick L, Di-Marzo-Veronese F, Schupbach J, et al. Intra-blood—brain-barrier synthesis of HTLV-III-specific IgG in patients with neurologic symptoms associated with AIDS or AIDS-related complex. N Engl J Med 1985; 313:1498-1504.
12. Holland JC, Tross S. The psychosocial and neuropsychiatric sequelae of the acquired immunodeficiency syndrome and related disorders. Ann Intern Med 1985; 103:760-4.
13. Wolcott DL, Fawzy FI, Pasnau RO. Acquired immune deficiency syndrome (AIDS) and consultation-liaison psychiatry. Gen Hosp Psychiatry 1985; 7:280-92.
14. Ochitill HN, Dilley JW. The neuropsychiatric aspects of AIDS. In: Rosenblum ML, Levy RM, Bredeson DE, eds. AIDS and the nervous system. New York: Raven Press, 1987.
15. Bach MC, Boothby JA. Dementia associated with human immunodeficiency virus with a negative ELISA. N Engl J Med 1986; 315:891-2.

Altered Mental States: Treatment Issues

Jay Baer, M.D., James Dilley, M.D., Alicia Boccellari, Ph.D., and Herbert Ochitill, M.D.

This chapter provides a general overview of the treatment issues surrounding patients with HIV-related altered mental states. It identifies psychiatric syndromes — delirium, dementia, depression, and psychosis — and provides pharmacologic information on treating AIDS/HIV patients based upon experiences at San Francisco General Hospital. The chapter also discusses non-pharmacologic interventions and psychiatric hospitalization, and concludes with guidelines for inpatient care of the HIV-infected psychiatric patient.

Many psychiatric symptoms in AIDS patients are caused by reversible organic insults, including iatrogenic factors (e.g., drug-induced delirium) and some central nervous system (CNS) opportunistic infections. Central nervous system infection by human immunodeficiency virus (HIV) is unfortunately not treatable at this time, although its course can wax and wane. If possible, the underlying cause of the altered mental state should be treated.

Even if the underlying cause cannot be treated, symptoms are often amenable to treatment with psychoactive medication. Patients without marked cognitive impairment can usually tolerate and benefit from standard medication dosing. This is not the case for patients with obvious impairment or dementia, however. These patients should be medicated with lower dosages than those used in healthy age-matched subjects to minimize side effects and avoid further cognitive compromise.[1] Drug regimens with minimal anticholinergic side effects should be used when possible.

■ PSYCHIATRIC SYNDROMES AND PHARMACOLOGIC INTERVENTIONS

DELIRIUM

The first interventions for delirium are: (1) a vigorous review of the patient's medical problems — this may yield possible reversible causes of the delirium (e.g., hypoxia); and (2) the removal of drugs that may cause or exacerbate central nervous system compromise. Psychotropics should not be added unless the patient's safety is compromised by the delirium (e.g., severe panic in response to hallucinations). In this instance, treatment with low-dose antipsychotics is indicated (e.g., haloperidol 0.5 or 1 mg qhs or bid) and should be maintained until the dangerous behavior subsides.

DEMENTIA

Patients with this syndrome sometimes require medication for agitation and/or psychotic symptoms. They are susceptible to unusually severe side effects, including extrapyramidal syndromes caused by antipsychotic medication. Thus, patients receiving antipsychotics must be closely monitored.

At San Francisco General Hospital, the majority of such side effects have occurred with haloperidol, so agitated or psychotic demented patients (or both) are given mid-range potency antipsychotic agents as the first line of pharmacologic treatment.

Dosages should start low and be increased cautiously if the drug effect is inadequate and if the drug tolerance is adequate. Sample agents and dosages include perphenazine (4 to 8 mg po qhs or bid), thiothixene (2 to 5 mg po qhs or bid), and trifluoperazine (2 to 5 mg po qhs or bid).

When antipsychotic medications are used, low-dose antiparkinsonian agents may be given prophylactically (e.g., benztropine 0.5 or 1 mg bid; diphenhydramine 25 mg po bid). It can be difficult to distinguish some drug side effects from advanced neurologic signs of central nervous system HIV infection.

While many patients respond effectively to this medication approach, others fail to respond to or tolerate it. Benzodiazepines should be tried in these patients. However, clinicians should be aware that these agents tend to yield worsening cognitive performance, disinhibition, or other forms of toxicity (e.g., worsening ataxia) in HIV-demented patients. Lorazepam has been cited as such an offender in several cases at San Francisco General Hospital.

We recommend alprazolam (beginning at 0.125 to 0.25 mg po bid-tid). Like the medications discussed above, alprazolam dosing may be increased cautiously if the response is inadequate and side effects are tolerable.

When antipsychotic and benzodiazepine treatments fail, other agents may be tried (e.g., clonidine, lithium, carbamazepine, and β-blockers such as propranolol), though none of these agents has yet established a consistent track record.

Although there is no cure for HIV dementia, some preliminary studies suggest that psychostimulants (methylphenidate 30 to 60 mg/day, D-amphetamine 30 to 40 mg/day) can improve the cognitive performance of HIV-infected patients with *moderate* intellectual deficits.[2] However, our attempts at treating a small number of *markedly* impaired (i.e., demented) individuals with low-dose stimulants (methylphenidate 5 mg qam or D-amphetamine 5 to 10 mg qam) failed due to drug-induced irritability. Zidovudine (AZT) was recently shown to yield improvement in neuropsychologic test scores in moderately impaired patients[5]; its efficacy in the long-term course of dementia is unknown.

The clinician who medicates an HIV-demented patient must consider the constantly changing condition of the patient's central nervous system. These constant changes can often result in the need for changes in medication as well.[3] For example, a patient receiving an antipsychotic for agitation often requires less medication — and sometimes none at all — after several weeks of treatment.

DEPRESSION

Antidepressants are helpful in depressed HIV patients and should be considered when a patient manifests symptoms of major depression for more than two weeks (as well as after treatment for reversible organic etiologies). Usually, HIV patients require similar dosages to those used for non-HIV infected patients. Cognitively compromised patients must be carefully watched for side effects, however.

Anticholinergic load should be reduced as much as possible in the medications chosen for treatment. The more sedating medications should be avoided unless a patient has a depression with marked anxiety or agitation. Dosages should be built up gradually over 7 to 10 days to minimize side effects. Preferred medications and target dosages include nortryptyline (50 to 75 mg po qhs) and desipramine (150 mg po qhs). Patients who fail to respond after three weeks of consistent therapy, as well as those who have unusually severe side effects, may have serum levels checked to determine if dosage levels are outside the recommended therapeutic range.

PSYCHOSIS

As explained above, HIV-infected patients may exhibit psychotic symptoms in conjunction with a number of syndromes. For psychotic patients who are not delirious or demented, antipsychotic medications are indicated, tolerated, and effective in dosages similar to those used in non-HIV infected patients with psychotic disorders.

Reasonable starting regimens include haloperidol (5 to 10 mg po qhs or bid), perphenazine (8 to 16 mg po qhs or bid), and thiothixene (5 to 10 mg po qhs or bid). Prophylaxis with antiparkinsonian agents (e.g., benztropine 1 mg po bid) is recommended. Antipsychotic drug dosages can be increased moderately if effect is inadequate and if side effects do not prohibit this.

■ NONPHARMACOLOGIC INTERVENTIONS

Patients may require assistance with a host of physical problems; consultation with internists, nursing specialists, and physical therapists should be sought out and used.

Psychosocial interventions are essential and useful. AIDS patients frequently struggle with feelings of alienation, rejection, and loss of control over their lives. Special attention should be paid to how an individual is coping with terminal illness. Patients' coping skills vary tremendously, but a clinician's offer to simply be with a dying person can be of inestimable value.

Particular delicacy is required in the clinician's handling of a diagnosis of AIDS dementia. For some patients, this aspect of HIV disease is the most horrifying — the loss of the personality, psychological self, or soul is worse than the loss of the body. The clinician must balance the importance of making or discussing a diagnosis of dementia with the individual patient's ability to tolerate the diagnosis.

Patients also require assistance from a variety of social service agencies. Their loved ones often require help, including education (e.g., about personal risk and contagion of HIV and about managing a demented person) and treatment for particularly severe and disruptive bereavement.

It is crucial to discuss a patient's feelings about continued medical treatment of his or her HIV-related illnesses, including resuscitation in the event of cardiopulmonary arrest. Ideally, such a discussion occurs before there is significant cognitive compromise. Patients should be encouraged to designate medical power of attorney to trusted individuals who can then act on the patient's wishes, if needed.

■ PSYCHIATRIC HOSPITALIZATION

Some behavioral disturbances in patients with HIV-related illness necessitate psychiatric hospitalization. These include suicide attempts or escalating ideation, psychosis, and severe dementia with behavioral disturbance. The introduction of patients with a communicable life-threatening disease to the inpatient psychiatric setting is a substantial but manageable problem. The following guidelines may help to make it more manageable.[2,4]

- The staff must be kept up to date on AIDS information. This can be accomplished through literature surveillance and in-service presentations.

- Staffing level must expand its capacity in order to manage AIDS patients' medical problems. The needs of patients can become labor-intensive as well as emotionally draining. A source of competent medical consultation is essential.

- In a supportive atmosphere, staff must be allowed to express and discuss feelings provoked by working with AIDS patients. Staff members may need help in confronting their own profound feelings about death, contagion, and sexuality.

- Patient confidentiality must be respected.

- The non-HIV patient group, which constantly changes, must receive ongoing, clear, concise information about AIDS — especially about the current understanding of HIV transmission. This group of predominantly psychotic individuals requires reassurance that all is safe.

- Like the staff, the patient group must be given opportunities to discuss their feelings about AIDS in a supportive atmosphere.

REFERENCES

1. Wolcott DL, Fawzy FI, Pasnau RO. Acquired immune deficiency syndrome (AIDS) and consultation-liaison psychiatry. Gen Hosp Psychiatry 1985; 7:280-92.
2. Baer JW, Hall JM, Holm K, Lewitter-Koehler S. Challenges in developing an inpatient psychiatric program for patients with AIDS and ARC. Hosp Community Psychiatry 1987; 38:1299-1303.
3. Fernandez F, Adams F, Levy JK, et al. Cognitive impairment due to AIDS-related complex and its response to psychostimulants. Psychosomatics 1988; 29:38-46.
5. Schmitt FA, Bigley JW, McKinnis R, et al. Neuropsychological outcome of zidovudine (AZT) treatment of patients with AIDS and AIDS-related complex. N Engl J Med 1988; 319:1573-8.
4. Amchin J, Polan HJ. A longitudinal account of staff adaptation to AIDS patients in a psychiatric unit. Hosp Community Psychiatry 1986; 37:1235-8.
5. Schmitt FA, Bigley JW, McKinnis R, et al. Neuropsychological outcome of zidovudine (AZT) treatment of patients with AIDS and AIDS-related complex. N Engl J Med 1988; 319:1573-8.

Neuropsychologic Assessment in HIV-Related Disorders

Alicia Boccellari, Ph.D., James Dilley, M.D., Jay Baer, M.D., and Herbert Ochitill, M.D.

Neuropsychologic testing consists of evaluating patients using standardized tests sensitive to the behavioral, emotional, and cognitive components of cerebral dysfunction. The evaluation may be useful at any stage of the diagnostic process — such as detecting and characterizing a brain disorder when first suspected, or for assessing a patient's functional state long after signs, symptoms, and laboratory studies have confirmed a diagnostic impression.[1] This chapter describes the role of neuropsychologic testing and reviews neuropsychiatric studies of HIV dementia.

■ STRENGTHS AND LIMITATIONS OF NEUROPSYCHOLOGIC TESTING

As diagnostic tools, neuropsychologic tests have advantages over traditional clinical interviews or mental-status exams. A neuropsychologic test battery is administered in a standardized fashion, and the results are interpreted in relation to a standard set of values derived from individuals assumed to be normal. In general, cognitive abilities and behavioral presentation can be scored quantitatively and then used as a baseline for comparisons over time as well as for planning patient care. Many of the tests adjust results for both age and education — two factors that can influence a patient's test performance. However, cultural variables are not fully controlled for in neuropsychologic test batteries. This limitation should be considered during test interpretation.

■ ROLE OF NEUROPSYCHOLOGIC TESTING

Neuropsychiatric studies of HIV-infected patients have provided evidence that cognitive, behavioral, and other neurologic changes do frequently occur in individuals with AIDS and ARC. Some preliminary data suggest that a smaller number of otherwise asymptomatic HIV-positive subjects may experience similar changes. Longitudinal studies are needed to determine the natural history and course of neuropsychiatric abnormalities in HIV infection.

Neuropsychologic testing has proven to be sensitive even during the early stages of central nervous system (CNS) dysfunction — when neurologic exams, laboratory tests, and neuroradiologic procedures are often normal. Memory problems, psychomotor retardation, and cognitive deficits may herald the initial stage of an insidious, dementing process, and may be mistaken for a reactive depression. In some patients with AIDS, neurologic illness will manifest itself in an acute psychotic episode or in some other form of psychiatric symptomatology.[2] Testing can help differentiate between a functional and an organic disorder.

In addition to characterizing the neuropsychologic deficits of patients with AIDS and related disorders, testing can help the clinician understand how the patient is coping with disability. It can also be helpful in treatment and discharge planning. Recommendations based on neuropsychologic testing can aid caregivers in the day-to-day management of the patient with cerebral dysfunction. Our experience with this population would certainly support the usefulness of neuropsychologic assessment in the care of AIDS patients.

Neuropsychologic testing may be helpful in patient management in four ways.

- Documentation of the presence or absence of cerebral dysfunction.
- Clarification of the nature of the disorder (i.e., whether the condition is acute or chronic, progressive or static, focal or diffuse), as well as the quantitative assessment of the severity or degree of cerebral impairment.
- Provision of baseline estimates for comparison in follow-up evaluation, to help determine the natural course of the disease or the recovery process in a given patient.
- Documentation of the patient's cognitive strengths and weaknesses, and mental status, to allow for more effective treatment planning and patient management.

■ PRACTICAL CONSIDERATIONS IN TESTING

Neuropsychologic testing involves considerable patient time (generally one to four hours) and cooperation. Patients selected for neuropsychologic testing at San Francisco General Hospital are interviewed and tested for fine motor speed, verbal fluency, attention, concentration, memory, and problem-solving skills.

We find that the majority of patients fatigue easily, so the testing approach must be limited, brief, and focused.

■ REVIEW OF RESULTS OF NEUROPSYCHIATRIC STUDIES OF HIV DEMENTIA

Tross et al.[3] used a brief neuropsychologic screening battery in a study of two groups of AIDS patients. One group of 30 patients had described neurologic complaints and indications for CNS pathology. The other group consisted of 26 newly diagnosed AIDS patients without signs or symptoms of CNS pathology. Both groups of patients were found to have notable cognitive deficits in the following areas:

- Slowing on timed tasks;
- Verbal and visual–spatial short-term memory problems;
- Language fluency and naming problems;
- Visual–spatial constructional impairment;
- Complex sequential problem-solving impairment;
- Difficulty performing novel tasks.

In patients with suspected CNS pathology, 48 percent had impairment in four or more cognitive areas. In patients without suspected CNS pathology, 88 percent had cognitive impairment in at least one area. Impaired test performance was defined as poor ability when compared to nationally based norms for individuals of similar age and educational backgrounds. Hence, even a single area of impairment is meaningful.

These results were particularly disturbing for those patients not suspected of having neurologic illness; they also show that CNS pathology in AIDS patients is common — even when no neurologic diagnosis has been established. In addition, only 4 of the 26 patients in this group were diagnosed as having a major depression. Thus, the results were not attributable to depression alone.

Ayers et al.[4] performed a neuropsychologic evaluation on 60 individuals: 15 subjects with a diagnosis of ARC (ARC Group), 15 subjects with an AIDS diagnosis of less than three months (AIDS Recent Group), 15 subjects with an AIDS diagnosis of at least one year (AIDS Prolonged Group), and a control group of 15 HIV-negative individuals. All subjects were given the Luria Nebraska Neuropsychological Battery (LNNB) as well as two psychiatric measures: the Beck Depression Inventory (BDI) and the Minnesota Multiphasic Personality Inventory (MMPI).

The results suggested that while none of the HIV-negative subjects was impaired on the LNNB, 27 percent of the ARC Group, 33 percent of the AIDS Recent Group, and 33 percent of the AIDS Prolonged Group were impaired on at least 3 of the 11 LNNB clinical scales. Impairment was particularly noted on measures of motor and tactile abilities, receptive speech, expressive speech, reading, and memory. Ayers et al. also explored whether psychologic factors (such as depression) were influencing and confounding neuropsychologic testing. Intercorrelational analysis among the LNNB, MMPI, and BDI measures demonstrated that there were no associations between the psychologic measures and neuropsychologic performance. The authors concluded that there did not appear to be a relationship between psychologic reaction to AIDS and the degree of neuropsychologic impairment demonstrated.

In a similar fashion, Grant et al.[5] performed neuropsychologic evaluations on 15 subjects with AIDS, 13 subjects with ARC, 16 HIV-positive subjects, and a control group of 11 HIV-negative subjects. In addition, a subset of the AIDS and ARC subjects was evaluated with magnetic resonance imaging (MRI) scans. On the basis of this evaluation, Grant et al. concluded that 87 percent of the AIDS group, 54 percent of the ARC group, 44 percent of the HIV-positive group, and 9 percent of the HIV-negative group were abnormal on neuropsychologic testing. The AIDS subjects were particularly impaired on measures of attention, abstract reasoning, and speed of information processing. Magnetic resonance imaging results were abnormal in 9 of the 13 AIDS subjects (69 percent) and 5 of the 10 subjects with ARC (50 percent). The most common abnormality was sulcal and ventricular enlargement. Bilateral patchy areas of high-signal intensity in the white matter were also noted. The authors concluded that "CNS involvement by HIV may begin early in the course of AIDS and cause mild cognitive deficits in otherwise asymptomatic persons." This study is limited, however, by its small sample size.

Janssen et al.[6] evaluated 39 HIV-positive men with lymphadenopathy syndrome (LAS) and 38 HIV-negative controls. All subjects were given a complete neuropsychologic battery, MRI, and immunologic tests. Nine of 18 LAS patients (50 percent) and 2 of the 26 controls (8 percent) were found to have mild abnormalities on neuropsychologic testing. Abnormalities were particularly noted in the areas of verbal fluency, memory, motor speed, and visual-scanning abilities. Magnetic resonance imaging scans were abnormal in one LAS patient and in one control patient. Neither neurologic nor neuropsychologic abnormalities correlated with duration of LAS, absolute T-helper lymphocyte count, or T-helper/T-suppressor lymphocyte ratio. The authors concluded that mild neurologic abnormalities in individuals with LAS are common and suggested that HIV may directly or indirectly cause these abnormalities.

At San Francisco General Hospital, the Neuropsychology Service has found cognitive deficits in individuals with HIV dementia similar to those described above. In particular, the following characteristics have proven to be clinically important.

- An increase in impulsiveness, poor judgment, difficulty in planning, poor organizational abilities, and loss of mental flexibility (sufficient to interfere with daily affairs).

- Apathy and anosognosia (denial of cognitive problems), along with a decreased awareness of the impact of one's behavior on other people.

- Cognitive and motoric slowing.

- Difficulty on 30-minute delayed memory tasks. (Delayed memory being more impaired than immediate memory.)

- Visual–spatial abstract reasoning difficulties.

- Verbal fluency problems and slowing on speech production.

REFERENCES

1. Lezak MD. Neuropsychological assessment. New York: Oxford Press, 1976:152.
2. Holland JC, Tross S. The psychosocial and neuropsychiatric sequelae of the acquired immune deficiency syndrome and related disorders. Ann Intern Med 1985; 103:760-4.
3. Tross S, Price R, Siotis J, et al. Neuropsychological complications of AIDS [Abstract]. American College of Neuropharmacology Meeting Abstracts 1985:28.
4. Ayers MR, Abrams DI, Newell TG, Friedrich F. Performance of individuals with AIDS in the Luria-Nebraska neuropsychological battery. Int J Clin Neuropsychology 1987; 10:101-5.
5. Grant I, Atkinson JH, Hesselink JR, et al. Evidence for early central nervous system involvement in the acquired immunodeficiency virus (HIV) infections: studies with neuropsychologic testing and magnetic resonance imaging. Ann Intern Med 1987; 107:828-36.
6. Janssen RS, Saykin AJ, Kaplan JE, et al. Neurological complications of human immunodeficiency virus infections in patients with lymphadenopathy syndrome. Ann Neurol 1988; 23:49-55.

Clinical Evaluation of Early HIV Dementia

Sharone Abramowitz, M.D.

P atients with HIV dementia can have affective, cognitive, motor, and behavioral abnormalities.[1,2] At San Francisco General Hospital's Psychiatric Consultation Service, we have found that clinicians can incorporate an understanding of these neuropsychological deficits into a modified bedside mental-status evaluation that permits a more accurate assessment of the patient's state. This is important, because the results of unmodified cognitive mental-status exams given to HIV-infected patients are often normal. However, when many of these same patients are later evaluated by our service — using a modified mental-status exam — they exhibit abnormalities that are characteristic of early HIV dementia. The purpose of this chapter is to outline the SFGH Psychiatry Service's approach to the mental-status evaluation of HIV-infected patients.

Early HIV dementia can be subtle and difficult to diagnose. Although formal neuropsychologic testing is required to confirm its diagnosis, a careful bedside evaluation using the recent findings of AIDS neuropsychologic research can help the clinician make an initial assessment. This is important at the outset of treatment for a number of reasons.

A diagnosis of HIV dementia influences management decisions — for example, whether to start the patient on zidovudine (AZT) or psychostimulants. It may also contraindicate the use of benzodiazepines and suggest the conservative use of other psychotropic medications, since benzodiazepines and other psychotropic medications can worsen the mildly HIV-demented patient's already-compromised cognitive functioning. Assessing the extent of dementia can help the clinician determine the appropriate level for communicating with a patient whose cognitive abilities are compromised. Finally, early diagnosis of HIV dementia can spur needed discussions with the patient about resuscitation, durable power-of-attorney, home care, and other plans for eventual disability and death.

■ MODIFIED BEDSIDE MENTAL-STATUS EVALUATION FOR HIV DEMENTIA

History. A good mental-status evaluation begins when the clinician first comes in contact with the patient. While obtaining the patient's medical and social history, the clinician should note whether the patient:

1. seems to answer questions slowly;
2. has difficulty recalling specific information;
3. appears affectively subdued and emotionally non-responsive;
4. has trouble tracking the conversation;
5. appears to mishear or misinterpret questions.

Since these are subjective rather than quantitative impressions, it may be difficult to determine whether the patient's behaviors are "baseline" or are indicative of early HIV dementia. Besides subjective impressions, the clinician should seek both the patient's and other caregivers' assessments of any changes in the patient's behavior. The clinician should ask if they have noticed:

1. worsening memory;
2. difficulties in following conversations or in reading;
3. problems keeping up at work;
4. clumsiness or other motor difficulties;
5. trouble with frequently misplacing things or with getting lost;
6. personality changes.

Our experience corresponds to that of Price et al., who found that:

> *Early in the illness, patients frequently report that they must keep lists in order to carry out their normal activities and that complex but formerly routine mental tasks take longer and need to be consciously broken down into component steps.*[3]

Unfortunately, apathy and denial of these deficits commonly occur among HIV-demented patients, making it more difficult to obtain accurate assessments of the patient's abilities. In addition, some HIV-infected patients have no social support system, so evaluation and confirmation of progressive deficits is difficult to obtain.

As part of the history, the patient's highest level of education and his or her work history should be obtained. These are useful in assessing declines in skill levels. For example, if a patient who was a computer analyst can now perform only simple calculations very slowly, this is probably a more significant sign of decline than it would be in a patient who dropped out of high school. The patient's psychiatric history must also be reviewed.

Level of Consciousness.   The patient with early HIV dementia usually appears alert and shows no fluctuations in level of consciousness. If these abnormalities are present, however, then delirium is likely. In our experience at SFGH, the patient with early HIV dementia is at increased risk for medical delirium induced by drugs, hypoxia, and metabolic abnormalities.

Orientation.   Patients with early HIV dementia should not be disoriented. Disorientation can occur secondary to acute delirium in mildly HIV-demented patients,[1] but it is common only in patients with advanced dementia.

Attention.   Patients with early HIV dementia are usually good at performing simple tasks that call for attention, such as repeating six numbers forward, but they often perform more complex tasks (such as serial sevens or repeating numbers in reverse order) awkwardly. These patients can also exhibit apathetic inattention.

Neuromotor Function.   Clumsiness (with rapid alternating-movement tests of the hands), ataxia (with tandem gait), progressive leg weakness, and mild tremor are not unusual in early HIV-dementia patients. The patient's handwriting is often impaired and should be tested.[1,2,3]

Psychomotor Function and Affect.   These patients are slow to answer questions, even when they come up with the correct answers. Their speech rate is often slowed as well. Their range of facial expressions and voice tone can seem unanimated, and create the impression that their blunted, affective presentation is secondary to depression. Depending on their ability to tolerate frustration, some of these patients become irritable while struggling to perform cognitive tasks that in the past came easily to them.

Visual–Spatial Function.   This area of brain functioning is often impaired early in the course of HIV dementia. Two simple bedside tests can help the clinician assess the level of impairment.

1. Ask the patient to construct a clock face reading a specific time.
2. Have the patient dial a phone number.

Frequently the patient with early HIV dementia can correctly perform these tasks, but only slowly, clumsily, or after repeated attempts.

Thought Process.   A psychotic process is not part of early HIV dementia, although it can be seen in patients suffering from late stages of dementia.[1,2] In early HIV dementia, the patient's thought process tends to be goal-directed, although slow and lumbering, as if the patient's mind were made up of slow-moving cogs.

Memory.   Initially, visual–spatial memory can be more impaired than verbal memory. Therefore, the early HIV-dementia patient often performs well on routine five-minute (short-term) verbal-memory tasks. If this is the only test performed, the clinician may mistakenly feel that no dementia is present, since in cortical dementias (such as Alzheimer's), short-term verbal memory is frequently impaired. When tested in the usual bedside manner (such as by asking historical questions), long-term verbal memory in early HIV dementia is not usually grossly impaired.

Language.   If patients are asked to perform simple three-step commands, their comprehension is frequently found to be mildly impaired. Patients with early HIV dementia often ask for the three-step instructions to be repeated, or they will perform the steps slowly. It is common for patients to perform only two of the three steps correctly. The naming of whole objects (such as "a pen" and "a telephone") is frequently unimpaired, but when asked to name the parts of a pen (such as "the tip" or "the cap"), patients frequently struggle for the answer. One useful test is to ask the patient to read a paragraph out loud (if he or she was functionally literate at baseline). Gross aphasia is generally not seen in early HIV dementia.

Calculations.   Patients with early HIV dementia can frequently solve simple arithmetic problems, although they often do so slowly.

Abstraction.   Generally, abstracting ability is not a useful differentiating bedside test in these patients. Although some patients answer concretely, many others can abstract fairly well.

Insight and Judgment.   Apathy and denial can occur in these patients, causing some impairment in insight and judgment. Usually, however, the early HIV-dementia patient does not have moderate-to-severe deficiencies in these areas.

■ EARLY HIV DEMENTIA VERSUS DEPRESSION

The patient with early HIV dementia may display apathy, mental slowing, psychomotor slowing, and affective blunting. These signs can easily be misdiagnosed as depression.[3] But unlike typically depressed patients, these individuals do not subjectively feel depressed. They do not exhibit suicidal ideation, guilt, and severe anhedonia. Unfortunately, depression often coexists in patients facing early HIV dementia; this is also true for patients with other subcortical dementias.[4]

REFERENCES

1. Navia B, Price R. Dementia complicating AIDS. Psych Annals 1986; 16:158-66.
2. Navia B, Jordan B, Price R. The AIDS dementia complex: I. Clinical features. Ann Neurol 1986; 19:517-24.
3. Price RW, Brew B, Sidtis J, et al. The brain in AIDS: central nervous system HIV-1 infection and AIDS dementia complex. Science 1988; 239:586-92.
4. Cummings JL, Benson DF. Subcortical dementia. Review of an emerging concept. Arch Neurol 1984; 41:874-9.

5.14

Rheumatologic Aspects

Myositis in HIV-Infected Patients

David Chernoff, M.D.

A clinical syndrome resembling polymyositis has been observed in patients with HIV infection. Several case-reports document a clinical syndrome characterized by the subacute onset of proximal muscle weakness associated with myalgias and extreme fatigue.[1-4] The clinical presentation in these HIV-infected individuals is indistinguishable from idiopathic polymyositis in non-HIV-infected persons. A recent report reviewed the clinical presentations in 11 patients with HIV-associated myositis.[5]

■ CLINICAL PRESENTATION

Physical examination revealed proximal muscle weakness, tenderness, and muscle atrophy. Laboratory data showed elevated muscle enzymes, including creatine kinase, aldolase and SGOT (serum glutamic-oxaloacetic transaminase). Electromyograms revealed myopathic changes. Nerve-conduction studies were normal.

Muscle biopsies revealed muscle fiber necrosis with minimal interfascicular inflammatory infiltrates consisting of macrophages, lymphocytes, and occasional polymorphonuclear neutrophil leukocytes. One patient with HIV-associated myositis had multinucleated giant cells found on muscle biopsy.[6]

Immunocytochemical examination of muscle biopsies have yielded variable results. Some samples have stained positively for HIV in the cellular infiltrates but not in the muscle fibers. This is not surprising, since macrophages are known to harbor HIV within their cytoplasm. Electron microscopy failed to reveal viral particles in the myofibrils. Extensive serologic evaluation for infectious agents other than HIV have been negative in the approximately 40 patients studied.

■ TREATMENT

Forty patients who presented with a polymyositis-like illness were treated with steroids. Most responded with a decrease in creatine kinase levels and a gradual resolution of muscle weakness. The long-term infectious risks of corticosteroid therapy in HIV-infected individuals are unknown. The decision to use steroids must therefore depend on the severity of the myositis.

■ ZIDOVUDINE-ASSOCIATED MYOSITIS

Recent case reports have implicated the antiviral agent zidovudine (AZT) as a cause of myositis in HIV-infected individuals.[7,8] A polymyositis-like illness was observed in four patients taking AZT for more than six months.[7] All of the patients had subacute onset of myalgias, muscle tenderness, and proximal weakness. Creatine kinase elevation was noted in all of the patients and elec-tromyograms revealed myopathic changes. Muscle biopsies showed myofibril necrosis with scant inflammation. When AZT was discontinued, symptomatic improvement was observed; creatine kinase levels fell to normal.

A subsequent report[8] revealed that 8 of 113 patients receiving AZT devel-oped a polymyositis-like illness. When the drug was discontinued, gradual clinical improvement was noted and creatine kinase levels returned to normal. In patients in whom the AZT dose was reduced rather than discontinued, neither clinical nor biochemical improvement was observed.

The pathogenesis of AZT-associated myositis is unclear. The drug itself may be directly myotoxic when given for prolonged periods. Patients receiving AZT should be observed for signs of myopathy and have their creatine kinase levels routinely monitored for myotoxicity. If creatine kinase levels are elevated but no clinical symptoms are reported, current indications suggest that the patient can continue with AZT therapy.

■ ANIMAL MODELS OF HIV-ASSOCIATED MYOSITIS

A clinical syndrome resembling polymyositis has been observed in rhesus mon-keys infected with simian AIDS virus.[9] Approximately 50 percent of the in-fected animals develop weakness and muscle wasting. Of those animals who develop a wasting illness, roughly 50 percent will show evidence of myositis on muscle biopsy. Creatine kinase levels can rise to 5 to 10 times normal in these monkeys.

Muscle biopsies from these animals showed interfascicular infiltrates similar to those observed in human biopsy specimens. Immunocytochemistry was positive for retrovirus in the inflammatory cell infiltrates but not in the muscle fibers. In tissue cultures, virus could be seen in myocytes but cytopathic changes were not observed.

REFERENCES

1. Dalakas MC, Pezeshkpour GH, Gravell M, Sever JL. Polymyositis associated with AIDS retrovirus. JAMA 1986; 256:2381-3.
2. Stern R, Gold J, DiCarlo EF. Myopathy complicating the acquired immunodeficiency syndrome. Muscle Nerve 1987; 10:318-22.
3. Simpson DM, Bender AN. HTLV-III-associated myopathy. Neurology 1987; 37:319.
4. Gonzalez MF, Olney RK, So YT, et al. Subacute structural myopathy associated with human immuno-deficiency virus infection. Arch Neurol 1988; 45:585-7.
5. Simpson DM, Bender AN. Human immunodeficiency virus-associated myopathy: analysis of 11 pa-tients. Ann Neurol 1988; 24:79-84.
6. Bailey RO, Turok DI, Jaufmann BP, Singh JK. Myositis and acquired immunodeficiency syndrome. Hum Pathol 1987; 18:749-51.
7. Bessen LJ, Greene JB, Louie E, et al. Severe polymyositis-like syndrome associated with zidovudine therapy of AIDS and ARC. N Engl J Med 1988; 318:708.
8. Gorard DA, Henry K, Guiloff RJ. Necrotizing myopathy and zidovudine. Lancet 1988; 1:1050-1.
9. Dalakas MC, London WT, Gravell M, Sever JL. Polymyositis in an immunodeficiency disease in monkeys induced by a type D retrovirus. Neurology 1986; 36:569-72.

HIV-Associated Salivary-Gland Disease (Sjögren's Syndrome)

David Chernoff, M.D.

O ral manifestations of HIV infection occur frequently. Enlargement of the parotid glands is seen in children but has been reported only rarely in adults.[1]

Recent reports describe a Sjögren's-like syndrome in HIV-infected individuals.[2-5] Parotid-gland enlargement associated with xerostomia and keratoconjunctivitis has been observed. HIV-associated salivary-gland disease may represent an autoimmune phenomenon associated with viral infection of the salivary glands.

■ CLINICAL PRESENTATION

Ten patients were reported as having a Sjögren's-like syndrome. These patients presented with dry eyes, dry mouths, salivary-gland enlargement, and arthralgias. An evaluation of the majority of these patients included:

1. Schirmer's test to assess lacrimation;

2. rose bengal staining to assay for keratoconjunctivitis;

3. salivary-gland scintigraphy;

4. serologic profile;
   antinuclear antibodies (ANA),
   rheumatoid factor (RF),
   cryoglobulins, and

5. minor salivary-gland biopsies.

The majority of patients had positive Schirmer's tests and corneal staining with rose bengal dye, indicating inadequate lacrimation. Salivary-gland biopsies revealed intense lymphocytic infiltration of the glandular parenchyma. In some cases, the lymphocytic infiltrate resulted in destruction of the normal gland architecture and the formation of myoepithelial islands characteristic of Sjögren's syndrome.

Serologic evaluation failed to detect RF, ANA, or cryoglobulins. The absence of serologic markers differs from the profile seen in non-HIV-associated Sjögren's syndrome, in which autoimmune markers (such as RF) are present in up to 70 percent of cases.

■ PATHOGENS

In some patients with HIV-associated salivary-gland disease, diffuse extraglandular lymphocytic infiltrates were noted in a variety of sites (liver, spleen, lung, lymph nodes). Two of the patients had a histologic diagnosis of lymphocytic interstitial pneumonitis, a common finding in HIV-infected children.[1] The association of salivary-gland disease with lymphocytic pneumonitis is of interest because the two processes may suggest a spectrum of autoimmune responses to HIV infection. HIV has been isolated from salivary-gland tissue.[6] The pathogenic role of HIV or other viruses, such as Epstein–Barr virus (EBV) and cytomegalovirus (CMV), is unknown.

■ DIFFERENTIAL DIAGNOSIS

The differential diagnosis of salivary gland enlargement in HIV-infected patients includes bacterial sialadenitis, viral infections (mumps, EBV, possibly HIV), tumors, and occasionally salivary-gland enlargement due to lymphadenopathy within the salivary glands.[7]

Evaluation of patients complaining of dry eyes or dry mouths should include a careful drug history (tricyclic antidepressants and antihistamines may be at fault) in order to rule out iatrogenic illness.

The identification of a Sjögren's-like illness in a young patient with atypical or uncommon clinical features should suggest the possibility of HIV-associated salivary-gland disease. Clinical and laboratory features suggesting this condition include the following: (1) young age (less than 40); (2) high-risk group (gay, bisexual, intravenous drug user, transfusion recipient, hemophiliac); (3) male (79 percent of non-HIV-related Sjögren's occurs in females); (4) generalized lymphadenopathy; and (5) negative autoimmune serologies.

■ TREATMENT

The treatment of HIV-associated Sjögren's is mostly symptomatic. Artificial saliva is used to reduce symptoms of dry mouth. Sugar should be avoided because of the high incidence of cavities and periodontal disease associated with inadequate salivary flow. Artificial tears are used to prevent corneal ulcerations.

Whether antiviral agents will play a role in the treatment of HIV-associated salivary-gland disease remains to be seen. Anecdotal reports suggest that lymphocytic interstitial pneumonitis responds to zidovudine. If the glandular disease results from an autoimmune response to viral infection, immunomodulating agents (such as steroids) may play a role in treatment.

REFERENCES

1. Pahwa S, Kaplan M, Fikrig S, et al. Spectrum of human T-cell lymphotropic virus type III infection in children. Recognition of symptomatic, asymptomatic, and seronegative patients. JAMA 1986; 255:2299-305.
2. Ulirsch RC, Jaffe ES. Sjögren's syndrome-like illness associated with the acquired immunodeficiency syndrome-related complex. Hum Pathol 1987; 18:1063-8.
3. Couderc LJ, D'Agay MF, Danon F, et al. Sicca complex and infection with human immunodeficiency virus. Arch Intern Med 1987; 147:898-901.
4. DeClerck LS, Coultenye MM, DeBroe ME, Stevens WJ. Acquired immunodeficiency syndrome mimicking Sjögren's syndrome and systemic lupus erythematosus. Arthritis Rheum 1988; 31:272-5.
5. Gordon JJ, Golbus J, Kurtidis ES. Chronic lymphadenopathy and Sjögren's syndrome in a homosexual man. N Engl J Med 1984; 311:1441-2.
6. Lecatsas G, Houff S, Marker A, et al. Retrovirus-like particles in salivary glands, prostate and testes of AIDS patients. Proc Soc Exp Biol Med 1985; 178:653-5.
7. Ryan JR, Ioachim HL, Marmer J, Loubeau JM. Acquired immune deficiency syndrome — related lymphadenopathies presenting in the salivary gland lymph nodes. Arch Otolaryngol 1985; 111:554-6.

5.15

Diagnostic Imaging

Radiographic Assessment of AIDS

Michael P. Federle, M.D., and Philip C. Goodman, M.D.

The role of radiologists and specialists in nuclear medicine varies among the main institutions caring for AIDS patients. Some make extensive use of gallium scanning for patients with *Pneumocystis carinii* pneumonia; some enthusiastically recommend barium studies of the gastrointestinal (GI) tract. Others insist that magnetic resonance imaging (MRI) is essential in the evaluation of AIDS patients with neurologic symptoms. Although not in total agreement on the exact role of imaging studies in the evaluation of AIDS, most authorities have reached similar conclusions about the strengths and weaknesses of different methods. Availability of equipment and expertise, along with philosophic differences, will continue to influence referral patterns, while increasing experience may settle certain debates.

Radionuclide scanning has its primary utility in gallium scanning of AIDS or ARC patients. Gallium scanning of the lungs appears to be the most sensitive imaging method for diagnosing and monitoring patients with *Pneumocystis carinii* pneumonia; sensitivity of over 90 percent and specificity of 75 to 80 percent have been reported.[1,2] Gallium scanning may obviate or help direct biopsy or bronchoscopy. Moreover, some researchers have recommended scanning over the abdomen for abnormal uptake of gallium, since gallium localization may indicate an infectious or neoplastic process.

Plain radiography has been most useful in the evaluation of patients with suspected pulmonary, mediastinal, or hilar pathology. Barium studies of the GI tract have revealed a variety of infectious and neoplastic processes. Abdominal imaging is described later in this chapter.

Computed tomography (CT) has been used extensively in AIDS patients for evaluating the central nervous system and abdomen. MRI is emerging as an important tool for assessing lesions of the central nervous system as well. CT or MRI of the brain is indicated for the evaluation of dementia or focal neurologic symptoms. Indications for abdominal CT in AIDS patients include the evaluation of suspected visceral or nodal infection with *M. avium-intracellulare* or of pelvic abscesses. It is also useful for diagnosis and staging of abdominal neoplasms, such as Kaposi's sarcoma (KS) and lymphoma. In patients with localized symptoms such as right upper quadrant pain, sonography is often an initial screening method, and on occasion it may reveal subtle hepatic lesions difficult to image by CT. Because of the frequency of mesenteric and retroperitoneal nodal disease in AIDS, CT remains the primary method for evaluation in most patients. Although chemotherapy for AIDS-related neoplasms is often limited in its effectiveness, repeat abdominal CT is often useful to assess the course of therapy.[3]

As discussed more completely in subsequent sections of this chapter that deal with specific pathologic conditions, imaging tests have certain limitations in the setting of AIDS. Because of the bewildering number and variety of infectious and neoplastic processes to which AIDS patients are prone and the many similar morphologic and pathologic features these processes share, imaging studies are rarely sufficient to provide a specific histologic diagnosis. Rather, they can be used in conjunction with clinical and laboratory findings to support or rule out certain diagnoses. Often, radiographic studies are used to detect a focal lesion and to direct biopsy techniques to establish a specific diagnosis.

■ RADIOGRAPHIC FINDINGS

PULMONARY INFECTIONS

Pneumocystis carinii **Pneumonia (PCP).**   PCP is the most frequently encountered opportunistic pneumonia in patients with AIDS.[4-8,26,27] Although the radiographic findings in patients with PCP vary, the vast majority of patients show bilateral, fairly symmetric, fine, reticular, interstitial infiltrates. As the disease worsens, density increases and air space consolidates. At times, a coarser linear nodular pattern may be seen. A miliary picture may be seen as well.

Occasionally, unilateral or unilobar involvement has been observed. Hilar or mediastinal adenopathy, as well as pleural fluid, have been observed in a very small number of patients. Approximately 5 percent of the patients with subsequently proven PCP have had normal chest films, however, radiographic resolution of PCP in AIDS patients may be prolonged. Interstitial fibrosis has been observed in these patients, as have air-filled cystic spaces and spontaneous pneumothorax. Approximately four days after beginning intravenous Septra therapy (trimethoprim/sulfamethoxazole), patients may present with worsened chest radiographs. This is probably due to pulmonary edema; the condition generally resolves in one to two days with diuresis.

In one series of patients, gallium lung scanning showed a sensitivity of 100 percent and a specificity of 90 percent for PCP infection.[1] In individuals with suspected infection but normal chest-film findings, this technique may provide additional information by obviating or helping to direct biopsy or bronchoscopy.

Cytomegalovirus (CMV).   In most patients, CMV infection coexists with other opportunistic infections, particularly PCP. In the few individuals with only CMV pneumonia, the chest films show bilateral, reticular, interstitial disease.[4,8] Radiographic differentiation of this infection from other opportunistic pneumonias is not possible. A few normal chest films have been noted in patients with CMV infections. Pleural fluid has not been reported.

Mycobacterial Infections.   The most frequently diagnosed mycobacterial organism in AIDS patients is *Mycobacterium avium-intracellulare* (MAI). The usual radiographic picture is of bilateral, diffuse, reticular, interstitial infiltrates. No specific pattern of distribution has been noted. Hilar and mediastinal adenopathy are only rarely noted with radiography. Cavitation has not been reported.[7] A normal chest film may be seen in 15 percent of patients with MAI pneumonia.[8]

Mycobacterium tuberculosis has a similar bilateral, reticular, interstitial pattern. Although no specific tendency for upper-lobe distribution has been observed, focal infiltrates have been reported. Pleural fluid has been reported rarely. Hilar and mediastinal adenopathy have been more commonly noted. Cavitation has not been described.[9]

Mycobacterium xenopi has been isolated from some patients with AIDS. Reticular, interstitial infiltrates were noted in the bases of one patient's lungs. Another patient's chest-film findings were normal.[10]

Fungi.   AIDS patients who live in regions of the country where certain fungi are endemic may contract the diseases caused by these organisms. Patients with histoplasmosis have chest films that predominantly show bilateral, diffuse, interstitial, reticular, and linear infiltrates. Alveolar consolidation, hilar adenopathy, cavitation, and normal radiographic findings have also been described in patients with proven histoplasmosis.[11]

A small number of patients have been reported with coccidioidomycosis. The chest films have shown diffuse, interstitial infiltrates and cavitation. A chest CT scan has shown hilar adenopathy in at least one case.[12,13]

Candida and cryptococcus have been isolated from several patients with AIDS. In general, these fungi are usually seen when other opportunistic organisms are present. The chest films reveal bilateral interstitial infiltrates, alveolar infiltrates, or both.

Other Organisms.   Conventional bacterial pneumonias are reported with increased frequency in patients with AIDS. Among the organisms responsible for these pneumonias are *Streptococcus pneumoniae* and clostridium, salmonella, and klebsiella species. The chest films in these patients usually reveal unilobar or multilobar air-space consolidation — typical of the pictures caused by these pathogens in non-HIV-infected individuals. Occasionally, adult respiratory distress syndrome may result in diffuse interstitial or alveolar consolidation, or both.

Nocardia has been found in patients with AIDS.[28] It caused a pneumonia in one of our patients who had a right middle-lobe infiltrate.

Pulmonary toxoplasmosis has also been reported in patients with AIDS.[29] We have seen it cause poorly defined nodules scattered throughout the lungs of a patient.

NEOPLASMS

Kaposi's Sarcoma.   Two basic radiographic patterns have been observed in patients with Kaposi's sarcoma. One is a pattern of poorly-defined nodular densities scattered throughout both lungs. The second is a diffuse, coarse, linear, interstitial pattern. Hilar adenopathy has been reported in patients with KS. A very high percentage of these patients' chest films may show the presence of pleural fluid. Usually, the chest-film abnormalities in KS patients are seen late in the course of disease, although there have been a few reported instances of pulmonary KS manifestations occurring before the lymphocutaneous manifestations.[14-18,30]

Lymphoma.   In a report of one series, the lung parenchyma was involved by either Hodgkin's or non-Hodgkin's lymphoma in 10 percent of patients.[19] Hodgkin's disease in this group may be unusual. Another report indicates no mediastinal adenopathy in a patient with bibasilar infiltrates. Pleural fluid, as well as hilar and mediastinal adenopathy, have been reported in other cases, however.[20,21]

I have now seen several cases of lymphoma in which a single well-defined nodule (or multiple well-defined nodules) has been present on chest radiographs. These areas of parenchymal lymphoma have shown rapid enlargement and have measured from as small as 1 cm to as large as 8 cm in diameter (see plates 5.15.1.a and b).

PRIMARY LUNG CARCINOMA

One small-cell carcinoma and one adenosquamous-cell carcinoma of the lung have been reported in AIDS patients.[22,23] These may be coincidental findings, but they may relate to the abnormal immune function seen in these patients. The chest radiographs in these patients have shown a small mass and a right lower-lobe cavitary process.

MISCELLANEOUS DISEASES

Castleman's Disease.   Two patients in whom KS subsequently developed were initially reported as having Castleman's disease. One patient's chest-film findings were normal, whereas the other's showed bilateral hilar adenopathy. This lymph-node hyperplasia, which is usually benign, has been recently reported to express itself more aggressively in the setting of AIDS.[24]

Lymphoid Interstitial Pneumonitis.   Several AIDS patients are suspected of having lymphoid interstitial pneumonitis. The chest radiographs have shown bilateral, diffuse, interstitial disease, usually in the lower lobes.[25]

Lymphadenopathy Syndrome.   Patients with lymphadenopathy syndrome usually show subdiaphragmatic lymphadenopathy and splenomegaly. No patients having this symptom alone have been observed with either hilar or mediastinal adenopathy on chest film or at CT scanning. The presence of hilar or mediastinal adenopathy in a patient with the lymphadenopathy syndrome should suggest the possibility of lymphoma or KS. Occasionally, an enlarged spleen may be seen on the chest films.

■ ABDOMINAL RADIOGRAPHIC FINDINGS

INFECTIONS

Candida.   *Candida albicans* is the opportunistic organism that most frequently affects the GI tract in patients with AIDS and AIDS-related complex (ARC). The radiographic findings of candida (monilial) esophagitis range from mild mucosal irregularity of the proximal to mid-esophagus to diffuse nodularity with extensive plaque formation and occasional deep ulceration. Large fungus balls and bezoars have rarely been reported. Invasive candidiasis can mimic primary or secondary tumor of the esophagus, causing luminal narrowing and mass-like thickening of the esophageal wall.[31]

Cytomegalovirus (CMV).   Cytomegalovirus and other herpesviruses may cause esophagitis that is radiographically indistinguishable from candida on contrast studies. More characteristic, however, are shallow ulcerations with a surrounding halo of edema or deep, longitudinally oriented ulcers. Nodular or vertical linear plaques are also encountered. Cases of CMV gastritis have also been reported with radiographic features similar to other forms of gastritis, shallow ulcers, and enlarged folds[32] (see plate 5.15.1.c).

CMV is also a recognized cause of colitis that clinically, radiographically, and pathologically may simulate idiopathic inflammatory bowel disease or ischemic colitis.[33] Contrast studies may reveal superficial erosions, granular mucosa, spasm, and prominent submucosal nodular indentations (2 to 4 mm) representing lymphoid nodular hyperplasia in mild-to-moderate disease, while severe infection may be characterized by frank ulceration, submucosal hemorrhage ("thumbprinting"), and perforation. The findings may be diffuse or focal; cecal involvement predominates in some series.

Cryptosporidiosis.   The radiographic manifestations of cryptosporidiosis in contrast studies are nonspecific and varied, and range from diffuse regular thickening of duodenal and jejunal folds to a more disorganized, irregular fold pattern. Increased secretions are often evident in the small bowel and, less commonly, in the colon, radiographically recognized as dilution and flocculation of the intraluminal barium. A pattern of diffuse colitis has been reported when parasitic infestation has persisted for a period of several months.[31,34]

Patients with AIDS who are referred for radiographic examination of the GI tract have a high incidence and a wide spectrum of abnormal findings. In general, contrast radiography is relatively sensitive but not specific in the detection of GI infections and tumors, although patients may have endoscopically confirmed GI infection and a normal barium study. A potentially important observation is the existence of multifocal areas of involvement of the GI tract, seen in most patients with AIDS.[31] Multifocal abnormalities (e.g., duodenum, plus small bowel or colon) are uncommon in the general population, regardless of the nature of the GI pathology. In AIDS, multifocal abnormalities may be due to multiple foci of Kaposi's sarcoma, widely distributed opportunistic infection, multiple opportunistic infections, coexistent tumor and infection, or even coexisting tumors (e.g., KS and lymphoma).

The detection of multifocal GI abnormalities may be an important indicator of the syndrome in patients at risk for AIDS. In patients already diagnosed with AIDS, barium radiography of the GI tract can aid in the selection of those who might need endoscopy and can help direct the selection of sites for biopsy. Barium radiography is also valuable in detecting easily treatable non-AIDS-related conditions, such as peptic-ulcer disease, that may coexist in these patients.

Mycobacterium avium-intracellulare (**MAI**).   AIDS patients have an increased incidence of infections with atypical mycobacteria, particularly *M. avium-intracellulare*. Since *M. avium* and *M. intracellulare* are difficult to distinguish by the usual laboratory methods and because differentiation is usually not clinically important, they are referred to as a single group. Patients with disseminated MAI associated with AIDS often complain of systemic and abdominal symptoms, particularly night sweats, abdominal pain, diarrhea, and weight loss. Barium studies of the GI tract and abdominal computed tomography are often obtained in this setting. Barium studies of the upper GI tract may reveal esophageal ulceration or small-bowel pathology marked by thickened, distorted folds and increased secretions.[35] Abdominal CT frequently (>80 percent) demonstrates large, bulky, retroperitoneal and mesenteric adenopathy, often with characteristic central necrosis.[36] CT-guided biopsy is definitive in most cases, showing large, foamy macrophages filled with acid-fast bacteria. The intracellular, rod-like organisms may also test positive on periodic acid–Schiff (PAS) stain. This latter feature, the clinical presentation, and radiographic and CT findings are very similar to findings in Whipple's disease, leading to the designation of abdominal MAI as "pseudo-Whipple's disease," and suggesting that the gut may be one portal of entry in disseminated MAI.[35,37]

NEOPLASMS

Kaposi's Sarcoma.   AIDS-related KS is similar in clinical presentation to the aggressive and disseminated form seen in African adolescents. Early lymph node and visceral involvements are the predominant features. Gastrointestinal lesions are common, occurring in 50 percent of patients. Late in the course of the disease, widespread lesions may be found involving virtually all organ systems. Occasionally the lesions are present in unusual sites.[16,38]

The radiologic diagnosis of gastrointestinal lesions in KS has been described. KS can affect any part of the GI tract from the pharynx to the anus. Most individuals with lesions are asymptomatic, although more advanced KS may involve GI bleeding, obstruction, perforation, and diarrhea. Nearly 50 percent of patients with mucocutaneous KS have evidence of gastrointestinal KS on endoscopy, although barium radiography reveals only a minority of these lesions.[38] The most common manifestations of gastrointestinal KS are submucosal plaques, some with central ulceration ("target" or "bull's eye" lesions). Larger polypoid masses are relatively common; circumferential and diffusely spreading lesions are rare.

Initial reports of CT findings in AIDS-related KS emphasized the overlap between this entity and the lymphadenopathy syndrome.[39] Splenomegaly and mild retroperitoneal and mesenteric nodal enlargement are common to both, and do not necessarily indicate widespread involvement with KS. This is particularly true when the lymph nodes are less than 1.5 cm in greatest diameter. However, bulky nodal enlargement may be the only CT evidence of abdominal KS. Indeed, a purely lymphadenopathic form of AIDS-related KS is being recognized with increasing frequency. This is an interesting clinical correlate to the growing histochemical evidence of the origin of KS from lymphatic endothelial cells. Bulky adenopathy in AIDS-related KS cannot be distinguished from lymphoma or infections such as *Mycobacterium avium-intracellulare* unless determined by fine-needle aspiration biopsy.[3]

Although the characteristic "target" lesions of KS seen on air-contrast studies of the gastrointestinal tract are rarely seen on CT studies, larger focal masses may be identified by mural thickening. The CT demonstration of focal hepatic or splenic lesions of KS in AIDS is uncommon. As with retroperitoneal adenopathy, this sarcoma has a nonspecific CT appearance and can only be distinguished from other neoplastic or infectious causes by fine-needle aspiration biopsy. In our experience, fine-needle biopsy has proven reliable in diagnosing AIDS-related KS. Cohesive clusters of bland spindle cells are arranged in characteristic slit-like spaces. Because KS can involve virtually any organ in the body, it may produce unusual intra-abdominal lesions that can readily be detected and biopsied under CT guidance.

Lymphoma.   In addition to KS, a variety of aggressive B-cell lymphomas (without primary central nervous system involvement) have been associated with AIDS. To date, non-Hodgkin's lymphoma, including the Burkitt type, has been the most common lymphoma in patients with AIDS. However, Hodgkin's disease has also been described.

In some patients, lymphoma may occur before the onset of full-blown AIDS. In evaluating non-Hodgkin's lymphoma in 90 homosexual men, Ziegler et al. emphasized several unique manifestations within this subgroup of patients, including a dramatic increase in extranodal involvement in AIDS-related lymphoma, in which the brain and bone marrow, as well as abdominal, visceral, and mucocutaneous sites, were affected (see plate 5.15.1.d). Of the 90 patients reported by these investigators, 88 had extranodal sites of involvement. In addition, patients with AIDS-related lymphoma typically had highly malignant histologic subtypes of non-Hodgkin's lymphoma and advanced stages of disease. In their series, 58 percent of patients had stage III (or greater) lymphoma, and 62 percent had high grade malignant histologic cell types.[19]

When compared with patients with non-Hodgkin's lymphoma without AIDS, the response to treatment has been poor, and these cases with AIDS generally have an unfavorable prognosis.

A significant percentage of patients with AIDS-related lymphoma demonstrate focal hepatic and splenic lesions (see plate 5.15.1.e). In our series of 19 AIDS-related lymphomas, 26 percent of patients with non-Hodgkin's lymphoma had biopsy-proven focal hepatic lesions compared with 4 to 6 percent of patients without AIDS who had the lesions.[40] In patients with relatively diffuse hepatic involvement with lymphoma, smaller microscopic foci (less than 1 cm) may occasionally be difficult to recognize on contrast-enhanced CT. We have noted on several occasions that sonography may be useful in depicting disorganized hepatic echogenicity with small hypoechoic foci in patients with hepatomegaly and no obvious focal lesions on CT. The overall sensitivity for CT and sonography in diagnosing hepatic involvement with AIDS-related lymphoma is not known, but it is likely that many cases of microscopic disease will escape detection by current imaging.

AIDS-related Hodgkin's disease appears to be substantially less common than non-Hodgkin's lymphoma. However, features of this disease are distinctive in the AIDS population. Patients typically appear with advanced stages of Hodgkin's disease (clinical stage III or IV), with mixed cellularity or nodular sclerosing histology. In addition, unusual manifestations of Hodgkin's disease include involvement of the skin overlying involved lymph nodes and bone marrow involvement without splenic lesions. In our series of 10 patients with AIDS-related Hodgkin's disease studied at San Francisco General Hospital, two patients (20 percent) had bulky mesenteric nodal masses with Hodgkin's disease, an uncommon feature in the non-AIDS population. In addition, noncontiguous sites of nodal involvement were identified by CT in which pelvic adenopathy without paraaortic involvement was present.

We make extensive use of CT-guided percutaneous needle biopsy of enlarged lymph nodes in lymphoma patients. Although the technique is somewhat controversial and requires considerable cytologic skill, fine-needle biopsy has allowed diagnosis and subtyping of most AIDS-related lymphomas in our institution. If there is any question about the histologic subtype, surgical biopsy is recommended.

■ BRAIN IMAGING IN AIDS

Neurologic signs and symptoms occur frequently in AIDS patients, owing to a variety of central nervous system infections and tumors. Computed tomography scanning and magnetic resonance imaging are important tools for early diagnosis and treatment of these processes, although precise diagnosis remains difficult and the ultimate prognosis is grave.[41-43]

TOXOPLASMOSIS

The most frequent CT appearance of untreated toxoplasma encephalitis consists of multiple deep and superficial lesions in both cerebral hemispheres, associated with edema and mass effect. The most characteristic locations of the lesions are the corticomedullary junction and the basal ganglia. The lesions typically are enhanced, after intravenous administration of contrast material, in a ring, nodular, or mixed pattern. Enhancement and lesion detectability are accentuated by a "double dose" of contrast medium (100 ml of 76 percent contrast medium or 36 g iodine) and a delay of one hour before scanning.[43]

The CT appearance of toxoplasma encephalitis is not pathognomonic, but it directs appropriate therapy in most cases and is effective in monitoring response. Serial CT scans show progressive diminution of enhancing lesions, edema, and mass effect, beginning within two to four weeks after institution of therapy. Clinical improvement is expected within one week. With continuous and long-term medical therapy, healing does occur, as evidenced by the return to normal of some scans and the appearance on others of areas of encephalomalacia. Because of the persistent cellular immune defects in AIDS patients, however, this healing process may be reversed when medical therapy is interrupted. When this occurs, CT is a reliable indicator of recurrence. Recurrent lesions have the same appearance as the original lesions.

If the clinical status and CT scan fail to show a satisfactory response to medical therapy, biopsy of CNS lesions may be warranted to exclude other infectious and neoplastic processes that may simulate toxoplasmosis. Choosing a biopsy site likely to lead to the least damage to normal brain tissue is important. Magnetic resonance imaging appears to be more sensitive than CT in detection of AIDS-related CNS pathology. If CT, preferably double-dose delayed CT, fails to reveal a lesion accessible to biopsy, then MRI is a useful adjunct. Some researchers believe that MRI is the method of choice for all AIDS-related CNS pathology and, where available, obviates CT scanning.

OTHER INFECTIONS

CT usually detects other CNS parenchymal infections if they cause focal masses. Brain abscesses caused by *M. tuberculosis* and *Candida albicans* are indistinguishable from toxoplasmosis by CT criteria alone. After failure of empirical anti-toxoplasma medical therapy, repeat CT is indicated for guiding needle aspiration and for culture of such lesions. Herpes encephalitis may cause focal lesions, but usually with a hemorrhagic component that is detectable by CT or MRI.

CT seems to be less sensitive in the early detection of infections that are diffuse and infiltrative in nature (such as CMV encephalitis and progressive multifocal leukoencephalopathy (PML) caused by the papovavirus) than in the detection of focal lesions. In CMV encephalitis, CT may be normal or show white matter disease manifested by diffuse low-density lesions, or gray-matter disease manifested by enhancing cortical nodules. Subependymal involvement has also been reported, seen on CT as diffuse enhancement of the borders of the lateral ventricles. MRI appears to be more sensitive in detecting CMV encephalitis and PML.

PML may be difficult to detect by CT, but characteristically shows central and/or convolutional white-matter low densities, often in a parieto-occipital location and with negligible mass effect. It has also been reported in the cerebellum, where it appeared as a large, low-density lesion.

In contradistinction to parenchymal infection, meningitis is infrequently diagnosed by CT. Occasional findings of communicating hydrocephalus, dilated cerebrospinal fluid spaces, and meningeal enhancement are nonspecific. Parenchymal involvement is seen infrequently. CSF analysis, however, is usually diagnostic. The most common organism causing meningitis in AIDS is *Cryptococcus neoformans*; *Escherichia coli* and other bacteria have rarely been found. The value of CT lies in excluding any superimposed parenchymal diseases that might make lumbar puncture dangerous and in detecting communicating hydrocephalus that might require shunting.

CNS NEOPLASMS

CT is sensitive, though nonspecific, in detecting AIDS-related CNS neoplasms.[41-43] Most appear as ring-enhancing or homogeneously enhancing focal parenchymal mass lesions. Both large-cell and Burkitt-type lymphomas have been reported. Primary brain lymphomas are considered a hallmark of AIDS, since they occur rarely in populations other than those with suppressed immune systems. Kaposi's sarcoma is the other CNS tumor reported in AIDS, again appearing as an enhancing focal mass(es). Because lymphomas and KS are indistinguishable from CNS parenchymal infections, biopsy is necessary for diagnosis. Early biopsy is performed when there is a relatively low clinical suspicion of infection, or when empirical medical treatment for toxoplasmosis has been unrewarding.

REFERENCES

1. Coleman DL, Hattner RS, Luce JM, et al. A correlation between gallium lung scans and fiberoptic bronchoscopy in patients with *Pneumocystis carinii* pneumonia and the acquired immune deficiency syndrome. Am Rev Resp Dis 1984; 130:1166-9.

2. Barron TF, Birnbaum NS, Shane LB, et al. *Pneumocystis carinii* pneumonia studied by gallium-67 scanning. Radiology 1985; 154:791-3.

3. Jeffrey RF Jr, Nyberg DA, Bottles K, et al. Abdominal CT in acquired immunodeficiency syndrome. AJR 1986; 146:7-13.

4. Goodman PC, Broaddus CV, Hopewell PC. Chest radiographic patterns in the acquired immunodeficiency syndrome. Am Rev Resp Dis 1984; 129:A36. abstract.

5. Gottlieb MS. Pulmonary disease in the acquired immune deficiency syndrome. Chest 1983; 86(Suppl 3); 295-315.

6. Murray JF, Felton CP, Garay SM, et al. Pulmonary complications of the acquired immunodeficiency syndrome. N Engl J Med 1984; 310:1682-8.

7. Hopewell PC, Luce JM. Pulmonary involvement in the acquired immunodeficiency syndrome. Chest 1985; 87:104-12.

8. Stover DE, White DA, Romano PA, et al. Spectrum of pulmonary diseases associated with the acquired immune deficiency syndrome. Am J Med 1985; 78:429-37.

9. Pitchenik AE, Rubinson HA. The radiographic appearance of tuberculosis in patients with the acquired immune deficiency syndrome (AIDS) and pre AIDS. Am Rev Resp Dis 1985; 131:393-6.

10. Tecson-Tumang FT, Bright JL. *Mycobacterium xenopi* and the acquired immunodeficiency syndrome. Ann Intern Med 1984; 100:461.

11. Wheat LJ, Slama TG, Zeckel ML. Histoplasmosis in the acquired immune deficiency syndrome. Am J Med 1985; 78:203-10.

12. Abrams DI, Robia M, Blumenfeld W, et al. Disseminated coccidioidomycosis in AIDS. N Engl J Med 1984; 310:986-7.

13. Kovacs A, Forthal DN, Kovacs JA, et al. Disseminated coccidioidomycosis in a patient with acquired immune deficiency syndrome. West J Med 1984; 140:447-9.

14. Brown RKJ, Huberman RP, Vanley G. Pulmonary features of Kaposi's sarcoma. AJR 1982; 139:659-60.

15. Friedman-Kien AE, Laubenstein LJ, Rubinstein P, et al. Disseminated Kaposi's sarcoma in homosexual men. Ann Intern Med 1983; 96:693-700.

16. Hill CA, Harle TS, Mansell PWA. The prodrome: Kaposi's sarcoma and infections associated with acquired immunodeficiency syndrome: radiologic findings in 39 patients. Radiology 1983; 149:393-9.

17. Kornfeld H, Axelrod JL. Pulmonary presentation of Kaposi's sarcoma in a homosexual patient. Am Rev Resp Dis 1983; 127:248-9.

18. Ognibene FP, Steis RG, Macher AM, et al. Kaposi's sarcoma causing pulmonary infiltrates and respiratory failure in the acquired immunodeficiency syndrome. Ann Intern Med 1985; 102:471-5.

19. Ziegler JL, Beckstead JA, Volberding PA, et al. Non-Hodgkin's lymphoma in 90 homosexual men. N Engl J Med 1984; 311:565-70.

20. Schoeppel SL, Hoppe RT, Dorfman RF, et al. Hodgkin's disease in homosexual men with generalized lymphadenopathy. Ann Intern Med 1985; 102:68-70.

21. Cohen BA, Pomeranz S, Rabinowitz JG, et al. Pulmonary complications of AIDS: radiologic features. AJR 1984; 143:115-22.

22. Irwin LE, Begandy MK, Moore TM. Adenosquamous carcinoma of the lung in the acquired immunodeficiency syndrome. Ann Intern Med 1984; 100:158.

23. Nusbaum NJ. Metastatic small-cell carcinoma of the lung in a patient with AIDS. N Engl J Med 1985; 312:1706.

24. Lachant NA, Sun MCJ, Leong LA, et al. Multicentric angiofollicular lymph node hyperplasia (Castleman's disease) followed by Kaposi's sarcoma in two homosexual males with the acquired immunodeficiency syndrome (AIDS). Am J Clin Pathol 1985; 83:27-33.

25. Solal-Celigny P, Couderac LJ, Herman D, et al. Lymphoid interstitial pneumonitis in acquired immunodeficiency syndrome related complex. Am Rev Resp Dis 1985; 131:956-60.

26. Naidich DP, Garay SM, Goodman PC, et al. Pulmonary manifestations of AIDS. In: Federle MP, Megibow AJ, Naidich DP. Radiology of AIDS. New York: Raven Press, 1988; 47-75.

27. Jeffrey RB Jr, Goodman PC, Olsen WL, Wall SD. Radiologic imaging of AIDS. Curr Probl Diagn Radiol 1988; 17:73-117.

28. Rodriguez JL, Barrio JL, Pitchenik AE. Pulmonary nocardiosis in the acquired immunodeficiency syndrome. Diagnosis with bronchoalveolar lavage and treatment with non-sulfur containing drugs. Chest 1986; 90:912-4.

29. Mendelson MH, Finkel LJ, Meyers BR, et al. Pulmonary toxoplasmosis in AIDS. Scand J Infect Dis 1987; 19:703-6.

30. Kaplan LD, Hopewell PC, Jaffe H, et al. Kaposi's sarcoma involving the lung in patients with the acquired immunodeficiency syndrome. J Acquir Immune Defic Syndr 1988; 1:23-40.

31. Wall SD, Ominski S, Altman DF, et al. Multifocal abnormalities of the gastrointestinal tract in AIDS. AJR 1986; 146:1-5.

32. Balthazar EJ, Megibow AJ, Hulnick DH. Cytomegalovirus esophagitis and gastritis in AIDS. AJR 1985; 144:1201-4.

33. Balthazar EJ, Megibow AJ, Fazzini E, et al. Cytomegalovirus colitis in AIDS: radiographic findings in 11 patients. Radiology 1985; 155:585-9.

34. Berk RN, Wall SD, McArdle CB, et al. Cryptosporidiosis of the stomach and small intestine in patients with AIDS. AJR 1984; 143:549-54.

35. Vincent ME, Robbins AH. *Mycobacterium avium intracellulare* complex enteritis: pseudo-Whipple disease in AIDS. AJR 1985; 144:921-2.

36. Nyberg DA, Federle MP, Jeffrey RB, et al. Abdominal CT findings of disseminated *Mycobacterium avium intracellulare* in AIDS. AJR 1985; 145:297-9.

37. Roth RI, Owen RL, Keven DF. AIDS with *Mycobacterium avium-intracellulare* lesions resembling those of Whipple's disease. N Engl J Med 1983; 309:1324-5.

38. Rose HS, Balthazar EJ, Megibow AJ, et al. Alimentary tract involvement in Kaposi's sarcoma: radiographic and endoscopic findings in 25 homosexual men. AJR 1982; 139:661-6.

39. Moon KL Jr, Federle MP, Abrams DI, et al. Kaposi's sarcoma and lymphadenopathy syndrome: limitations of abdominal CT in acquired immunodeficiency syndrome. Radiology 1984; 150:479-83.

40. Nyberg DA, Jeffrey RB Jr, Federle MP. Abdominal CT of AIDS-related lymphomas. Radiology 1986; 159:59-63.

41. Whelan MA, Kricheff II, Handler M, et al. Acquired immunodeficiency syndrome: cerebral computed tomographic manifestations. Radiology 1983; 149:477-84.

42. Kelly WM, Brant-Zawadzki M. Acquired immunodeficiency syndrome: neuroradiologic findings. Radiology 1983; 149:485-91.

43. Post MJ, Kwisunoglu SJ, Hensley GT, et al. Cranial CT in acquired immunodeficiency syndrome: spectrum of diseases and optimal contrast enhancement technique. AJR 1985; 145:929-40.

6

INFECTIONS ASSOCIATED WITH AIDS

EDITORS

Constance B. Wofsy, M.D., and Merle A. Sande, M.D.

6.1

Pyogenic Bacterial Infections

6.1.1

Salmonella

Richard E. Chaisson, M.D., Merle A. Sande, M.D., and J. Louise Gerberding, M.D.

■ EPIDEMIOLOGY

Nontyphoidal salmonellosis is an opportunistic infectious complication of AIDS. Early reports of opportunistic infections in AIDS patients or people at risk for AIDS (Haitians,[1] Africans,[2,3] children of high-risk parents,[4] and homosexual men[5]) included cases of unusually severe bacteremic salmonellosis. Since then, it has become apparent that disseminated infection with *Salmonella typhimurium, S. enteritidis, S. arizona, S. dublin*, and other salmonella serotypes occurs in AIDS patients at a prevalence greatly exceeding that of the general population.[6-12] Nontyphoidal salmonella infections are mild and self-limited. Gastroenteritis is a common manifestation. More severe disease, including bacteremia, is associated with immunocompromised hosts.[13] Salmonella infections in AIDS patients are usually systemic and disseminated, tend to relapse despite effective antimicrobial agents, and fail to demonstrate foci of persistent infection.

Salmonellosis may occur in patients with a pre-existing AIDS diagnosis or may be the presenting illness in patients who later develop AIDS.[7,10] Since 4 percent to 6 percent of nontyphoidal salmonellosis is associated with bacteremia in the general population,[14] a diagnosis of salmonella sepsis alone does not constitute a diagnosis of AIDS. However, in a person from an AIDS risk group, the diagnosis of salmonellosis, particularly with septicemia, suggests the possibility of underlying cell-mediated immune dysfunction and AIDS.

Unlike *S. typhi*, which is found only in humans, nontyphoidal salmonella is found in many lower animals, and animal products are the major source of most human outbreaks. The usual route of infection is oral, and food and drink are reliably identified as sources for clusters. Salmonella can be isolated from chicken and other fowl, livestock, domestic pets, and turtles. Food sources of salmonella include unpasteurized milk,[12] eggs, meat, and many processed foods. Moreover, virtually any food product can be contaminated by rodents or insects harboring salmonella organisms. Animal products such as bone meal and meat by-products are also sources of infection for both humans and animals.

Salmonellosis in AIDS patients is infrequent and probably accounts for less than 5 percent of all opportunistic infections. Nonetheless, its incidence in San Francisco's AIDS patients has been estimated as 20-fold greater than in the city's general population.[18] Sources of salmonella in patients with AIDS do not appear to differ from those affecting the rest of the population, but the distribution of disease type is clearly atypical — bacteremia and relapsing infection are the rule in AIDS patients, while gastroenteritis is less common. Reports of salmonellosis associated with pet turtles,[15] raw milk,[12] and contaminated animal-skin products are evidence of nonhuman sources of infection in AIDS patients. Reports of salmonellosis are more frequent among AIDS patients who are IV drug users, Haitians, Africans, or children of urban risk-group members, suggesting that low socioeconomic status may confer greater risk of exposure to salmonella. Salmonellosis is not a common sexually transmitted enteric disease of homosexual men[16] and does not appear to occur more frequently in this population.

PATHOPHYSIOLOGY

Nontyphoidal salmonellas, particularly *S. typhimurium* and *S. enteritidis*, are common isolates from human sources and are seen frequently in AIDS patients. Salmonellae are nonspore-forming, aerobic and facultatively anaerobic, motile, gram-negative bacilli. Over 2000 serotypes have been identified based on the O and H antigens. Identification in the laboratory is based on fermentation of glucose and the inability to ferment lactose or sucrose. *S. typhi* is the cause of enteric fever and has not been associated with AIDS.

Cell-mediated immunity is an essential component of host defenses against infection with salmonella species.[14] Patients with defects in cell-mediated immunity, such as those with Hodgkin's disease, leukemia, lymphoma, renal transplantations, and those undergoing corticosteroid therapy, are particularly susceptible to severe infections with *S. typhimurium*. Salmonella may persist intracellularly despite adequate humoral immunity and antimicrobial therapy in the presence of altered T-cell function.[14] Introduction of salmonella is usually by the oral route; occurrence of disease depends on inoculum size, serotype, and host factors. The bacteria pass through the stomach to the small intestine and multiply. Fecal excretion, with or without symptoms, then follows. Small inocula of salmonella are inactivated by gastric pH but may survive in patients taking antacids or in patients who have had a gastrectomy. Larger inocula may overwhelm gastric protective mechanisms. Normal enteric flora may inhibit salmonella growth and pathogenesis. Previous use of antibiotics may alter intestinal flora, permitting growth of salmonella, as in a recent outbreak in many states.[17]

CLINICAL PRESENTATION

Most salmonella infections in the general population are manifested by gastro-enteritis alone. Invasion of the intestinal wall and hematogenous dissemination may occur in 4 percent to 6 percent of infected individuals, resulting in either bacteremia or localized infection, such as mycotic aneurysms, endocarditis, or abscesses. One-quarter of patients with recurrent infections have a localized site of persistence identified, frequently the gallbladder. However, in AIDS, no sequestered reservoir of infection appears to be necessary for recurrence. Recurrent salmonella infections have been reported in patients with hemolytic anemias, particularly sickle-cell disease, although this may reflect asplenia more than hemolysis. Jacobs and associates,[6] however, found a Coomb's-positive anemia in 5 patients with AIDS-related salmonellosis. Access of the organisms to the bloodstream in AIDS patients is more prevalent and is clinically associated with disruption of gastrointestinal mucosa by coexisting infectious agents, including cytomegalovirus (CMV), herpes simplex virus, cryptosporidium, and candida.[6,8] Once blood-borne, salmonella may reach any organ. At autopsy, *S. typhimurium* has been cultured from the lungs, heart, brain, liver, spleen, kidneys, and bone marrow.[6]

Salmonella infections typically present in stereotypic syndromes. The majority of symptomatic patients have a mild, self-limited enterocolitis that resolves without treatment. A bacteremic syndrome occurs in approximately 5 percent of cases and is associated with underlying illnesses such as malignancy, hemolytic diseases, corticosteroid use, or sickle-cell disease. Recurrent episodes of bacteremia may occur in such patients owing to persistent foci of infection (often the gallbladder), or to the release of organisms from intracellular sites in the reticuloendothelial system. Focal infections outside the gastrointestinal system include mycotic aneurysms, intra-abdominal abscesses, endocarditis, pneumonia, urinary tract infection, and osteomyelitis.

Patients with AIDS or ARC and salmonellosis may initially have generalized sepsis, localized infection (such as brain abscess or endocarditis), or other opportunistic infections. In 41 published cases of AIDS-related salmonellosis, 17 patients lacked CDC-defined surveillance criteria for AIDS at initial presentation.[1-11] Although enterocolitis is a frequent problem in patients with AIDS, salmonella is rarely the cause. The majority of patients first appear with signs and symptoms of sepsis and opportunistic infection but lack localizing signs for salmonella. Fever is universal in these patients; other constitutional symptoms, including chills, sweats, weight loss, diarrhea, and anorexia are common. Mucocutaneous candidiasis and herpes simplex infections may also be present.

Additional gastrointestinal derangements may be found concomitantly with salmonella, including cryptosporidiosis and CMV enteritis. These manifestations may provide a mechanism for systemic infection. Other manifestations of AIDS-related conditions, such as Kaposi's sarcoma, lymphadenopathy, aseptic meningitis, toxoplasmosis, or *Pneumocystis carinii* pneumonia, may be present. Patients treated for previous salmonella infections may appear with relapses either coincident with symptoms of other illnesses or with sepsis. A history of ingestion of raw milk, use of powders derived from snakeskins, or handling of pet turtles may be seen in some cases. Most signs and symptoms, however, are noncharacteristic, so the diagnosis is usually suggested after laboratory data have been obtained.

■ DIAGNOSIS

The diagnosis of salmonellosis is made by bacterial culture. Many AIDS patients with salmonellosis have bacteremia, and standard blood cultures provide the diagnosis. Stool cultures for salmonella are essential for patients presenting with gastrointestinal symptoms, and these cultures may identify the organism in patients with negative blood cultures. Cultures from patients previously treated with appropriate antibiotics may continue to yield the organism.

Other findings in nontypical salmonella septicemia may include a Coomb's-positive hemolytic anemia,[6] elevated transaminase levels, and an elevated sedimentation rate. The white blood-cell count may be normal or elevated. The classic leukopenia of enteric fever is usually not present in nontyphoidal salmonellosis, although AIDS patients frequently are neutropenic, lymphopenic, or pancytopenic. Evaluation of the biliary tree in AIDS patients with salmonellosis has been uniformly unrewarding.[6-8] Patients with brain abscesses containing salmonella have characteristic ring-enhancing lesions indistinguishable from cerebral toxoplasmosis by cerebral computed tomography (CT).[11] Diagnosis in these patients is established by brain biopsy. Patients with previous episodes of disseminated salmonella infections should have blood and stool cultures at the first sign of clinical symptoms that suggest relapse.

■ TREATMENT

Treatment of nontyphoidal salmonellosis in the normal host is supportive, consisting of fluids, antipyretics, and atropinic agents for severe abdominal symptoms. Antibiotics are not always advised for gastroenteritis, since they may prolong fecal excretion of organisms and lead to a chronic carrier state. Focal abscesses are treated with drainage and antibiotics. Bacteremic salmonellosis in the normal host is treated with antibiotics.

Treatment of AIDS-related salmonellosis with systemic antibiotics is mandatory, and frequent recurrences of salmonellosis may make lifelong therapy essential.[6-8] Episodes of drug-resistant salmonellosis in AIDS patients are increasing; organisms have been reported to acquire resistance during the course of treatment.[6] Initial treatment depends on drug sensitivities, but ampicillin or chloramphenicol are the time-honored drugs of choice (for trimethoprim and sulfamethoxazole, see below). Ampicillin is as effective as chloramphenicol in most instances, and for patients with endocarditis or mycotic aneurysms, ampicillin is preferred because of its bactericidal action. Long-term oral therapy with ampicillin or amoxicillin may be feasible, but relapses may occur during treatment. Chloramphenicol can be initially administered, but long-term therapy with chloramphenicol should be avoided, if possible, because of dose-related myelosuppression.

Trimethoprim and sulfamethoxazole are highly effective for treating salmonella infections, but their use in AIDS-related salmonellosis is problematic for two reasons. First, severe cutaneous and systemic toxicity to trimethoprim and sulfamethoxazole occurs in up to 50 percent of AIDS patients treated with these agents for *Pneumocystis carinii* pneumonia (PCP).[19-21] Second, trimethoprim and sulfamethoxazole remain one of two approved treatments for PCP and should be reserved for that indication in AIDS patients if possible.

Use of a third-generation cephalosporin and an aminoglycoside during initial therapy may be beneficial. Long-term suppressive therapy is recommended for all AIDS patients with recurrent bacteremic salmonellosis and may be achieved with amoxicillin or chloramphenicol. Studies are under way in several centers to determine the effectiveness of quinolones, including ciprofloxacin and norfloxacin, as chronic suppressive therapy.

The concomitant use of rifampin may enhance intracellular killing during the initial phase of treatment but cannot be recommended until further studies clarify its role in salmonellosis. Localized abscesses are treated by surgical drainage and antibiotics.

■ OUTCOME

Salmonella infections, like other opportunistic infections in AIDS patients, have a uniformly dismal outcome. The long-term mortality rate in any AIDS patient with an opportunistic infection is 100 percent; the median survival is 9 months.[22] Immediate mortality from sepsis has been observed, but more frequently, coexistent diseases such as PCP, cryptococcal disease, or toxoplasmosis contribute to death. Patients surviving initial episodes frequently relapse — some while on appropriate antibiotics — and these patients require repeat courses of intravenous therapy. Studies of long-term therapy with quinolones to suppress recurrent bacteremia are under way. Until effective immunorestorative and antiviral therapies for HIV infection are available, treatment of any opportunistic infection is likely to remain palliative.

■ PREVENTION

Prevention of salmonellosis in any population depends on public health and hygienic measures. Clean water and properly cooked and stored foods are the cornerstones of prevention in developing countries. Avoidance of contact with potentially contaminated foodstuffs is particularly important for immunosuppressed hosts. Persons with AIDS or in AIDS risk groups should avoid raw milk.[23] Pet turtles are a known source of salmonella, and bacteremia has been reported in an AIDS patient after handling a turtle.[15] Prevention of nosocomial infection relies on meticulous infection-control measures by hospital staff. Universal precautions for avoiding direct contact with blood, stool, and other body fluids should be followed by health-care workers caring for hospitalized patients with salmonellosis. Outpatients who are salmonella carriers should be educated about hygiene and effective means of handling soiled surfaces and linens in the home. AIDS patients with salmonellosis should undergo epidemiologic investigation by public-health authorities so that common-source outbreaks can be identified and effective control measures instituted.

REFERENCES

1. Pitchenik AE, Fischl MA, Dickinson GM, et al. Opportunistic infections and Kaposi's sarcoma among Haitians: Evidence of a new acquired immunodeficiency state. Ann Intern Med 1983; 98:277-84.

2. Clumeck N, Mascart-Lemone F, de Mauberuge J, et al. Acquired immune deficiency syndrome in black Africans. Lancet 1983; 1:642.

3. Offenstadt G, Pinta P, Hericord P, et al. Multiple opportunistic infection due to AIDS in a previously healthy black woman from Zaire. N Engl J Med 1983; 308:775.

4. Oleske J, Minnefor A, Cooper R, et al. Immune deficiency syndrome in children. JAMA 1983; 249:2345-9.

5. Probable transfusion associated acquired immune deficiency syndrome (AIDS) — California. MMWR 1982; 31:652.

6. Jacobs JL, Gold JWM, Murray HW, et al. Salmonella infections in patients with acquired immunodeficiency syndrome. Ann Intern Med 1985; 102:186-9.

7. Glaser JB, Morton Kute L, Berger SR, et al. Recurrent *Salmonella typhimurium* bacteremia associated with the acquired immunodeficiency syndrome. Ann Intern Med 1985; 102:189-93.

8. Smith PD, Macher AM, Bookman MA, et al. *Salmonella typhimurium* bacteremia in the acquired immunodeficiency syndrome. Ann Intern Med 1985; 102:207-9.

9. Profeta S, Forrester C, Eng RHK, et al. Salmonella infections in patients with acquired immunodeficiency syndrome. Arch Intern Med 1985; 145:670-2.

10. Bottone EJ, Wormser GP, Duncanson FP. Nontyphoidal salmonella bacteremia as an early infection in acquired immunodeficiency syndrome. Diagn Microbiol Infect Dis 1984; 2:247-50.

11. Sharer LR, Kapila R. Neuropathologic observations in acquired immunodeficiency syndrome. Acta Neuropathol 1985; 66:188-98.

12. Salmonella dublin and raw milk consumption — California. MMWR 1984; 33:196.

13. Wolfe MS, Armstrong D, Louria DB, et al. Salmonellosis in patients with neoplastic disease: a review of 100 episodes at Memorial Cancer Center over a 13 year period. Arch Intern Med 1971; 128:546-54.

14. Cherubin CE, Neu HC, Imperato PJ, et al. Septicemia with non-typhoid salmonella. Medicine 1974; 53:365-76.

15. Tauxe RV, Rigan Perez JG, Wells JG, et al. Turtle associated salmonellosis in Puerto Rico. JAMA 1985; 254:237-9.

16. Quinn TC, Stamm WE, Goodell SE, et al. The polymicrobial origin of intestinal infections in homosexual men. N Engl J Med 1983; 309:576-82.

17. Holmberg SD, Osterholm MT, Senger KA, et al. Drug-resistant salmonella from animals fed antimicrobials. N Engl J Med 1985; 311:617-22.

18. Celum CL, Chaisson RE, Rutherford GW, et al. Incidence of salmonellosis in patients with AIDS. J Infect Dis 1987; 156:998-1002.
19. Wharton M, Coleman DL, Fitz G, et al. Prospective, randomized trial of trimethoprim-sulfamethoxazole versus pentamidine for *Pneumocystis carinii* pneumonia in the acquired immunodeficiency syndrome. Am Rev Respir Dis 1984; 129:188a. abstract.
20. Jaffe HS, Abrams DI, Ammann AJ, et al. Complications of co-trimoxazole in treatment of AIDS associated *Pneumocystis carinii* pneumonia in homosexual men. Lancet 1983; 2:1109-11.
21. Gordin FM, Simon GL, Wofsy CB, Mills J. Adverse reactions to trimethoprim-sulfamethoxazole in patients with the acquired immunodeficiency syndrome. Ann Intern Med 1984; 100:495-9.
22. Moss AR, McCallum G, Volberding PA, et al. Mortality associated with mode of presentation in the acquired immunodeficiency syndrome. J Natl Cancer Inst 1984; 73:1281-4.
23. Probable transfusion-associated acquired immune deficiency syndrome (AIDS) — California. MMWR 1982; 31:652.

Encapsulated Bacteria

J. Louise Gerberding, M.D.

■ EPIDEMIOLOGY

The incidence of infection with encapsulated bacteria such as *Streptococcus pneumoniae, Haemophilus influenzae, Branhamella catarrhalis*, and *Neisseria meningitidis* increases in patients with AIDS.[1-5] Recent reports suggest that the incidence of infection with these pathogens may also be increased in patients with earlier stages of HIV infection[5] (Witt DJ: personal communication).

In 1985, the reported attack rate for community-acquired pneumococcal pneumonia in patients with AIDS was 17.9 per 1000 per year at Memorial Sloan–Kettering Cancer Hospital in New York.[1] The incidence of pneumococcal infection in patients with AIDS at San Francisco General Hospital appears to be increasing; the attack rate for pneumococcal pneumonia from 1983 through 1984 was 3.1 per 1000 per year but increased to 12.5 per 1000 per year by 1986.[5]

Four patients with AIDS and community-acquired pneumococcal pneumonia were identified at the New York Veterans Administration Medical Center in an 18-month period between January 1982 and June 1983.[2] Bacteremia was present in two of these patients. An additional patient with hospital-acquired pneumococcal pneumonia was also reported. This individual had been vaccinated with 14-valent pneumococcal vaccine 6 months before the onset of bacteremic pneumonia with type-4 *S. pneumoniae*.

Eighteen episodes of community-acquired pneumonia have been seen in 13 patients with AIDS treated at Memorial Sloan–Kettering Cancer Hospital since 1979.[1] In 16 of these episodes, a microbiologic diagnosis was established; *H. influenzae* was the etiologic agent in eight cases, *S. pneumoniae* in seven cases, and *B. catarrhalis* and Group B streptococcus in one case each. Bacteremia was present in four of these episodes. Of three patients with pneumococcal pneumonia who were tested for antibody titers, one developed a suboptimal increase in type-specific antibody to type-23 bacteremia and the other two patients showed no rise in antibody levels. Four patients had recurrent episodes of pneumonia with encapsulated bacteria. One patient had three consecutive episodes of *H. influenzae* pneumonia.

Preliminary reports from San Francisco General Hospital identified over 50 episodes of infection with encapsulated bacteria in 44 patients with HIV infection admitted between January 1981 and May 1986.[5] These episodes occurred in AIDS patients as well as in patients with mildly symptomatic and asymptomatic HIV infection. Pneumococcal pneumonia was the most common infection seen in this population, although several episodes of *H. influenzae* pneumonia also occurred.

■ CLINICAL MANIFESTATIONS

The clinical manifestations of pneumonia caused by encapsulated bacteria in patients with HIV infection are similar to those seen in other patient populations with community-acquired bacterial pneumonia. The majority of patients in all series reported to date manifest fever, productive cough, dyspnea, and evidence of pulmonary consolidation on physical examination. Pleuritic chest pain, hemoptysis, and tachypnea have also been described. The duration of symptoms before hospitalization is usually less than five days.

In most AIDS patients with encapsulated bacterial infections, the complete blood count shows a relative leukocytosis with increased immature forms, although the absolute white count is rarely greater than 15,000/cubic mm. Lymphopenia, anemia, and occasionally thrombocytopenia may be seen, but these manifestations usually reflect the severity of the underlying illness or coexistent opportunistic infections. Arterial blood-gas analysis is usually abnormal and correlates with the severity of pulmonary involvement in patients with pneumonia.

Chest x-rays in these patients are nearly always abnormal. Segmental, lobar, or multilobar consolidative changes are the most frequent abnormality, although interstitial infiltrates have been noted in some patients with documented bacterial pneumonias.

Gram's stain of the sputum often suggests the etiologic organism, if an adequate specimen is obtained. Sputum cultures are less helpful. Blood cultures should be performed in all patients with suspected infection. The incidence of bacteremia in patients with symptomatic HIV disease with pneumococcal pneumonia at San Francisco General Hospital from 1981 to mid-1986 was unusually high; over 75 percent of patients in this cohort had positive blood cultures.[5]

■ PATHOGENESIS

Immunologically normal hosts respond to infection with encapsulated bacteria (such as *S. pneumoniae*) in a two-step process. Initially, the alternate complement pathway is activated, which in conjunction with opsonins, promotes clearance of the offending organism by the neutrophils. Subsequently, the host produces specific antibodies that enhance phagocytosis by the neutrophils and the reticuloendothelial system. Defects in any of these processes predispose the host to persistent infection with encapsulated bacteria.

Abnormalities in the components of the humoral immune system have been described in patients with AIDS.[6-8] Preliminary studies have demonstrated that in vitro, B lymphocytes from patients with AIDS proliferate subnormally in response to B-cell-specific mitogens in a T-cell-depleted assay system. They become nonspecifically activated and secrete polyclonal antibodies. Mixing studies with normal T cells and B cells from AIDS patients also have shown subnormal immunoglobulin production in response to pokeweed mitogen. Abnormal T-cell function may also contribute to the impairment of the humoral immune response, since B cells are dependent upon T-cell activation. In AIDS patients, T4 lymphocytes do not proliferate normally in response to soluble antigen. Thus, defective antibody response to infection with *S. pneumoniae* may explain the tendency for recurrent infection[5] (Witt DJ: personal communication). The failure of Pneumovax to protect against infection has been documented in at least one patient with AIDS.[2]

The integrity of the complement system and the ability of the reticuloendothelial system to clear antigens in patients with HIV infection have not been systematically evaluated. Further study will be necessary to fully characterize these defects.

If AIDS patients cannot produce protective levels of type-specific antibody in response to infection, it is unlikely that immunization with Pneumovax will be very effective. Small numbers of AIDS patients have been immunized and appear to exhibit suboptimal responses to Pneumovax.[2,9] Whether patients with less severe manifestations of HIV infection will respond appropriately is not known, but preliminary evidence suggests that response rates correlate with the stage of infection. Because the potential benefit of Pneumovax outweighs the small risk associated with immunization, the CDC recommends vaccination of HIV-infected persons as early as possible.

■ TREATMENT, OUTCOME, AND PROGNOSIS

Despite the presence of underlying immunodeficiency and the high frequency of bacteremia, HIV-infected patients usually respond rapidly to standard doses of appropriate antimicrobial therapy for bacterial pneumonias[5,10] (Witt DJ: personal communication). Subjective improvement and defervescence occur in most patients after three to four days of therapy and are followed by complete resolution. Although most patients are initially hospitalized and treated with parenteral antibiotics, many complete therapy as outpatients. A few have been treated successfully as outpatients for the entire course. Most authorities recommend using trimethoprim/sulfamethoxazole when the etiology of the pneumonia is in doubt, since this regimen will be effective against both *S. pneumoniae* and *H. influenzae*, as well as *P. carinii*. The dose used for PCP is substantially greater than the dose for *S. pneumoniae* and *H. influenzae*.

Patients with bacterial pneumonia who fail to respond to appropriate antibiotic therapy may have coincident opportunistic infections, particularly *Pneumocystis carinii*. Several patients treated at San Francisco General Hospital developed clinically apparent pneumocystis pneumonia while undergoing treatment for documented pneumococcal pneumonia.[5] These patients failed to improve or clinically deteriorated, despite treatment regimens usually effective against *S. pneumoniae*. Similar cases have been reported in other series.[2]

The incidence of recurrent infections with encapsulated bacteria appears increased in patients infected with HIV[2,5] (Witt DJ: personal communication). Recurrent episodes with the same organism as well as multiple infections with more than one type of organism have been described. One patient with recurrent infection with the same serotype of pneumococcus (type 4) has been seen.[5] Guidelines for initiating antibiotic prophylaxis and immunization are currently undergoing evaluation. Pneumovax is now recommended for HIV-infected patients.

A consistent relationship between the onset of infection with encapsulated bacteria in patients with early symptomatic HIV disease and the subsequent development of AIDS has not been determined. Additional follow-up will be necessary to determine if patients with recurrent bacterial infections are more likely to develop AIDS or have a worse long-term prognosis.

REFERENCES

1. Polsky B, Gold JWM, Whimbey E, et al. Bacterial pneumonia in patients with the acquired immunodeficiency syndrome. Ann Intern Med 1986; 104:38-41.

2. Simberkoff MS, Sadr WE, Schiffman G, Rahal JJ. *Streptococcus pneumoniae* infections and bacteremia in patients with acquired immune deficiency syndrome with a report of a pneumococcal vaccine failure. Am Rev Respir Dis 1984; 130:1174-6.

3. White S, Tsou E, Waldhorn RE, Katz P. Life threatening bacterial pneumonia in male homosexuals with laboratory features of the acquired immunodeficiency syndrome. Chest 1985; 87:486-8.

4. Garbowit DL, Alsip AG, Griffin FM. *Hemophilus influenzae* bacteremia in a patient with immunodeficiency caused by HTLV-III. N Engl J Med 1986; 314:56.

5. Gerberding JL, Krieger J, Sande MA. Recurrent bacteremic infection with *S. pneumoniae* in patients with AIDS virus (AV) infection [Abstract]. New Orleans: Twenty-sixth Interscience Conference on Antimicrobial Agents and Chemotherapy, 1986; 177.

6. Pahwa S, Fikrig S, Menez R, Pahwa R. Pediatric acquired immunodeficiency syndrome: demonstration of B lymphocyte defects in vitro. Diagn Immunol 1986; 4:24-30.

7. Katz IR, Krown SE, Safai B, et al. Antigen specific and polyclonal B cell responses in patients with acquired immunodeficiency disease syndrome. Clin Immunol Immunopathol 1986; 39:359-67.

8. Lane HC, Masur H, Edgar LC, et al. Abnormalities of B-cell activation and immunoregulation in patients with the acquired immunodeficiency syndrome. N Engl J Med 1983; 309:453-8.

9. Ammann AJ, Schiffman G, Abrams D, et al. B cell immunodeficiency in acquired immune deficiency syndrome. JAMA 1983; 251:1447-9.

10. Polsky B, Gold JWM, Whimbey E, et al. Bacterial pneumonia in patients with the acquired immunodeficiency syndrome. Ann Intern Med 1986; 104:38-41.

6.2

Mycobacterial Infections

6.2.1

Mycobacterium avium Complex

Peter M. Small, M.D., and Philip C. Hopewell, M.D.

■ EPIDEMIOLOGY

Before the AIDS epidemic, disseminated infection with *Mycobacterium avium* complex (MAC) organisms was extremely uncommon. Comprehensive reviews by Wolinsky[1] in 1979 and Horsburgh and coworkers[2] in 1985 reported 30 and 37 instances, respectively, of disseminated *Mycobacterium avium* complex in non-AIDS patients. Many, but not all, of the patients in these series had identifiable immunologic defects. Their response to treatment was generally poor; mortality rates of 73 percent and 44 percent were reported in the two series.

The first reports of disseminated *Mycobacterium avium* complex infection in patients with AIDS were published in 1982.[3-5] Since then, it has been widely recognized as a frequent opportunistic pathogen in all parts of the United States and in all AIDS risk groups.[6]

The prevalence of disseminated disease caused by *Mycobacterium avium* complex is not well established. In the clinical literature, estimates vary from approximately 15 percent to 20 percent of patients, although autopsy series have reported a 21 percent to 50 percent prevalence.[6-9] Several factors cause underestimation of MAC in living patients: patients often have other infections that can account for symptoms and findings; *Mycobacterium avium* complex infections in AIDS patients generally do not involve the lungs and therefore commonly remain undetected in lung-derived specimens; detection often requires culture of blood, bone marrow, lymph nodes, or stool — sites that are not routinely cultured.

■ PATHOPHYSIOLOGY

The clinical significance of *Mycobacterium avium* complex infection in patients with AIDS is unclear. This organism is known to have a low pathogenicity and is found in high numbers in tissue without clinical evidence of damage,[15] which suggests that although the infection may contribute to the general discomfort and disability of AIDS patients, it may not be an important cause of specific organ failure.

The effect on mortality rates due to *Mycobacterium avium* complex is also unclear. There is inferential evidence that neither disseminated nor local infections influence outcome in patients with *P. carinii* pneumonia (PCP). Demopolus et al.[10] found no differences in number of hospitalized days, blood transfusions, or median survival time between patients with PCP who did and those who did not have *Mycobacterium avium* complex. These authors concluded that *Mycobacterium avium* complex was probably not an important pathogen in this group of patients and that patients died with, not from, *Mycobacterium avium* complex infection.[10] A more recent retrospective review of 2269 cases of nontuberculous mycobacterial infections in patients with AIDS reported to the Centers for Disease Control showed a 5.9-month shorter survival rate in AIDS patients with *Mycobacterium avium* complex than in AIDS patients with other opportunistic infections.[12] It is unclear how the retrospective design of this study may bias the results.[17]

■ CLINICAL PRESENTATION

In general, *Mycobacterium avium* complex infections occur relatively late in the course of HIV infection — often after other pathologic processes have been identified. The symptoms attributed to this infection are multiple and nonspecific. Fever, weight loss, weakness, and anorexia are seen in many AIDS patients, but they appear with greater frequency in patients with *Mycobacterium avium* complex. Abdominal pain and diarrhea are also common symptoms; these probably result from intra-abdominal adenopathy.[15] Other lymph nodes may be involved as well. Respiratory symptoms are uncommon — the process is not usually associated with significant lung involvement.

Physical and laboratory findings are also often difficult to ascribe to *Mycobacterium avium* complex alone. Abdominal lymph nodes may be palpable and hepatosplenomegaly may be noted. In patients with bone-marrow involvement, other symptoms may also occur, including anemia, leukopenia, and thrombocytopenia. Computed tomographic (CT) scanning of the abdomen may show very large lymph nodes. Although CT scanning cannot determine etiology, the finding of markedly variable intranodal density in the abdomen is thought to be highly suggestive of a mycobacterial process.[12]

■ DIAGNOSIS

The diagnosis of *Mycobacterium avium* complex is established by isolation of the organism. Although routine culture techniques are occasionally positive, yield is improved by using special media for mycobacteria. More rapid isolation from blood cultures is possible with radiometric (Bactec™) and lysis-centrifugation (Isolator™) systems. Isolation can be further expedited by the use of nucleic-acid probes.[18] Dissemination can be proven by isolating the organism from blood, bone marrow, liver biopsies, or lymph nodes. Positive cultures from these normally sterile sites are sensitive and specific for infection. In 46 patients reviewed retrospectively, blood cultures were positive in 98 percent of the patients, and bone marrow, liver, or lymph nodes were positive in 100 percent.[11] Stool cultures are commonly positive in patients with disseminated disease.[13] Biopsy specimens of involved tissues are remarkable for two features: weak inflammatory response to the organism and large number of organisms present.[7,9,15] The histologic examination of lymph nodes or bone marrow shows infiltration with foamy histiocytes. Granulomata, if present at all, are very poorly formed. Thus, the absence of granulomata cannot be used to exclude a mycobacterial infection. All biopsy specimens should be appropriately stained and cultured for these organisms.

■ TREATMENT

Even in persons with normal cell-mediated immunity, treatment of disease caused by *Mycobacterium avium* complex is not very successful. There is no standard procedure for determining the in vitro susceptibility of the organism.[19] Drug therapy for patients with pulmonary *Mycobacterium avium* complex disease has an overall cure rate of approximately 50 percent to 75 percent.[14] To achieve these rates of cure, treatment regimens (consisting usually of 4, 5, or 6 drugs) must be given for 18 to 24 months. It is not surprising, therefore, that response to treatment in patients with AIDS is very poor.[16,20] Hawkins et al.[11] reported the results of therapy in 29 patients, 26 of whom had bacteremia. None of the 29 responded to therapy. Only 2 of the 26 bacteremic patients cleared the organism from their bloodstreams with treatment, and one of those still had involvement in multiple organs at autopsy. Symptoms were persistent as well, despite antimycobacterial therapy. Hawkins et al. concluded that therapy with existing drugs, including ansamycin LM427 (rifabutin) and clofazimine, was largely ineffective.

Because questions concerning the importance of *Mycobacterium avium* complex infection and about effective, appropriate drug regimens remain unanswered, treatment recommendations are difficult to formulate. Because stains cannot reliably differentiate *Mycobacterium avium* complex from *M. tuberculosis*, it is frequently prudent to initiate standard anti-tuberculosis therapy in patients with positive acid-fast bacilli stains. A decision on further therapy can be made when the organism is identified. The basic therapeutic principle should be to treat patients whose symptoms are directly attributable to *Mycobacterium avium* complex with as benign a drug regimen as possible, given the very low likelihood of success. A reasonable regimen would be ansamycin (150 mg to 300 mg/day); clofazimine (100 mg/day); and ethambutol (800 mg/day). These drugs are well tolerated, and based on susceptibility testing, stand some chance of being effective.[16,18] *Mycobacterium avium* complex organisms are often susceptible to cycloserine and ethionamide as well, but intolerable side effects from these agents are common.

REFERENCES

1. Wolinsky E. Nontuberculous mycobacteria and associated diseases. Am Rev Respir Dis 1979; 119:107-59.
2. Horsburgh CR Jr, Mason US III, Farki DC, Iseman MD. Disseminated infection with *Mycobacterium avium-intracellulare*: a report of 13 cases and a review of the literature. Medicine 1985; 64:36-48.
3. Fainstein V, Bolivar R, Mavligit G, et al. Disseminated infection due to *Mycobacterium avium-intracellulare* in a homosexual man with Kaposi's sarcoma. J Infect Dis 1982; 145:586.
4. Greene JB, Sidhu GS, Lewin S, et al. *Mycobacterium avium-intracellulare*: a cause of disseminated life-threatening infection in homosexuals and drug abusers. Ann Intern Med 1982; 97:539-46.
5. Zakowski P, Fligiel S, Berlin OGW, et al. Disseminated *Mycobacterium avium-intracellulare* infection in homosexual men dying of acquired immunodeficiency. JAMA 1982; 248:2980-2.
6. Murray JF, Felton CP, Garay SM, et al. Pulmonary complications of the acquired immunodeficiency syndrome: report of a National Heart, Lung and Blood Institute workshop. N Engl J Med 1984; 310:1682-8.
7. Wilkes MS, Fortin A, Felix J, Godwin T, Thompson W. The utility of the autopsy in the acquired immunodeficiency syndrome [Abstract]. IV International Conference on AIDS. Stockholm, 1988; 2:307, #7530.
8. Wallace JM, Hannah J. Pulmonary disease found at autopsy in patients with the acquired immunodeficiency syndrome (AIDS). Am Rev Respir Dis 1985; 131:A222. abstract.
9. Armstrong D, Gold JWM, Dryjanski J, et al. Treatment of infections in patients with the acquired immunodeficiency syndrome. Ann Intern Med 1985; 103:738-43.

10. Demopulos P, Sande MA, Bryant C, et al. Influence of *Mycobacterium avium-intracellulare* (MAI) infection on morbidity and survival in patients with *Pneumocystis carinii* pneumonia (PCP) and the acquired immunodeficiency syndrome (AIDS). Program and abstracts of the Twenty-fifth Interscience Conference on Antimicrobial Agents and Chemotherapy. Minneapolis: American Society for Microbiology, 1985:230.

11. Hawkins CC, Gold JWM, Whimby E, et al. *Mycobacterium avium* complex infections in patients with the acquired immunodeficiency syndrome. Ann Intern Med 1986; 105:184-8.

12. Jeffrey RB Jr, Nyberg DA, Bottles K, et al. Abdominal CT in acquired immunodeficiency syndrome. Am J Radiol 1986; 146:7-13.

13. Kiehn TE, Edwards FF, Brannon P, et al. Infections caused by Mycobacterium avium complex in immunocompromised patients: diagnosis by blood culture and fecal examination, antimicrobial susceptibility tests, and morphological and seroagglutination characteristics. J Clin Microbiol 1985; 21:168-73.

14. Iseman MD, Corpe RF, O'Brien RJ, et al. Disease due to *Mycobacterium avium-intracellulare*. Chest 1985; 87(2 Suppl):139S-149S.

15. Wallace JM, Hannah JB. *Mycobacterium avium* complex infection in patients with the acquired immunodeficiency syndrome. A clinicopathologic study. Chest 1988; 93:926-32.

16. Horsburgh RC, Selik RM. The epidemiology of disseminated nontuberculous mycobacterial infections in AIDS. Am Rev Respir Dis 1989; 139:4-7.

17. Chaisson RE, Hopewell PC. Mycobacteria and AIDS mortality. Am Rev Respir Dis 1989; 139:1-3.

18. Drake et al. J Clin Microbiol 1987; 25:1442.

19. Inderlied CB, Young LS, Yamada JK. Determination of in vitro susceptibility of *Mycobacterium avium* complex isolates to antimycobacterial agents by various methods. Antimicrob Agents Chemother 1987; 31:1697-702.

20. Masur H, Tuazon C, Gill V, et al. Effect of combined clofazimine and ansamycin therapy on *Mycobacterium avium-Mycobacterium intracellulare* bacteremia in patients with AIDS. J Infect Dis 1987; 155:127-9.

6.2.2

Mycobacterium tuberculosis

Gisela F. Schechter, M.D., M.P.H.

■ EPIDEMIOLOGY AND INCIDENCE

One hundred years ago, tuberculosis (TB) was the chief infectious cause of death in the United States. Since then there has been a steady decline in tuberculosis morbidity, and this has accelerated since the introduction of effective chemotherapy in about 1950. Because of the decline in new infections, the mean age of persons with tuberculosis disease progressively increased until, by 1980, tuberculosis in the U.S. had become a disease of a limited number of high-risk groups — the elderly, the homeless, alcoholics, refugees and recent immigrants, and minority groups.

With the advent of HIV disease, the decline in TB has been halted; essentially the same number of cases were reported in 1985 as in 1984.[1] In 1986, the first increase in tuberculosis cases was seen in the U.S. since national reporting began in 1953.[12] In areas such as New York City and New Jersey, total tuberculosis cases have increased markedly.[1,2,13] The age distribution of cases has also changed, increasing in the young-adult age groups that are most heavily represented in reported cases of AIDS.

TABLE 1. U.S. TUBERCULOSIS MORBIDITY

YEAR	NUMBER OF CASES	CASE RATE (per 100,000)
1985	22,201	9.1
1986	22,768	9.3
1987	22,517	9.3

Tuberculosis among patients with HIV infection has occurred most frequently in those groups with historically high rates of tuberculosis infection and disease, such as Haitians, Hispanics, blacks, and intravenous drug users (IVDUs).[3,4,14] This pattern is prominent in Florida, New York, and New Jersey. In San Francisco, where AIDS is predominantly seen in white homosexual or bisexual males, the majority of patients with tuberculosis and AIDS are non-IVDU white males, but the incidence of patients with both diseases is much lower — about 2 percent versus about 20 percent in New Jersey.[4,5]

The overall prevalence of tuberculosis in the U.S. declined to 9.1 per 100,000 in 1985.[1] Certain immunocompromised groups have a higher incidence of active TB — specifically patients with lymphoreticular malignancies, patients on corticosteroid treatment or other immunosuppressive drugs, and those with renal failure or diabetes (especially insulin-dependent patients), but precise figures are unknown. The prevalence of TB in AIDS patients is several orders of magnitude higher than in the general population.

■ PATHOGENESIS

Mycobacterium tuberculosis is an obligate, aerobic, acid-fast bacillus. It is spread almost exclusively by the respiratory route. A person with pulmonary lesions can aerosolize droplets containing organisms by coughing, singing, or even talking. These droplets can condense and remain airborne for extended periods. When a susceptible individual inhales droplets from 6 to 10 microns in size, they lodge in the lung and can lead to infection.

Initially, the organisms multiply and are picked up by alveolar macrophages, which transport them to the regional lymph nodes. From there, hematologic dissemination occurs. At about this time (three to eight weeks after infection), the patient's cell-mediated immunity develops, a process crucial to halting further multiplication of the organism through the development of granulomas and caseation. Tissue macrophages are the cells most involved in halting the progression of infection. Because of the profound depression of cell-mediated immunity in AIDS patients, the organism cannot be held in check. Rapid multiplication occurs, often simultaneously at multiple organ sites. Patients with AIDS who come in close contact with persons with active pulmonary tuberculosis are unable to limit the multiplication of *M. tuberculosis* after initial dissemination and are prone to miliary disease.

■ CLINICAL PRESENTATION

Eighty-five percent of the tuberculosis cases in the U.S. are pulmonary, with disease usually concentrated in the upper lobes of the lungs. Extrapulmonary disease is uncommon in non-HIV-infected patients and is most frequently pleural or lymphatic. Extrapulmonary disease, however, has been seen in up to 72 percent of patients with tuberculosis and HIV disease,[3,4,6] including miliary tuberculosis as well as involvement of the lymphatics (including intrathoracic lymphatics), central nervous system (parenchymal and meningeal), soft tissue, bone marrow, genitourinary tract, liver, and blood.[3,4,6,15] The classical symptoms of tuberculosis (such as weight loss, fevers, night sweats, and fatigue) can be due to many other conditions in patients with AIDS and do not specifically suggest tuberculosis.

■ DIAGNOSIS

Diagnosing tuberculosis in AIDS patients is difficult. Only 10 percent to 30 percent of patients react to the PPD skin test.[3,6] Chest x-ray findings seldom show classic upper-lobe infiltrates; more often, they reveal diffuse, interstitial, or lower-lobe infiltrates, often with prominent hilar and paratracheal enlargement.[3,6,7] Only in a minority of cases is the sputum smear-positive, so invasive diagnostic procedures are usually necessary. Every bronchoscopy specimen and every biopsy specimen in an HIV-infected or HIV risk-group patient should be sent for an acid-fast bacilli (AFB) smear and culture.[8] Diagnosis may require culture of specimens from bone marrow, lymph nodes, brain tissue, cerebrospinal fluid, urine, stool, or blood.

■ TREATMENT

Tuberculosis in both HIV-infected and non-HIV-infected patients should always be treated with at least two drugs. There are two preferred treatment regimens: (1) a six-month regimen of two months daily isoniazid (INH), rifampin, and pyrazinamide, followed by four months of daily or twice weekly INH and rifampin; (2) a nine-month regimen of isoniazid and rifampin given daily for one or two months followed by daily or twice-weekly therapy.[9] Usual doses are INH 300 mg daily, rifampin 600 mg daily, and pyrazinamide 20 to 30 mg/kg daily. Ethambutol is often used initially as a companion drug when INH resistance is suspected. The most common toxicity is hepatic, occurring in approximately 0.5 percent of patients. Ninety-eight percent of patients are cured with these regimens.

There have been no treatment trials in HIV-infected patients with TB. In late 1987, a compliant patient failed on four-drug, six-month therapy.[16] The Centers for Disease Control (CDC) and the Advisory Committee for the Elimination of Tuberculosis (ACET) recommend that patients with tuberculosis and HIV disease receive a minimum of 9 to 12 months of chemotherapy.[17,18] Patients with HIV disease who are found to have positive acid-fast smears (on sputum or biopsy specimens) or whose cultures yield an acid-fast organism should be treated with therapy adequate for *M. tuberculosis* pending final culture results.[10] In some cases, *Mycobacterium avium-intracellulare* (MAI) will be the final diagnosis. Very limited data suggest that most HIV-infected patients with TB respond well to treatment, although side effects occur in about one-fourth of cases. Rash occurs most frequently, but thrombocytopenia and renal failure also occur.[6] Patients with tuberculosis should be assessed for HIV infection because of the implications for treatment of both infections and in order to enhance HIV prevention and control efforts.[18]

■ PREVENTION

Because an unknown percentage of HIV-infected persons will go on to develop full-blown AIDS, the CDC has recommended that all persons with antibody to HIV and a reactive PPD skin test of greater than or equal to 5 mm receive isoniazid prophylaxis for 12 months.[10,18] Because HIV infection causes immunosuppression and the risk of TB is high in persons with both TB and HIV infection, tuberculin reactions of greater than or equal to 5 mm induration should be considered evidence of TB infection. The efficacy of the treatment is unknown.

Patients with AIDS and TB who have positive sputum or bronchoscopy specimens are infectious, and their contacts should be screened for tuberculosis and given prophylaxis when indicated. Patients with AIDS and TB should not be isolated in a hospital or excluded from a work setting any longer than other TB patients; after one to two weeks on effective chemotherapy, patients can resume social contacts.[11]

The CDC reported that documented tuberculin skin-test conversions occurred in 17 of 70 staff members at a Florida clinic that began providing aerosolized pentamidine treatments in January, 1988, for people with AIDS and at risk for AIDS.[19] Because of concern about possible transmission of tuberculosis in the setting of aerosolized pentamidine treatment and the coughing it induces, the CDC recommends that patients considered for aerosolized pentamidine should be evaluated first for pulmonary tuberculosis with a chest x-ray. If this is abnormal, sputum smears should be obtained. If tuberculosis is suspected, treatment should begin before the patient starts on aerosolized pentamidine.

REFERENCES

1. Centers for Disease Control. Tuberculosis, United States, 1985, and the possible impact of HTLV-III/LAV infections. MMWR 1986; 35:74-6.

2. Stoneburner RL, Kristal A. Increasing tuberculosis incidence and its relationship to acquired immuno-deficiency syndrome in New York City. Atlanta: International Conference on AIDS, 1985:66.

3. Pitchenik AE, Cole C, Russell BW, et al. Tuberculosis, atypical mycobacteriosis, and AIDS among Haitian and non-Haitian patients in South Florida. Ann Intern Med 1984; 101:641-5.

4. Sunderam G, MacDonald RJ, Moniatis T, et al. Tuberculosis as a manifestation of AIDS. JAMA 1986; 256:362-6.

5. Schechter GF, Rutherford GW, Echenberg DF. Tuberculosis in AIDS patients in San Francisco, 1982-1985. Am Rev Resp Dis 1986; 133(Suppl A):184.

6. Chaisson RE, Schechter GF, Theur CP, et al. Tuberculosis in patients with the acquired immuno-deficiency syndrome. Clinical features, response to therapy, and survival. Am Rev Respir Dis 1987; 136:570-4.

7. Pitchenik AE, Rubinson HA. The radiographic appearance of tuberculosis in patients with AIDS and pre-AIDS. Am Rev Respir Dis 1985; 131:393-6.

8. Murray JF, Felton CP, Saray SM, et al. Pulmonary complications of AIDS: report of a National Heart, Lung and Blood Institute workshop. N Engl J Med 1984; 310:1682-8.

9. American Thoracic Society. Medical Section of the American Lung Association: treatment of tuber-culosis and tuberculosis infection in adults and children. Am Rev Respir Dis 1986; 134:355-63.

10. Centers for Disease Control. Diagnosis and management of mycobacterial infection and disease in persons with HTLV-III/LAV infection. MMWR 1986; 35:448-52.

11. Centers for Disease Control. Guidelines for prevention of TB transmission in hospitals. Atlanta, Geor-gia: U.S. Department of Health and Human Services, 1982. PHS publication no. (CDC) 82-8371.

12. Tuberculosis, final data — United States, 1986. MMWR 1988; 36:817-20.

13. Tuberculosis and acquired immunodeficiency syndrome — New York City. MMWR 1987; 36:785-90, 795.

14. Pitchenik AE, Fertel D, Bloch AB. Mycobacterial disease: epidemiology, diagnosis, treatment, and prevention. Clin Chest Med 1988; 9:425-41.

15. Moreno S, Pacho E, Lopez-Herce JA, et al. *Mycobacterium tuberculosis* visceral abscesses in the acquired immunodeficiency syndrome (AIDS). Ann Intern Med 1988; 109:437.

16. Sunderam G, Mangura BT, Lombardo JM, Reichman LB. Failure of "optimal" four-drug short-course tuberculosis chemotherapy in a compliant patient with human immunodeficiency virus. Am Rev Respir Dis 1987; 136:1475-8.

17. Mycobacterioses and the acquired immunodeficiency syndrome. Joint Position Paper of the American Thoracic Society and the Centers for Disease Control. Am Rev Respir Dis 1987; 136:492-6.

18. Tuberculosis and human immunodeficiency virus infection: recommendations of the Advisory Commit-tee for the Elimination of Tuberculosis (ACET). MMWR 1989; 38:236-8, 243-50.

19. *Mycobacterium tuberculosis* transmission in a health clinic — Florida, 1988. MMWR 1989; 38:256-64.

6.3

Fungal Infections

Aspergillosis

David Chernoff, M.D., and Merle A. Sande, M.D.

■ **EPIDEMIOLOGY**

Aspergillus species are ubiquitous and are found throughout the world. The fungus commonly grows in decaying vegetation and soil. Exposure to the fungus occurs through the inhalation of spores. Although more than 300 species of aspergillus exist, only a few have been implicated as causes of human disease. Most of the disease in humans is caused by *A. fumigatus*. Other important pathogens include *A. niger* and *A. flavus*. Exposure to aspergillus is universal, but disease is uncommon unless host defense has been altered by drugs, infection, or malignancy. Aspergillosis is usually seen in patients with hematologic malignancies such as leukemia or lymphoma. The infection commonly occurs when these patients have been made leukopenic with chemotherapeutic agents. Despite the overwhelming immunosuppression that results from infection with HIV, infection with aspergillus is relatively uncommon in AIDS patients.[1]

■ **PATHOGENESIS**

The major portal of entry for infection is the respiratory tract. Aspergillus may colonize and grow in bronchi, cysts, or cavities caused by previous infections, such as tuberculosis. In patients with invasive disease, hyphae are found in areas of abscess formation surrounded by epithelioid cells and multinucleated giant cells. Hyphae are easily missed on routine hematoxylin-eosin stained specimens. In disseminated disease, hyphae may be seen growing into vessels.

Host defense against infection appears to depend primarily on phagocytic cell function. Invasive and disseminated disease has been observed in patients with leukemia, renal and cardiac transplant patients, neutropenic patients, and in patients treated with large doses of steroids. The relative paucity of aspergillus infection in the setting of AIDS may be the result of primary T-cell dysfunction with relatively intact phagocytic cell function.

■ **CLINICAL PRESENTATION**

Aspergillus species produce a spectrum of pulmonary diseases whose expression depends primarily on the immune status of the infected host.[2] The pulmonary diseases can be divided into three distinct clinical syndromes:

1. Allergic bronchopulmonary aspergillosis. This disease occurs in individuals with a history of asthma and atopy and is characterized by the allergic response of the host to the fungus. Wheezing, eosinophilia, pulmonary infiltrates, and bronchial plugging are all manifestations of allergic bronchopulmonary aspergillosis.

2. Mycetoma or fungal ball. This infection usually occurs as a result of fungal colonization of a preexisting cavity. It is localized to the cavity and rarely disseminates.

3. Invasive aspergillosis. This form of infection almost always occurs in the setting of immunosuppression as a fulminating disease associated with widespread dissemination. The disease is characterized by high fevers, pulmonary consolidation, and hematogenous dissemination.

The organism is rarely detected in sputum samples despite extensive infection. After the lungs, the most common sites of isolation of the fungus are the gastrointestinal tract, brain, liver, and kidney. Uncommon manifestations of aspergillus infection include endocarditis, sinusitis, endophthalmitis, osteomyelitis, esophagitis, necrotizing skin ulcers, meningitis, and brain abscesses. These extrapulmonary forms of infection are almost exclusively seen in the severely leukopenic patient. Locally invasive forms of aspergillosis have also been observed in patients with serious underlying diseases.

As stated above, aspergillus infections are relatively uncommon in AIDS patients.[3] Most of the infections have occurred in the setting of multiple opportunistic infections rather than as an isolated fungal infection, in which case diagnosis of infection was usually made postmortem. Unusual manifestations of infection in AIDS patients have included maxillary sinusitis secondary to *A. niger* and skin abscesses secondary to *A. fumigatus*.[4,5] Pulmonary manifestations have included cavitary and invasive aspergillosis. A variant form of invasive pulmonary aspergillosis has been observed in several AIDS patients.[3,5] Postmortem examination of these patients revealed extensive plugging of bronchi and smaller airways by thick pseudomembranes containing hyphae. Extensive bronchial hemorrhage and invasion of the bronchial walls and vessels also were observed. Aspergillus endocarditis, esophagitis, and brain abscesses have also been reported in AIDS patients.[6-8]

■ DIAGNOSIS

The diagnosis of aspergillus infection can be made by the identification of the characteristic septate hyphae on biopsy specimens. Because aspergillus species are ubiquitous, it is difficult to determine whether culture of the fungus per se reflects actual disease. Whereas a positive sputum culture in a normal host may have no clinical significance, a positive sputum or nasal culture in a neutropenic patient is highly suggestive of disease. Between 10 percent and 30 percent of patients with invasive aspergillosis have positive sputum cultures. The appearance of hyphae on transbronchial biopsy in an AIDS patient should be taken as evidence of invasive disease. Culture of the fungus from sputum in this setting should also be treated as evidence of infection rather than contamination. The fungus is rarely isolated from blood, cerebrospinal fluid, or bone marrow.

■ TREATMENT

In patients without AIDS, localized forms of aspergillus infection such as mycetoma may be treated conservatively. Surgical excision of an aspergilloma is indicated for complications such as severe hemoptysis. Treatment of aspergillus infections in AIDS patients follows recommendations for treatment of invasive disease in other immunosuppressed patients. Amphotericin-B should be administered and rapidly increased until a dose of between 0.5 and 0.8 mg/kg/day is reached. Duration of therapy is not fixed, but most patients will require between 1 and 2 g of amphotericin-B. Because so few AIDS patients have completed standard courses of therapy, it is impossible to evaluate the response rate to therapy. Probably ketoconazole has no role in treating aspergillus infections because the fungus is relatively resistant to the drug. No evidence has been found that 5-flucytosine is synergistic with amphotericin-B in treating aspergillus infections. Furthermore, the combination of amphotericin-B and 5-flucytosine has been reported to be unsuccessful in treating aspergillus infections in leukemic patients and in renal-transplant patients.

■ OUTCOME

Because aspergillus infections in AIDS patients usually occur in the setting of multiple opportunistic infections, the response to therapy is usually poor. The disease is often widely disseminated by the time the diagnosis is made. Unlike cryptococcal infections, in which detection of circulating antigen reliably predicts disease, serologic tests that accurately diagnose infection with aspergillus are not yet available.

■ PREVENTION

Given the widespread distribution of aspergillus species, it is impossible to isolate AIDS patients from the organism. Aisner and colleagues suggest that nasal cultures are useful in predicting disease.[9] Obviously, the use of any drug that causes neutropenia might predispose AIDS patients to infection with aspergillus. The use of trimethoprim-sulfamethoxazole and pentamidine for treatment of *Pneumocystis carinii* pneumonia often causes severe neutropenia and might predispose patients to aspergillus infection. Nosocomial outbreaks of aspergillosis have occurred in air-conditioned hospital units as a result of contamination of the air-intake ducts with aspergillus spores. Meticulous attention to environmental contamination must be paid, given the possibility of nosocomial infection.

REFERENCES

1. Murray JF, Felton CP, Garay S, et al. Pulmonary complications of the acquired immunodeficiency syndrome: report of a National Heart, Lung and Blood Institute workshop. N Engl J Med 1984; 310:1682-8.
2. Young RC, Bennett JE, Vogel CL, et al. Aspergillosis: the spectrum of the disease in 98 patients. Medicine 1970; 49:147-73.
3. Marchevsky A, Rosen MJ, Chrystal G, Kleinerman J. Pulmonary complications of the acquired immunodeficiency syndrome: a clinicopathological study of 70 cases. Hum Pathol 1985; 16:659-70.
4. Hui AN, Koss MN, Meyer PR. Necropsy findings in acquired immunodeficiency syndrome: a comparison of premortem diagnoses and postmortem findings. Hum Pathol 1984; 15:670-6.
5. Pervez NK, Kleinerman J, Kattan M, et al. Pseudomembranous necrotizing bronchial aspergillosis. a variant of invasive aspergillosis in a patient with hemophilia and acquired immunodeficiency syndrome. Am Rev Respir Dis 1985; 131:961-3.
6. Henochowicz S, Mustafa M, Lawrinson WE, et al. Cardiac aspergillosis in acquired immunodeficiency syndrome. Am J Cardiol 1985; 55:1239-40.
7. Masuc H, Micheli MA, Greene J, et al. An outbreak of community-acquired P. carinii pneumonia. N Engl J Med 1981; 305:1431-8.
8. Britton CB, Mesa-Tejada R, Fengolio CM, et al. A new complication of AIDS: thoracic myelitis caused by herpes simplex virus. Neurology 1985; 35:1071-4.
9. Aisner J, Murillo J, Schimpff S, et al. Invasive aspergillosis in acute leukemia: correlation with nose culture and antibiotic use. Ann Intern Med 1979; 90:4-9.

Candidiasis

David Chernoff, M.D., and Merle A. Sande, M.D.

■ EPIDEMIOLOGY

C andida species are round-to-oval yeast that reproduce by budding. Although there are many species of candida, only a few are important pathogens in humans. Pathogenic species include *C. albicans*, *C. tropicalis*, *C. parapsilosis*, and several other less common isolates. The fungi are commensal organisms that, in humans, exist in the gastrointestinal (GI) tract, the female genital tract, the oropharynx, and on diseased skin. Infection usually results from the breakdown of barriers to infection (burned skin, indwelling catheters, etc.) or from suppression of the immune system, either by drugs or infectious agents such as HIV. *Candida albicans* is the most common fungus infecting patients with AIDS.[1,2]

■ PATHOGENESIS

The use of broad-spectrum antibiotics, which can cause changes in endogenous flora, may allow overgrowth and dissemination of the fungus. The widespread use of indwelling catheters (for hemodynamic monitoring, intravenous fluid administration, and measurement of urine output) provides a nidus for fungal colonization and an entry through the normal skin barrier. Agents that suppress the immune system (such as steroids, cytotoxic agents, or infectious agents such as HIV) also predispose patients to candida infections.

One of the major defenses against infection by candida species is an intact integument. Alterations in the skin caused by trauma, burns, maceration, or indwelling catheters may provide a portal of entry for the fungus.

The precise role of the T cell in the defense against candida infection is unknown. The widespread occurrence of mucosal infections in AIDS patients suggests that alterations in T-cell function and number predispose these patients to localized infections. Chronic mucocutaneous candidiasis — a syndrome characterized by T-cell dysfunction and persistent and recurrent candida infection of the skin, nails, and mucous membranes — provides an in vivo model for the role of the T cell in host-defense against fungal infection. A single defect in T-cell function has not been consistently found in patients with this syndrome. The most common abnormality is cutaneous anergy and failure to produce lymphokines in response to antigenic stimulation. Cutaneous anergy and abnormal T-cell proliferative responses are commonly observed immunologic abnormalities in patients with ARC and AIDS.[3]

■ CLINICAL PRESENTATION

Candida infections can be broadly divided into two general categories: mucocutaneous (a very common site of infection) and systemic (a rare site of infection).

MUCOCUTANEOUS INFECTION

Oral. Oral candidiasis (thrush) is characterized by creamy, curd-like patches on the tongue and buccal mucosa. The patches are pseudomembranes and consist of epithelial cells, leukocytes, yeast, and necrotic debris. Although relatively common in newborns (approximately 5 percent), thrush in adults usually involves some predisposing risk factor, such as steroid use, chronic illness (e.g., diabetes), immunodeficiency, and often, immunodeficiency-associated antibiotic use.[4]

Oral candidiasis is the most common fungal infection in patients with ARC or AIDS. Unexplained oral candidiasis in patients with risk factors for AIDS is often a harbinger of increasingly severe opportunistic infections. In one study, over 50 percent of patients with thrush and AIDS risk factors developed a major opportunistic infection or Kaposi's sarcoma within 18 months of the diagnosis of thrush. Patients with risk factors for AIDS who did not have thrush did not go on to develop severe opportunistic infections over a similar follow-up period.[5] The diagnosis of ARC or AIDS should be considered in any patient with unexplained thrush. Risk factors such as blood-product transfusions, IV drug use, or homosexual contact should be explored by the clinician.

Alimentary: Esophagitis. Gastrointestinal (GI) candidiasis most frequently involves the esophagus. Most cases of candidal esophagitis occur in patients with obvious risk factors for fungal infection. Only 50 percent of non-AIDS patients with esophagitis have oral thrush.[6] Thus, the absence of thrush does not rule out the diagnosis of candidal esophagitis. In ARC or AIDS patients with candidal esophagitis, however, oral thrush is almost always present.[8] The most common symptoms include painful swallowing (odynophagia), dysphagia, retrosternal pain, and nausea.[7] Extensive pseudomembrane formation may cause partial obstruction. Rarely, perforation occurs in the lower esophagus as a result of severe mucosal ulceration. The diagnosis of candidal esophagitis in a person infected with HIV establishes a diagnosis of AIDS.

Candida frequently infects the stomach and, less commonly, the small and large intestine.[9] Almost all cases of GI candida infections have occurred in patients treated with cytotoxic agents, steroids, or broad-spectrum antibiotics.

Other mucocutaneous infections due to candida include vaginitis, balanitis, folliculitis, onychomycosis, and intertrigo. In the setting of fungemia, cutaneous lesions may appear as pink macronodules.

SYSTEMIC INFECTION

Systemic candida infection is seldom encountered in patients with AIDS. From reports of other patient populations, it appears that virtually every organ system in the body can become infected as a result of hematogenous dissemination of candida.[10,11] The central nervous system, heart, kidneys, eyes, and vasculature are common sites of disseminated candida infection. Deep-organ infection can occur in the absence of fungemia. Candida infection of the kidneys may occur as a result of ascending infection in the presence of obstruction or a Foley catheter. Candidal peritonitis can occur in the setting of peritoneal dialysis because of the indwelling catheter. In many cases, candidal sepsis occurs as a terminal event in critically ill patients treated for malignancies with cytotoxic agents and broad-spectrum antibiotics.

■ DIAGNOSIS

Diagnosing candida infection depends on identifying the fungus in KOH-treated scrapings, histopathologic findings, or cultures from body fluids. The diagnosis of invasive disease is sometimes difficult because the distinction is not always clear between infection and colonization in a culture from the mouth, sputum, or urine. Even isolation of candida from the blood is not absolute proof of disseminated infection, because patients often have indwelling catheter lines — a known potential cause of candidemia in many patient populations. (Transient candidemia from an infected catheter often resolves without antifungal therapy when the line is removed.)

Despite tremendous interest and research concerning the serodiagnosis of candidiasis, no reliable (i.e., sensitive and specific) tests exist. Agglutinins and precipitins to *C. albicans* can be detected in patients with no clinical signs of fungal infection. Similar problems have been encountered with newer and more sensitive assays, such as radioimmunoassay (RIA) and ELISA.[12]

MUCOCUTANEOUS INFECTION

Thrush.   Oral candidiasis is diagnosed by identifying the yeast in oral scrapings treated with KOH. Cultures of oral lesions are not useful because candida can be found in the mouths of normal individuals. An outbreak of a new form of oral leukoplakia referred to as hairy leukoplakia has been observed in patients with risk factors for AIDS[13] and in patients with verified HIV infection. These lesions appear as white, hair-like plaques on the lateral borders of the tongue. They are often misdiagnosed as the plaques of thrush. These lesions have been shown to contain both papillomavirus and a herpes-group virus. They may also become colonized by candida.

Esophagitis.   Candidal esophagitis can be diagnosed presumptively by contrast radiography or definitively by esophagoscopy. In a patient with oral thrush and odynophagia or substernal chest pain, the most likely diagnosis is candidal esophagitis. Occasional patients are asymptomatic for oral thrush, so its absence does not rule out the diagnosis of candidal esophagitis.

Candidal esophagitis can be diagnosed indirectly by barium swallow. Because of superficial ulcerations, the barium pattern is irregular, shaggy, or cobblestoned in appearance. This pattern is not specific for candida and can also be seen in patients with herpes esophagitis. Mild infection may go undetected by the barium swallow. False-negative rates of 20 percent to 60 percent have been reported in several series using barium radiography.[7] Although patients with esophageal candidiasis usually present with diffuse infection, focal infections simulating ulcerating neoplasms have been observed in AIDS patients undergoing barium studies.[14]

The definitive diagnosis of candidal esophagitis is made by esophagoscopy. Characteristic endoscopic findings include patchy white plaques overlying a friable mucosa. Identifying spores and pseudohyphae in biopsy specimens with the use of KOH is the most reliable indicator of infection. Histopathologic evidence from biopsy specimens of fungal invasion of the mucosa is a reliable indicator of infection. Positive cultures from biopsy specimens are not definitive evidence of infection because the fungus is a commensal organism in the esophagus.

In patients with ARC or AIDS, candidal esophagitis is usually associated with oral thrush. In a small series of patients with AIDS and thrush, every patient had candidal esophagitis on endoscopy, whether they were symptomatic or not.[8] A presumptive diagnosis of candidal esophagitis is reasonable in a patient with AIDS and thrush who has esophageal complaints; in such cases, a trial of antifungal therapy is warranted. Esophagoscopy should be performed in patients with odynophagia (in the absence of thrush), in those for whom esophageal candida would establish an AIDS diagnosis, and in those patients who fail to respond clinically to antifungal therapy. Other infectious agents (such as herpes or CMV) can cause esophagitis and can be treated with specific antiviral agents, such as acyclovir for HSV and HZV or ganciclovir for CMV.

SYSTEMIC INFECTION

Unfortunately, disseminated candidiasis is often only diagnosed postmortem. Blood cultures are often negative before death because fungemia may be transient. It may be difficult to distinguish colonization or contamination from true infection when candida is recovered from the blood, urine, or sputum. Patients at greatest risk for disseminated infection include those with hematologic malignancies treated with cytotoxic agents, those treated with steroids, burn patients, and patients treated for prolonged periods with broad-spectrum antibiotics.[10,11] Despite the common occurrence of candida infections of the mucosa among AIDS patients, disseminated infection is quite rare unless other previously described risk factors are present. For example, only nine cases of cerebral candidiasis have been observed among 1300 patients who have been followed at the University of California-San Francisco.[15]

Candidal meningitis has been reported in an AIDS patient who presented with chronic headache and fevers. A computerized tomographic (CT) scan of the head revealed no abscesses; the cerebrospinal fluid showed a minimal neutrophilic pleocytosis. No organisms were seen on Gram's stain or India-ink preparations, but cultures were positive for *Candida albicans*.

■ TREATMENT

MUCOCUTANEOUS INFECTION

Thrush.   Several therapeutic choices are available for the treatment of thrush. Nystatin suspensions (containing 100,000 to 200,000 units/ml) can be used as a mouthwash several times a day. Alternatively, clotrimazole troches can be used (three to five times a day).[16]

Esophagitis.   Candidal esophagitis is often difficult to treat and eradicate in patients with AIDS. Some patients may respond to initial topical antifungal therapy that includes relatively high doses of nystatin (400,000 to 600,000 U, four to six times a day) as a swish-and-swallow suspension. Nystatin pastilles are an alternative preparation for patients who prefer their medication in lozenge or tablet form. Clotrimazole troches can also be used to treat candidal esophagitis (four to six troches a day).[17] Oral ketoconazole (200 to 400 mg/day) is the preferred therapy and should be used in those patients who fail to respond to topical antifungal agents. Treatment with ketoconazole for two weeks (or at least one week) after symptoms have resolved is usually necessary.[18] Ketoconazole-resistant *C. albicans* strains have been isolated from esophageal lesions in AIDS patients on long-term ketoconazole therapy. Although symptoms of dysphagia and odynophagia resolved with ketoconazole therapy, repeated esophagoscopy revealed persistent candidal esophagitis in several AIDS patients who were treated for over two months with ketoconazole.[8]

Patients failing to respond to either local therapy or ketoconazole may respond to short-term, low-dose intravenous amphotericin-B. Esophagoscopy should be performed in all patients being considered for amphotericin-B therapy to rule out other causes of esophagitis. Amphotericin-B is given at a relatively low dose (10 to 20 mg/day) for 10 to 14 days.[19]

SYSTEMIC INFECTION

Disseminated candidiasis is treated with standard doses of intravenous amphotericin-B (0.6 to 0.8 mg/kg/day) for six to eight weeks. There are no controlled studies documenting the efficacy of 5-flucytosine (5-FC) used in combination with amphotericin-B. 5-FC cannot be used as a single agent because of resistant strains of yeast and because it exacerbates pre-existing bone-marrow suppression in AIDS patients.

■ OUTCOME AND PREVENTION

In non-AIDS patients, mucocutaneous forms of candidiasis are usually cured with standard courses of antifungal agents. In AIDS patients, mucosal candidiasis is often readily suppressed but rarely cured because of the underlying immunodeficiency. Many patients must continue therapy indefinitely because of rapid relapse after therapy is discontinued.

Broad-spectrum antibiotics should be avoided when possible in patients with AIDS because of the risk of fungal dissemination. Scrupulous aseptic techniques should be used on hospitalized AIDS patients, particularly if central catheters are used. Fungal cultures should be obtained if unexplained fever develops in a patient with an indwelling line. Mucosal infections should be treated topically for two to four weeks. Patients can often titrate the appropriate suppressive dose of an antifungal agent by themselves.

REFERENCES

1. Edwards JE, Lehrer RI, Stiehm ER, et al. Severe candidal infections. Ann Intern Med 1978; 89:91-106.
2. Armstrong D, Gold J, Dryjanski J, et al. Treatment of infections in patients with the acquired immunodeficiency syndrome. Ann Intern Med 1985; 103:738-43.
3. Kirkpatrick CH. Host factors in defense against fungal infections. Am J Med 1984; 77:1-12.
4. Dreizen S. Oral candidiasis. Am J Med 1984; 77:28-33.
5. Klein RS, Harris CA, Small CB, et al. Oral candidiasis in high-risk patients as the initial manifestation of the acquired immunodeficiency syndrome. N Engl J Med 1985; 311:354-7.
6. Kodsi BE, Wickremsinghe PC, Kozinn PJ, et al. Candida esophagitis: a prospective study of 27 cases. Gastroenterology 1976; 71:715-9.
7. Mathieson R, Dutta SK. Candida esophagitis. Dig Dis Sci 1983; 28:365-70.
8. Tavitian A, Raufman JP, Rosenthal LE. Oral candidiasis as a marker of esophageal candidiasis in the acquired immunodeficiency syndrome. Ann Intern Med 1986; 104:54-5.
9. Trier JS, Bjorkman DJ. Esophageal, gastric, and intestinal candidiasis. Am J Med 1984; 77:39-43.
10. Young RC, Bennett JE, Geehoed GW, Levine AS. Fungemia with compromised host resistance. Ann Intern Med 1974; 80:605-12.
11. Menier-Carpentier F, Kiehn TE, Armstrong D. Fungemia in the compromised host. Am J Med 1981; 71:363-70.

12. Richardson D, Warnock DW. Serologic tests in the diagnosis and prognosis of fungal infection in the compromised host. In: Warnock DW, Richardson MD, eds. Fungal infection in the compromised patient. London: J. Wiley & Sons,1982:236-42.

13. Greenspan D, Greenspan J, Conant M, et al. Oral "hairy" leukoplakia in male homosexuals: evidence of association with both papillomavirus and a herpes group virus. Lancet 1984; 2:831-4.

14. Farman J, Tavitian A, Rosenthal LE, et al. Focal esophageal candidiasis in acquired immunodeficiency syndrome (AIDS). Gastrointest Radiol 1986; 11:213-7.

15. Levy RM, Bredesen DE, Rosenblum ML. Opportunistic central nervous system pathology in patients with AIDS. Ann Neurol 1988; 23:Suppl:7S-12S.

16. Schectman LB, Fumaro L, Robin T, et al. Clotrimazole treatment of oral candidiasis in patients with neoplastic disease. Am J Med 1984; 76:91-6.

17. Ehni WF, Ellison RT III. Spontaneous *Candida albicans* meningitis in a patient with the acquired immune deficiency syndrome. Am J Med 1987; 83:806-7.

18. Fazio RA, Wickremsinghe PC, Arsura EL. Ketoconazole treatment of candida esophagitis: a prospective study of 12 cases. Am J Gastroenterol 1983; 78:261-4.

19. Medoff G, Dismukes W, Meade R, Moses J. A new therapeutic approach to candida infection. Arch Intern Med 1972; 130:241-5.

Cryptococcosis

David Chernoff, M.D., and Merle A. Sande, M.D.

■ EPIDEMIOLOGY

Cryptococcus neoformans is a yeast-like fungus responsible for the majority of human cryptococcal infections. The organism is an encapsulated fungus found worldwide and without defined endemic regions. The most important environmental source of the fungus is soil contaminated with bird excrement. Exposure occurs when the organisms are aerosolized and inhaled. There is no evidence that infection is transmitted from human to human or animal to human. Although exposure to *C. neoformans* is quite common, infection is relatively rare unless the host has an underlying immune defect such as AIDS. Cryptococcal infection is almost always due to *C. neoformans*, although sporadic cases of disease due to other species of cryptococci such as *C. albidus* and *C. laurentii* have been reported.[1] Although localized candidiasis is the most common fungal infection in patients with HIV infection, cryptococcus is by far the most common life-threatening fungal pathogen in these patients.[2]

■ PATHOGENESIS

After inhalation, cryptococci are locally contained in the lung by neutrophils, monocytes, and macrophages — provided the host has a normal immune response. Alterations in host defense (such as those seen in patients with malignancies, transplant patients, AIDS patients, and patients treated with immunosuppressive agents such as steroids or cytotoxics) predispose these persons toward local proliferation of the fungus and subsequent widespread dissemination. Although immunosuppression predisposes the host to infection, about 50 percent of patients with cryptococcal infections have no obvious immune deficit.[3]

Host defense against cryptococcal infection depends on a complex interaction between cellular and humoral immune mechanisms. Animal models suggest that resistance to infection depends on macrophage activation by sensitized lymphocytes.[4] Activation of effector macrophages requires intact T-cell-mediated immunity. This T-cell-directed network is profoundly disrupted in AIDS patients because of HIV infection. Opsonization of the fungus by antibody and complement is also important in the clearance and killing of the organism by leukocytes. Humoral immunity is also abnormal in patients with AIDS because of altered regulation of antibody production consequent to T-cell destruction by HIV infection.[5] Cryptococcal infections in AIDS patients probably result from the progressive and relentless destruction of the immune system and reactivation of latent foci of infection.

■ CLINICAL PRESENTATION

In the normal host, initial pulmonary infection is usually asymptomatic. Cough, mild sputum production, and low-grade fever may be the only manifestations of initial exposure to cryptococcus. In the absence of an effective host immune response, infection with *C. neoformans* may progress to a widely disseminated and frequently fatal illness.

Cryptococcus is responsible for three major forms of disease: pulmonary, central nervous system (CNS), and disseminated infection. The most common clinical form of cryptococcal infection is a slowly progressive meningitis. *C. neoformans* has a predilection for localizing in the central nervous system, causing meningitis, encephalitis, and, less commonly, focal granulomas named cryptococcomas. The onset of cryptococcal meningitis is usually subtle; few localizing clues to the diagnosis are present. Patients often initially have non-specific complaints such as malaise, fever, headache, nausea, or vomiting. The headache is often described as frontal or temporal. Family members or friends often note subtle changes in personality or behavior. Less commonly, patients initially have cranial nerve palsies. Seizures are rare unless the infection has gone undetected for a substantial period. Focal neurologic deficits are occasionally observed when cryptococcomas are present.[6]

The majority of pulmonary infections due to cryptococcus go undetected because the initial exposure and infection are asypmtomatic or subclinical. Solitary or multiple subpleural nodules may be the only roentgenographic evidence of previous infection. Pulmonary infections may resolve spontaneously without therapy. Invasive pulmonary disease almost always occurs in the setting of chronic illness or immunosuppression. Nodules or infiltrates may be seen on chest roentgenograms in patients with invasive pulmonary infection. Cryptococcal pneumonia does not necessarily imply disseminated infection.[7]

Cryptococci can infect other organs and tissues besides the CNS and respiratory tract. Painless skin lesions occur in 5 percent to 10 percent of patients with disseminated disease. These lesions can appear as macules, papules, pustules, shallow cutaneous ulcers, or subcutaneous swellings.[8] Other organs, such as the heart, pericardium, kidney, adrenals, bone, and lymph nodes, can also be infected when the fungus disseminates.

Cryptococcal disease accounts for approximately 5 percent to 8 percent of all opportunistic infections in patients with AIDS. Although less common than *Pneumocystis carinii* pneumonia or localized candidiasis, cryptococcus is the most common fungal pathogen causing life-threatening illness in these patients.[9] In contrast to a fungal disease such as histoplasmosis (which is usually seen only in endemic regions), cryptococcosis has been observed in AIDS patients in the United States, Europe, Africa, and Haiti. This geographic distribution reflects the ubiquitous nature of the fungus.

As in non-AIDS patients, the clinical presentation of cryptococcal infection, particularly meningitis, may be subtle in AIDS patients; few localizing signs or symptoms may be present. The most common complaint is severe headache and fever. Behavioral changes, memory loss, and confusion are also commonly observed. Signs of meningeal irritation, such as nuchal rigidity or meningismus, are uncommon. Focal neurologic deficits, cranial-nerve palsies, and seizures occur in a minority of AIDS patients with CNS infection. Cryptococcomas are occasionally seen in AIDS patients with CNS infection.[10]

AIDS patients may have extraneural forms of cryptococcal infection. Subacute disease may be detected by routine screening of serum, urine, or sputum for cryptococcal antigen. Cryptococcemia without meningitis and isolated pulmonary disease have been reported in patients with AIDS. In the three published series of cryptococcal infections in AIDS patients, meningitis was the most common form of infection.[9-11] Of the patients with meningitis, 15 percent to 40 percent had positive cryptococcal blood cultures. Evidence of disseminated disease was detected in over 50 percent of patients with meningitis. Unusual manifestations of disseminated cryptococcal infection, such as myocarditis with acute heart failure, have been observed in patients with AIDS.[16] Other unusual presentations of extraneural cryptococcal infection in AIDS patients include mediastinal involvement mimicking lymphoma, isolated pleural effusion, and massive peripheral and mediastinal lymph-node infection.[17-19] Cryptococcal disease was often the first opportunistic infection observed in the patients in these studies.

The diagnosis of AIDS should be seriously considered in any patient with risk factors for HIV infection (such as drug use, homosexual activity, or history of blood-product transfusions) who has cryptococcal infection. Since cryptococcal meningitis can occur in normal hosts and HIV is now more prevalent in populations without obvious risks, an HIV serologic test should be performed to confirm or exclude the AIDS diagnosis if doubt exists.

■ **DIAGNOSIS**

Diagnosis of cryptococcal infection has been greatly facilitated by assay systems that rapidly detect the presence of cryptococcal capsular antigen in various body fluids. Commercial kits, most often using latex agglutination assays, can detect cryptococcal antigen at concentrations as low as 10 to 20 ng/ml. The definitive diagnosis of infection depends on culturing and identifying the organism. False-positive latex agglutination tests have been reported when rheumatoid factor was present in the fluid. Internal controls have been incorporated in the commercial kits to control for false-positive reactions.[12]

Diagnosis of cryptococcal meningitis can be made by using any of the following methods: (1) visualizing the fungus in cerebrospinal fluid (CSF), using India ink; (2) detecting cryptococcal antigen; or (3) culturing the fungus. Cryptococci can be visualized in CSF with India ink because the ink forms a dark halo around the cryptococcal capsule. Care must be taken when interpreting the India-ink test so that lymphocytes or erythrocytes are not confused with cryptococci.[13] Poorly encapsulated forms of the fungus may not be visualized with India ink, however. The test is extremely useful because it can rapidly establish the diagnosis of meningitis before antigen or culture results are available. In non-AIDS patients with meningitis, about 60 percent have positive India-ink tests.[6] In patients with AIDS and meningitis, the rate of India-ink positivity is 75 percent to 85 percent.[9-11]

In patients without AIDS, the CSF formula in cryptococcal meningitis suggests a chronic, lymphocytic meningitis. The opening pressure is usually elevated (approximately 65 percent), CSF protein is almost always elevated (approximately 90 percent), and CSF glucose is low (approximately 75 percent). Almost all cases show a predominately lymphocytic pleocytosis (<150 cells/ml).[6] The CSF formula in patients with AIDS and cryptococcal meningitis is variable but often completely normal. All published series report minimal changes in the CSF. The most common finding is a minimal pleocytosis (<5 cells/ml), normal protein, and normal glucose.[9-11] A normal CSF formula in an AIDS patient with suspected meningitis in no way rules out the diagnosis of cryptococcal meningitis.

Cryptococcal antigen is detected in CSF in greater than 95 percent of cases of culture-proven meningitis. Detection of antigen is presumptive evidence of infection. Occasionally, antigen will be detected in culture-negative CSF.[14]

Patients with antigen-positive and culture-negative CSF have responded to treatment; headache and CSF abnormalities have resolved. Rare cases of meningitis have been reported with negative antigen and positive cultures. These unusual cases probably represent poorly encapsulated fungi or serotype variants that react poorly with the serotypes used to prepare the latex agglutination reagents. An increased incidence of poorly encapsulated strains of cryptococci has been reported in patients with AIDS and meningitis.[15] There have also been anecdotal reports of AIDS patients with cryptococcal antigen-negative and culture-positive CSF. Early detection of asymptomatic meningeal infection may account for some of these cases. With the widespread availability and use of antigen detection assays, patients with no clinical evidence of meningitis may undergo a lumbar puncture when antigen is detected in urine or serum. CSF should be routinely cultured for fungus in any AIDS patient undergoing a lumbar puncture, even if cryptococcal antigen is not detected in the CSF.

All AIDS patients in whom cryptococcal antigen is detected in urine, serum, or CSF should be rigorously evaluated for evidence of disseminated disease. Blood, urine, and CSF should be sent for fungal culture. A computerized tomographic (CT) scan of the head should be obtained to rule out hydrocephalus or focal lesions such as cryptococcomas. A careful ophthalmologic examination and skin examination should be conducted to rule out ocular or cutaneous infection. Cutaneous cryptococcal infection has been observed within Kaposi's sarcoma lesions in AIDS patients.[20] Chest roentgenogram abnormalities may represent cryptococcal pneumonia, especially if sputum or bronchoscopic specimens are culture-positive. The interpretation of these abnormalities is often complicated because other organisms (such as *P. carinii*) may be simultaneously detected in sputum samples. As in other immunosuppressed patients, cryptococcal pneumonia in AIDS patients will probably disseminate if not treated promptly.[7]

■ TREATMENT

The treatment of choice for cryptococcal infections is amphotericin-B. Cryptococcal meningitis has been treated with amphotericin-B at a dose of 0.6 to 0.8 mg/kg/day to a usual total dose of 1.5 to 2.5 g over a period of six to eight weeks. The duration of therapy is not fixed and depends on the clinical response of the patient.

The combination of amphotericin-B and 5-flucytosine (5-FC) has been shown to be synergistic against cryptococci in vitro. Clinical trials evaluating the efficacy and toxicity of combination therapy took place before the AIDS epidemic began. A large, multicenter, randomized, prospective study demonstrated the efficacy of combination therapy in patients with cryptococcal meningitis; none of the patients had AIDS.[21] The response rate was 67 percent in patients treated with low-dose amphotericin-B (0.3 mg/kg/day) plus 5-FC (150 mg/kg/day) compared to a response rate of 47 percent in the group treated with amphotericin-B alone at a higher dose (0.4 mg/kg/day). The results of this study must be interpreted with caution because patients who were unable to tolerate combination therapy were excluded from analysis and subsequently cured with amphotericin-B alone. There is no conclusive evidence that combination therapy is more efficacious than amphotericin-B alone at the somewhat higher standard doses now used (0.6 to 0.8 mg/kg/day).[6]

5-FC cannot be used as a single agent in the treatment of cryptococcal infections, because of the rapid emergence of drug resistance. It can cause significant marrow suppression, and the dosage may be decreased (to 50 to 100 mg/kg/day) or withdrawn completely if significant marrow-suppression results. Toxicity can be a serious problem for AIDS patients because many of them are already leukopenic due to HIV infection. AIDS patients with cryptococcal infections should be treated with standard-to-high doses of amphotericin-B (0.6 to 0.8 mg/kg/day) for a period of four to eight weeks with the option of adding 5-FC at modified doses if the patient can tolerate it.

Other agents (such as miconazole) cannot be recommended unless amphotericin-B cannot be given because of severe toxicity or allergy. Isolated case reports document miconazole's efficacy, but numerous failures and toxicities have also been reported.[22,23] Ketoconazole cannot be recommended as a single agent because of its poor penetration into the cerebrospinal fluid.[24]

Intrathecal amphotericin-B has usually been reserved for patients who are failing standard courses of intravenous amphotericin-B.[25] There are many problems associated with the use of intrathecal therapy. Intrathecal amphotericin-B can cause a severe arachnoiditis and acute myelopathy. The Ommaya reservoir, the common route for administering the drug, can become infected, clogged, or displaced.[26] A recent report suggests that the early use of combined intrathecal and intravenous therapy significantly improves outcome when compared to intravenous therapy alone in patients with cryptococcal meningitis.[27] The risks and benefits of intrathecal amphotericin-B therapy must be considered in each patient for whom its use is contemplated. In the limited number of AIDS patients treated with intrathecal amphotericin-B, outcome has been uniformly poor; there have been no long-term survivors. Intrathecal therapy cannot be routinely recommended in AIDS patients with cryptococcal meningitis.

Despite the fact that cryptococcal isolates from AIDS patients are often poorly encapsulated, no difference in drug sensitivity has been noted. Ninety percent of cryptococcal isolates were inhibited by achievable serum levels of amphotericin-B, ketoconazole, miconazole, and flucytosine.[29]

■ OUTCOME

Untreated cryptococcal infections such as meningitis or cryptococcemia are invariably fatal. Before the AIDS epidemic, about 65 percent of patients with cryptococcal meningitis were cured with standard doses of amphotericin-B.[6] About half of these "cured" patients, however, were left with permanent neurologic sequelae. The most important predictor of response to therapy (and of survival) was the presence or absence of a major predisposing illness. In non-AIDS patients with cryptococcal meningitis, predictors of poor outcome included the following: positive India-ink test, high opening pressure, minimal pleocytosis (<20 cells/ml), positive extraneural cultures, and serum antigen >1:32.

Relapse was more common if the following laboratory parameters were present: positive extraneural cultures, persistent hypoglycorrhachia, and serum or CSF antigen titers of >1:80.[3]

In patients with AIDS and cryptococcal meningitis, these predictors of outcome and relapse probably do not apply. Cryptococcal meningitis is temporarily suppressed during therapy and is probably never completely cured in these patients. Relapses are extremely common despite intensive and prolonged courses of therapy. Cerebrospinal fluid antigen titers, which can be extraordinarily high (>1:1,000,000), fall with therapy and cultures usually become sterile within one to two weeks after initiation of amphotericin-B therapy.

Serum and CSF antigen titers do not appear to have prognostic value in these patients, with the possible exception of a good outcome if titers are low and then turn negative.

There does not seem to be a difference in outcome between patients treated with amphotericin-B alone and those treated with the combination of low-dose amphotericin-B and 5-flucytosine. About 30 percent of patients with AIDS have toxic reactions to 5-flucytosine (marrow suppression, transaminase elevation, nausea, and vomiting) that require discontinuing the drug. These patients are already frequently leukopenic and do not seem to tolerate standard doses of 5-FC. A small number of patients in whom initial therapy failed were retreated with a combination of intravenous and intrathecal amphotericin-B. All of these patients had toxic reactions to intrathecal therapy (arachnoiditis, bacterial infection associated with the Ommaya reservoir), and all died despite aggressive therapy.

Because relapse is so common in AIDS patients, various regimens are being tested in an effort to suppress indolent infection. A small group of AIDS patients have been followed prospectively after initial therapy for cryptococcal infection. Of the patients who completed therapy and who were not treated with outpatient suppressive therapy, 50 percent relapsed within one year.[30] There were no relapses in a small group of patients treated with weekly amphotericin-B (100 mg/week).[10]

Some patients have been treated with various doses of ketoconazole in an effort to prevent relapse. There have been many anecdotal reports of patients relapsing despite high and often toxic doses of ketoconazole. Because of its poor penetration into the CSF, ketoconazole is not likely to be valuable as a single suppressive agent. There is experimental evidence that the combination of ketoconazole and 5-FC is synergistic in animal models of cryptococcal meningitis.[28] The combination of ketoconazole and 5-FC might be useful as an outpatient suppressive regimen in these patients. Given the high rate of relapse in these patients, some form of suppressive therapy should be considered. Intermittent doses of amphotericin-B (0.6 to 1 mg/kg) given weekly or biweekly are a reasonable method of outpatient suppressive therapy. Relapses of cryptococcal meningitis have occurred despite maintenance therapy with amphotericin-B.[37]

The use of experimental imidazoles that penetrate the blood–brain barrier represents a promising approach to effective suppressive therapy. Fluconazole is effective in the animal model of cryptococcal meningitis and has excellent penetration of the central nervous system.[31,32] It is given at a dosage of 200 to 400 mg/day. Both fluconazole and itraconazole have been used with promising results as primary therapy for cryptococcal meningitis in patients with AIDS.[38-40] AIDS patients who have failed or relapsed on amphotericin-B have been successfully treated with fluconazole.[33,34] Trials are now in progress to evaluate the effectiveness of fluconazole as a suppressive agent in AIDS patients with cryptococcal meningitis. Itraconazole, despite poor penetration of the central nervous system, has been used to prevent CNS relapse in a small number of AIDS patients with cryptococcal meningitis.[35,36,38] On the basis of these preliminary results, a prospective randomized trial is under way to compare fluconazole with amphotericin-B (with or without 5-flucytosine) for primary therapy of cryptococcal meningitis.[41] A prospective randomized trial of oral fluconazole (200 mg/day) versus intravenous amphotericin-B (1.0 mg/kg/week) is now under way in patients who have completed primary therapy and who are culture-negative. The purposes of the trial are to determine the effect of fluconazole and amphotericin-B on prevention of relapse and on the overall survival rate of patients in the trial. Eligible patients can be enrolled by contacting Dr. Patrick Robinson, Associate Director, Pfizer Research (203/441-4100).

■ PREVENTION

Because of the widespread distribution of cryptococcus, it is impossible to prevent patients from being exposed to the fungus. Most infections are probably the result of reactivating old latent pulmonary foci. Nevertheless, individuals at risk for AIDS should avoid situations where exposure to the fungus is likely (i.e., heavily contaminated soil, bird roosts, etc). Early detection of occult infection may alter the prognosis and outcome in AIDS patients. The use of screening assays for cryptococcal antigen makes it possible to detect asymptomatic infection so therapy can begin at an earlier stage.

REFERENCES

1. Hay RJ. Clinical manifestations and management of cryptococcosis in the compromised patient. In: Winock DW, Richardson MD, eds. Fungal infection in the compromised patient. New York: J. Wiley & Sons, 1982:93-114.
2. Grant I, Armstrong D. Management of infectious complications in acquired immunodeficiency syndrome. Am J Med 1986; 81(Suppl 1A):59-72.
3. Diamond RD, Bennett JE. Prognostic factors in cryptococcal meningitis. Ann Intern Med 1974; 80:176-81.
4. Fung PYS, Murphy JW. In vitro interactions of immune lymphocytes and *Cryptococcus neoformans*. Infect Immun 1982; 36:1128-34.
5. Lane HC, Masur H, Edgar LC, et al. Abnormalities of B-cell activation and immunoregulation in patients with the acquired immunodeficiency syndrome. N Engl J Med 1983; 309:453-8.
6. Sabetta JR, Andriole VT. Cryptococcal infection of the central nervous system. Med Clin North Am 1985; 69:333-44.
7. Kerkering TM, Duma RJ, Shadomy S. The evolution of pulmonary cryptococcosis. Ann Intern Med 1981; 94:611-16.
8. Schupach CW, Wheeler CE, Briggaman RA, et al. Cutaneous manifestations of disseminated cryptococcosis. Arch Dermatol 1976; 112:1734-40.
9. Kovacs JA, Kovacs AA, Polis M, et al. Cryptococcosis in the acquired immunodeficiency syndrome. Ann Intern Med 1985; 103:533-8.
10. Zuger A, Louie E, Holtzman R, et al. Cryptococcal disease in patients with the acquired immunodeficiency syndrome. Ann Intern Med 1986; 104:234-40.
11. Eng RH, Bishberg E, Smith SM, Kapila R. Cryptococcal infections in patients with the acquired immunodeficiency syndrome. Am J Med 1986; 81:19-23.
12. Goodman JS, Kaufman L, Koenig MG. Diagnosis of cryptococcal meningitis. N Engl J Med 1971; 285:434-6.
13. Portnoy D, Richards GK. Cryptococcal meningitis: misdiagnosis with India ink. Can Med Assoc J 1981; 124:891-2.
14. Snow RM, Dismukes WE. Cryptococcal meningitis. Diagnostic value of cryptococcal antigen in CSF. Arch Intern Med 1975; 135:1155-7.
15. Bottone EJ, Toma M, Johansson BE, Wormser GP. Poorly encapsulated *Cryptococcus neoformans* from patients with AIDS. I: Preliminary observations. AIDS Res 1986; 2:211-8.
16. Lafont A, Wolff M, Marche C, et al. Overwhelming myocarditis due to *Cryptococcus neoformans* in an AIDS patient. Lancet 1987; 2:1145-6.
17. Newman TG, Soni A, Acaron S, Huang CT. Pleural cryptococcosis in the acquired immune deficiency syndrome. Chest 1987; 91:459-61.
18. Witt D, McKay D, Schwam L, et al. Acquired immune deficiency syndrome presenting as bone marrow and mediastinal cryptococcosis. Am J Med 1987; 82:149-50.
19. Torres RA. Cryptococcal mediastinitis mimicking lymphoma in the acquired immune deficiency syndrome. Am J Med 1987; 83:1004-5.
20. Libow LF, Robert D, Sibulkin D. Co-existent cutaneous cryptococcosis and Kaposi's sarcoma in patients with AIDS. Cutis 1988; 41:159-62.
21. Bennett JE, Dismukes WE, Duma RJ, et al. A comparison of amphotericin-B alone and combined with flucytosine in the treatment of cryptococcal meningitis. N Engl J Med 1979; 301:126-31.

22. Weinstein L, Jacoby I. Successful treatment of cerebral cryptococcoma and meningitis with miconazole. Ann Intern Med 1980; 93:569-71.

23. Hay RJ. Miconazole in cryptococcosis. In: Royal Society of Medicine International Congress and Symposium Series, Vol. 45. The role of intravenous miconazole in the treatment of systemic mycoses. London: Academic Press, 1982:43-7.

24. Perfect JR, Durack DT, Hamilton JD, Gallis HA. Failure of ketoconazole in cryptococcal meningitis. JAMA 1982; 247:3349-51.

25. Diamond RD, Bennett JE. A subcutaneous reservoir for intrathecal therapy of fungal meningitis. N Engl J Med 1973; 288:186-8.

26. Schnheyder H, Thestrup-Pedersen K, Esmann V, Stenderup A. Cryptococcal meningitis: complications due to intrathecal treatment. Scand J Infect Dis 1980; 12:155-7.

27. Polsky B, Depman MR, Gold JW, et al. Intraventricular therapy of cryptococcal meningitis via a subcutaneous reservoir. Am J Med 1986; 81:24-8.

28. Craven PC, Graybill JR. Combination of oral flucytosine and ketoconazole as therapy for experimental cryptococcal meningitis. J Infect Dis 1984; 149:584-90.

29. Poon M, Cronin DC II, Wormser GP, Bottone EJ. In vitro susceptibility of *Cryptococcus neoformans* isolates from patients with acquired immunodeficiency syndrome. Arch Pathol Lab Med 1988; 112:161-2.

30. Nonviral infections of the central nervous system. In: Levy RM, Bredesen DE, Rosenblum ML, eds. AIDS and the nervous system. New York: Raven Press, 1988:263-88.

31. Perfect JR, Savani DV, Durack DT. Comparison of itraconazole and fluconazole in treatment of cryptococcal meningitis and candida pyelonephritis in rabbits. Antimicrob Agents Chemother 1986; 29:579-83.

32. Perfect JR, Durack DT. Penetration of imidazoles and triazoles into cerebrospinal fluid of rabbits. J Antimicrob Chemother 1985; 16:81-6.

33. Dupon B, Drouhet E. Cryptococcal meningitis and fluconazole. Ann Intern Med 1987; 106:778.

34. Byrne WR, Wajszczuk CP. Cryptococcal meningitis in the acquired immunodeficiency syndrome (AIDS): successful treatment with fluconazole after failure of amphotericin-B. Ann Intern Med 1988; 108:384-5.

35. de Gans J, Eeftinck-Schattenkerk JK, van Ketel RJ. Itraconazole as maintenance treatment for cryptococcal meningitis in the acquired immune deficiency syndrome. Br Med J 1988; 296:339.

36. Viviani MA, Tortorano AM, Giani PC, et al. Itraconazole for cryptococcal infection in the acquired immunodeficiency syndrome. Ann Intern Med 1987; 106:166.

37. Zuger A, Schuster M, Sinberhoff M, et al. Maintenance amphotericin-B for cryptococcal meningitis in the acquired immunodeficiency syndrome (AIDS). Ann Intern Med 1988; 109:592-3.

38. Cryptococcosis and AIDS. Lancet 1988; 1:1434-6.

39. Stern JJ, Hartman BJ, Sharkey P, et al. Oral fluconazole therapy for patients with acquired immunodeficiency syndrome and cryptococcosis: experience with 22 patients. Am J Med 1988; 85:477-80.

40. Sugar AM, Saunders C. Oral fluconazole as suppressive therapy of disseminated cryptococcosis in patients with acquired immunodeficiency syndrome. Am J Med 1988; 85:481-9.

41. Dismukes WE. Cryptococcal meningitis in patients with AIDS. J Infect Dis 1988; 157:624-8.

6.3.4

Histoplasmosis

David Chernoff, M.D.

■ EPIDEMIOLOGY

Histoplasma capsulatum exists in its mycelial form in soil contaminated by bird droppings or other organic material. The major endemic area is the central United States. Large numbers of spores are dispersed into the air when contaminated soil is disturbed; exposure occurs when spores are inhaled. The initial infection is commonly asymptomatic in the normal host. Disseminated disease usually occurs in immunosuppressed patients or in patients with chronic illnesses. Patients with AIDS who live in endemic areas are at increased risk for disseminated disease because of frequent environmental exposure.

■ PATHOGENESIS

After inhalation, the spores germinate into the pathogenic yeast form. The yeast proliferate locally and disseminate hematogenously. In the lung, the yeast are ingested by alveolar macrophages, which accumulate at sites of infection. A granulomatous inflammatory response occurs at these sites and results in focal infiltrates. These areas may later undergo necrosis and calcification, forming "buck-shot" lesions that appear on chest x-ray. A normal host acquires lifelong cell-mediated immunity within 10 to 14 days after exposure. In the immunologically normal host, heavy re-exposure to *H. capsulatum* spores may result in a transient pulmonary infection.

The two most important factors that appear to determine the outcome of infection are the host's immune status and, to a lesser extent, the size of the inoculum. In normal individuals with previous exposure to *H. capsulatum*, viable organisms probably exist intracellularly throughout the person's life. When cell-mediated immunity is impaired, reactivation of infection may occur. Cell-mediated immunity is profoundly suppressed in patients with AIDS. Thus, patients with AIDS must be considered at high risk for disseminated histoplasmosis in endemic areas.

■ CLINICAL PRESENTATION

In the normal host, initial infection is usually asymptomatic. The primary infection appears as a flu-like illness in 5 percent to 10 percent of patients. Scattered infiltrates and hilar adenopathy are seen in up to 25 percent of patients with primary infection. Unusual manifestations of initial infection include erythema multiforme and erythema nodosum.[1]

In the absence of effective cell-mediated immunity, infection with *H. capsulatum* may progress to fulminating and often fatal illness. Disseminated infection has been observed in patients with hematologic malignancies, patients treated with steroids, and patients treated with cytotoxic agents.[2,3] Less commonly, disseminated disease has been observed in patients without obvious immunologic deficit. These patients are often elderly and have some form of chronic disease, such as renal failure, diabetes, alcoholism, or pulmonary disease.[4]

Signs and symptoms of disseminated histoplasmosis include high fever, weight loss, respiratory complaints, hepatomegaly, splenomegaly, lymphadenopathy, and anemia. Less common manifestations include gastrointestinal bleeding secondary to mucosal ulcerations, cutaneous lesions, cerebritis, and meningitis. Chest x-rays are normal in up to 30 percent of patients with disseminated infection. In two recent outbreaks of histoplasmosis, approximately 8 percent of infected individuals had disseminated disease.[3]

The frequency of histoplasmosis in patients with AIDS is unknown. Autopsy series rarely document infection with *H. capsulatum*.[5] The number of cases reported[5] is small compared with reports of other fungal pathogens such as *Cryptococcus neoformans* or *Candida albicans*. The relative infrequency of infection is probably a reflection of the geographic epidemiology of AIDS: the majority of cases of AIDS have occurred in large cities such as San Francisco, New York City, and Los Angeles, outside of *H. capsulatum*—endemic areas.

In endemic areas such as Indiana, where relatively small numbers of AIDS patients have been seen, disseminated histoplasmosis is common. Of the first 15 AIDS patients seen in Indianapolis, 6 had disseminated histoplasmosis.[6] The clinical syndrome in these patients was more severe than in other immunocompromised patients with disseminated infection. Of these six AIDS patients, four had a clinical syndrome resembling sepsis that included disseminated intravascular coagulation, leukopenia, adult respiratory distress syndrome, and acute renal failure. Other case reports document fatal disseminated histoplasmosis in patients with AIDS.[7-11]

■ DIAGNOSIS

The definitive diagnosis of histoplasmosis depends on the identification and culture of the fungus in tissue specimens. In non-AIDS patients with disseminated infection, histopathologic and culture diagnoses are most often made by examination of biopsies from the lung, bone marrow, lymph nodes, and liver. Occasionally, examination of the peripheral smear or buffy coat smear will reveal intracellular yeast, providing a rapid means of diagnosis. A small percentage of patients (approximately 5 percent) initially have cutaneous lesions, ranging from plaques to ulcers, from which *H. capsulatum* can be identified.

Disseminated histoplasmosis in patients with AIDS has been diagnosed by examination of the bone marrow, blood cultures, peripheral smear, transbronchial biopsy, lymph node biopsy, and biopsy of cutaneous lesions. In an AIDS patient suspected of having histoplasmosis, examination of biopsy specimens from the lung, bone marrow, or lymph node should reveal evidence of infection. Peripheral smears should also be examined because they may provide evidence of infection and eliminate the need for invasive procedures.[8] Blood and urine should also be cultured for fungus.

Unusual manifestations of disseminated histoplasmosis have been observed in patients with AIDS. These include chorioretinitis, meningitis, and brain abscesses.[17,18] Space-occupying lesions resembling toxoplasmosis or central nervous system (CNS) lymphoma have been observed on brain computed tomographic (CT) scans in AIDS patients with CNS histoplasmosis. In devising a therapy plan, it is important to document CNS involvement, since agents such as ketoconazole, which has poor CNS penetration, are less likely to prevent relapse.

The most reliable serologic method for diagnosing histoplasmosis is checking complement-fixation titers against mycelial and yeast antigens.[12] Titers of greater than 1:32 are highly suggestive but not diagnostic of infection. Agar immune-diffusion assays, which detect M and H precipitin bands, can also be used to detect infection. In patients with disseminated disease, complement fixation titers may be negative in up to 20 percent of cases.[3] Furthermore, when the complement-fixation titers are positive, they are often present in low titers (less than 1:32). Recently, a radioimmunoassay has been developed that detects *H. capsulatum* polysaccharide antigen.[13] In patients with disseminated infection, the assay was positive in greater than 90 percent of cases. Such assays, which detect antigen rather than antibody response, should provide a means for rapid diagnosis of infection.

In the small number of cases of disseminated histoplasmosis reported in AIDS patients, complement-fixation titers have been positive in almost all cases. One patient, however, had negative serologies, including a negative complement-fixation titer in the cerebrospinal fluid (CSF) despite widespread infection.[8] Positive serologies provide an early clue to the diagnosis of histoplasmosis in patients with AIDS and may permit prompt initiation of antifungal therapy pending identification and culture of the fungus from tissue specimens.

Skin testing with histoplasmin has no role in the diagnosis of histoplasmosis. A positive skin test is meaningless in an endemic region because of residents' widespread exposure. Furthermore, cutaneous anergy is frequently observed in patients with AIDS, making skin testing useless for diagnostic purposes.

■ TREATMENT

Acute histoplasmosis in the normal host is a self-limited disease that does not require therapy. Amphotericin-B is the treatment of choice for patients with disseminated disease or for immunosuppressed patients with limited infection. The dose of amphotericin-B is rapidly increased to 0.6 mg/kg/day. Duration of therapy and total dose are not fixed. Most patients require a minimum total dose of 30 mg/kg of amphotericin-B.[3]

Ketoconazole has been successfully used in pulmonary and disseminated histoplasmosis in patients without serious underlying disease or immunosuppression.[14] It has, however, been ineffective in treating immunosuppressed patients with disseminated infection,[3] so its use as primary therapy in AIDS patients with disseminated histoplasmosis is precluded.

■ OUTCOME

Untreated disseminated histoplasmosis is almost always fatal.[15] Mortality has been reduced to less than 10 percent when adequate doses of amphotericin-B are given. Non-AIDS patients who have disseminated histoplasmosis rarely relapse when treated with a minimum total of 30 mg/kg of amphotericin-B. The response to therapy in AIDS patients, however, is extremely poor. Data from two small series of AIDS patients with disseminated histoplasmosis show a 100 percent relapse rate in five patients despite treatment with at least 30 mg/kg of amphotericin-B.[6,7] One patient treated with ketoconazole alone for disease limited to the lymph nodes relapsed with disseminated disease when the ketoconazole was discontinued.[6] After completion of initial therapy, serious consideration should be given to suppressive outpatient therapy.

There are two options for preventing relapse. One is to give ketoconazole indefinitely; the second involves intermittent infusions of amphotericin-B. Weekly doses of 100 mg of amphotericin-B appear to be effective in preventing relapse in AIDS patients with cryptococcal infections.[16] However, the relative efficacy and toxicity of ketoconazole at 200 to 400 mg/day versus weekly amphotericin-B to prevent relapse are unknown.

Central nervous system histoplasmosis mandates the prolonged use of amphotericin-B. Central nervous system relapses have occurred in patients taking ketoconazole.

■ PREVENTION

Given the ubiquity of *H. capsulatum* in endemic areas, a reduction in environmental exposure is extremely difficult. Patients with AIDS in endemic regions may reactivate latent infections as a consequence of their underlying immunosuppression. Disseminated histoplasmosis is not contagious, and thus protective isolation is not necessary.

REFERENCES

1. Goodwin RA, Loyd JE, Des Prez RM. Histoplasmosis in normal hosts. Medicine 1981; 60:231-66.
2. Goodwin RA, Shapiro JL, Thurman GH, et al. Disseminated histoplasmosis: clinical and pathologic correlations. Medicine 1980; 59:1-31.
3. Sathapatayavongs B, Batteiger BE, Wheat J, et al. Clinical and laboratory features of disseminated histoplasmosis during two large urban outbreaks. Medicine 1983; 62:263-70.
4. Wheat JL, Slama TG, Norton JA, et al. Risk factors for disseminated or fatal histoplasmosis. Ann Intern Med 1982; 96:159-63.
5. Marchevsky A, Rosen MJ, Chrystal G, Kleinerman J. Pulmonary complications of the acquired immunodeficiency syndrome: a clinicopathologic study of 70 cases. Hum Pathol 1985; 16:659-70.
6. Wheat JL, Slama TG, Zeckel ML. Histoplasmosis in the acquired immunodeficiency syndrome. Am J Med 1985; 78:203-10.
7. Bonner JR, Alexander WJ, Dismukes WE, et al. Disseminated histoplasmosis in patients with the acquired immunodeficiency syndrome. Arch Intern Med 1984; 144:2178-81.
8. Henochowicz S, Sahovic E, Pistole M, et al. Histoplasmosis diagnosed on peripheral blood smear from a patient with AIDS. JAMA 1985; 253:3148.
9. Pasternak J, Bolivar R. Histoplasmosis in acquired immunodeficiency syndrome (AIDS): diagnosis by bone marrow examination. Arch Intern Med 1983; 143:2024.
10. Gerstein HC, Fanning MM, Read SE, et al. AIDS in a patient with hemophilia receiving mainly cryoprecipitate. Can Med Assoc J 1983; 131:45-7.
11. Taylor MN, Baddour LM, Alexander JR. Disseminated histoplasmosis associated with the acquired immune deficiency syndrome. Am J Med 1984; 77:579-80.
12. Wheat J, French ML, Kohler RB, et al. The diagnostic laboratory tests for histoplasmosis. Ann Intern Med 1982; 97:680-5.
13. Wheat JL, Kohler RB, Tewari RP. Diagnosis of disseminated histoplasmosis by detection of *Histoplasma capsulatum* antigen in serum and urine specimens. N Engl J Med 1986; 314:83-8.
14. NIAID Mycosis Study Group. Treatment of blastomycosis and histoplasmosis with ketoconazole. Ann Intern Med 1985; 103:861-72.
15. Furcolow ML. Comparison of treated and untreated severe histoplasmosis. JAMA 1983; 183:823-6.
16. Zuger A, Lovie E, Holtzman R, et al. Cryptococcal disease in patients with acquired immunodeficiency syndrome. Ann Intern Med 1986; 104:234-40.
17. Macher A, Rodrigues MM, Kaplan W, et al. Disseminated bilateral chorioretinitis due to *Histoplasma capsulatum* in a patient with the acquired immunodeficiency syndrome. Ophthalmology 1985; 92:1159-64.
18. Anaissie E, Fainstein V, Samo T, et al. Central nervous system histoplasmosis. An unappreciated complication of the acquire [sic] immunodeficiency syndrome. Am J Med 1988; 84:215-7.

6.4

Viral Infections

Varicella–Zoster Virus

Kim S. Erlich, M.D., and John Mills, M.D.

Varicella–zoster virus (VZV), a herpesvirus, is responsible for both varicella ("chickenpox") and zoster ("shingles"). The illness was initially described in the ninth century by Rhazes, who noted that a "mild form of smallpox" did not protect against epidemic smallpox. The contagious nature of the varicella rash was first demonstrated by Steiner in 1875, but it was not until 1932 that Bruusgaard presented evidence that varicella could be transmitted by a patient with herpes zoster.

As with other herpesviruses, VZV causes both an acute illness and a lifelong latent infection. The acute primary infection (varicella) commonly occurs during childhood. In a child with normal cellular immunity, primary VZV infection is relatively benign and self-limiting. In adults, however, varicella infection can be more severe; systemic manifestations and occasional visceral dissemination occur. Recurrent VZV infection (zoster) may occur as a result of decreased specific humoral or cellular-mediated immunity. Zoster usually presents as a localized cutaneous eruption occurring along one or more contiguous dermatomes. During a zoster recurrence, immunocompetent patients occasionally develop cutaneous or visceral dissemination, with multiple lesions occurring outside the primary dermatomal pattern.[1,2]

AIDS patients and other immunocompromised individuals may develop severe illnesses from either primary or recurrent VZV infection. Progressive primary varicella, a syndrome in which new lesions continually form and disseminate to the viscera, can be life-threatening and can occur in AIDS patients with primary infection. Zoster eruptions in AIDS patients can be extensive, locally destructive, and secondarily infected. They may disseminate and involve visceral organs.[3,4]

Management of VZV infections in AIDS patients often requires the administration of acyclovir (an antiviral agent with activity against VZV) and may require hospitalization.[5,6] Although varicella–zoster immune globulin (VZIG) may be effective as prophylaxis in AIDS patients with known recent exposure to an infectious individual,[7,8] no data on its efficacy in this circumstance are available.[7]

■ EPIDEMIOLOGY

Humans are the only natural host for VZV. Transmission occurs through direct contact with infectious lesions or mucous membrane contact with aerosolized infected droplets. The virus can be easily transmitted; secondary cases of varicella in susceptible household contacts of patients with varicella or zoster are common. Infectivity usually begins one to two days before the onset of rash and persists until all vesicular lesions are dried and crusted.[1,2] Lesions in AIDS patients with VZV infection may heal slowly and can remain infectious for several weeks.

In temperate climates, varicella is a disease of childhood, thus most AIDS patients born in the US and Europe have had previous primary VZV infection.

For reasons that are not completely understood, varicella in tropical and sub-tropical areas occurs with greater frequency in adults. Therefore, AIDS patients from Africa, Haiti, and other equatorial areas may be more susceptible to primary VZV infection.

In the normal host, the risk of developing recurrent VZV (zoster) increases with age. The greatest incidence of zoster in the non-HIV-infected population occurs between ages 50 and 80. Zoster in AIDS patients, however, occurs more frequently than would be expected in the age groups studied.[8,9] Recurrent zoster eruption also occurs occasionally in AIDS patients — this is rare in the non-HIV-infected population.

■ PATHOGENESIS

Like other herpesviruses, VZV has a double-stranded DNA nucleoprotein core surrounded by a protein capsid and contained within a lipoprotein membrane envelope. Infection usually occurs through direct inoculation of the virus onto mucous membranes.

After inoculation, VZV replication probably occurs in tonsillar or lymphoid tissue. A primary viremia develops four to seven days after infection with virus seeding of internal organs. A secondary, more prolonged viremia occurs approximately 14 days after the initial infection. This results in the spread of the virus to the skin and the development of the characteristic vesicular rash of varicella. Successive crops of vesicles typically occur during the acute illness, attesting to the intermittent episodes of viremia. In the non-HIV-infected host, new lesions develop for one to four days; lesion formation ceases with the onset of circulating serum antibody. Continued viremia and prolonged new lesion formation can occur in immunocompromised patients.[1-3]

The mechanisms responsible for VZV latency and recurrent infection with recrudescence in a dermatomal pattern are incompletely understood. It is likely that during the initial varicella infection, the virus enters the cutaneous endings of sensory nerves and migrates along nerve fibers to reach the sensory ganglia. At this point, the virus interacts with the host ganglia and becomes latent in the host ganglionic tissue. Although the mechanisms responsible for recurrent infection are incompletely understood, reactivation with clinical illness may occur when the host resistance falls owing to either advancing age or immunosuppression. Virus reactivation produces inflammation of the sensory ganglion and the descending spread of virus along sensory nerves to the cutaneous dermatome, which corresponds to the ganglia initially infected. The characteristic vesicular eruption of herpes zoster usually remains confined to the primary dermatome(s), though secondary dissemination may infrequently occur in the AIDS patient with herpes zoster.[1-3]

■ CLINICAL PRESENTATION

The rash of primary VZV infection (varicella or "chickenpox") usually appears 14 days after infection (range: 10 to 23 days). Common prodromal symptoms occur in adults one to two days before the appearance of the rash and include malaise, low-grade fever, and myalgia. Cutaneous lesions begin as small erythematous macules and progress over 12 to 36 hours to become papules and vesicles. Vesicles are variable in size and shape and are filled with straw-colored fluid. They rest on an erythematous base and resemble "a dewdrop on a rose petal." They umbilicate rapidly, dry completely, and eventually crust, forming scabs. New vesicles continue to develop for the first several days of the illness so that lesions in all stages of development are characteristic of varicella infection; they tend to be most numerous on the trunk, neck, face, and proximal extremities (historically, this helped to differentiate "chickenpox" from smallpox). Zoster is more common in AIDS patients than in non-HIV-infected hosts.

New lesion formation is prolonged and the risk of visceral dissemination is higher in AIDS patients with primary varicella infection than in normal hosts. This is also true for other immunocompromised patients with primary VZV infection[1-3] (see Complications and Sequelae, below).

Recurrent VZV infection (zoster or "shingles") usually appears as a localized or segmented erythematous, maculopapular eruption along a single dermatome. The lesions evolve over one to two days to form true vesicles, pustules, and crusts. Vesicles often become confluent, and bullae may form. In the non-HIV-infected host, zoster often remains localized and resolves spontaneously, but in AIDS patients the virus may disseminate to cutaneous and visceral sites.[3-5] Many patients with localized zoster have few (less than 20) isolated vesicles outside the dermatomal pattern. This is not cutaneous dissemination. In contrast, extensive cutaneous dissemination may result in hundreds of vesicles outside the dermatome; this may be distinguishable from primary varicella infection.[3]

Pain is common during acute zoster infection, and it is often described as burning, stabbing, or as a deep aching. Such pain usually resolves as the skin lesions heal, but post-herpetic neuralgia, a prolonged pain syndrome, can be a severe and disabling complication. It occurs most frequently in elderly patients and is unusual in non-HIV-infected patients under 40 years of age. Post-herpetic neuralgia is not known to be more frequent in AIDS patients[6,8] than in non-AIDS patients with zoster, although it is often a more severe and debilitating problem for AIDS patients. The exact etiology of this complication is unknown.[1,2]

■ COMPLICATIONS AND SEQUELAE

Complications from varicella–zoster virus infection may produce a prolonged illness with significant morbidity. Dissemination during either primary infection (varicella) or recurrent infection (zoster) is associated with a mortality rate of 6 percent to 17 percent. Visceral involvement with resultant pneumonia, hepatitis, or encephalitis may cause the patient's death.[1-3]

Despite their impaired immune systems, the majority of AIDS patients with zoster do not develop life-threatening complications from zoster infection. Several reports describe AIDS patients who have had benign and uncomplicated courses following recurrent VZV infection.[8,9] We have also seen AIDS patients with extensive cutaneous and visceral dissemination during VZV recurrences.

Primary varicella pneumonia occurs in up to one-third of non-HIV-infected adults with clinical chickenpox. Symptoms are variable; most of these patients suffer only a mild respiratory illness. Severe pulmonary involvement (with hypoxemia, cyanosis, and death) occurs rarely. In such cases, radiographic abnormalities are usually out of proportion to clinical signs or symptoms. Diffuse nodular densities that coalesce are frequently present; pleural effusions are also occasionally seen.

Encephalitis rarely occurs in association with VZV infection, but when it does, it usually develops from three to eight days after the primary varicella rash or one to two weeks after herpes zoster. AIDS patients, however, have developed progressive VZV neurologic disease up to three months after an episode of localized zoster.[13] Cerebellar findings are typical; ataxia, tremors, and dizziness are prominent symptoms. Corticocerebral involvement (with headache, vomiting, and lethargy) also occurs. Cerebrospinal fluid usually reveals a mild mononuclear pleocytosis with an elevated protein level, but viral cultures are invariably negative.

Zoster of the ophthalmic division of the trigeminal nerve occurs in about one-third of patients with VZV. Vesicles on the tip of the nose may correlate with eye involvement. Anterior uveitis, corneal scarring, visual loss, and severe postherpetic eye neuralgia can result.[1-3,9]

■ DIAGNOSIS

Varicella–zoster virus (VZV) infection in AIDS is often suspected based on the patient's clinical presentation. The characteristic primary rash of varicella can be confused with other exanthems, but the centripetal distribution and the presence of lesions in all stages of development usually suggest VZV as the etiologic agent. Zoster eruptions, when they are confined to dermatomal patterns, are often easily diagnosed. Dissemination of recurrent zoster outside the dermatomal pattern can make diagnosis difficult, however, and it must occasionally be confirmed by laboratory means. Disseminated herpes simplex virus (HSV) infection can be confused with VZV infection, but it is easily differentiated by virus culture.[1,2]

Scrapings of cutaneous lesions from either varicella or zoster can be stained with specific fluorescein-conjugated monoclonal antibodies to confirm the presence of VZV. This technique is rapid, relatively inexpensive, and reliable for differentiating suspected lesions from those caused by HSV. Scrapings can also be stained with Giemsa stain to demonstrate multinucleated giant cells (Tzanck preparation), although this test is less sensitive than immunofluorescence and cannot differentiate between VZV and HSV.

Diagnosis using virus culture is less sensitive for VZV than for HSV. VZV remains cell-associated, and unlike HSV, is not released in high titers into tissue culture media. Cytopathic effects develop slowly, often over 10 days to 2 weeks, if at all. Obtaining virus cultures in suspected VZV infection is useful primarily to exclude HSV as the etiologic agent.

■ TREATMENT

Treatment of severe or disseminated VZV infections in AIDS patients often requires hospitalization and the administration of intravenous acyclovir. Not all AIDS patients with either primary varicella or recurrent zoster will be ill enough to require hospitalization, however, so the decision to institute systemic antiviral therapy should be based on the extent and severity of the infection, the immune status of the host, and whether visceral or cutaneous dissemination has occurred.[3-6]

Both vidarabine and acyclovir have been shown to be superior to placebo in treating severe or disseminated VZV infections in the immunocompromised host.[5,6] Early administration of these agents decreases the duration of viral shedding, the extent of new lesion formation, the incidence of dissemination, and patient mortality. A recent study comparing acyclovir and vidarabine in treating VZV infections in immunocompromised patients demonstrated that acyclovir is clearly superior.[6] Acyclovir treatment, when compared to vidarabine, shortened the duration of viral shedding (4 vs. 7 days), new lesion formation (3 vs. 6 days), time until pain was decreased (4 vs. 7 days), time to crusting of all lesions (7 vs. 17 days), and time to complete healing of all lesions (17 vs. 28 days). In patients with localized dermatomal infection, cutaneous dissemination of VZV occurred in 50 percent of those treated with vidarabine but in none of those treated with acyclovir. This study did not address the issue of post-herpetic neuralgia.

Serum levels of acyclovir necessary to inhibit the replication of VZV are about 10 times greater than those needed to inhibit HSV, so the dosage of acyclovir must be greater than that used for HSV. Acyclovir is primarily eliminated by glomerular filtration, and adequate hydration should be maintained to prevent crystallization of the drug in the renal tubules. Dosage must be adjusted for renal dysfunction (see Table 1).

TABLE 1. DOSAGE ADJUSTMENT OF INTRAVENOUS ACYCLOVIR IN PATIENTS WITH RENAL DYSFUNCTION

CREATININE CLEARANCE (ml/min/1.73 m^2)	PERCENT OF STANDARD DOSE*	DOSING INTERVAL (hours)
>50	100	8
25 to 50	100	12
10 to 25	100	24
0 to 10	50	24

*   *10 mg/kg recommended for varicella–zoster infections requiring hospitalization.*

Oral acyclovir in a standard dose (200 mg 5 times daily) results in steady state serum levels of 2.0 to 3.0 micromoles per liter. These levels are lower than those needed to inhibit VZV (the 50 percent inhibitory dose is 2.0 to 10.0 micromoles per liter) and should not be substituted for intravenous therapy. High doses of oral acyclovir (600 to 800 mg 5 times daily) may result in adequate serum levels to treat VZV infection (steady state levels of 5 to 10 micromoles per liter). This regimen has been effective in the treatment of acute VZV infection and has the advantage of outpatient treatment, but it is expensive and may cause intolerable gastrointestinal side effects.[10] Current studies have suggested that this regimen is effective in preventing dissemination of VZV infection and may decrease the incidence of post-herpetic neuralgia.[11,12]

SPECIFIC TREATMENT RECOMMENDATIONS

HIV-infected patients who are immunocompromised (e.g., with an AIDS diagnosis or T4-helper lymphocyte count below 200/cubic mm, or history of thrush, anergy, or hairy leukoplakia) should be treated with oral or intravenous acyclovir for VZV infections.

Hospitalization is indicated for HIV-infected patients with either primary varicella complicated by visceral involvement, ophthalmic zoster, or disseminated zoster (cutaneous or visceral). These patients should be treated with intravenous acyclovir (10 mg/kg every 8 hours, with dosage adjustment for impaired renal function).

HIV-infected patients with severe dermatomal zoster may also benefit from hospitalization and intravenous therapy. Alternatively, they may be treated with oral acyclovir (600 to 800 mg 5 times daily, with dose adjustments for impaired renal function).

HIV-infected patients with dermatomal zoster and no indication of immunocompromise may also be treated with oral acyclovir. However, some clinicians would initiate oral acyclovir therapy for these patients only if the clinical manifestations are unusual (e.g., lesions are slow to heal, pain is severe, extensive areas of skin are involved).

Pain control is an important aspect of managing zoster; narcotic analgesics are often required.

Some reports suggest that steroid therapy may be effective in preventing post-herpetic neuralgia in elderly patients if administered early in the course of the illness, although studies have reported conflicting results.[1-3] Steroid therapy should be avoided in AIDS patients with zoster, however, owing to the potential immunosuppressive effect.

Since secondary infection with bacterial or fungal pathogens can occur, local care of cutaneous lesions is important in the AIDS patient with either varicella or zoster. Lesions should be kept clean and dry whenever possible. Necrotic areas can be gently debrided with "wet-to-dry" dressing changes (use Domeboro's solution). Empiric antibacterial or antifungal therapy is not indicated, but areas suspected of being secondarily infected should be gram-stained and cultured for bacteria and fungi. Therapy can be instituted, if necessary, based on the identification of other organisms.

REFERENCES

1. Weller TH. Varicella and herpes zoster: changing concepts of the natural history, control, and importance of a not-so-benign virus (first of two parts). N Engl J Med 1983; 309:1362-8.

2. Weller TH. Varicella and herpes zoster: changing concepts of the natural history, control, and importance of a not-so-benign virus (second of two parts). N Engl J Med 1983; 309:1434-40.

3. Dolin R, Reichman RC, Mazur MH, Whitley RJ. Herpes zoster varicella infections in immunosuppressed patients. Ann Intern Med 1978; 89:375-88.

4. Quinnan GV Jr, Masur H, Rook AH, et al. Herpesvirus infections in the acquired immune deficiency syndrome. JAMA 1984; 252:72-7.

5. Balfour HH, Bean B, Laskin OL, et al. Acyclovir halts progression of herpes zoster in immunocompromised patients. N Engl J Med 1983; 308:1448-53.

6. Shepp DH, Dandliker PS, Meyers JD. Treatment of varicella–zoster virus infection in severely immunocompromised patients: a randomized comparison of acyclovir and vidarabine. N Engl J Med 1986; 314:208-12.

7. Centers for Disease Control. Varicella–zoster immune globulin for the prevention of chickenpox: recommendations of the Immunization Practices Advisory Committee. Ann Intern Med 1984; 100:859-65.

8. Cone LA, Schiffman MA. Herpes zoster and the acquired immunodeficiency syndrome. Ann Intern Med 1984; 100:462.

9. Sandor E, Croxson TS, Millman A, Mildvan D. Herpes zoster ophthalmicus in patients at risk for AIDS. N Engl J Med 1984; 310:1118-9.

10. McKendrick MW, McGill JI, White JE, Wood MJ. Oral acyclovir in acute herpes zoster. Br Med J 1986; 293:1529-32.

11. Wood MJ, Ogan PH, McKendrick MW, et al. Efficacy of oral acyclovir treatment of acute herpes zoster. Am J Med 1988; 85:79-83.

12. Huff JC, Bean B, Balfour HH Jr, et al. Therapy of herpes zoster with oral acyclovir. Am J Med 1988; 85:84-9.

13. Ryder JW, Croen K, Kleinschmidt-DeMasters BK, et al. Progressive encephalitis three months after resolution of cutaneous zoster in a patient with AIDS. Ann Neurol 1986; 19:182-8.

Herpes Simplex Virus

Kim S. Erlich, M.D., and John Mills, M.D.

Herpes simplex virus (HSV) infections have afflicted mankind throughout most of recorded history. The earliest reference to HSV orolabial eruptions date from the time of Hippocrates in the fifth century BC, although genital HSV infections were not described until the 1700s.[1,19] Both orolabial and genital HSV infections continue to plague populations throughout the world. AIDS patients are infected at an equal or greater frequency than members of the general population.[2] Often only an uncomfortable and mildly debilitating infection in the immunocompetent host, HSV infection in AIDS patients may produce extensive, locally destructive, and sometimes life-threatening disseminated lesions.[3]

Management of HSV infections in AIDS patients is a difficult challenge. Rates of recurrence and severity of eruptions can change as the immune status of the AIDS patient changes. The occasional atypical clinical presentation can result in an inaccurate diagnosis, leading to a delay in initiating appropriate therapy.

The recent development of effective antiviral agents provides safe and effective therapy for many HSV infections. Two intravenous agents, vidarabine and acyclovir, are demonstrably superior to placebo in the treatment of severe HSV infections in both immunocompetent and immunocompromised individuals. The availability of acyclovir capsules makes successful management of HSV infections possible in the outpatient setting.

■ EPIDEMIOLOGY

The herpes simplex virus requires a moist environment for survival. As there is no known animal vector, human-to-human spread is the only important mode of transmission. The prevalence of HSV infection in the general population is high, but depends on the social and demographic characteristics of the population studied. Precise data on the prevalence rates of HSV infections in AIDS patients have not been determined, but evidence suggests that the rate parallels or exceeds that of the general population. Of 50 homosexual AIDS patients closely evaluated in 1983, all patients had serum antibodies to HSV, as did 95 percent of their nonsexual household contacts.[4]

HSV type 1 (HSV-1) and HSV type 2 (HSV-2) classically have been associated with infection of the orolabial and genital areas, respectively; these anatomic associations are not absolute, however, and infection with either virus type may occur at any site.

HSV-1

Serologic studies indicate that HSV-1 exposure commonly occurs during childhood (between the ages of 6 months and 5 years).[5] The risk of HSV-1 infection increases with low socioeconomic status and crowded living conditions. Prevalence rates can approach 80 percent to 100 percent in some populations and are probably due to close person-to-person contact.

Prevalence rates for orolabial HSV-1 in the general population vary widely. Many seropositive individuals have no recollection of a clinical outbreak, whereas other apparently immunocompetent people suffer from frequently recurring symptomatic eruptions. Recurrences can be triggered by several well-described external events, such as sunlight, febrile illnesses, menstruation, and stress. Although factors in the variability of individual recurrence rates are poorly understood, subtle alterations in the host's immune status or the presence of unrecognized external triggering events may explain this difference.

Once infected with HSV, immunocompromised HIV-seropositive individuals have an increased likelihood of having recurrences, as has been demonstrated in bone-marrow transplant recipients[6] and in individuals with other forms of deficient cell-mediated immunity.[7] Many AIDS patients have serologic evidence of previous exposure to HSV-1, and the immunosuppression induced by HIV infection may lead to an increased incidence of HSV clinical recurrences. In a study of 34 patients with AIDS, 8 showed clinical or virologic evidence of active HSV recurrences at the time of screening.[8] Many AIDS patients report frequent and severe orolabial HSV recurrences. These may become more severe as immunosuppression increases.[3]

HSV-2

Infection with HSV-2 follows a different pattern from that of HSV-1. Except for infants born to mothers with genital HSV infections, individuals run the highest risk of infection with HSV-2 at the onset of sexual activity.[4] Transmission is usually through sexual contact, and as with other sexually transmitted diseases, the risk of infection increases with the number of sexual partners. Prevalence rates vary from 10 percent to 70 percent, depending upon sexual activity and socioeconomic level.[5] Sexually active homosexual males are at an especially high risk of becoming infected with HSV-2. Ninety-one percent of 254 healthy homosexual males studied had serologic evidence of HSV-2 infection.[5] Other groups at risk for HIV infection may have prevalence rates similar to those of the general population. As with HSV-1, recurrence rates for HSV-2 are variable but may increase with immunosuppression. Unlike persons with orolabial HSV-1 infection, however, most individuals with HSV-2 genital infection are symptomatic during their primary episode and develop symptomatic recurrences thereafter.[9]

Anorectal HSV-2 infection is a frequent cause of proctitis in homosexual men. In one study of 102 homosexual men with proctitis, 23 patients (23 percent) were infected with HSV-2.[10] Subclinical recurrences of HSV-2 proctitis may also occur infrequently — e.g., 3 of 75 homosexual men without symptoms (4 percent) in the same study had active HSV-2 rectal infection.[11]

■ PATHOGENESIS

The structure and mode of replication of HSV are similar to those of other herpesviruses. A double-stranded DNA nucleoprotein core is surrounded by an icosahedral protein capsid and enclosed in a lipid and glycoprotein outer membrane. Transmission occurs by direct inoculation of infected droplets onto a susceptible mucosal surface or by entry of the virus through a break in the normally protective skin surface.[7]

After resolution of the acute infection, the virus becomes latent in neural tissues, usually in the trigeminal or sacral ganglia.[12] Early in the course of infection (possibly during the incubation period and prior to the onset of symptoms), viral particles travel from the site of inoculation along sensory nerves to the corresponding dorsal nerve-root ganglia or to the trigeminal ganglia. At this point, viral DNA can be demonstrated in the ganglion cells by in situ hybridization techniques, although viral antigens and complete virions are not produced.[7]

Once viral latency has been established, the virus may "reactivate" at any time by mechanisms that are incompletely understood. During reactivation, viral replication occurs in the sensory ganglia. Viral particles then travel peripherally along sensory nerves to mucosal or epithelial surfaces and cause active, acute HSV infection.[7]

Infection with one HSV type induces the development of cell-mediated immunity and the production of type-common and type-specific antibodies. Although these immune mechanisms do not affect the underlying state of viral latency, they probably play important roles in regulating the number of clinical recurrences and minimizing viral replication at the epithelial surface.

Antibodies elicited by previous HSV-1 infection cannot completely protect the host against subsequent infection with HSV-2. It appears, however, that this immune response results in a milder clinical course than that occurring in an HSV-1-seronegative individual experiencing a primary HSV-2 infection.[9]

The relative frequency of HSV proctitis in homosexual males corresponds to the high incidence of anal intercourse in this population.[10] Most cases of symptomatic proctitis due to HSV occur in previously seronegative individuals, indicating a primary infection.[11] The incidence and pathogenesis of recurrences of HSV proctitis are undetermined.

■ CLINICAL PRESENTATION

Both initial and recurrent episodes of herpes simplex virus (HSV) infections in AIDS patients are different from infections in the normal host. The severity of each episode depends on several factors, including the degree of immunosuppression, the site of initial viral infection, and whether pre-existing cross-reacting anti-HSV antibodies are present at the time of initial infection.[13] Both HSV-1 and HSV-2 are capable of causing infection at any mucocutaneous site, although HSV-1 is more often associated with orolabial infection and HSV-2 with genital and anorectal infection.[9]

OROLABIAL INFECTION

After an incubation period of 2 to 12 days, orolabial infection with HSV can result in a gingivostomatitis. Symptoms may be mild enough to go unnoticed or may take the form of a painful vesicular eruption occurring on the lips, tongue, or buccal mucosa.[14] As many as 20 distinct vesicles appear, rapidly coalesce, and rupture to form shallow ulcers covered with a whitish-yellow necrotic material. If the pharynx and tonsils are involved,[15] fever and cervical lymphadenopathy may be present.

In the normal host, primary herpetic lesions heal by reepithelialization over a 7- to 10-day period.[13] In AIDS patients and other immunocompromised individuals, the clinical course can be more protracted. Lesions may persist for several weeks with minimal evidence of tissue repair. Continued viral replication, local progression of cutaneous lesions, extensive tissue destruction, and occasional viral dissemination to distant sites may also occur.[3,16]

Recurrences of orolabial HSV-1 infection occur spontaneously or in association with poorly understood external triggering events — e.g., sunlight, febrile illnesses, stress, or menstruation. Immunosuppression may also increase an infected patient's risk of developing a clinical recurrence. Recurrent eruptions are often preceded by a 1- to 2-day prodrome consisting of paresthesias at the area of impending eruption. The eruptions tend to occur in the same general area as the initial primary infection. In the normal host, orolabial recurrences are usually milder than the primary infection.[14]

AIDS patients may develop clinical recurrences of orolabial disease spontaneously or in association with other external stimuli, such as an unrelated opportunistic infection or the administration of systemic chemotherapy. Recurrent HSV-1 infection in AIDS patients may be mild and indolent (showing minimal inflammation), or severe and persistent (exhibiting large ulcerative lesions and extensive tissue destruction).[3] Dissemination of orolabial HSV-1 infection to distant sites during recurrent episodes has not been clearly documented in AIDS patients.

GENITAL INFECTION

Many individuals infected with HSV-2 through sexual contact have circulating polyclonal cross-reactive anti-HSV antibodies from a previous HSV-1 orolabial infection. These "nonprimary" infections are somewhat less severe than the "primary" infections that occur in patients with no previous exposure to either HSV type.[13] Both HSV types can cause genital infection, although 65 percent to 95 percent of genital isolates from patients with primary infections are HSV-2[9] and most rectal infections are also caused by HSV-2.[10]

After an incubation period of 2 to 12 days, primary genital infection in normal hosts causes local symptoms in 95 percent of men and 99 percent of women (Table 1).

TABLE 1. SIGNS AND SYMPTOMS PRESENT DURING PRIMARY GENITAL HSV INFECTION IN THE NORMAL HOST*

Clinical Findings	FREQUENCY (%)	
	Men (63 patients)	Women (126 patients)
Local pain	95	99
Tender inguinal lymphadenopathy	80	81
Dysuria	44	83
Urethral or vaginal discharge	27	85
Systemic symptoms (fever, headache, myalgias, malaise)	39	68
Findings of meningitis	11	36

* *Modified with permission from* Ann Intern Med *1983; 98:958-72.*

Typical HSV lesions begin as small papules and rapidly develop into painful vesicles. The vesicles typically rest on an erythematous base and are often tender to palpation. They ulcerate rapidly and heal by crusting and re-epithelialization. In the normal host, a primary infection heals in an average of 16.5 days in men and 19.7 days in women,[13] although infections take longer to heal completely; signs and symptoms can occasionally last as long as four to six weeks. Systemic symptoms, consisting of fever, headache, myalgias, and malaise, occur in about one-third of men and more than two-thirds of women with primary genital herpes. These symptoms usually resolve by the end of the first week of illness.[13]

Primary HSV infection in homosexual men usually occurs before the development of AIDS, so most genital HSV eruptions in AIDS patients are recurrences.[2,17] When a primary HSV infection occurs in an AIDS patient, it parallels the presentation seen in other immunocompromised individuals: more severe local infection, prolonged healing time, increased risk of viral dissemination, and more severe systemic symptoms.[16] Most important, the occurrence of a primary genital infection implies ongoing direct sexual contact and therefore a lack of "safe sex" practices. Counseling in this situation is essential.

In contrast to "primary" HSV infection, recurrent genital eruptions in AIDS patients frequently occur and can be a major source of morbidity.[3] In all patients, genital HSV is more likely to recur if the initial infection was caused by HSV-2 instead of HSV-1.[9] Many patients report prodromal symptoms, such as paresthesias, itching, or tingling, at the area of impending eruption. These symptoms may begin as long as 48 hours before the development of visible lesions. Occasionally patients will have "false prodromes" (symptoms not followed by clinical outbreak).[13]

During a clinical recurrence in the normal host, the number of vesicles, degree of discomfort, and duration of viral shedding are less than during initial infection. In some AIDS patients, however, recurrences of genital HSV can become more frequent and more severe as HIV-induced immunosuppression progresses. Progressive genital ulcerations accompanied by severe local pain and prolonged viral shedding are frequently seen among AIDS patients.[3] Secondary infection of macerated genital ulcers by bacterial or fungal pathogens can also occur. Alternatively, recurrent HSV infections in AIDS patients may be clinically mild and indolent. Small, shallow ulcerations may be the only evidence of a clinical recurrence, although viral shedding may continue for days to weeks.

ANORECTAL INFECTION

Severe, chronic ulcerative HSV lesions of the perianal area were reported as one of the first opportunistic infections in patients with AIDS.[18] Since that time, HSV has been recognized as the most frequent cause of nongonococcal proctitis in sexually active homosexual men.[10] Most clinically apparent episodes of true HSV proctitis are probably due to primary infection with HSV-2, although HSV-1 infection and subacute HSV-2 recurrences can occur.[10,11]

Anorectal pain, perianal ulcerations, constipation, and tenesmus are prominent symptoms of HSV proctitis. Other frequent symptoms include fever, inguinal adenopathy, rectal discharge, hematochezia, sacral paresthesias, and difficulty in initiating urination. Neurologic symptoms in the distribution of the sacral plexus help to differentiate HSV proctitis from proctitis caused by other etiologic agents (see Table 2).

**TABLE 2.   SIGNS AND SYMPTOMS IN PATIENTS WITH HSV
PROCTITIS AND PROCTITIS DUE TO OTHER CAUSES***

	FREQUENCY (%)	
Clinical Finding	HSV Proctitis (23 patients)	Non-HSV Proctitis (79 patients)
Anorectal pain‡	100	77
Tenesmus‡	100	77
Anal discharge	91	82
Constipation‡	78	41
Perianal lesions‡	70	8
Inguinal lymphadenopathy	57	11
Fever‡	48	16
Neurologic symptoms‡	52	13
Hematochezia	61	41
Abdominal pain	9	22

*   *Modified with permission from* N Engl J Med *1983; 308:868-71.*
‡   *Significant difference (P) by Fisher exact test.*

Anorectal and sigmoidoscopic examinations usually reveal a friable mucosa with vesicular or pustular lesions and diffuse mucosal ulceration.[11]

Recurrent HSV eruptions in the perianal area are common in previously infected AIDS patients. Local pain, itching, and painful defecation are prominent symptoms. Shallow ulcerative lesions are typically present on examination. In AIDS patients, an indolent fissure-like ulceration of the gluteal crease is particularly common and may not be accompanied by perianal lesions. Viral shedding can be prolonged during these recurrences and healing may not occur without aggressive antiviral treatment.[3]

■ DIAGNOSIS

The Centers for Disease Control has recently revised the diagnostic criteria for AIDS to include chronic mucocutaneous herpes simplex virus infection. Large ulcerative HSV lesions (without visceral or cutaneous dissemination) are a frequent occurrence in HIV-infected patients. Ulcerative HSV infection present for longer than one month in an individual with no other cause for underlying immunodeficiency or with laboratory evidence of HIV infection is now diagnostic of AIDS.[21]

The appearance of characteristic lesions often raises suspicion of genital HSV infection. Multiple, tender, bilaterally distributed, ulcerative lesions are typical of primary infection; in recurrent infection, only a few small lesions in a single area may be present.[13,20] Other causes of genital ulceration (both infectious and non-infectious) must be considered in the differential diagnosis of AIDS patients with suspicious lesions (see Table 3). The definitive diagnosis of genital HSV infection often requires laboratory confirmation.

TABLE 3. DIFFERENTIAL DIAGNOSIS OF GENITAL ULCERATION*

Herpes simplex virus
Primary, secondary syphilis
Chancroid
Lymphogranuloma venereum
Granuloma inguinale
Scabies
Traumatic ulceration
Venereal warts
Molluscum contagiosum
Behçet's syndrome
Contact dermatitis
Fixed drug eruption
Recurrent VZV (shingles)

* *This differential diagnosis is valid for non-HIV infections and HIV infections.*

Proctitis due to HSV often appears similar to proctitis from other causes, but the presence of anorectal pain, perianal ulcerations, difficult urination, and sacral neurologic findings help to identify HSV as the etiologic agent.[11] Diagnosis should be suspected in a sexually active homosexual male on clinical grounds but should always be confirmed by culture if possible. Findings on sigmoidoscopy include diffuse, shallow, ulcerative lesions with occasional intact vesicles and a friable mucosa.[11] Nonhealing, fissure-like ulcerations in the gluteal crease or perirectal area are common and may be debilitating. In very slender or cachetic patients, these HSV lesions may be misdiagnosed as sacral decubiti. Any genital or perirectal lesion in an AIDS patient should be cultured for HSV to assure rapid diagnosis and early institution of therapy.

Encephalitis due to HSV is usually caused by reactivation of previously latent HSV-1 infection, although HSV-2 encephalitis in AIDS patients has been reported.[23,24] Diagnosis of HSV encephalitis on clinical grounds is impossible, since many AIDS patients have an atypical presentation.[24,25] Lumbar puncture findings are nonspecific; cerebrospinal fluid (CSF) examination reveals elevated protein, a lymphocytic pleocytosis, and occasional erythrocytes. Viral cultures of CSF are usually negative. Computed tomographic (CT) scanning or electroencephalographic studies are abnormal in the majority of cases and can be helpful in locating areas of involvement for diagnostic biopsy.[23] Recent studies have demonstrated the diagnostic value of detecting HSV antibody in the CSF, but these techniques have not been evaluated in AIDS patients.[32] Definitive diagnosis of HSV encephalitis in patients with AIDS can be made only by identifying the virus in cerebral tissue obtained through brain biopsy. The typical histopathology seen in normal hosts with HSV encephalitis — hemorrhagic cortical necrosis and lymphocytic infiltration — is often not present in the AIDS patient.[24,25]

Diagnostic brain biopsy should be considered early for AIDS patients with suspected HSV encephalitis. Effective treatment is available, and early institution of therapy is associated with a more favorable outcome than delayed treatment. An empiric trial of antiviral chemotherapy is occasionally warranted in individuals with clinical presentation consistent with HSV encephalitis who refuse brain biopsy.

DIAGNOSTIC LABORATORY PROCEDURES

Many methods for laboratory diagnosis of HSV infection are currently available, but direct culture of suspected lesions remains the optimal method. Viral culture has been shown to be more sensitive and specific than other methods. (These include demonstration of multinucleated giant cells or inclusion bodies by the Tzanck smear, direct staining by immunofluorescence or immunoperoxidase, or detection of viral particles by electron microscopy.[26-28]) Material for a viral culture is obtained by gently scraping the erythematous base of an ulcerative lesion with a dacron- or cotton-tipped applicator or by unroofing an intact vesicle and then swabbing the base or carefully aspirating the fluid with a small-bore needle. Rectal mucosal specimens should be obtained directly during proctoscopy. Care should be taken to avoid introducing stool, blood, alcohol, soap, or detergent into the material to be cultured, since these substances can inactivate the virus and result in a negative culture. Moreover, because drying destroys the virus, specimens should be kept moist during transport. The virus may not be detectable by culture of lesions that are dried and partially healed. Commercially available viral-transport media can maintain the virus without serious loss of infectivity for up to 72 hours if refrigerated at 4°C.[29]

Material to be cultured is usually inoculated into one or more continuous tissue-culture cell lines. Typical changes in the cell morphology and cytopathic effects are usually observed within 24 to 48 hours, progressing rapidly as virus is released into the media through cell lysis. Both HSV-1 and HSV-2 produce similar cytopathology in infected cell cultures and cannot be differentiated reliably by culture alone.

If differentiation between HSV and varicella–zoster virus (VZV) cannot be made clinically because of an atypical presentation, virus culture and antigen detection (by immunofluorescence) can accurately diagnose the causative pathogen.

HSV TYPING

Because relapse rates for HSV-1 and HSV-2 vary for different anatomic sites, differentiation between the two may have prognostic implications.[9] Typing is usually performed with commercially available fluorescein-conjugated monoclonal antibodies. More sophisticated techniques, such as restriction-endonuclease fingerprinting of the virus DNA, can identify differences in strains within the same HSV type or confirm that isolates from two individuals are identical strains. In the clinical setting, identifying such strains suggests case-to-case transmission.[30] For practical purposes, however, strain typing has little utility in the clinical management of AIDS patients with herpes infections.

SEROLOGIC STUDIES

HSV serology is rarely useful in the clinical setting because prevalence rates for HSV antibodies in AIDS patients are high.[2] Moreover, most currently available techniques cannot reliably differentiate between antibodies to HSV-1 and HSV-2.[31] Routine antibody studies can be useful, however, following a suspected initial infection when both acute and convalescent sera are available.[23] A fourfold or greater increase in measured antibody titer over a period of several weeks is indicative of a first-episode infection. The presence of detectable antibody in the acute sample followed by a fourfold or greater increase in titer implies that the infection is "nonprimary" — i.e., that the patient has been previously infected with the other HSV type. Recurrent HSV eruptions are only rarely associated with a rise in antibody titer.

■ COMPLICATIONS AND SEQUELAE

Herpes simplex virus encephalitis occurs infrequently but remains the most severe and life-threatening complication of the infection. Encephalitis may occur either as a complication of primary HSV infection or from reactivation of previously latent orolabial disease. Both HSV-1 and HSV-2 have been implicated as etiologic agents of encephalitis in AIDS patients. Occasional patients have had central nervous system infection with both HSV and cytomegalovirus and have had minimal inflammatory response noted at autopsy.[24,33] The virus preferentially infects the orbitofrontal and temporal lobes, possibly as the result of ascending spread along nerve fibers from the trigeminal ganglia to the anterior and middle fossae.[34]

The most common clinical presentation in otherwise normal (nonimmunocompromised) hosts is acute encephalitis. Nonspecific findings (fever, headache, nausea, confusion, and meningismus) and temporal lobe findings (focal seizures, aphasia, or olfactory hallucinations) are characteristic. Localizing neurologic signs, such as transient hemiparesis and cranial-nerve defects, are also frequently present. If left untreated, the illness progresses rapidly, resulting in obtundation, generalized seizures, coma, and death. Examination of cerebrospinal fluid reveals increased intracranial pressure, elevated protein, lymphocytic pleocytosis, and the occasional presence of erythrocytes. Viral cultures of CSF are usually negative.[35]

The presentation of HSV encephalitis in AIDS patients can be highly atypical. Many AIDS patients develop only subtle neurologic abnormalities indicative of a subacute form of encephalitis.[36] Diagnosis of HSV encephalitis based on clinical findings can be extremely difficult because of its similarities to HIV encephalopathy and other opportunistic infectious agents. Noninvasive diagnostic methods may suggest the diagnosis of HSV encephalitis, but definitive diagnosis often requires brain biopsy.[23]

The electroencephalogram is frequently abnormal early in the course of the illness, showing spikes and slow-wave abnormalities localized to the area of cerebral involvement. CT scans are frequently normal early in the illness but may later reveal localized edema, low-density focal lesions, mass effect, contrast enhancement, and hemorrhage.[37] Recent studies have suggested the diagnostic value of measuring anti-HSV antibody in the CSF, but this technique has not been evaluated in AIDS patients.[32]

Aseptic meningitis is a frequent complication of primary genital and rectal HSV infection in immunocompetent hosts, occurring in about one-third of men and over two-thirds of women.[13] Headache, photophobia, and meningismus are frequent complaints, but most nonimmunocompromised patients are not ill enough to require hospitalization. Examination of the CSF shows a slightly elevated opening pressure, elevated protein level, normal or slightly low glucose level, and lymphocytic pleocytosis. Viral cultures are usually negative.[38]

Herpes simplex virus can occasionally be isolated from the CSF of AIDS patients with meningitis.[36,39] Both HSV types have been recovered and may be associated with either primary or recurrent genital or anorectal eruptions.

Autonomic nervous system dysfunction can occur in association with genital or anorectal HSV infection. Neurogenic bladder, constipation, impotence, and sacral anesthesia are the probable results of sacral-nerve root involvement.[13,11] Ascending myelitis[40] and Mollaret's meningitis[41] have also been reported.

Extragenital lesions are often found during the initial HSV infection and may arise by neural spread (zosteriform herpes), blood-borne dissemination, or autoinoculation. Extensive dissemination can cause a presentation similar to chickenpox or shingles. Laboratory differentiation may be necessary for definitive diagnosis.

■ TREATMENT

Prompt therapy for herpes simplex virus (HSV) infections helps to minimize the morbidity and mortality associated with the illness in patients with AIDS and HIV infection. Treatment should be tailored to each patient and should be based on the location and severity of the infection, immune status of the host, episode (first or recurrent), and the patient's degree of illness — most specifically whether he or she requires hospitalization.

ANTIVIRAL CHEMOTHERAPY: ACYCLOVIR

Specific antiviral chemotherapy is effective in managing HSV infections in the immunocompromised host.[1-9] Acyclovir (9-[(2-hydroxyethoxy) methyl] guanine), an acyclic nucleoside analogue of guanosine, is the drug of choice for treating HIV-related HSV infections. Its activity against HSV-infected cells results from selective monophosphorylation by the viral but not the host enzyme, thymidine kinase. Acyclovir monophosphate is subsequently converted to the triphosphate form by host cellular kinases.

Acyclovir triphosphate, the active antiviral, is a selective inhibitor of viral DNA polymerase that causes early termination of viral DNA synthesis. The drug is slightly more active against HSV-1 than HSV-2. Acyclovir reaches all tissues, including the brain and cerebrospinal fluid, and is cleared from the bloodstream by the kidney. The serum half-life in patients with normal renal function is two to three hours. The intravenous dose should be adjusted in patients with compromised renal function (see Table 4).

Acyclovir is available in intravenous, oral, and topical forms. The route, amount, and duration of therapy determine the patient's serum acyclovir level and his or her clinical response.

TABLE 4. DOSAGE ADJUSTMENT OF INTRAVENOUS ACYCLOVIR IN PATIENTS WITH RENAL DYSFUNCTION

CREATININE CLEARANCE (ml/min/1.73 m^2)	PERCENT OF STANDARD DOSE*	DOSING INTERVAL (hours)
>50	100	8
25 to 50	100	12
10 to 25	100	24
0 to 10	50	24

* Usually 5 mg/kg; 10 mg/kg employed for HSV central nervous system infections and in some instances for varicella–zoster infection.

Intravenous Acyclovir

Many studies show that intravenous acyclovir shortens the clinical illness in both normal and immunosuppressed patients with primary or recurrent HSV infection.[16,42,49] Treatment with IV acyclovir (15 mg/kg/day for 5 days) results in a marked reduction in the duration of viral shedding, reduced symptoms, fewer numbers of new lesions, and promotes more rapid healing of external lesions in normal patients with first-episode infection.[50] Immunosuppressed patients with chronic mucocutaneous HSV infections also respond well to intravenous acyclovir.[16,42,43] In a study evaluating 34 bone-marrow transplant patients with severe HSV infections, IV acyclovir treatment (750 mg per square meter of body surface area per day for 7 days) was associated with fewer symptoms, decreased viral shedding, and faster healing of lesions than placebo.[1] After completion of therapy, however, patients receiving acyclovir had a shorter interval before their next HSV outbreak; these outbreaks were more severe than those in the placebo group.

Acyclovir is also effective in treating HSV encephalitis and is superior to vidarabine. In a recent multicenter study, patients receiving acyclovir (30 mg/kg/day for 10 days) had a lower mortality rate (28 percent vs. 54 percent) and lower incidence of severe sequelae (63 percent vs. 86 percent) than patients treated with vidarabine (15 mg/kg/day for 10 days).[51] An additional study produced similar results.[52]

Intravenous acyclovir is also useful in preventing recurrences of HSV in immunosuppressed patients with latent HSV infection.[45,46] For example, bone-marrow transplant recipients with serologic evidence of HSV infection who received acyclovir (750 mg per square meter per day for 21 days) at the time of marrow transplantation had a lower incidence of recurrent infection during therapy than patients receiving placebo.[45] As in other studies, many of these acyclovir-treated patients developed HSV recurrences when the drug was stopped.

Oral Acyclovir

In immunocompetent patients with primary genital HSV infection, oral acyclovir (200 mg 5 times daily for 10 days) produced a shorter duration of viral shedding, less subjective discomfort, and fewer new lesions than in placebo-treated controls.[53] The drug also has a beneficial, if less dramatic, effect in patients with recurrent genital HSV infection.[54]

Immunosuppressed patients with acute recurrent HSV infections also respond to oral acyclovir. Although the clinical response does not appear to be as dramatic as with intravenous acyclovir, no controlled comparative studies have been done.[16,44]

Continuously administered oral acyclovir also prevents HSV recurrences in immunocompetent[55,56] and immunocompromised[47-49] patients with frequently recurring HSV infections. Recurrences during therapy are shorter and milder than those occurring while patients are on placebo. Although continuous acyclovir therapy for prevention of HSV recurrences is approved for only 6 months, patients have been maintained on chronic administration of the drug for up to 48 months with no observed toxic effects. Serum IgG antibody to HSV decreases slightly with prolonged acyclovir therapy.[62] Although the clinical importance of this finding is unknown, discontinuing long-term suppressive acyclovir therapy may result in a severe initial recurrence due to the patient's waning immune response.

Topical Acyclovir

Acyclovir ointment (5 percent solution in polyethylene glycol) has a modest beneficial effect when applied to immunocompetent patients with primary genital HSV[57] or to immunosuppressed patients with chronic mucocutaneous lesions.[58] The topical drug reduces subjective symptoms and viral shedding but has no effect on healing lesions or preventing formation of new ones. Topical acyclovir also has no effect on healing recurrent herpes in immunocompetent patients.

Acyclovir Resistance

Over the past few years, reports have appeared of acyclovir-resistant HSV strains that cause severe and progressive mucocutaneous disease in AIDS patients.[59,60,63] Most of the strains have developed in AIDS patients who had been treated successfully with acyclovir in the past, suggesting that clinically significant resistance may develop as a result of drug usage. In most cases, resistance is due to the emergence and overgrowth of mutant strains lacking the enzyme thymidine kinase [TK(–)]. These TK(–) strains do not phosphorylate acyclovir to an active antiviral agent and render the drug ineffective. Although most (but not all) of these strains are less virulent than wild-type HSV in animal models of infection, they appear to be quite virulent in patients with AIDS and can produce severe mucocutaneous disease in immunocompromised hosts.[59,60,63,64]

Of 12 acyclovir-resistant HSV strains (isolated from patients with AIDS) that have been fully characterized in our laboratory, all 12 were also resistant in vitro to ganciclovir — a nucleoside analogue that also requires thymidine kinase—induced phosphorylation for antiviral activity.[63] In contrast, all of the acyclovir-resistant strains studied from AIDS patients have retained in vitro susceptibility to two other antiviral drugs — vidarabine and foscarnet. Both of these agents are direct inhibitors of viral DNA polymerase and do not require viral thymidine kinase for activity.

Treatment of Acyclovir-Resistant HSV.   Clinical experience with vidarabine and foscarnet for the treatment of acyclovir-resistant, mucocutaneous HSV infection in patients with AIDS is limited. We have observed a good clinical response to foscarnet (60 mg/kg IV for 14 to 21 days) in four patients.[22] A randomized trial comparing these two agents in AIDS patients with acyclovir-resistant HSV infections is planned.

■ MANAGEMENT OF HSV INFECTIONS IN PATIENTS WITH AIDS

MUCOCUTANEOUS INFECTIONS

AIDS patients with recurrent mucocutaneous HSV infections due to acyclovir-susceptible virus can usually be managed as outpatients. Although localized mucocutaneous herpes infections may not contribute to mortality, they are painful and should be treated. As soon as infection is diagnosed, oral acyclovir (200 mg 5 times daily) should be administered and continued until all external lesions have crusted. Topical acyclovir should not be used unless the patient is unable to tolerate either oral or intravenous systemic treatment.

Severe or life-threatening mucocutaneous HSV infections should be initially treated with intravenous acyclovir in the hospital. Fifteen mg/kg/day in divided doses (5 mg/kg every 8 hours) with adjustments for renal dysfunction (see

Table 4) should be used and continued until complete crusting of all lesions has occurred. Patients who require prolonged therapy can be switched to oral acyclovir (200 mg 5 times daily or 400 mg 2 to 3 times daily) when they are discharged from the hospital. Treatment should be continued until all lesions are healed.

Frequently recurring or chronic, indolent HSV infections should be treated with oral acyclovir as suppressive therapy. Patients should be started on acyclovir (200 mg 3 times a day or 400 mg twice daily). The dose can be adjusted as needed, based on the patient's clinical response. Patients who continue to develop HSV eruptions while on suppressive therapy may benefit from a higher dose, since their gastrointestinal absorption of the drug may be limited. A reduction of the suppressive dose can be tried in patients who demonstrate a good clinical response to the oral regimen.

Topical acyclovir should be reserved for patients who cannot be managed parenterally. For those patients who are not ill enough to require hospitalization for intravenous therapy and who are unable to tolerate or absorb the oral drug because of nausea, vomiting, or diarrhea, topical acyclovir (four to five times daily) can be used although it produces fewer beneficial effects than oral or IV medication.

LOCAL CARE OF EXTERNAL LESIONS

Local care of the AIDS patient's cutaneous and mucosal lesions is important for comfort and prevention of secondary infection. External HSV-infected areas should be kept clean and dry when possible. Use gentle cleansing with mild soap and water for perianal lesions and other areas subject to frequent contamination. Extensive lesions with large areas of tissue necrosis can be gently debrided by wet-to-dry dressing changes.

PALLIATIVE MEASURES

Pain and discomfort due to mucocutaneous HSV lesions can be severe, so analgesics should be administered as needed. Acetaminophen with codeine is effective for pain control in most patients, but some individuals require parenteral narcotics. Because codeine can cause constipation, care must be taken to keep bowel movements soft, particularly in patients with rectal HSV.

HSV ENCEPHALITIS

Treatment of HSV encephalitis in AIDS patients should be started as soon as diagnosis is made. Ideally, patients with suspected HSV encephalitis should undergo diagnostic brain biopsy to confirm the diagnosis, since many other CNS infections can mimic the symptoms of HSV encephalitis (e.g., toxoplasmosis, HIV). In many instances, however, a brain biopsy cannot be obtained. In these cases, the clinician may need to treat the patient empirically for HSV encephalitis with high-dose IV acyclovir. Current studies evaluating the use of CSF antibody for diagnosis of HSV encephalitis have not addressed the issue in patients with AIDS.

Acyclovir (30 mg/kg/day) in divided doses (10 mg/kg every 8 hours) with adjustments for renal dysfunction (see Table 4) is the therapy of choice.[51,52] An alternate regimen of vidarabine (15 mg/kg/day) is less effective[51,52] but is better than no treatment.[35] Therapy should last at least 10 days but can be prolonged if necessary.

TREATMENT FAILURE

The development of HSV acyclovir resistance should be suspected in patients who do not respond to systemic acyclovir therapy and in those patients who had been previously well-controlled on acyclovir but who develop progressive disease while still on suppressive therapy. First, it is essential to be sure that the patient is actually complying with the recommended dose. Second, serum acyclovir levels can be measured to document adequate virus inhibitory levels. Third, virus isolates should be promptly assessed for in vitro susceptibility to acyclovir and alternate antiviral agents. Patients with HSV isolates that are demonstrably resistant to acyclovir should discontinue acyclovir therapy. If systemic therapy of HSV infection due to acyclovir-resistant virus is necessary, vidarabine (15 mg/kg/day) or foscarnet (60 mg/kg IV every eight hours, if available) can be substituted.[62,64] Serial virus isolates should be obtained and assessed for acyclovir susceptibility, since resistant strains may revert to susceptibility after the drug is withdrawn.[35,61]

REFERENCES

1. Hutfield DC. History of herpes genitalis. Br J Vener Dis 1966; 42:263-8.

2. Rogers MF, Morens DM, Stewart JA, et al. National case control study of Kaposi's sarcoma and *Pneumocystis carinii* pneumonia in homosexual men. Part 2. Laboratory results. Ann Intern Med 1983; 99:151-8.

3. Armstrong D, Gold JWM, Dryjanski BJ, et al. Treatment of infections in patients with the acquired immunodeficiency syndrome. Ann Intern Med 1985; 103:738-43.

4. Nerurkar L, Goedert J, Wallen W, et al. Study of antiviral antibodies in sera of homosexual men. J Fed Proc 1983; 42:6109.

5. Nahmias AJ, Josey WE. Herpes simplex viruses 1 and 2. In: Evans A, ed. Viral infections of humans: epidemiology and control. 2nd ed. New York: Plenum Press, 1982:351-72.

6. Meyers JD, Fluornoy N, Thomas ED. Infection with herpes simplex virus and cell-mediated immunity after marrow transplant. J Infect Dis 1980; 142:338-46.

7. Nahmias AJ, Roizman B. Infection with herpes simplex viruses 1 and 2. N Engl J Med 1973; 289:667-74, 719-25, 781-9.

8. Quinnan GV, Masur H, Rook AH, et al. Herpes virus infections in the acquired immune deficiency syndrome. JAMA 1984; 252:72-7.

9. Reeves WC, Corey L, Adams HG, et al. Risk of recurrence after first episodes of genital herpes: relation to HSV type and antibody response. N Engl J Med 1981; 305:315-9.

10. Quinn TC, Corey L, Chaffee RG, et al. The etiology of anorectal infections in homosexual men. Am J Med 1981; 71:395-406.

11. Goodell SE, Quinn TC, Mkrtichian E, et al. Herpes simplex virus proctitis in homosexual men: clinical, sigmoidoscopic, and histopathological features. N Engl J Med 1983; 308:868-71.

12. Baringer JR, Swoveland P. Recovery of herpes simplex virus from human trigeminal ganglions. N Engl J Med 1972; 288:648-50.

13. Corey L, Adams HG, Brown ZA, Holmes KK. Genital herpes simplex virus infections: clinical manifestations, course, and complications. Ann Intern Med 1983; 98:958-72.

14. Spruance SL, Overall JC, Kern ER, et al. The natural history of recurrent herpes simplex labialis: implications for antiviral therapy. N Engl J Med 1977; 297:69-75.

15. Glezen WP, Fernald GW, Lohr JA. Acute respiratory disease of university students with special reference to the etiologic role of herpesvirus hominis. Am J Epidemiol 1975; 101:111-21.

16. Straus SE, Smith HA, Brickman C, et al. Acyclovir for chronic mucocutaneous herpes simplex virus infection in immunosuppressed patients. Ann Intern Med 1982; 96:270-7.

17. Nerurkar L, Goedert J, Wallen W, et al. Study of antiviral antibodies in sera of homosexual men. J Fed Proc 1983; 42:6109.

18. Siegel FP, Lopez C, Hammer GS, et al. Severe acquired immunodeficiency in male homosexuals, manifested by chronic perianal ulcerative herpes simplex lesions. N Engl J Med 1981; 305:1439-44.

19. Wildy P. Herpes: history and classification. In: Kaplan AS, ed. The Herpesviruses. New York: Academic Press, 1973:1.

20. Chapel T, Brown WJ, Jeffries C, Stewart JA. The microbiological flora of penile ulcerations. J Infect Dis 1978; 137:50-7.

21. Centers for Disease Control. Revision of the CDC surveillance case definition for AIDS. MMWR 1987; 36:Suppl:1S-15S.

22. Erlich KS, Jacobson MA, Koehler JE, et al. Foscarnet therapy of severe acyclovir-resistant herpes simplex virus infections in patients with the acquired immunodeficiency syndrome. (unpublished)

23. Nahmias AJ, Whitley RJ, Visintine AN, et al. Herpes simplex virus encephalitis: laboratory evaluations and their diagnostic significance. J Infect Dis 1982; 146:829-36.

24. Dix RD, Waitzman DM, Follansbee S, et al. Herpes simplex virus type 2 encephalitis in two homosexual men with persistent lymphadenopathy. Ann Neurol 1985; 17:203-6.

25. Dix RD, Bredeson DE, Davis RL, Mills J. Herpesvirus neurologic diseases associated with AIDS: recovery of viruses from central nervous system (CNS) tissues, peripheral nerve, and cerebral spinal fluid (CSF) [Abstract]. Atlanta: International Conference on AIDS, 1985; 43.

26. Corey L, Holmes KK. Genital herpes simplex virus infections: current concepts in diagnosis, therapy, and prevention. Ann Intern Med 1983; 98:973-83.

27. Brown ST, Jaffee HW, Zaidi A, et al. Sensitivity and specificity of diagnostic tests for genital infections with herpesvirus hominis. Sex Transm Dis 1979; 6:10-3.

28. Moseley RC, Corey L, Benjamin D, et al. Comparison of viral isolation, direct immunofluorescence, and indirect immunoperoxidase techniques for detection of genital herpes simplex virus infection. J Clin Microbiol 1981; 13:913-8.

29. Yeager AS, Moris JE, Prober CG. Storage and transport of cultures for herpes simplex virus, type 2. Am J Clin Pathol 1979; 72:977-9.

30. Buchman TG, Roizman B, Adams G, Stover BH. Restriction endonuclease fingerprinting of herpes simplex virus DNA: a novel epidemiological tool applied to a nosocomial outbreak. J Infect Dis 1978; 138:488-98.

31. McClurg H, Seth P, Rawls WE. Relative concentrations in human sera of antibodies to cross-reacting and specific antigens of herpes simplex virus types 1 and 2. Am J Epidemiol 1976; 104:192-201.

32. Kahlon J, Chatterjee S, Lakeman FD, et al. Detection of antibodies to herpes simplex virus in the cerebrospinal fluid of patients with herpes simplex encephalitis. J Infect Dis 1987; 155:38-44.

33. Dix RD, Bredeson DE, Davis RL, Mills J. Herpesvirus neurological diseases associated with AIDS: recovery of viruses from CNS tissues, peripheral nerve and CSF [Abstract]. Atlanta: International Conference on AIDS, 1985; M-82.

34. Davis LE, Johnson RT. An explanation for the localization of herpes simplex encephalitis. Ann Neurol 1979; 5:2-5.

35. Whitley RJ, Soong SJ, Dolin R, et al. Adenine arabinoside therapy of biopsy-proved herpes simplex encephalitis: National Institute of Allergy and Infectious Diseases collaborative antiviral study. N Engl J Med 1977; 297:289-94.

36. Dix RD, Bredeson DE, Erlich KS, Mills J. Recovery of herpesviruses from cerebrospinal fluid of immunodeficient homosexual men. Ann Neurol 1985; 18:611-4.

37. Whitley JR, Soong SJ, Linneman C, et al. Herpes simplex encephalitis: clinical assessment. JAMA 1982; 247:317-20.

38. Hevron JE. Herpes simplex virus type 2 meningitis. Obstet Gynecol 1977; 49:622-4.

39. Heller M, Dix RD, Baringer JR, et al. Herpetic proctitis and meningitis: recovery of two strains of herpes simplex virus type 1 from cerebrospinal fluid. J Infect Dis 1982; 146:584-8.

40. Klastersky J, Cappel R, Snoeck JM, et al. Ascending myelitis in association with herpes simplex virus. N Engl J Med 1972; 287:182-4.

41. Steel JG, Dix RD, Baringer JR. Isolation of herpes simplex virus type 1 in recurrent (Mollaret) meningitis. Ann Neurol 1982; 11:17-21.

42. Wade JC, Newton B, McLaren C, et al. Intravenous acyclovir to treat mucocutaneous herpes simplex virus infection after marrow transplantation. Ann Intern Med 1982; 96:265-9.

43. Mitchell CD, Gentry SR, Boen JR, et al. Acyclovir therapy for mucocutaneous herpes simplex infections in immunocompromised patients. Lancet 1981; 1:1389-94.

44. Shepp DH, Newton BA, Dandliker PS, et al. Oral acyclovir therapy for mucocutaneous herpes simplex virus infections in immunocompromised marrow transplant recipients. Ann Intern Med 1985; 102:783-5.

45. Saral R, Burns WH, Laskin OL, et al. Acyclovir prophylaxis of herpes simplex virus infections. N Engl J Med 1981; 305:63-7.

46. Saral R, Ambinder RF, Burns WH, et al. Acyclovir prophylaxis against herpes simplex virus infection in patients with leukemia. Ann Intern Med 1983; 99:773-6.

47. Gluckman E, Devergie A, Melo R, et al. Prophylaxis of herpes infections after bone marrow transplantation by oral acyclovir. Lancet 1983; 2:706-8.

48. Wade JC, Newton B, Flournoy N, Meyers JD. Oral acyclovir for prevention of herpes simplex virus reactivation after marrow transplantation. Ann Intern Med 1984; 100:823-8.

49. Straus SE, Seidlin M, Takiff H, et al. Oral acyclovir to suppress recurring herpes simplex virus infections in immunodeficient patients. Ann Intern Med 1984; 100:522-4.

50. Corey L, Fife KH, Benedetti JK, et al. Intravenous acyclovir for the treatment of primary genital herpes. Ann Intern Med 1983; 98:914-21.

51. Whitley RJ, Alford CA, Hirsch MS, et al. Vidarabine versus acyclovir therapy in herpes simplex encephalitis. N Engl J Med 1986; 314:144-9.

52. Skoldenberg B, Alestig K, Burman L, et al. Acyclovir versus vidarabine in herpes simplex encephalitis. Lancet 1984; 2:707-11.

53. Bryson YJ, Dillon M, Lovett M, et al. Treatment of first episodes of genital herpes simplex virus infection with oral acyclovir. N Engl J Med 1983; 308:916-21.

54. Reichman RC, Badger GJ, Mertz GJ, et al. Treatment of recurrent genital herpes simplex infections with oral acyclovir. JAMA 1984; 251:2103-7.

55. Straus SE, Takiff JE, Mindell S, et al. Suppression of frequently recurring genital herpes. N Engl J Med 1984; 310:1545-50.

56. Douglas JM, Critchlow C, Benedetti J, et al. Double-blind study of oral acyclovir for suppression of recurrences of genital herpes simplex virus infection. N Engl J Med 1984; 310:1551-6.

57. Corey L, Nahmias AJ, Guinan ME, et al. A trial of topical acyclovir in genital herpes simplex virus infections. N Engl J Med 1982; 306:1313-9.

58. Whitley RJ, Levin M, Barton N, et al. Infections caused by herpes simplex virus in the immunocompromised host: natural history and topical acyclovir therapy. J Infect Dis 1984; 150:323-9.

59. Crumpacker CS, Schnipper LE, Marlowe SI, et al. Resistance to antiviral drugs of herpes simplex virus isolated from a patient treated with acyclovir. N Engl J Med 1982; 306:343-6.

60. Schnipper LE, Crumpacker CS, Marlowe SI, et al. Drug resistant herpes simplex virus in vitro and after acyclovir treatment in an immunocompromised patient. Am J Med 1982; 73:387-92.

61. Whitley RJ, Spruance S, Hayden FJ, et al. Vidarabine therapy for mucocutaneous herpes simplex virus infections in the immunocompromised host. J Infect Dis 1984; 149:1-8.

62. Erlich KS, Hauer L, Mills J. Effects of long-term acyclovir chemosuppression on serum IgG antibody to herpes simplex virus. J Med Virol 1988; 26:33-9.

63. Erlich KS, Mills J, Chatis P, et al. Acyclovir-resistant herpes simplex virus infections in patients with the acquired immunodeficiency syndrome. N Engl J Med 1989; 320:293-6.

64. Norris SA, Kessler HA, Fife KH. Severe, progressive herpetic whitlow caused by an acyclovir-resistant virus in a patient with AIDS. J Infect Dis 1988; 157:209-10.

Cytomegalovirus: Epidemiology

W. Lawrence Drew, M.D., Ph.D., and Kim S. Erlich, M.D.

The incidence of cytomegalovirus (CMV) infection among patients with AIDS is high[1] and CMV is a major cause of morbidity and mortality in this group.[2] The infection can take many forms, including asymptomatic virus shedding, retinitis,[1,3] pneumonia,[1] colitis,[4] and other syndromes.

■ EPIDEMIOLOGY

Neonates. CMV is a common cause of congenital viral infection in the United States; nearly 1 percent of all babies are born infected.[5,6] Additionally, 5 percent to 10 percent of babies become asymptomatically infected with CMV as a result of exposure to the virus in the maternal cervix during birth.[7] Breast milk has also been implicated as an important vehicle for neonatal transmission.[8,9]

Young Adults. Children who escape congenital and perinatal CMV infection may avoid infection for many years. In the United States, for example, only 10 percent to 15 percent of adolescents are infected. During young adulthood, the rate of seropositivity increases rapidly; by age 35, approximately 50 percent of the population shows serologic evidence of infection.[16] In poor populations or underdeveloped countries, however, childhood infection is common because of crowded living conditions and frequent transmission by breast milk.

Adults. Approximately 50 percent of the adult population in developed countries have been infected with CMV.[10] The virus is transmitted sexually, but it can also be spread by close personal contact, blood, and organ transplantation.[11] In CMV-infected immunocompromised patients, the virus may "reactivate," causing febrile illness, hepatitis, pneumonia, neurologic disturbances, and even death.[12-15]

There is convincing evidence that many CMV infections during adulthood are sexually transmitted.

1. CMV does not spread readily among adults by ordinary, non-sexual, person-to-person contact,[17] even with prolonged exposure to individuals who are excreting the virus.[18,19]

2. CMV has been isolated from the cervix of 13 percent to 23 percent of women attending STD clinics[20,21] versus 1 percent of women undergoing routine pelvic examination in other settings. The virus has also been isolated from semen.[22]

3. The prevalence of CMV antibody more than doubles during the years of highest sexual activity — ages 15 to 35.[10,16]

4. CMV mononucleosis developed in two men after sexual contact with a CMV-infected woman.[23] Evidence of recent CMV infection was found in another female sexual contact of one of the two male patients, whereas their roommates (who were not their sexual partners) had no evidence of CMV infection.

Homosexual Men.   Homosexual men have a high prevalence rate of CMV infection. We have observed urinary excretion of CMV in 14 of 90 (7.4 percent) homosexual men, but in none of 101 heterosexual men attending the same STD clinic ($p < 0.005$). Antibody to CMV was detected in 130 of 139 (93.5 percent) homosexual men, but in only 38 of 70 (54.3 percent) heterosexual men ($p < 0.005$).[24]

In a prospective study of 237 homosexual men participating in a hepatitis vaccine trial, CMV IgG serum antibody was found in 206 of 237 participants (86.9 percent).[25] Of the 31 men who did not have CMV antibody on initial testing, 22 seroconverted within nine months of follow-up, making an overall attack rate of 71 percent during this period. During follow-up (mean, 14.3 months; range, 2 to 20 months), 66 of the 206 initially seropositive men (32 percent) excreted CMV in their urine. Urine and semen specimens were obtained during a single visit from 52 of the participants, and although CMV was recovered from 18 semen specimens, the virus was isolated from only 3 of the 18 corresponding urine samples. Only one individual had CMV cultured from urine but not from semen. Semen, therefore, appears to be a more sensitive index than urine for detecting the presence of CMV. The widespread occurrence of CMV viruria and "virusemenia" in this population makes exposure to the virus through multiple sexual contacts almost inevitable and probably accounts for the extraordinarily high attack rate of CMV infections in seronegative homosexual men.

The high prevalence of CMV IgM antibody suggests that homosexual men experience repeated exposures to CMV. IgM antibody to CMV has been detected on one or more occasions in sera of over 90 percent of homosexual men followed over time.[25] In contrast, IgM antibody to CMV was detected in only 2.8 percent of 103 random serum specimens from volunteer male blood donors. There was no temporal correlation between serum IgM antibody and the presence of CMV viruria. CMV IgM antibody was detected in a higher proportion of men already seropositive for CMV (67 percent of 1135 samples) than in seroconverters (53 percent of 86 samples) (see Table 1).

TABLE 1.   PRESENCE OF CMV IgM ANTIBODY IN 237
LONGITUDINALLY FOLLOWED HOMOSEXUAL MEN

Group	SUBJECTS no. positive/no. tested (%)	SUBJECTS' SERUM SAMPLES no. positive/no. tested (%)
Seronegatives	0/9 (0)	0/54 (0)
IgG Seropositives	196/206 (95)	765/1136 (67)
IgG Seroconverters	20/22 (91)	46/86 (53)*

* *Samples obtained after seroconversion.*

The higher prevalence of CMV IgM antibody in longstanding seropositive men may also suggest that this group is continually re-exposed to (and possibly reinfected with) exogenous strains of CMV. We have recently shown that AIDS patients may be infected with more than one strain of CMV. Using a restriction enzyme technique to distinguish different isolates, we found from autopsy organ cultures that all four AIDS patients had at least two different isolates.[26]

Double infections with CMV do occur in patients with AIDS. These may represent terminal CMV superinfections in patients already severely immuno-compromised or exogenous reinfections prior to the development of AIDS.[26]

Of numerous sexual practices evaluated by questionnaire, only receptive anal intercourse correlated with an increased presence of CMV antibody or CMV seroconversion. CMV antibody was present in 96.6 percent of 59 men who engaged in receptive anal intercourse, but in only 73.7 percent (14 of 19 men) who did not engage in this practice ($p < 0.01$) (see Table 2).

TABLE 2.   PREVALENCE OF CMV ANTIBODY AMONG HOMOSEXUAL MEN

GROUP*	NO. OF MEN	NO. WHO WERE CMV SEROPOSITIVE (%)
1. Homosexual men: anal receptive intercourse	59	57 (96.6)
2. Homosexual men: no anal receptive intercourse	19	14 (73.7)
3. Heterosexual men	70	38 (54.3)

*   *1 vs 3: $p < 0.01$; 1 vs 2: $p < 0.001$; 2 vs 3: not statistically significant.*

It is likely that exposure of the anorectal mucosa to CMV-infected semen is the major route of infection in homosexual men, as the antibody prevalence rates among heterosexual men attending a venereal disease clinic and homosexual men not having anal-receptive sex do not differ significantly.

REFERENCES

1. Lerner CW, Tapper ML. Opportunistic infection complicating acquired immune deficiency syndrome: clinical features of 25 cases. Medicine (Baltimore) 1984; 63:155-64.
2. Macher AM, Reichert CMV, Straus SE, et al. Death in the AIDS patient: role of cytomegalovirus. N Engl J Med 1983; 309:1454.
3. Palestine AG, Rodrigues MM, Macher AM, et al. Ophthalmic involvement in acquired immuno-deficiency syndrome. Ophthalmology (Rochester) 1984; 91:1092-9.
4. Meiselman MS, Cello JP, Margaretten W. Cytomegalovirus colitis: report of the clinical, endoscopic, and pathologic findings in two patients with the acquired immune deficiency syndrome. Gastroenterology 1985; 88:171-5.
5. Birnbaum G, Lynch JI, Margileth AM, et al. Cytomegalovirus infections in newborn infants. J Pediatr 1969; 789-95.
6. Starr JG, Bart RD, Gold E. Inapparent congenital cytomegalovirus infection: clinical and epidemiologic characteristics in early infancy. N Engl J Med 1970; 282:1075-8.
7. Reynolds DW, Stagno S, Hosty TS, et al. Maternal cytomegalovirus excretion and perinatal infection. N Engl J Med 1973; 289:1-5.
8. Leinikki P, Heinonen K, Pettay O. Incidence of cytomegalovirus infections in early childhood. Scand J Infect Dis 1972; 4:1-5.

9. Stagno S, Beynolds DW, Pass RF, Alford CA. Breast milk and the risk of cytomegalovirus infection. N Engl J Med 1980; 302:1073-6.

10. Stern H, Elek SD. The incidence of infection with cytomegalovirus in a normal population: a serological study in Greater London. J Hyg Camb 1965; 63:79-87.

11. Betts RF, Freeman RB, Douglas RG Jr, et al. Transmission of cytomegalovirus infection with renal allograft. Kidney Int 1975; 8:387-94.

12. Betts RF, Freeman RB, Douglas RG Jr, Talley TE. Clinical manifestations of renal allograft derived primary cytomegalovirus infection. Am J Dis Child 1977; 131:759-63.

13. Fine RN, Grushkin CM, Malekzadeh M, Wright HT. Cytomegalovirus syndrome following renal transplantation. Arch Surg 1972; 105:564-70.

14. Hill RB Jr, Rowlands DT Jr, Rifkind D. Infectious pulmonary disease in patients receiving immunosuppressive therapy for organ transplantation. N Engl J Med 1964; 271:1021-7.

15. Peterson PK, Balfour HH Jr, Marker SC, et al. Cytomegalovirus disease in renal allograft recipients: a prospective study of the clinical features, risk factors and impact on renal transplantation. Medicine 1980; 59:283-300.

16. Wentworth BB, Alexander ER. Seroepidemiology of infections due to members of the herpesvirus group. Am J Epidemiol 1971; 94:496-507.

17. Wenzel RP, McCormick DP, Davies JA, et al. Cytomegalovirus infection: a seroepidemiologic study of a recruit population. Am J Epidemiol 1973; 97:410-4.

18. Betts RF, Cestero RVM, Freeman RB, Douglas RG. Epidemiology of cytomegalovirus infection in end stage renal disease. J Med Virol 1979; 4:89-96.

19. Tolkoff-Rubin NE, Rubin RH, Keller EE, et al. Cytomegalovirus infection in dialysis patients and personnel. Ann Intern Med 1978; 89:625-8.

20. Jordan MC, Rousseau WE, Noble GR, et al. Association of cervical cytomegalovirus with venereal disease. N Engl J Med 1973; 288:932-4.

21. Wentworth BB, Bonin P, Holmes KK, et al. Isolation of viruses, bacteria and other organisms from venereal disease clinic patients: methodology and problems associated with multiple isolations. Health Lab Sci 1973; 10:75-81.

22. Lang DJ, Kummer JF, Hartley DP. Cytomegalovirus in semen: persistence and demonstration in extracellular fluids. N Engl J Med 1974; 291:121-3.

23. Chretien JH, McGinniss CG, Muller A. Venereal causes of cytomegalovirus mononucleosis. JAMA 1977; 238:1644-5.

24. Drew WL, Mintz L, Miner RC, et al. Prevalence of cytomegalovirus infection in homosexual men. J Infect Dis 1981; 143:188-92.

25. Mintz L, Drew WL, Miner RC, Braff EH. Cytomegalovirus infections in homosexual men: an epidemiologic study. Ann Intern Med 1983; 99:326-9.

26. Drew WL, Sweet E, Miner RC, Mocarski ES. Multiple infections by CMV in patients with acquired immunodeficiency syndrome: documentation by southern blot. J Infect Dis 1984; 150:952-3.

Cytomegalovirus as a Cofactor in AIDS

W. Lawrence Drew, M.D., Ph.D., and Kim S. Erlich, M.D.

Although HIV infection appears to be a prerequisite for the development of AIDS, that there are other "cofactors" in the progression from asymptomatic infection to true disease remains a possibility. Virtually all patients with AIDS have been infected with cytomegalovirus (CMV), but exceptions have occurred. Therefore, if CMV is a cofactor, it is not absolutely necessary but rather may be one of several, albeit one of the most important, cofactors involved in HIV disease. Several lines of evidence suggest that CMV infection may be a cofactor in the development of AIDS.

CMV is highly prevalent in homosexual men and in patients with AIDS. From a mechanistic standpoint, CMV may infect the same cells that are infected with HIV. Prior infection with CMV may facilitate subsequent infection by HIV. Alternately, CMV infection of cells could reactivate a latent HIV infection.

T-cell dysfunction commonly occurs during acute CMV mononucleosis. Suppression of both T-helper lymphocytes and mitogen responses occur during acute infection but both return to normal after resolution of the acute infection and convalescence.[1,2] These immunologic abnormalities have been well described.[3]

In vitro studies have shown that lymphocytes, natural killer cells, and monocytes can be infected with CMV.[4] Viral expression is limited to the synthesis of immediate or early CMV polypeptides, however, and complete viral replication does not occur. "Wild" virus strains are more infective to blood cells than laboratory-adapted viruses. These data suggest that laboratory strains of CMV are highly adapted to fibroblasts, while wild strains are more lymphotropic. Mononuclear cells from immunocompetent individuals infected with CMV have diminished mitogen and antigen responses, suggesting that acute CMV infection is associated with decreased lymphocyte proliferation and defects in the cytotoxic T-cell response.[5-7]

We have investigated the relationship between CMV serology and T-cell imbalance in homosexual men who were seronegative for HIV.[8] Normal ratios (>1.0) of helper/suppressor cells (H/S) were found in 40 of 42 homosexual men lacking antibodies to cytomegalovirus. In contrast, H/S ratios were normal (>1.0) in only 34 of 67 (51 percent) homosexual men with antibodies to CMV (p < 0.001).[8]

To determine if asymptomatic primary infection induces immunologic abnormalities, 32 of 42 CMV-seronegative men were followed prospectively to trace the relationship between seroconversion and H/S ratio. During an average follow-up of 13.6 months, 12 patients (35 percent) underwent CMV seroconversion. All 12 of these patients had normal H/S ratios (greater than or equal to 1.0) in the month before seroconversion, but the ratios all dropped below 1.0 from one to three months after seroconversion (average nadir, 0.62). None of these patients seroconverted for HIV infection. The H/S ratios have remained less than or equal to 1.0 for an average of 9.6 months; of the seven seroconverters who have been followed for at least 12 months, three have ratios that remained less than 1.0. These data are summarized in Table 1.

TABLE 1.   H/S RATIOS BEFORE AND AFTER CMV SEROCONVERSION*

	NO. PERSONS FOLLOWED	NO. WITH H/S >1.0	NO. WITH H/S <1.0
<1 month before seroconversion	12	12	0
3 months after seroconversion	12	0	12
12 months after seroconversion	7	4	3

*   *Compiled by the authors.*

Of 20 seronegative men with initially normal H/S ratios who have remained seronegative, only one has developed an H/S ratio below 1.0. In patients who seroconverted, the H/S ratio's degree of abnormality did not correlate with the degree of symptoms. Three of the 12 CMV seroconverters have developed antibodies to HIV. The immunologic profiles of these three men do not differ from those of men who are not HIV-infected.

These results suggest that cytomegalovirus is responsible for at least some of the immunologic abnormalities occurring in homosexual men. Even asymptomatic CMV infection induces profound disturbances in the ratio of helper/suppressor lymphocytes. These abnormalities may persist for prolonged periods, appearing before, and independent of, infection by HIV.

In conclusion, it is possible that cytomegalovirus is a cofactor in the acquisition of HIV infection and/or a cofactor for the clinical expression of HIV infection.

REFERENCES

1. Rinaldo CR, Carney WP, Richter BS, et al. Mechanisms of immunosuppression in cytomegaloviral mononucleosis. J Infect Dis 1980; 141:488-95.
2. Carney WP, Rubin RH, Hoffman RA, et al. Analysis of T lymphocyte subsets in cytomegalovirus mononucleosis. J Immunol 1981; 126:2114-6.
3. Hirsch MS, Felsenstein D. Cytomegalovirus induced immunosuppression. In: Selikoff IJ, Teirstein AS, Hirschman SZ, eds. Acquired immune deficiency syndrome. Ann NY Acad Sci 1984:437:8-15.
4. Rice GPA, Schrier RD, Oldstone MBA. Cytomegalovirus infects human lymphocytes and monocytes: Virus expression is restricted to immediate early gene products. Proc Natl Acad Sci USA 1984; 81:6134-8.
5. Rinaldo CR, Black PH, Hirsch MS. Virus leukocyte interactions in cytomegalovirus mononucleosis. J Infect Dis 1977; 136:667-8.
6. Levin MJ, Rinaldo CR, Leary PL, et al. Immune response to herpes virus antigens in adults with acute cytomegalovirus mononucleosis. J Infect Dis 1979; 140:851-7.
7. Carney WP, Iacoviello V, Hirsch MS. Functional properties of T lymphocytes and their subsets in cytomegalovirus mononucleosis. J Immunol 1983; 130:390-3.
8. Drew WL, Mills J, Levy J, et al. Cytomegalovirus infection and abnormal T lymphocyte subset ratios in homosexual men. Ann Intern Med 1985; 103:61-3.

Cytomegalovirus: Role in
P. carinii Pneumonia and
in Kaposi's Sarcoma

W. Lawrence Drew, M.D., Ph.D., Mark A. Jacobson, M.D., and Kim S. Erlich, M.D.

■ ROLE OF CMV IN *PNEUMOCYSTIS CARINII* PNEUMONIA

Early in the AIDS epidemic, we reported that CMV might be a cofactor in AIDS-related *Pneumocystis carinii* pneumonia (PCP).[1,2] The virus was recovered from lung tissue in seven of the eight cases in which viral cultures were obtained, suggesting an association between CMV and PCP. In several instances, we could infer that the virus was present in extremely high titers, since the virus culture displayed cytopathogenic effects in one to two days.

Subsequently, CMV isolation has been reported from pulmonary specimens in 13 percent to 37 percent of AIDS-associated PCP cases.[8,22]

Although coexistent CMV and PCP infections have been described, the nature of their relationship is unclear. Animal models suggest that CMV may predispose individuals to PCP. Both human and murine alveolar macrophages can be infected with CMV.[3,4] Cytomegalovirus infection impairs bacterial phagocytosis,[4] and histologic studies suggest that the macrophage is important in the host response to *P. carinii*.[5] One hypothesis is that CMV infection of alveolar macrophages impairs the host's ability to remove *P. carinii* by impairing cell-mediated immunity.

It is unclear whether CMV co-infection predicts poor clinical outcome in PCP; clinical trials have reported conflicting results. In one study, mortality was 92 percent in 13 patients with PCP and CMV co-infection, compared to 14 percent in 22 patients with PCP and negative CMV respiratory cultures.[22] Another group of investigators reported that CMV was isolated from bronchoalveolar lavage fluid in only 38 percent of 16 patients who survived PCP without mechanical ventilation versus all 6 patients who did require mechanical ventilation.[23] On the other hand, there is at least one retrospective study in which no significant difference in survival was observed among patients with PCP, whether or not CMV was isolated from their pulmonary specimens at the time of PCP diagnosis.[24]

■ ROLE OF CMV IN KAPOSI'S SARCOMA

Numerous AIDS-related cases of malignant KS have been reported since the beginning of the AIDS epidemic. Several lines of evidence suggest that CMV may be a cofactor in causing KS in AIDS patients:

1. Cytomegalovirus can stimulate DNA and RNA synthesis in host cells,[6] transforming human fibroblasts to sarcomatous tumors when transplanted to immunosuppressed mice.[7] The transforming segment of the CMV genome was recently identified.[7]

2. Cytomegalovirus nucleic acids and antigens have been demonstrated in KS tumor biopsies. Additionally, CMV early antigens have been identified in tumor tissues from patients with classic and endemic forms of KS.[9,10] In a similar study, we detected CMV early antigens in six of nine KS biopsy specimens from homosexual men with AIDS[11] and later found this antigen in an additional 9 of 18 cases, even though their cultures were negative. Biopsies of normal skin from 21 of 22 patients were negative for CMV by culture. The presence of CMV early antigens without the presence of late antigens or whole virus in biopsy specimens suggests that the CMV genome is present in a nonreplicative (and possibly oncogenic) state.[10,11] The presence of only early antigen implies that the presence of virus does not result simply from disseminated infection or from a tropism of CMV for dermal or tumor tissue.

   Additionally, Boldogh et al.[9] have detected CMV DNA in 6 of 12 and RNA in 3 of 9 biopsies from African patients with KS. Epstein–Barr virus and HSV-2 nucleic-acid sequences were not detected. CMV RNA has been detected by in situ hybridization in two of three KS biopsies from homosexual men whose tumor cultures were negative for replicating virus.[11] More recently, Spector et al.[12] detected CMV DNA through in situ hybridization in tumor cells from KS tissue specimens. They used probes composed of subgenomic fragments of CMV DNA that had been shown to not cross-hybridize with human DNA. This technique enabled them to detect CMV genetic sequences in tumor cells from 6 of 10 evaluable KS specimens but not from sections of uninvolved skin.[12]

3. Renal transplant patients and homosexual men with AIDS share the twin features of immunosuppression-related KS and extremely high rates of active CMV infection. There are at least 36 reports of KS developing between 16 and 36 months after transplantation,[13-16] suggesting an approximate incubation period for the development of the tumor in immunocompromised patients. It is estimated that KS accounts for more than 3 percent of all malignancies occurring in organ transplant recipients.[14] Renal transplant recipients, who are immunosuppressed during the post-transplant period, are also subject to extremely high rates of primary or reactivated CMV infection.[17]

   We have evaluated 57 homosexual men with KS for evidence of CMV infection. All 57 patients have antibody to CMV. Of 39 secretion cultures from these patients, 24 (62 percent) were positive for virus. The average age of these patients was 36 years; these patients had been homosexual for an average of 17 years. A quantitative estimate of the extent of CMV exposure among gay men can be inferred from the finding that, even on a single sample, the semen of 25 percent of homosexual men is CMV culture-positive.[19]

   An additional epidemiologic clue linking CMV to KS is the marked discrepancy in the incidence of KS cases among homosexual and heterosexual AIDS patients. In New York City, KS occurs in 45 percent of homosexual men with AIDS but in only 8 percent of heterosexual men with AIDS.[20] It is probable that this discrepancy is related to a cofactor present in homosexual men but not in heterosexuals. This cofactor may be CMV, since heterosexual IV drug users do not have high rates of CMV infection. Of 143 IV drug users in San Francisco and New York City, only 92 (64 percent) had IgG antibody to CMV, a rate similar to that observed in the general population.[21]

The development of Kaposi's sarcoma in homosexual men is clearly a complication of their immunocompromised state. Indeed, whether or not CMV is a cofactor in the pathogenesis of AIDS, the evidence suggests that the virus may make a contribution to the development of KS. Additional evidence for an etiologic role for CMV in the genesis of KS would require demonstration that a CMV vaccine afforded protection against KS.

REFERENCES

1. Drew WL, Mintz L. Cytomegalovirus infection in healthy and immunodeficient homosexual men. In: Ma P, Armstrong D, eds. The acquired immune deficiency syndrome and infections of homosexual men. New York: Yorke Medical Books, 1983:117-23.

2. Follansbee SE, Busch DF, Wofsy CB, et al. An outbreak of *Pneumocystis carinii* pneumonia in homosexual men. Ann Intern Med 1982; 96:705-13.

3. Drew WL, Mintz L, Hoo R, Finley TN. Growth of herpes simplex and cytomegalovirus in cultured human alveolar macrophages. Am Rev Respir Dis 1979; 119:287-91.

4. Shanley JD, Pesanti EL. Replication of murine cytomegalovirus in lung macrophages: effect on phagocytosis of bacteria. Infect Immun 1980; 29:1152-9.

5. Hughes WT. *Pneumocystis carinii*. In: Mandell GL, Douglas RG, Bennett JE, eds. Principles and practice of infectious diseases. New York: John Wiley & Sons, 1979:2137-42.

6. St. Jeor SC, Albrecht TB, Frank FD, Rapp R. Stimulation of cellular DNA synthesis with human cytomegalovirus. J Virol 1974; 13:353-62.

7. Geder L, Lausch R, O'Neill F, Rapp F. Oncogenic transformation of human embryo lung cells by human cytomegalovirus. Science 1976; 192:1134-7.

8. Murray JF, Felton CP, Garay SM, et al. Pulmonary complications of the acquired immunodeficiency syndrome: report of a National Heart, Lung, and Blood Institute workshop. N Engl J Med 1984; 310:1682-8.

9. Boldogh I, Beth E, Huang E-S, et al. Kaposi's sarcoma. IV. Detection of CMV DNA, CMV RNA and CMNA in tumour biopsies. Int J Cancer 1981; 28:469-74.

10. Giraldo G, Beth E, Huang E-S. Kaposi's sarcoma and its relationship to cytomegalovirus (CMV). III. CMV DNA and CMV-early antigens in Kaposi's sarcoma. Int J Cancer 1980; 26:23-9.

11. Drew WL, Miner RC, Ziegler JL, et al. Cytomegalovirus and Kaposi's sarcoma in young homosexual men. Lancet 1982; 2:125-7.

12. Spector DH, Shaw SB, Hock LJ, et al. Association of human cytomegalovirus with Kaposi's sarcoma. In: Gottlieb MS, Groopman JE, eds. Acquired immune deficiency syndrome. New York: Alan R. Liss, Inc., 1984:109-26.

13. Myers BD, Kessler E, Levi J, et al. Kaposi's sarcoma in kidney transplant recipients. Arch Intern Med 1974; 133:307-11.

14. Penn I. Kaposi's sarcoma in organ transplant recipients. Transplantation 1979; 27:8-11.

15. Gange RW, Jones EW. Kaposi's sarcoma and immunosuppressive therapy: an appraisal. Clin Exp Dermatol 1978; 3:135-46.

16. Harwood AR, Osoba D, Hofstader SL, et al. Kaposi's sarcoma in recipients of renal transplants. Am J Med 1979; 67:759-65.

17. Fiala M, Payne JE, Berne TV, et al. Epidemiology of cytomegalovirus infection after transplantation and immunosuppression. J Infect Dis 1975; 132:421-32.

18. Zur Hausen H. The role of viruses in human tumors. Adv Cancer Res 1980; 33:77-107.

19. Mintz L, Drew WL, Miner RC, Braff EH. Cytomegalovirus infections in homosexual men: an epidemiologic study. Ann Intern Med 1983; 99:326-9.

20. Marmor M, Friedman-Kien AE, Laubenstein L, et al. Risk factors for Kaposi's sarcoma in homosexual men. Lancet 1982; 1:1083-6.

21. Brodie HR, Drew WL, Maayan S. Prevalence of Kaposi's sarcoma in AIDS patients reflects differences in rates of cytomegalovirus infection in high risk groups. AIDS Memorandum 1984; 1:12.

22. Stover DE, White DA, Romano PA, et al. Spectrum of pulmonary diseases associated with the acquired immunodeficiency syndrome. Am J Med 1985; 78:429-37.

23. Minozzi C. Cytomegalovirus in bronchoalveolar lavage of AIDS patients with *Pneumocystis carinii* pneumonia [Abstract]. 27th Interscience Conference on Antimicrobial Agents and Chemotherapy. New York, 1987; 835.

24. Brodie HR, Broaddus C, Blumenfield W, et al. Is cytomegalovirus a cause of lung disease in patients with AIDS? Clin Res 1985; 33:396A. abstract.

Cytomegalovirus: Clinical Presentations

W. Lawrence Drew, M.D., Ph.D., Mark A. Jacobson, M.D., and Kim S. Erlich, M.D.

Infection with cytomegalovirus (CMV) is common in HIV-infected patients and can result in several clinical syndromes, including chorioretinitis, pneumonitis, encephalitis, adrenalitis, colitis, esophagitis, sclerosing cholangitis, laryngitis, and hepatitis.[1,9,15-18] Not all patients with blood, urine, or tissue cultures positive for CMV have clinical illness caused by CMV. With the exception of chorioretinitis, a definitive diagnosis of clinically significant CMV infection requires tissue biopsy to demonstrate histologic evidence of CMV-mediated damage.

■ CHORIORETINITIS

Ocular disease due to CMV occurs only in patients with severe immunodeficiency; it is particularly common in patients with AIDS, occurring in approximately 5 percent.[19] Painless loss of vision, visual field cuts, or floaters are common complaints, and funduscopic examination reveals large yellowish-white granular areas with perivascular exudates and hemorrhages (see color plate 6.4.6.a). These abnormalities initially may be found at the periphery of the fundus but often progress if untreated to involve the macula and optic disc. Histologically, coagulation necrosis and microvascular abnormalities are present.[2,3] CMV retinitis may be complicated by retinal detachment.

Differentiation between CMV retinitis and cotton-wool spots is essential. Cotton-wool spots are common in AIDS patients but are asymptomatic, may regress spontaneously, and have an excellent prognosis. On ophthalmologic examination, cotton-wool spots appear as fluffy white lesions with distinct margins and are not usually associated with hemorrhages.[2,3]

Immediate ophthalmologic examination with pupillary dilatation is advised for patients with AIDS who have any new visual complaints. Patients with suspected or confirmed CMV chorioretinitis should be considered for treatment with ganciclovir (9-(1,3-dihydroxy-2-propoxymethyl) guanine, DHPG), especially if the lesions are in or near the macule. Recently licensed by the FDA, ganciclovir has shown a salutary effect on CMV chorioretinitis.[20] Lesions recur once therapy is discontinued, however, so maintenance therapy is necessary.[4,5,16,19,20] For patients who cannot tolerate ganciclovir because of myelosuppression, or for those who have ganciclovir-resistant CMV isolates, therapy with foscarnet should be considered.[21,22]

■ GASTROINTESTINAL INFECTION

Histologic and culture evidence of CMV esophagitis and enterocolitis has been reported. Colonic ulceration, lower-gastrointestinal bleeding, persistent rectal ulcers, and esophagitis have been described in the presence of positive CMV cultures and histopathology suggestive of CMV infection.[12-14,17,19]

Patients with CMV colitis experience diarrhea, weight loss, anorexia, and fever. Differential diagnosis includes other gastrointestinal pathogens (e.g., cryptosporidium, isospora, giardia, *Entamoeba histolytica*, shigella, and campylobacter). Sigmoidoscopy reveals diffuse submucosal hemorrhages and diffuse mucosal ulcerations. Biopsy specimens often reveal vasculitis with neutrophilic infiltration, CMV-infected endothelial cells, and nonspecific inflammation. Cytomegalovirus esophagitis resembles esophagitis caused by herpes simplex or candida, but it may be less painful. Ganciclovir may be effective in treating CMV colitis, but no controlled studies have yet been reported.[17,19]

■ PNEUMONIA

Cytomegalovirus frequently can be isolated from AIDS patients' pulmonary secretions or lung tissue during bronchoscopy, but a true pathogenic role for the virus is not always apparent. Many patients with pulmonary disease in whom CMV has been isolated are infected with other pathogens, especially *Pneumocystis carinii*. Many respond to therapy directed at *Pneumocystis carinii* pneumonia (PCP) alone, raising the question of whether CMV is a true pulmonary pathogen in these cases. Diagnostic bronchoscopy in some patients with CMV infection and pulmonary disease reveals no other pathogens, suggesting the possibility of invasive CMV pneumonia. Diagnosis of CMV pneumonitis, therefore, relies upon a combination of factors, including the presence of pathognomonic cells with intranuclear or intracytoplasmic inclusion bodies, or the demonstration of CMV antigen or DNA in lung tissue, positive CMV culture from lung tissue, and the absence of other pathogenic organisms.[6,7]

When CMV causes pulmonary disease in immunocompromised patients with AIDS, the presenting syndrome resembles an interstitial pneumonia: gradually worsening shortness of breath, dyspnea on exertion, and a dry, nonproductive cough. The heart and respiratory rate are elevated, and auscultation of the lungs is often unrevealing, with no evidence of consolidation. Chest x-ray shows diffuse interstitial infiltrates similar to those present in PCP. Hypoxemia is often present.[1,8]

Ganciclovir has been less effective for pulmonary CMV than for CMV retinitis, although rare patients with CMV pneumonia have responded to treatment.[23] Therapy should be considered if CMV is the only identifiable pulmonary pathogen in a patient whose pulmonary function is progressively deteriorating.[8,23]

■ CENTRAL NERVOUS SYSTEM INFECTION

Subacute encephalitis caused by CMV probably occurs in patients with AIDS, but recent evidence suggests that most cases of AIDS-related encephalitis are probably due to neural invasion by HIV. Cytomegalovirus is not considered a neurotropic virus, although occasional reports of its isolation from brain tissue or cerebrospinal fluid support the hypothesis that CMV can, on occasion, infect the CNS.[9-11]

The clinical presentation of CMV encephalitis in patients with AIDS is similar to that seen in subacute encephalitis caused by other agents: personality changes, difficulty in concentrating, headaches and somnolence are frequent findings. Diagnosis can be confirmed only by brain biopsy, with evidence of periventricular necrosis, giant cells, intranuclear and intracytoplasmic inclusions, and isolation or other identification of the virus.[9]

No effective treatment for confirmed CMV encephalitis has been established. Administration of ganciclovir can be considered, but specific protocols are not yet developed and no data on its efficacy are available. Polyradiculopathy/myelopathy with severe flaccid paraparesis in patients with AIDS has also been attributed to CMV, based on positive CSF cultures, CMV nucleic acids, or the presence of CSF polymorphonuclear pleocytosis. Reported cases to date suggest that ganciclovir therapy is ineffective.

REFERENCES

1. Armstrong D, Gold JWM, Dryjanski J, et al. Treatment of infections in patients with the acquired immunodeficiency syndrome. Ann Intern Med 1985; 103:738-43.

2. Teich S, Orellana J. Retinal lesions in cytomegalovirus infection. Ann Intern Med 1986; 104:132.

3. Akula SK, Mansell PWA, Ruiz R. Complications of the acquired immunodeficiency syndrome. Ann Intern Med 1986; 104:726-7.

4. Felsenstein D, D'Amico DJ, Hirsch MS, et al. Treatment of cytomegalovirus retinitis with 9-[2-hydroxy-1-(hydroxymethyl) ethoxymethyl] guanine. Ann Intern Med 1985; 103:377-80.

5. Bach MC, Bagwell SP, Knapp NP, et al. 9-(1,3-dihydroxy-2- propoxymethyl) guanine for cytomegalovirus infections in patients with the acquired immunodeficiency syndrome. Ann Intern Med 1985; 103:381-2.

6. Macher AM, Reichert CM, Straus SE, et al. Death in the AIDS patient: role of cytomegalovirus. N Engl J Med 1983; 309:1454.

7. Emanuel D, Peppard J, Stover D, et al. Rapid immunodiagnosis of cytomegalovirus pneumonia by bronchoalveolar lavage using human and murine monoclonal antibodies. Ann Intern Med 1986; 104: 476-81.

8. Shepp DH, Dandliker PS, de Miranda P, et al. Activity of 9-[2-hydroxy-1-(hydroxymethyl) ethoxymethyl] guanine in the treatment of cytomegalovirus pneumonia. Ann Intern Med 1985; 103:368-73.

9. Hawley DA, Schaefer JF, Schulz DM, Muller J. Cytomegalovirus encephalitis in acquired immunodeficiency syndrome. Am J Clin Pathol 1983; 80:874-7.

10. Dix RD, Bredesen DE, Erlich KS, Mills J. Recovery of herpesviruses from cerebrospinal fluid of immunodeficient homosexual men. Ann Neurol 1985; 18:611-4.

11. Wiley CA, Nelson JA. Role of human immunodeficiency virus and cytomegalovirus in AIDS encephalitis. Am J Pathol 1988; 133:73-81.

12. Meiselman MS, Cello JP, Margaretten W. Cytomegalovirus colitis: report of the clinical, endoscopic, and pathologic findings in two patients with the acquired immune deficiency syndrome. Gastroenterology 1985; 88:171-5.

13. Knapp AB, Horst DA, Eliopoulos G, et al. Widespread cytomegalovirus gastroenterocolitis in a patient with acquired immunodeficiency syndrome. Gastroenterology 1983; 85:1399-1402.

14. Gertler SL, Pressman J, Price P, et al. Gastrointestinal cytomegalovirus infection in a homosexual man with severe acquired immunodeficiency syndrome. Gastroenterology 1983; 85:1403-6.

15. Schneiderman DJ, Cello JP, Laing FC. Papillary stenosis and sclerosing cholangitis in the acquired immunodeficiency syndrome. Ann Intern Med 1987; 106:546-9.

16. Treatment of serious cytomegalovirus infections with 9-(1,3-dihydroxy-2-propoxymethyl) guanine in patients with AIDS and other immunodeficiencies. Collaborative DHPG Treatment Study Group. N Engl J Med 1986; 314:801-5.

17. Chachoua A, Dieterich D, Krasinski K, et al. 9-(1,3-Dihydroxy-2-propoxymethyl) guanine (ganciclovir) in the treatment of cytomegalovirus gastrointestinal disease with the acquired immune deficiency syndrome. Ann Intern Med 1987; 107:133-7.

18. Small PM, McPhaul LW, Sooy CD, et al. Cytomegalovirus infection of the laryngeal nerve presenting as hoarseness in patients with acquired immunodeficiency syndrome. Am J Med 1989; 86:108-10.

19. Jacobson MA, O'Donnell JJ, Porteus D, et al. Retinal and gastrointestinal disease due to cytomegalovirus in patients with the acquired immune deficiency syndrome: prevalence, natural history, and response to ganciclovir therapy. Quart J Med 1988; 67:473-86.

20. Jacobson MA, O'Donnell JJ, Brodie HR, et al. Randomized prospective trial of ganciclovir maintenance therapy for cytomegalovirus retinitis. J Med Virol 1988; 25:339-49.

21. Erice A, Chou S, Biron KK, et al. Progressive disease due to ganciclovir-resistant cytomegalovirus in immunocompromised patients. N Engl J Med 1989; 320:289-93.

22. Jacobson MA, O'Donnell JJ, Mills J. Foscarnet treatment of cytomegalovirus retinitis in patients with the acquired immunodeficiency syndrome. Antimicrob Agents Chemother 1989; 33:736-41.

23. Masur H, Lane HC, Palestine A, et al. Effect of 9-(1,3-dihydroxy-2-propoxymethyl) guanine on serious cytomegalovirus disease in eight immunosuppressed homosexual men. Ann Intern Med 1986; 104:41-4.

Cytomegalovirus: Diagnosis

W. Lawrence Drew, M.D., Ph.D., and Kim S. Erlich, M.D.

■ GENERAL CONSIDERATIONS

Diagnosis of cytomegalovirus (CMV) infection is confirmed by either positive virus culture from any site or by CMV seroconversion. The diagnosis of CMV disease is far more difficult, and requires identifying inclusion bodies or positive culture from a specific end organ, or both, in the absence of other infectious agents in the tissue.

Patients may excrete CMV in urine, semen, or cervix for years after infection and still have no evidence of clinical illness. Thus, a positive secretion culture does not prove that CMV is the causative agent of symptoms in an infected patient. Recovery of the virus from blood is, however, suggestive of active CMV disease, although some patients may be asymptomatic even when viremic. Recovery of the virus from lung culture supports the diagnosis of CMV pneumonitis if characteristic viral inclusions are present in tissue sections. In the absence of viral inclusions, a positive lung culture may not explain a clinical pneumonia. If no other pathogen or pathologic process is identified and if CMV is recovered from lung but no inclusions are present, CMV may be the cause of the pneumonia. Sorting out a contributing role for CMV in pneumonia is frequently complicated by the identification of other opportunistic pathogens such as *Pneumocystis carinii*. Indeed, these two particular agents are found together frequently and a synergistic relationship has been suggested but not proven.

Similar interpretive problems arise when CMV is recovered from intestinal and esophageal biopsy specimens. If no other pathogen is identified, CMV may explain colitis or esophagitis, especially if viral inclusions are present. When CMV is recovered from other organs, such as the brain, liver, and the adrenal glands, the virus is also likely to be responsible for clinical disease, especially when inclusions are also seen in histologic sections. Viral inclusions may not be seen, even when disease is truly present, because of sampling error, which allows them to be missed.

■ VIRUS ISOLATION

CMV may require four or more weeks to induce cytopathic effects recognizable by standard tissue-culture procedures. Recently, excellent correlation has been reported using a 24- to 48-hour tissue culture method.[1] With this rapid method, specimens are inoculated by centrifuging a shell vial containing a coverslip seeded with diploid fibroblast cells. After 24 to 48 hours of culture, the coverslip cells are stained with a specific CMV monoclonal antibody and the slide is examined with a fluorescent microscope. This procedure offers a practical method for rapidly identifying CMV in clinical specimens, especially urine.[1] Further tests will be needed to determine if this technique is equally effective for cultures from other sites.

■ OTHER METHODS OF VIRAL DETECTION

CMV antigen can be detected in tissue from clinical specimens with monoclonal antibodies.[2] This method is specific but not as sensitive as virus culture. Additionally, detection of CMV genome in blood and urine by DNA-DNA hybridization has been described.[3,4] The sensitivity, specificity, and clinical relevance of these procedures remain to be established.

■ SEROLOGY

Development of CMV antibody in previously seronegative patients indicates primary CMV infection. Cytomegalovirus antibody titers may fluctuate, so low-level increases of antibody are not diagnostic of active viral infection.

The presence of IgM antibody to CMV may be helpful in the diagnosis of recent or active infection, especially if seroconversion has occurred by the time the first serum specimen is obtained. In primary CMV infection, IgM antibody generally develops and disappears over a period of six to nine months. Theoretically, IgM antibody develops only during primary CMV infection, but in fact it may reappear during CMV reactivation. CMV IgM antibody is common in the sera of homosexual men,[5] probably as a result of viral reactivation or repetitive exposure to different strains of CMV. Therefore this test is not an indicator of primary infection in this patient population.

REFERENCES

1. Gleaves CA, Smith TF, Shuster EA, Pearson GR. Rapid detection of cytomegalovirus in MRC-5 cells inoculated with urine specimens by using low-speed centrifugation and monoclonal antibody to an early antigen. J Clin Microbiol 1984; 19:917-9.
2. Goldstein LC, McDougall J, Hackman R, et al. Monoclonal antibodies to cytomegalovirus: rapid identification of clinical isolates and preliminary use in diagnosis of cytomegalovirus pneumonia. Infect Immun 1982; 38:273-81.
3. Chou S, Merigan TC. Rapid detection and quantitation of human cytomegalovirus in urine through DNA hybridization. N Engl J Med 1983; 308:921-5.
4. Spector SA, Rua JA, Spector DH, McMillan R. Detection of human cytomegalovirus in clinical specimens by DNA-DNA hybridization. J Infect Dis 1984; 150:121-6.
5. Mintz L, Drew WL, Miner RC, Braff EH. Cytomegalovirus infections in homosexual men: an epidemiological study. Ann Intern Med 1983; 99:326-9.

Cytomegalovirus: Treatment

W. Lawrence Drew, M.D., Ph.D., Mark A. Jacobson, M.D., and Kim S. Erlich, M.D.

■ GANCICLOVIR

Ganciclovir (also known as DHPG) is an acyclic nucleoside structurally related to another antiviral agent, acyclovir. Activation of ganciclovir occurs by cellular and possibly viral tri-phosphorylation. The resulting phosphorylated compound is a potent inhibitor of cytomegalovirus (CMV) replication in vitro.[1-3] Ganciclovir undergoes phosphorylation 10 times more readily in virus-infected cells than in normal ones, affording some selective antiviral activity. Ganciclovir triphosphate competitively inhibits the binding of deoxyguanosine triphosphate to DNA polymerase, resulting in an inhibition of DNA synthesis and termination of DNA elongation. Oral absorption of the drug is poor, and treatment of CMV infections requires intravenous administration.[12]

Uncontrolled studies evaluating ganciclovir in treating AIDS patients with invasive CMV infection have produced some encouraging results. Patients with retinal, gastrointestinal, or pulmonary disease have shown clinical improvement, disease stabilization, or slowing of disease progression following ganciclovir therapy. The drug has a definite antiviral effect in vitro, with a reduction in virus-shedding occurring on therapy.[19-25] To date, the only AIDS-associated CMV disease for which ganciclovir therapy has been carefully studied is retinitis.[13,14] Several small trials involving serial retinal examinations of ganciclovir-treated patients have demonstrated a beneficial effect in halting retinal destruction. Unfortunately, however, disease progression typically resumes after therapy stops, so a treatment regimen involving lifelong maintenance therapy is usually required after response to initial therapy. In June 1989, the FDA licensed ganciclovir for treatment of sight-threatening CMV retinitis. Treatment of other CMV end-organ diseases with ganciclovir is still considered investigational.

Administration. Induction therapy: 5 mg/kg IV every 12 hours for 10 to 14 days. Maintenance therapy: 5 to 6 mg/kg 5–7 days/week.

Toxicity. Ganciclovir undergoes renal elimination, so dose-reduction in renal insufficiency is indicated. Toxicity is manifested as neutropenia in up to one-third of patients. This may limit widespread use of the drug.[13]

Azoospermia has been reported in animal studies and is likely to complicate human therapy. Thrombocytopenia occurs in up to 5 percent of human recipients. Rarely, gastrointestinal distress, central nervous system abnormalities, and rash have been associated with ganciclovir therapy.

Two strategies to maximize ganciclovir efficacy and minimize toxicity are currently being investigated. One involves direct delivery of the drug to the eye by intravitreal injection. Since very small amounts of drug are used, systemic toxicity can be avoided.[15,16] The other strategy is to add granulocyte-macrophage colony-stimulating factor (GM-CSF) to ganciclovir therapy in order to reverse bone-marrow suppression. The National Institute of Allergy and Infectious Diseases is sponsoring experimental studies of these two strategies.

■ FOSCARNET

Foscarnet (trisodium phosphonoformate) is a pyrophosphate analog with in vitro antiviral activity against all human herpes viruses and HIV.[26,27] Unlike ganciclovir, foscarnet does not require intracellular phosphorylation to inhibit viral DNA polymerase. Oral absorption is poor and oral administration is poorly tolerated, so treatment must be given intravenously.

Uncontrolled studies evaluating foscarnet in treating AIDS patients with CMV retinitis have been encouraging.[28,29] Ophthalmologic evaluation of these patients has demonstrated stabilization of retinitis during induction foscarnet therapy. However, disease progression typically has occurred after therapy stops. A Phase I study to determine the most effective, well-tolerated long-term maintenance dose of this drug is nearing completion.

Availability.   A salvage protocol using foscarnet therapy for CMV retinitis patients is now in use. Patients must be unable to tolerate ganciclovir therapy because of neutropenia or because of clinical or virologic evidence of ganciclovir resistance.[30] Trials are under way at many centers participating in the NIAID's AIDS Clinical Trials Group (phone number 1-800-TRIALS-A).

Toxicity.   The most common serious toxicity caused by foscarnet is azotemia.[28,29,31] Since foscarnet clearance is exclusively renal, careful and precise dosage adjustment must be made at frequent intervals according to estimated creatinine clearance. Abnormalities in serum phosphorus and calcium concentrations also occur frequently during foscarnet therapy.[28] Life-threatening hypocalcemia has rarely been reported.[32] Because the risk of hypocalcemia may correlate with the rate of infusion, foscarnet administration, unlike ganciclovir, must be controlled with an intravenous infusion pump. Other less common adverse effects associated with foscarnet therapy include nausea and central nervous system abnormalities.

■ INTERFERON

Leukocyte (α) interferon is part of the human body's natural response to many viral infections.[4] Administration of exogenous α interferon is effective for prevention and treatment of a variety of viral infections. A double-blind, placebo-controlled trial of interferon in preventing cytomegalovirus infections was performed in patients receiving immunosuppressive therapy with or without antithymocyte globulin.[5] A decreased incidence of CMV viremia occurred in the patients receiving interferon, but this was limited to patients who did not receive antithymocyte globulin. A delay in the onset of CMV viruria occurred in both groups. Alpha interferon therapy was also studied in four patients with CMV retinitis, but a clear benefit was not demonstrated.[6] Three of these patients suffered from AIDS and one had Hodgkin's disease. Bone-marrow transplant patients with CMV pneumonia showed no clinical improvement when treated with interferon[7] or combined vidarabine and interferon.[8] Interferon is not presently used in routine care and treatment of CMV-infected persons.

■ CMV IMMUNE GLOBULIN

CMV immune globulin (derived from plasma with a high titer of CMV antibody) has been used effectively to prevent CMV infection in CMV-seronegative patients undergoing bone-marrow transplants. Patients receiving granulocyte transfusion from CMV-seropositive donors were not protected,[9] although patients not receiving granulocyte transfusion were protected when compared with controls. Other investigators have reported success with CMV immune globulin or high-dose human gamma globulin in treating patients with CMV infection, but these trials have been uncontrolled.[10,11] Recently, the combination of ganciclovir and immune globulin has been reported as more effective than ganciclovir alone in treating CMV pneumonitis in bone-marrow transplant patients.[33]

REFERENCES

1. Field AK, Davies ME, DeWitt C, et al. 9([2-hydroxy-1(hydroxymethyl)-ethoxyl]methyl) guanine: a selective inhibitor of herpes group virus replication. Proc Natl Acad Sci 1983; 80:4139-43.

2. Mar EC, Cheng YC, Huang ES. Effect of 9(1,3-dihydroxy-2-propoxymethyl) guanine on human cytomegalovirus replication in vitro. Antimicrob Agents Chemother 1983; 24:518-21.

3. Tocci MJ, Levelli TJ, Perry HC, et al. Effects of the nucleoside analog 2'-nor-2'-deoxyguanosine on human cytomegalovirus replication. Antimicrob Agents Chemother 1984; 24:247-52.

4. Finter NB, ed. Interferons and interferon inducers. New York: American Elsevier, 1973:363-90.

5. Cheeseman SH, Rubin R, Stewart J, et al. Controlled clinical trial of prophylactic human-leukocyte interferon in renal transplantation. N Engl J Med 1979; 300:1345-9.

6. Chou S, Dylewski J, Gaynon M, et al. Alpha-interferon administration in cytomegalovirus retinitis. Antimicrob Agents Chemother 1984; 25:25-8.

7. Meyers JD, McGuffin R, Neiman P, et al. Toxicity and efficacy of human leukocyte interferon for the treatment of cytomegalovirus pneumonia after marrow transplantation. J Infect Dis 1980; 141:555-62.

8. Meyers JD, McGuffin R, Bryson Y, et al. Treatment of cytomegalovirus pneumonia after marrow transplant with combined vidarabine and human leukocyte interferon. J Infect Dis 1982; 146:80-4.

9. Condie RM, Hall BL, Howard RJ, et al. Treatment of life threatening infections in renal transplant recipients with high dose intravenous IgG. Transplantation Proc 1979; 11:66-8.

10. Meyers JD, Leszczynski J, Zaia JA, et al. Prevention of cytomegalovirus infection by cytomegalovirus immune globulin after marrow transplantation. Ann Intern Med 1983; 98:442-6.

11. Nicholls AJ, Brown CB, Edward N, et al. Hyperimmune immunoglobulin for cytomegalovirus infections. Lancet 1983; 1:532-3.

12. Jacobson MA, de Miranda P, Cederberg DM, et al. Human pharmacokinetics and tolerance of oral ganciclovir. Antimicrob Agents Chemother 1987; 31:1251-4.

13. Jacobson MA, O'Donnell JJ, Porteus D, et al. Retinal and gastrointestinal disease due to cytomegalovirus in patients with the acquired immune deficiency syndrome: prevalence, natural history, and response to ganciclovir therapy. Quart J Med 1988; 67:473-86.

14. Jacobson MA, O'Donnell JJ, Brodie HR, et al. Randomized prospective trial of ganciclovir maintenance therapy for cytomegalovirus retinitis. J Med Virol 1988; 25:339-49.

15. Ussery FM III, Conklin R, Stool E, et al. Ganciclovir by intravitreal injection in the treatment of AIDS-associated cytomegalovirus (CMV) retinitis [Abstract]. IV International Conference on AIDS. Stockholm, 1988; 1:7178.

16. Cantrill HL, Henry K, Knobloch WH, et al. Treatment of CMV retinitis with intravitreal ganciclovir — long-term results [Abstract]. IV International Conference on AIDS. Stockholm, 1988; 1:7188.

17. Jacobson MA, de Miranda P, Gordon SM, et al. Prolonged pancytopenia due to combined ganciclovir and zidovudine therapy. J Infect Dis 1988; 158:489-90.

18. Hochster H, Dieterich D, Laverty M, et al. Toxicity of coadministered AZT and ganciclovir (DHPG) for CMV infection: (AIDS Treatment Evaluation Unit #004) [Abstract]. IV International Conference on AIDS. Stockholm, 1988; 2:3666.

19. Bach MC, Bagwell SP, Knapp NP, et al. 9-(1,3-dihydroxy-2-propoxymethyl) guanine for cytomegalovirus infections in patients with the acquired immunodeficiency syndrome. Ann Intern Med 1985; 103:381-2.

20. Shepp DH, Dandliker PS, de Miranda P, et al. Activity of 9-(1,3-dihydroxy-2-propoxymethyl) guanine in the treatment of cytomegalovirus pneumonia. Ann Intern Med 1985; 103:368-73.

21. Felsenstein D, D'Amico DJ, Hirsch MS, et al. Treatment of cytomegalovirus retinitis with 9-(1,3-dihydroxy-2-propoxymethyl)guanine. Ann Intern Med 1985; 103:377-80.

22. Collaborative DHPG Treatment Study Group. Treatment of serious cytomegalovirus infections with 9-(1,3-dihydroxy-2-propoxymethyl) guanine in patients with AIDS and other immunodeficiencies. N Engl J Med 1986; 314:801-5.

23. Chachoua A, Dieterich D, Krasinski K, et al. 9-(1,3-dihydroxy-2-propoxymethyl) guanine (ganciclovir) in the treatment of cytomegalovirus gastrointestinal disease with the acquired immunodeficiency syndrome. Ann Intern Med 1987; 107:133-7.

24. Laskin OL, Stahl-Bayliss CM, Kalman CM, Rosecan LR. Use of ganciclovir to treat serious cytomegalovirus infections in patients with AIDS. J Infect Dis 1987; 155:323-7.

25. Cytomegalovirus infection and treatment with ganciclovir: a conference. San Francisco, 21–22 May 1987. Proceedings. Rev Infect Dis 1988; 10(Suppl 3):S457-S572.

26. Oberg B. Antiviral effects of phosphonoformate (PFA, foscarnet sodium). Pharmacol Ther 1982; 19:387-415.

27. Sandstrom EG, Kaplan JC, Byington RE, Hirsch MS. Inhibition of human T-cell lymphotropic virus type III in vitro by phosphonoformate. Lancet 1985; 1:1480-2.

28. Jacobson MA, O'Donnell JJ, Mills J. Foscarnet treatment of cytomegalovirus retinitis in patients with the acquired immunodeficiency syndrome. Antimicrob Agents Chemother 1989; 33:736-41.

29. Walmsley SL, Chew E, Read SE, et al. Treatment of cytomegalovirus retinitis with trisodium phosphonoformate hexahydrate (foscarnet). J Infect Dis 1988; 157:569-72.

30. Erice A, Chou S, Biron KK, et al. Progressive disease due to ganciclovir-resistant cytomegalovirus in immunocompromised patients. N Engl J Med 1989; 320:289-93.

31. Cacoub P, Deray G, Baumelou A, et al. Acute renal failure induced by foscarnet: four cases. Clin Nephrol 1988; 29:315-8.

32. Youle M, Clarbour J, Gazzard B, Chanas A. Possible drug interaction between foscarnet and pentamidine in AIDS patients [Abstract]. IV International Conference on AIDS. Stockholm, 1988; 2:3590.

33. Reed EC, Bowden RA, Dandliker PS, et al. Treatment of cytomegalovirus pneumonia with ganciclovir and intravenous cytomegalovirus immunoglobulin in patients with bone marrow transplants. Ann Intern Med 1988; 109:783-8.

Epstein–Barr Virus

Kim S. Erlich, M.D., and John Mills, M.D.

Infection with Epstein–Barr virus (EBV), one of the herpes viruses, is a frequent finding in AIDS patients. Epstein–Barr virus is endemic in human populations and serologic studies have shown that most AIDS patients are infected.[1] The initial infection may be either asymptomatic or acute, and it is followed by lifelong latency. The virus preferentially infects B lymphocytes, incorporating its viral genome within the infected cells, thereby producing an immortalized B-lymphocyte subpopulation.

Initial infection with EBV results in a range of clinical findings. Primary infection in childhood is often asymptomatic. Primary infection in adolescence and adulthood usually results in an acute mononucleosis-like illness characterized by fever, pharyngitis, lymphadenopathy, splenomegaly, and lymphocytosis with atypical lymphocytes and the development of heterophile antibodies. Signs and symptoms associated with primary infection usually resolve spontaneously and without complications over a two- to three-week period, but oropharyngeal virus shedding may persist for 12 to 18 months. Intermittent shedding of EBV from the oropharynx and recovery of EBV from peripheral blood lymphocytes persist for life in infected individuals.

There is abundant evidence associating EBV with malignancies. Seroepidemiologic data suggest that EBV is associated with African Burkitt's lymphoma and nasopharyngeal carcinoma. More recently, direct evidence has suggested a relationship between EBV in AIDS and the development of B-cell lymphomas, central nervous system (CNS) lymphomas, and oral hairy leukoplakia.[2,3] A cause-and-effect relationship has not been established, but the detection of EBV DNA in malignant tissue of non-AIDS patients strongly suggests an etiologic role for the virus in these syndromes.[4]

AIDS patients have an atypical serologic profile to EBV. Most AIDS patients have abnormally high antibody titers to viral capsid antigen, as well as antibody to both early antigen and EBV nuclear antigen.[1] The significance of this pattern is unclear but may indicate ongoing active viral replication or chronic infection.

The immune mechanisms responsible for controlling EBV are abnormal in AIDS patients; their B lymphocytes produce abnormally low numbers of immunoglobulin-secreting cells when cultured in the presence of EBV.[5] Additionally, autologous cocultures of T cells with EBV-activated B cells from AIDS patients result in enhancement of immunoglobulin production. The normal hosts' T cells suppress the production of EBV-activated B-cell immunoglobulin.

The role of EBV in the development of B-cell lymphomas in AIDS patients is incompletely understood.[6,7] Undifferentiated lymphomas similar to Burkitt's lymphoma frequently occur in patients with AIDS, and these lymphomas have been shown to contain EBV DNA. Chromosomal translocations similar to those present in endemic African Burkitt's lymphoma have also been demonstrated.[8-11] The incidence of high-grade lymphomas in patients with AIDS appears to be increasing. Most AIDS patients presenting with lymphomas have extranodal sites of involvement.[6] These patients with lymphoma respond poorly to therapy; their mortality rates exceed those of the general population with lymphomas.

Primary lymphoma of the central nervous system occurs infrequently in AIDS and also may be related to EBV.[2,12] The EBV genome has been demonstrated in lymphoma tissue from AIDS patients, including tissue from a CNS lymphoma.[2] Some patients with CNS lymphoma have serologic evidence of ongoing EBV infection, suggesting an etiologic role for the virus. The clinical presentation of CNS lymphoma can mimic other CNS illnesses and must be diagnosed by brain biopsy.

Oral hairy leukoplakia, a lesion in AIDS patients frequently misdiagnosed as candidiasis, may be related to EBV infection.[3,13] The white lesions typically appear on the lateral border of the tongue and occasionally on the buccal mucosa. They are slightly raised, poorly demarcated, and have a corrugated or hairy appearance. They usually produce no symptoms and range in size from a few millimeters to 3.5 by 2 cm. They do not rub off and, unlike thrush, do not reveal abundant fungal elements on Gram's stain or KOH preparation.

A study designed to identify viruses in tissue biopsies of hairy leukoplakia revealed EBV genome in 100 percent and papillomavirus core antigen in 73 percent of specimens tested.[3] Large quantities of EBV DNA, usually 200 or more molecules per cell, were found in leukoplakia lesions but not in normal buccal mucosa. EBV capsid antigen was also detected in the leukoplakia lesions, suggesting an ongoing permissive epithelial cell infection. The frequent finding of both EBV and papillomavirus in hairy leukoplakia suggests an interaction between the two viruses, but the exact relationship that produces leukoplakia remains to be determined.

Effective treatment for EBV infections in AIDS is not yet available. The acute mononucleosis-like illness is treated conservatively and usually resolves spontaneously. Antiviral chemotherapy (e.g., acyclovir) is of limited benefit for acute EBV infection and has not been shown to be effective in treating malignancies related to EBV.[14] Non-Hodgkin's and CNS lymphomas in AIDS patients respond poorly to conventional therapy and are often fatal.[6] Oral hairy leukoplakia usually causes no symptoms and does not require therapy. It must be differentiated from oral candidiasis, a treatable condition. Conservative management of leukoplakia by frequent gargling and swishing of dilute hydrogen peroxide can be implemented but is not of documented benefit.

A recent open-label study demonstrated that five of six seropositive individuals with hairy leukoplakia had regression of oral lesions when treated with oral acyclovir (3.2 grams per day for 20 days). All patients had a clinical recurrence when the medication was discontinued, however.[15]

REFERENCES

1. Rogers MF, Morens DM, Stewart JA, et al. National case control study of Kaposi's sarcoma and *Pneumocystis carinii* pneumonia in homosexual men. Part 2. Laboratory results. Ann Intern Med 1983; 99:151-8.

2. Hochberg FH, Miller G, Schooley RT, et al. Central nervous system lymphoma related to Epstein–Barr virus. N Engl J Med 1983; 309:745-8.

3. Greenspan JS, Greenspan D, Lennette ET, et al. Replication of Epstein–Barr virus within the epithelial cells of oral "hairy" leukoplakia, an AIDS-associated lesion. N Engl J Med 1985; 313:1564-71.

4. Andiman W, Gradoville L, Heston L, et al. Use of cloned probes to detect Epstein–Barr viral DNA in tissues of patients with neoplastic and lymphoproliferative diseases. J Infect Dis 1983; 148:967-77.

5. Birx DL, Redfield RR, Tosato G. Defective regulation of Epstein–Barr virus infection in patients with acquired immunodeficiency syndrome (AIDS) or AIDS related disorders. N Engl J Med 1986; 314:874-9.

6. Ziegler JL, Beckstead JA, Volberding PA, et al. Non-Hodgkin's lymphoma in 90 homosexual men. N Engl J Med 1984; 311:565-70.

7. Levine AM, Meyer PR, Begandy MK, et al. Development of B cell lymphoma in homosexual men. Ann Intern Med 1984; 100:7-13.

8. Ziegler JL, Miner RC, Rosenbaum E, et al. Outbreak of Burkitt's-like lymphoma in homosexual men. Lancet 1982; 2:631-3.

9. Chaganti RSK, Jhanwar SC, Koziner B, et al. Specific translocations characterize Burkitt's-like lymphoma of homosexual men with the acquired immunodeficiency syndrome. Blood 1983; 61:1269-72.

10. Magrath I, Erikson J, Whang-Peng J, et al. Synthesis of kappa light chains by cell lines containing an 8; 22 chromosomal translocation derived from a male homosexual with Burkitt's lymphoma. Science 1983; 222:1094-8.

11. Petersen JM, Tubbs RR, Savage RA, et al. Small noncleaved B cell Burkitt-like lymphoma with chromosome t(8; 14) translocation and Epstein-Barr virus nuclear-associated antigen in a homosexual man with acquired immunodeficiency syndrome. Am J Med 1985; 78:141-8.

12. Snider WD, Simpson DM, Aronyk KE, Nielsen SL. Primary lymphoma of the nervous system associated with acquired immunodeficiency syndrome. N Engl J Med 1983; 308:45.

13. Greenspan D, Greenspan JS, Conant M, et al. Oral "hairy" leukoplakia in male homosexuals: evidence of association with both papillomavirus and a herpes group virus. Lancet 1984; 2:831-4.

14. Andersson J, Britton S, Ernberg I, et al. Effect of acyclovir on infectious mononucleosis: a double blind, placebo controlled study. J Infect Dis 1986; 153:283-9.

15. Resnick L, Herbst JS, Ablashi DV, et al. Regression of oral hairy leukoplakia after orally administered acyclovir therapy. JAMA 1988; 259:384-8.

6.5

Protozoan Infections

Pneumocystis carinii Pneumonia: Epidemiology, Microbiology, and Pathophysiology

Gifford S. Leoung, M.D., and Philip C. Hopewell, M.D.

P*neumocystis carinii* is an extracellular parasite ubiquitous in nature. It was first isolated in 1909–1910 by Chagas and Carini in São Paulo, Brazil; they found the parasite in rats infected with *Trypanosoma cruzi* and *T. lewisi* and originally thought it to be part of the trypanosome's life cycle. However, in 1912, Delanoes identified the organism in rats and guinea pigs that were not infected with trypanosomes and named it *Pneumocystis carinii*.[1] Since then, the organism has been found in other rodents, monkeys, foxes, humans, a variety of domestic animals including dogs, cats, sheep, and goats, and on every continent in the world.[2,3] The organism causes disease almost exclusively in immunodeficient hosts, where its prolonged survival allows it to grow to sufficient numbers to cause disease.

■ EPIDEMIOLOGY

Pneumocystis carinii pneumonia (PCP) is a disease that occurs almost exclusively in immunodeficient hosts.[1,4] In immunocompetent hosts, infection occurs but is asymptomatic, presumably because of the organism's low virulence. A number of serologic studies have shown that 65 percent to 100 percent of children (both normal and immunosuppressed) have acquired antibodies to *P. carinii* by 2 to 4 years of age.[4,5]

The first human hosts identified were premature or debilitated infants.[1-3] These children had a pneumonia characterized by plasma-cell infiltrates, so the process was termed "plasma-cell interstitial pneumonia." Epidemics of the disease occurred in Europe during and after World War II but were limited to orphanages in which malnutrition and overcrowding were common. Since then, outbreaks have occurred in orphanages in the Middle East.[6] "Classic" outbreaks in institutionalized, premature infants usually appeared at two to six months of age; peak onset was three to four months. In these settings, transmission of the organisms was thought to be airborne and perhaps interpersonal. There was no evidence of vertical transmission.

Before the AIDS epidemic in the United States, cases in both children and adults were sporadic, usually occurring in association with neoplastic disease or its therapy. Children with congenital immunodeficiency syndromes (B-cell or T-cell defects, or both) were also found to be particularly susceptible to the parasite. The most common underlying conditions associated with PCP were leukemia, Hodgkin's disease and other lymphomas, primary immunodeficiencies, and organ transplants.[7] Antecedent or concomitant use of corticosteroids also appeared to increase risk of PCP.

The recent increase in incidence of PCP is a direct result of the HIV/AIDS epidemic. Pneumocystis pneumonia alone accounts for 43 percent of all opportunistic infections in AIDS patients, and alone or with Kaposi's sarcoma (KS), it is the index diagnosis in 62 percent of patients. Thus, it is the most common infection occurring in AIDS patients.[8] Data collected since the beginning of the epidemic show that the incidence of PCP has continued to increase relative to other reported opportunistic infections in persons with AIDS[9-11]; approximately 85 percent of all AIDS patients have PCP at some time in the course of their disease. In U.S. children with AIDS, the percentage with PCP was once as high as 77 percent but has declined to 58 percent.[7,8] As the epidemic continues, the number of patients who have both KS and PCP is declining, but this is because the incidence of KS is decreasing while the incidence of PCP is not.

■ MICROBIOLOGY AND PATHOPHYSIOLOGY

The protozoan *Pneumocystis carinii* has cystic and extracystic forms. The cysts are oval or round, approximately 5 to 8 microns in diameter, and contain four to eight intracystic organisms (sporozoites). The sporozoites are nucleated and measure approximately 1 to 2 microns in diameter. The extracystic form (trophozoite) measures 2 to 5 microns in diameter. It is pleomorphic in shape and often has an eccentric nucleus. In bronchoalveolar lavage specimens and lung tissue, trophozoites and cysts are associated with an eosinophilic and faintly PAS-positive "foamy" matrix in which the organisms are embedded. The organisms are abundant in pulmonary exudate, a feature that suggests they may be transmitted from the lungs by aerosol.

The cyst walls are faintly PAS-positive but may be poorly seen against the exudate, which also stains with PAS. They are easily seen (appearing black) using the Gomori methenamine-silver stain. In addition, the walls stain purple-violet with toluidine blue O. The individual trophozoites and sporozoites can be seen with Giemsa, Gram, or Wright stains. The nuclei of both forms take up hematoxylin. The morphology of trophozoites can be clearly seen on touch preparations of tissue using the Giemsa stain.[1,2,6]

The life cycle of *P. carinii* is not well understood, mainly because the organism cannot be maintained in cell culture. For reasons not yet understood, it does not survive repeated passage. It has been cultured on a variety of cell lines, including human embryonic lung fibroblasts, chick embryonic epithelial lung, and African green monkey kidney cells.[7] There are four stages in the life cycle: precyst, cyst, sporozoites within the cysts, and free-standing trophozoites. The most commonly accepted modes of reproduction are endogeny and fission. Recent evidence suggests meiosis at the precyst stage.[12] The organism's natural reservoir is unknown.

Although there has been past controversy over whether *P. carinii* should be in the phylum Protozoa or Fungi, it has generally been accepted as a protozoan. Recent data showing a high degree of homology between the ribosomal RNA sequence of *P. carinii* and the fungi *Saccharomyces cerevisiae* and *Neurospora crassa* may revive the controversy.[13]

Because seropositivity to *P. carinii* occurs as early as age four, it is possible that the organisms may reside in the lungs as an asymptomatic infection. Several autopsy studies have been done in an attempt to answer this question. In asymptomatic patients with malignancy, there was approximately a 5 percent incidence of *P. carinii*; in infants, prematures, and stillborns, the incidence was 1 percent. In 245 autopsies (excluding the above-mentioned groups), there were no organisms found.[14,15] A study at the National Institutes of Health examined 25 asymptomatic HIV-infected men for *P. carinii* using sputum induction and bronchoscopy and found no evidence of infection.[16] Although it is presumed that active disease occurs as a result of reactivation, de novo infection or reinfection are at least hypothetical possibilities.

In early stages of the infestation, cysts may be seen in small numbers without provoking any inflammatory response. Multiplication of the organisms is predominantly extracellular. As the infestation grows, more alveoli become filled with organisms and exudative material, causing defects in host gas exchange. There is hypertrophy of the Type 1 and Type 2 alveolar cells along with a predominantly mononuclear cell infiltration. Eventually, the alveolar cells desquamate and the extensive monocellular infiltrate causes thickening on the alveolar walls. As a result of organism proliferation and host-tissue reaction, pneumonitis appears and symptoms begin, evolving into the clinical entity of *P. carinii* pneumonia.

REFERENCES

1. Frenkel JK. Pneumocystis. In: Binford CH, Connor DH, eds. Pathology of tropical and extraordinary diseases. Washington, D.C.: Armed Forces Institute of Pathology, 1976; 303-7.

2. Hughes WT. *Pneumocystis carinii*. In: Mandel GL, Douglas RG, Bennett JE, eds. Principles and practice of infectious diseases. New York: John Wiley & Sons, 1985:1549-52.

3. Brown HW. Blood and tissue protozoa of man. In: Basic clinical parasitology. New York: Appleton-Century-Croft, 1975:73.

4. Pifer LL, Hughes WT, Stagno S, Woods D. *Pneumocystis carinii* infection: evidence for high prevalence in normal and immunosuppressed children. Pediatrics 1978; 61:35-41.

5. Meuwissen JH, Tauber I, Leeuwenberg AD, et al. Parasitologic and serologic observations of infection with pneumocystis in humans. J Infect Dis 1977; 136:43-9.

6. Young LS. Introduction and historical perspective. In: Young LS, ed. *Pneumocystis carinii* pneumonia. New York: Marcel Dekker, 1984:1-6.

7. Walzer PD, Perl DP, Krogstad DJ, et al. *Pneumocystis carinii* pneumonia in the U.S.: epidemiologic, diagnostic, and clinical features. In: Robbins JB, DeVita VU Jr, Dutz W, eds. Symposium on *Pneumocystis carinii* pneumonia. Bethesda, Md.: Dept. of Health, Education and Welfare, 1976. National Cancer Institute monograph no. 43. DHEW publication no. NIH 76:930.

8. Update: Acquired immunodeficiency syndrome — United States. MMWR 1986; 35:17-21.

9. Update: Acquired immunodeficiency syndrome (AIDS) — United States. MMWR 1984; 32:688-91.

10. Update: Acquired immunodeficiency syndrome (AIDS) — United States. MMWR 1984; 33:337-9.

11. Update: Acquired immunodeficiency syndrome (AIDS) — United States. MMWR 1985; 34:245, 248.

12. Matsumoto Y, Yoshida Y. Sporogony in *Pneumocystis carinii*: synaptonemal complexes and meiotic nuclear divisions observed in precysts. J Protocol 1984; 31:420-8.

13. Edman JC, Kovacs JA, Masur H, et al. Ribosomal RNA sequence shows *Pneumocystis carinii* to be a member of the fungi. Nature 1988; 344:519-22.

14. Esterly JA. *Pneumocystis carinii* in lungs of adults at autopsy. Am Rev Respir Dis 1988; 97; 935-7.

15. Hamlin WB. *Pneumocystis carinii*. JAMA 1968; 204:173-4.

16. Ognibene FP, Masur H, Suffredini AF. Asymptomatic human immunodeficiency virus (HIV) seropositive individuals have bronchoscopic evidence of interstitial pneumonitis (IP) but no *Pneumocystis carinii* (PC) [Abstract]. Los Angeles: Twenty-eighth Interscience Conference on Antimicrobial Agents and Chemotherapy. 1988:1115.

Pneumocystis carinii Pneumonia: Clinical Presentation and Diagnosis

Gifford S. Leoung, M.D., and Philip C. Hopewell, M.D.

■ CLINICAL PRESENTATION

In early stages of infestation with *Pneumocystis carinii*, the patient experiences no symptoms because of the paucity of organisms. Cyst forms line the alveoli but provoke little or no inflammatory response. As the organisms proliferate, symptoms begin.[1] Although usually slow and insidious, the disease can cause acute symptoms, with abrupt onset of fevers, chills, sweats, cough, and dyspnea on exertion.[2] The cough is either non-productive or produces thin, clear mucus. Accompanying the worsening cough and dyspnea is a steadily progressing, often profound fatigue. In a review of *P. carinii* pneumonia (PCP) before the AIDS epidemic, Walzer described the characteristics of 194 patients with PCP.[3] Dyspnea was the most common symptom, occurring in 91 percent of all patients. Fever and cough occurred much less often — 66 percent and 47 percent, respectively. Only 7 percent of all patients had a productive cough. The mean duration of symptoms before diagnosis was 19.7 days (range, 3 to 120 days), testifying to the slow progression in some patients.

Corticosteroid therapy does not lead to a more abrupt onset, and indeed it may suppress the initial manifestations of disease. In non-AIDS patients, a flare of the respiratory symptoms may coincide with a reduction or discontinuation of steroid therapy, presumably due to elimination of the steroid's antiinflammatory effects.[3]

In AIDS patients, the clinical presentation is often insidious, with slow but steady progression of fatigue, fever, chills, sweats, and exertional dyspnea.[4-7] In a comparison of AIDS and non-AIDS patients with PCP, Kovacs et al.[6] showed similarities in the disease's presentation, but the median duration of symptoms before diagnosis was much longer for AIDS patients (28 vs. 5 days; p <0.0002).

Extrapulmonary *P. carinii* infection was recognized prior to the AIDS epidemic. It has occurred only very rarely in AIDS patients; only 14 cases have been reported in the literature compared to the over 65,000 cases of pulmonary disease reported to the CDC. In AIDS patients, extrapulmonary sites have included the eye, ear, skin, esophagus, bone marrow, liver, spleen, adrenals, small intestine, and thyroid.[21-33] With the more widespread use of aerosolized pentamidine for prophylaxis and treatment, we can expect to see a rise in the number of extrapulmonary cases.

■ PHYSICAL FINDINGS

AIDS patients with PCP may initially exhibit minimal symptoms and signs, but they often appear ill from several weeks of fever and cough. Tachypnea may be pronounced; respiratory rates may be over 30, and patients may be so dyspneic that they are unable to speak without stopping to catch their breath. Circumoral, acral, and mucous membrane cyanosis may be evident. Although rales were found in 33 percent of immunocompromised patients without AIDS,[3] in AIDS patients chest findings often are minimal despite advanced signs and symptoms. Prominent adventitious sounds suggest an etiology other than PCP.

■ LABORATORY FINDINGS

Complete blood counts and sedimentation rates show no characteristic pattern in this disease. Serum chemistries are not particularly helpful; however, serum lactate dehydrogenase (LDH) concentrations are frequently elevated in patients with PCP.[8] A study of 62 patients (54 with AIDS) showed that only 7 percent of those with documented PCP had normal serum LDH levels; the mean LDH level in patients with PCP was 362 International Units (IU). The mean initial level of surviving patients (74 percent) was 340 IU versus 447 IU for the non-survivors. Seventy-five percent of the survivors showed a consistent decrease in the LDH with treatment; 19 percent showed an increase before the levels finally decreased. In contrast, 75 percent of the non-survivors showed increasing levels before death. These values were comparable whether or not the patient's PCP was AIDS-related. There was no correlation between serum LDH levels and respiratory rate, resting A-aDO$_2$ serum albumin or lymphocyte count.[34] Medina et al. evaluated 78 AIDS patients with PCP and found that the mean initial LDH level in patients with good outcomes (survival without respiratory failure) was 355 IU versus 710 IU in patients with poor outcomes (respiratory failure or death). All survivors showed a decline in LDH level at one week; non-survivors showed progressive increases.[35] Serum LDH levels are probably a nonspecific indicator of lung parenchymal damage instead of an indicator for PCP; however, they may be useful for predicting which patients will do well.

Arterial blood-gas measurements (with the patient breathing room air) generally show a moderate hypoxemia, although oxygen-tension values vary widely depending on the severity of the process. Up to 25 percent of patients may have arterial oxygen tensions of 80 mm Hg or above.[6] The blood-gas pattern usually shows an uncompensated respiratory alkalosis with an increased alveolar-arterial oxygen tension difference.[5-7,9]

Serologic testing for *P. carinii* has shown that the organism is more prevalent in the general population than previously thought, but its use as a diagnostic test has been disappointing. In an examination of patients with PCP using acute and convalescent sera and a "normal" titer up to 1:32, 18 of 21 patients were considered to have converted (fourfold or greater rise in titer). However, eight had a convalescent titer less than the "normal" titer of 1:32, and 56 percent of controls had titers up to 1:32.[10] More recently, Pifer has examined the usefulness of an ELISA for IgG antibody to *P. carinii* and a latex agglutination for *P. carinii* antigen (there are no data on IgM antibodies). While mean IgG antibody titers of patients with and without acute PCP were not statistically different, antigen titers were found to be both sensitive and specific in identifying patients with acute PCP. In addition, antigen titers appeared to parallel the patients' clinical course during therapy.[36,37] Thus, although antibody testing is helpful as an epidemiologic tool, it has no place in the diagnosis of acute PCP. Antigen testing may prove to be a useful adjunct to other tests presently used, but it needs further evaluation before being recommended as a routine diagnostic test.

■ PULMONARY FUNCTION TESTS

Most patients are able to complete pulmonary function tests (PFT) in spite of their dyspnea. The most consistent finding is a marked decrease in the single-breath diffusing capacity for carbon monoxide (DLCO). Other typical findings include a modest reduction in the vital capacity (VC) and the total lung capacity (TLC). Often the DLCO is reduced out of proportion to the volume reductions. The forced expiratory volume at 1 second (FEV1), forced vital capacity (FVC) and their ratio (FEV1/FVC) are only mildly reduced.[4,7] Curtis et al.[11] reported that the sensitivity for PCP of an abnormal TLC was 71 percent; of VC, 85 percent; and of DLCO, 89 percent. While these findings are not specific for PCP, in combination with chest x-ray and gallium scans, they are highly suggestive of a diagnosis.

After therapy for PCP, pulmonary function can be expected to return toward normal. Many patients will return to baseline, but some may have a mild restrictive pattern with or without a reduced DLCO.

■ RADIOGRAPHIC PRESENTATION

A diffuse interstitial or perihilar pattern, occasionally with peripheral sparing, is the most common radiographic presentation of PCP, occurring in 75 percent of AIDS patients with the disease.[9,12] However, all of the following presentations have been seen: abscesses, cavitation or cystic lesions, lobar consolidation, nodular lesions, effusions, pneumothorax, and a normal chest film[1,4,13,38-45] (see color plates 6.5.2.a–f).

Radiographic presentation with patchy upper-lobe consolidation imitating tuberculosis or hilar enlargement has been reported but is rare.[14,41] There is a single case report of PCP occurring as an endobronchial mass in a patient with concomitant tuberculosis and a chest film showing a hilar mass that upon subsequent radiography evolved into a cavitary lesion. Transbronchial biopsy confirmed the presence of *P. carinii* organisms, but the pathogenesis of the evolving radiographic lesions remained unclear.[46]

Local patchy interstitial infiltrates, including unilateral disease, are also reported.[41] Although relapses were seen before the use of aerosolized pentamidine, they have been increasingly reported as upper-lobe infiltrates occurring in patients on prophylactic aerosolized pentamidine.[43] Lowery reported that approximately 60 percent of relapsing patients who were receiving aerosolized pentamidine for secondary prophylaxis presented with infiltrates in a predominantly upper-lobe distribution. This may have been a result of poor deposition of the aerosol into the upper lobes (as measured by radionuclide studies).[48] Slow, even intake of breath from residual volume during prophylactic therapy should result in a more even distribution of the pentamidine droplets.

Pleural effusions are very uncommon in patients with PCP alone. When present, particularly if they are large, they should raise suspicions of pulmonary Kaposi's sarcoma, lymphoma, tuberculosis or other bacterial or fungal infections.[4] Finally, 5 percent to 10 percent of patients may have normal chest films,[11,16] although in some small series, up to 25 percent of patients were reported to have normal radiographic examinations.[10]

Pneumatoceles and spontaneous pneumothoraces in patients with PCP are uncommon. However, they are increasingly being reported both in the acute presentation and after successful completion of therapy.[15,41,49-51] A review of 100 consecutive patients with PCP at San Francisco General Hospital showed that 10 percent of all cases had pneumatoceles. There was no predilection for any particular lobe of the lung. In eight of the cases, the cysts were present at the time of diagnosis; cysts developed in two other cases while on therapy. Five patients had resolution of the cysts (one while still on therapy); one cyst was present but decreasing in size after four months; two patients died and two were lost to follow-up.[52,53] Of these 10 pneumatoceles, 3 were associated with spontaneous pneumothoraces. The cause of the increased number of spontaneous pneumothoraces is unclear; however, several factors may play a role. Since the number of cases of PCP is increasing, we may be simply seeing a larger absolute number of pneumothoraces. In addition, since patients are surviving longer and we are seeing more patients with multiple episodes of PCP, the parenchymal damage from prior episodes may increase the likelihood of pneumothorax. Finally, the incidence of spontaneous pneumothorax in the population at large is highest in young men. Because AIDS occurs most frequently in young men, the increase in spontaneous pneumothoraces may be an artifact of the patients' average age.

It is common for the radiographic appearance of PCP to worsen early in the course of therapy; in the more severe cases, there may be progression to airspace consolidation. However, if the deterioration continues beyond 7 to 10 days, failure of therapy should be considered.[7,17]

A diffuse interstitial pattern can also be seen in other infections common to AIDS patients, including cytomegalovirus, coccidioidomycosis, histoplasmosis, tuberculosis, and *Mycobacterium avium-intracellulare* infections.[4,18] It is important to remember that interstitial reticular and reticulonodular infiltrates can also be present in noninfectious complications (such as lymphoid interstitial pneumonitis).[4] In studies surveyed by the National Institutes of Health, clinical pneumonitis was seen in up to 38 percent of patients, but no specific etiology was found in 32 percent of those episodes. These cases of pneumonitis were clinically indistinguishable from cases of PCP, although the radiographic abnormalities were generally less serious (half of the patients with nonspecific pneumonitis had normal chest x-rays) and histologically showed less alveolar damage than those in patients with PCP.[54,55]

■ GALLIUM SCANNING

Evaluation of the lung using 67 gallium and scanning at 48 to 72 hours is very sensitive (90 to 100 percent) for PCP,[11,19,20] but the specificity is as low as 20 percent. However, if the abnormal scans were graded in terms of the degree of uptake and if the scans were considered positive only when the lung uptake was equal to or greater than that in the liver, the specificity was increased to 90 percent.[19] Using these criteria to define a positive scan, Curtis et al. found a positive predictive value of 92 percent and a negative predictive value of 58 percent.[18] Gallium scans begin to show resolution while the patient is undergoing therapy but it may be weeks after therapy is completed before a return to normal is seen.

Other organisms in the lungs of AIDS patients found to have abnormal gallium scans include *Cryptococcus neoformans*, *Mycobacterium avium* complex and (most frequently) cytomegalovirus (CMV).

REFERENCES

1. Hughes WT. *Pneumocystis carinii*. In: Mandel GL, Douglas RG, Bennett JE, eds. Principles and practice of infectious diseases. New York: John Wiley & Sons, 1978:1549-52.

2. Young LS. Clinical aspects of pneumocystosis in man: epidemiology, clinical manifestations, diagnostic approaches, and sequelae. In: Young LS, ed. *Pneumocystis carinii* pneumonia. New York: Marcel Dekker, 1984:139-74.

3. Walzer PD, Perl DP, Krogstad DJ, et al. *Pneumocystis carinii* pneumonia in the United States. Ann Intern Med 1974; 80:83-93.

4. Hopewell PC, Luce JM. Pulmonary manifestations of the acquired immunodeficiency syndrome. (unpublished.)

5. Grant IH, Armstrong D. Management of infectious complications in acquired immunodeficiency syndrome. Am J Med 1986; 81(Suppl 1A):59-72.

6. Kovacs JA, Hiemenz JW, Macher AM, et al. *Pneumocystis carinii* pneumonia: a comparison between patients with the acquired immunodeficiency syndrome and patients with other immunodeficiencies. Ann Intern Med 1984; 100:663-71.

7. Wharton JM, Coleman DL, Wofsy CB, et al. Trimethoprim-sulfamethoxazole or pentamidine for Pneumocystis carinii pneumonia in the acquired immunodeficiency syndrome. Ann Intern Med 1986; 105:37-44.

8. Silverman BA, Rubinstein A. Serum lactate dehydrogenase levels and children with acquired immune deficiency syndrome (AIDS) and AIDS-related complex: possible indicator of B-cell lymphoproliferation and disease activity. Am J Med 1985; 78:728-36.

9. Rosen MJ, Tow TW, Teirstein, et al. Diagnosis of pulmonary complications of the acquired immune deficiency syndrome. Thorax 1985; 40:571-5.

10. Nowosklawski A, Brzosko WJ. Indirect immunoflorescence test for serodiagnosis of *Pneumocystis carinii* infection. Bull Acad Polon Sci 1964; 12:143-7.

11. Curtis JL, Goodman P, Hopewell PC. Noninvasive tests in the diagnostic evaluation for *Pneumocystis carinii* pneumonia in patients with or suspected of having the acquired immunodeficiency syndrome. Am Rev Respir Dis 1986; 133:A-182. abstract.

12. Marchevsky A, Rosen MJ, Chrystal G, Kleinerman J. Pulmonary complications of the acquired immunodeficiency syndrome: a clinicopathologic study of 70 cases. Hum Pathol 1985; 16:659-70.

13. Mones JM, Saldana MJ, Oldham SA. Diagnosis of *Pneumocystis carinii* pneumonia. Chest 1986; 89:522-6.

14. Milligan SA, Stulbarg MS, Gamsu G, Golden JA. *Pneumocystis carinii* pneumonia radiographically simulating tuberculosis. Am Rev Respir Dis 1985; 132:1124-6.

15. Goodman PC, Daley C, Minagi H. Spontaneous pneumothorax in AIDS patients with *Pneumocystis carinii* pneumonia. Am Roent Ray Soc 1986; 147:29-31.

16. Heron CW, Hine AL, Pozniak AL, et al. Radiographic features in patients with pulmonary manifestations of the acquired immune deficiency syndrome. Clin Radiol 1985; 36:583-8.

17. Leoung GS, Mills J, Hopewell P, et al. Dapsone trimethoprim is effective treatment for *Pneumocystis carinii* pneumonia in patients with the acquired immune deficiency syndrome. Ann Intern Med 1986; 105:45-8.

18. Wheat LJ, Slama TG, Zeckel ML. Histoplasmosis in the acquired immune deficiency syndrome. Am J Med 1985; 78:203-10.

19. Coleman DL, Hattner RS, Luce JM, et al. Correlation between gallium lung scans and fiberoptic bronchoscopy in patients with suspected *Pneumocystis carinii* pneumonia and the acquired immune deficiency syndrome. Am Rev Respir Dis 1984; 130:1166-9.

20. Tuazon CU, Delaney MD, Simon GL, et al. Utility of gallium scintigraphy and bronchial washings in the diagnosis and treatment of *Pneumocystis carinii* pneumonia in patients with acquired immune deficiency syndrome. Am Rev Respir Dis 1985; 132:1087-92.

21. Kwok S, O'Donnell JJ, Wood IS. Retinal cotton-wool spots in a patient with *Pneumocystis carinii* infection. N Engl J Med 1982; 307:184-5.

22. Rossi JF, Dubois A, Bengler C, et al. *Pneumocystis carinii* in bone marrow. Ann Intern Med 1985; 102:868.

23. Macher AM, Bardenstein DS, Zimmerman LE, et al. *Pneumocystis carinii* choroiditis in a male homosexual with AIDS and disseminated pulmonary and extrapulmonary *P. carinii* infection. N Engl J Med 1987; 316:1092.

24. Coulman CU, Green I, Archibald RW. Cutaneous pneumocystosis. Ann Intern Med 1987; 106:396-8.

25. Breda SD, Hammerschlag PE, Gigliotti F, Schinella R. *Pneumocystis carinii* in the temporal bone as a primary manifestation of the acquired immunodeficiency syndrome. Ann Otol Rhinol Laryngol 1988; 97:427-31.

26. Grimes MM, LaPook JD, Bar MH, et al. Disseminated *Pneumocystis carinii* infection in a patient with acquired immunodeficiency syndrome. Hum Pathol 1987; 18:307-8.

27. Carter TR, Cooper PH, Petri WA, et al. *Pneumocystis carinii* infection of the small intestine in a patient with acquired immune deficiency syndrome. Am J Clin Pathol 1988; 89:679-83.

28. Heyman MR, Rasmussen P. *Pneumocystis carinii* involvement of the bone marrow in acquired immunodeficiency syndrome. Am J Clin Pathol 1987; 87:780-3.

29. Gherman CR, Ward RR, Bassis ML. *Pneumocystis carinii* otitis media and mastoiditis as the initial manifestation of the acquired immunodeficiency syndrome. Am J Med 1988; 85:250-2.

30. Pilon VA, Echols RM, Celo JS, Elmendorf SL. Disseminated Pneumocystis carinii infection in AIDS. N Engl J Med 1987; 316:1410-1.

31. Schinella RA, Breda SD, Hammerschlag PE. Otic infection due to *Pneumocystis carinii* in an apparently healthy man with antibody to the human immunodeficiency virus. Ann Intern Med 1987; 106:399-400.

32. Gallant JE, Enriquez RE, Cohen KL, Hammers LW. *Pneumocystis carinii* thyroiditis. Am J Med 1988; 84:303-6.

33. Unger PD, Rosenblum M, Krown SE. Disseminated *Pneumocystis carinii* infection in a patient with acquired immunodeficiency syndrome. Hum Pathol 1988; 19:113-6.

34. Zaman MK, White DA. Serum lactate dehydrogenase levels and *Pneumocystis carinii* pneumonia. Diagnostic and prognostic significance. Am Rev Respir Dis 1988; 137:796-800.

35. Medina I, Mills J, Wofsy C. Serum lactate dehydrogenase levels (LDH) in *Pneumocystis carinii* pneumonia (PCP) in AIDS: possible indicator and predictor of disease activity [Abstract]. III International Conference on AIDS. Washington, D.C., 1987; 109,W.5.5.

36. Pifer LL, Wood DR, Edwards CC, et al. *Pneumocystis carinii* serologic study in pediatric acquired immunodeficiency syndrome. Am J Dis Child 1988; 142:36-9.

37. Pifer LL, Wolf BL, Weems JJ Jr, et al. *Pneumocystis carinii* antigenemia in acquired immunodeficiency syndrome. J Clin Microbiol 1988; 26:1357-61.

38. Blumenfeld W, Basgoz N, Owen WF Jr, Schmidt DM. Granulomatous pulmonary lesions in patients with the acquired immunodeficiency syndrome (AIDS) and *Pneumocystis carinii* infection. Ann Intern Med 1988; 109:505-7.

39. Bleiweiss IJ, Jagirdar JS, Klein MJ, et al. Granulomatous *Pneumocystis carinii* pneumonia in three patients with the acquired immune deficiency syndrome. Chest 1988; 94:580-3.

40. de los Santos Sastre S, Capote F, Pereira A. Atypical roentgenographic manifestations of *Pneumocystis carinii* pneumonia in AIDS. Chest 1988; 94:219-20.

41. DeLorenzo LJ, Huang CT, Maguire GP, Stone DJ. Roentgenographic patterns of *Pneumocystis carinii* pneumonia in 104 patients with AIDS. Chest 1987; 91:323-7.

42. Suster B, Akerman M, Orenstein M, Wax MR. Pulmonary manifestations of AIDS: review of 106 episodes. Radiology 1986; 161:87-93.

43. Rankin JA, Collman R, Daniele RP. Acquired immune deficiency syndrome and the lung. Chest 1988; 94:155-64.

44. Barrio JL, Suarez M, Rodriguez JL, et al. *Pneumocystis carinii* pneumonia presenting as cavitating and noncavitating solitary pulmonary nodules in patients with the acquired immunodeficiency syndrome. Am Rev Respir Dis 1986; 134:1094-6.

45. Hopewell PC. *Pneumocystis carinii* pneumonia: diagnosis. J Infect Dis 1988; 157:1115-9.

46. Gagliardi AJ, Stover DE, Zaman MK. Endobronchial *Pneumocystis carinii* infection in a patient with the acquired immune deficiency syndrome. Chest 1987; 91:463-4.

47. Abd AG, Nierman DM, Ilowite JS, et al. Bilateral upper lobe *Pneumocystis carinii* pneumonia in a patient receiving inhaled pentamidine prophylaxis. Chest 1988; 94:329-31.

48. Lowery WS, Fallat RJ, Montgomery AB, et al. Changing radiologic patterns of *Pneumocystis carinii* pneumonia in patients on aerosol pentamidine prophylaxis (unpublished).

49. Fleisher AG, McElvaney G, Lawson L, et al. Surgical management of spontaneous pneumothorax in patients with acquired immunodeficiency syndrome. Ann Thorac Surg 1988; 45:21-3.

50. Afessa B, Green WR, Williams WA, et al. *Pneumocystis carinii* pneumonia complicated by lymphadenopathy and pneumothorax. Arch Intern Med 1988; 148:2651-6.

51. Sherman M, Levin D, Breidbart D. Pneumocystis carinii pneumonia with spontaneous pneumothorax. A report of three cases. Chest 1986; 90:609-10.

52. Sandhu J, Goodman PC. Pulmonary cysts associated with *Pneumocystis carinii* pneumonia in patients with the acquired immunodeficiency syndrome [Abstract]. Seventy-fourth Scientific Assembly and Annual Meeting. Chicago 1988:877.

53. Sandhu J, Goodman PC. Pulmonary cysts associated with *Pneumocystis carinii* pneumonia in patients with the acquired immunodeficiency syndrome. Radiology 1989 (submitted for publication).

54. Suffredini AF, Ognibene FP, Lack EE, et al. Nonspecific interstitial pneumonitis: a common cause of pulmonary disease in the acquired immunodeficiency syndrome. Ann Intern Med 1987; 107:7-13.

55. Simmons JT, Suffredini AF, Lack EE, et al. Nonspecific interstitial pneumonitis in patients with AIDS: radiologic features. AJR 1987; 149:265-8.

Pneumocystis carinii Pneumonia: Diagnostic Tissue Examination and Diagnostic Algorithm

Gifford S. Leoung, M.D., and Philip C. Hopewell, M.D.

■ DIAGNOSTIC PROCEDURES

Traditionally, the diagnosis of *P. carinii* pneumonia was made by open-lung biopsy.[1,2] Since the widespread use of fiberoptic bronchoscopy, transbronchial biopsy has become the gold standard by which other diagnostic procedures are evaluated. Reports of the sensitivity of transbronchial biopsy for *P. carinii* pneumonia have ranged from 66 percent to 98 percent using both fixed tissue and touch preparation.[3-7] When touch preparations were evaluated alone, the sensitivity ranged from 74 percent to 88 percent.[3,4,7] Bronchial brushings, when evaluated separately, have had a sensitivity of 20 percent to 78 percent.[3-7,17]

More recently, bronchoalveolar lavage (BAL) has been found to have a 55 percent to 98 percent sensitivity.[4-9] In most reports, sensitivity has been approximately 90 percent. In this procedure, the bronchoscope is wedged into a distal bronchus and 100 to 120 ml of saline is instilled in 20 ml aliquots, and then aspirated to retrieve at least 50 ml. Gal et al. found that bronchoalveolar lavage cell block (made from the sediment of the aspirated material) yields a slightly higher sensitivity than bronchoalveolar lavage fluid (95 percent vs. 88 percent) and that bronchial brushings are the least sensitive of all the bronchoscopic specimens (78 percent).[17] In general, reports have indicated that bronchoalveolar lavage and transbronchial biopsy have an additive sensitivity that approaches 100 percent.

Nonbronchoscopic bronchoalveolar lavage may be performed using a control-tipped reusable catheter.[10] This technique is less costly and it appears promising, but more experience is needed before its full value can be assessed.

Bronchoscopy, although generally safe, does carry a small risk of complications. In a review by Broaddus et al., approximately 9 percent of patients undergoing transbronchial biopsy developed a pneumothorax and 5 percent required a chest-tube placement.[4,10] An obvious advantage of lavage is that it avoids this complication entirely and may also be performed in patients with bleeding diatheses.

The least invasive mode of "tissue" diagnosis is the examination of sputum, which is induced by inhalation of hypertonic saline. The procedure involves inhalation of a 3 percent to 5 percent saline mist generated by an ultrasonic nebulizer and collection of the subsequent expectorated sputum. Early results from two centers showed that sputum induction had a sensitivity of 55 percent, allowing one center to reduce the need for bronchoscopy by 44 percent.[11-13] However, the negative predictive value of sputum induction was only 39 percent. Since then, further experience at San Francisco General Hospital has raised the sensitivity of induced sputum examination for PCP to 79 percent and its negative predictive value to 61 percent.[24] Zaman et al. reported a concentration technique that raised the sensitivity to 78 percent with a concomitant negative predictive value of 71 percent.[18] Because of sputum induction's low negative predictive value, patients producing a negative specimen should also undergo invasive diagnostic procedure.

Advantages of sputum induction include lower cost, lower morbidity, less patient discomfort, and reduced demands for bronchoscopy. The main disadvantage of this procedure is that patients with a lower organism load may expectorate few or no organisms. Moreover, evaluating the slides requires more time and more experienced laboratory personnel. The delay in bronchoscopy while awaiting sputum induction results is not significant.

One new method of detection that could potentially increase the rapidity and accuracy of sputum and bronchoalveolar lavage examinations is the use of mouse monoclonal antibodies directed against human *P. carinii*.[14] Kovacs et al. utilized the mouse monoclonal antibodies in an indirect immunofluorescent stain and compared the results with those of a Giemsa-type stain and toluidine blue O in one series, and against toluidine blue O in another.[19] In the first series, 92 percent of 49 patients with documented PCP were positive by immunofluorescence, 76 percent by Diff-Quik, and 80 percent by toluidine blue O. In the second series, 23 of 25 patients diagnosed with PCP were positive by immunofluorescence compared to 21 of 25 by toluidine blue O. All specimens positive by immunofluorescence were confirmed by a second method and there was only one false-negative. Elvin et al. showed that immunofluorescent staining of sputum was only 57 percent as sensitive as using lavage specimens but did not induce all their sputum specimens.[20] Development of a highly sensitive and specific direct immunofluorescent stain is in progress and shows promise in decreasing the background fluorescence, thus making interpretation easier.

Open-Lung Biopsy.   Open-lung biopsy, which was the preferred means of diagnosis before the advent of AIDS, should now be reserved for very selected patients. The above procedures have such a high rate of success that few additional diagnoses of PCP would be obtained.[15] In addition, open-lung biopsy carries a significant morbidity. Candidates for the procedure include patients with progressive pulmonary disease in whom the above procedures are unsuccessful, patients who have a bleeding diathesis, patients in whom sputum and lavage examinations are nondiagnostic, and finally, patients on mechanical ventilation, for whom biopsy would be imprudent and lavage has been unsuccessful.

Needle-Aspiration Biopsy.   Needle-aspiration biopsy was reported in one study to have a 90 percent sensitivity in PCP. However, both pneumothorax and bleeding were frequent (44 percent and 13 percent, respectively).[16] This has no place in the routine diagnostic evaluation for PCP.

■ DIAGNOSTIC ALGORITHM

The initial evaluation of patients suspected of having PCP should begin with a chest film. If the chest film is normal in a symptomatic patient, pulmonary function tests and gallium scanning should be done. Patients with abnormal findings at any of these steps should forego the remaining diagnostic steps and progress immediately to sputum induction (if available) or to bronchoscopy.[21-24]

Diagnostic Algorithm for PCP

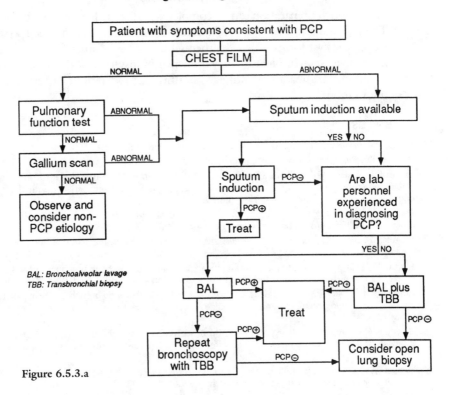

Figure 6.5.3.a

Sputum specimens collected by induction that reveal *P. carinii* should also be stained for acid-fast organisms and fungi, as well as cultured for mycobacteria and cytomegalovirus. Patients whose sputum examinations do not show *P. carinii* or another pathogen should undergo bronchoscopy, at which time specimens for other pathogens should be collected.

When sputum induction is not available or if it is negative, bronchoscopy is the procedure of choice. In institutions where personnel are experienced in diagnosing PCP, it may be sufficient to perform bronchoalveolar lavage without using transbronchial biopsy as the initial invasive procedure, since the sensitivity of lavage alone is high. Should the lavage be negative, repeat transbronchial biopsy would increase the yield for PCP.[24] If transbronchial biopsy is avoided on every patient during initial bronchoscopy, the risk of pneumothorax would be limited to only those patients who may require it for diagnosis.

An aliquot of lavage fluid should be centrifuged and the sediment stained for *P. carinii*, acid-fast organisms, and fungi. Fluid should also be cultured for mycobacteria and fungi and inoculated onto cell culture for viral isolation. Touch imprints should be made from tissue specimens and stained for *P. carinii*. Tissue should then be cultured for mycobacteria and fungi. Fixed tissue should also be stained for *P. carinii* as well as acid-fast organisms and fungi.

Only if all procedures are nondiagnostic and the lung disease is progressive should patients be considered for open-lung biopsy (as described above). It should be remembered, however, that findings from open-lung biopsies often are no more revealing than findings from transbronchial biopsy. Specimens obtained by open-biopsy should be evaluated like those obtained by transbronchial biopsy.

Giemsa staining of the bronchoalveolar lavage fluid and the transbronchial biopsy touch preparation can be completed and ready for viewing in one hour. The individual trophozoites stain darkly using Giemsa, as do the sporozoites within the cyst forms. The cysts themselves are best visualized using methenamine silver stain applied to transbronchial biopsy tissue. The cyst walls stain black and are readily identified, but this method requires overnight tissue preparation.

REFERENCES

1. Hughes W. *Pneumocystis carinii* pneumonia. Chest 1984; 85:810-3.
2. Winston DJ. *Pneumocystis carinii* pneumonia. Pul Med 1981; 7:41-8.
3. Mones JM, Suldana MJ, Oldham SA. Diagnosis of *Pneumocystis carinii* pneumonia: roentgenographic-pathologic correlates based on fiberoptic bronchoscopy specimens from patients with the acquired immunodeficiency syndrome. Chest 1986; 84:522-6.
4. Harcup C, Baier HJ, Pitchenik AE. Evaluation of patients with the acquired immunodeficiency syndrome (AIDS) by fiberoptic bronchoscopy. Endoscopy 1985; 17:217-20.
5. Hartman B, Koss M, Hui A, et al. *Pneumocystis carinii* pneumonia in the acquired immunodeficiency syndrome (AIDS). Chest 1985; 87:603-7.
6. Murray JF, Felton CP, Garay SM, et al. Pulmonary complications of the immunodeficiency syndrome: report of a National Heart, Lung and Blood Institute workshop. N Engl J Med 1984; 310:1682-8.
7. Coleman DL, Dodek PM, Luce JM, et al. Diagnostic utility of fiberoptic bronchoscopy in patients with *Pneumocystis carinii* pneumonia and the acquired immune deficiency syndrome. Am Rev Respir Dis 1983; 128:795-9.
8. Broaddus C, Dake MD, Stulbarg MS, et al. Bronchoalveolar lavage and transbronchial biopsy for the diagnosis of pulmonary infections in the acquired immune deficiency syndrome. Ann Intern Med 1985; 102:747-52.
9. Golden JA, Hollander H, Stulbarg MS, Gamsu G. Bronchoalveolar lavage as the exclusive diagnostic modality for *Pneumocystis carinii* pneumonia. Chest 1986; 90:18-22.
10. Caughey G, Wong H, Gamsu G, Golden J. Nonbronchoscopic bronchoalveolar lavage for the diagnosis for *Pneumocystis carinii* pneumonia in the acquired immunodeficiency syndrome. Chest 1985; 88:659-62.
11. Pitchenik AE, Ganjei P, Torres A, et al. Sputum examination for the diagnosis of *Pneumocystis carinii* pneumonia in the acquired immunodeficiency syndrome. Am Rev Respir Dis 1986; 133:226-9.
12. Bigby TD, Margolskee D, Curtis JL, et al. The usefulness of induced sputum in the diagnosis of *Pneumocystis carinii* pneumonia in patients with the acquired immunodeficiency syndrome. Am Rev Respir Dis 1986; 133:515-8.
13. Luce JM. Sputum induction in the acquired immunodeficiency syndrome. Am Rev Respir Dis 1986; 133:513-4.
14. Kovacs JA, Swan JC, Shelhamer J, et al. Prospective evaluation of a monoclonal antibody in diagnosis of *Pneumocystis carinii* pneumonia. Lancet 1986; 2:1-3.
15. Pass HI, Potter D, Shelhammer J, et al. Indications for and diagnostic efficacy of open-lung biopsy in the patient with acquired immunodeficiency syndrome (AIDS). Ann Thorac Surg 1986; 41:307-12.
16. Wallace JM, Batra P, Gong H Jr. Percutaneous needle lung aspiration in patients with AIDS. Am Rev Resp Dis 1985; 131:389-92.
17. Gal AA, Klatt EC, Koss MN, et al. The effectiveness of bronchoscopy in the diagnosis of *Pneumocystis carinii* and cytomegalovirus pulmonary infections in acquired immunodeficiency syndrome. Arch Pathol Lab Med 1987; 111:238-41.
18. Zaman MK, Wooten OJ, Suprahmanya B, et al. Rapid noninvasive diagnosis of *Pneumocystis carinii* from induced liquefied sputum. Ann Intern Med 1988; 109:7-10.
19. Kovacs JA, Ng VL, Masur H, et al. Diagnosis of *Pneumocystis carinii* pneumonia: improved detection in sputum with use of monoclonal antibodies. N Engl J Med 1988; 318:589-93.
20. Elvin KM, Bjorkman A, Linder E, et al. *Pneumocystis carinii* pneumonia: detection of parasites in sputum and bronchoalveolar lavage fluid by monoclonal antibodies. Br Med J 1988; 297:381-4.
21. Murray JF, Garay SM, Hopewell PC, et al. NHLBI workshop summary. Pulmonary complications of the acquired immunodeficiency syndrome: an update. Report of the second National Heart, Lung and Blood Institute workshop. Am Rev Respir Dis 1987; 135:504-9.
22. Rankin JA, Collman R, Daniele RP. Acquired immune deficiency syndrome and the lung. Chest 1988; 94:155-64.
23. Stover DE, White DA, Romano PA, et al. Spectrum of pulmonary diseases associated with the acquired immune deficiency syndrome. Am J Med 1985; 78:429-37.
24. Hopewell PC. *Pneumocystis carinii* pneumonia: diagnosis. J Infect Dis 1988; 157:1115-9.

Pneumocystis carinii Pneumonia: Therapy and Prophylaxis

Gifford S. Leoung, M.D., and Philip C. Hopewell, M.D.

Before pentamidine was recognized as an effective treatment for *Pneumocystis carinii* pneumonia (PCP), the mortality rate of the disease was approximately 50 percent in malnourished and immunocompromised infants and 90 percent to 100 percent in children and adults. Treatment with pentamidine reduced the mortality to 3 percent in infants and 25 percent in children and adults.[1,2] In 1974, trimethoprim/sulfamethoxazole (TMP/SMX) was found to be effective against PCP, and because it produced fewer adverse reactions, it replaced pentamidine as the drug of choice.[1]

Survival in AIDS patients from the first episode of PCP was initially reported to be 60 percent to 70 percent, with mortality rates higher for subsequent episodes. Patients with Kaposi's sarcoma have a 90 percent first-episode survival rate, whereas patients with other prior AIDS-defining opportunistic infections have a survival rate of only 50 percent to 70 percent.[3] More recently, perhaps due to more experience in treating the disease, the mortality for first-episode PCP has declined to 10 percent to 15 percent (Montgomery A: unpublished data). Since the beginning of the epidemic, data from San Francisco show that mean survival after the first episode of PCP has increased from 8 months to 18 months (Chaisson R: unpublished data). There has been only one reported case of an AIDS patient who was documented to have PCP and who improved with essentially no therapy.[34] That patient took only two doses of oral trimethoprim/sulfamethoxazole before treating himself with garlic therapy; the patient had a documented improvement over a two week period and relapsed after another month. Although allium sativum, a garlic extract, has known antifungal efficacy, it is unclear what role it played in this patient's course, particularly in light of the latest data regarding the possibility that *P. carinii* may be a fungus.

■ TRIMETHOPRIM/SULFAMETHOXAZOLE

Trimethoprim/sulfamethoxazole (TMP/SMX) is most often used as initial therapy for PCP. The dose initially used in AIDS patients was 20 mg/kg/day of trimethoprim plus 100 mg/kg/day of sulfamethoxazole given either orally or intravenously (divided every six or every eight hours daily). The usual length of therapy is 14 to 21 days. For reasons that are unclear, the rate of adverse effects is higher in AIDS patients (65 percent) than in previously studied populations (12 percent).[2] Because of the high incidence and severity of adverse effects, only 35 percent to 45 percent of patients who start therapy with TMP/SMX are able to complete a 14- to 21-day course.[4-9] Twenty percent to 30 percent of patients fail to respond to TMP/SMX as initial therapy and require a change in therapy.[4,5,9] Unfortunately, patients who do not respond to TMP/SMX tend not to respond to pentamidine. In several series, survival was only 11 percent in those who required a change in therapy because of drug failure.[3,8,9]

Wharton and colleagues[6] reported adverse effects in all patients treated with TMP/SMX, including rash (33 percent), elevation of liver-function tests (LFT) (44 percent), nausea and vomiting (50 percent), anemia (40 percent), creatinine elevation (33 percent), and hyponatremia (94 percent). The most common adverse reactions that necessitated a change in therapy were neutropenia (15 percent) and severe rash (15 percent). These reactions occurred after a mean of 11.5 days of treatment (range, 6 to 18). Both Gordin et al.[5] and Kovacs et al.[4] reported a lower rate of overall adverse effects, but a greater number of patients required a change of therapy for rash (33 percent) and neutropenia (28 percent). Drug-induced neutropenia usually does not occur prior to one week's duration of therapy and usually will respond to a discontinuation of the medication. Fortunately, neutropenia induced by TMP/SMX does not appear to be further affected by subsequently administered pentamidine and vice versa.[35] Less common adverse reactions to TMP/SMX include tremor[36] and ataxia.[37]

Since the initial studies, there has been controversy over the optimal dose of trimethoprim/sulfamethoxazole. In a noncrossover study comparing TMP/SMX to pentamidine, Sattler et al.[38] treated patients with TMP/SMX at a lower dose of 15 mg/kg/day and 75 mg/kg/day, respectively, and tailored their doses to maintain a trimethoprim level of 5 to 8 micrograms/ml. Despite the lower initial dose, 25 of 36 patients required further reductions to keep within the prescribed TMP level (average final dose: 12 mg/kg/d). There was an 86 percent survival rate but adverse reactions remained common (rash, 44 percent; anemia, 39 percent; neutropenia, 72 percent; LFT elevation, 22 percent). Neutrophil counts rose when the TMP/SMX dosage was lowered. At many institutions, this lower dosing regimen has become standard.

The suggested therapeutic concentrations for trimethoprim and sulfamethoxazole range from 3 to 10 micrograms/ml and 100 to 150 micrograms/ml, respectively.[39,40] McLean showed that lowering the sulfamethoxazole dose did not affect the frequency of adverse reactions in 11 patients, implying that TMP may be more the culprit.[40] However, measurements of drug levels are not widely available and are not standard of care at most institutions.

In an abstract reporting cross-reactions to various sulfa medications, three patients with previously documented allergic reactions to TMP/SMX during PCP therapy were rechallenged during a subsequent episode and were able to complete 21-day courses, although two had the same reaction (rash and fever) during the subsequent course.[44]

■ PENTAMIDINE

Pentamidine is the alternative drug most commonly used for patients who have adverse reactions or fail to respond to TMP/SMX. The usual dose of pentamidine is 4 mg/kg/day given intramuscularly or intravenously once daily, although lower doses are being studied (see below). Because of the incidence of sterile abscesses, most physicians administer pentamidine intravenously. The usual length of therapy is also 14 to 21 days. Approximately 45 percent of patients started on pentamidine require a change to another agent because of adverse effects.[4,6,42] As in those treated with TMP/SMX, up to 33 percent of patients initially treated with pentamidine will not respond and will require therapy with another drug.[2] Contrary to Wharton's findings,[6] Sattler[38] found that patients begun on pentamidine had a lower survival rate than those started on TMP/SMX (61 percent vs. 86 percent); this was true both for patients with first and repeat episodes.

Wharton[6] reported adverse effects in all patients treated with pentamidine, including anemia (33 percent), creatinine elevation (60 percent), LFT elevation (63 percent), and hyponatremia (56 percent). The most common adverse effect requiring a change in therapy was neutropenia (32 percent). Adverse effects requiring a change in therapy occurred after a mean of 10.4 days on therapy (range, 6 to 16). Gordin,[5] Kovacs,[4] and Sattler[38] all reported similar adverse effects but at somewhat different rates. Uncommon reactions included one case of renal failure associated with myoglobinemia and myoglobinuria; creatinine kinase elevation has also been reported.[59] Four cases of cardiac arrhythmias (resulting in two deaths) have been reported in patients receiving pentamidine; in several of those cases, the rhythm was torsade de pointes.[35]

Conte et al. studied a dose of 3 mg/kg/day in nine patients; eight patients improved and six patients completed the course of therapy.[44] Therapy was discontinued in two patients due to neutropenia and hepatotoxicity; minor toxicity occurred in four patients. This small preliminary study suggests that a lower dose of pentamidine may not substantially change the therapeutic outcome or toxicity, although further confirmatory studies are needed.

Pancreatitis and dysglycemia are unique to pentamidine. In a review of AIDS patients treated with pentamidine dispensed by the CDC, Waskin et al. found that 57 percent of all patients had dysglycemic reactions (abnormal serum glucose levels).[45] There have been at least three cases of fatal pancreatitis attributed to pentamidine in which the autopsy revealed extensive pancreatic necrosis.[46,47] Prior studies have shown that pentamidine directly affects the pancreatic islet cells. Both hyperglycemia and hypoglycemia have resulted from treatment with pentamidine. The risk of hypoglycemia increases with duration and dosage of therapy[45]; however, it may occur precipitously — early during the course of therapy or after completion of therapy. In one patient, hypoglycemia occurred one week after the last intramuscular dose[10,11]; four known cases of fatal hypoglycemia have been reported.[38,45] Hyperglycemia may not be noted until several months after treatment is completed. Diabetes has been known to occur as late as 150 days after therapy.[45]

Several studies have shown that parenteral pentamidine is distributed widely in the body, particularly in kidneys, adrenal glands, spleen, and liver.[39,42,48] Lung levels are lower, and at a dosing interval of 24 hours, they do not begin to accumulate until the fourth dose. In fact, lung levels of pentamidine were not detected until patients had received approximately 1 gram.[48,49] Based on animal data, Donnelly has suggested that a concentration of 30 micrograms per gram of lung tissue is required to treat PCP. This level is not achieved by parenteral administration until five doses have been administered.[48] Conte et al. have shown that peak plasma concentrations of pentamidine after IM and IV administration were 209 ng/ml and 612 ng/ml, respectively. Because renal clearance was only 5.0 percent and 2.5 percent of plasma clearance after IM and IV administration, respectively, dosage adjustments are not required in patients with creatinine clearances above 35 ml/min. Neither peritoneal dialysis nor hemodialysis appear to alter plasma concentrations. The plasma half-life of pentamidine after IV administration is approximately 6.5 hours.[50,51]

■ **DAPSONE/TRIMETHOPRIM**

Dapsone (100 mg/day once daily) plus trimethoprim (20 mg/kg/day in four divided doses, both given orally) (DS/TMP) was studied in 15 patients with first-episode PCP and was found to be effective in all 15.[18] Fourteen patients experienced adverse effects, including nausea and vomiting, rash, and LFT elevation. Only two patients required change to another drug, both because of a rash that did not respond to dipheniramine and a 50 percent reduction in the trimethoprim dose; however, both patients were improving at the time of the change. The adverse reactions that occurred were milder than those observed in patients treated with conventional therapy. This is now the most widely used outpatient regimen for PCP in the San Francisco community.

A subsequent open study evaluating dapsone (100 mg/day as a single daily dose orally) without trimethoprim found that 11 of 18 (61 percent) first-episode PCP patients responded. Of the 11 patients who responded, six (55 percent) had adverse reactions; however, none was severe enough to require switching therapy. Although a 39 percent failure rate is high compared to existing therapy, dapsone as single-agent therapy (possibly at higher doses) may be considered as an alternate regimen for patients unable to tolerate conventional therapy or as prophylaxis.[19,52]

A 60-patient, double-blind randomized trial at San Francisco General Hospital compared DS/TMP to TMP/SMX and confirmed that the efficacy of DS/TMP was equal to that of TMP-/MX (two and three failures, respectively); there was only one death (on the TMP/SMX arm).[20,53] Although 57 of the 60 patients experienced adverse effects of some nature, only 9 and 17 patients required a change of therapy in the DS/TMP and TMP/SMX arms, respectively. In the TMP/SMX group, the rates of LFT elevation (p = 0.05) and neutropenia (p = 0.08) were higher and more severe. Asymptomatic methemoglobinemia occurred in 20 of 30 DS/TMP treated patients but only one patient required discontinuation of therapy due to a methemoglobin level of 21 percent (at day nine of therapy). The methemoglobinemia responded promptly to administration of methylene blue. Asymptomatic hyperkalemia was also noted to be significantly more frequent in the DS/TMP group. The majority of the adverse reactions occurred after the first week of therapy.

Because of the risk of hemolysis, patients being considered for dapsone treatment should be tested for G6PD deficiency. Patients who are G6PD-deficient should be treated with other regimens. If G6PD-deficient patients are unable to tolerate other regimens and are treated with DS/TMP, physicians should be prepared to support them should hemolysis occur. All patients treated with DS/TMP should be monitored for methemoglobinemia twice weekly for the duration of therapy, beginning the second week. If the methemoglobin level reaches 20 percent and the patient is symptomatic, therapy should be changed and the patients treated with methylene blue.

Lee et al. evaluated serum levels from 18 patients treated with dapsone alone and 30 patients treated with DS/TMP. They found that patients who were treated with combination therapy had significantly higher dapsone levels than those treated with dapsone alone (2.1 vs 1.5 micrograms/ml), significantly higher rates of methemoglobinemia (67 percent vs. 11 percent), adverse reactions requiring a change in therapy (30 percent vs. 0 percent), and rash (40 percent vs. 17 percent; not significant).[54] Compared to 30 patients treated with TMP/SMX, the 30 patients on DS/TMP had 48 percent higher trimethoprim levels but fewer patients required a change in therapy for adverse reactions (30 percent vs. 57 percent). Thus, both dapsone and trimethoprim affect each other's metabolism, causing higher levels of both drugs than otherwise would be expected. Although dapsone is eliminated from the body by acetylation and oxidative metabolism, acetylation status (rapid vs. slow) appears to have no relationship to the rates of toxicity seen in patients. However, there was a higher proportion of rapid acetylators seen in the study patients than in the general population, raising the possibility that drug metabolism in AIDS patients may be altered.

Cross-toxicity of dapsone (a sulfone) to sulfa drugs is not firmly established; four patients with hypersensitivity reactions to TMP/SMX were treated with dapsone without deleterious effect.[21] In another series, of 21 patients who had adverse reactions to TMP/SMX during initial treatment for PCP and were treated with DS/TMP for their second episodes, only 6 had adverse reactions. Conversely, of nine who had prior reactions to DS, none had problems when taking TMP/SMX for their second episodes.[41]

■ DIFLUOROMETHYLORNITHINE

Difluoromethylornithine (DFMO) has been successful in some patients in whom conventional agents have failed.[25,55,56] The dose ranges from 6 grams/square meter orally to 400 mg/kg/day intravenously, in divided doses. The survival rate of those in whom it is used is approximately 40 percent. Toxicity includes marrow suppression and gastrointestinal disturbances. Relapse after completed therapy is common. Because it has been used only as a salvage regimen, its true efficacy is difficult to assess and its role in treating PCP remains unclear.

■ TRIMETREXATE AND PIRITREXIM

Trimetrexate, a dihydrofolate reductase (DHFR) inhibitor orders of magnitude more efficient than trimethoprim, is presently under investigation.[26] Allegra et al. used trimetrexate (30 mg/square meter given intravenously once daily for 21 days) with leucovorin (20 mg/square meter IV or PO q6h for 23 days) in 49 patients divided into three groups: as salvage regimen in patients failing or intolerant of conventional therapy; as initial therapy in patients with sulfa intolerance; and in patients as initial therapy (along with sulfadiazine 1 gram orally q6h).[57] The response rate was 63 percent in the second group and 70 percent in the others; there were 11 deaths (22 percent). Neutropenia or thrombocytopenia occurred in 12 patients (25 percent), requiring dosage reduction in 9 patients. Renal and hepatic toxicity were uncommon, occurring in two and five patients, respectively (one patient had both). Of the nine patients who had a rash, eight were receiving sulfadiazine. Of concern, 7 of 38 survivors had a documented relapse within three months of therapy. A dose ranging study evaluating various combinations of trimetrexate and leucovorin showed that 45 mg/square meter plus 80 mg/square meter, respectively, was the best combination. Fever, rash, and LFT elevation occurred in 19 percent, 21 percent, and 31 percent of patients, respectively. Overall survival was 85 percent but the relapse rate was 36 percent within 66 days.[58]

Piritrexim, another DHFR inhibitor, is also being considered as a therapeutic agent. This lipid-soluble antifolate has activity against both *P. carinii* and *T. gondii*. It is available in an oral formulation. Its ability to inhibit the *P. carinii* DHFR is slightly better than that of trimetrexate (both are three orders of magnitude more effective than trimethoprim). As with trimetrexate, leucovorin must be administered concomitantly.[59] Studies are presently under way.

■ AEROSOLIZED PENTAMIDINE

At San Francisco General Hospital, a study of 15 patients with first-episode PCP showed that 600 mg of pentamidine administered daily through an aerosol device is effective treatment.[60] All patients had initial arterial oxygen tensions of 50 mm Hg or better. Thirteen of the 15 patients successfully completed the 21-day course of therapy; 1 patient who was also being treated for tuberculosis died of respiratory failure after switching to TMP/SMX. Another patient was switched to TMP/SMX after only one aerosol treatment because he required mechanical ventilation. (The aerosol device was not designed for use in conjunction with mechanical ventilation.)

Twelve patients reported cough as the only adverse local reaction; there were no systemic reactions reported. Serum pentamidine levels ranged from <10 to 32 ng/ml compared to peak levels above 600 ng/ml observed in patients given the standard 4 mg/kg intravenous dose.[42,50] Patients who underwent bronchoscopy 18 to 24 hours after a single aerosol treatment were found to have pentamidine levels of 23 ng/ml and 705 ng/ml in bronchoalveolar lavage supernatant and sediment, respectively, compared to levels of 2.6 ng/ml and 9.3 ng/ml, respectively, in patients who had received intravenous pentamidine.[61] The lack of systemic absorption through the aerosol route may contribute to the low incidence of adverse reactions. A multicenter, double-blind, randomized study of aerosolized pentamidine versus TMP/SMX is now under way.

Conte et al. administered aerosolized pentamidine by weight (4 mg/kg) instead of using a fixed dosage in 13 patients.[44] Excluding 3 patients who had less than four days of therapy, 9 of 10 patients had a successful outcome. Neutropenia occurred in two patients who were taking zidovudine concomitantly. Cough and reversible bronchospasm were the only other adverse reactions reported. Thirteen patients studied by Godfrey-Faussett did poorly when treated by aerosolized pentamidine, but this may have been due to the nebulizer system used (see below).[62,63] Subsequent attempts using the RespirGard II nebulizer by the same group have been more successful (Montgomery B: personal communication). Reports of adverse reactions have included hemoptysis, hypoglycemia, and bronchospasm; the bronchospasm is usually relieved by pretreating with aerosolized bronchodilators.[64,65]

Ten additional patients were treated with aerosolized pentamidine after failing or developing intolerance to conventional therapy, including seven patients who were intolerant to parenteral pentamidine (one patient both failed and was intolerant). All 10 patients successfully completed therapy with aerosolized pentamidine; the only adverse reaction was a cough that responded to metaproterenol (6 patients).[66]

A special word of caution must be added for those administering aerosolized pentamidine for acute PCP therapy. The low rate of systemic absorption (which probably accounts for the low rate of systemic adverse reactions) also precludes any therapeutic benefit in patients who may have extrapulmonary pneumocystis, which is increasingly being reported.

Delivery Systems and Particle Size.   Because aerosolized therapy is a new and radical departure from standard therapy, controversy over the best nebulizer, the optimum dose, the duration of therapy, and other issues continues. Although the "best" nebulizer may not yet be identified, certain characteristics of the aerosolized particles have been identified as important in determining which devices should be used. Studies show that almost all particles with a mass median aerodynamic diameter of greater than 10 microns become impacted in the oropharynx. Most particles of greater than 5 microns do not reach the lower airways. Conversely, 80 percent of particles 0.1–0.5 microns remain suspended in the airways and do not impact in the alveoli. Thus, the optimum device to maximize alveolar deposition should generate particles between 1 and 2 microns in size with a narrow distribution of greater than 90 percent of particles being less than 4 microns (measured at the mouthpiece).[67] The RespirGard II nebulizer used in the study cited above corresponds to these specifications and is estimated to deliver approximately 5 percent to 10 percent of the drug into the alveolar space (30 to 60 mg of the 600 mg in the chamber). Because the amount of pentamidine deposited in the alveoli is a function of the efficiency of the nebulizer output and the fraction of the aerosol that is of appropriate size, various nebulizers may deliver the same amount of drug by varying the initial amount introduced into the chamber. Particle generation by an ultrasonic mechanism (as opposed to those requiring an air source) is desirable, since this permits portability; however, ultrasonic devices are more costly and their ability to generate a uniform particle size may become degraded as the crystal is used repeatedly. Comparison studies of various nebulizers are under way.[63,67]

Because larger particle sizes result in more impaction in the oropharynx or in the larger airways, they may produce coughing and bronchospasm in the patient. Other factors affecting alveolar deposition include the patient's position during therapy, inspiratory flow rates, depth and frequency of respiration, and breath-holding. Pulmonary factors affecting deposition include bronchospasm, emphysema, mucus, and other alveolar-filling processes.

■ CORTICOSTEROID THERAPY

Because of sporadic reports in which patients with PCP inadvertently received corticosteroids and improved, it has been suggested that these agents may be of benefit.[22,23,68,69] In a number of small series, patients treated with corticosteroids in conjunction with routine therapy were compared with patients treated without corticosteroids. Although the steroid-treated groups were usually more severely ill and often required mechanical ventilation, their mortality, time to clinical and radiographic improvement, number of adverse effects, and relapse rate were generally improved over the non-steroid-treated groups.[24,70-74] Survival of steroid-treated patients was increased to levels seen in less severely ill patients. However, some patients were studied retrospectively; the steroid regimens were not standardized and the studies were often small. Preliminary analysis of the first 50 patients in an ongoing randomized, double-blinded study of steroids for patients who responded poorly on conventional therapy at San Francisco General Hospital does not suggest significant advantages in the steroid-treated group (Clement M: unpublished data).

■ PROGNOSTIC INDICATORS

Several studies show that patients with mean serum lactate dehydrogenase (LDH) levels less than 350 International Units (IU) at the time of diagnosis had a better survival rate than those with higher serum LDH levels.[75-77] Most survivors also showed a decline in LDH levels by four to seven days after initiation of therapy. Improved arterial oxygen tensions also correlated with survival.[77] Brenner et al. showed that alveolar–arterial oxygen gradients (A-aDO$_2$) greater than 30 mm Hg were associated with a higher mortality rate and that long-term survival correlated with the severity of interstitial edema seen on initial transbronchial biopsy specimen.[78] The persistence of *P. carinii* organisms on follow-up transbronchial biopsy specimen did not influence the outcome of that particular episode of PCP, but it was associated with decreased long-term survival.

■ THERAPEUTIC STRATEGY

Initial therapy for PCP should be either trimethoprim/sulfamethoxazole or pentamidine. Because the clinical response may be delayed for three to five days in a substantial proportion of patients despite appropriate and effective therapy, patients should be maintained on their initial regimen for five to seven days before a determination of clinical failure is made. Therapeutic failure should be determined on the basis of clinical deterioration and worsening arterial oxygenation.

Adverse effects from both trimethoprim/sulfamethoxazole and pentamidine appear most often during the second week of therapy. Patients experiencing major adverse effects should be switched to the alternative regimen. Some patients unable to tolerate both regimens have been successfully treated with dapsone plus trimethoprim, but clinical trials of DS/TMP as a salvage regimen have not been undertaken. The usual course of treatment is two to three weeks. Although most clinicians prefer the longer course, there has been no randomized study comparing these two lengths of therapy. When patients are switched to an alternate regimen because of therapeutic failure, a minimum of two weeks of effective therapy is desirable.

In San Francisco, dapsone plus trimethoprim has been widely used as initial therapy for mild-to-moderate disease, and with good success. It is preferred by a number of physicians because it appears to have fewer and milder adverse effects than conventional therapy. However, this is not yet widely accepted outside San Francisco as first-line therapy. Because of the drug's availability and the attraction of being able to deliver a drug to "its site of action," aerosolized pentamidine is rapidly becoming popular despite the controversies over optimum dosage and the best nebulizer for drug delivery.[79] Its apparent lack of systemic adverse reactions is attractive; however, its overall efficacy remains unproven. Experience with other alternative regimens is even more limited.

Despite a completed course of therapy and clinical improvement, a patient may still harbor *P. carinii* organisms. This has been documented in bronchial lavage specimens in several studies.[12-17,78] Organisms are seen in approximately 65 percent of patients evaluated after a mean of three weeks of therapy. There has been a single report of a patient who completed therapy for PCP, underwent thoracotomy for a bronchopleural fistula repair, and was found to have negative methenamine-silver and Diff-Quik examinations, although under electron microscopic examination he was found to have trophozoites.[80] The significance of the persistence of these organisms is unclear. Although some clinicians continue to treat patients, repeat bronchoscopy in some asymptomatic patients shows clearance without further therapy. Currently, most clinicians would not administer additional therapy unless the patient's clinical condition warranted it.

■ RESPIRATORY FAILURE

Analyzing 478 episodes of PCP that occurred in San Francisco General Hospital over a five-year period, Wachter et al. found that 11 percent of the patients were admitted to an intensive care unit because of respiratory failure.[27] The mortality rate was 86 percent in 45 patients who required mechanical ventilation; 5 of 9 ICU patients who did not require mechanical ventilation also died in the hospital. The mortality rate was similar whether it was the patient's first episode or subsequent episode of PCP. Of the 54 patients admitted to the ICU because of PCP, only 5 were still alive six months after discharge.

Clinically and physiologically, respiratory failure in AIDS patients with PCP is indistinguishable from adult respiratory distress syndrome (ARDS).[28] Pathologic changes are similar except for the absence of hyaline membranes and hemorrhage in AIDS patient with PCP. Patients with HIV-related acute respiratory failure should be treated in the same fashion as patients with AIDS and counseled with respect to possible outcomes and alternatives.

■ PROPHYLAXIS

Because approximately 40 percent of all AIDS patients have a second episode of PCP (usually in the 12- to 18-month period after the first episode), major efforts have been made to prevent or delay subsequent episodes. Data from 201 patients with first-episode PCP who were followed at San Francisco General Hospital for two years showed that median survival after the first episode was 9.8 months. Eighteen percent of those surviving to six months developed a second episode of PCP. Forty-six percent of the patients surviving to 9 months and 65 percent of those surviving to 18 months developed a second episode of PCP.[81,82]

Trimethoprim/Sulfamethoxazole.   TMP/SMX (1 double strength tab, bid) has been tried by many investigators, but most patients are unable to tolerate the regimen because of nausea, vomiting, rash, fever, or marrow toxicity.[29] Only Fischl and Shafer have been able to maintain 80 percent to 90 percent of their study patients on this regimen.[30,31] In the only completed and published study, Fischl randomized 60 patients with Kaposi's sarcoma to either TMP/SMX twice daily plus leucovorin or nothing.[83] No patient randomized to TMP/SMX developed PCP while on therapy; 4 of 5 developed PCP after stopping the drug because of adverse reactions; 16 of 30 developed PCP in the control group. Fifty percent of the patients on TMP/SMX had an adverse reaction; four of those who stopped had severe erythroderma, and the last had persistent neutropenia.

Fansidar.   Although not used as PCP therapy, Fansidar (25 mg pyrimethamine, 500 mg sulfadoxine) once weekly for prophylaxis has been studied by Hardy at UCLA.[33,84] After a mean follow-up time of 11 months (range, 3 to 27 months) in 60 patients, only 5 patients had a second episode of PCP; 3 had undetectable sulfa levels measured at the time of diagnosis. All recurrences happened in the first nine months of follow-up; in 5 patients the drug was discontinued because of rash. Fischl evaluated 30 patients, of whom 7 failed and 10 experienced adverse reactions. Five patients stopped taking medication;

four because of rash (one with Stevens–Johnson syndrome) and one because of anemia.[85] Five of 21 other patients had recurrences on Fansidar with rashes occurring in 3 patients.[86,87] A single fatality from Fansidar-associated toxic epidermal necrolysis has been reported to the CDC along with four cases of nonfatal Stevens–Johnson syndrome.[88] These reports, along with those of severe cutaneous adverse reactions in non-AIDS patients taking Fansidar as malaria prophylaxis, may have dampened investigators' enthusiasm for this regimen. Gottlieb reported successful administration of Fansidar to patients with previous hypersensitivity reactions by beginning prophylaxis with a half-tablet initially. Details were not included.[89]

Dapsone.   Dapsone alone, although not an appropriate regimen for acute therapy at 100 mg daily (see above), has been suggested as a prophylactic regimen in doses ranging from 25 mg to 100 mg daily. Metroka et al. used 25 mg by mouth four times a day in 221 HIV-infected patients as both primary and secondary prophylaxis.[90] Only two patients receiving prophylaxis developed PCP, in contrast to 19 of 26 patients who refused prophylaxis. Adverse reactions included anemia, LDH elevation, methemoglobinemia, nausea, and skin rash. Because the patient population was mixed, quantitative efficacy was difficult to assess, but the regimen appears promising and studies are ongoing.

Parenteral Pentamidine.   Pentamidine (4 mg/kg monthly, IM or IV) has been used as prophylaxis with promising results in patients who had previously received pentamidine for treatment.[32] Only 2 of 10 treated patients had a recurrence, compared with 7 of 12 patients who had no prophylaxis. Three patients experienced adverse effects not clearly related to its use, but their participation in the study was nonetheless discontinued.

Aerosolized Pentamidine.   Recently, aerosolized pentamidine has gained enormous popularity as potential prophylactic therapy. Since the first report of its use in 1987, a number of trials to evaluate aerosol devices and dosage regimens have begun.

There are no completed aerosol prophylaxis studies published to date; all reports are in abstract form. Dosages used in trials under way range from 30 mg to 300 mg, administered at intervals of two to four weeks; some centers also incorporate an initial loading regimen. From the information available in nine studies, a total of 1252 patients have participated in some form of aerosolized pentamidine prophylaxis.[91-99] At least 563 patients had one or more episodes of PCP before entering the study; the remainder had either symptomatic HIV infection or AIDS with no history of PCP. Evaluable data from these studies suggest that treatment with aerosolized pentamidine at any dose significantly reduces the relapse rate when compared to the relapse rate in patients receiving no prophylaxis. Paulson reports in a letter that at eight months, patients' recurrence rate was 10 percent using aerosolized pentamidine at 2 mg/kg via a Bird aerosol device.[100] However, the optimum regimen has still not been determined.

At San Francisco General Hospital, a community-based trial of aerosolized pentamidine involving 408 patients (256 patients with prior PCP) has been under way for 18 months.[94] Patients were randomized to 30 mg every two weeks, 150 mg every two weeks, or 300 mg every four weeks. Interim results showed a significant difference in the relapse rate among patients with prior PCP (secondary prophylaxis) compared to historical controls (10 percent vs.

45 percent of patients at risk at six months). The most common adverse effects were cough, mild bronchospasm, and a metallic taste in the mouth. There were two reports of rash and a possible hypoglycemic episode that may have been related to the treatments. The rate of pneumothoraces in patients with PCP was not exacerbated by aerosol treatments; available PFT data also did not suggest long-term toxicity.

Interim analysis of data from that trial showed that the 300 mg every four weeks dose regimen was significantly better than the other two arms in reducing the rate of relapse in patients who had prior episodes of PCP. The number of patients remaining in the study and available for follow-up was too small to evaluate efficacy of prophylaxis in patients with no prior episode of PCP. After reviewing the data, the Food and Drug Administration (FDA) concluded that there was sufficient evidence to stop the study and announce a treatment IND for PCP prophylaxis using aerosolized pentamidine. The treatment IND targets HIV infected individuals who have had a history of PCP or have a T-cell count <200/cubic mm. Patients enrolled into the treatment IND will be treated with 300 mg of aerosol pentamidine every four weeks using a RespirGard II (or equivalent) nebulizer.

Although this is the first prophylaxis regimen recognized by the FDA as efficacious for PCP prophylaxis, a number of studies evaluating a variety of oral agents that may prove to be equally or more efficacious are presently under way.

REFERENCES

1. Hughes WT. *Pneumocystis carinii* pneumonia. N Engl J Med 1977; 297:1381-3.
2. Hughes WT. *Pneumocystis carinii*. In: Mandel GL., Douglas RG, eds. Principles and practice of infectious diseases. New York: John Wiley & Sons, 1978; 1549-52.
3. Grant IH, Armstrong D. Management of infectious complications in acquired immunodeficiency syndrome. Am J Med 1986; 81(Suppl 1A):59-72.
4. Kovacs JA, Hiemenz JW, Macher AM, et al. *Pneumocystis carinii* pneumonia: a comparison between patients with the acquired immunodeficiency syndrome and patients with other immunodeficiencies. Ann Intern Med 1984; 100:663-71.
5. Gordin FM, Simon GL, Wofsy CB, Mills J. Adverse reactions to trimethoprim-sulfamethoxazole in patients with the acquired immunodeficiency syndrome. Ann Intern Med 1984; 100:495-9.
6. Wharton JM, Coleman DL, Wofsy CB, et al. Trimethoprim/sulfamethoxazole or pentamidine for *Pneumocystis carinii* pneumonia in the acquired immunodeficiency syndrome. Ann Intern Med 1986; 105:37-44.
7. Masur H. The acquired immunodeficiency syndrome. DM 1983; 30:3-48.
8. Murray JF, Felton CP, Garay SM, et al. Pulmonary complications of the acquired immunodeficiency syndrome: report of a National Heart, Lung, and Blood Institute workshop. N Engl J Med 1984; 310:1682-8.
9. Small CB, Harris CA, Friedland GH, Klein RS. The treatment of *Pneumocystis carinii* pneumonia in the acquired immunodeficiency syndrome. Arch Intern Med 1985; 145:837-40.
10. Waskin H, Sattler FR. Pentamidine-associated dysglycemia [Abstract]. Program and Abstracts of the Twenty-sixth Interscience Conference on Antimicrobial Agents and Chemotherapy. New Orleans: American Society for Microbiology, 1986; 225.
11. Stahl-Bayliss CM, Kalman CM, Laskin OL. Pentamidine induced hypoglycemia in patients with the acquired immune deficiency syndrome. Clin Pharmacol Ther 1986; 39:271-5.
12. DeLorenzo LJ, Maguire GP, Wormser GP, et al. Persistence of *Pneumocystis carinii* pneumonia in the acquired immunodeficiency syndrome. Chest 1985; 88:79-83.
13. Tuazon CU, Delaney MD, Simon GL, et al. Utility of gallium scintigraphy and bronchial washings in the diagnosis and treatment of *Pneumocystis carinii* pneumonia in patients with the acquired immune deficiency syndrome. Am Rev Respir Dis 1985; 132:1087-92.
14. Catterall JR, Potasman I, Remington JS. *Pneumocystis carinii* pneumonia in the patient with AIDS. Chest 1985; 88:758-62.
15. Hartman B, Koss M, Hui A, et al. *Pneumocystis carinii* pneumonia in the acquired immunodeficiency syndrome (AIDS). Chest 1985; 87:603-7.
16. Coleman DL, Hattner RS, Luce JM, et al. Correlation between gallium scanning and fiberoptic bronchoscopy in patients with *P. carinii* pneumonia and AIDS. Am Rev Respir Dis 1984; 130:1166.

17. Shelhamer JH, Ognibene FP, Macher AM, et al. Persistence of *Pneumocystis carinii* in lung tissue of acquired immunodeficiency syndrome patients treated for pneumocystis pneumonia. Am Rev Resp Dis 1984; 130:1161-5.

18. Leoung GS, Mills J, Hopewell P, et al. Dapsone trimethoprim is effective treatment for *Pneumocystis carinii* pneumonia in patients with the acquired immune deficiency syndrome. Ann Intern Med 1986; 105:45-8.

19. Mills J, Leoung G, Medina I, et al. Dapsone is less effective than standard therapy for pneumocystis pneumonia in AIDS patients. Annual Meeting of the American Thoracic Society. Kansas City, 1986; A:184. abstract.

20. Medina I, Leoung G, Mills J, et al. Oral therapy for Pneumocystis carinii pneumonia in AIDS. A randomized double blind trial of trimethoprim/sulfamethoxazole (S) versus dapsone trimethoprim (D) for first-episode Pneumocystis carinii pneumonia in AIDS [Abstract]. III International AIDS Conference. Washington, D.C., 1987; 208.

21. Edelson PJ, Metroka CE, Friedman-Kien A. Dapsone, trimethoprim-sulfamethoxazole, and the acquired immunodeficiency syndrome. Ann Intern Med 1985; 103:963.

22. Foltzer MA, Hannan SE, Kozak AJ. Pneumocystis pneumonia: response to corticosteroids. JAMA 1985; 253:979.

23. MacFadden DK, Edelson JD, Rebuck AS. *Pneumocystis carinii* pneumonia in the acquired immune deficiency syndrome: Response to inadvertent steroid therapy. Can Med Assoc J 1985; 132: 1161-3.

24. Walmsley S, Salit IE, Brunton J, Krajden S. Corticosteroid therapy for pneumocystis pneumonia in AIDS [Abstract]. Program and abstracts of the Twenty-sixth Interscience Conference on Antimicrobial Agents and Chemotherapy. American Society for Microbiology. New Orleans 1986; 224.

25. Golden JA, Sjoerdsma A, Santi DV. *Pneumocystis carinii* pneumonia treated with ∝-difluoromethylornithine. A prospective study among patients with the acquired immunodeficiency syndrome. West J Med 1984; 141:613-23.

26. Allegra CJ, Drake J, Swan J, et al. Preliminary results of a phase I-II trial for the treatment of *Pneumocystis carinii* pneumonia (PCP) using a potent lipid-soluble dihydrofolate reductase (DHFR) inhibitor, trimetrexate (TMTX) [Abstract]. Twenty-sixth Interscience Conference on Antimicrobial Agents and Chemotherapy. New Orleans 1986; 224.

27. Wachter RM, Luce JM, Turner J, et al. Intensive care of patients with the acquired immunodeficiency syndrome: outcome and changing patterns of utilization. Am Rev Respir Dis 1986; 134:891-6.

28. Maxfield RA, Sorkin JB, Fazzini EP, et al. Respiratory failure in patients with acquired immunodeficiency syndrome and *Pneumocystis carinii* pneumonia. Crit Care Med 1986; 14:443-9.

29. Kaplan LD, Wong R, Wofsy C, Volberding PA. Trimethoprim sulfamethoxazole (TMP-SMZ) prophylaxis of *Pneumocystis carinii* pneumonia (PCP) in AIDS [Abstract]. Second International Conference on AIDS. Paris, 1986; 53.

30. Fischl MA, Dickinson GM. Trimethoprim-sulfamethoxazole prophylaxis of *Pneumocystis carinii* pneumonia in the acquired immunodeficiency syndrome [Abstract]. Twenty-fifth Interscience Conference on Antimicrobial Agents and Chemotherapy. Minneapolis 1985; 171.

31. Shafer RW, Seitzman PA, Tapper ML. Successful prophylaxis of pneumocystis pneumonia with trimethoprim-sulfamethoxazole in AIDS patients with previous allergic reactions [Abstract]. Second International Conference on AIDS. Paris, 1986; 54.

32. Busch DF, Follansbee SE. Continuation therapy with pentamidine isethionate for prevention of relapse of Pneumocystis carinii pneumonia in AIDS [Abstract]. Second International Conference on AIDS. Paris, 1986; 38.

33. Hardy D, Wolfe PR, Gottlieb MS, et al. Fansidar prophylaxis for *Pneumocystis carinii* pneumonia (PCP) [Abstract]. First International Conference on Acquired Immunodeficiency Syndrome. Atlanta, 1985; 25.

34. Hurley P, Weikel C, Temeles D, et al. Unusual remission of *Pneumocystis carinii* pneumonia in a patient with the acquired immune deficiency syndrome. Am J Med 1987; 82:645-8.

35. Wofsy CB. Use of trimethoprim-sulfamethoxazole in the treatment of *Pneumocystis carinii* pneumonitis in patients with acquired immunodeficiency syndrome. Rev Infect Dis 1987; 9(Suppl 2):S184-S94.

36. Borucki MJ, Matzke DS, Pollard RB. Tremor induced by trimethoprim-sulfamethoxazole in patients with the acquired immunodeficiency syndrome (AIDS). Ann Intern Med 1988; 109:77-8.

37. Liu LX, Seward SJ, Crumpacker CS. Intravenous trimethoprim-sulfamethoxazole and ataxia. Ann Intern Med 1986; 104:448.

38. Sattler FR, Cowan R, Nielsen DM, Ruskin J. Trimethoprim-sulfamethoxazole compared with pentamidine for treatment of *Pneumocystis carinii* pneumonia in the acquired immunodeficiency syndrome. A prospective, noncrossover study. Ann Intern Med 1988; 109:280-7.

39. Wordell CJ, Hauptman SP. Treatment of *Pneumocystis carinii* pneumonia in patients with AIDS. Clin Pharm 1988; 7:514-27.

40. McLean I, Lucas CR, Mashford ML, Harman PJ. Modified trimethoprim-sulfamethoxazole doses in *Pneumocystis carinii* pneumonia. Lancet 1987; 2:857-8.

41. Medina I, Feigal D, Wofsy C. Cross-allergy to sulfonamides/sulfones (Sulfa), and folic antagonists in AIDS [Abstract]. III International Conference on AIDS. Washington, D.C., 1987; 208,F.3.1.

42. Salamone FR, Cunha BA. Update on pentamidine for the treatment of *Pneumocystis carinii* pneumonia. Clin Pharm 1988; 7:501-10.

43. Sensakovic JW, Suarez M, Perez G, et al. Pentamidine treatment of *Pneumocystis carinii* pneumonia in the acquired immunodeficiency syndrome. Association with acute renal failure and myoglobinuria. Arch Intern Med 1985; 145:2247.

44. Conte JE Jr, Hollander H, Golden JA. Inhaled or reduced-dose intravenous pentamidine for *Pneumocystis carinii* pneumonia. A pilot study. Ann Intern Med 1987; 107:495-8.

45. Waskin H, Stehr-Green JK, Helmick CG, Sattler FR. Risk factors for hypoglycemia associated with pentamidine therapy for pneumocystis pneumonia. JAMA 1988; 260:345-7.

46. Salmeron S, Petitpretz P, Katlama C, et al. Pentamidine and pancreatitis. Ann Intern Med 1986; 105:140-1.

47. Zuger A, Wolf BZ, el-Sadr W, et al. Pentamidine-associated fatal acute pancreatitis. JAMA 1986; 256:2383-5.

48. Donnelly H, Bernard EM, Rothkotter H, et al. Distribution of pentamidine in patients with AIDS. J Infect Dis 1988; 157:985-9.

49. Donnelly H, Bernard EM, Rothkotter HE, et al. Distribution of pentamidine in humans [Abstract]. Twenty-Sixth Interscience Conference on Antimicrobial Agents and Chemotherapy. New Orleans 1986; 696.

50. Conte JE Jr, Upton RA, Phelps RT, et al. Use of a specific and sensitive assay to determine pentamidine pharmacokinetics in patients with AIDS. J Infect Dis 1986; 154:923-9.

51. Conte JE Jr, Upton RA, Lin ET. Pentamidine pharmacokinetics in patients with AIDS with impaired renal function. J Infect Dis 1987; 156:885-90.

52. Mills J, Leoung G, Medina I, et al. Dapsone treatment of *Pneumocystis carinii* pneumonia in the acquired immunodeficiency syndrome. Antimicrob Agents Chemother 1988; 32:1057-60.

53. Medina I, Mills J, Leoung G, et al. Oral therapy for *Pneumocystis carinii* pneumonia in AIDS: a randomized double blind trial comparing trimethoprim and sulfamethoxazole with dapsone and trimethoprim (submitted for publication).

54. Lee BL, Medina I, Benowitz NL, et al. Dapsone, trimethoprim and sulfamethoxazole plasma levels during treatment of Pneumocystis pneumonia in patients with acquired immunodeficiency syndrome: evidence of drug interactions. Ann Intern Med 1989; 110:606-11.

55. Gilman TM, Paulson YJ, Boylen CT, et al. Eflornithine treatment of *Pneumocystis carinii* pneumonia in AIDS. JAMA 1986; 256:2197-8.

56. McLees BD, Barlow JLR, Kuzma RJ, et al. Studies on successful eflornithine treatment of *Pneumocystis carinii* pneumonia (PCP) in AIDS patients failing conventional therapy [Abstract]. III International Conference on AIDS. Washington, D.C., 1987; 155,TH.4.2.

57. Allegra CJ, Chabner BA, Tuazon CU, et al. Trimetrexate for the treatment of *Pneumocystis carinii* pneumonia in patients with the acquired immunodeficiency syndrome. N Engl J Med 1987; 317:978-85.

58. Sattler F, Allegra C, Tuazon C, et al. Trimetrexate and leucovorin for *Pneumocystis carinii* pneumonia (PCP) [Abstract]. IV International Conference on AIDS. Stockholm, 1988; 1:422, 7177.

59. Kovacs JA, Allegra CJ, Swan JC, et al. Potent antipneumocystis and antitoxoplasma activities of piritrexim, a lipid-soluble antifolate. Antimicrob Agents Chemother 1988; 32:430-3.

60. Montgomery AB, Debs RJ, Luce JM, et al. Aerosolised pentamidine as sole therapy for *Pneumocystis carinii* pneumonia in patients with acquired immunodeficiency syndrome. Lancet 1987; 2:480-3.

61. Montgomery AB, Debs RJ, Luce JM, et al. Selective delivery of pentamidine to the lung by aerosol. Am Rev Respir Dis 1988; 137:477-8.

62. Godfrey-Faussett P, Miller RF, Semple SJ. Nebulised pentamidine. Lancet 1988; 1:645-6.

63. O'Doherty MJ, Thomas S, Page C, et al. Differences in relative efficiency of nebulisers for pentamidine administration. Lancet 1988; 2:1283-5.

64. Jesuthasan AJ, Datta AK, Hamilton R, et al. Aerosolised pentamidine. Lancet 1987; 2:971-2.

65. Karboski JA, Godley PJ. Inhaled pentamidine and hypoglycemia. Ann Intern Med 1988; 108:490.

66. Montgomery AB, Debs RJ, Luce JM, et al. Aerosolized pentamidine as second-line therapy in patients with the acquired immunodeficiency syndrome and *Pneumocystis carinii* pneumonia. Chest 1989; 95:747-50.

67. Corkery KJ, Luce JM, Montgomery AB. Aersolized pentamidine for treatment and prophylaxis of *Pneumocystis carinii*: an update. Respir Care 1988; 33:676-86.

68. Rankin JA, Pella JA. Radiographic resolution of *Pneumocystis carinii* pneumonia in response to corticosteroid therapy. Am Rev Respir Dis 1987; 136:182-3.

69. Foltzer MA, Hannan SE, Kozak AJ. Pneumocystis pneumonia: response to corticosteroids. JAMA 1985; 253:979.

70. Mottin D, Denis M, Dombret H, et al. Role for steroids in treatment of *Pneumocystis carinii* pneumonia in AIDS. Lancet 1987; 2:519.

71. MacFadden DK, Edelson JD, Hyland RH, et al. Corticosteroids as adjunctive therapy in treatment of *Pneumocystis carinii* pneumonia in patients with acquired immunodeficiency syndrome. Lancet 1987; 1:1477-9.

72. Lambertus MW, Goetz MB. Treatment of pneumocystis pneumonia in AIDS. N Engl J Med 1988; 318:988-90.

73. Skorde J, Heise W, L'Age M. Steroids in treatment of severe *Pneumocystis carinii* pneumonia in AIDS [Abstract]. IV International Conference on AIDS. Stockholm, 1988; 1:418, 7163.

74. Jubran A, Matzke D, Pollard RB. Effect of corticosteroids on immediate survival from *Pneumocystis carinii* pneumonia (PCP) in patients with acquired immunodeficiency syndrome (AIDS) [Abstract]. III International Conference on AIDS. Washington, D.C., 1987; 133,WP.140.

75. Zaman MK, White DA. Serum lactate dehydrogenase levels and *Pneumocystis carinii* pneumonia. Diagnostic and prognostic significance. Am Rev Respir Dis 1988; 137:796-800.

76. Medina I, Mills J, Wofsy C. Serum lactate dehydrogenase levels (LDH) in *Pneumocystis carinii* pneumonia (PCP) in AIDS: possible indicator and predictor of disease activity [Abstract]. III International Conference on AIDS. Washington, D.C., 1987; 109,W.5.5.

77. Kales CP, Murren JR, Torres RA, Crocco JA. Early predictors of in-hospital mortality for *Pneumocystis carinii* pneumonia in the acquired immunodeficiency syndrome. Arch Intern Med 1987; 147:1413-7.

78. Brenner M, Ognibene FP, Lack EE, et al. Prognostic factors and life expectancy of patients with acquired immunodeficiency syndrome and *Pneumocystis carinii* pneumonia. Am Rev Respir Dis 1987; 136:1199-206.

79. Armstrong D, Bernard E. Aerosol pentamidine. Ann Intern Med 1988; 109:852-4.

80. El-Sadr W, Sidhu G. Persistence of trophozoites after successful treatment of *Pneumocystis carinii* pneumonia. Ann Intern Med 1986; 105:889-90.

81. Rainer CA, Feigal DW, Leoung G, et al. Prognosis and natural history of *Pneumocystis carinii* pneumonia: Indicators for early and late survival [Abstract]. III International Conference on AIDS. Washington, D.C., 1987; 189,THP.154.

82. Feigal DW, Edison R, Leoung GS, et al. Recurrent *Pneumocystis carinii* pneumonia (PCP) in 201 patients before AZT or prophylaxis: implications for clinical trials [Abstract]. IV International Conference on AIDS. Stockholm, 1988; 1:416, 7153.

83. Fischl MA, Dickinson GM, La Voie L. Safety and efficacy of sulfamethoxazole and trimethoprim chemoprophylaxis for *Pneumocystis carinii* pneumonia in AIDS. JAMA 1988; 259:1185-9.

84. Hardy D, Wolfe PR, Gottlieb MS, et al. Long-term follow-up of Fansidar prophylaxis for *Pneumocystis carinii* pneumonia (PCP) in patients with AIDS [Abstract]. III International Conference on AIDS. Washington, D.C., 1987; 202,THP.232.

85. Fischl MA, Dickinson GM. Fansidar prophylaxis of pneumocystis pneumonia in the acquired immunodeficiency syndrome. Ann Intern Med 1986; 105:629.

86. Gottlieb MS, Knight S, Mitsuyasu R, et al. Prophylaxis of *Pneumocystis carinii* infection in AIDS with pyrimethamine-sulfadoxine. Lancet 1984; 2:398-9.

87. Frissen PH, Stronkhorst A, Eeftinck-Schattenkerk JK, Danner SA. Fansidar and *Pneumocystis carinii* pneumonia. Ann Intern Med 1988; 108:638-9.

88. Fansidar-associated fatal reaction in an HIV-infected man. MMWR 1988; 37:571-2, 577.

89. Gottlieb MS, Young LS. Adverse reactions to pyrimethamine-sulfadoxine in context of AIDS. Lancet 1985; 1:1389.

90. Metroka CE, Braun N, Josefberg H, Jacobus D. Successful chemoprophylaxis for *Pneumocystis carinii* pneumonia with dapsone in patients with AIDS and ARC [Abstract]. IV International Conference on AIDS. Stockholm, 1988; 1:417, 7157.

91. Bernard E, Schmitt H, Pagel L, et al. Safety and effectiveness of aerosol pentamidine for prevention of PCP in patients with AIDS [Abstract]. Twenty-seventh Interscience Conference on Antimicrobial Agents and Chemotherapy. New York 1987; 944.

92. Smith DE, Herd DA, Hawkins DA, et al. *Pneumocystis carinii* pneumonia prophylaxis with inhaled pentamidine [Abstract]. IV International Conference on AIDS. Stockholm, 1988; 1:418, 7164.

93. Conte JE Jr, Chernoff D, Feigal D, et al. Once-monthly inhaled pentamidine for the prevention of *Pneumocystis carinii* pneumonia (PCP) [Abstract]. IV International Conference on AIDS. Stockholm, 1988; 1:419, 7165.

94. Leoung GS, Montgomery AB, Abrams DA, et al. Aerosol pentamidine for *Pneumocystis carinii* (PCP) pneumonia: a randomized trial of 439 patients [Abstract]. IV International Conference on AIDS. Stockholm, 1988; 1:419, 7166.

95. Gabin SJ, Poscher HL. Nebulized pentamidine isethionate for prophylaxis of *Pneumocystis carinii* pneumonia [Abstract]. IV International Conference on AIDS. Stockholm, 1988; 1:419, 7168.

96. Bernard EM, Schmitt HJ, Lifton A, et al. Prevention of *Pneumocystis carinii* pneumonia with aerosol pentamidine [Abstract]. IV International Conference on AIDS. Stockholm, 1988; 1:420, 7169.

97. Van Gundy KP, Akil B, Bill R, Boylen CT. The effect of inhaled pentamidine on the suppression of *Pneumocystis carinii* pneumonia in patients with the acquired immunodeficiency syndrome (AIDS) [Abstract]. IV International Conference on AIDS. Stockholm, 1988; 1:420, 7170.

98. Van Gundy KP, Boylen CT, Weisman J, et al. Community study of the effect of inhaled pentamidine on the prevention of *Pneumocystis carinii* pneumonia in HIV-positive patients [Abstract]. IV International Conference on AIDS. Stockholm, 1988; 1:420, 7171.

99. Girard PM, Lepretre A, Michon C, et al. Aerosolized pentamidine (PM) for prophylaxis of pneumocystosis (PCP) in AIDS patients [Abstract]. IV International Conference on AIDS. Stockholm, 1988; 1:420, 7172.

100. Lin GA, Paulson YJ, Boylen CT, et al. Chemoprophylaxis for *Pneumocystis carinii* pneumonia in AIDS. JAMA 1988; 260:921-5.

Cryptosporidiosis

Constance B. Wofsy, M.D.

C ryptosporidium is a coccidian parasite that produces chronic profuse watery diarrhea in immunocompromised individuals, including AIDS patients, and serves as a diagnostic marker for AIDS if infection is present for four weeks or longer. Diagnosis in stool requires special laboratory techniques such as acid-fast stain, iodine wet preparation, or a modified sugar flotation technique. Diagnosis may be established on bowel biopsy as well. No effective treatment has been identified either in vitro or in human or animal trials. Treatment is therefore largely supportive.

■ EPIDEMIOLOGY

Cryptosporidium is an intestinal protozoan parasite of the subclass Coccidia, well described in the literature as a cause of self-limited diarrheal disease in a wide variety of vertebrate animals, including mammals, birds, and reptiles.[1] Interspecies and intraspecies spread of infection is well documented experimentally.[1] The first human case of cryptosporidiosis was reported in 1975. By 1983, there were 27 published case reports, excellently summarized by Navin in 1984.[2] Since then, the parasite has gained increased recognition as a cause of diarrhea in adults and children.[30] The first human cases were diagnosed primarily by bowel biopsy in individuals with severe diarrhea and immunosuppressive disorders.[3,4]

In the early 1980s, with the identification of cryptosporidium in homosexual men with AIDS,[5] a less invasive means of diagnosis was needed, and a variety of laboratory techniques were perfected to allow detection of the oocysts in stool specimens.[6] Thereafter, many institutions reported their experiences with cryptosporidium in homosexual men and others with AIDS.[3,7,8] Because of AIDS, laboratories became prepared to evaluate stool for cryptosporidium, and reports from Finland, Australia, Massachusetts, and South Carolina showed that cryptosporidium is actually a very frequent cause of diarrhea in immunologically normal individuals.[9-12]

In Finland, 9 percent of hospitalized, immunologically normal patients evaluated for cryptosporidium were actually infected with this intestinal parasite. All of these patients had self-limited disease with an incubation period of 4 to 12 days. All gave a history of travel.[9] In Australia in 1983, Tzipori reviewed 884 hospitalized patients with gastroenteritis. Thirty-six (4.1 percent) were excreting cryptosporidium oocysts, only five of whom also had another enteric pathogen.[10] In 1983, all stool specimens submitted for ova and parasite examination at Massachusetts General Hospital were scrutinized for cryptosporidium; 2.8 percent of 2821 stools were positive. Of the 47 patients whose stools revealed cryptosporidium, all but 4 were otherwise healthy hosts. Thirty-four patients were index cases and 13 had secondary infection.[11] In 1986, at the Medical University of South Carolina, cryptosporidium was found in 42 percent of stools showing any parasitic infection.[12] In these studies, transmission patterns showed spread within families, nursery schools, and from person to person.

Transmission from animal to human is well documented in a report of self-limited cryptosporidium infection after experimental exposure to infected calves.[13] A researcher exposed to a coughing, experimentally-infected rabbit developed a self-limited diarrhea five days after exposure.[14] A waterborne outbreak of cryptosporidium with an attack rate of 34 percent occurred in normal persons after contamination of the community water supply by an artesian well.[15] In 1985, cryptosporidium was recognized as a cause of a traveler's diarrhea after return from Mexico.[16] Most disturbingly, nosocomial transmission was reported in 1985 when 31 percent of hospital workers with close contact with a cryptosporidium-infected AIDS patient developed symptoms or laboratory evidence of infection. In contrast, only 3 of 18 control personnel had antibody to cryptosporidium, and none had symptoms.[17] This study documented transmission from person to person in the hospital setting among a population expected to be following excellent infection-control techniques. It also noted serologic evidence of widespread infection among hospital personnel in general.[17]

Cryptosporidium is a frequent cause of infection in patients who already have an AIDS diagnosis, usually occurring late in the course of disease. It constitutes the initial diagnosis of AIDS if at least four weeks of chronic diarrhea occurs in a person without any other reason for immunodeficiency.[6,18]

■ MICROBIOLOGY AND PATHOPHYSIOLOGY

Cryptosporidium is a member of the general family of organisms including *Toxoplasma gondii* and isospora. It was first described in 1907 and was initially thought to be host-specific for the various vertebrate animals that are infected. Subsequent studies show that there is considerably less host specificity than was once thought. The life cycle is similar to that of other organisms in the class Sporozoa. Hardy oocysts are shed in the feces of infected animals and are immediately infectious to others. In humans, the organisms can be found in the pharynx, esophagus, stomach, duodenum, jejunum, ileum, appendix, colon, and rectum.[2] Various case reports of patients with AIDS describe infection in the gallbladder[19-21] and lung.[22-25] The organism is 4 to 5 micrometers in diameter, about the size of a yeast, with which it is most frequently confused on routine stool examination. On light microscopy of hematoxylin-and-eosin-stained intestinal biopsies, the darkly staining organisms are located extracellularly, lined up at the tips of the microvilli of the epithelial brush border.[7,19]

Electron microscopy has been helpful in revealing the life cycle of the organism and in defining changes in villus architecture. Even with severe infection, the villus structure remains nearly normal. Cryptosporidial forms in all stages of development may be seen at the surface of the villus epithelium. A modification of the epithelial surface membrane of the microvillus encloses the parasite in a parasitic vacuole at the attachment pole.[26] At the attachment site, secretory granules are seen, and unique tubuloreticular structures of unknown function are observed on electron microscopy in numerous patients with AIDS, even in the absence of cryptosporidium. These structures are not found in non-AIDS patients with other chronic inflammatory intestinal disorders.[27]

Although the mechanism for the profound watery diarrhea has not been found, the lack of structural abnormalities[26,27] supports the hypothesis of a cholera-like enterotoxin.[2] The full extent of immunologic deficits that lead to the development of cryptosporidiosis has not been described. However, the disease has occurred in individuals with isolated defects in either cellular or humoral immune function.[4] The persistence of symptoms in immunosuppressed individuals suggests that symptoms and chronicity are related to the degree of immunocompromise[6] and that cryptosporidium can undergo multiple cycles of its life cycle in the bowel of the immunodeficient host.[2] Despite production of antibodies, sustained immunity does not occur.[28]

The lack of a suitable animal model for chronic cryptosporidiosis has impeded studies of this infection. However, the in vitro isolation of cryptosporidium was recently achieved in cultured human fetal lung cells. This development will lead the way to the in vitro study of cell cycles and the evaluation of therapeutic agents.[29]

■ CLINICAL PRESENTATION

In otherwise healthy hosts, the clinical presentation of cryptosporidiosis is well described.[1,2,11] The disease is highly infectious; it is transmitted from person to person or animal to person and has an incubation period of 5 to 14 days. Infection results in a self-limited diarrhea that lasts from 4 to 20 days and is associated with abdominal pain and cramping, nausea and vomiting, low-grade fever, and anorexia. Short-term carriage of cryptosporidium in asymptomatic individuals is known to occur.[2]

Cryptosporidiosis was first reported in AIDS patients in November 1982, when the disease was described in 21 males.[5] Patients had chronic profuse watery diarrhea, a stool frequency of 6 to 26 bowel movements per day, and stool volumes of 1 to 17 liters per day (mean: 3.6 liters). Diagnosis was established by small-bowel biopsy, large-bowel biopsy, or microscopic stool examination. Since then, series of 2 to 10 patients with cryptosporidiosis have been reported at various institutions seeing large numbers of AIDS patients.[6-8,19,31,32] Cryptosporidiosis tends to appear late in the course of AIDS, when many other opportunistic infections or Kaposi's sarcoma are also present.

Although cryptosporidiosis is typically associated with a severe, profuse, usually chronic diarrhea, the degree of symptomatology is highly variable. Spontaneous cures have been described. Abdominal pain and cramping, along with anorexia, nausea, vomiting, weight loss or profound wasting, are common. Low-grade fever may be present. Malabsorption, documented by abnormal D-xylose and abnormalities of 72-hour fecal fat, is frequently described.[6,7,31] The situation is confused, however, by the finding of similar malabsorption associated with chronic inflammation of the lamina propria in AIDS patients with no evidence of intestinal parasites or enteric pathogens.[33] Thus, malabsorption cannot always be attributed to cryptosporidiosis. Despite the usual severity of the disease, asymptomatic cryptosporidium may occur even in patients with AIDS.[34]

Symptoms of cryptosporidiosis are exactly mimicked by infection with another coccidian parasite, *Isospora belli*, which can also be identified by special stool examination.[7] A unique feature of cryptosporidiosis in AIDS, compared with that in immunocompetent hosts, is that cryptosporidium bowel infection may be associated with simultaneous infections of the intestinal mucosa by other organisms, including cytomegalovirus (CMV)[6,34] or giardia.[33] In addition to infection at multiple sites along the entire gastrointestinal tract, cryptosporidium cholecystitis has been reported in a number of patients with AIDS.[19-21]

Biliary tract disease can be characterized symptomatically by severe abdominal pain and fever and radiographically by dilation of the biliary tree and stenosis of the papilla of Vater, along with laboratory evidence of cholestasis. Biliary cryptosporidiosis is diagnosed by finding the parasite in histologic sections of the gallbladder.[20] Concomitant CMV infection may play a role in symptomatology.[34] Cryptosporidium may also cause symptomatic interstitial pulmonary infection indistinguishable from pneumocystis. Organisms can be found in respiratory secretions and on the mucosal surface of epithelium.[22-25] Cryptosporidium is a unique pathogen because it can establish the diagnosis of AIDS in certain patients, is associated with profound symptomatology, and may be seen outside of the intestine, specifically in the gallbladder and respiratory tree. Disseminated disease to other organs has not been described.

■ DIAGNOSIS

Diagnosis can be established by biopsy of the large or small bowel, although the infection is more readily identified in the small bowel.[5] Hematoxylin-and-eosin-stained specimens reveal darkly staining structures several microns in diameter at the tips of intestinal microvilli.[1,2,7,19] Stool testing is less invasive than bowel biopsy and is preferred for screening. Because the 4- to 5-mm oocysts are about the same size as a yeast and cannot be distinguished by routine ova and parasite testing, a variety of special techniques has been developed for detecting oocysts in the stool of infected individuals (see color plates 6.5.5.a and b).

A three-step stool examination is recommended because of the need to screen large numbers of susceptible individuals. This includes: (1) a preliminary differential determination by an iodine-stained wet mount in which cryptosporidia are colorless and yeast are brown; (2) a modified Kinyoun acid-fast stain in which the oocysts stain red and yeast stain green; and (3) the Sheathers sugar cover-slip flotation method, a more laborious test that concentrates oocysts and allows quantitation of oocysts per high-power field.[35] Other techniques include formalin concentration, Giemsa, trichrome, periodic acid–Schiff (PAS), acridine orange, auramine–rhodamine, and a variety of modifications of various acid-fast techniques.[24,35,36] Garcia compared 15 methods for detecting cryptosporidium oocysts and evaluated ease of recognition, organism morphology, and organism quantification. The modified Ziehl–Neelsen carbol-fuchsin stain on 10 percent formalin-preserved stool received the highest overall recommendation.[36] Some cryptosporidial infections are characterized by production of atypical oocysts that require entirely different techniques for identification.[39] The clinician must make a special request in most hospital microbiology laboratories for proper screening tests for cryptosporidium.

Serologic techniques have recently been developed to detect antibodies to cryptosporidium by indirect immunofluorescence. Seroconversion accompanies recovery from infection in immunocompetent individuals; titers remain high at 1:40 or 1:640 for at least one year. The antibody is presumably not protective and has very little or no cross-reactivity with other coccidia, such as toxoplasma or isospora.[37] Serologic techniques were used to evaluate nosocomial transmission in hospital personnel caring for an AIDS patient actively excreting cryptosporidium in 1985, and 31 percent of personnel directly exposed had an antibody titer of 1:10 or greater, in contrast to 17 percent of control personnel with little exposure.[17] Serologic testing is not useful in the diagnosis of acute cryptosporidiosis because antibodies may not be present in persons with deficiencies of humoral immunity and the antibody does not appear until some time after infection. It should be used only for retrospective diagnosis or epidemiologic studies.

Contrast radiographic studies are likewise not diagnostic. However, 13 of 16 individuals with cryptosporidiosis showed abnormalities in barium studies of the stomach or small intestine, including prominence of mucosal folds and moderate or marked dilation of the small intestine. The radiographic changes are nonspecific.[38] Other routine laboratory tests, such as complete blood count and liver function, are not helpful in establishing a diagnosis of cryptosporidiosis.

■ TREATMENT

The response to treatment of cryptosporidium infection has been abysmal among AIDS patients. In fact, no effective treatment has been established in animal studies or in vitro, or in human clinical trials. In animal studies, none of 25 different compounds that might be expected to show efficacy in coccidian infections was useful in treating cryptosporidial disease.[1] In 1984, Navin summarized the response to treatment of 40 immunodeficient patients with cryptosporidiosis who had received a total of 20 different agents. The most commonly used drugs were trimethoprim/sulfamethoxazole in 21 patients, furazolidone in 15 patients, metronidazole in 9 patients, and pyrimethamine and sulfa in 7. Out of 79 treatment courses in 40 patients, only 6 courses resulted in improvement, and only 2 courses resulted in recovery. There was no consistency in medication leading to improvement or recovery in the small number who responded.[2] Other published series confirm the lack of response to therapy.[6-8,19,31]

Treatment has therefore focused on supportive care and symptomatic relief, using fluid and electrolyte replacement, antispasmodics, antidiarrheals, antiemetics, and, in the case of severe biliary obstruction, occasional T-tube placement.

The only drug that has shown a glimmer of promise is spiramycin. Spiramycin is a macrolide antibiotic closely related to erythromycin. It has little toxicity. It is used in Europe and Canada for the treatment of a variety of infections, including toxoplasmosis. It is manufactured by Rhone Poulenc and is available in the United States solely for investigational use. In 1982, the Centers for Disease Control reported results of spiramycin treatment in 21 AIDS patients with cryptosporidiosis.[5] Three out of 13 were cured after three to four weeks of spiramycin (given as 1 g three or four times a day). These patients remained free of symptoms or evidence of cryptosporidium after not taking spiramycin for a period of six to seven months. All three had AIDS diagnoses (one with Kaposi's sarcoma, and the other two with pneumocystis pneumonia). Three others showed symptomatic improvement but continued to shed oocysts in their stools.

Portnoy described 10 patients with AIDS who responded to treatment with spiramycin. Five patients had complete resolution of symptoms and four had partial resolution.[40] In New York, 10 episodes of diarrhea in seven AIDS and three symptomatic HIV-infected patients were treated with spiramycin (4 g per day for three weeks). Two of the AIDS patients had a microbiologic response but persistent diarrhea; five had persistent infection. Two of the three symptomatic, non-AIDS patients had both a microbiologic and symptomatic response, but four of five who remained untreated also had spontaneous resolution.[41] A double-blinded prospective study comparing spiramycin to placebo in 39 malnourished South African children with cryptosporidial diarrhea demonstrated no therapeutic benefit of spiramycin.[44] These data demonstrate the inconsistency of results and point out the need for controlled trials.

No in vitro studies suggest the mechanism of resistance to therapy. Failure to respond is not simply a consequence of severe immunologic impairment, because none of the numerous therapeutic options succeeds in vitro or prevents the acquisition of infection in exposed, immunologically competent animals.[1] Total parenteral nutrition has been used in patients with very serious diarrheal illness and malabsorption due to persistent cryptosporidiosis,[6,31] but its usefulness has not been examined in a consistent, prospective fashion. A long-acting somatostatin analog, SMS 201-995, provided substantial relief in one very symptomatic patient.[45] Further studies of it are under way.

Treatment of cryptosporidiosis consists of supportive care, including nutritional supplementation like Ensure™. The role of parenteral nutrition is unproven. Effective antimicrobials are being sought. Spiramycin is currently undergoing clinical trials and is available on an experimental basis only.

■ OUTCOME

In otherwise healthy individuals, cryptosporidium causes a relatively benign, self-limited infection. Clinical and parasitologic clearing occurs no longer than one month after infection. Cryptosporidiosis accounts for the initial diagnosis of AIDS in 4 percent of patients.[42] It occurs more frequently as the unrelenting immunologic deterioration underlying AIDS progresses. Patients probably die with, rather than of, cryptosporidiosis. There is no proven therapeutic intervention for it beside making the patient as comfortable as possible. In HIV-infected patients with lymphadenopathy or other early stages of HIV infection, cryptosporidium may produce a self-limited infection.[41] Cryptosporidium infection does not constitute a diagnosis of AIDS unless it is present with chronic diarrhea of greater than four weeks' duration in a person with no other reason to be immunocompromised.[18]

■ PREVENTION

Prophylaxis has not been effective in studies of animal infection, nor are there any instances of prophylaxis in humans. It is well documented that infection is passed from person to person, probably by the fecal-oral route. It is particularly common in homosexual men, perhaps as a consequence of anilingus.[6,11,12] Prevention, therefore, rests with preventing transmission through good hygiene, hand washing, and awareness of the risks of direct fecal-oral exposure.

The nosocomial transmission of cryptosporidium infection to hospital personnel is a public-health concern. The hospital is an environment in which reasonable infection-control measures should be in place.[17] When nosocomial cryptosporidium infection is identified, hospital personnel should follow infection-control precautions for enteric infections. In the laboratory, oocysts are very resistant to the usual antiseptic techniques, including iodophor, cresylic acid, sodium hypochlorite, benzalkonium chloride, and sodium hydroxide. However, their infectivity is destroyed by ammonium, formol saline, freeze-drying, and exposure to temperatures below freezing and above 65°C for 30 minutes.[1] Oocysts are also inactivated by a combination of 50 percent sodium hypochlorite and 70 percent ethanol.[43] Caution must be taken in the laboratory because of the risk of laboratory transmission from infected samples.

Cryptosporidiosis is not a reportable disease. Nonetheless, public-health measures support educating all persons infected with or exposed to the infection about the risk of transmission and the need for hygienic precautions. AIDS is a reportable disease, including that subset of patients who have an AIDS diagnosis established because of cryptosporidial diarrhea of four or more weeks' duration.

REFERENCES

1. Tzipori S. Cryptosporidiosis in animals and humans. Microbiol Rev 1983; 47:84-96.

2. Navin TR, Juranek DD. Cryptosporidiosis: clinical, epidemiologic, and parasitologic review. Rev Infect Dis 1984; 6:313-27.

3. Pitlik SD, Fainstein V, Garza D, et al. Human cryptosporidiosis: spectrum of disease. Report of six cases and review of literature. Arch Intern Med 1983; 143:2269-75.

4. Miller RA, Holmberg RE Jr, Clausen CR. Life-threatening diarrhea caused by cryptosporidium in a child undergoing therapy for acute lymphocytic leukemia. J Pediatr 1983; 103:256-9.

5. Centers for Disease Control. Cryptosporidiosis: assessment of chemotherapy of males with acquired immune deficiency syndrome (AIDS). MMWR 1982; 31:589-92.

6. Soave R, Danner RL, Honig CL, et al. Cryptosporidiosis in homosexual men. Ann Intern Med 1984; 100:504-11.

7. Whiteside ME, Barkin JS, May RG, et al. Enteric coccidiosis among patients with the acquired immunodeficiency syndrome. Am J Trop Med Hyg 1984; 33:1065-72.

8. Wong B. Parasitic diseases in immunocompromised hosts. Am J Med 1984; 76:479-86.

9. Jokipii L, Pohjola S, Jokipii AMM. Cryptosporidium: a frequent finding in patients with gastrointestinal symptoms. Lancet 1983; 2:358-61.

10. Tzipori S, Smith M, Birch C, et al. Cryptosporidiosis in hospital patients with gastroenteritis. Am J Trop Med Hyg 1983; 32:931-4.

11. Wolfson JS, Richter JM, Waldron MA, et al. Cryptosporidiosis in immunocompetent patients. N Engl J Med 1985; 312:1278-82.

12. Holley HP Jr, Dover C. Cryptosporidium: a common cause of parasitic diarrhea in otherwise healthy individuals. J Infect Dis 1986; 365-8.

13. Current WL, Reese NC, Ernst JV, et al. Human cryptosporidiosis in immunocompetent and immunodeficient persons: studies of an outbreak and experimental transmission. N Engl J Med 1983; 308:1252-7.

14. Blagburn BL, Current WL. Accidental infection of a researcher with human cryptosporidium. J Infect Dis 1983; 148:772-3.

15. D'Antonio RG, Winn RE, Taylor JP, et al. A waterborne outbreak of cryptosporidiosis in normal hosts. Ann Intern Med 1985; 103:886-8.

16. Sterling CR, Seegar K, Sinclair NA. Cryptosporidium as a causative agent of traveler's diarrhea. J Infect Dis 1986; 153:380.

17. Koch KL, Phillips DJ, Aber RC, Current WL. Cryptosporidiosis in hospital personnel: evidence for person-to-person transmission. Ann Intern Med 1985; 102:593-6.

18. Centers for Disease Control. Update on acquired immune deficiency syndrome AIDS — United States. MMWR 1982; 31:507-14.

19. Guarda A, Stein SA, Cleary KA, Ordonez NG. Human cryptosporidiosis in the acquired immune deficiency syndrome. Arch Pathol Lab Med 1983;107:562-6.

20. Blumberg RS, Kelsey P, Perrone T, et al. Cytomegalovirus- and cryptosporidium-associated acalculous gangrenous cholecystitis. Am J Med 1984; 76:1118-23.

21. Pitlik SD, Fainstein V, Rios A, et al. Cryptosporidial cholecystitis. N Engl J Med 1983; 308:967-8.

22. Forgacs P, Tarchis A, Pearl MA, et al. Intestinal and bronchial cryptosporidiosis in an immunodeficient homosexual man. Ann Intern Med 1983; 99:793-4.

23. Chiampi NP, Sundberg RD, Klompus JP, Wilson AJ. Cryptosporidial enteritis and pneumocystis pneumonia in a homosexual man. Hum Pathol 1983; 14:734-7.

24. Ma P, Villanueva TG, Kaufman D, Gillooley JF. Respiratory cryptosporidiosis in the acquired immune deficiency syndrome. JAMA 1984; 252:1298-1301.

25. Brady EM, Margolis ML, Korzeniowski OM. Pulmonary cryptosporidiosis in acquired immune deficiency syndrome. JAMA 1984; 252:89-90.

26. Lefkowitch JH, Krumholz S, Kuo-Ching F, et al. Cryptosporidiosis of the human small intestine: a light and electron microscopic study. Hum Pathol 1984; 15:746-52.

27. Dobbins WO III, Weinstein WM. Electron microscopy of the intestine and rectum in acquired immunodeficiency syndrome. Gastroenterology 1985; 88:738-49.

28. Campbell PN, Current WL. Demonstration of serum antibodies to cryptosporidium sp. in normal and immunodeficient humans with confirmed infections. J Clin Microbiol 1983; 18:165-9.

29. Current WL, Haynes TB. Complete development of cryptosporidium in cell culture. Science 1984; 224:603-5.

30. Katz M, Despommier DD, Deckelbaum RJ. Cryptosporidiosis or an Aesop fable for modern times. Pediatr Infect Dis J 1987; 6:619-21.

31. Modigliani R, Bories C, Le Charpentier Y, et al. Diarrhoea and malabsorption in acquired immune deficiency syndrome: a study of four cases with special emphasis on opportunistic protozoan infestations. Gut 1985; 26:179-87.

32. Gillin JS, Shike M, Alcock N, et al. Malabsorption and mucosal abnormalities of the small intestine in the acquired immunodeficiency syndrome. Ann Intern Med 1985; 102:619-22.

33. Zar F, Geiseler PJ, Brown VA. Asymptomatic carriage of cryptosporidium in the stool of a patient with acquired immunodeficiency syndrome. J Infect Dis 1985; 151:195-6.

34. Weinstein L, Edelstein M, Madara JL, et al. Intestinal cryptosporidiosis complicated by disseminated cytomegalovirus infection. Gastroenterology 1981; 81:584-91.

35. Ma P, Soave R. Three step stool examination for cryptosporidiosis in 10 homosexual men with protracted watery diarrhea. J Infect Dis 1983; 147:824-8.

36. Garcia LS, Bruckner DA, Brewer TC, Shimizu RY. Techniques for the recovery and identification of cryptosporidium oocysts from stool specimens. J Clin Microbiol 1983; 18:185-90.

37. Campbell PN, Current WL. Demonstration of serum antibodies to cryptosporidium sp. in normal and immunodeficient humans with confirmed infections. J Clin Microbiol 1983; 18:165-9.

38. Berk RN, Wall SD, McArdle CB, et al. Cryptosporidiosis of the stomach and small intestine in patients with AIDS. AJR 1984; 143:549-54.

39. Baxby D, Blundell N. Recognition and laboratory characteristics of an atypical oocyst of Cryptosporidium. J Infect Dis 1988; 158:1038-45.

40. Portnoy D, Whiteside ME, Buckley E III, MacLeod CL. Treatment of intestinal cryptosporidiosis with spiramycin. Ann Intern Med 1984; 101:202-4.

41. Agins B, El-Sadr W, Simberkoff MS, Rahal JJ. Evaluation of efficacy of spiramycin in intestinal cryptosporidiosis. Atlanta: Program of the First International Conference on Acquired Immunodeficiency Syndrome, 1985:78.

42. Centers for Disease Control. Acquired immunodeficiency syndrome, United States. MMWR 1986; 35:17-21.

43. Ma P. Cryptosporidium and the enteropathy of immune deficiency. J Pediatr Gastroenterol Nutr 1984; 4:488-9.

44. Wittenberg DF, Miller NM, van den Ende J. Spiramycin is not effective in treating cryptosporidium diarrhea in infants: results of a double-blind randomized trial. J Infect Dis 1989; 159:131-2.

45. Robinson EN Jr, Fogel R. SMS 201-995, a somatostatin analogue, and diarrhea in the acquired immunodeficiency syndrome (AIDS). Ann Intern Med 1988; 109:680-1.

Toxoplasmosis

*Catherine Reinis-Lucey, M.D., Merle A. Sande, M.D.,
and J. Louise Gerberding, M.D.*

Toxoplasma gondii, an obligate intracellular protozoan, is now recognized as a major cause of neurologic morbidity and mortality among patients with the acquired immunodeficiency syndrome (AIDS). Like other opportunistic pathogens, *T. gondii* causes asymptomatic or mildly symptomatic infections in normal hosts, but it causes rapidly progressive, fatal disease in immunosuppressed patients.

Toxoplasmosis is a zoonosis with an infectious reservoir encompassing all animals. The domestic cat appears to be a major culprit in transmitting it to other animals, including humans. Transmission to humans occurs primarily in two ways: (1) eating meat containing cysts (it is estimated that 25 percent of pork and lamb are contaminated),[1] and (2) vertical transmission from mother to fetus during an acute infection. Rarer forms of transmission that have become more important in recent years include transmission via organ transplantation[2] and granulocyte transfusion.[3] Laboratory workers have contracted toxoplasmosis after accidental inoculation of substances containing viable tachyzoites.

Toxoplasma gondii can cause a wide spectrum of disease after infecting a new host. Acute acquired toxoplasmosis is most commonly asymptomatic but can range from mildly symptomatic in the normal host to fulminant and fatal in the immunocompromised host. After an appropriate immunologic response to the initial acute infection, most normal hosts contain the infection. This leads to a latent asymptomatic phase of the disease characterized by the presence of tissue cysts. Chronic, symptomatic toxoplasmosis has rarely been reported in some normal hosts.

Acute reactivated toxoplasmosis occurs in the immunocompromised host and is characterized by symptomatic dissemination of the once-dormant parasite. Congenital toxoplasmosis results from transmission in utero, and may not become clinically recognized for months or even years. Finally, toxoplasmic chorioretinitis can occur as a sequela of congenital toxoplasmosis (usually bilaterally) or as a complication of acute acquired or acute reactivated toxoplasmosis (more commonly unilateral).

■ EPIDEMIOLOGY

The prevalence of seropositivity for toxoplasmosis varies with geographic location and nationality. Overall, seroprevalence increases with age. In the United States, it is estimated that approximately 50 percent of all adults have been previously infected with toxoplasmosis.[4] Over 90 percent of citizens in El Salvador, Tahiti, and France have positive serologies for toxoplasma by their fourth decade.[1] In 1956, Feldman and Miller found a seropositivity rate of 30 percent among normal Haitians[5]; CDC data from 1982 demonstrate a seropositivity rate of 76 percent in Port-au-Prince,[6] comparable to rates found in other populations.

Seroprevalence of toxoplasma antibodies in AIDS patients is similar to that in other populations. Wong et al. noted that 22 to 45 percent of AIDS patients without clinical evidence of disease had serologic evidence of infection with *Toxoplasma gondii*.[7] Even though the rate of infection with toxoplasma among AIDS patients appears to be no higher than in other populations, AIDS patients are unusually susceptible to severe disease caused by this parasite.

T. gondii has been recognized as an opportunistic pathogen for more than 20 years, primarily in connection with collagen vascular diseases, reticuloendothelial malignancies, and organ transplantation. Despite profound immunosuppression, the incidence of toxoplasmosis in these populations ranges from 2 to 5 percent.[8,9] In contrast, the overall incidence of clinical toxoplasmosis among all AIDS patients with neurologic disease is approximately 25 percent to 30 percent.[10,11] Fifty-five percent of Haitian AIDS patients have toxoplasmosis at the time of autopsy.[12] Among 34 cases of toxoplasmosis reported to the CDC in 1982, 50 percent occurred in Haitians, despite the fact that they accounted for only 5.6 percent of the AIDS cases. The reason for this disproportionate incidence of toxoplasmosis among Haitians is unclear, but it does not appear to be solely related to an increased incidence of exposure to the organism.[6]

■ MICROBIOLOGY

Toxoplasma is a sporozoan of the subclass Coccidia. The only species is gondii. It exists in three forms: tachyzoites (trophozoites), tissue cysts, and oocysts.

The tachyzoite, formerly known as the trophozoite, is the form of *T. gondii* capable of invasion, proliferation, and cell destruction. All mammalian cells, with the exception of the mature erythrocyte, are susceptible to infection with tachyzoites. They enter the cell most probably through an energy-dependent process — a cross between phagocytosis and mechanical invasion.[13] The tachyzoite can also reverse the process. Once inside the cell, the envacuolated tachyzoite multiplies by endogeny and eventually either destroys the host cell, or, if contained by host defenses, forms a tissue cyst.

Tissue cysts serve as a reservoir of tachyzoites and are therefore responsible for disease transmission and latent infection. When raw or undercooked meat is ingested, the cysts are lysed by digestive juices, and release anywhere from 100 to 3000 tachyzoites. The tachyzoites then invade intestinal epithelial cells and disseminate hematogenously. Cysts are most commonly found in brain, heart, and skeletal muscle. Despite the frequency of lymphadenopathy as a primary manifestation of toxoplasmosis, cysts are rarely found in lymph nodes.

Oocysts are formed only in the cat. Tachyzoites invade the epithelial cells lining the cat's intestine and replicate by gametogeny, and eventually form oocysts. These oocysts are excreted in feces and can survive for months in moist soil. Contamination of food with dirt containing oocysts can result in disease transmission.

■ HISTOPATHOLOGY

The histopathology of toxoplasmosis varies with the immune status of the host. In normal hosts with acquired toxoplasmosis, the characteristic histopathology of the lymph node is considered diagnostic, despite the relative paucity of organisms present. Typical findings include reactive follicular hyperplasia, irregular clusters of histocytes encroaching on the margins of germinal centers, and focal distension of sinuses with monocytoid cells. Necrosis and vasculitis are not observed.[1] At autopsy, tissue cysts are noted as incidental findings in the skeletal muscle and myocardium of normal hosts but invoke little inflammatory response.

In immunodeficient patients and children with severe congenital toxoplasmosis, tachyzoite proliferation is accompanied by tissue necrosis and an intense, usually monocytic, inflammatory response. In over 90 percent of patients with disseminated toxoplasmosis, central nervous system involvement is present.[4] The pathology ranges from focal abscesses to diffuse meningoencephalitis. In AIDS and other acquired immunodeficiency states, examination of the brain shows a well demarcated, necrotizing encephalitis that involves primarily the white matter or white-gray matter interface.[14,15] In AIDS patients, there appears to be a special predilection for the basal ganglia.

Microscopical examination of a toxoplasma abscess shows a center of necrotic debris with occasional fragments of organisms. Surrounding this zone of necrosis is an area of mononuclear inflammation with arteritis and thrombosis of vessels. Vascular wall necrosis is present. Free and intracellular tachyzoites are seen in this area.[1,12,16-19] Normal brain tissue surrounding the inflammation characteristically shows edema and toxoplasma tissue cysts. Variations on this characteristic histopathology have been documented in autopsy series of some AIDS patients. Luft and colleagues noted the unusual presence of a granulocytic inflammatory response in some patients, and granuloma formation in others.[18] Necrotizing granulomas with minimal inflammation have been seen in some AIDS patients.[20]

In addition to the brain, the same necrotizing inflammation is seen when toxoplasma involves the myocardium, lungs, and skeletal muscle in immunosuppressed patients. Toxoplasmic involvement of these organs occasionally dominates the clinical picture[21]; more commonly, however, myocardial and lung involvement are incidental in a patient with symptoms of encephalitis.

Chorioretinitis in congenital or acquired toxoplasmosis also causes necrotizing inflammation that involves the retina and the posterior chamber. Granulomas are commonly seen. Although organisms are identified in the retina and vitreous, at least part of the necrotizing inflammation is due to a hypersensitivity reaction to toxoplasma antigens rather than to proliferation of the organisms.

Identifying *T. gondii* in tissue samples may be extremely difficult, and may require special staining techniques. Gram, hematoxylin and eosin, and PAS stains can usually identify tissue cysts appropriately, but cysts are rare in areas of inflammation and necrosis. It is estimated that up to 50 percent of hematoxylin and eosin stains will miss free tachyzoites.[18] Many laboratories now rely on immunofluorescent stain to identify tachyzoites in unfixed tissue.[29] An immunofluorescent antiperoxidase antibody stain (IFA) developed by Conley and colleagues has a high sensitivity rate for free tachyzoites as well as for parasitized cells, and the stain can be performed on formalin-fixed, paraffin-embedded tissue.[17] Since IFA is simpler to use than peroxidase antiperoxidase, it should be used initially to document free tachyzoites in tissue samples. Peroxidase antiperoxidase may be helpful when initial stains of tissue from a patient with necrotizing encephalitis are negative or when the diagnosis of toxoplasmosis is not considered until after the specimen has been embedded in plastic.

■ HOST DEFENSE MECHANISMS

The Defect in AIDS.   The cellular immune system is primarily responsible for defense against *T. gondii*, an intracellular parasite. Effective host defense is dependent on the interaction between normally functioning T cells and mononuclear phagocytes. Lymphokines also play a critical role in this interaction.

The murine model of toxoplasmosis can explain the mechanisms of defense against *T. gondii*.[22,23] The activated monocyte is essential for microbicidal activity against this parasite. In mice previously exposed to *T. gondii*, infection leads to parasitization of the inactivated monocyte. Protozoal replication then proceeds unchecked and leads to lysis of the cell. Lysis is followed by the release of tachyzoites, and subsequent parasitization of adjacent cells. In mice rendered immune to *T. gondii* by previous exposure, rechallenge with the organism stimulates previously sensitized lymphocytes to secrete lymphokines. Effector mononuclear phagocytes are activated by exposure to these lymphokines and to Fc fragments of antibody-coated organisms. Gamma interferon appears to be a key component of this interaction.[23]

When phagocytosis of *T. gondii* by an activated monocyte occurs, an oxidative burst is triggered. This respiratory burst is responsible for the production of hydrogen peroxide, superoxide, and other toxic oxygen metabolites. The magnitude of this respiratory burst correlates directly with toxoplasmicidal activity. These metabolites are produced in large enough quantities to overcome the relative resistance of *T. gondii* to oxygen metabolites.[24]

Although *T. gondii* inhibits phagolysosomal formation, phagolysosomes are readily formed when the organism is coated with specific antibody.[25] Nonetheless, lysosomal products only play a minor role in the intracellular killing of *T. gondii*.[24,26] When normal host defenses are present, 90 percent or more of the organisms are killed. Replication of those surviving is inhibited and the organisms eventually become encysted. This leads to the formation of the dormant tissue cyst.

In AIDS patients, defects in both cellular and humoral immune systems render the patients susceptible to overwhelming disease caused by intracellular pathogens such as *T. gondii*. Despite a polyclonal hypergammaglobulinemia, patients with AIDS have a decreased ability to produce a specific antibody after exposure to a foreign antigen.[27] This defective antibody synthesis may explain the unusual lack of serologic response to acute toxoplasma infection in AIDS patients. The absence of specific antibody may also result in ineffective phagolysosomal formation. T-helper cell defects may prevent activation of macrophages by a suboptimal production of lymphokines.

Murray and colleagues suggest that the defect in toxoplasmicidal activity in AIDS patients is due to the absence of lymphokine activation of monocytes rather than to an abnormality of the oxidative system of the activated macrophage.[28] T lymphocytes from AIDS patients failed to produce lymphokines after specific (toxoplasma or candida) or nonspecific mitogen. Lymphocytes from only 1 of 14 patients formed gamma interferon after specific microbial antigen stimulation. However, when *T. gondii* was added to cell cultures of AIDS monocytes stimulated with exogenously derived gamma interferon, an appropriate and effective respiratory burst was initiated and the toxoplasma organisms were destroyed. This study successfully localized a specific defect in cell-mediated immunity leading to the decreased ability of AIDS patients to fight infection by *T. gondii*.

In a murine model of toxoplasmosis, mice treated with anti-CD4 monoclonal antibody experienced reactivated central nervous system toxoplasmosis despite high titers of circulating antitoxoplasma antibody.[30]

In summary, the effective killing of intracellular *T. gondii* requires the following: (1) the presence of type-specific antibody against *T. gondii*; (2) the production of gamma interferon or other lymphokines by sensitized T lymphocytes; and (3) an effective oxidative burst by mononuclear phagocytes. The susceptibility of AIDS patients to severe toxoplasmosis may be explained by defective antibody and lymphokine production.

■ CLINICAL PRESENTATION

Toxoplasmosis in the Normal Host. The most common form of symptomatic acute toxoplasmosis is lymphadenopathy. Typically, this lymphadenopathy is painless, firm, and confined to one chain of nodes, most commonly cervical. Less commonly, the adenopathy can be diffuse and associated with a mononucleosis-like syndrome of rash, arthralgias, myalgias, fever, sore throat, and hepatosplenomegaly accompanied by slightly abnormal liver-function tests. Although the disease is usually benign and self-limited, the symptoms may persist for 12 months. Symptomatic chronic disease occurs rarely in normal hosts. Acute acquired toxoplasmosis may cause unilateral chorioretinitis in the normal host. Patients complain of pain, visual disturbances, photophobia, and scotomata. Antitoxoplasma treatment is usually indicated for this form of the disease to minimize retinal damage.[1]

Congenital Toxoplasmosis. Congenital toxoplasmosis occurs when a pregnant woman becomes infected during gestation and transmits the infection transplacentally to the fetus during an episode of parasitemia. Women who are infected with *Toxoplasma gondii* before conception do not transmit the disease to their offspring.

Although the sequelae of in utero infection with *Toxoplasma gondii* may be present at birth, often they are not seen until months to years later. The clinical manifestations of congenital toxoplasmosis range from lymphadenopathy hepatosplenomegaly syndrome in the infant to bilateral chorioretinitis in the preschooler. Severe psychomotor and mental retardation, epilepsy, encephalitis, and pneumonitis are the most dreaded sequelae. Patients with this constellation of symptoms are frequently born premature and become symptomatic at birth or soon after.[31]

Toxoplasmosis in the Immunocompromised Host. Disseminated toxoplasmosis, rarely seen in the normal host, is now recognized as a serious complication in immunosuppressed patients.[8-10,12,17,32-36] Disease- and drug-induced changes in cellular immunity can lead to a fulminant course of acute acquired toxoplasmosis or to an increased incidence of reactivation toxoplasmosis. Disseminated disease was initially recognized in patients receiving organ transplantation, or in those with collagen vascular diseases or both hematologic and solid neoplasms.[32] It is seen with increasing frequency in patients with AIDS.

Clinical Presentation of Toxoplasmosis in AIDS Patients. As with other immunocompromised patients, the majority of AIDS patients with toxoplasmosis present with central nervous system (CNS) complaints suggestive of encephalitis or focal processes. Ironically, despite the severity of the infection, the symptoms are often vague and nonspecific and can easily be ignored. Headache, usually dull and constant, is an almost universal symptom. Severe incapacitating headaches are more suggestive of cryptococcal meningitis. An alteration in mental status is also common and may be extremely subtle. Despite the fact that most AIDS patients with toxoplasmosis have focal brain abscesses,[10] only 30 percent have focal neurologic findings; somewhere between 15 percent and 30 percent have seizures.[7,10-12,18,34] Seizures in an AIDS patient are more often due to toxoplasmosis than to any other opportunistic infection.

Levy et al.[10] found that most patients with seizures or focal neurologic deficits gave histories of: (1) altered mental status lasting from weeks to months, (2) disturbances of cognitive function, or (3) headaches. Since early therapeutic intervention in AIDS patients with toxoplasmosis may prevent progression of lesions, it clearly benefits the patient to have the diagnosis made before the development of hemiparesis, seizures, or profound mental status aberrations. Involvement of other organ systems, such as lung, heart, and muscle, may be seen at autopsy, but patients rarely have symptoms referable to these organs.

■ DIFFERENTIAL AND NON-SEROLOGIC DIAGNOSIS

Unfortunately, the clinical presentation of toxoplasmosis in AIDS patients is nonspecific. Many other opportunistic infections and neoplastic processes clinically mimic toxoplasmosis. The presence of associated chorioretinitis can be a clue to toxoplasmosis, but it can also be seen with cytomegalovirus (CMV) and cryptococcal disease. Other viruses causing similar CNS symptoms include papovavirus (progressive multifocal leukoencephalopathy), herpes simplex, and human immunodeficiency virus (HIV). Both *Mycobacterium avium-intracellulare* and *Mycobacterium tuberculosis* have been found in the brains of AIDS patients. Fungal abscesses secondary to infection with aspergillus, cryptococcus, candida, and coccidioidomycosis have been seen. Neoplastic diseases affecting the CNS in AIDS patients include primary CNS lymphoma, secondary CNS lymphoma, and rarely, metastatic Kaposi's sarcoma. In addition, cerebrovascular accidents secondary to hypoxia, emboli from marantic endocarditis, and hemorrhage are seen with increased frequency in this population.[10-12]

Despite the lengthy differential diagnosis, toxoplasmosis is probably the most frequently identified secondary CNS pathogen among AIDS patients. It was responsible for 104 of 315 cases of neurologic dysfunction in Levy's series.[10] In Haitian populations with AIDS, it is responsible for almost 50 percent of CNS pathology.[12] Even though toxoplasmosis is the most common cause of neurologic abnormalities among AIDS patients, it is probably more responsive to treatment than any other cause of CNS dysfunction in AIDS patients.

It is crucial that physicians caring for AIDS patients with toxoplasmosis:

1. be aware of the disease and its subtle presentations;
2. understand the limitations of radiographic and serologic tests in diagnosing toxoplasmosis in AIDS patients; and
3. be prepared to use invasive procedures when appropriate.

DIAGNOSTIC PROCEDURES AND TESTS

Computerized Tomographic (CT) Scanning. The CT scan is useful in suggesting the diagnosis of toxoplasmosis. It can also guide stereotactic biopsy and follow response to therapy. The CT scan in patients with toxoplasmosis is almost always abnormal, although 2 of 103 patients in Levy's series had normal CT scans despite also having biopsy-proven disease.[10] Multiple lesions are more frequent than solitary lesions.[14-16,37] Lesions are most common in the basal ganglia, white matter, or gray-white matter interface.[15,38] Three patterns of hypodense lesions are typically seen: ring enhancement with edema, nodular enhancement with edema, and focal edema with enhancement.[14,37] Unlike congenital toxoplasmosis, brain calcifications are rarely seen. Delayed scanning after a double dose of iodine appears to give the maximal yield.[14,37]

Magnetic Resonance Imaging (MRI) Scanning. Patients with normal CT scans may have lesions demonstrable by MRI scanning. MRI may demonstrate lesions in areas of the brain more accessible to biopsy than those shown by CT scanning. It should be emphasized that neither technique can be used to definitively diagnose toxoplasmosis. Roentgenographically similar lesions can be seen in CNS lymphoma and other infectious processes.

Lumbar Puncture. Lumbar puncture is a valuable diagnostic technique because it excludes other opportunistic infections as the cause of altered mental status. Whenever feasible, it should not be done before CT scanning, even in the absence of focal neurologic deficits or clinical evidence of increased intracranial pressure. Analysis of the cerebrospinal fluid in patients with toxoplasmic encephalitis almost always shows a normal glucose level. Protein levels are slightly elevated in about half the patients. In contrast to congenital toxoplasmosis, extremely high protein levels are rarely seen. Approximately 15 percent of patients show a mild mononuclear pleocytosis.[10] Some authors have reported a pleocytosis in as many as 70 percent of their patients.[7] The deepseated nature of the lesions may explain the relative paucity of cerebrospinal-fluid abnormalities.

Culture and Isolation. Toxoplasma cannot be isolated from specimens by using conventional microbial culture methods. Isolation involves inoculation of the specimen into the peritoneal cavities of mice. The peritoneal fluid is then examined 7 to 10 days after inoculation. If no organisms are found, the mouse antibodies against toxoplasma are checked. If the mouse demonstrates serologic evidence of toxoplasma infection, it is then killed and histopathologic evidence of the infection is sought.[1,31]

Alternatively, tissue cultures can be inoculated and then examined for the presence of *T. gondii*. This is generally considered a less reliable procedure. Acute reactivation toxoplasmosis was recently diagnosed, however, in three patients with allogenic bone-marrow transplants, and in one patient with AIDS, after tissue cultures were inoculated with their sera. Growth took 5 to 39 days.[38,39] Obviously, these isolation methods are too cumbersome, expensive, and time-consuming for reliable, rapid, or routine diagnosis of toxoplasmosis. They may be helpful, however, in identifying toxoplasmosis in very selected patients whose clinical pictures, serologies, and biopsy results are nondiagnostic.

■ SEROLOGIC DIAGNOSIS

Given the difficulty of isolating *Toxoplasma gondii*, serologic studies are relied upon to support the diagnosis of toxoplasmosis. These studies are reliable in the normal host but lose their sensitivity when used in the immunologically compromised host. In AIDS patients, serologic studies are rarely helpful in establishing a diagnosis of acute toxoplasmosis. Even with severe toxoplasmosis, it is unusual for a patient with AIDS to demonstrate a diagnostic four-fold rise in IgG titer. The absence of antibody against *T. gondii* is strong presumptive evidence against a diagnosis of toxoplasmosis, although isolated reports of negative antibody titers in AIDS patients with biopsy-proven toxoplasmosis have occurred. IgM titers are seen in some AIDS patients in areas with a high prevalence of toxoplasmosis, such as France, and suggest recently acquired primary infection.

The methods and merits of a number of available serologic tests, all of which identify the presence of toxoplasma-specific antibody in the patient's serum, are described below.[1,31,40,41]

SEROLOGIC TESTS

The Sabin–Feldman Dye Test.   This is one of the most commonly used serologic tests. Live tachyzoites are incubated with the patient's serum. If specific antibody is present, the tachyzoites will lyse and not stain when methylene blue is added. The test titer is reported as the dilution of serum at which half of the organisms present are stained. The measured IgG antibody appears one to two weeks after infection or reactivation, and peaks at six to eight weeks. Titers gradually decline over two to three years but may persist at low levels for life. Intrathecal antibody titer can also be measured in the Sabin–Feldman dye test (SFDT). If the value [(CSF dye test reciprocal titer/total CSF IgG) multiplied by the (total sum IgG/serum dye test reciprocal titer)] is greater than 1, active CNS toxoplasmosis should be suspected.[53]

The Indirect Fluorescent Antibody Test.   The IFA is the most widely available serologic test for toxoplasmosis and measures the same antibody as the SFDT, but it is somewhat less reliable. Killed organisms are incubated with test serum and the mixture is then washed. Fluorescein-tagged anti-IgG is then added to identify the toxoplasma-specific IgG bound to the organisms. False-positive results are occasionally seen when high titers of antinuclear antibodies are present.

Agglutination Tests.   These tests involve the incubation of preserved whole parasites with the test serum. The presence of specific IgG causes visible agglutination. False positives are seen in patients with rheumatoid factors and other causes of nonspecific elevations of IgM. The addition of 1-mercapto-ethanol to the test serum can eliminate these false positives. Agglutination tests are not widely available in the United States.

Complement Fixation and Indirect Hemagglutination Tests.   These tests measure the presence of an IgG that appears and peaks later (three to six weeks postinfection) than the antibody measured by the Sabin Feldman and the indirect fluorescent antibody tests. If the diagnosis of toxoplasmosis is not considered until after the peak of SFDT/IFA has occurred, complement fixation and indirect hemagglutination may demonstrate a rising titer suggestive of recent infection.

The IgM-IFA, IgM-ELISA, and DS-IgM-ELISA Tests.   These tests measure the presence of IgM in the serum. A high titer of IgM suggests recent infection, since the IgM response to a foreign antigen is usually quicker and more short-lived than the IgG response. Of the three IgM tests available, the

DS-IgM-ELISA appears to be the most sensitive and specific.[41] In the ELISA technique, patient serum is added to a test well that is coated with a soluble parasitic extract. A solution of an enzyme-linked (usually the enzyme is alkaline phosphatase) anti-IgM antibody is then added and the mixture is washed. Enzyme activity is assayed by noting a color change of the solution. Although there is close agreement between IgM-IFA and IgM-ELISA titers, IgM ELISA titers are generally higher than IgM-IFA titers.[41] Unlike the titers from DS-IgM-ELISA, both of these tests are subject to false-positive results in the presence of rheumatoid factor or positive antinuclear-antibody tests.

SEROLOGY IN NORMAL HOSTS

A diagnosis of acute toxoplasmosis is made when the results of a previously negative IFA or SFDT convert to positive in the appropriate clinical setting, or when a fourfold rise in titer is seen in serum samples taken three weeks apart. Over 90 percent of patients with lymphadenopathic toxoplasmosis have an SFDT of greater than 1:1024.[10] A single high SFDT or IFA titer does not establish a diagnosis of acute toxoplasmosis, however, since titers occasionally remain high for months to years after an acute infection. If a single high IgG titer is present in association with a high IgM titer, acute toxoplasmosis is the likely diagnosis.[1]

SEROLOGY IN (NON-AIDS) IMMUNOCOMPROMISED HOSTS

Before the advent of AIDS, serologic studies were relied upon to aid in the diagnosis of toxoplasmosis in the immunocompromised host, although the sensitivity of the studies was somewhat less than in normal hosts. Luft reported in 1984 that 12 of 15 patients with CNS toxoplasmosis and immunosuppressive disease other than AIDS demonstrated a positive DS-IgM-ELISA test.[18] Hakes and associates in 1983 reviewed 25 cases of toxoplasmosis in immunocompromised hosts; 18 of 25 patients demonstrated a diagnostic fourfold rise in their SFDT titers, CSF titers, or both. Four others did not exhibit a rise in titer but had single high SFDT titers of greater than 1:4096. Only 2 of the 25 patients had insignificant SFDT, IFA, and IgM titers.[9]

SEROLOGY IN AIDS

Unfortunately, formal studies and clinical reports of toxoplasmosis in AIDS patients have suggested that serologies are unreliable diagnostic indicators in this particular immunocompromised population. A review of the literature reveals that AIDS patients with toxoplasmosis rarely show positive IgM titers, appropriate increases in IgG titers, or even stable high-titer SFDT results.[10,34,42,43] In fact, absence of antibody is good evidence against toxoplasmic infection.

Luft and colleagues studied the serologic response of 37 AIDS patients to CNS toxoplasmosis. Only 1 of the 37 patients demonstrated a positive IgM-ELISA.[18] None of the seven AIDS patients in Wong's series on toxoplasmosis had positive IgM titers as evidence of recent infection.[7] In all reports, the Sabin–Feldman dye test is uniformly positive but of low titer, an unexpected finding in the setting of acute toxoplasmosis. Only 22 percent of AIDS patients demonstrated an SFDT of greater than 1:1024.[7,18]

Interestingly, 35 of Luft's 37 patients had positive agglutination tests. Two-thirds of these tests showed titers disproportionately high in comparison to the low SFDT. Luft suggests that the ratio of AGG:SFDT titers may be a clue to the presence of CNS toxoplasmosis in AIDS patients with low SFDT results. Agglutination titers 5 to 20 times greater than simultaneous SFDT titers were found in 50 percent to 75 percent of AIDS patients with CNS toxoplasmosis.[18,43] The ratio was much lower in immunologically normal hosts with toxoplasmosis or in AIDS patients without toxoplasmic encephalitis.

ANTIGEN DETECTION

Methods to detect toxoplasma antigens in blood CSF and other body fluids of AIDS patients are undergoing clinical evaluation.[54] If these tests prove to be sensitive and specific, they may greatly facilitate noninvasive diagnosis when serologic tests are unreliable.

■ TREATMENT

The mainstay of therapy for acute toxoplasmosis is sulfadiazine combined with pyrimethamine.[32,44] Although in combination these drugs are effective against free and intracellular tachyzoites, they are not useful against tissue cysts. Therefore, short-term administration cannot be expected to eradicate latent infection. Sulfadiazine or any trisulfapyrimidine acts synergistically with pyrimethamine against *T. gondii* in mice. Both drugs are folic acid antagonists. The dosage of sulfadiazine is a 75 mg/kg load (2 to 4 grams), then 100 mg/kg/day (6 to 8 grams) in two to four divided doses. Sulfadiazine has good central nervous system (CNS) penetration with a cerebrospinal fluid (CSF) to serum ratio of 1:2 (0.4:0.8). Side effects include neutropenia, nausea, vomiting, diarrhea, rash, fever, and interstitial nephritis. These may limit therapy. Pyrimethamine is known mostly for its use in Fansidar, in which it is combined with sulfadoxine. The recommended dose of pyrimethamine for immunocompromised patients, including those with HIV disease, is 100 mg/day in two divided doses for two days as a load and then 75 to 100 mg/day. Pyrimethamine penetrates the cerebrospinal fluid (CSF) moderately well, and produces peak CSF levels equal to 10 percent to 25 percent of simultaneous serum levels. Side effects include pancytopenia, headache, and gastrointestinal upset. The duration of therapy varies,[45] as discussed below.

Normal Hosts.   In normal hosts, antitoxoplasma therapy is usually reserved for those patients with prolonged symptomatic lymphadenopathy or chorioretinitis. Women who contract toxoplasmosis during pregnancy should be treated in an attempt to decrease the likelihood of transmission to their offspring. Because of its teratogenicity, pyrimethamine cannot be used in the first trimester. Alternative drugs such as spiramycin and clindamycin may be used.

Immunocompromised Hosts, Including AIDS Patients.   All immunocompromised patients, including those with AIDS, should be treated whenever toxoplasmosis occurs, whether as a newly acquired or a reactivated infection. The efficacy of therapy with sulfadiazine and pyrimethamine has been documented retrospectively. Ruskin and Remington reviewed 81 cases of toxoplasmosis in non-AIDS compromised hosts and found that 80 percent of those patients treated either improved clinically or were cured, whereas only 30 percent of untreated patients with acute toxoplasmosis survived.[32] In AIDS patients, the data are less extensive but also support the use of pyrimethamine and sulfadiazine for toxoplasmic encephalitis. Wong and colleagues reported a response in six of seven patients (documented by improvement in symptoms, resolution of CT findings, or both).[7] The one patient who failed to respond was comatose when the therapy began. Handler and colleagues published a report on a series of five AIDS patients, four of whom improved on antitoxoplasma therapy.[15] In AIDS patients, symptomatic improvement usually appears between days 8 and 10. Resolution of CT abnormalities occurs between the first and fourth weeks of therapy.

Duration of Therapy.   The optimal duration of primary therapy for toxoplasmosis in AIDS patients is unknown. Relapse after discontinuation of therapy is the rule rather than the exception, even if CT scan and clinical abnormalities have totally disappeared. Thus, suppressive therapy is recommended for the life of the patient. No large-scale studies on the success of antitoxoplasma therapy in AIDS patients have been done, thus making statements about the standard duration for the therapy impossible. One small series in the literature documents relapse after apparent cure in patients whose therapy was discontinued at or before six weeks.[7] Relapse did not occur when one patient was treated with nine weeks of antitoxoplasma therapy. Another treated patient relapsed and was then given six months of additional therapy; no further relapse occurred. Given the limited information available, it is recommended that AIDS patients with CNS toxoplasmosis be treated with full-strength therapy for a minimum of nine weeks or until all CT evidence of toxoplasmosis has resolved. Beyond that, low-dose suppressive therapy should be continued for the life of the patient. Possible choices of therapy include pyrimethamine at 25 mg/day with or without sulfadiazine (2 to 4 grams per day as tolerated). This regimen may be fraught with drug toxicity, but given the irreversible immune suppression and our inability to eradicate the reservoir of encysted organisms, prolonged therapy appears to be a necessary evil. Studies of the efficacy of this regimen are under way.

Adjuvant Therapy.   Adjuvant therapy for patients with toxoplasmic encephalitis may include: (1) decadron (on a tapering dosage schedule) for abscesses associated with severe mass effect, (2) dilantin for infection-induced seizures, and (3) folinic acid to decrease the incidence of drug-induced pancytopenia. Administration of folinic acid does not negate the beneficial effect of the therapy, since *T. gondii* is unable to use folinic acid. The optimal dose is not established — dosages ranging from 1 to 10 mg/day have been used. Future therapeutic strategies may include the use of gamma interferon or in vitro-stimulated macrophages. The impact of antiviral therapy (including the use of such agents as zidovudine [AZT]) on the clinical course of toxoplasmosis has not yet been defined.

Alternate Regimens.   The high incidence of adverse reactions to sulfa drugs in AIDS patients, particularly neutropenia and rash, occasionally necessitates altering antitoxoplasma therapy. If neutropenia develops during dilantin therapy, a switch to an alternative anti-seizure medication such as phenobarbital might be prudent.

Unfortunately, no other drugs have been proven to be clinically effective in toxoplasmic encephalitis. Clindamycin concentrates in the choroid plexus and has been used successfully to treat chorioretinitis.[46] However, it has minimal CSF penetration. There have been several animal studies showing that clindamycin is a useful drug, even in CNS disease.[47,48] Clindamycin is not recommended as primary therapy. However, anecdotal experience and preliminary results in an ongoing clinical trial suggest that clindamycin in combination with pyrimethamine may be effective treatment in some patients. A retrospective review of cases showed a clinical or radiologic response in 11 of 15 AIDS patients with toxoplasmic encephalitis after treatment with intravenous clindamycin, 1.2 to 4.8 grams per day administered every six to eight hours, either alone or in combination with pyrimethamine.[55-57]

Spiramycin, a drug analogous to clindamycin but with better CNS penetration, has been used to treat pregnant women in their first trimester — a time when pyrimethamine is contraindicated. It is not currently available in the United States but has been used in Europe. The clinical efficacy of spiramycin in humans has not been established, but anecdotal data suggest it is not usually effective for treating encephalitis. Most animal studies demonstrate that it is inferior to regimens containing sulfa (including trimethoprim/sulfamethoxazole and sulfadiazine/pyrimethamine).[49,50] In one study of toxoplasmosis in squirrel monkeys, there were no survivors in the group treated with spiramycin.[50] Trimetrexate, a dihydrofolate reductase inhibitor with a higher affinity than pyrimethamine, is a promising investigational drug that may prove useful.[52]

Pyrimethamine by itself is effective in mouse toxoplasmosis and may be an option (in doses of 50 mg or more) for a patient whose therapeutic side effects seem to be related to sulfadiazine.[44]

The use of trimethoprim and sulfamethoxazole is controversial. In animal studies, both trimethoprim and sulfamethoxazole are less active than their counterparts, sulfadiazine and pyrimethamine. Wong and colleagues did treat one patient successfully with trimethoprim and sulfamethoxazole.[7] Because the incidence of side effects with trimethoprim and sulfamethoxazole is likely to be similar to that with sulfadiazine and pyrimethamine and because no clinical data support the use of trimethoprim and sulfamethoxazole, they are not recommended as primary therapy.

It is difficult to determine the exact mortality rate from CNS toxoplasmosis in AIDS patients, since the simultaneous presence of other opportunistic infections greatly influences survival. In a combined study, half the deaths of AIDS patients with toxoplasmosis were directly related to the toxoplasmosis.[7] Twenty percent of the patients in a small study by Wong and colleagues died as a result of their toxoplasmosis.[7]

Summary of Therapeutic Strategy.   A controversy remains about whether or not all AIDS patients presenting with signs, symptoms, and CT findings suggestive of CNS toxoplasmosis should undergo immediate biopsy or should be treated empirically and undergo biopsy if no therapeutic response is achieved. Levy and colleagues favor biopsy, and cite the finite occurrence of mixed CNS infections in their study (5 of 315), the difficulty in distinguishing a CNS lymphoma from a toxoplasma abscess, and the relatively low morbidity from brain biopsy in their treatment center.[10,51] Others favor empiric therapy for a defined group of patients for several reasons: first of all, other CNS opportunistic pathogens (CMV, papovavirus, MAI) are unlikely to respond to therapy; a two-week delay in therapy of CNS lymphoma is not likely to alter the outcome; and finally, brain biopsy in critically ill patients, many with thrombocytopenia and coagulation abnormalities, may not be a benign procedure — especially in centers that do not perform this procedure frequently.

For these reasons, we recommend the following diagnostic and therapeutic strategy.

Patients should have immediate biopsies if:

- they carry no CDC-defined AIDS diagnosis (HIV infection is insufficient);
- they have substantially increased intracranial hypertension that could respond to surgical decompression;
- their CT findings are atypical for toxoplasmosis;
- they have evidence of disseminated fungal, mycobacterial, or bacterial disease; and
- they have a disseminated lymphoma.

Empiric therapy with sulfadiazine and pyrimethamine and folinic acid should be undertaken if the above criteria are not met or if the patient is not a candidate for biopsy because of thrombocytopenia, inaccessibility of the lesion to biopsy, or because of noncompliance. If the patient deteriorates on therapy, a biopsy should be performed immediately. A biopsy should also be performed after two weeks if clinical or CT improvement, or both, is not evident.

If no clinical change is noted but CT improvement is evident, therapy should be continued. If a biopsy is performed and is nondiagnostic, empiric antitoxoplasma therapy should be given and a clinical response sought. If there is no response after four weeks of empiric therapy and no other diagnosis emerges, most clinicians would discontinue therapy for toxoplasmosis.

■ PREVENTION AND PROPHYLAXIS

Since the immune deficit seen in AIDS patients cannot be reversed, it is unlikely that dissemination of latent toxoplasmosis can be prevented in these patients. Preventive measures must be directed at those AIDS patients who have no serologic evidence of latent toxoplasmosis. This group of AIDS patients needs instruction on ways to avoid exposure to *T. gondii*.

Pregnant women, as well as AIDS and ARC patients, should avoid contact with cat feces. Litter boxes should be cleaned daily (using gloves). Established pets within the household need not be removed. Additionally, all meat should be well cooked, and reach an internal temperature of 60°C for at least 10 minutes to kill any *T. gondii* cysts that may be present. Physicians caring for AIDS patients should be aware that leukocyte transfusions have been associated with transmission of toxoplasma.[2,3]

In addition to recognizing possible modes of transmission, it is important to know the ways in which *T. gondii* is not transmitted. Isolation of the patient with toxoplasmosis is unnecessary, since there is no evidence that casual contact can transmit the disease.

As with most serious infectious diseases, once preventive measures have failed, prompt diagnosis and treatment of disease maximizes the patient's chances of survival without chronic sequelae. Toxoplasmosis is unique among opportunistic infections in AIDS patients because most patients respond to therapy; thus, treatment of the minimally symptomatic patient may prevent the development of severe neurologic abnormalities.

Physicians should consider banking baseline serum samples from AIDS patients as a future aid in serologic diagnosis of toxoplasmosis. When symptoms occur, these baseline specimens and acute serum samples should be assayed simultaneously to determine whether a diagnostic increase in titer has occurred. Alternatively, it might be appropriate to test patient sera on a regular basis to identify an asymptomatic rise in titers. This could allow for the recognition of early reactivation of toxoplasmosis before neurologic morbidity occurs. The discovery of a positive test for antitoxoplasma antibodies with stable titers in an otherwise asymptomatic patient is not an indication for prophylactic therapy, since the cyst stage of toxoplasmosis does not respond to any known antitoxoplasma therapy.

REFERENCES

1. McCabe RE, Remington JS. *Toxoplasma gondii*. In: Mandell GL, Douglas RG, Bennett JE, eds. Principles and practices of infectious diseases. New York: John Wiley & Sons, 1985:1540-9.
2. Ryning FW, McLeod R, Maddox JC, et al. Probable transmission of *Toxoplasma gondii* by organ transplantation. Ann Intern Med 1979; 90:47-9.
3. Siegel SE, Lunde MN, Gelderman AH, et al. Transmission of toxoplasmosis by leukocyte transfusion. Blood 1971; 37:388-94.
4. Krick JA, Remington JS. Toxoplasmosis in the adult — an overview. N Engl J Med 1978; 298:550-3.
5. Feldman HA, Miller LT. Serological study of toxoplasmosis prevalence. Am J Hyg 1956; 64:320-35.
6. Moskowitz LB, Kory P, Chan JC, et al. Unusual causes of death in Haitians residing in Miami. High prevalence of opportunistic infections. JAMA 1983; 250:1187-91.
7. Wong B, Gold JW, Brown AE, et al. Central nervous system toxoplasmosis in homosexual men and parenteral drug abusers. Ann Intern Med 1984; 100:36-42.
8. Chernik NL, Armstrong D, Posner JB. Central nervous system infections in patients with cancer. Medicine 1973; 52:563-81.
9. Hakes TB, Armstrong D. Toxoplasmosis: problems in diagnosis and treatment. Cancer 1983; 52:1535-40.
10. Levy RM, Bredeson DE, Rosenblum MC, et al. Neurological manifestations of the acquired immune deficiency syndrome: experience at UCSF and review of the literature. J Neurosurg 1985; 62:475-95.
11. Snider WD, Simpson DM, Nielson S, et al. Neurologic complications of acquired immune deficiency syndrome: analysis of 50 patients. Ann Neurol 1983; 14:403-18.
12. Moskowitz LB, Hensley GT, Chan JC, et al. The neuropathy of acquired immunodeficiency syndrome. Arch Pathol Lab Med 1984; 108:867-72.
13. Werk R. How does *Toxoplasma gondii* enter host cells? Rev Infect Dis 1985; 7:449-57.
14. Whelan MA, Kricheff II, Handler M, et al. Acquired immunodeficiency syndrome: cerebral computed tomographic manifestations. Radiology 1983; 149:477-84.
15. Handler M, Ho V, Whelan M, Budziolovich G. Intracerebral toxoplasmosis in patients with acquired immune deficiency syndrome. J Neurosurg 1983; 59:994-1001.
16. Post MJ, Chan JC, Hensley GT, et al. Toxoplasma encephalitis in Haitian adults with acquired immunodeficiency syndrome: a clinical pathologic CT correlation. AJR 1983; 140:861-8.
17. Conley FK, Jenkins KA, Remington JS. *Toxoplasma gondii* infection of the central nervous system. Use of the peroxidase antiperoxidase method to demonstrate toxoplasma in formalin fixed, paraffin embedded tissue sections. Hum Pathol 1981; 12:690-8.
18. Luft BJ, Brooks RG, Conley FK, et al. Toxoplasma encephalitis in patients with acquired immune deficiency syndrome. JAMA 1984; 252:913-7.
19. Millard PR. AIDS: histopathological aspects. J Pathol 1984; 143:223.
20. Sher JH. Cerebral toxoplasmosis. Lancet 1983; 1:1225.
21. Marchevsky A, Rosen MJ, Chrystal G, Kleinerman J. Pulmonary complications of the acquired immunodeficiency syndrome: a clinicopathologic study of 70 cases. Hum Pathol 1985; 16:659-70.
22. McLeod R, Wing EJ, Remington JS. Lymphocytes and macrophages in cell mediated immunity. In: Mandell GL, Douglas RG, Bennett JE, eds. Principles and practice of infectious diseases. New York: John Wiley & Sons, 1985:72-91.
23. Frenkel JK, Taylor DW. Toxoplasmosis in immunoglobulin M suppressed mice. Infec Immun 1982; 38:360-7.
24. Nathan CF, Murray HW, Cohn ZA. The macrophage as an effector cell. N Engl J Med 1980; 303:622-6.
25. Edelson PJ. Intracellular parasites and phagocytic cells: cell biology and pathophysiology. Rev Infec Dis 1982; 4:124-35.
26. Unanue ER. Cooperation between mononuclear phagocytes and lymphocytes in immunity. N Engl J Med 1980; 303:977-85.
27. Lane HC, Masur H, Edgar LC, et al. Abnormalities of B-cell activation and immunoregulation in patients with the acquired immunodeficiency syndrome. N Engl J Med 1983; 309:453-8.

28. Murray HW, Rubin BY, Masur H, Roberts RB. Impaired production of lymphokines and immune (gamma) interferon in the acquired immunodeficiency syndrome. N Engl J Med 1984; 310:883-9.

29. Sun T, Greenspan J, Tenenbaum M, et al. Diagnosis of cerebral toxoplasmosis using fluorescein-labeled antitoxoplasma monoclonal antibodies. Am J Surg Path 1986; 10:312-6.

30. Vollmer TL, Waldor MK, Steinman L, Conley FK. Depletion of T-4+ lymphocytes with monoclonal antibody reactivates toxoplasmosis in the central nervous system: a model of superinfection in AIDS. J Immunol 1987; 128:3737-41.

31. Remington JS, Desmonts G. Toxoplasmosis. In: Remington JS, Klein JO, eds. Infectious diseases of the fetus and newborn infant. Philadelphia: W.B. Saunders, 1983:143-263.

32. Ruskin J, Remington JS. Toxoplasmosis in the compromised host. Ann Intern Med 1976; 193-9.

33. Hooper DL, Pruitt A, Rubin H. CNS infection in the chronically immunosuppressed. Medicine 1982; 61:166-88.

34. Horowitz SL, Bentson JR, Benson F, et al. CNS toxoplasmosis in acquired immunodeficiency syndrome. Arch Neurol 1983; 40:649-52.

35. Wong B. Parasitic diseases in immunocompromised hosts. Am J Med 1984; 76:479-86.

36. Britt RH, Enzmann DR, Remington JS. Intracranial infection in cardiac transplant recipients. Ann Neurol 1981; 107-19.

37. Kelly W, Brant-Zawadzki M. Acquired immunodeficiency syndrome: neuroradiologic findings. Radiology 1983; 149:485-91.

38. Shepp DH, Hackman RC, Conley FK, et al. *Toxoplasma gondii* reactivation by detection of parasitemia in tissue culture. Ann Intern Med 1985; 103:218-21.

39. Hofflin JM, Remington JS. Tissue culture isolation of toxoplasma from blood of a patient with AIDS. Arch Intern Med 1985; 145:925-6.

40. Anderson SE, Remington JS. The diagnosis of toxoplasmosis. South Med J 1975; 68:1433-43.

41. Camargo ME, Ferreira AW, Mineo JR, et al. Immunoglobulin G and immunoglobulin M enzyme-linked immunosorbent assays and defined toxoplasmosis serologic patterns. Infect Immun 1978; 21:55-8.

42. Luft BJ, Conley F, Remington JS, et al. Outbreak of central nervous system toxoplasmosis in western Europe and North America. Lancet 1983; 1:781-4.

43. McCabe RE, Gibbons D, Brooks RG, et al. Agglutination test for diagnosis of toxoplasmosis in AIDS. Lancet 1983; 2:680.

44. Eyles DE, Coleman N. An evaluation of the curative effects of pyrimethamine and sulfadiazine alone and in combination on experimental mouse toxoplasmosis. Antibiot Chemother 1955; 5:529-39.

45. Zinner SH, Mayer KH. Sulfonamides and trimethoprim. In: Mandell GL, Douglas RG, Bennett JE, eds. Principles and practices of infectious diseases. New York: John Wiley & Sons, 1985:237-43.

46. Lakhanpal V, Schockett SS, Niranker VS. Clindamycin in the treatment of toxoplasmic retinochoroiditis. Am J Ophthalmol 1983; 95:605-13.

47. Araujo FG, Remington JS. Effect of clindamycin on acute and chronic toxoplasmosis in mice. Antimicrob Agents Chemother 1974; 5:647-51.

48. Hofflin JM, Remington JS. Clindamycin in a murine model of toxoplasmic encephalitis. Antimicrob Agents Chemother 1987; 31:492-6.

49. Nguyen RT, Stadtsbaeder S. Comparative effects of cotrimoxazole and spiramycin in pregnant mice infected with *Toxoplasma gondii* (Beverly strain). Br J Pharmacol 1985; 3:713-6.

50. Harper JS III, London WT, Sever JL. Five drug regimens for treatment of acute toxoplasmosis in squirrel monkeys. Am J Trop Med Hyg 1985; 34:50-7.

51. Levy RM, Pons VG, Rosenblum ML. Intracerebral mass lesions in the acquired immunodeficiency syndrome (AIDS). N Engl J Med 1983; 309:1454-5.

52. Luft BJ, Remington JS. Toxoplasmic encephalitis. J Infect Dis 1988; 157:1-6.

53. Potasman I, Resnick L, Luft BJ, Remington JS. Intrathecal production of antibodies against *Toxoplasma gondii* in patients with encephalitis and the acquired immunodeficiency syndrome (AIDS). Ann Intern Med 1988; 108:49-51.

54. Araujo FG, Remington JS. Antigenemia in recently acquired acute toxoplasmosis. J Infect Dis 1980; 141:144-50.

55. Dannemann BR, Israelski DM, Remington JS. Treatment of toxoplasmic encephalitis with intravenous clindamycin. Arch Intern Med 1988; 148:2477-82.

56. Westblom TU, Bleshe RB. Clindamycin therapy of cerebral toxoplasmosis in an AIDS patient. Scand J Infect Dis 1988; 20:561-3.

57. Rolston KV. Clindamycin in cerebral toxoplasmosis. Am J Med 1988; 85:285.

Isospora belli

Constance B. Wofsy, M.D.

The coccidian parasite *Isospora belli* is an infrequent cause of severe watery diarrhea in a small number of patients with AIDS. Chronic isospora-induced diarrhea in conjunction with a positive antibody test for the human immunodeficiency virus (HIV) serves as a specific diagnosis of AIDS. Transmission is thought to occur by the fecal-oral route. Diagnosis can be made using special laboratory tests on stool specimens, including acid-fast stain or iodine preparation. Detection is enhanced by analyzing duodenal contents. Some patients have had a striking response to treatment with high doses of trimethoprim/sulfamethoxazole or pyrimethamine/sulfadiazine. Long-term suppression can be achieved with lower-dose maintenance therapy.

■ EPIDEMIOLOGY

Isospora belli is a protozoan of the subclass Coccidia, previously described as an infrequent cause of acute or chronic diarrhea in humans. From 1948 to 1974, about 500 cases of gastrointestinal isospora infection were reported.[1] Most cases were in South America or the tropics. With increasing numbers of patients with AIDS, episodic reports of *Isospora belli* as a cause of debilitating diarrhea with wasting and malabsorption were reported.[2-4] In Haiti, isospora infection occurred in 15 percent of AIDS patients.[5] Person-to-person transmission has not been confirmed, but a history of direct oral-anal contact in several infected patients strongly suggests fecal-oral transmission.[4]

■ MICROBIOLOGY AND PATHOPHYSIOLOGY

Isospora is a large protozoan with elliptical oocysts. Isospora cysts can be distinguished from the more frequently encountered cryptosporidial cysts by their larger size (25 micrometers in contrast to 5 micrometers) and their intracellular location during other stages of the life cycle. On light microscopy, the organisms appear within the cytoplasm of villus epithelium when stained with hematoxylin and eosin. Electron microscopy reveals all phases of the sexual and asexual life cycle within the enterocyte. Cryptosporidium, by contrast, is attached extracytoplasmically by a thin membrane to the very tip of the epithelial brush border. In both coccidian infections, the oocysts are shed into the gut lumen and then evacuated.

Infection results in a nonbloody watery diarrhea lacking fecal leukocytes. Electron microscopy reveals mucosal alterations, including shortened villus and eosinophilic infiltration of the lamina propria, particularly in the proximal small intestine.[6] After successful treatment, villus architecture may return to normal. Malabsorption has been well described,[2,3,6] even in a patient who maintained normal villus architecture. The specific immunologic deficits leading to chronic infection have not been described.

■ CLINICAL FEATURES

Clinical features are indistinguishable from those of cryptosporidium infection. Symptoms include a particularly cramping abdominal pain and profuse watery diarrhea of 8 to 10 stools per day, along with weight loss (which may be profound), weakness, anorexia, and occasional low-grade fever.[3] Unlike cryptosporidium, which frequently results in asymptomatic infection, particularly in patients with non-AIDS symptomatic HIV infection, asymptomatic *Isospora belli* infection has not been reported. Unlike cryptosporidium, which has been identified in the lung and biliary tree, isospora infection has thus far been found only in the bowel.

■ DIAGNOSIS

Biopsy of the villus epithelium, particularly of the small bowel, is diagnostic but cumbersome to perform. It may require electron microscopy of biopsy material for definitive diagnosis.[3] Characteristic isospora oocytes can occasionally be found in concentrated stool by means of special flotation or sedimentation techniques, which are less invasive than biopsy. The oocysts do not stain readily with iodine and are best seen under reduced illumination as elongated oval structures of approximately 30×15 micrometers, tapering at the end (see color plate 6.5.7.a). Oocysts may be difficult to find in stool, even in individuals known to be infected. The Entero™ test, (registered trademark) or duodenal aspirate may be particularly helpful. In one series of three patients strongly positive on duodenal aspirate, two showed only rare oocytes on stool examination and one of these required a sugar flotation method for detection. The third patient, who was strongly positive on the Entero™ test, had six negative stool examinations.[3] In another case of mixed isospora and cryptosporidium infection, isospora was not identified on routine ova and parasite examination but was readily found using the acid-fast technique for cryptosporidium.[7] There are no serologic means of detection of isospora infection. Recently developed antibody tests for cryptosporidium infection show very little or no cross-reactivity with other coccidia, including isospora.[8]

■ TREATMENT

There have been very few treatment trials of isospora infection in AIDS. In individual cases and series of two or three patients, the most promising response occurred after treatment with trimethoprim/sulfamethoxazole (160/800 mg four times a day for 10 days and then twice daily for three weeks — three out of three patients responding); furazolidone (100 mg four times a day for 10 days — one out of two responding); and pyrimethamine/sulfadiazine (one response out of three treated patients).[3] Twenty Haitian patients all responded to oral trimethoprim/sulfamethoxazole within 48 hours of treatment but 47 percent relapsed. In other series, after therapy ended relapse followed within weeks to months. The relapses often responded, however, to a repeat course of the same therapy.[5] One patient who failed to respond to multiple forms of therapy responded to pyrimethamine (50 mg daily) and sulfadiazine (4.5 g daily) with resolution of severe malabsorption, a weight gain of 23 kg, and elimination of *Isospora belli* from stool, duodenal aspirate, and duodenal biopsy.[2] The patient relapsed, however, when taken off the medication but responded again to a repeat course of pyrimethamine and sulfadiazine. The largest treatment trial was conducted in Haiti. Thirty-two symptomatic *Isospora belli*-infected AIDS patients were treated with trimethoprim/sulfamethoxazole (160/800 mg orally four times a day for 10 days) and then randomized to trimethoprim/sulfamethoxazole (160/800 mg three times a week) or sulfadoxine (500 mg) and pyrimethamine (25 mg) or placebo once a week. All 32 patients responded clinically to the initial trimethoprim/sulfamethoxazole therapy and all achieved microbiologic cure. Recurrent disease was prevented by ongoing prophylaxis with either trimethoprim/sulfamethoxazole or sulfadoxine/pyrimethamine. Fifty percent of the 10 patients given placebo after initial cure relapsed at a mean of 1.6 months.[9]

Strikingly, 21 Haitian patients who received trimethoprim/sulfamethoxazole for *Isospora belli* or cryptosporidium infection showed no evidence of hypersensitivity reaction[10] in contrast to the 50 percent likelihood of severe hypersensitivity occurring in homosexual men treated with trimethoprim/sulfamethoxazole for pneumocystis pneumonia.[11] Two patients with severe hypersensitivity reactions to sulfa drugs were treated successfully with pyrimethamine alone (75 mg/day). Recurrences were prevented with daily pyrimethamine (25 mg/day).[13] Roxithromycin, a macrolide licensed in Europe, was used effectively in one French patient who failed to respond to trimethoprim/sulfamethoxazole.[14] Spiramycin, a drug that may be effective for treating cryptosporidium, was totally ineffective when it was used in one reported case to treat *Isospora belli*.[12]

■ PREVENTION

Although no nosocomial transmission has been reported, meticulous attention to handwashing and secretion precautions is essential because the fecal-oral route is suspected as the means of transmitting *Isospora belli*. Isospora are host-specific and no evidence of animal-to-human transmission has been reported.[15]

REFERENCES

1. Weinstein L, Edelstein SM, Madara JL, et al. Intestinal cryptosporidiosis complicated by disseminated cytomegalovirus infection. Gastroenterology 1981; 81:584-91.

2. Modigliani R, Bories C, LeCharpentier Y, et al. Diarrhea and malabsorption in acquired immune deficiency syndrome: a study of four cases with special emphasis on opportunistic protozoan infestations. Gut 1985; 26:179-87.

3. Whiteside ME, Barkin JS, May RG, et al. Enteric coccidiosis among patients with the acquired immunodeficiency syndrome. Am J Trop Med Hyg 1984; 33:1066-72.

4. Forthal DN, Guest SS. *Isospora belli* enteritis in three homosexual men. Am J Trop Med Hyg 1984; 33:1060-4.

5. De Hovitz JA, Pape JW, Boncy M, Johnson WO. Clinical manifestations and therapy of *Isospora belli* infection in patients with the acquired immunodeficiency syndrome. N Engl J Med 1986; 315:87-90.

6. Trier JS, Moxey PC, Schimmel EM, Robles E. Chronic intestinal coccidiosis in man: intestinal morphology and response to treatment. Gastroenterology 1974; 66:923-35.

7. Ng E, Markell EK, Fleming RL, Fried M. Demonstration of *Isospora belli* by acid-fast stain in a patient with acquired immune deficiency syndrome. J Clin Microbiol 1984; 3:384-6.

8. Campbell PN, Current WL. Demonstration of serum antibodies to cryptosporidium sp. in normal and immunodeficient humans with confirmed infections. J Clin Microbiol 1983; 18:165-9.

9. Pape JW, Verdier RI, Johnson WD Jr. Treatment and prophylaxis of *Isospora belli* infection in patients with the acquired immunodeficiency syndrome. N Engl J Med 1989; 320:1044-7.

10. DeHovitz JA, Johnson WD, Pape JW. Cutaneous reactions to trimethoprim sulfamethoxazole in Haitians. Ann Intern Med 1985; 103:479-80.

11. Gordin FM, Simon GL, Wofsy CB, Mills J. Adverse reactions to trimethoprim sulfamethoxazole in patients with the acquired immunodeficiency syndrome. Ann Intern Med 1984; 100:495-9.

12. Gaska JA, Tietze KJ, Cosgrove EM. Unsuccessful treatment of enteritis due to *Isospora belli* with spiramycin: a case report. J Infect Dis 1985; 152:1336-8.

13. Weiss LM, Perlman DC, Sherman J, et al. *Isospora belli* infection: treatment with pyrimethamine. Ann Intern Med 1988; 109:474-5.

14. Musey KL, Chidiac C, Beaucaire G, et al. Effectiveness of roxithromycin for treating *Isospora belli* infection. J Infect Dis 1988; 158:646.

15. Kirkpatrick CE. Animal reservoirs of Cryptosporidium spp. and *Isospora belli*. J Infect Dis 1988; 158:909-10.

6.6

Spirochetal Infections

6.6.1

Syphilis in Non-HIV-Infected Hosts

Gail Bolan, M.D.

This chapter briefly discusses the epidemiology, diagnosis, and treatment of syphilis in non-HIV-infected hosts. Because HIV status is important in managing syphilitic patients, all patients with syphilis should be tested for HIV. If testing is not possible, patients should be managed as if they might be HIV-infected. HIV testing should be accompanied by pre- and post-test counseling and the confidentiality of all test results should be assured. Issues peculiar to syphilis in HIV-infected hosts are discussed in two subsequent chapters.

The spirochete *Treponema pallidum* causes syphilis, a complex systemic illness divided into the following stages:

1. An incubation period averaging three weeks;

2. A primary stage characterized by a chancre (a painless skin lesion) associated with regional lymphadenopathy;

3. A secondary stage characterized by a diffuse body rash, mucous-membrane lesions, generalized lymphadenopathy, and constitutional symptoms;

4. A latent period of asymptomatic infection divided into two categories:
   a. early latent — syphilis of less than one year's duration and
   b. late latent — syphilis of more than one year's, or indeterminate duration;

5. A tertiary stage characterized by disease involving the skin, bones, central nervous system, and viscera, particularly the heart and great vessels.

Because it is difficult to readily grow *T. pallidum* in vitro, diagnosing syphilis must rely on patient history, clinical findings, dark-field examination of specimens from primary or secondary lesions, and serologic testing. Penicillin is currently the treatment of choice for syphilis, although doses and routes of administration vary with different stages of disease.

■ EPIDEMIOLOGY

Syphilis continues to be a disease of considerable medical importance, ranking third among reportable communicable diseases in the United States in 1986.[1] Because approximately 95 percent of all syphilis is acquired by sexual contact with an infectious lesion, syphilis occurs predominantly among the most sexually active age group — persons 15 to 35 years old. The incidence of early syphilis is higher among men (especially homosexual and bisexual men), persons of color, and persons living in urban centers.[2]

Although the total number of syphilis cases reported in the United States in recent years is substantially less than the 600,000 reported in 1943, the total continues to wax and wane. For example, between 1977 and 1982, the number of primary and secondary syphilis cases increased 64 percent — from 20,399 to 33,613[3] — and then decreased steadily to 27,599 in 1986.[4] Recent decreases in syphilis morbidity occurred primarily among males and presumably reflect changes in sexual practices among homosexual and bisexual men seeking to reduce their risk of HIV infection.[5,6] In the 1970s, 50 percent to 70 percent of reported syphilis cases were estimated to occur among homosexual and bisexual men living in areas reporting high rates of syphilis infection.[2] This percentage decreased to 10 percent to 20 percent in 1986.[6] In contrast, a 23 percent increase in heterosexual cases of primary and secondary syphilis was observed in the United States in the first quarter of 1987.[6]

While homosexual or bisexual men are at increased risk for both syphilis and HIV infection, it is not known whether those with HIV infection are at a higher risk for syphilis. Epidemiologic studies demonstrate that a history of a sexually transmitted disease (STD) (including syphilis) is associated with increased risk for HIV infection and AIDS among both homosexuals[7-10] and heterosexuals,[11,12] presumably because sexual behaviors that increase the risk for acquiring other STDs also increase the risk for acquiring HIV. Furthermore, STDs that cause genital ulcerations are implicated as cofactors for acquiring HIV infection.[12-14] Therefore, cases of early syphilis among any population may presage future HIV-related morbidity and mortality.

■ PATHOGENESIS AND CLINICAL COURSE

The clinical manifestations of syphilis in the normal host have been well described.[15,16] *Treponema pallidum* enters the body through mucous membranes or abraded skin, multiplies locally, and disseminates within hours to any organ via the lymphatics or bloodstream or both. After an incubation period of 3 to 90 days (mean, approximately three weeks), a chancre, the classic lesion of primary syphilis, may appear at the site of inoculation. These lesions may be single or multiple.[17] They characteristically begin as painless papules that quickly ulcerate and become indurated. Regional lymph nodes are usually enlarged, firm, and nontender. Chancres typically heal spontaneously within 3 to 6 weeks (range, 1 to 12 weeks), even in the absence of therapy, as the normal host's immune system is able to clear most of the spirochetes from the lesion site.

Secondary syphilis, which results from proliferation of the disseminated organisms, begins after an incubation period of 2 to 12 weeks (mean, approximately 6 weeks). The clinical manifestations of secondary syphilis are widespread and commonly include a diffuse body rash that may be macular, papular, follicular, and/or pustular, and usually involves the palms and soles. Other manifestations include condyloma lata, mucous patches, generalized lymphadenopathy, and constitutional symptoms such as fever, malaise, anorexia, weight loss, and arthralgias. Central nervous system (CNS) involvement (i.e., neurosyphilis) during this stage is not uncommon; increased cerebrospinal fluid (CSF) protein and lymphocytes are found in up to 35 percent of these patients and acute aseptic meningitis in up to 2 percent.[18-20] Spirochetes have been isolated from the CSF of secondary syphilis patients with and without CNS symptoms or CSF abnormalities.[20,21] Less common clinical manifestations of secondary syphilis include anterior uveitis, glomerulonephritis, nephrotic syndrome, hepatitis, synovitis, and osteitis. Signs and symptoms of secondary syphilis may last for days to months until an immune response from the host develops to control the proliferation of spirochetes.

CSF examination is not recommended for patients with syphilis of less than one year's duration and no neurologic symptoms or signs. If the CSF is examined in these patients, abnormalities are commonly found (including cells, increased proteins, and a positive CSF-VDRL test), but they do not require therapy with regimens recommended for neurosyphilis. These abnormalities usually resolve after standard therapy for early syphilis. CSF examination is recommended for patients with syphilis of less than one year's duration if clinical signs and symptoms of neurologic involvement exist (e.g., optic, auditory, cranial nerve, or meningeal signs or symptoms).

After the manifestations of secondary syphilis resolve, the infection enters a latent period, during which the patient is asymptomatic and the CSF is normal. Signs and symptoms of secondary syphilis, especially mucocutaneous manifestations, may recur in approximately 25 percent of cases during this stage. Ninety percent of these relapses occur within the first year of infection and 100 percent within four years.[22] Therefore, patients with latent syphilis of greater than four years' duration generally are considered to be noninfectious (unless they are pregnant or donate blood) and resistant to reinfection. For treatment purposes and for distinguishing the majority of infectious cases from noninfectious cases, latent syphilis has been divided into two categories: early latent (syphilis of less than one year's duration) and late latent (syphilis of more than one year's duration).

Tertiary or late syphilis follows latent syphilis in approximately 15 percent of untreated patients.[22,23] This stage is a progressive inflammatory disease that can affect any organ. It eventually produces clinical manifestations 5 to 30 years after the initial infection. Tertiary syphilis is generally divided into three clinical categories: neurosyphilis, cardiovascular syphilis, and/or gummatous syphilis.

The least common type of tertiary syphilis diagnosed in the pre-antibiotic era was neurosyphilis. Although CNS involvement, or "neurosyphilis," may occur at any stage of syphilis, the later stage of neurosyphilis is the result of obliterative endarteritis affecting the small blood vessels of the meninges, brain, and spinal cord. This endarteritis can cause meningovascular neurosyphilis (with symptoms of meningitis, seizures, and strokes) or parenchymatous neurosyphilis (with symptoms of general paresis and tabes dorsalis). Meningovascular syphilis, which was less common than parenchymatous neurosyphilis in the pre-antibiotic era, usually occurs 5 to 10 years after the onset of infection.[20] General paresis usually occurs 15 to 20 years after infection and tabes dorsalis after 25 to 30 years.[20] Approximately 30 percent of untreated patients with neurosyphilis are asymptomatic but have one or more CSF abnormality, including pleocytosis, elevated protein level, or a positive CSF-VDRL (Venereal Disease Research Laboratory) test.[20] Cardiovascular syphilis is the result of obliterative endarteritis of the aortic vasa vasorum, commonly causing aortic aneurysms or aortic insufficiency or both. Gummatous syphilis, the most common type of tertiary syphilis diagnosed in the pre-antibiotic era, results from a nonspecific granulomatous lesion — the gumma — that may occur singly or multiply in any tissue. It is most commonly found in skin, mucous membranes, and bones.

■ **DIAGNOSIS**

The diagnosis of syphilis should be based on the following: the patient's history, clinical findings, examination of material from lesions or tissue for spirochetes, and/or serologic testing. A careful history of prior treatment for syphilis, recent sexual exposure, and suspicious lesions, rashes, and/or symptoms should be obtained. The patient should be examined for any clinical manifestations of primary, secondary, or tertiary syphilis. Among the laboratory tests available, dark-field examination of exudate from suspicious lesions is the test of choice for primary syphilis because it is rapid and generally sensitive and specific if performed by personnel with a high level of expertise.[24]

A positive dark-field examination removes the uncertainty that may occur if a suspicious lesion is treated empirically in a patient who has not yet become seropositive for syphilis. It also allows a definitive diagnosis of syphilis to be made early so that proper measures can be initiated to assure identification and treatment of sexual contacts and proper follow-up for the patient.

As visualized in the dark-field microscope, *Treponema pallidum* is a corkscrew-shaped organism, slightly longer than the diameter of an erythrocyte, which moves in a spiraling motion with a characteristic undulation about its midpoint. If the patient has used local or systemic antibiotics, or if an inadequate specimen was collected, dark-field examination of exudate from suspicious lesions may be insensitive. Because of this possibility, a lesion is considered dark-field-negative only after three negative examinations. Problems with specificity can result if saprophytic spirochetes inhabiting the mouth, anus, and genital region are mistakenly identified as *T. pallidum*. For this reason, examination of specimens from oral lesions is not recommended and specimens from anal lesions should be interpreted with caution. *Treponema pallidum* may be visualized by dark-field examination of some secondary lesions, such as condyloma lata, thus aiding the diagnosis of secondary syphilis.

The direct fluorescent antibody (DFA) test on lesions or tissue is another definitive method for diagnosing early syphilis. This test, if available, is more sensitive and specific than dark-field examination and is particularly useful if the diagnosis is uncertain and a dark-field microscope is not available or if the exudate is from an oral or anal lesion.

Serologic tests for syphilis include nontreponemal tests, which detect antibodies directed against a cardiolipin-lecithin-cholesterol antigen, and treponemal tests, which detect antibodies directed against *T. pallidum*. The most common of the nontreponemal tests are the VDRL and the RPR (rapid plasma reagin) test.[24-26] These tests are nonspecific but convenient for screening large numbers of serum samples and are also helpful for following disease activity. Nontreponemal antibody test results should be reported quantitatively and titered out to a final end point rather than reported as greater than an arbitrary cutoff. When following disease activity, the same nontreponemal test should be used and it should be run by the same laboratory. These tests usually become reactive at some time during primary syphilis. The titer rises rapidly, remains peaked during the first year of infection, and then falls steadily to low levels in late syphilis, at which time 25 percent of patients may be nonreactive. After treatment, the titer falls at a rate related to the prior duration of untreated infection. Biologic false-positives are not uncommon with nontreponemal tests.[27] Tests may be transiently false-positive after a variety of febrile illnesses or immunizations and persistently false-positive in intravenous drug users and persons with autoimmune disease and chronic infections such as leprosy. A false-positive nontreponemal test can be verified as such and syphilis excluded as a diagnosis by obtaining a negative treponemal test.

The two most common treponemal tests are the FTA-abs (fluorescent treponemal antibody-absorbed) and the MHA-TP (microhemagglutination-*Treponema pallidum*). These tests are more specific than the nontreponemal tests, usually become reactive in primary syphilis, and remain reactive for life despite therapy.[24-26] Treponemal antibody titers do not correlate with disease activity and should be reported as positive or negative. False-positives are rare, although they can occur.[28] Both nontreponemal and treponemal tests are also reactive in persons with other spirochetal illnesses, such as yaws and pinta.

The sensitivities of the serologic tests in untreated syphilis vary with the type of test and duration of illness. For the RPR/VDRL, FTA-abs, and MHA-TP tests, sensitivities are shown in Table 1.[24,29] The specificity of these tests varies with the population being tested. In general, the specificity of all tests in healthy volunteers is approximately 99.5 percent to 100 percent, but it decreases to 75 percent to 85 percent in sick persons.[24]

TABLE 1.   SENSITIVITIES OF TESTS FOR SYPHILIS

TEST	STAGE OF SYPHILIS			
	Primary	Secondary	Latent	Tertiary
RPR/VDRL	59–87%	100%	73–91%	37–99%
FTA-abs	86–100%	99–100%	96–99%	90–100%
MHA-TP	64–87%	96–100%	96–100%	99–100%

Diagnosis of Neurosyphilis.   The diagnosis of syphilis should be based on examination of the CSF for cells (usually lymphocytes), on protein concentration, and on a CSF-VDRL. The CSF-VDRL is highly specific but lacks sensitivity.[24] Sensitivity ranges from 10 percent to 89 percent,[30-32] depending on the type of neurosyphilis; it is highest for meningitic, meningovascular, and paretic neurosyphilis, and lowest for asymptomatic neurosyphilis and tabes dorsalis. Therefore, a positive CSF-VDRL is considered diagnostic of neurosyphilis, but a negative CSF-VDRL cannot be used to exclude the diagnosis of neurosyphilis in any patient. The CSF-FTA-abs test may be more sensitive than the VDRL, but problems with specificity and interpretation have limited its usefulness,[30,33] so the diagnosis of neurosyphilis should not be based solely on a positive CSF-FTA-abs test. However, a negative CSF-FTA-abs test provides evidence against neurosyphilis. Better diagnostic tests for neurosyphilis are needed. Other tests, such as measurement of plasma cells and immunoglobulins, have been suggested but have not been studied adequately to date.[24]

■ EXAMINATION OF THE CEREBROSPINAL FLUID

The Centers for Disease Control (CDC) currently recommends examination of the CSF in all patients with any stage of syphilis and neurologic symptoms and/or signs.[34] Cerebrospinal fluid examination has been considered desirable in all patients with syphilis of greater than one year's duration. However, questions have been raised about the benefit of examining the CSF of older, asymptomatic individuals with syphilis of greater than one year's duration because the VDRL test cannot exclude the diagnosis of neurosyphilis and the outcome with standard penicillin therapy is generally good.[35] CSF examination is clearly indicated in persons with syphilis of more than one year's duration when (1) serum nontreponemal antibody titer is ≥1:32, (2) HIV-antibody test is positive, (3) nonpenicillin therapy is planned, (4) treatment for early syphilis has failed, (5) neurologic signs or symptoms are present, or (6) other evidence of active syphilis such as aortitis, gummas, or iritis is present. Routine CSF examination in patients without neurologic symptoms or signs and with early syphilis of less than one year's duration is not indicated because the frequent abnormalities at this stage of disease appear to be transient[18] and the outcome with standard penicillin therapy is excellent.[36-38]

■ HIV TESTING IN PATIENTS DIAGNOSED WITH SYPHILIS

Because the management of syphilis in HIV-infected patients may be different from that in patients without HIV infection, all sexually active persons with syphilis should be tested for HIV (with informed consent of the patient).[53] If testing is not possible, they should be managed as if they might be HIV-infected. HIV testing should be accompanied by pre- and post-test counseling and the confidentiality of all test results should be assured. Management of syphilis in HIV-infected patients is discussed in a subsequent chapter.

■ TREATMENT OF SYPHILIS

Although the drug of choice for treating syphilis remains parenteral penicillin (either benzathine penicillin G, aqueous procaine, or crystalline penicillin G), there have never been well-controlled prospective studies to determine the optimal dose or duration of therapy.[39] To further confuse matters, case reports of patients who failed to respond to standard treatment periodically appear.[40-43] The CDC currently recommends that incubating, primary, secondary, or latent syphilis of less than one year's duration and no clinical evidence of neurologic involvement be treated with 2.4 million units of benzathine penicillin G (administered intramuscularly at a single session).[34] Clinical and/or serologic failure rates for this treatment schedule have been reported to range from less than 1 percent to 2 percent.[44] Penicillin-sensitive, non-pregnant patients can be treated with doxycycline (100 mg orally 2 times a day for 2 weeks) or tetracycline hydrochloride (500 mg orally 4 times a day for 2 weeks). In penicillin-sensitive, non-pregnant patients who cannot tolerate tetracycline, erythromycin can be given, if compliance and follow-up are assured. All syphilis patients should be warned about the possibility of a Jarisch–Herxheimer reaction before any treatment is given.

   All patients with syphilis of greater than one year's duration should have a careful clinical examination and CSF examination, if indicated. If findings consistent with neurosyphilis are found by physical or CSF examination, patients should be treated with a neurosyphilis regimen. Otherwise, syphilis of greater than one year's duration (i.e., latent syphilis of indeterminate or more than one year's duration, cardiovascular syphilis, or gummatous syphilis) should be treated with 7.2 million units of benzathine penicillin G total (administered as 3 doses of 2.4 million units by intramuscular injection weekly for 3 successive weeks). Some experts also treat cardiovascular syphilis patients with a neurosyphilis regimen. Penicillin-sensitive, non-pregnant patients with syphilis of greater than one year's duration can be given doxycycline (100 mg orally 2 times a day for 4 weeks) or tetracycline hydrochloride (500 mg orally 4 times a day for 4 weeks).

While tetracycline and erythromycin seem to be effective in treating syphilis, they have been evaluated less extensively than penicillin. Problems with gastrointestinal intolerance and patient compliance are significant among patients treated with these antibiotics. Therefore, close follow-up of these patients is essential. If compliance and close follow-up cannot be assured, the patient should be desensitized to penicillin and managed in consultation with an expert. Other antibiotics, such as ceftriaxone (250 mg by intramuscular injection daily for 10 days), have also been used in treating early syphilis. Again, no long-term follow-up studies of significant numbers of patients are available for these antibiotics and careful follow-up is mandatory if used. Although it is theoretically possible that strains of *T. pallidum* could acquire resistance to antimicrobial agents via plasmids,[45] there is no evidence available to date suggesting that penicillin-resistance is a significant problem among these organisms.

Treatment of Neurosyphilis. Treatment of neurosyphilis remains controversial. Until recently, benzathine penicillin G (7.2 million units over 3 weeks) had been considered acceptable treatment for neurosyphilis, especially asymptomatic CNS infection in patients with syphilis of greater than one year's duration, despite documented treatment failures[43] and the fact that benzathine penicillin G cannot guarantee treponemicidal levels in the CSF.[46-48] More recently, the CDC has recommended that all cases of symptomatic and asymptomatic neurosyphilis in patients with syphilis of greater than one year's duration be treated with aqueous crystalline penicillin G (12 to 24 million units IV per day, i.e., 2 to 4 million units every 4 hours for 10 to 14 days).[34] If outpatient compliance can be ensured, procaine penicillin (2.4 million units by intramuscular injection daily) and probenecid (500 mg orally 4 times a day) for 10 to 14 days is the alternative regimen for neurosyphilis. Many experts also recommend the addition of benzathine penicillin G (2.4 million units IM weekly for 3 successive weeks) after completion of these neurosyphilis regimens. In penicillin-sensitive patients, the allergy should be confirmed. The patient should be managed in consultation with an expert and desensitized to penicillin. Studies comparing the efficacy of these two neurosyphilis regimens have not been done. Preliminary data suggest that ceftriaxone may be an alternative antibiotic for the treatment of neurosyphilis.[49] Other antibiotics, such as doxycycline, amoxicillin, and chloramphenicol, may be useful in special cases. Better studies are needed to determine the optimal therapy for neurosyphilis.

■ ASSESSING THERAPEUTIC CURE IN NON-HIV-INFECTED PATIENTS

Determining therapeutic cure of syphilis after standard treatment regimens is problematic because no simple test is available to determine cure. Moreover, clinical symptoms and signs of early syphilis resolve even without treatment. Treatment-failure rates for all types of syphilis have been estimated to range from less than 1 percent to 7 percent[50] and are based on any of the following findings in a patient who has been treated:

1. persistence or recurrence of clinical signs or symptoms of syphilis;

2. fourfold (two dilutions) increase in the titer of nontreponemal tests;

3. failure of the initially high nontreponemal test titer in patients with primary syphilis to decrease fourfold (two dilutions) and eightfold (four dilutions) at three- and six-month follow-up tests, respectively, and in patients with secondary syphilis to decrease fourfold at six months.[51,52]

Treatment failures determined by the above criteria may occur for a variety of reasons. Reinfection is most likely, but it is also the most difficult to document. Such patients should be retreated for early syphilis if either clinical evidence of early syphilis or infected contacts are identified. Unfortunately, it is often difficult to exclude the possibility of reinfection because patients fail to return for follow-up serologic testing after treatment and imprecise histories of sexual contacts may be obtained. Increasing or persistently high titer on the nontreponemal test due to a febrile illness or vaccination may be a confounding event, causing a false-positive on the nontreponemal test. These patients should be followed closely because most false-positive reactions are transient. If the titer does not eventually decrease, then a true treatment failure is possible.

If there is no evidence for reinfection or an event that would produce a false-positive result in an otherwise healthy person, then a true treatment failure must be considered (persons with HIV infection are discussed in subsequent chapters). In patients with early syphilis who appear to be true treatment failures, an HIV-antibody test and a CSF examination should be done, treatment for syphilis of greater than one year's duration should be given (assuming evidence of neurosyphilis and/or HIV infection is not found), and close follow-up should continue. In patients who are treated for latent syphilis, the absence of a serologic response to therapy is not an indication for retreatment. Evidence of disease activity by clinical findings or a rising nontreponemal titer is an indication for further evaluation as outlined above for patients with early syphilis and retreatment in such patients. Patients with neurosyphilis should have follow-up CSF examinations every six months until the cell count is normal. If the initial CSF pleocytosis has not decreased at six months or is not normal by two years then retreatment with a neurosyphilis regimen is recommended.

REFERENCES

1. Summary of notifiable diseases, United States, 1986. MMWR 1986; 1-57.

2. Fichtner RR, Aral SO, Blount JH, et al. Syphilis in the United States: 1967-1979. Sex Transm Dis 1983; 10:77-80.

3. Annual Summary 1984. Reported morbidity and mortality in the United States. MMWR 1986; 33:57-9.

4. Summary — case specified notifiable diseases, United States. MMWR 1987; 35:813.

5. Syphilis — United States 1983. MMWR 1984; 33:433-6, 441.

6. Increases in primary and secondary syphilis — United States. MMWR 1987; 36:393-7.

7. Jaffe HW, Choi K, Thomas PA, et al. National case-control study of Kaposi's sarcoma and *Pneumocystis carinii* pneumonia in homosexual men. Part 1. Epidemiologic results. Ann Intern Med 1983; 99:145-51.

8. Rogers MF, Morens DM, Stewart JA, et al. National case-control study of Kaposi's sarcoma and *Pneumocystis carinii* pneumonia in homosexual men. Part 2. Laboratory results. Ann Intern Med 1983; 99:151-8.

9. Darrow WW, Echenberg DF, Jaffe HW, et al. Risk factors for human immunodeficiency virus (HIV) infections in homosexual men. Am J Public Health 1987; 77:479-83.

10. Moss AR, Osmond D, Bacchetti P, et al. Risk factors for AIDS and HIV seropositivity in homosexual men. Am J Epidemiol 1987; 125:1035-47.

11. Risk factors for AIDS among Haitians residing in the United States. Evidence of heterosexual transmission. The Collaborative Study Group of AIDS in Haitian-Americans. JAMA 1987; 257:635-9.

12. Cameron DW, Plummer FA, Simonsen JW, et al. Female-to-male heterosexual transmission of HIV infection in Nairobi [Abstract]. Washington, D.C.: III International Conference on AIDS, 1987:25.

13. Greenblatt RM, Lukehart SA, Plummer FA, et al. Genital ulceration as a risk factor for human immuno-deficiency virus infection. AIDS 1988; 2:47-50.

14. Holmberg SD, Stewart JA, Gerber AR, et al. Prior herpes simplex virus type 2 infection as a risk factor for HIV infection. JAMA 1988; 259:1048-50.

15. Stokes JH, Beerman H, Ingraham NR. Modern clinical syphilology: diagnosis, treatment, case study. 3rd ed. Philadelphia: W.B. Saunders, 1944.

16. Kampmeier RH. Essentials of syphilology. Philadelphia: J.B. Lippincott, 1944.

17. Chapel TA. The variability of syphilitic chancres. Sex Transm Dis 1978; 5:68-70.

18. Mills CH. Routine examination of the cerebrospinal fluid in syphilis: its value in regard to more accurate knowledge, prognosis, and treatment. Br Med J 1927; 2:527-32.

19. Chesney AM, Kemp JE. Incidence of *Spirochaeta pallida* in cerebrospinal fluid during early stage of syphilis. JAMA 1924; 83:1725-8.

20. Simon RP. Neurosyphilis. Arch Neurol 1985; 42:606-13.

21. Tramont EC. Persistence of *Treponema pallidum* following penicillin G therapy. JAMA 1976; 236:2206-7.

22. Clark EG, Danbolt N, Chapel TA. The Oslo study of untreated syphilis: an epidemiologic investigation based on a restudy of the Boeck–Bruursgaard material. Med Clin North Am 1964; 48:613-23.

23. Rockwell DH, Yobs AR, Moore MB. The Tuskegee study of untreated syphilis: the 30th year of observation. Arch Int Med 1964; 114:792-8.

24. Hart G. Syphilis tests in diagnostic and therapeutic decision making. Ann Intern Med 1986; 104:368-76.

25. Jaffe HW. The laboratory diagnosis of syphilis. New concepts. Ann Intern Med 1975; 83:846-50.

26. Felman YM, Nikitas JA. Syphilis serology today. Arch Dermatol 1980; 116:84-9.

27. Moore JE, Mohr CF. Biologically false-positive serologic tests for syphilis: type, incidence, and cause. JAMA 1952; 150:467.

28. Tuffanelli DL, Wuepper KD, Bradford LL, Wood RM. Fluorescent treponemal-antibody absorption tests. Studies of false-positive reactions to tests for syphilis. N Engl J Med 1967; 276:258-62.

29. Jaffe HW. Management of reactive serology. In: Holmes KK, Mardh PA, Sparling PF, Wiesner PJ, eds. Sexually transmitted diseases. New York: McGraw-Hill, 1984:313-8.

30. Larsen SA, Hambie EA, Wobig GH, Kennedy EJ. Cerebrospinal fluid test for syphilis: treponemal and nontreponemal tests. In: Moriset R, Kurstak E, eds. Advances in sexually transmitted diseases. Utrecht: VNU Science Press, 1985:157-62.

31. Hooshmand H, Escobar MR, Kopf SW. Neurosyphilis: a study of 241 patients. JAMA 1972; 219:726-9.

32. Bracero L, Wormser GP, Bottone EJ. Serologic tests for syphilis: a guide to interpretation in various stages of disease. Mt Sinai J Med (NY) 1979; 46:289-92.

33. Jaffe HW, Larsen SA, Peters M, et al. Tests for treponemal antibody in CSF. Arch Intern Med 1978; 138:252-5.

34. 1989 STD treatment guidelines. MMWR 1989; 38(Suppl 8):5S-15S.

35. Wiesel J, Rose DN, Silver AL, et al. Lumbar puncture in asymptomatic late syphilis. An analysis of the benefits and risks. Arch Intern Med 1985; 145:465-8.

36. Smith CA, Kamp M, Olansky J, et al. Benzathine penicillin G in the treatment of syphilis. Bull WHO 1956; 15:1087-96.

37. Hahn RD, Cutler JL, Curtis AC, et al. Penicillin treatment in asymptomatic central nervous system syphilis: probability of progression to symptomatic neurosyphilis. AMA Arch Dermatol 1956; 74:355-66.

38. Rothenberg R. Treatment of neurosyphilis. J Am Vener Dis Assoc 1976; 3:153-8.

39. Idsoe O, Guthe T, Willcox RR. Penicillin in the treatment of syphilis. The experience of three decades. Bull WHO 1972; 47:1-68.

40. Berry CD, Hooton TM, Collier AC, Lukehart SA. Neurologic relapse after benzathine penicillin therapy for secondary syphilis in a patient with HIV infection. N Engl J Med 1987; 316:1587-9.

41. Bayne LL, Schmidley JW, Goodin DS. Acute syphilitic meningitis. Its occurrence after clinical and serologic cure of secondary syphilis with penicillin G. Arch Neurol 1986; 43:137-8.

42. Markovitz DM, Beutner KR, Maggio RP, Reichman RC. Failure of recommended therapy for secondary syphilis. JAMA 1986; 255:1767-8.

43. Greene BM, Miller NR, Bynum TE. Failure of penicillin G benzathine in the treatment of neurosyphilis. Arch Intern Med 1980; 140:1117-8.

44. Schroeter AL, Lucas JB, Price EV, Falcone VH. Treatment for early syphilis and reactivity of serologic tests. JAMA 1972; 221:471-6.

45. Stapleton JT, Stamm LV, Bassford PJ Jr. Potential for development of antibiotic resistance in pathogenic treponemes. Rev Infect Dis 1985; Suppl 2:S314-S317.

46. Mohr JA, Griffiths W, Jackson R, et al. Neurosyphilis and penicillin levels in cerebrospinal fluid. JAMA 1976; 236:2208-9.

47. Dunlop EM, Al Egaily SS, Houang ET. Penicillin levels in blood and CSF achieved by treatment of syphilis. JAMA 1979; 241:2538-40.

48. Ducas J, Robson HG. Cerebrospinal fluid penicillin levels during therapy for latent syphilis. JAMA 1981; 246:2583-4.

49. Hook EW III, Baker-Zander SA, Moskovitz BL, et al. Ceftriaxone therapy for asymptomatic neurosyphilis. Case report and Western blot analysis of serum and cerebrospinal fluid IgG response to therapy. Sex Transm Dis 1986:(Suppl 3):185S-188S.

50. Brown S. Update on recommendations for the treatment of syphilis. Rev Infect Dis 1982; 4:Suppl: 837S-841S.

51. Brown ST, Zaidi A, Larsen SA, Reynolds GH. Serologic response to syphilis treatment. A new analysis of old data. JAMA 1985; 253:1296-9.

52. Guinan ME. Treatment of primary and secondary syphilis: defining failure at three- and six-month follow-up. JAMA 1987; 257:359-60.

53. Recommendations for diagnosing and treating syphilis in HIV-infected patients. MMWR 1988; 37:600-2, 607-8.

Syphilis in HIV-Infected Hosts

Gail Bolan, M.D.

T he interaction of syphilis and HIV infection is an increasingly complex problem. Epidemiologic studies have demonstrated that a history of sexually transmitted diseases (STDs), including syphilis, is associated with increased risk for HIV infection and AIDS among sexually active persons, and that STDs causing genital ulceration might be cofactors for acquiring HIV infection.[1-8] More recently, isolated case reports have suggested that coexistent HIV infection may alter the natural history of syphilis and/or the dosage or duration of treatment required to cure syphilis.[9,10] Also, reports of false-negative serologic tests for syphilis in HIV-infected persons raise questions regarding the sensitivity of serologic diagnoses in such patients.[11] Questions about such issues as the efficacy of therapy for neurosyphilis and the significance of cerebrospinal fluid (CSF) abnormalities in early syphilis may assume greater importance in the presence of HIV infection.[23,24]

Because data are not yet available to answer many of these questions, definitive recommendations for managing HIV-infected patients with syphilis are currently limited. Management options are presented here for clinicians to consider until more definitive recommendations can be made. Options to consider in HIV-infected patients include: (1) evaluating CSF for evidence of neurosyphilis earlier in the course of infection; (2) obtaining biopsies of suspicious lesions and using special stains for spirochetes in patients with serologic tests negative for syphilis; and (3) testing syphilitic patients for antibodies to HIV and testing HIV-infected patients for syphilis.

■ EPIDEMIOLOGY

Epidemiologic studies demonstrate that a history of an STD, including syphilis, is associated with increased risk for HIV infection and AIDS among both homosexuals[1-4] and heterosexuals,[5,6] presumably because sexual behaviors that increase the risk for acquiring other STDs also increase the risk for acquiring HIV. Furthermore, STDs causing genital ulcerations have been implicated as cofactors for acquiring HIV infection in Africa.[7,8] Therefore, increases in the incidence of early syphilis in any population may presage future HIV-related disease.

Since 1982, the significant decreases seen in syphilis morbidity in the U.S. have occurred primarily among men. In areas reporting high rates of syphilis infection, the percentage of early syphilis cases occurring among homosexual and bisexual men decreased from 50 percent to 70 percent in the late 1970s[12] to 10 percent to 20 percent in 1986.[13] These data presumably reflect changes in sexual practices that reduce the risk of HIV infection among homosexual and bisexual men. They suggest that education efforts encouraging safer-sex practices have been effective among gay men. However, because many patients with syphilis are not routinely tested for neurosyphilis or HIV infection, and because these conditions (if diagnosed) are not reportable in many areas, the incidence of syphilis — especially neurosyphilis — in HIV-infected patients is unknown. In addition, it is not known whether patients with HIV infection are at higher risk for syphilis than persons without HIV infection.

■ PATHOGENESIS

It is plausible that impairment of both cell-mediated and humoral immunity by HIV[14] could limit the host's defenses against *Treponema pallidum*, thereby altering the clinical manifestations and/or natural course of syphilis infection. Host immunity, especially cell-mediated immunity, plays an important role in protecting the host against syphilis.[15,16] In animal models, selective impairment of cell-mediated immunity alters the host response to syphilis infection. Incubation time is shorter, lesions are more numerous and widespread, and healing time is slower.[17] Furthermore, HIV-induced meningeal inflammation may facilitate penetration of spirochetes into the central nervous system (CNS) and thus contribute to the development of symptomatic neurosyphilis.

■ CLINICAL MANIFESTATIONS AND COURSE

Recent case reports have suggested that the clinical manifestations of syphilis may be unusual and the course more rapid in patients with HIV infection. These anecdotal reports have led to the hypothesis that in patients co-infected with HIV and *T. pallidum*, symptomatic neurosyphilis may be more likely to develop, the latency period before development of meningovascular syphilis may be shorter, and the efficacy of standard therapy for early syphilis may be reduced.

Several cases of neurosyphilis have been reported in patients with HIV infection.[9] One patient presented with a diffuse maculopapular rash, hepatomegaly, and a unilateral facial palsy. Laboratory data were remarkable for transient elevation of serum transaminases, an RPR (rapid plasma reagin) titer of 1:512, and a positive fluorescent treponemal antibody-absorbed (FTA-abs) test. Cerebrospinal fluid examination revealed mononuclear pleocytosis (66 cells/cubic mm), an elevated protein level (182 mg/dl), and a CSF-VDRL (Venereal Disease Research Laboratory) titer of 1:4. This case is consistent with secondary syphilis accompanied by acute syphilitic meningitis and cranial-nerve involvement.

Another patient presented with a pure motor hemiplegia that appeared after a two-month prodrome of fatigue, malaise, and headache. No previous history of syphilis or chancre was reported. Laboratory data were remarkable for transient elevation of serum transaminases, an RPR titer of 1:256, and a positive FTA-abs. Cerebrospinal examination revealed lymphocytic pleocytosis (234 cells/cubic mm), an elevated protein level (94 mg/dl), hypoglycorrhachia (glucose 33 mg/dl), and a CSF-VDRL titer of 1:1. This case is consistent with meningovascular syphilis. A third patient presented with posterior uveitis, neurosensory hearing loss, and meningovascular syphilis (pure motor hemiparesis) four months after the diagnosis of primary syphilis.

Other atypical clinical findings in HIV-infected patients with syphilis include syphilitic blindness,[18] retrobulbar neuritis,[19] chorioretinitis,[20,21] and keratoderma.[21] Lukehart et al. found viable treponemes in the CSF of two of three HIV-infected patients with secondary syphilis three to six months after treatment with a single dose of 2.4 million units of benzathine penicillin G (as recommended by the Centers for Disease Control [CDC]).[23] In these two patients, no signs or symptoms of neurologic relapse were reported, CSF-VDRL titers had seroreverted, CSF-WBC count decreased, and serum VDRL titers decreased. In another HIV-infected patient with early syphilis who was treated with a single dose of benzathine penicillin, serum and CSF-VDRL titers were found to be increased but no treponemes were isolated at eight months following therapy. This patient also had no signs or symptoms of neurologic relapse. Long-term studies on larger numbers of patients are needed to know whether this phenomenon is common and reflects inadequate therapy, or whether the common course after therapy is to eventually clear the CSF of organisms, albeit slowly.

Several cases of neurologic relapse after benzathine penicillin therapy for early syphilis have been reported in patients with HIV infection.[9,10] One patient presented with eye pain, double vision, dizziness, and headache; two weeks later he was found in a stuporous state with a hemiparesis, homonymous hemianopsia, and expressive aphasia. Cerebrospinal fluid evaluation revealed mononuclear pleocytosis (32 cells/cubic mm), elevated protein level (92 mg/dl), and a CSF-VDRL titer of 1:4. This case is consistent with meningovascular syphilis. This patient had been treated for secondary syphilis five months before this neurological event and his serum VDRL titer had decreased from 1:256 to 1:16. Although a serum VDRL titer around the time of the stroke was 1:256, careful contact-tracing and close follow-up after the initial treatment suggested that reinfection did not occur.

Asymptomatic neurosyphilis (serum RPR titer of 1:8, normal CSF indices, and CSF-VDRL titer of 1:4) was also diagnosed in a patient with AIDS who was hospitalized for *Pneumocystis carinii* pneumonia. This patient had been treated for secondary syphilis five years before admission.

Both neurologic relapse following penicillin therapy and optic, auditory, and neurologic signs and symptoms in early syphilis are not unique to HIV-infected patients, but they are uncommon in non-HIV-infected patients.[22] In addition, a short latency period before the development of meningovascular syphilis has been reported in several cases,[22] but the four- or five-month incubation period is an unusually short interval, especially after benzathine penicillin therapy. Additional studies are needed to evaluate the clinical manifestations and natural history of syphilis in HIV-infected patients and to determine patient responses to currently recommended therapy.

■ DIAGNOSIS OF SYPHILIS IN HIV-INFECTED PATIENTS

The diagnosis of syphilis may be more complicated in HIV-infected patients because of false-negative serologic tests and atypical clinical presentations in the presence of HIV infection. The diagnosis should be based on a number of factors, including the patient's history, clinical findings, direct examination of lesion material for spirochetes, and serologic tests for syphilis. The importance of a careful clinical examination of HIV-infected patients with syphilis cannot be overstated. Central nervous system disease may occur during any stage of syphilis. Clinical evidence of neurologic involvement warrants CSF examination.

Dark-field examination or direct fluorescent antibody (DFA) staining of exudate from suspicious lesions of primary syphilis should always be done if feasible, because in a patient with suspicious lesions but negative serologies, a positive dark-field examination or DFA stain will be diagnostic. Dark-field examination or DFA staining of selected secondary lesions should also be used in establishing the diagnosis of secondary syphilis. It is important to confirm by direct fluorescent antibody (DFA) that the treponema seen in dark-field-positive oral and anal lesions are *T. pallidum*, since nontreponemal spirochetes may be found in the gastrointestinal tract.

Serologic tests for syphilis continue to be the cornerstone in diagnosing untreated syphilis infection — even in HIV-infected patients. Serum samples should be obtained from any patient in whom the diagnosis of syphilis is suspected. All patients with known HIV infection should also be screened for possible untreated syphilis infection. Nontreponemal antibody test results should be reported quantitatively and titered out to a final end point.

A negative RPR or VDRL test result may not rule out syphilis in patients with HIV infection. While the sensitivity of these serologic tests in diagnosing secondary syphilis is generally very high, the recent case report of seronegative secondary syphilis in a patient with HIV infection[11] suggests that some patients may fail to develop normal antibody responses to *T. pallidum*. Even though this patient eventually seroconverted, more data are needed on the serologic response to *T. pallidum* in HIV-infected patients.

When clinical syndromes compatible with primary or secondary syphilis occur, and when dark-field examinations and serologic tests are negative, the "prozone phenomenon" (nontreponemal serologic test read as falsely negative because the specimen was not tested after sufficient dilution and thus the high concentration of antigen did not allow detectable antigen–antibody complex formation) should be ruled out. Suspicious lesions should be biopsied. Such biopsies should be evaluated for spirochetes using special stains or isolation techniques or both. A silver stain, such as the Steiner stain,[32] has been used. Specific DFA stains for *T. pallidum* can also be used, but they are not commonly available. Because *T. pallidum* cannot be grown on artificial media, inoculation of laboratory animals (usually rabbit testes) is the only method currently available to isolate the organism. This method is available only in a few research laboratories.

Clinicians should consult with infectious disease specialists or pathologists about special tests available in their areas. If spirochetes are not demonstrated on biopsy material, or if special techniques are not available to identify spirochetes but clinical suspicion of syphilis remains high, clinicians may wish to presumptively treat HIV-infected patients for early syphilis. Such patients should be followed closely with serial serologic testing at one month, two months, three months, and six months to detect any delayed antibody response.

Diagnosis of Neurosyphilis in HIV-Infected Patients. The diagnosis of neurosyphilis is based on the cerebrospinal fluid findings of cells, elevated protein concentration, and a positive CSF-VDRL. Even if the CSF-VDRL test is negative, the finding of increased CSF leukocytes (>5 per cubic mm) and protein (>0.4 mg/ml) requires consideration of a diagnosis of neurosyphilis. If the CSF-VDRL test is negative, the diagnosis of neurosyphilis is complicated by the lack of another reliable diagnostic test and the difficulty of distinguishing between neurologic disease caused by *T. pallidum* and that caused by HIV or other CNS pathogens found in patients with AIDS. Better diagnostic tests for neurosyphilis are needed. Measurement of immunoglobulins or treponemal antigens and isolation of treponemes have been suggested, but they have not yet been adequately studied.[25]

Indications for CSF Examination. It is currently unclear when to examine the CSF in patients with syphilis and concurrent HIV infection. Examination of

CSF for evidence of neurosyphilis certainly should be performed in all HIV-infected patients (or patients at risk for HIV infection) who have any unexplained behavioral abnormalities, psychologic dysfunction, or ocular, auditory, or other neurologic symptoms or signs — especially those consistent with neurosyphilis. Patients should also have their CSF examined for signs of neurosyphilis if they fail treatment for early syphilis (e.g., if the titer does not decrease appropriately: fourfold [two dilutions] decrease by three months for primary syphilis or by six months for secondary syphilis; or if a substantial fourfold [two dilutions] or greater increase occurs); or if they are HIV-infected patients diagnosed with syphilis of greater than one year's duration.

Because of recent case reports of neurosyphilis or isolation of *T. pallidum* from the CSF of HIV-infected patients who had completed standard therapy for early syphilis, some experts believe that routine CSF examination in HIV-infected patients with syphilis of less than one year's duration is now indicated and that therapy for neurosyphilis (see below) should be offered to those patients with a positive CSF-VDRL test.[23,33] Other experts, however, believe that these isolated case reports do not yet justify the need for routine CSF examinations in early syphilis, and that additional studies are needed to determine the significance of these worrisome reports.[34] Until data are available to address the need for evaluating CSF in early syphilis, patients should be informed of the current dilemma and their available treatment options should be discussed.

Indications for Screening for HIV Infection. Many of the diagnostic options discussed above (such as routine lumbar punctures in patients with early syphilis), and the therapeutic options discussed below, are recommended only for patients with coexisting HIV infection. Therefore, it is important to know the HIV-antibody status of patients with syphilis when choosing diagnostic and therapeutic options. All patients with syphilis should be tested for HIV antibodies and counseled. If HIV antibody testing is not possible, the clinician should manage the patient from the perspective that HIV co-infection may be present.

■ TREATMENT

The recent isolated case reports discussed above have also raised questions regarding the efficacy of current treatment recommendations for syphilis in the HIV-infected patient. Until further studies determine the optimal therapeutic regimen for early syphilis and neurosyphilis in HIV-infected patients and the significance of abnormal CSF findings in early syphilis, treatment in such patients will remain controversial. The CDC currently recommends that penicillin regimens should be used whenever possible for all stages of syphilis in HIV-infected patients.[26] Also, no proven alternative therapies to penicillin are available for treating patients with neurosyphilis, congenital syphilis, and syphilis in pregnancy. Therefore, confirmation of penicillin allergy and desensitization is recommended for these patients.

Treatment of Non-Neurologic Syphilis of Less Than One Year's Duration. A careful clinical examination to rule out clinical evidence of neurologic involvement (e.g., optic and auditory symptoms, cranial-nerve palsies) must be done before treatment of HIV-infected patients with syphilis of less than one year's duration. For HIV-infected patients with incubating, primary, secondary, or latent syphilis of less than one year's duration and no clinical evidence of neurologic involvement, the same treatment regimen as for patients without HIV infection is recommended: 2.4 million units of benzathine penicillin G administered intramuscularly at a single session.[26,34] In penicillin-sensitive, non-pregnant patients, allergy should be confirmed. If compliance and close follow-up are assured, doxycycline (100 mg orally 2 times a day for 2 weeks) or tetracycline hydrochloride (500 mg orally 4 times a day for 2 weeks) may be given. However, no data are available on the efficacy of tetracyclines in treating syphilis in HIV-infected patients and if compliance and close follow-up cannot be assured in patients taking tetracyclines, then desensitization to penicillin and management in consultation with an infectious disease expert is recommended.

Treatment of Non-Neurologic Syphilis of More Than One Year's Duration. A careful clinical examination and CSF examination should precede and guide treatment of HIV-infected patients with syphilis of greater than one year's duration or of indeterminate age. If a CSF examination is not possible, patients should be treated for presumed neurosyphilis. If the CSF examination yields no evidence of neurosyphilis, then 7.2 million units of benzathine penicillin G total (administered as 3 doses of 2.4 million units by intramuscular injection weekly for 3 successive weeks) is recommended.[26] In penicillin-sensitive, non-pregnant patients, allergy should be confirmed. If doxycycline (given as 100 mg orally 2 times a day for 4 weeks) or tetracycline hydrochloride (given as 500 mg orally 4 times a day for 4 weeks) is used, compliance and careful follow-up are mandatory. All patients should be warned about the possibility of a Jarisch–Herxheimer reaction before any treatment is given. In addition, HIV-infected patients should be informed that currently recommended regimens may be less effective for them than for patients without HIV infection and that close follow-up is therefore essential.

Neurosyphilis. For HIV-infected patients with any type of symptomatic neurosyphilis (including ocular or auditory syphilis), aqueous crystalline penicillin G is the treatment of choice (12 to 24 million units IV per day, i.e., 2 to 4 million units every 4 hours for 10 to 14 days).[34] Penicillin-sensitive patients should be desensitized to penicillin.

If hospitalization is imposslble, then aqueous procaine penicillin G is another option (2.4 million units intramuscularly daily plus probenecid 500 mg by mouth 4 times daily for 10 days). However, these injections are painful and patient compliance may be difficult to ensure. Many experts also recommend the addition of benzathine penicillin G (2.4 million units IM weekly for 3 successive weeks) after completion of aqueous crystalline or aqueous procaine penicillin G. Other outpatient regimens have been used in the treatment of neurosyphilis in patients with normal immune function. These regimens include amoxicillin (2 g with probenecid 500 mg by mouth 3 times daily for 14 days),[27,28] doxycycline (200 mg by mouth twice a day for 21 days),[29] and ceftriaxone (1 g intramuscularly daily for 14 days).[35] The efficacy of these regimens for treating syphilis in HIV-infected patients is unknown.

For HIV-infected patients with asymptomatic neurosyphilis and syphilis of greater than one year's duration, aqueous penicillin therapy is the treatment of choice.[34] Any of the other regimens outlined above for treatment of symptomatic neurosyphilis could also be considered.

Because of concerns regarding neurologic relapse and persistence of treponemes in the CSF of HIV-infected patients treated with benzathine penicillin for early syphilis, some experts feel that until better data are available, HIV-infected patients with syphilis of less than one year's duration and an abnormal

CSF with a positive VDRL titer (i.e., asymptomatic neurosyphilis) should be offered treatment regimens of longer duration, higher doses, and better CSF penetration (e.g., the antibiotic regimens for neurosyphilis outlined above) (personal communication, CDC panel on syphilis and HIV, March 1988). Other experts emphasize that HIV-infected patients treated for syphilis who fail to respond (as defined below) to standard benzathine penicillin therapy should also be offered antibiotic regimens of higher doses, longer duration, and better CSF penetration, such as those described above for neurosyphilis (personal communication, CDC panel on syphilis and HIV, March 1988).

Follow-up.   Until the efficacy of treatment regimens is better defined, the importance of closely following HIV-infected patients with syphilis cannot be overstated. All patients should be watched carefully for persistent or recurrent symptoms and for any signs of neurologic involvement.

Patients treated for syphilis of less than one year's duration should be examined and retested with a quantitative nontreponemal test at 1 to 2 weeks and at 1, 2, 3, 6, 9, and 12 months after treatment. The reasons for the follow-up intervals include: verifying that the level of the nontreponemal test peaks and then falls; identifying the peak level for comparison in six months; documenting a Jarisch–Herxheimer reaction; and assuring compliance with treatment, effective partner notification, and safe-sex practices. More frequent follow-up may be necessary to characterize the peak level in some cases. Patients should be followed longer if any questions about the adequacy of their clinical or serologic response exist. Patients must be followed using the same nontreponemal test because titers from the VDRL and RPR tests are not interchangeable. In the absence of HIV infection and no previous history of *T. pallidum* infection, treatment usually produces seronegativity within one year in patients with primary syphilis and within two years in patients with secondary syphilis. The serologic response in HIV-infected patients is unknown.

Determining what constitutes the therapeutic cure of syphilis is problematic because no simple test is available. Moreover, clinical symptoms and signs of early syphilis may resolve even without treatment. Criteria for treatment failure are currently based on curves of serologic response to treatment established in patients with normal immune function. These include the following findings: (1) persistence or recurrence of clinical signs or symptoms of syphilis; (2) fourfold (two dilutions) increase in the titer of nontreponemal tests; or (3) failure of the initially high nontreponemal test titer in patients with early syphilis to decrease fourfold (two dilutions) by three months for primary syphilis and by six months for secondary syphilis.[30,31]

Until additional data on the serologic response in HIV-infected patients are available, the above criteria should also be used for determining treatment failures in HIV-infected patients.

For patients with neurosyphilis, repeat serologic testing as described above and CSF examination at six-month intervals is recommended until the findings have stabilized. Abnormal CSF white blood cell counts and protein levels should decrease by six months if no coexisting CNS infections are present, but CSF-VDRL tests may not return to nonreactivity. If the CSF white blood cell count is not normal by 2 years, retreatment using an antibiotic regimen for neurosyphilis is recommended.

Treating Sexual Contacts.   It is important that an effort be made to identify and treat any possible contacts of patients with early syphilis. In patients with primary syphilis, all contacts for three months prior to the appearance of the chancre should be evaluated clinically and serologically. In patients with secondary syphilis and no history of a chancre, contacts for six months prior should be evaluated clinically and serologically. In patients with early latent syphilis and no history of symptoms or signs suggestive of primary or secondary syphilis, contacts for 12 months prior should be evaluated clinically and serologically. Efforts should be made to establish a diagnosis of syphilis by history, clinical findings, and serologic testing before treating such contacts. However, persons exposed to a patient with early syphilis within the previous three months may be infected yet seronegative and, therefore, should be treated presumptively for early syphilis even without an established diagnosis.

Follow-up serologic tests should also be done at one week and three months to establish the diagnosis of syphilis in these contacts, especially if they are at risk of HIV infection. All cases of infectious syphilis (primary, secondary, and early latent) must be reported to local health departments. In addition, some state and local health departments, such as San Francisco's, require that healthcare providers notify the Director of STD Control of HIV-infected patients who have (1) neurosyphilis confirmed by CSF examination (i.e., positive CSF-VDRL) or histopathology (DFA or special stains of biopsy material); (2) negative serologic tests for syphilis (nontreponemal [VDRL, RPR] or treponemal [FTA-abs, MHA-TP] tests during secondary syphilis diagnosed by dark-field microscopy or histopathology of lesion material); or (3) failed treatment for syphilis as defined above.

■ EDUCATION

All patients with syphilis and their contacts must be given education and counseling to reduce their risk of future STDs, including HIV. Formal HIV counseling and testing should be discussed and offered along with appropriate discussion of confidentiality issues and anonymous testing options. Safer-sex messages should include reducing the numbers of sexual partners, knowing the health status of partners (if possible), avoiding unsafe sexual practices, and using condoms.

REFERENCES

1. Jaffe HW, Choi K, Thomas PA, et al. National case-control study of Kaposi's sarcoma and *Pneumocystis carinii* pneumonia in homosexual men. Part 1. Epidemiologic results. Ann Intern Med 1983; 99:145-51.

2. Rogers MF, Morens DM, Stewart JA, et al. National case-control study of Kaposi's sarcoma and *Pneumocystis carinii* pneumonia in homosexual men. Part 2. Laboratory results. Ann Intern Med 1983; 99:151-8.

3. Darrow WW, Echenberg DF, Jaffe HW, et al. Risk factors for human immunodeficiency virus (HIV) infections in homosexual men. Am J Public Health 1987; 77:479-83.

4. Moss AR, Osmond D, Bacchetti P, et al. Risk factors for AIDS and HIV seropositivity in homosexual men. Am J Epidemiol 1987; 125:1035-47.

5. Risk factors for AIDS among Haitians in the United States. Evidence of heterosexual transmission. The Collaborative study group of AIDS in Haitian-Americans. JAMA 1987; 257:635-9.

6. Cameron DW, Plummer FA, Simonsen JW, et al. Female-to-male heterosexual transmission of HIV infection in Nairobi [Abstract]. Washington, D.C.: III International Conference on AIDS, 1987; 25.

7. Greenblatt RM, Lukehart SA, Plummer FA, et al. Genital ulceration as a risk factor for human immunodeficiency virus infection. AIDS 1988; 2:47-50.

8. Holmberg SD, Stewart JA, Gerber AR, et al. Prior herpes simplex virus type 2 infection as a risk factor for HIV infection. JAMA 1988; 259:1048-50.

9. Johns DR, Tierney M, Felsenstein D. Alteration in the natural history of neurosyphilis by concurrent infection with the human immunodeficiency virus. N Engl J Med 1987; 316:1569-72.

10. Berry CD, Hooten TM, Collier AC, Lukehart SA. Neurologic relapse after benzathine penicillin therapy for secondary syphilis in a patient with HIV infection. N Engl J Med 1987; 316:1587-9.

11. Hicks CB, Benson PM, Lupton GP, Tramont EC. Seronegative secondary syphilis in a patient infected with the human immunodeficiency virus (HIV) with Kaposi's sarcoma. A diagnostic dilemma. Ann Intern Med 1987; 107:492-5.

12. Fichtner RR, Aral SO, Blount JH, et al. Syphilis in the United States: 1967-1979. Sex Transm Dis 1983; 10:77-80.

13. Increases in primary and secondary syphilis — United States. MMWR 1987; 36:393-7.

14. Musher D, Baugh RE. Syphilis. In: Samter M, ed. Immunological disease. 3rd ed. Boston: Little, Brown, 1978:639-50.

15. Pavia CS, Folds JD, Baseman JB. Cell-mediated immunity during syphilis: a review. Br J Vener Dis 1978; 54:144-50.

16. Pacha N, Metzger M, Smogor W, et al. Effects of immunosuppressive agents on the course of experimental syphilis in rabbits. Archivum immunologiae et therapiae experimentalis. 1979; 27:45-51.

17. Bowen DL, Lane HC, Fauci AS. Immunopathogenesis of the acquired immunodeficiency syndrome. Ann Intern Med 1985; 103:704-9.

18. Zambrano W, Perez GM, Smith JL. Acute syphilitic blindness in AIDS. J Clin Neuro Ophthalmol 1987; 7:1-5.

19. Zaidman GW. Neurosyphilis and retrobulbar neuritis in a patient with AIDS. Ann Ophthalmol 1986; 18:260-1.

20. Stoumbos VD, Klein ML. Syphilitic retinitis in a patient with acquired immunodeficiency syndrome-related complex. Am J Ophthalmol 1987; 103:103-4.

21. Radolph JD, Kaplan RP. Unusual manifestations of secondary syphilis and abnormal humoral immune response to *Treponema pallidum* antigens in a homosexual man with asymptomatic human immunodeficiency virus infection. J Am Acad Dermatol 1988; 18:423-8.

22. Merritt HH, Admas RD, Soloman HC. Neurosyphilis. New York: Oxford University Press, 1946.

23. Lukehart SA, Hook EW III, Baker-Zander SA, et al. Invasion of the central nervous system by *Treponema pallidum*: implications for diagnosis and treatment. Ann Intern Med 1988; 109:855-62.

24. Musher DM. How much penicillin cures early syphilis? Ann Intern Med 1988; 109:849-51.

25. Hart G. Syphilis tests in diagnostic and therapeutic decision making. Ann Intern Med 1986; 104:368-76.

26. 1989 sexually-transmitted diseases treatment guideline. MMWR 1989; 38(Suppl 8):5S-15S.

27. Morrison RE, Harrison SM, Tramont EC. Oral amoxicillin, an alternative treatment for neurosyphilis. Genitourin Med 1985; 61:359-62.

28. Faber WR, Bos JD, Reitra PJ, et al. Treponemicidal levels of amoxicillin in cerebrospinal fluid after oral administration. Sex Transm Dis 1983; 10:148-50.

29. Yim CW, Flynn NM, Fitzgerald FT. Penetration of oral doxycycline into the cerebrospinal fluid of patients with latent or neurosyphilis. Antimicrob Agents Chemother 1985; 28:347-8.

30. Brown ST, Zaidi A, Larsen SA, Reynolds GH. Serological response to syphilis treatment. A new analysis of old data. JAMA 1985; 253:1296-9.

31. Guinan ME. Treatment of primary and secondary syphilis: defining failure at three- and six-month follow-up. JAMA 1987; 257:359-60.

32. Swisher BL. Modified Steiner procedure for microwave staining of spirochetes and non-filamentous bacteria. J Histotechnology 1987; 10:241-3.

33. Tramont EC. Syphilis in the AIDS era. N Engl J Med 1987; 316:1600-1.

34. Recommendations for diagnosing and treating syphilis in HIV-infected patients. MMWR 1988; 37:600-2, 607-8.

35. Hook EW III, Baker-Zander SA, Moskovitz BL, et al. Ceftriaxone therapy for asymptomatic neurosyphilis. Case report and Western blot analysis of serum and cerebrospinal fluid IgG response to therapy. Sex Transm Dis 1986:(Suppl 3):185S-188S.

MALIGNANCIES
ASSOCIATED
WITH
AIDS

EDITOR

Paul A. Volberding, M.D.

7.1

Kaposi's Sarcoma

Non-HIV Kaposi's Sarcoma:
African KS

Paul A. Volberding, M.D., James O. Kahn, M.D., and David M. Heyer, M.D.

K aposi's sarcoma (KS) is a common tumor in black Africans. Its clinical features vary widely, depending upon the presence or absence of underlying infection with the human immunodeficiency virus (HIV).

Kaposi's sarcoma was recognized as common in Africans even before the AIDS epidemic.[1] Both this endemic form of KS and cases related to the new HIV epidemic in Africa are concentrated in the same central region of the continent.[1] There are, however, many important differences between endemic KS and HIV-related KS. This chapter briefly reviews endemic non-AIDS-related KS in black Africans.

■ CLINICAL FEATURES OF AFRICAN KS

Four types of African KS are recognized from their clinical features; these are summarized below.[1,2]

Nodular KS. This form is most common in adults. Nodules or plaques of pigmented cutaneous lesions are seen. The clinical course is relatively indolent and early visceral spread is uncommon. Nodular KS is also the most common variant seen in elderly non-African men (classical KS) and in AIDS patients, but the clinical course in these populations varies widely.

Florid KS. This form of Kaposi's sarcoma is also common in African adults. Lesions are usually larger and less numerous than in nodular KS. Florid Kaposi's sarcoma tumors are frequently exophytic and have eroded surfaces. This form infiltrates locally and often extends into the underlying bone.

Infiltrating KS. This form is similar to the florid form. Aggressive, spreading local tumors and painful bone involvement are seen, but tumors are less often exophytic; rather, a diffuse tissue infiltration is typical.

Lymphadenopathic KS. In contrast to other types of KS in Africa, this form is most common in children and young adults. Lymph-node enlargement (often massive) is typical. Cutaneous involvement, although common, is usually not extensive. Lymphadenopathic KS disseminates quickly to visceral organs and is rapidly fatal.

■ ETIOLOGY OF AFRICAN KS AND LIMITATIONS OF PUBLISHED STUDIES

Several studies have suggested that African KS follows immune dysfunction, infection with cytomegalovirus, or both.[3,4] These studies, however, are inconclusive. A role for CMV cannot be established, because infection with this virus is so common in endemic areas of Africa. Results of immune function testing show minor defects in cutaneous antigen reactivity in African KS, but the ratio of CD4+/CD8+ T cells is normal.[16]

■ THERAPY OF AFRICAN KS

Chemotherapy and radiation therapy have been used to treat African KS.[5-8] The results have depended largely upon the clinical type of KS; responses have been highest in local (nodular) disease and lowest in the lymphadenopathic disease. Interpreting the many published series is problematic, however, because patient numbers are small and clinical evaluation inadequate. Also, in contrast to AIDS-related cases of KS, the underlying immune system in non-AIDS-related African KS patients is intact, and infections as a complication of therapy have been infrequent. Therefore, direct extrapolation of results to AIDS-related KS is not possible.

Radiation Therapy.   No controlled trials of radiation therapy for African KS have been published, but some local control of the tumor has been reported with several doses and schedules of radiation.[9]

Chemotherapy.   Drugs with activity in African KS include BCNU, bleomycin, DTIC, actinomycin D, ICRF-159, and vincristine. Although the response rates with these drugs were high, the duration of response and survival were not specified.[8]

Despite the limitations described, these studies may be helpful in designing experimental therapeutic strategies for patients with AIDS-related KS.

■ CURRENT AFRICAN KS: ITS RELATIONSHIP TO AIDS

A more aggressive form of KS was observed when HIV appeared in central Africa.[10,11] Unlike those with endemic KS, African patients infected with HIV are immunodeficient and many develop KS.[12-15] The disease follows the same clinical course seen in other AIDS risk groups. The current cases of AIDS-related KS in Africa are a new phenomenon.

REFERENCES

1. Safai B, Good RA. Kaposi's sarcoma: a review and recent developments. Cancer 1981; 31:2-12.
2. Templeton C, Bhana D. Prognosis in Kaposi's sarcoma. J Natl Cancer Inst 1975; 55:1301-4.
3. Master SP, Taylor JF, Kyalwazi SK, Ziegler JL. Immunological studies in Kaposi's sarcoma in Uganda. Br Med J 1970; 1:600-2.
4. Giraldo G, Beth E, Huange E-S. Kaposi's sarcoma and its relationship to cytomegalovirus (CMV) III. CMV DNA and CMV early antigens in Kaposi's sarcoma. Int J Cancer 1980; 26: 23-9.
5. Ketiku KK, Durosinmi-Etti A. The treatment of Kaposi's sarcoma by combination chemotherapy in Nigeria. Clin Radiol 1984; 35:155-8.
6. Kyalwazi SK, Bhana D, Master SP. Actinomycin D in malignant Kaposi's sarcoma. E African Med J 1971; 48:16-26.
7. Vogel CL, Clements D, Wanume AK, et al. Phase II clinical trials of BCNU (NSU-409962) and bleomycin (NSC-125066) in the treatment of Kaposi's sarcoma. Cancer Chemother Rep 1973; 57: 325-33.
8. Volberding P, Conant MA, Stricker RB, Lewis BJ. Chemotherapy in advanced Kaposi's sarcoma. Am J Med 1983; 74:652-6.
9. Duncan JTK. Radiotherapy in the management of Kaposi's sarcoma in Nigeria. Clin Radiol 1977; 28:503-9.
10. Bayler AC. Aggressive Kaposi's sarcoma in Zambia, 1983. Lancet 1984; 1:1318-20.
11. Serwadda D, Carswell W, Ayuko WO, et al. Further experience with Kaposi's sarcoma in Uganda. Br J Cancer 1986; 53:497-500.
12. Bayley AC, Cheingsong-Popov R, Dalgleish AG, et al. HTLV-III serology distinguishes atypical and endemic Kaposi's sarcoma in Africa. Lancet 1985; 1:359-61.

13. Downing RG. African Kaposi's sarcoma and AIDS. Lancet 1984; 1:478-80.

14. Van de Perre P, Lepage P, Kestelyn P, et al. Acquired immunodeficiency syndrome in Rwanda. Lancet 1984; 2:62-9.

15. Clumeck N, Sonnet J, Taelman H, et al. Acquired immunodeficiency syndrome in African patients. N Engl J Med 1984; 310:492-7.

16. Kestens L, Melbye M, Biggar RJ, et al. Endemic African Kaposi's sarcoma is not associated with immunodeficiency. Int J Cancer 1985; 36:49-54.

Non-HIV Kaposi's Sarcoma: Classic KS and KS Associated with Immunosuppression

Paul A. Volberding, M.D.

■ CLASSIC KAPOSI'S SARCOMA (KS)

Kaposi's sarcoma was originally described by Moritz Kaposi in 1872 as an indolent cutaneous tumor of elderly men.[1] In this population, KS typically consists of painless nonpruritic nodules on the feet and distal lower extremities. Infiltration of bone is distinctly uncommon and necrosis of the surface of the tumor is rare. Tumor progression is usually slow, and visceral or lymph-node involvement occurs only very late in the disease process. Survival of 8 to 15 years is common — with or without therapy — and death is usually not caused by KS itself.[1] Patients with classic KS are not severely immune deficient and are not infected by the human immunodeficiency virus (HIV).

Etiology of Classic KS. Although not related to AIDS, classic KS may be a consequence of immune attrition, since the median age of patients at diagnosis is 70 to 80 years.[1] An association between classic KS and cytomegalovirus has been proposed on the basis of seroepidemiologic studies, but a direct causal link has not been made. Because classic KS is relatively more common in people from the Mediterranean basin (and in Ashkenazic Jews), a genetic predisposition is also possible, but unlikely.

Treatment of Classic KS. Classical KS is rare even in the elderly, and no large controlled clinical trials have been reported. Radiation therapy using a wide variety of sources and doses is effective in local control of KS,[2,3] and surgery is useful for palliation of some lesions. Chemotherapy for KS has not been adequately studied, but vinblastine and other cytotoxic agents have been used.[4,5]

Vinblastine is used as either a systemic or local treatment for classic KS. Doses of 5 mg to 10 mg have been successful as systemic treatment when given on a weekly schedule.[4] Local control can also be attempted with direct intralesion injection of dilute vinblastine. Bleomycin, adriamycin, and vincristine also are active against classic KS.[3,5] These drugs are used systemically in conventional doses and schedules. Combinations of chemotherapeutic drugs have rarely been used in classic KS.

■ KS ASSOCIATED WITH IMMUNOSUPPRESSION

In the early 1970s, Kaposi's sarcoma was reported to be associated with iatrogenic immunosuppression, generally in the setting of organ transplantation. Kaposi's sarcoma has been associated most commonly with renal transplantation but also with chronic immunosuppression due to the treatment of various auto-immune diseases. Most often, patients have been chronically treated with corticosteroids, especially prednisone, and often with azathioprine as well.

The intervals from first use of immunosuppressive medications to diagnosis of KS in this patient population ranges from 15 to 24 months.[6-9] Apart from the use of immunosuppressive medications, there is no evidence that these patients are suffering from underlying immunosuppression. Cases of KS in this patient population have been reported since the early 1970's, whereas HIV did not appear in the United States until the late 1970s.

Clinical Course and Diagnosis.   Kaposi's sarcoma in the immunosuppressed, non-HIV-infected patient follows a clinical course not unlike that seen in HIV-infected patients.[6-9] The tumor in this population is usually nodular in appearance. All areas of the body, including the internal organs, can be affected. Disease progression is often rapid. Kaposi's sarcoma is diagnosed the same way in these patients as in other populations. Biopsy of malignant lesions reveals a histologic profile typical of KS in other settings.

Treatment.   From the perspective of a clinician interested in HIV disease, the therapy of KS in non-HIV-infected, immunodeficient patients is of great interest. Although not many cases of non-HIV-related, immunosuppression-related KS have been fully documented, several reports of response to radiation therapy and chemotherapy highlight the generally responsive nature of this tumor to conventional treatments.[6,8,10,11] Of far greater interest, however, are the numerous reports that in the non-HIV-immunosuppressed population, KS can respond to the withdrawal of immunosuppressive medications. In nearly 50 percent of reported cases, KS, even in advanced stages of development, regressed completely after discontinuation of prednisone and azathioprine and reinstitution of hemodialysis (in the case of transplant-related KS).[6,9,10,11] The obvious implication for current cases of HIV-related KS is that if immunosuppression could be reversed, KS would regress. This is the basis for including patients with HIV-related Kaposi's sarcoma in many experimental trials of immunomodulatory and antiretroviral drugs.

REFERENCES

1. Safai B, Good RA. Kaposi's sarcoma: a review and recent developments. Cancer 1981; 31:2-12.

2. Holecek MJ, Harwood AR. Radiotherapy of Kaposi's sarcoma. Cancer 1978; 41:1733-8.

3. Hainsworth J, Oldham RK, Sismani AR, et al. Treatment of the syndrome of inappropriate secretion of antidiuretic hormone in small cell lung cancer. Proc Am Assoc Cancer Res, Am Soc Clin Oncol 1980; 21:627. abstract.

4. Scott WP, Voight JA. Kaposi's sarcoma. Management with vincaleucoblastine. Cancer 1966; 19:557-64.

5. Lanzotti VJ, Campos LT, Sinkovics JG, Samuels ML. Chemotherapy for advanced Kaposi's sarcoma. Arch Dermatol 1975; 111:1331-3.

6. Myers BD, Kessler E, Levi J, et al. Kaposi's sarcoma in kidney transplant recipients. Arch Intern Med 1974; 133:307-11.

7. Stribling J, Weitzner S, Smith GV. Kaposi's sarcoma in renal allograft recipients. Cancer 1978; 42:442-6.

8. Meyers AM, Rice GC, Kaye S, et al. Kaposi's sarcoma in an immunosuppressed renal allograft recipient. S Afr Med J 1976; 50:1299-1300.

9. Little PH, Khader AA, Farthing CF, et al. Kaposi's sarcoma in a patient after renal transplantation. Postgrad Med J 1983; 59:325-6.

10. Zisbrod Z, Haimov M, Schanzer H, et al. Kaposi's sarcoma after kidney transplantation. Report of complete remission of cutaneous and visceral involvement. Transplantation 1980; 30:383-4.

11. Hardy MA, Goldfarb P, Levine S, et al. De novo Kaposi's sarcoma in renal transplantation. Cancer 1976; 38:144-8.

HIV-Related Kaposi's Sarcoma

David M. Heyer, M.D., James O. Kahn, M.D., and Paul A. Volberding, M.D.

■ ETIOLOGY

Despite the clinical importance of HIV-related Kaposi's sarcoma (KS), surprisingly little is understood about the etiology of this tumor. Several possible etiologies have been proposed, however, and among those under investigation are the following: (1) the use of potentially carcinogenic recreational drugs; (2) an association with viral infections common in HIV risk populations, particularly cytomegalovirus; (3) a general breakdown in the system of immune surveillance; (4) a direct association with and cellular transformation by human immunodeficiency virus (HIV); and (5) the presence of circulating factor(s) responsible for endothelial proliferation.

RECREATIONAL DRUG THEORY

One of the first theories proposed for the etiology of HIV-related KS was that one or more of the recreational drugs commonly used by at-risk populations might be carcinogenic or immunosuppressive. The principal suspect was inhaled nitrites or "poppers."[1,2] These drugs, in common use at the time AIDS was first noted, have been the subject of ongoing epidemiologic and laboratory-based investigations, none of which have been conclusive. No convincing carcinogenic potential has been found in any of the inhaled nitrites, although trace contamination of largely unregulated drugs by carcinogens or their contamination (or both) after purchase, remain possibilities. Epidemiologic studies have shown no association between the development of AIDS and the use of these recreational drugs, but some studies have found that they were used more frequently by AIDS patients diagnosed with Kaposi's sarcoma.[1] Further studies of these drugs are clearly needed to establish a relationship to KS, but it seems prudent to recommend discontinuing recreational use of these drugs in all populations, as the U.S. Surgeon General did in February 1989.

CMV COFACTOR THEORY

Another early proposal for the pathogenesis of HIV-related KS was a direct or cofactor effect caused by another known virus, such as cytomegalovirus (CMV). Cytomegalovirus is present in many populations, but there is a particularly high incidence of infection among homosexual men.[3] Studies of AIDS patients show that nearly 100 percent have previous evidence of CMV exposure, and antibody profiles in patients with AIDS show evidence of CMV reactivation.[4,5] There are also reports of an association between CMV and KS in non-AIDS populations.[6] The fact that the prevalence of KS in AIDS patients declined from 1981 to 1985, in parallel with a decline in CMV seroconversion in a cohort of initially CMV-negative homosexual men, provides further evidence in support of CMV as a cofactor.[10]

Studies of CMV in AIDS patients have not established a conclusive relation to KS, however. While some reports have indicated that CMV can contain a transforming genome,[7] some AIDS patients with KS show no evidence of previous or current infection with CMV. Studies of KS lesions themselves have shown no integration of CMV genomes into the malignant cells.[4] Furthermore, CMV infection is common in many populations affected by AIDS in whom KS is infrequently seen.

IMMUNE SURVEILLANCE THEORY

It may appear that KS and other tumors in patients with AIDS are direct proof of the existence of the long-proposed system of immune surveillance. Proponents of this theory argue that KS must represent a commonly-appearing, spontaneous neoplasm and that in AIDS it is the recognition and elimination of these spontaneously-appearing malignant clones that is the primary defect.

While it is clear that lymphocytes are markedly reduced in patients infected with HIV, this theory does not adequately explain why this particular malignancy is so common, nor does it help us design rational therapeutic strategies. Although at present a role for defective immune surveillance in the appearance of KS is unproven, it probably contributes to the rapid progression and dissemination of this tumor.

HIV THEORY

A direct etiologic relationship between KS and HIV was proposed very early in the epidemic on the grounds that HIV might have direct oncogenic potential. Human immunodeficiency virus core protein and viral particles have been found in epidermal Langerhan's cells of the skin.[11] However, Southern blot analysis of KS tumor biopsies are negative for HIV DNA.[12] Recently, Vogel et al. found that introducing the HIV *tat* gene into the germ cells of mice could induce dermal lesions resembling KS in adult mice. The *tat* gene was expressed in the skin of these transgenic mice, but *tat* mRNA was not found in tumor cells themselves by Northern blot analysis.[13]

CIRCULATING ENDOTHELIAL "GROWTH FACTORS" THEORY

A final and intriguing theory of KS pathogenesis proposes that this tumor is not a true malignancy but rather a widespread cellular proliferation in response to a circulating substance or substances.[8,9] This theory postulates that HIV infection either directly or secondarily induces the production of growth factors for lymphatic endothelial cells. The continued progression of KS depends upon ongoing stimulation by these factors. In support of this theory, Nakamura et al. recently found that media conditioned by retrovirus-infected transformed T cells supported the growth of KS cells in culture. This "growth factor" only temporarily supported the growth of normal vascular endothelial cells and was distinct from other known endothelial growth-promoting factors or lymphokines.[14] Robert Gallo et al. established cells derived from lung biopsies and pleural effusions from AIDS patients with KS in long-term cultures and found that these AIDS-KS cells produced factors supporting their own growth (autocrine) as well as the growth of other cells (paracrine); these cells also expressed potent angiogenic activity.[15] While not conclusive, the growth-factor hypothesis is attractive, since it may help to explain the multicentric nature of KS and the relative paucity of mitotic figures found in KS tissue. The presence of HIV gene products in skin but not in the tumor cells is consistent with this theory.

■ HISTOPATHOLOGY

Histologic variants of Kaposi's sarcoma, including anaplastic, spindle-cell, and mixed-cell forms, have been reported in each of the populations affected by this tumor. In anaplastic and spindle-cell KS variants, one cell population predominates. In the anaplastic form, disordered, malignant-appearing cells are seen,[16] whereas the spindle-cell variant consists of a proliferation of rather similar, normal-appearing, uniformly sized spindle cells.[16] Both the anaplastic and spindle variants are uncommon in HIV-related KS. The third variant — the mixed cellular form — is by far the most common in HIV-related KS.[16] In the mixed-cell variant of KS, three features are commonly seen.[16] These include: (1) a proliferation within the tumor of vascular structures and slits, often lined by abnormally large, malignant-appearing endothelial cells; (2) a proliferation of surrounding spindle-shaped cells; and (3) an often striking extravasation of erythrocytes. Together, these features are diagnostic of KS.

CELL OF ORIGIN

The cell origin of KS has long been controversial.[17] Although the vascular nature of the tumor has been obvious to most observers, it has been difficult to prove conclusively that the tumor is of endothelial or supportive-cell origin. Recent studies have suggested that lymphatic endothelial cells are the cells of origin,[18,24] but others suggest a vascular endothelial cell origin,[19] or that both cell types are involved.[25] A lymphatic origin is consistent with the clinical distribution of KS lesions along cutaneous lymphatic drainage channels, as well as with the frequently associated lymphedema, especially in patients with HIV-related KS.

■ NATURAL HISTORY

The natural history of AIDS-related KS is complex and incompletely understood. The most common presenting sites of disease and patterns of spread are reviewed below.

INITIAL PRESENTATION OF AIDS-RELATED KS

Kaposi's sarcoma should be considered a multicentric process, affecting lymphatic endothelium at any site, including internal organs. Nevertheless, it is most often first detected in external sites, including the skin and oral cavity.[20,21] The first lesions often appear on the face, head, and in the oral cavity. Early KS lesions can be subtle. In most cases they are pigmented (red to blue), palpable, and asymptomatic.[20,21] Initial lesion size varies from 0.5 cm to more than 2 cm in diameter. To make an early diagnosis, it is imperative to examine the patient's entire skin surface, including the sides of the feet, the groin, and the oral cavity.

PATTERNS OF SPREAD

The natural history of AIDS-related KS is only now beginning to be understood. Although a few patients have had spontaneous remissions or stable disease for several years, the vast majority of cases of AIDS-related KS are characterized by continued and often rapid progression. Shortly after the first lesions are seen, new ones develop, but not necessarily in a pattern suggesting metastatic deposition. Rather, AIDS-related KS is a multicentric process. Lesions may appear on any body surface or in the viscera.

For the newly diagnosed patient, it is most important to estimate the prognosis of KS. Some clinical observations (most of them not validated prospectively) may help in this process. The best prognosis is seen in those patients with only a few small nodular lesions, especially if the lesions were present for at least several months before diagnosis. Prognosis is also better for those with no previous serious infection and for those with no recent weight loss, fevers, or night sweats (i.e., "B" symptoms).[26] A relatively high proportion (but not the majority) of these patients will have very slow progression of their KS.

In contrast, patients with many lesions involving multiple anatomic regions, "B" symptoms, or previous opportunistic infections, will probably not do well and additional lesions will develop relentlessly.

An interesting trend has been noted recently at San Francisco General Hospital: KS patients diagnosed after 1983 have had a significantly shorter survival time than those patients diagnosed before 1983. The reasons for this temporal trend of worsening survival are unclear, but the patients who developed KS after 1983 had more immunologic impairment, suggesting later development of KS in the course of their HIV disease.[26]

In patients with progressing AIDS-related KS, new lesions appear at variable rates anywhere on or in the body. Some sites are characteristic, however. These include the tip of the nose, the eyelid, the hard palate and posterior pharynx, the glans penis, and the sole of the foot. A common problem is the appearance of large clusters of innumerable lesions in the thigh against an ecchymotic background.

The site of cutaneous involvement has not appeared particularly important in determining a prognosis,[22] although a recent retrospective analysis described better survival in patients whose initial lesions were on the lower extremities.[27] The presence or absence of lymph-node involvement appears to have no effect on prognosis.[22] Visceral KS does, however, imply a poor prognosis.[22] Several studies report a somewhat reduced survival rate in patients with gastrointestinal KS. Patients with pulmonary KS have a high short-term mortality rate; their median survival period is 2 months.[23]

■ CLINICAL MANIFESTATIONS

Patients with AIDS-related KS range from those with minimal and stable disease to those with rapid tumor progression and tumor-related fatality. What follows is a review of methods for recognizing important clinical variants of KS. Typical patterns of disease spread are discussed elsewhere.

CUTANEOUS KS

Most patients with HIV-related KS have subcutaneous, painless, nonpruritic tumor nodules.[29-32] These are usually pigmented (red to blue) and nonblanching, but the pigmentation may be inapparent in deeper lesions. Kaposi's sarcoma lesions are almost always palpable. Exophytic tumor masses with breakdown of overlying skin are rarely seen in HIV-related KS and are exceptions to the general rule that the lesions are painless. Exophytic tumors, especially in areas exposed to frequent trauma, can necrose, bleed, and be moderately to severely painful when present on the feet or lower extremities.

TUMOR PLAQUES OF KS

Although less common than discrete tumor nodules, tumor plaques are seen more often than exophytic masses. Plaques of cutaneous KS are often seen on the thigh and the sole of the foot. They are uncommon in other areas of the body. Involvement of the superficial skin is common in all forms of AIDS-related KS, but fixation to deeper structures and infiltration of underlying bone are distinctly rare. Although nodular KS is generally painless, tumor plaques often cause chronic moderate pain. When present in the thigh, plaques of KS are often associated with underlying lymphedema. The clinical management of both problems can be difficult. In general, both exophytic KS tumors and KS plaques should be managed with local radiation therapy.

KS-ASSOCIATED LYMPHEDEMA

Lymphedema is common in patients with AIDS-related KS.[33] Probably because of the diffuse lymphatic involvement of this tumor, lymphedema may occur out of proportion to the extent of visible cutaneous disease. Usually, however, lymphedema is seen in patients with obvious cutaneous lesions as a late-stage manifestation of AIDS-related KS.

Body regions primarily affected by KS-associated lymphedema include the face, penis, scrotum, and the lower extremities. Edema of the chest and upper extremities is uncommon. The patient generally becomes aware of edema before it is obvious to the examining physician, especially in the case of lower-extremity involvement. The consistency of the collecting fluid is usually very firm and nonpitting. In the case of lower-extremity lymphedema, swelling may be limited to the distal lower extremity, but more commonly it involves the entire extremity. Associated edema of the scrotum and penis is common, in some cases extending to the level of the diaphragm. Facial lymphedema, like edema of the lower extremities, is rarely concentrated in one region but rather involves the entire face. Lymphedema in both face and lower extremities can be striking and rapidly progressive.

Management most frequently involves radiation therapy, which is most effective in reducing facial edema.[34] Lymphedema in the lower extremities responds less often to this management strategy. Diuretic therapy (furosemide 10 to 40 mg/day as needed) is of some value. In addition, chemotherapy is often used to improve the lymphedema. At San Francisco General Hospital, adriamycin (15 mg/square meter, IV/week) has been well tolerated and beneficial.

■ DIAGNOSIS

In most cases, Kaposi's sarcoma lesions are readily recognized. The physician should be suspicious of any pigmented cutaneous lesion in a patient known to be in a high-risk group for HIV infection. Irrespective of clinical appearance and probability of HIV infection, biopsy should be performed to establish histologic diagnosis. Biopsy confirmation is most important if the patient is not known to be at risk or if the clinical appearance of the lesion is unusual.

Most early KS lesions are not striking in their clinical appearance. They are typically nodular with obvious red-to-blue pigmentation, even early in the disease. Occasionally (particularly in cases of rapidly progressing disease), surrounding ecchymosis is apparent. The differential diagnosis of KS includes other pigmented cutaneous processes, such as dermatofibromas, granuloma annulare, insect-bite reactions, pyogenic granuloma, and stasis dermatitis.[28] Recently, angiomatous nodules caused by the cat-scratch bacillus have been described in HIV-infected patients. These lesions are remarkably similar in appearance to KS.[35] This differential diagnosis makes biopsy essential.

TECHNIQUES FOR DIAGNOSING KS

An adequate biopsy specimen is obtained with a 4 mm to 6 mm punch biopsy, although even a 2 mm biopsy may suffice. It is helpful to include unaffected (normal-appearing) adjacent skin in the punch specimen. This biopsy can be readily performed in the outpatient setting under local anesthesia. Skin biopsies collected in this way are preserved and stained by conventional methods.[28] Recently, fine-needle aspiration (FNA) biopsy has been used in diagnosing KS with a high degree of sensitivity and specificity.[36,37] Intraoral and intraabdominal lesions were diagnosed accurately with FNA, as were cutaneous lesions and lymph nodes.[37] Parenchymal lesions of the pulmonary tree viewed endoscopically should not be biopsied because of the low yield of such procedures and the increased likelihood of hemorrhage.

■ ROLE OF LABORATORY TESTING IN DIAGNOSIS AND PROGNOSIS

The Centers for Disease Control (CDC) surveillance criteria for AIDS are fulfilled if KS is diagnosed in an otherwise healthy person under 60 years of age.[38] Laboratory studies are useful, however, for estimating disease severity and hence its prognosis. They can also help exclude other treatable medical disorders. In exceptional cases, testing for evidence of human immunodeficiency virus (HIV) infection may help clarify the relationship of KS to AIDS.

TESTING TO ESTIMATE DISEASE SEVERITY AND PROGNOSIS

The natural history of HIV-related KS is complex, and laboratory test-results are of limited value in determining prognosis. Routine studies of probable value include complete blood count (CBC), erythrocyte sedimentation rate (ESR), and multitest chemistry profiles.[39,40] Leukopenia, anemia, and thrombocytopenia carry a poor prognosis. Isolated leukopenia or thrombocytopenias are seen frequently and may predate the development of opportunistic infections.[22,39,41] Lymphocytopenia is common but of uncertain prognostic significance.

In addition to the CBC, the ESR is useful.[42] Survival is decreased when the patient's ESR is over 40 mm/hr. Abnormalities common in AIDS patients on chemistry panels include low cholesterol and albumin and elevated globulins.[40] These are of uncertain prognostic value.

Immunologic tests are not needed to establish an AIDS diagnosis and are not essential to patient management unless they are used in making a decision about prophylaxis for *Pneumocystis carinii* pneumonia (PCP) and prescribing zidovudine (AZT). This is worth stressing, given the expense of many immunologic assays and the difficulty in interpreting them. However, tests of some prognostic value that should be done include skin testing to antigen panels and enumerating T-lymphocyte populations. Cutaneous anergy is seen in almost all AIDS patients.[42] Depression of the T-helper (CD4+ or Leu3) subtype of lymphocytes is also almost universally seen.[42-44] Most investigators have found a particularly poor prognosis in patients with absolute T-helper-cell numbers less than 100 cells per cubic millimeter.[45,46] The ratio of helper to suppressor T lymphocytes is probably less valuable as a predictor than the absolute T-helper-cell number. Because of variations in suppressor- as well as helper-cell numbers, ratios may be relatively normal, even in patients with diagnosed AIDS.

Tests for evidence of HIV infection are of almost no value in diagnosing or managing KS. Antibodies to HIV are present in almost all persons less than 60 years of age with KS,[47-49] and no antibody profile of prognostic significance has been found. The virus can be isolated from 50 percent to 70 percent of patients with HIV-related KS,[50,51] but its presence has no known value in estimating prognosis. There is some evidence that the presence of p24 antigen may be a useful prognostic factor,[26] but detailed analyses have not been done. The only definite use for HIV testing in the presence of KS is in those few patients whose risk-group status is unusual. This could include an elderly homosexual man with KS who may (despite the CDC surveillance definition) have AIDS or a low-risk person less than 60 years of age who may not be infected and who thus cannot be considered to have AIDS.

It is important to emphasize that although a diagnosis of HIV-related KS is ultimately a mortal one, patients diagnosed with it have on average longer lives than those diagnosed with other HIV-related illnesses.

In summary, the prognosis for HIV-related KS patients can be relatively good. Laboratory testing in most patients is almost never needed for diagnosis, but it may help in establishing prognosis and be useful for management decisions such as AZT therapy and PCP prophylaxis. Test results that imply a poor prognosis are leukopenia, anemia, thrombocytopenia, an elevated ESR, a low absolute T-helper-cell number, low T4/T8 ratio, and presence of p24 antigen. With rare exceptions, testing for HIV infection is not clinically indicated.

■ GASTROINTESTINAL KAPOSI'S SARCOMA

Unlike Kaposi's sarcoma in most other populations, KS in patients with AIDS commonly involves the viscera. The diagnosis of visceral KS is relatively straightforward, but its management is often very difficult.

The most common sites of diagnosed visceral KS are the gastrointestinal (GI) tract and the lungs. Intrapharyngeal and laryngeal KS, also common, are discussed in another document.

DIAGNOSIS

Lesions are found in the GI tract in 40 percent of KS cases at the time of initial diagnosis and in almost 80 percent of cases at autopsy.[52-54] Gastrointestinal KS is more likely if extensive cutaneous disease is present,[52,60] but gastrointestinal KS was diagnosed in six patients who had no evidence of cutaneous KS.[61] Any portion of the GI tract can be affected, but the most common sites are the stomach and the duodenum. Diagnosis is usually made by visualizing lesions endoscopically. Typically, the lesions are red, raised, and not ulcerated. Their size usually varies from 0.5 cm to 2 cm in diameter. Biopsy of lesions is not contraindicated but is often nondiagnostic (23-percent yield of characteristic lesions)[52] because the actual lesion, although easily visible, is often submucosal and not reached by the biopsy forceps. Kaposi's sarcoma lesions can sometimes be visualized radiographically. On contrast barium studies, they appear as smooth round masses protruding into the intestinal lumen.[53,54] Computed tomographic (CT) scan is not a useful diagnostic tool for gastrointestinal KS[55]; it may show intra-abdominal lymphadenopathy, but this finding is most indicative of lymphoma or *Mycobacterium avium* infection, especially if nodes are extremely enlarged.

TREATMENT

Kaposi's sarcoma in the GI tract is rarely symptomatic and seldom requires specific management.[52] Very rarely, one sees obstruction or bleeding that may require surgical palliation or local radiation therapy. A protein-losing enteropathy attributed to intestinal KS has been described in both classic and AIDS-related KS.[62,63] Gastrointestinal involvement with KS has been correlated in several series with a worse prognosis[22,52,56] and thus has been used to justify a more rapid initiation of systemic chemotherapy. Because gastrointestinal KS rarely causes death,[52] the value of screening patients for it is uncertain. It is not our practice at San Francisco General Hospital to screen patients for gastrointestinal involvement. If involvement is found, however, we generally recommend early initiation of systemic chemotherapy.

■ PULMONARY KS

DIAGNOSIS

Of all visceral KS sites, the lung is clinically the most significant. Pulmonary KS can cause severe symptoms, including bronchospasm, intractable coughing, and progressive respiratory insufficiency.[23,57-59] Fatality from pulmonary KS is not unusual and is often rapid.[23,57-59] Evaluation is complicated by the difficulty in distinguishing pulmonary KS from an opportunistic infection, especially *Pneumocystis carinii* pneumonia (PCP). Pulmonary KS and PCP have similar symptoms.[23,57] In both, the chest x-ray typically shows diffuse interstitial infiltrates, but in pulmonary KS, pulmonary nodules and pleural effusions are more common.[23] Pulmonary function testing is not helpful in the differential diagnosis, except for the carbon monoxide diffusing capacity (DLCO), which is rarely <80 percent predictive in pulmonary KS without opportunistic infection,[23] whereas it is often low in PCP. Pulmonary gallium scanning is also helpful; gallium uptake is minimal.[23] Probably the most direct diagnostic test is bronchoscopy. Endoscopic visualization of characteristic vascular lesions in the bronchial tree and negative exams for PCP are sufficient. Biopsy is not usually performed because of the potential for hemorrhaging and inadequate sample size. Open-lung biopsy is rarely indicated.[57,58]

TREATMENT

The prognosis of pulmonary KS is poor, and early initiation of aggressive, systemic chemotherapy is recommended.[23,57] However, the value of chemotherapy in prolonging survival has not been proven. The role of radiation therapy is also uncertain, although some reports suggest a benefit.[57] We have attempted chemotherapy with multiple agents when pulmonary KS is documented. Because bronchospasm is frequent, empiric bronchodilators are also used. Despite these measures, disease progression and rapid fatality are to be expected.

■ INTRAORAL KS

DIAGNOSIS

Intraoral KS is the initial site of 15 percent of AIDS-related KS.[64,65] Kaposi's sarcoma is usually clinically silent in the pharynx, but discomfort can occur as a result of superficial ulceration of palatal lesions or dental displacement in gingival KS. Intraoral KS may involve any tissue, but the most frequent site is the palate, where lesions are pigmented but not initially palpable.

Diagnosis of intraoral KS by biopsy is straightforward in most cases. Biopsy is required if the oral cavity is the initial or sole site of disease. It is not essential if the diagnosis has been previously established from other sites.[66] Histology is typical of KS in other sites.

TREATMENT

If the patient is asymptomatic, oral KS requires no specific treatment. When clinical problems occur, radiation therapy is useful. Complete or substantial partial-tumor regression follows moderate-dose (2000 rad) external-beam radiation.[67] Toxicities are common, however, particularly mucositis, which may take two or more weeks to resolve. Patients beginning radiation treatment of the oral cavity should be cautioned to maintain scrupulous oral hygiene to prevent secondary infection. Prophylactic treatment of oral candida should be considered. Besides radiation therapy, other measures to control intraoral KS include surgical excision of lesions, intralesional chemotherapy injection, and laser excision. Each of these approaches avoids toxicity to normal mucosa and should be considered when symptomatic KS lesions are small.

■ LYMPHATIC KAPOSI'S SARCOMA

Kaposi's sarcoma involving the lymph nodes is seen in large numbers of AIDS patients.[68] In AIDS-related KS this site of disease may not imply a worse prognosis, as it does in African KS. Because symptoms from localized lymph-node enlargement are uncommon, therapy is not often needed. Lymphedema is common in AIDS-related KS. Edema is due to diffuse small-lymphatic obliteration, not to localized obstruction.

In any HIV-infected patient, lymph-node size should be carefully monitored. Biopsy is not commonly required, but rather should be reserved for rapid or asymmetric nodal enlargement. Fine-needle aspirate cytology is often diagnostic of KS, infection, or lymphoma, but should be performed and interpreted by experts; the diagnosis is a difficult one and requires training.[36]

LYMPHEDEMA ASSOCIATED WITH AIDS-RELATED KS

Kaposi's sarcoma arises from the lymphatic endothelium and is multi-centric in most cases. Lesions are often somewhat linear and follow cutaneous lymphatic drainage.[69] Given widespread tumor distribution, lymphedema from lymphatic obstruction is frequent. KS-associated lymphedema is common in the face, lower extremities, scrotum, and abdomen, but rare in other regions. In most cases, it is associated with advanced cutaneous KS, although it may occur with minimal evidence of external disease.

The management of KS-related lymphedema is far from satisfactory. Elevation of affected lower extremities is only minimally helpful. Diuretic therapy with 40 to 80 mg/day of furosemide is occasionally useful. Local radiation therapy to regional nodal groups is not useful, but more extensive radiation therapy is occasionally effective. For facial edema, the entire face, neck, and supraclavicular fields are treated. For lower-extremity edema, the field usually includes the proximal leg from knee or below to thigh and entire groin. Moderate doses (in the range of 2000 rad) are usually sufficient.[66]

Despite this treatment, edema often persists. Systemic chemotherapy after local/regional radiation therapy can occasionally help, but the benefit is almost never complete.

■ TREATMENT OF HIV-RELATED KS

Many options exist for treating HIV-related Kaposi's sarcoma. Treatment options can be grouped into "conventional" and experimental modalities. A discussion of when therapy is appropriate appears later in this chapter.

CONVENTIONAL MODALITIES

Surgery

Surgical excision of KS lesions may be useful for initial diagnosis, although punch biopsies are sufficient in most cases. If the patient has only one lesion, excision may offer sufficient, although not curative, therapy.

The usual role for surgery in KS management is to eliminate lesions that protrude, are uncomfortable, or bleed due to repeated friction against clothes or shoes. In these cases, excision can provide relief. Local infection is infrequent and surgical wounds heal well.

Patients with slowly progressing KS may want repeated excision of lesions for cosmetic reasons, especially on exposed areas of the skin. Usually this is not a successful strategy over time, given the relentless progression typical of most KS cases.

Surgery is rarely needed for relief of major visceral KS. Pulmonary KS is almost always a diffuse process not amenable to surgery; gastrointestinal KS seldom causes luminal obstruction or symptomatic bleeding.

Radiation Therapy

Radiation therapy has a major role in KS management. The tumor is often locally symptomatic and is responsive to radiation. Optimal dosing schedules have not been determined, but 2500 to 3000 rad often induces prompt regression; even lower doses are sometimes effective.[34,83] Recent experience with single-fractioned dosing at 8 Gy is another promising treatment strategy.

Radiation therapy is most useful for the following clinical problems:

Extensive Intraoral or Pharyngeal KS.   Oropharyngeal KS may cause local discomfort from partial obstruction or necrosis, causing pain, dysphonia, dysphagia, and chronic superficial infection. Radiation can be extremely useful and should be recommended. Patients should be advised that mucositis is a common side effect and may be severe, requiring two to three weeks to heal. Scrupulous oral hygiene and control of oral candida may ameliorate this problem.

Painful Cutaneous KS.   KS lesions can be painful, especially those on the soles of the feet. Pain is also common in very large, long-standing cutaneous lesions. Although these lesions often respond incompletely to radiation, pain is usually relieved.[83] Tender erythema is an expected but temporary toxicity and is not severe.

Lymphedema.   Radiation therapy is useful for managing lymphedema, including that of the face or extremities. It can be recommended for both.

Chemotherapy

Aggressive combination chemotherapy has been avoided until recently because treatment-induced immunosuppression may hasten the development of fatal opportunistic infections. Clinicians have therefore used single-agent regimens most frequently. Recent reports suggest that chemotherapy treatments do not decrease survival of KS patients, compared to KS patients not treated with these drugs.[84] Although much more information needs to be developed, some agents are in common use.

Vinblastine.   Vinblastine is administered as a weekly intravenous bolus. At San Francisco General Hospital, we begin therapy at 0.1 mg/kg intravenously every week, monitoring the total leukocyte and absolute neutrophil counts once weekly, since leukopenia is the usual dose-limiting toxicity. We try to maintain patients so that total neutrophil count is at least 1000 cells per cubic millimeter. Patients seldom tolerate more than 8 mg per week; therapy is much less effective if less than 4 mg per week is given. Using a similar regimen, we found a 25 percent complete and partial remission rate in a prospective study of 38 patients; 50 percent of the remaining patients had stable disease after single-dose vinblastine.[70]

Vinblastine toxicity is minimal. Leukopenia is common, but nausea and alopecia are rare. The lack of controlled studies makes firm conclusions on the relative rate of opportunistic infections in patients receiving vinblastine impossible, but our impression is that they are no more frequent than in patients not receiving treatment.

Vincristine.   Vincristine has been reported as extremely effective in AIDS patients with KS and thrombocytopenia. A 75 percent objective response rate was reported in one series; no severe neurotoxicity was reported. In this study, weekly intravenous bolus injections of 1.4 mg to 2 mg were used.[71]

Our own experience (unpublished) with vincristine as a single agent was based on a small patient group and produced less favorable results. We observed substantial, dose-limiting peripheral neuropathy. Therefore, we tend to avoid its use except when HIV-related myelosuppression demands it or when it is combined with other drugs.

Alternating Vinblastine/Vincristine.   To reduce the dose-limiting toxicities of vinca alkaloids in AIDS patients with KS, we began using vinblastine and vincristine intravenously in a weekly regimen of alternating single agents. We begin with 2 mg of vincristine every other week and give vinblastine at a dose of 0.1 mg/kg in the alternating weeks. Dose modifications in each drug are made as needed. For example, we hold vinblastine if the absolute neutrophil count falls below about 1000 cells per cubic millimeter. As the neutrophil count reduces to the 1500 to 1000 level, we decrease vinblastine to 75 percent of the dose. The vincristine dose is reduced for moderate paresthesias and discontinued if detectable muscle weakness or severe paresthesias occur. With this flexible approach, we observed a 45 percent overall response rate with few toxic side effects (12 percent detectable muscle weakness, 8 percent severe neutropenia).[84] This is now our "standard" chemotherapy for KS at San Francisco General Hospital.

VP-16.   The podophyllotoxin VP-16-213, or etoposide, was one of the first agents reported active against HIV-related KS. In an early series from New York, VP-16 was given to patients in a dose of 150 mg per square meter of body surface area on three consecutive days every four weeks. An objective response rate of over 75 percent was reported using this regimen.[72] However, the lack of a control group in this study limits conclusions regarding immunotoxicity. Subjective toxicity with VP-16 is minimal and nausea is rarely reported. Alopecia is common. Myelosuppression, although not often severe, is frequent.

VP-16 given orally is a more convenient alternative for patients. It is given in a dose of 150 mg per square meter of body surface area divided into two doses on three consecutive days every four weeks. No more than 150 mg can be given at any one time because of increased absorption at higher doses.

We consider VP-16 a somewhat more aggressive agent than the vinca alkaloids and generally reserve it for more advanced cutaneous disease that is not responsive to vinca therapy.

Other Single Agents.   Studies are under way to expand our repertoire of cytotoxic agents. Preliminary reports suggest that low-dose weekly adriamycin is active against KS. In a study of 32 patients given adriamycin at a dose of 15 mg per square meter of body surface area intravenously each week, 16 percent had a partial anti-tumor response and another 39 percent responded by resolution of edema or flattening of lesions.[85] Neutropenia was a major dose-limiting toxicity.

Preliminary reports also suggest that moderate-dose methotrexate and bleomycin are active against KS. Although these reports must be confirmed, the drugs can be considered in some cases. Agents that are reported as ineffective include vinzolidine, ICRF-159, and mitoxantrone.[73,74]

Combination Chemotherapy.   Aggressive combinations have usually been avoided in HIV-related KS because of potential immunotoxicity. Recently, however, several centers have reported results of combination therapy trials.[72,86] Laubenstein et al. used adriamycin, bleomycin, and vinblastine in relatively advanced KS and achieved a 75 percent objective response rate.[72] However, the rate of life-threatening opportunistic infections seemed much higher in this group than expected. Gill et al. recently reported a randomized trial of adriamycin, bleomycin, and vincristine (ABV) versus adriamycin alone in 53 patients with advanced KS.[86,87] They found an 87 percent overall objective response rate in the ABV group versus a 39 percent overall response rate in the adriamycin group. The median time to progression of KS on therapy was longer in the ABV group (12 months versus 4 months). There was no difference in the number of opportunistic infections or in median survival. The ABV group did have a substantial incidence of neuropathy.[86]

At San Francisco General Hospital, we generally reserve aggressive combination chemotherapy for patients with extensive disease.

Alpha Interferon.   One of the first experimental drugs tested on AIDS patients was recombinant human ∝ interferon. Testing began in AIDS patients with KS in 1982 on the hypothesis that ∝ interferon might act as an antiviral, an immune stimulator, and an antineoplastic agent, all of which are potentially valuable effects in treating these patients. Testing was conducted at several centers using slightly different formulations of ∝ interferon and using different doses, schedules, and routes of administration. Despite the many variables, many similar conclusions can be drawn. The first is that ∝ interferon has a certain amount of activity against KS. Objective response rates of 25 percent to 40 percent have been reported from several studies.[75-78] The second conclusion is that response to ∝ interferon requires large doses, generally more than 20 million units daily. A third is that some subsets of patients are more responsive than others. Patients with histories of previous opportunistic infections and lymphoma-like B symptoms have a lower response rate. Daily intramuscular or subcutaneous injections are convenient and provide clinically useful results.

Human ∝ interferon is not demonstrably useful in measurably augmenting immunity. If it is used, serial immunologic studies are not essential. The in vivo activity of the drug against HIV is being investigated and may offer a rationale for wider use in this and other HIV-infected populations.[79]

EXPERIMENTAL THERAPIES

Topical/Intralesional Therapy
Increasingly, topical and intralesional therapies are being investigated for treating individual lesions. Liquid nitrogen has been used at San Francisco General Hospital to treat several patients. This therapy involves applying liquid nitrogen directly to the tumor until a halo of surrounding erythema is observed. This causes a mild inflammatory response, after which the tumor flattens or disappears completely (Tappero J: personal communication). Larger lesions may require repeated treatments and may leave a residual area of hyperpigmentation.

Individual lesions can also be treated with intralesional injections of dilute chemotherapy. Newman treated 190 KS lesions from 15 patients with intralesional vinblastine.[88] He injected 0.01 to 0.02 milligrams of vinblastine in 0.1 ml of saline directly into the lesions every two weeks (up to a maximum of three injections). He achieved complete resolution in 25 lesions and a partial response in 149 lesions (flattening and depigmentation) for a total overall response rate of 92 percent. Mean duration of response was 4.5 months. The only complications were local pain and skin irritation; there was no evidence of systemic effects.

Intralesional recombinant tumor necrosis factor (rTNF) has also been used as local therapy against KS. A Phase I trial at San Francisco General Hospital demonstrated tumor regression and occasional complete resolution of lesions when 25 micrograms per square meter of body surface area of rTNF was injected directly into lesions.[89] However, systemic side effects (fever, chills, nausea) were frequent.

AIDS patients with KS have often been used as subjects in clinical trials of immune augmentation to study such approaches as recombinant interleukin-2, thymic hormones, and bone-marrow transplantation. Some KS patients have also been included in early trials of anti-HIV agents, such as suramin, HPA 23, and AZT.[80-82] Despite much effort, little benefit has yet been shown when objective KS response is the criterion of success. Recently, several groups treated patients with a combination of ∝ interferon and AZT.[90,91] Fischl et al. found that the combination of 9 million units of intramuscular ∝ interferon daily and 100 milligrams of AZT every four hours was well tolerated over time, resulting in major tumor regression in over 50 percent of patients.[90]

The newest investigations involve studying combination chemotherapy with AZT. The rationale for this therapy is obvious, but additive or synergistic myelosuppression may make it difficult to administer. At San Francisco General Hospital, we are currently investigating alternating vincristine/vinblastine with AZT in a prospective trial.

TREATMENT GUIDELINES

It is difficult and dangerous to be dogmatic about the most appropriate therapy for HIV-related KS. The natural history of the tumor is not completely known and our available modalities are not yet the most rational or effective. Nevertheless, clinicians need to make decisions. What follows are one institution's (San Francisco General Hospital) current guidelines for the management of KS in AIDS. Other physicians may well have different recommendations. In our guidelines, we stress the need for flexibility in recognizing the many unresolved questions. Part of the difficulty in comparing management strategies is the lack of an agreed-upon staging system. We will not attempt to impose any such unvalidated system here but rather will base recommendations on the broad clinical status of the patient.

Treatment Guidelines for Recently Diagnosed KS

Early in the disease, the patient demands education about prognosis and therapeutic options. This discussion should be extensive, often divided into several clinic visits, and should be as frank as possible with the goal of making the patient an effective participant in planning therapy.

Patients with recent KS will often have one or several lesions. Especially if they have other factors suggesting better prognosis (such as a lack of previous opportunistic infections), it is reasonable to follow the disease without specific therapy. This allows the patient and physician to estimate the disease's tempo, which if slow or stable may permit prolonged observation. When progression is seen, especially when it is rapid, therapy can still be initiated promptly.

Some patients prefer active therapy from the outset and are anxious about "just watching" the lesions. In this circumstance, the physician can recommend specific therapies against HIV and KS lesions.

Intervention in the recently diagnosed KS patient can be local if the disease is limited; for example, intralesional injection of dilute vinblastine or topically applied liquid nitrogen. When systemic therapy is used in the patient with early

KS, aggressive (i.e., multi-agent) chemotherapy should be avoided. Single-agent vinca alkaloids or alternating weekly vinblastine/vincristine are suggested for patients with early disease. Alternatively, moderate-to-high dose parenteral ∝ interferon may be used.

In the recently diagnosed patient with a high probability of rapid progression (for example, patients with rapidly appearing lesions in multiple anatomic regions), systemic therapy should be recommended immediately. Spontaneous remission or prolonged stability are uncommon in this situation and control of KS is probably easier before further progression.

Treatment Guidelines for Established KS

In patients with a longer history of KS, treatment guidelines are similar to those for the recently diagnosed patient, but very few patients have stable disease. The majority will have extensive KS, often with visceral involvement and symptoms related to these features. Previous therapy should be continued if it has resulted in tumor control without excess toxicity. This recommendation should, in general, extend even to those patients whose previous therapy is not what the current physician might have recommended. If new therapy is needed, more aggressive single agents such as VP-16 are used, including less-established ones like low-dose weekly adriamycin or moderate-dose methotrexate.

Pulmonary KS.   Pulmonary KS represents a particular challenge. Agents such as VP-16 should be used immediately, especially if respiratory symptoms are seen in a patient with endobrachial lesions. This is one situation in which combination chemotherapy, such as adriamycin (15 mg/square meter), bleomycin (10 units/square meter), and vincristine (2.0 mg every two weeks with dose adjustment based on absolute neutrophil count) can be attempted. Whole-lung radiation therapy has been used, but like chemotherapy, its role has not been fully established in pulmonary KS.

Treatment Guidelines in KS Patients with an Intercurrent Opportunistic Infection

We have repeatedly observed a rapid progression of KS in patients responding to systemic chemotherapy in whom treatment is discontinued because of an intercurrent opportunistic infection, such as *Pneumocystis carinii*. We do recognize that antibiotic therapy may require this interruption, but we stress that chemotherapy should be reinitiated as rapidly as possible.

Special Considerations for Inclusion of KS Subjects in Experimental Drug Testing

KS patients are ideal candidates for experimental drug testing, insofar as their KS status potentially offers a direct means to assess immunologic reconstitution. Nevertheless, KS presents problems because many drug trials are placebo controlled and KS usually progresses rapidly without therapy. In addition, the use of an experimental agent precludes simultaneous administration of systemic antineoplastic drugs.

Including carefully selected patients with minimal KS in placebo-controlled trials can be justified, assuming that the patients are fully educated about the goals of the trial. More advanced KS patients may be better used in early Phase I trials of limited duration.

A summary of treatment guidelines appears in Table 1.

TABLE 1.   TREATMENT GUIDELINES FOR HIV-RELATED KS

CLINICAL SITUATION	RECOMMENDED ACTION
Recent Diagnosis	
Minimal Disease	Observation Local therapy (surgical excision, intralesional chemotherapy)
Extensive Disease (multiple sites)	Systemic therapy (vinca alkaloids or $\propto$ interferon)
Opportunistic Infection (OI)	Systemic therapy for underlying infection
Established Disease	
Stable	Continue previous strategy, including observation or nontraditional treatment, if ethical

Progressing KS
  Cutaneous
  Gastrointestinal
  Pulmonary
	Systemic therapy (more aggressive chemotherapy; e.g., VP-16, combination chemotherapy)

HIV/KS with intercurrent OI	Discontinue therapy as briefly as possible and reinstitute as soon as OI is controlled.

REFERENCES

1. Marmor M, Laubenstein L, William DC, et al. Risk factors for Kaposi's sarcoma in homosexual men. Lancet 1982; 1:1084-6.
2. Jaffe HW, Keewhan C, Thomas PA, et al. National case control study of Kaposi's sarcoma and *Pneumocystis carinii* pneumonia in homosexual men: Part 1, epidemiologic results. Ann Intern Med 1983; 99:145-51.
3. Drew WL, Mills J, Levy J, et al. Cytomegalovirus infection and abnormal T lymphocyte subset ratios in homosexual men. Ann Intern Med 1985; 103:61-3.
4. Drew WL, Miner RC, Ziegler JL, et al. Cytomegalovirus and Kaposi's sarcoma in young homosexual men. Lancet 1982; 2:125-7.
5. Urmacher C, Myskowski P, Ochoa Jr M, et al. Outbreak of Kaposi's sarcoma with cytomegalovirus infection in young homosexual men. Am J Med 1982; 72:569-75.
6. Giraldo G, Beth E, Huang E-S. Kaposi's sarcoma and its relationship to cytomegalovirus (CMV) III, CMV DNA and CMV early antigens in Kaposi's sarcoma. Int J Cancer 1980; 26:23-9.
7. Spector DH, Spector SA. The oncogenic potential of human cytomegalovirus. Prog Med Virol 1984; 29:45-89.
8. Levy JA, Ziegler JL. Acquired immunodeficiency syndrome is an opportunistic infection and Kaposi's sarcoma results from secondary immune stimulation. Lancet 1983; 2:78-80.
9. Warner TFCS, O'Loughlin S. Kaposi's sarcoma: A byproduct of tumor rejection. Lancet 1975; 2:687-8.
10. Drew WL, Mills J, Hauer LB, et al. Declining prevalence of Kaposi's sarcoma in homosexual AIDS patients paralleled by fall in cytomegalovirus transmission. Lancet 1988; 1:66.
11. Tschachler E, Groh V, Popovic M, et al. Epidermal Langerhans cells — a target for HTLV-III/LAV infection. J Invest Dermatol 1987; 88:233-7.
12. Delli Bovi P, Donti E, Knowles DM 2d, et al. Presence of chromosomal abnormalities and lack of AIDS retrovirus DNA sequences in AIDS-associated Kaposi's sarcoma. Cancer Res 1986; 46:6333-8.
13. Vogel J, Hinrichs SH, Reynolds RK, et al. The HIV *tat* gene induces dermal lesions resembling Kaposi's sarcoma in transgenic mice. Nature 1988; 335:606-11.
14. Nakamura S, Salahuddin SZ, Biberfeld P, et al. Kaposi's sarcoma cells: long-term culture with growth factor from retrovirus-infected CD4+ T cells. Science 1988; 242:426-30.
15. Salahuddin SZ, Nakamura S, Biberfeld P, et al. Angiogenic properties of Kaposi's sarcoma-derived cells after long-term culture in vitro. Science 1988; 242:430-3.
16. Taylor JF, Templeton AC, Vogel CL, et al. Kaposi's sarcoma in Uganda: A clinicopathological study. Int J Cancer 1971; 8:122-35.

17. Dorfman RF. Kaposi's sarcoma revisited. Hum Pathol 1984; 15:1013-7.

18. Beckstead JH, Wood GS, Fletcher V. Evidence for the origin of Kaposi's sarcoma from lymphatic endothelium. Am J Pathol 1985; 119:294-300.

19. Rutgers JL, Wieczorek R, Bonetti F, et al. The expression of endothelial cell surface antigens by AIDS associated Kaposi's sarcoma. Am J Pathol 1986; 122:493-9.

20. Amberson JB, DiCarlo EF, Metroka CE, et al. Diagnostic pathology in the acquired immunodeficiency syndrome. Arch Pathol Lab Med 1985; 109:345-51.

21. Niedt GW, Schinella RA. Acquired immunodeficiency syndrome. Arch Pathol Lab Med 1985; 109:727-34.

22. Volberding PA, Kaslow K, Bilk M, et al. Prognostic factors in staging Kaposi's sarcoma in the acquired immune deficiency syndrome. Proc Am Soc Clin Oncol 1984; 3:51. abstract.

23. Kaplan LD, Hopewell PC, Jaffe H, et al. Kapsosi's sarcoma involving the lung in patients with the acquired immunodeficiency syndrome. J Acquir Immune Defic Syndr 1988; 1:23-30.

24. Dorfman RF. Kaposi's sarcoma: evidence supporting its origin from the lymphatic system. Lymphology 1988; 21:45-52.

25. Facchetti F, Lucini L, Gavazzoni R, Callea F. Immunomorphological analysis of the role of blood vessel endothelium in the morphogenesis of cutaneous Kaposi's sarcoma: a study of 57 cases. Histopathology 1988; 12:581-93.

26. Volberding PA, Kusick P, Feigal DW. HIV antigenemia at diagnosis with Kaposi's sarcoma: predictors of shortened survival [Abstract]. IV International Conference on AIDS. Stockholm, 1988; 2:2644.

27. Myskowski PL, Niedzwiecki D, Shurgot BA, et al. AIDS-associated Kaposi's sarcoma: variables associated with survival. J Am Acad Dermatol 1988; 18:1299-306.

28. McNutt NS, Fletcher V, Conant MA. Early lesions of Kaposi's sarcoma in homosexual men. Am J Pathol 1983; 111:62-79.

29. Friedman-Kien AE, Laubenstein LJ, Rubinstein P, et al. Disseminated Kaposi's sarcoma in homosexual men. Ann Intern Med 1982; 96:693-700.

30. Mitsuyasu RT, Taylor JMG, Glaspy J, Fahey JL. Heterogeneity of epidemic Kaposi's sarcoma. Cancer 1986; 57:1657-61.

31. Centers for Disease Control. Kaposi's sarcoma and pneumocystis pneumonia among homosexual men — New York City and California. MMWR 1981; 30:305-8.

32. Fauci AS, Macher AM, Longo DL, et al. Acquired immunodeficiency syndrome: Epidemiologic, clinical, immunologic, and therapeutic considerations. Ann Intern Med 1984; 100:92-106.

33. Volberding P. Therapy of Kaposi's sarcoma in AIDS. Semin Oncol 1984; 11:60-7.

34. Harris JW, Reed TA. Kaposi's sarcoma in AIDS: The role of radiation therapy. In: Veath JM, ed. Frontiers of radiation therapy and oncology. Basel: Karger, 1985:126-32.

35. Koehler JE, LeBoit PE, Egbert BM, et al. Cutaneous vascular lesions and disseminated cat-scratch disease in patients with the acquired immunodeficiency syndrome (AIDS) and AIDS-related complex. Ann Intern Med 1988; 109:449-55.

36. Bottles K, McPhaul LW, Volberding P. Fine-needle aspiration biopsy of patients with acquired immunodeficiency syndrome (AIDS): experience in an outpatient clinic. Ann Intern Med 1988; 108:42-5.

37. Hales M, Bottles K, Miller T, et al. Diagnosis of Kaposi's sarcoma by fine-needle aspiration biopsy. Am J Clin Pathol 1987; 88:20-5.

38. Centers for Disease Control. Update: Acquired immunodeficiency syndrome — United States. MMWR 1986; 35:17-21.

39. Abrams DI, Chinn EK, Lewis BJ, et al. Hematologic manifestations in homosexual men with Kaposi's sarcoma. Am J Clin Pathol 1984; 81:13-8.

40. Rogers M, Morens DM, Stewart JA, et al. National case control study of Kaposi's sarcoma and *Pneumocystis carinii* pneumonia in homosexual men: part 2, laboratory results. Ann Intern Med 1983; 99:151-8.

41. Abrams DI, Kiprov DD, Goedert JJ, et al. Antibodies to human T lymphotropic virus type III antibodies and development of acquired immunodeficiency syndrome in homosexual men presenting with immune thrombocytopenia. Ann Intern Med 1985; 104:47-50.

42. Fauci AS. Immunologic abnormalities in the acquired immunodeficiency syndrome (AIDS). Clin Res 1984; 32:491-9.

43. Stites DP, Casavant CH, McHugh TM, et al. Flow cytometric analysis of lymphocyte phenotypes in AIDS using monoclonal antibodies and simultaneous dual immunofluorescence. Clin Immunol Immunopathol 1986; 38:161-77.

44. Lane HC, Masur H, Gelmann EP, et al. Correlation between immunologic function and clinical subpopulations of patients with the acquired immune deficiency syndrome. Am J Med 1985; 78:417-22.

45. Taylor J, Afrasiabi R, Fahey J, et al. Prognostically significant classification of immune changes in AIDS with Kaposi's sarcoma. Blood 1986; 67:666-71.

46. Vadhan-Raj S, Wong G, Gnecco C, et al. Immunologic variables as predictors of prognosis in patients with Kaposi's sarcoma and the acquired immune deficiency syndrome. Cancer Res 1986; 46:417-25.

47. Weiss SH, Goedert JJ, Sarngadharan MG, et al. Screening test for HTLV-III (AIDS agent) antibodies. JAMA 1985; 253:221-5.

48. Carlson JR, Bryant ML, Hinrichs SH, et al. AIDS serology testing in low and high risk groups. JAMA 1985; 253:3405-8.

49. Safai B, Groopman JE, Popovic M, et al. Seroepidemiologic studies of human T lymphotropic retrovirus type III in acquired immunodeficiency syndrome. Lancet 1984; 1:1438-40.

50. Levy JA, Shimabukuro J. Recovery of AIDS associated retroviruses from patients with AIDS or AIDS related conditions and from clinically healthy individuals. J Infect Dis 1985; 152:734-8.

51. Levy JA, Hoffman AD, Kramer SM, et al. Isolation of lymphocytopathic retroviruses from San Francisco patients with AIDS. Science 1984; 225:840-2.

52. Friedman SL, Wright TL, Altman DF. Gastrointestinal Kaposi's sarcoma in patients with acquired immunodeficiency syndrome. Gastroenterology 1985; 89:102-8.

53. Rose HS, Balthazar EJ, Megibow AJ, et al. Alimentary tract involvement in Kaposi's sarcoma: Radiographic and endoscopic findings in 25 homosexual men. AJR 1982; 139:661-6.

54. Frager DH, Grager JD, Brandt LJ, et al. Gastrointestinal complications of AIDS: Radiologic features. Radiology 1986; 158:597-603.

55. Moon KL, Federle MP, Abrams DI, et al. Kaposi's sarcoma and lymphadenopathy syndrome: limitations of abdominal CT in acquired immunodeficiency syndrome. Radiology 1984; 150:479-83.

56. Krigel RL, Laubenstein LJ, Muggia FM. Kaposi's sarcoma: a new staging classification. Cancer Treat Rep 1983; 67:531-4.

57. Ognibene FP, Steis RG, Macher AM, et al. Kaposi's sarcoma causing pulmonary infiltrates and respiratory failure in the acquired immunodeficiency syndrome. Ann Intern Med 1985; 102:471-5.

58. Pitchenik AF, Fischl MA, Saldana MJ. Kaposi's sarcoma of the tracheobronchial tree. Clinical, bronchoscopic, and pathologic features. Chest 1985; 87:122-4.

59. Kornfeld H, Axelrod JL. Pulmonary presentation of Kaposi's sarcoma in a homosexual patient. Am Rev Respir Dis 1983; 127:248-9.

60. Saltz RK, Kurtz RC, Lightdale CJ, et al. Kaposi's sarcoma. Gastrointestinal involvement correlation with skin findings and immunologic function. Dig Dis Sci 1984; 29:817-23.

61. Barrison IG, Foster S, Harris JW, et al. Upper gastrointestinal Kaposi's sarcoma in patients positive for HIV antibody without cutaneous disease. Br Med J 1988; 296:92-3.

62. Laine L, Politoske EJ, Gill P. Protein-losing enteropathy in acquired immunodeficiency syndrome due to intestinal Kaposi's sarcoma. Arch Intern Med 1987; 147:1174-5.

63. Perrone V, Pergola M, Abate G, et al. Protein-losing enteropathy in a patient with generalized Kaposi's sarcoma. Cancer 1981; 47:588-91.

64. Sooy CD. Otolaryngologic manifestations of acquired immunodeficiency syndrome. West J Med 1984; 141:674.

65. Gnepp DR, Chandler W, Hyams V. Primary Kaposi's sarcoma of the head and neck. Ann Intern Med 1984; 100:107-14.

66. Green TL, Beckstead JH, Lozada-Nur F, et al. Histopathologic spectrum of oral Kaposi's sarcoma. Oral Surg 1984; 58:306-14.

67. Harris JW, Reed TA. Kaposi's sarcoma in AIDS: The role of radiation therapy. Radiat Ther Oncol 1985; 19:126-32.

68. Moskowitz LB, Hensley GT, Gould EW, Weiss SD. Frequency and anatomic distribution of lymphadenopathic Kaposi's sarcoma in the acquired immunodeficiency syndrome: an autopsy series. Hum Pathol 1985; 16:447-56.

69. Volberding PA. Kaposi's sarcoma in AIDS. Med Clin North Am 1986; 70:665-75.

70. Volberding P, Abrams DI, Conant M, et al. Vinblastine therapy for Kaposi's sarcoma in the acquired immunodeficiency syndrome. Ann Intern Med 1985; 103:335-8.

71. Mintzner DM, Real FX, Joving L, Krown SE. Treatment of Kaposi's sarcoma and thrombocytopenia with vincristine in patients with the acquired immunodeficiency syndrome. Ann Intern Med 1985; 100:200-2.

72. Laubenstein L, Krigel R, Odajnyk SM, et al. Treatment of epidemic Kaposi's sarcoma with etoposide or a combination of doxorubicin, bleomycin and vinblastine. J Clin Oncol 1984; 2:1115-20.

73. Kaplan L, Volberding PA. Failure and danger of mitozantrone in AIDS-related Kaposi's sarcoma. Lancet 1985; 2:396.

74. Volberding P, Abrams D, Kaplan L, et al. Therapy of AIDS related Kaposi's sarcoma (KS) with ICRF-159. Proc Am Soc Clin Oncol 1985; 4:4. abstract.

75. Krown SE, Real FX, Cunningham-Rundles S, et al. Preliminary observations on the effect of recombinant leukocyte A interferon in homosexual men with Kaposi's sarcoma. N Engl J Med 1983; 308:1071-6.

76. Groopman JE, Gottlieb MS, Goodman J, et al. Recombinant α 2 interferon therapy for Kaposi's sarcoma associated with the acquired immunodeficiency syndrome. Ann Intern Med 1984; 100:671-6.

77. Real FX, Oettgen HF, Krown SE. Kaposi's sarcoma and the acquired immunodeficiency syndrome: Treatment with high and low doses of recombinant leukocyte A interferon. J Clin Oncol 1986; 4:544-51.

78. Gelmann EP, Preble OT, Steis R, et al. Human lymphoblastoid interferon treatment of Kaposi's sarcoma in the acquired immune deficiency syndrome. Am J Med 985; 78:737-41.

79. Ho DD, Rota TR, Kaplan JC, et al. Recombinant human interferon ∝-A suppresses HTLV-III replication in vitro. Lancet 1985; 1:602-4.

80. Broder S, Collins JM, Markham PD, et al. Effects of Suramin on HTLV III/LAV infection presenting as Kaposi's sarcoma or AIDS-related complex: Clinical pharmacology and suppression of virus replication in vivo. Lancet 1985; 2:627-30.

81. Rozenbaum W, Dormont D, Spire B, et al. Antimoniotungstate (HPA 23) treatment of three patients with AIDS and one with prodrome. Lancet 1985; 1:450-1.

82. Yarchoan R, Weinhold KJ, Lyerly HK, et al. Administration of 3′-azido-3′deoxythymidine, an inhibitor of HTLV-III/LAV replication, to patients with AIDS or AIDS related complex. Lancet 1986; 1:575-80.

83. Chak LY, Gill PS, Levine AM, et al. Radiation therapy for acquired immunodeficiency syndrome-related Kaposi's sarcoma. J Clin Oncol 1988; 6:863-7.

84. Kaplan L, Abrams D, Volberding P. Treatment of Kaposi's sarcoma in acquired immunodeficiency syndrome with an alternating vincristine–vinblastine regimen. Cancer Treat Rep 1986; 70:1121-2.

85. Fischl M, Krown S, O'Boyle K, et al. Weekly doxorubicin in the treatment of patients with AIDS-related Kaposi's sarcoma [Abstract]. IV International Conference on AIDS. Stockholm, 1988; 2:4564.

86. Gill P, Krailo M, Slater L, et al. ABV in advanced KS. Proc Am Soc Clin Oncol 1988. abstract.

87. Gill P, Krailo M, Slater L, et al. Results of a randomized trial of ABV (adriamycin, bleomycin, vincristine) vs. A in advanced epidemic Kaposi's sarcoma (KS) [Abstract]. IV International Conference on AIDS. Stockholm, 1988; 2:7596.

88. Newman S. Treatment of epidemic Kaposi's sarcoma with intralesional vinblastine injection. Proc Am Soc Clin Oncol 1988:19. abstract.

89. Kahn J, Kaplan L, Jaffe H, et al. Intralesional recombinant tumor necrosis factor for AIDS related Kaposi's sarcoma [Abstract]. IV International Conference on AIDS. Stockholm, 1988; 2:7598.

90. Krown S, Bundow D, Gansbacher B, et al. Interferon-∝ plus zidovudine: a phase I trial in AIDS-associated Kaposi's sarcoma (KS) [Abstract]. IV International Conference on AIDS. Stockholm, 1988; 2:3627.

91. Fischl M, Reese J, Dearmas L, et al. Phase I study of interferon-∝ and AZT in patients with AIDS-related Kaposi's sarcoma [Abstract]. IV International Conference on AIDS. Stockholm, 1988; 1:3133.

Kaposi's Sarcoma: Management and Nursing Interventions

Gayling Gee, R.N., M.S.

K aposi's sarcoma (KS), a cancer of the blood vessel (endothelial cell) wall, is the most common oncologic disease presentation in HIV disease. In early disease, KS may appear as small multifocal skin lesions located on various parts of the body; these lesions are occasionally confused with bruises, nevi, or insect bites. In advanced disease, the lesions may become darker, larger, and more raised, often with two or more individual lesions coalescing into one large tumor. AIDS-related KS may be slow growing, consisting of small skin lesions limited to one anatomic area; or it may be a highly aggressive tumor that grows rapidly and involves many internal organs.[1,2]

Nurses who are evaluating people at high risk for HIV infection should examine the skin closely for lesions on the face, extremities, trunk, oral cavity (especially the hard palate), or soles of the feet. Identifying lesions suspicious for KS can lead to a diagnostic skin-punch biopsy, oral surgery biopsy, endoscopy, sigmoidoscopy, or lymph-node biopsy.

■ MANAGEMENT

KS is most commonly managed in an ambulatory-care setting, including the diagnostic evaluation, treatment, and follow-up care. The majority of patients are ambulatory even in more advanced cases. Hospitalization of a KS patient is indicated primarily for treatment of opportunistic infections (usually *Pneumocystis carinii* pneumonia) or the consequences of advanced KS disease (or both). These include severe respiratory compromise resulting from extensive KS pulmonary involvement; blockage and severe edema of the head, extremities, or both, due to extensive lymph-node involvement; and eating or swallowing difficulties due to oral mucosal tumors or extensive gastrointestinal (GI) involvement. Severe nausea and vomiting can occur, and infrequently, bleeding or ulceration in the GI tract.

■ GENERAL NURSING INTERVENTIONS

KNOWLEDGE DEFICIT

In the absence of any opportunistic infection, when first diagnosed with KS, the patient generally feels quite well. The patient with KS may only have unexplained fevers or weight loss, but usually has no physical limitations and does not experience any reduction in the usual activities of daily living during the early disease stages. The patient should be offered treatment options; the decision on whether to treat will be determined by the extent and stability of the disease.

The patient undergoing drug therapy, whether standard or investigational, should have a basic understanding of the drug being administered: its action, dosage, method of administration, and side effects. Patients in clinical trials need the same information, as well as assurance of close clinical monitoring by the investigator. All patients require counseling on the need for practicing safer sex techniques and avoiding unnecessary exposure to other infections. Other general-education topics include appropriate home-care infection-control precautions, good nutrition, adequate rest, and stress reduction.

NUTRITION

As KS progresses, the patient begins to experience more and more alterations in nutrition because of the obstructive and compressive nature of the tumor. Extensive tumor involvement in the mouth and along the GI tract may interfere with eating and absorption, resulting in anorexia, diarrhea, or both. Radiation therapy effectively shrinks localized lesions in the mouth; however, such measures are often temporary and palliative.

Regular weight and nutrition monitoring (including a food diary or calorie counts) are useful. Nutritional counseling may be indicated, especially for patients with early KS, to begin a good nutritional plan. Small, frequent, high-protein, high-calorie meals are appropriate for patients experiencing anorexia and weight loss. Liquid food supplements or high-protein milk shakes may be suggested for patients with obstructive oral lesions. Good oral hygiene is always indicated to maintain mucosal integrity. Soft toothbrushes or toothettes can minimize abrasions to the mucosa. Petroleum jelly applied to the lips can keep the skin moist. Regular monitoring of patient history for nausea, vomiting, diarrhea, or anorexia, intake and output, and orthostatic blood pressures are helpful in assessing dehydration and the need for intravenous fluid replacement.

SKIN INTEGRITY

Skin integrity is compromised by cutaneous KS lesions. Although most cutaneous KS lesions are non-ulcerative, lymph-node blockage due to the tumor invasion can cause chronic edema, resulting in ulceration of the lesions or of the surrounding skin. KS involvement of the lymph nodes in the groin, axilla, and neck can cause local blockage, leading to severe edema of the head, arms, and lower extremities. Radiation therapy to the obstructed lymph nodes is very effective in relieving local edema; however, tumor recurrence is common, with resulting edema. Weight loss, malnourishment, and progressive debilitation due to disease also contribute to the impairment of skin integrity.

The patient should be checked carefully for skin integrity, including skin color, moisture, temperature, and edema. Pressure sores, skin breakdowns, and ulcerations should be reported and an appropriate nursing-care plan devised to restore skin integrity. The skin should be kept clean and dry; lotions may be applied to prevent drying or cracking of skin. The patient should be monitored for incontinence and drenching night sweats. Patients with these conditions should be cleaned and dried regularly and repositioned frequently if bed- or wheelchair-bound. Rectal areas should be protected with ointments; lamb's wool, heel protectors, and egg-crate mattress should be used as appropriate.

The patient's nutritional status should also be checked. Adequate nutrition and hydration are essential for maintaining skin integrity. Elevating the edematous extremities or head or using support stockings may give the patient some relief from edema.

RESPIRATORY DISTRESS

Pulmonary KS may cause serious respiratory distress and is a poor prognostic indicator. It usually occurs late in the course of illness among patients who die from KS.

Assessing the patient's respiratory status includes evaluating chest sounds, cough, respiratory rate and pattern, skin color, nail beds, chest x-ray, blood gases, temperature, and vital signs. Additional evaluation may be required to distinguish between pulmonary KS and opportunistic lung infections. A worsening pulmonary status may require hospitalization. If the patient can still be treated as an outpatient, the home should be assessed for its suitability for oxygen and other ventilatory equipment.

IMPAIRED PHYSICAL MOBILITY

Extensive KS involvement of the lymph nodes can cause severe edema, which limits the patient's physical mobility. Pulmonary KS also limits the patient's functional status; disease progression and systemic symptoms (such as fevers, fatigue, and weight loss) may make physical activity difficult or impossible.

Careful history taking or home visits are needed to assess the patient's activity and functional status. Depending on the patient's competencies and the availability of home-care help, home-attendant services may be needed for some patients and hospitalization for others.

SELF CONCEPT

The KS patient experiences body-image changes when lesions on the face and extremities are highly visible. Severe weight loss can produce an emaciated, cachectic look; severe edema of the face and extremities can also cause the patient great distress in body image. Patients who have previously been independent and self-sufficient may have difficulty adjusting to a dependent, "sick" role.

A supportive, accepting atmosphere can be provided both in the clinic and at the patient's home. Helping patients express and ventilate feelings, fears, and frustrations may help them to identify and begin to resolve crucial issues. Incorporating the patient, lover and family in the care plan can restore control to the patient and promote independence. It is equally important to use the psychosocial team members to help identify crisis issues, pathology, and appropriate care plans.

More detailed information about nursing interventions has been published elsewhere.[1-20]

■ TREATMENT OPTIONS

Treatment options for KS include antineoplastic chemotherapy, radiation therapy, and immunomodulators.[2,21] Occasionally, in extensive disease, chemotherapy and radiation therapy are administered concurrently. Such combined modality therapy may increase the severity of side effects and presents the nurse with challenging care issues.

SIDE EFFECTS OF CHEMOTHERAPY

Chemotherapeutic agents used in the treatment of KS include bleomycin, doxorubicin, vinblastine, vincristine, and etoposide. Combination chemotherapy with doxorubicin, bleomycin, and vincristine is too toxic for the patient and often induces an opportunistic infection. Etoposide given in three daily doses on a 21-day cycle has shown some signs of success in treatment.[22-24] Single-agent vinblastine or vincristine given on a weekly basis has resulted in good response without debilitating toxicities.[25,26] Vincristine and vinblastine have also been used on an alternating weekly basis, thus minimizing bone-marrow suppression and vincristine-induced peripheral neuropathy.[27] Bleomycin, doxorubicin, vincristine and vinblastine are usually administered as intravenous "push" medications, and etoposide is given by intravenous "drip" over one to two hours.

Specific side effects of each of the drugs are discussed below, followed by a discussion of nursing interventions for the most common ones: bone-marrow depression, nausea and vomiting, and drug extravasation. More detailed information about chemotherapeutic drugs and nursing interventions has been published.[1,27-29]

Bleomycin.   Test doses of bleomycin are given before the first full dose to check for anaphylactic reactions. Fever, chills, and skin rashes are frequent side effects of this drug. Interstitial pneumonitis or pulmonary fibrosis may occur in patients receiving a cumulative dose greater than 400 units. KS patients receiving bleomycin who have had pneumocystis pneumonia should have their pulmonary status monitored regularly. Nausea and vomiting, stomatitis, and alopecia have also been observed.

Doxorubicin (Adriamycin).   Alopecia, bone-marrow depression, and nausea and vomiting are the most common side effects of this drug. Doxorubicin is also a vesicant drug, so tissue necrosis occurs if the drug extravasates during administration. Vein discoloration, stomatitis, dose-related cardiomyopathies, fever, chills, urticaria, anaphylaxis, and red-colored urine are other side effects.

Etoposide (Vepesid, VP16-213).   Alopecia, nausea, vomiting, anorexia, diarrhea, and bone-marrow depression are the most common side effects of etoposide. Hypotension may occur if the drug is infused too rapidly. Stomatitis, acute hypersensitivity reactions, and hepatotoxicity may also result from use of this drug.

Vinblastine (Velban).   Bone-marrow depression and nausea or vomiting are common side effects. Vinblastine is also a vesicant agent and can cause phlebitis or tissue necrosis if extravasation occurs. Neurotoxicity is a major side effect. KS patients appear to be very sensitive to its neurotoxic effects. Initial complaints consist primarily of paresthesias or numbness in the fingers or hands. Alopecia and stomatitis are other possible side effects.

Vincristine (Oncovin).   Peripheral, cranial nerve, and central nervous system neuropathy are commonly seen with vincristine treatment. KS patients are extremely sensitive to its neurotoxic effects. Common complaints initially include paresthesias of the fingers and hand, difficulty walking or climbing steps, and jaw pain. Extravasation of vincristine, like vinblastine, cause local tissue necrosis. Alopecia, nausea, or vomiting may occur. Mild bone-marrow depression may be seen, primarily in the white blood cell count. Vincristine seems to be a platelet-sparing chemotherapeutic agent and is substituted when vinblastine-induced thrombocytopenia occurs.

Bone-Marrow Depression.   Chemotherapeutic agents are toxic to rapidly dividing blood cells, including platelets, white cells, and red cells. Major side effects of doxorubicin, vincristine, vinblastine, and etoposide are thrombocytopenia or leukopenia (or both), due to the cytotoxic effects on the bone-marrow reserve. They are commonly seen 7 to 14 days after these drugs are administered. Blood counts should be done routinely before drug administration so that dosage levels may be adjusted or held according to the degree of bone-marrow depression. Patient with white blood counts of less than 2000 or total granulocyte counts of less than 1000 are at greater risk for developing infection. Patient with platelet counts below 50,000 are in danger of bleeding or hemorrhaging. Spontaneous bleeding usually occurs when the platelet count is less than 20,000.[29]

Nursing Interventions.   Preventing infections and recognizing early signs and symptoms of infection are critical to the care of leukopenic patients. If the patient does not require hospitalization, appropriate measures should be reviewed with the patient and family. These include:

- avoiding public places or visitors who may have respiratory or other communicable infections;
- avoiding raw fruits and vegetables and eating only cooked or processed foods;
- removing cut flowers from the household;
- stressing cleanliness and regular bathing and hand washing;
- using toothbrushes with soft bristles and sponge tips;
- avoiding anal sexual activities or other sexual practices that may cause trauma to the skin;
- keeping a temperature chart and reporting temperature elevations greater than 101°F;
- reporting to a nurse or physician any dizziness or orthostasis, tachycardia, mental-status changes, hyperventilation, dysuria, upper-respiratory infections, or skin ulcerations or infections.

Hospitalization of the leukopenic patient permits appropriate protective isolation measures and treatment of fever and infection.

Thrombocytopenic nursing care includes teaching the patient and family to:

- watch for signs and symptoms of bleeding, such as bruises, bleeding gums, hematuria, black emesis or stools, or epistaxis;
- avoid falls, cuts, or bruises;
- shave only with an electric razor;
- avoid the use of aspirin;
- brush the teeth gently, using soft bristles or sponge toothbrushes; and postpone dental work;
- eat a soft diet and avoid alcoholic beverages;
- use a stool softener if necessary to avoid straining during bowel movements;
- blow the nose gently.

If the patient requires hospitalization, appropriate bleeding precautions and platelet transfusions can be initiated.

Nausea and Vomiting.   Patients on chemotherapy frequently experience nausea. KS patients receiving combination chemotherapy (doxorubicin, bleomycin, and vincristine) or single-agent etoposide may experience mild-to-severe nausea or vomiting, or both. Most patients receiving single-agent vincristine or vinblastine experience only mild-to-moderate nausea, possibly because of the relatively low doses administered.

Assess the patient for nausea and vomiting, including onset, severity, and duration. Administer antiemetics prior to chemotherapy, then every four to six hours as needed. Assess the effectiveness of the agent used. If the patient is vomiting, antiemetics can be given in intramuscular or suppository form. Patients receiving outpatient chemotherapy should be given a prescription for antiemetics for home use. Suggest dietary changes such as small frequent snacks that include soda crackers or dry toast. A liquid diet or supplement may be indicated if the patient is experiencing nausea or vomiting. Fluid intake should be encouraged. If vomiting is severe or prolonged, the nurse should evaluate the patient for signs of dehydration.

Chemotherapy Extravasation.   The potential for injury caused by chemotherapy extravasation is of particular concern when administering doxorubicin, vincristine, and vinblastine. These drugs are known vesicants that can cause severe tissue necrosis. The damage caused is in direct relation to the amount of drug extravasated.

Although most institutions have established drug extravasation protocols listing antidotes for these and other vesicants, the protocols lack proven clinical trials that demonstrate the antidote's effectiveness. For this reason, the best way to manage extravasation is to avoid it by careful, meticulous administration of the drug.

The infusion site should be observed closely and continuously for pain, burning, a warm sensation, or "bleb" formation. A sluggish or absent blood return from the IV on aspiration, red "streaking," or pain along the individual vein extending from the IV site may also signal an extravasation. In such cases, the infusion must be stopped and the established procedure for managing extravasation must be implemented. The patient should be educated about the possibility of extravasation and should actively participate in observing the infusion so that he or she knows if an extravasation has occurred.

SIDE EFFECTS OF RADIATION THERAPY

Radiation therapy is indicated for treatment of bulky, localized KS lesions, especially oropharyngeal lesions, those causing lymphatic obstruction or painful compression on the face or extremities. Large, bulky lesions of the oral cavity, painful lesions of the feet, and blocked lymph nodes resulting in severe edema of the face or lower extremities are often effectively treated with doses of 1800 to 3000 rads. Four cases of hemibody irradiation in the treatment of extensive KS have been documented.[24] Although the response rate is rapid and dramatic in most cases, tumor progression often continues once radiotherapy is stopped.[2,21] Generalized side effects of radiation therapy include fatigue, malaise, headache, nausea, vomiting, and anorexia. The severity of these symptoms is related to the area of tissue treated and dose of radiation administered.

The symptoms are probably due to tumor cell lysis and absorption of cellular debris.[30]

Skin Integrity.   Irradiated skin may develop erythema, followed by a tanned appearance that does not fade. Dry skin with itching, flaking, or cracking follows.

Care of the skin includes keeping it clean and dry with warm water and mild soap, avoiding sun exposures, extreme temperatures caused by hot water, heating pads, or ice packs, wearing loose clothing, avoiding the use of irritating creams, shampoos, cosmetics, lotions, or other topicals, not using adhesive tape or dressing on irradiated skin, and reporting skin infections or breakdowns to the nurse or doctor. Patients can be taught to avoid friction or trauma to the skin by patting it dry and avoiding scratching or massaging. Shaving should be done with an electric shaver rather than a razor. Cornstarch can be applied to the skin to absorb moisture; Vaseline or A&D ointment can be applied to dry skin.[28,30]

Mucositis.   Radiation, especially to oral KS lesions, may lead to mucositis, resulting in pain, taste alterations, salivary-gland alterations, and possible nutrition and fluid imbalances.

Patients with mucositis should be told to avoid oral irritants, such as alcohol, tobacco, and spicy foods. Soft, bland, nutritious meals should be encouraged. Patients with reduced salivary-gland function can use artificial saliva or sugarless hard candy. Good oral hygiene, including gentle mouth rinsing and use of sponge-tipped toothbrushes, should be encouraged. Oral "swish" solutions containing xylocaine may reduce mouth pain. If the patient experiences nausea and vomiting, appropriate interventions include antiemetics, small frequent meals, increased fluids, and assessment for dehydration. If severe dysphagia results, hospitalization for tube feedings or hyperalimentation may be necessary.[30]

Bone-Marrow Suppression.   Extensive radiation to KS lesions may result in bone-marrow suppression, causing thrombocytopenia, leukopenia, or anemia.

SIDE EFFECTS OF IMMUNOTHERAPY

Alpha interferon has been used in clinical trials to treat KS. However, further clinical trials are needed to asses the role of interferons in KS treatment.[21,23,24,31] Until then, the use of ∝ interferon in KS patients remains limited. Major side effects of the drug are dose-dependent. They include mild-to-severe fevers (up to 106°F), chills, flu-like symptoms, myalgias, and headaches. Anorexia, fatigue, and weight loss have also been reported. Leukopenia, thrombocytopenia, and hepatotoxicity are also dose-related and reversible when the drug is discontinued.[32,33]

The nursing care of patients on immunotherapy focuses on symptom management and emotional support. Management of fevers and flu-like symptoms include administering acetaminophen for fevers and monitoring for vital signs, intake and output, and signs and symptoms of dehydration. Sponge baths or other cooling measures can be initiated for prolonged fevers; hospitalization must be considered for persistent temperatures greater than 104°F. The patient's nutrition and hydration should be monitored frequently and appropriate nursing measures should be used. Blood counts and liver-function tests should also be monitored. The nurse should assist and provide emotional support to patients as they readjust their activities to the fatigue that follows administration of interferon.

REFERENCES

1. Moran TA. Cancers in HIV infection. In: Gee G, Moran TA, eds. AIDS: concepts in nursing practice. Baltimore: Williams and Wilkins, 1988:123-40.

2. Volberding P, Kaposi's sarcoma in AIDS. In: Levy JA, ed. AIDS: pathogenesis and treatment. New York: Marcel Dekker, 1989:345-58.

3. Ake JM, Perlstein LM. AIDS: impact on neuroscience nursing practice. J Neurosci Nurs 1987; 19:300-4.

4. Beckham MM, Rudy EB. Acquired immunodeficiency syndrome: impact and implication for the neurologic system. J Neurosci Nurs 1986; 18:5-10.

5. Carr GS, Gee G. AIDS and AIDS-related conditions: screening for populations at risk. Nurs Pract 1986; 11:25-6, 29, 32-6.

6. Crocker KS. AIDS-related GI dysfunction: rationale for nutrition support. Crit Care Nurs 1988; 8:43-5.

7. Howes AD. Nursing diagnoses and care plans for ambulatory care patients with AIDS. Top Clin Nurs 1984; 6:61-6.

8. LaCamera DJ, Msur H, Henderson DK. The acquired immunodeficiency syndrome. Nurs Clin North Am 1985; 20:241-56.

9. Lillard J, Lotspeich P, Gurich J, et al. Acquired immunodeficiency syndrome (AIDS) in home care: Maximizing helpfulness and minimizing hysteria. Home Healthc Nurs 1984; 2:11-6.

10. Cummings D. Caring for the HIV-infected adult. Nurs Pract 1988; 13:28, 31, 34.

11. Gee G, Moran TA, eds. AIDS: concepts in nursing practice. Baltimore: Williams and Wilkins, 1988.

12. Robinson L. Acquired immunodeficiency syndrome (AIDS) — an update. Crit Care Nurs 1984; 4:75-83.

13. Jordan KS. Assessment of the person with acquired immunodeficiency syndrome in the emergency department. JEN 1987; 13:342-5.

14. Lovejoy NC. The pathophysiology of AIDS. Oncol Nurs Forum 1988; 15:563-71.

15. Sunder JA. AIDS: A neurological nursing challenge. Top Clin Nurs 1984; 6:67-71.

16. McArthur JH, McArthur JC. Neurological manifestations of acquired immunodeficiency syndrome. J Neurosci Nurs 1986; 18:242-9.

17. Perlstein LM, Ake JM. AIDS: an overview for the neuroscience nurse. J Neurosci Nurs 1987; 19:296-9.

18. Pheifer WG, Houseman C. Bereavement and AIDS. A framework for intervention. J Psychosoc Nurs Ment Health Serv 1988; 26:21-6.

19. Saunders JM, Buckingham SL. Suicidal AIDS patients: when the depression turns deadly. Nursing 1988; 18:59-64.

20. Schietinger H. AIDS beyond the hospital. A home care plan for AIDS. Am J Nurs 1986; 86:1021-8.

21. Krigel RL, Friedman-Kien AE. Kaposi's sarcoma in AIDS. In: De Vita VT Jr, Hellman S, Rosenberg SA, eds. AIDS: etiology, diagnosis, treatment, and prevention. Philadelphia: JB Lippincott, 1985; 185-211.

22. Laubenstein LJ, Krigel R, Odajnyk CM, et al. Treatment of epidemic Kaposi's sarcoma with etoposide or a combination of doxorubicin, bleomycin, and vinblastine. J Clin Oncol 1984; 2:115-20.

23. Volberding P. Therapy of Kaposi's sarcoma in AIDS. Semin Oncol 1984; 11:60-7.

24. Mitsuyasu RT, Groopman JE. Biology and therapy of Kaposi's sarcoma. Semin Oncol 1984; 11:53-9.

25. Volberding PA, Abrams DI, Conant M, et al. Vinblastine therapy for Kaposi's sarcoma in the acquired immunodeficiency syndrome. Ann Intern Med 1985; 103:335-8.

26. Mintzer DM, Real FX, Jovino L, Krown SE. Treatment of Kaposi's sarcoma and thrombocytopenia with vincristine in patients with the acquired immunodeficiency syndrome. Ann Intern Med 1985; 102:200-2.

27. Kaplan LD, Abrams DI, Volberding PA. Treatment of Kaposi's sarcoma in acquired immunodeficiency syndrome with an alternating vincristine-vinblastine regimen. Cancer Treat Rep 1986; 70:1121-2.

28. Swearington PL, ed. Manual of nursing therapeutics: Applying nursing diagnoses to medical disorders. Menlo Park: Addison Wesley, 1986.

29. Sarna LP. Concepts in the nursing management of patients receiving cancer chemotherapy and immunotherapy. In: Vredevo DL, Derdiarian A, Sarna LP, et al., eds. Concepts of oncology nursing. Englewood Cliffs, NJ: Prentice Hall, 1981; 81-153.

30. Sarna LP. Concepts of nursing care for patients receiving radiation therapy. In: Vredevoe DL, Derdiarian A, Sarna LP, et al., eds. Concepts of oncology nursing. Englewood Cliffs, NJ: Prentice-Hall, 1981:154-205.

31. Groopman JE, Gottlieb MS, Goodman J, et al. Recombinant alpha-2 interferon therapy for Kaposi's sarcoma associated with the acquired immunodeficiency syndrome. Ann Intern Med 1984; 100:671-6.

32. Mayer DK, Smalley RV. Interferon: Current status. Oncol Nurs Forum 1983; 10:14-19.

33. Wong RJ. Pharmacologic treatment of HIV infection. In: Gee G, Moran TA, eds. AIDS: concepts in Nursing Practice. Baltimore: Williams and Wilkins, 1988:324-50.

7.2

Lymphomas and Other Malignancies

HIV-Associated Non-Hodgkin's Lymphoma

Lawrence D. Kaplan, M.D.

T he first large series indicating a relationship between AIDS and high-grade non-Hodgkin's lymphoma (NHL) was a study of lymphomas in homosexual men reported by Ziegler et al. in 1984.[1] Since that time, many cases of aggressive lymphomas have been reported in HIV-infected patients, including those in several large series.[2-5] In June 1985, the Centers for Disease Control amended their case definition of AIDS to include patients with high-grade, B-cell non-Hodgkin's lymphoma in the setting of documented HIV infection.[12]

■ NON-HODGKIN'S LYMPHOMA IN NON-HIV INFECTED IMMUNOCOMPROMISED PATIENTS

Non-Hodgkin's lymphoma has been frequently observed in association with abnormal cell-mediated immunity. Patients with primary immunodeficiency disorders, such as the Wiskott-Aldrich syndrome or ataxia-telangiectasia, have developed high-grade B-cell NHL. Immunoblastic lymphoma has been the most prevalent histologic pattern. A striking feature in these patients has been marked generalized lymphadenopathy, often present for several years before lymphoma was diagnosed. Lymph-node biopsies in these patients frequently show a pattern of reactive hyperplasia.[6] A similar pattern has been observed in post-renal transplant patients receiving immunosuppressive medications. This group has a 35-fold increased risk of developing NHL, often at unusual sites. In 33 percent of NHL cases associated with renal transplantation, disease confined to the central nervous system (CNS) has been observed.[7] Lymphoproliferative disease in these patients may appear as an invasive polyclonal proliferation or as an aggressive monoclonal large-cell non-Hodgkin's lymphoma.[8] Furthermore, a renal-transplant recipient has been described in whom a high-grade immunoblastic lymphoma has evolved out of a polyclonal lymphoproliferative process.[9]

Circumstantial evidence supports a role for Epstein–Barr virus (EBV) in the etiology of these lymphomas.[10] A majority of patients with these disorders demonstrate serologic evidence for either acute or reactivated EBV infection. Southern blot hybridization has revealed multiple copies of the EBV genome within the cells of many of these lymphomas.[10]

■ NON-HODGKIN'S LYMPHOMA IN HIV-INFECTED PATIENTS

Cases of HIV-associated non-Hodgkin's lymphoma bear a striking resemblance to those described in association with other immunodeficiency states. The histologic appearance of HIV-associated lymphoma has generally included both intermediate- and high-grade large-cell varieties as well as high-grade small noncleaved-cell varieties (Burkitt's and non-Burkitt's), which are not seen in transplant patients. Immunologically, these are B-cell malignancies. Chromosomal translocations similar to those observed in patients with Burkitt's lymphoma[14] have been observed in patients with HIV-associated Burkitt's-like lymphoma.[15] Epstein—Barr virus nuclear antigen (EBNA) has been identified in some of these tumors and most patients have shown evidence of previous EBV infection.[11] In anecdotal reports, EBV DNA sequences have been identified in cells from some of these tumors.[16,18] At San Francisco General Hospital, however, we have found them in only approximately one-third of tumors isolated from HIV-infected individuals with NHL.[13,22] Similar observations have been made by Subar et al.[30] These investigators identified EBV genome in only 6 of 16 tumors.

Many of the HIV-infected patients with NHL had previous histories of persistent generalized lymphadenopathy; lymph-node biopsies revealed follicular hyperplasia. Ziegler et al.'s 1984 report described 90 homosexual men with non-Hodgkin's lymphoma.[1] Of 77 patients diagnosed, 33 had a prodrome of generalized lymphadenopathy, 15 had previous opportunistic infections, 9 had Kaposi's sarcoma, and 5 had both opportunistic infections and Kaposi's sarcoma before developing NHL. Similarly, of 14 homosexual patients with aggressive NHL reported by Kalter, 8 had a preceding diagnosis of AIDS and 5 had other symptomatic HIV disease.[2]

CLINICAL FEATURES OF NON-HODGKIN'S LYMPHOMA IN HIV-INFECTED PATIENTS

The most prominent clinical feature of NHL in the setting of HIV infection is the frequent occurrence of extranodal disease. In Ziegler's series,[1] all but two patients had extranodal disease; 42 percent of patients had CNS disease, and 33 percent had bone-marrow involvement. In a series of 89 patients diagnosed at New York University,[4] 87 percent had extranodal disease. The most common sites included the gastrointestinal tract (24 patients), CNS (19 patients), bone marrow (19 patients), and liver (14 patients). In a Memorial Hospital series of 43 patients,[5] 65 percent had extranodal disease. Bone marrow and meninges were the most common sites of involvement; the lung, stomach, liver, small intestine, large intestine, and pleura were also involved.

Unusual extranodal presentations are not uncommon in patients with HIV-associated lymphoma. Rectal lymphomas have been reported[22,23] and may appear as perirectal abscess. Four cases of NHL involving the heart have been described.[24,25] These patients have presented with respiratory symptoms or superventricular tachyarrhythmias. Lymphomatous pericarditis[22] presenting with chest pain, dyspnea, or hypotension may be confused with infectious etiologies such as viral or mycobacterial pericarditis. Other unusual sites include gingiva,[4,22] soft tissue,[4,5,22] Waldeyer's ring,[5,22] and the bile duct.[26]

Lymphoma confined to the CNS accounts for up to 25 percent of the reported cases of HIV-associated NHL.[1,16,17,27] Clinical presentation and radiographic findings in these patients are often indistinguishable from those of cerebral toxoplasmosis. Confusion, lethargy, memory loss, hemiparesis, aphasia, seizures, cranial nerve palsies, and headache are common presenting symptoms. However, in one series,[5] less than half the patients had demonstrable focal neurologic abnormalities. The most common findings on computed axial tomographic (CT) scan of the brain are single or multiple discrete hypo- or isodense contrast-enhancing lesions.

DIAGNOSIS

As suggested by the previous discussion, lymphoma should be suspected in a wide variety of situations. At our institution, we do not routinely biopsy lymph nodes in HIV-infected individuals with generalized lymphadenopathy. Biopsy of a peripheral node is reserved for patients with asymmetrical lymphadenopathy and rapidly enlarging or bulky nodes in the absence of other symptoms. Biopsy should also be considered in patients with persistent, unexplained constitutional symptoms and generalized lymphadenopathy.

In the patient without peripheral lymphadenopathy who has persistent unexplained fevers, an abdominal CT scan should be considered in order to identify enlarged nodes that might be accessible to fine-needle aspiration.

Intrahepatic and periportal involvement are common in the HIV-infected patient and should be considered when there is unexplained evidence of intra- or extra-hepatic obstruction. In these cases, imaging studies of the liver should be performed. Focal lesions can be sampled using fine-needle aspiration. If no focal lesions are found, percutaneous liver biopsy may be appropriate.

Anorectal lymphoma should be considered in HIV-infected patients with persistent anorectal complaints. Perirectal abscess is often the preoperative diagnosis in these patients but lymphoma may be present along with an abscess.[22]

Gastrointestinal symptoms should be thoroughly investigated, especially if accompanied by any evidence of bleeding. In patients with Kaposi's sarcoma (KS), GI bleeding should not be presumed to be a consequence solely of gastrointestinal KS.

In any of these circumstances, if isolated lactic dehydrogenase elevation or elevation out of proportion to that of other liver function studies is found, the clinician should suspect non-Hodgkin's lymphoma.

The diagnosis of primary central nervous system lymphoma deserves particular attention. Patients with central nervous system abnormalities (e.g., changes in mental status, seizures, focal neurologic findings, or persistent headache) should undergo prompt CT or magnetic resonance imaging (MRI) of the head as well as lumbar puncture (if imaging of the brain does not reveal a contraindicating mass lesion). Serum and spinal fluid should be assayed for cryptococcal antigen.

The CT or MRI scan (or both) cannot reliably distinguish focal CNS lesions caused by NHL from those caused by toxoplasma or less common entities such as bacterial, mycobacterial, or fungal abscesses. It is unusual for patients with negative toxoplasma serologic studies to develop toxoplasma encephalitis.[28] Therefore, if focal intracerebral lesions are found, toxoplasma serologic studies should be obtained and antitoxoplasma therapy should be administered. If toxoplasma serology is positive, toxoplasma therapy should be continued and a follow-up brain-imaging study done in 10 to 14 days. If the patient improves clinically and the CNS lesions diminish, a presumptive diagnosis of CNS toxoplasmosis is justified and a brain biopsy can be avoided. If toxoplasma serology is negative, or if the patient worsens or does not improve with anti-toxoplasma therapy, a biopsy of the brain is necessary to identify potentially treatable conditions other than toxoplasmosis. At San Francisco General Hospital, 72 percent of patients with CNS toxoplasmosis showed radiographic evidence of response to therapy within two weeks (Clement M: personal communication).

Efforts should be directed towards early diagnosis of central nervous system lymphoma. CNS lymphoma may be an aggressive and rapidly progressive malignancy, and if therapy is delayed until the patient has severe neurologic dysfunction, it may have little benefit.

TREATMENT AND PROGNOSIS

Ziegler et al.[1] reported the first group of patients with HIV-associated NHL. In this series, 53 percent of 66 evaluable patients achieved complete responses to a variety of aggressive combination chemotherapy regimens. This response rate was significantly worse than that for immunocompetent patients suffering from the same high-grade lymphomas. Fifty-four percent of patients having a complete response subsequently relapsed. While the prognosis was poor in all groups, morbidity and mortality were directly related to the severity of the patients' previous HIV-related diagnosis. Patients with asymptomatic HIV infection at the time of diagnosis had the best treatment results. Those with a history of persistent generalized lymphadenopathy fared less well, while 21 patients with a previous AIDS diagnosis had the worst outcome. Thirty-eight of the 66 evaluable patients had died at the time of reporting — half from progressive lymphoma and half from opportunistic infections. Patients with a previous diagnosis of AIDS or with primary CNS lymphoma had the highest morbidity and mortality.

Levine et al.[3] treated 7 patients with either cyclophosphamide, doxorubicin, vincristine and prednisone (CHOP), or with bleomycin, doxorubicin, cyclophosphamide, vincristine, and prednisone (BACOP). Two patients had complete responses; one subsequently relapsed. The same investigators subsequently reported that 7 of 13 (54 percent) patients attained complete remission after treatment with methotrexate, bleomycin, doxorubicin, cyclophosphamide, dexamethasone, and leucovorin (M-BACOD).[29] Two of these patients subsequently relapsed, while the remaining 5 remained free of disease 15 to 16 months after diagnosis. In comparison, only 3 of 9 (33 percent) patients receiving a more aggressive, novel chemotherapeutic regimen achieved complete remission. This intensive combination chemotherapy was associated with significant risk of early death from opportunistic infection.

A New York University series reported that 26 percent of patients with small noncleaved cell lymphoma responded completely to therapy (median survival = 5.5 months), as did 21 percent of those with immunoblastic lymphoma (median survival = 2.0 months), and 52 percent of patients with large noncleaved cell lymphoma (median survival = 7.5 months).[4]

In a series of 84 patients with HIV-associated NHL treated with a variety of therapeutic regimens, the median survival was only 4.5 months.[22] However, significantly improved survival was observed within subgroups. Total CD4-positive lymphocyte counts were the most important predictor of survival. Those patients with total CD4-positive lymphocyte counts greater than 100 cells/cubic mm had a median survival of 24 months, while those with a CD4 count of less than 100 cells/cubic mm had a median survival of 4.1 months. Other factors did not add prognostic information to CD4-positive lymphocyte counts. In the absence of CD4-positive lymphocyte counts, other factors predictive of improved survival included the absence of a prior AIDS diagnosis (median survival = 8.3 months), Karnofsky performance score of 70 percent or better (median survival = 6.8 months), and the absence of an extranodal site of disease (median survival = 12.2 months).

In the San Francisco General Hospital series,[22] 26 patients were treated with a variety of standard chemotherapeutic regimens and 38 were treated with a novel regimen consisting of cyclophosphamide, vincristine, methotrexate, etoposide, and cytosine arabinoside (COMET-A). Although patients treated with COMET-A had a slightly higher complete-response rate, they had a significantly shorter median survival (5.2 months) than those treated with standard chemotherapy (11.3 months). Furthermore, patients receiving chemotherapy regimens containing 1.0 g/square meter of body surface area or more of cyclophosphamide had significantly shorter median survival (4.6 months) than those treated with regimens containing less than 1 g/square meter of cyclophosphamide (12.2 months). These data support the earlier suggestion[29] that patients treated with more aggressive chemotherapy regimens may have shortened survival. The cause of death was advanced NHL in 9 of 25 (36 percent) patients treated with COMET-A, 6 of 16 patients (37 percent) treated with other regimens, and all 6 patients who received no treatment. Twenty-eight percent of COMET-A patients and 37 percent of standard chemotherapy patients died of opportunistic infection. Regardless of the cause of death, a majority of treated patients had active NHL at the time of death.

RECOMMENDATIONS FOR THERAPY

Deciding whether to treat a patient with HIV-related NHL is difficult. An individual with a low total CD4-positive lymphocyte count and poor performance status who develops NHL after a long and complicated history of AIDS is generally not likely to benefit from chemotherapy. Cytotoxic therapy in such a patient is unlikely to prolong survival and may produce severe toxicity. On the other hand, the patient with more than 100 CD4-positive lymphocytes and a good performance score who is diagnosed with AIDS because of NHL may live a longer and better life if treated with standard-combination chemotherapy. Other patients fall somewhere between these extremes. In such cases, clinical judgment and patient preference must shape treatment decisions. Highly aggressive chemotherapeutic regimens (particularly those in which the cyclophosphamide dose is greater than 1 g/square meter) should be avoided because they may reduce the benefits of therapy. Clinical trials are currently underway to evaluate the efficacy of lower-dose chemotherapeutic regimens. These may provide additional guidelines for the treatment of NHL in HIV-infected individuals.

TREATMENT OF CNS LYMPHOMA

Standard therapy should consist of whole-brain irradiation with approximately 3000 to 3500 cGy and a 1000 cGy boost to the primary site. If possible, patients should be referred to centers where clinical trials are available.

The prognosis for patients with primary CNS lymphoma and AIDS is very poor in most cases. Despite therapy with partial resection and whole-brain irradiation, only 1 of 6 patients reported by Gill et al. remains alive 28 months after diagnosis.[16] This lone surviving patient had a plasmacytoid lymphocytic lymphoma rather than the typical high-grade immunoblastic histologic pattern observed in most patients. Other than this patient, the longest-surviving patient died of progressive CNS lymphoma after 16 months. A total of two patients in this series died of progressive lymphoma, while two others died as a result of opportunistic infection. Similarly, So et al. at the University of California—San Francisco reported a mean survival of 2.7 months in 7 patients treated with whole-brain irradiation.[17] Their survival was not significantly longer than that of patients who received no therapy at all. In a subsequent San Francisco series,[25] patients responded well to radiation therapy but their survival continued to be short because of intercurrent opportunistic infection. The poor survival in these patients is not surprising in view of the high incidence of relapse in immunocompetent patients.[19,20]

With widespread use of zidovudine (AZT) and prophylaxis for *Pneumocystis carinii* pneumonia (PCP), HIV-infected patients are surviving longer. More patients with primary CNS lymphoma may benefit from adequate primary therapy for their malignancy. This is particularly true in patients with minimal neurologic impairment. Thus, early diagnosis and prompt therapeutic intervention are warranted.

REFERENCES

1. Ziegler JL, Beckstead JA, Volberding PA, et al. Non Hodgkin's lymphoma in 90 homosexual men. N Engl J Med 1984; 311:565-70.
2. Kalter SP, Riggs SA, Cabanillas F, et al. Aggressive non Hodgkin's lymphomas in immunocompromised homosexual males. Blood 1985; 66:655-9.
3. Levine AM, Gill PS, Meyer PR, et al. Retrovirus and malignant lymphoma in homosexual men. JAMA 1985; 254:1921-5.
4. Knowles DM, Chamulak GA, Subar M, et al. Lymphoid neoplasia associated with the acquired immunodeficiency syndrome (AIDS). The New York University Medical Center experience with 105 patients (1981-1986). Ann Intern Med 1988; 108:744-53.
5. Lowenthal DA, Straus DJ, Campbell SW, et al. AIDS-related lymphoid neoplasia. Cancer 1988; 61:2325-37.
6. Frizzera G, Rosai J, Dehner LP, et al. Lymphoreticular disorders in primary immunodeficiencies. Cancer 1980; 46:692-9.
7. Hoover R, Fraumeni JF Jr. Risk of cancer in renal transplant recipients. Lancet 1973; 55-7.
8. Frizzera G, Hanto DW, Gajl-Peczalska KJ, et al. Polymorphic diffuse B cell hyperplasias and lymphomas in renal transplant recipients. Cancer Res 1981; 41:4262-79.
9. Hanto DW, Frizzera G, Gajl-Peczalska KJ, et al. Epstein Barr virus induced B cell lymphoma after renal transplantation. Med Intell 1982; 306:913-8.
10. Hanto DW, Frizzera G, Purtilo DT, et al. Clinical spectrum of lymphoproliferative disorders in renal transplant recipients and evidence for the role of Epstein Barr virus. Cancer Res 1981; 41:4253-61.
11. Ziegler JL, Drew WL, Miner RC, et al. Outbreak of Burkitt's like lymphoma in homosexual men. Lancet 1982; 631-3.
12. Revision of the case definition of acquired immunodeficiency syndrome for national reporting — United States. MMWR 1985; 34:373-5.
13. Feigal EG, Lekas P, Beckstead JH, et al. Evidence for coinfection with HTLV-I and HIV in AIDS risk-group patients with high-grade non-Hodgkin's lymphoma. In: Human retroviruses, cancer and AIDS — Approaches to prevention and therapy. Bolognesi D, ed. UCLA Symposium on molecular and cellular biology 1988; 71:213-28.
14. Zech L, Hagland U, Nilsson K, Klein G. Characteristic chromosomal abnormalities in biopsies and lymphoid-cell lines from patients with Burkitt and non-Burkitt lymphomas. Int J Cancer 1976; 17:47-56.
15. Whang-Peng J, Lee EC, Sieverts H, Magrath IT. Burkitt's lymphoma in AIDS: Cytogenetic study. Blood 1984; 63:818-22.
16. Gill PS, Levine AM, Meyer PR, et al. Primary central nervous system lymphoma in homosexual men. Am J Med 1985; 78:742-8.
17. So YT, Beckstead JH, Davis RL. Primary central nervous system lymphoma in acquired immune deficiency syndrome: A clinical and pathological study. Ann Neurol 1986; 20:566-72.
18. Groopman JE, Sullivan JL, Mulder C, et al. Pathogenesis of B cell lymphoma in a patient with AIDS. Blood 1986; 67:612-5.
19. Henry JM, Heffner RR Jr, Dillard SH, et al. Primary malignant lymphomas of the central nervous system. Cancer 1974; 34:1293-1302.
20. Loeffler JS, Ervin TJ, Mauch P, et al. Primary lymphomas of the central nervous system: Patterns of failure and factors that influence survival. J Clin Oncol 1985; 3:490-4.
21. Petersen JM, Tubbs RR, Savage RA, et al. Small noncleaved B cell Burkitt-like lymphoma with chromosome t(8; 14) translocation and Epstein-Barr virus nuclear-associated antigen in a homosexual man with acquired immune deficiency syndrome. Am J Med 1985; 78:141-8.

22. Kaplan LD, Abrams DI, Feigal E, et al. AIDS-associated non-Hodgkin's lymphoma in San Francisco. JAMA 1989; 261:719-24.

23. Burkes RL, Meyer PR, Gill PS, et al. Rectal lymphoma in homosexual men. Arch Intern Med 1986; 146:913-5.

24. Balasubramanyam A, Waxman M, Kazal HL, Lee MH. Malignant lymphoma of the heart in acquired immune deficiency syndrome. Chest 1986; 90:243-6.

25. Guarner J, Brynes RK, Chan WC, et al. Primary non-Hodgkin's lymphoma of the heart in two patients with the acquired immunodeficiency syndrome. Arch Pathol Lab Med 1987; 111:254-6.

26. Kaplan LD, Kahn J, Jacobson M, et al. Primary bile duct lymphoma in the acquired immunodeficiency syndrome. Ann Intern Med 1989; 110:161-2.

27. Rosenblum ML, Levy RM, Bredesen DE, et al. Primary central nervous system lymphomas in patients with AIDS. Ann Neurol 1988; 23(suppl):S13-S16.

28. Israelski DM, Remington JS. Toxoplasmic encephalitis in patients with AIDS. Infect Dis Clin North Am 1988; 2:429-45.

29. Gill PS, Levine AM, Krailo M, et al. AIDS-related malignant lymphoma: results of prospective treatment trials. J Clin Oncol 1987; 5:1322-8.

30. Subar M, Neri A, Inghirami G, et al. Frequent c-myc oncogene activation and infrequent presence of Epstein-Barr virus genome in AIDS-associated lymphoma. Blood 1988; 72:667-71.

Hodgkin's Disease and AIDS

Lawrence D. Kaplan, M.D.

Although Hodgkin's disease in the setting of human immunodeficiency virus (HIV) infection does not presently constitute a diagnosis of AIDS, a number of such cases have recently been reported. Like the AIDS related non-Hodgkin's lymphomas, Hodgkin's disease in this setting is associated with an unfavorable histology, advanced stage, and poor therapeutic outcome, along with a high incidence of associated opportunistic infections.

A total of 14 homosexual men with Hodgkin's disease were evaluated at Stanford University (4 patients)[1] and San Francisco General Hospital (10 patients).[2] Twelve had a previous history of persistent generalized lymphadenopathy, biopsy proven in 4. No patient had a previous history of opportunistic infection or Kaposi's sarcoma. The predominant histologic pattern was mixed-cellularity, observed in 10 cases. A nodular sclerosis pattern was found in 3 cases, and 1 case was unclassified. Eleven patients had pathologic stage IV disease; 2, stage III; and 1, stage II disease. Extranodal sites of disease were present in 11 patients, and included bone marrow in 8, liver in 5, and skin in 1 patient. HIV was confirmed in all 6 patients evaluated for the presence of the virus.

The single patient with stage II disease was treated with total lymphoid radiation and died 5 years later from disseminated cytomegalovirus and *Mycobacterium avium* infections. The remaining 13 patients were treated with either nitrogen mustard, vincristine, procarbazine, and prednisone (MOPP), or MOPP alternating with doxorubicin, bleomycin, vinblastine, and DTIC (ABVD). *P. carinii* pneumonitis developed in 7 of these patients while they received chemotherapy. Of 7 patients who had complete responses, 3 remained disease free at 10, 11, and 21 months; and 1 has developed new lymphadenopathy after 21 months but refuses biopsy. Three patients who had complete responses have died of *Pneumocystis carinii* pneumonitis, and 1 of recurrent Hodgkin's disease. One of 4 patients who had a partial response to treatment is alive at 5 months; 1 died of progressive Hodgkin's disease, 1 of *P. carinii* pneumonia, and 1 of disseminated *M. avium*. One patient is not yet evaluable for response.

Biggar and colleagues reported an increase in the incidence of Hodgkin's disease in single men aged 20 to 49 years in San Francisco in the year 1984.[3] This was a sudden change over previous years and of borderline statistical significance. Registry data for subsequent years will be needed to confirm any new trend.

While the presently available epidemiologic information cannot confirm an increased incidence of Hodgkin's disease in patients infected with HIV, the natural history of Hodgkin's disease appears to be altered in the presence of HIV infection. When compared with national registry data for the general population,[4] these patients have an unusually high prevalence of mixed-cellularity histology and advanced stage at diagnosis. Comparisons with historical data show the incidence of opportunistic infection to be very high and the rate of survival poor.

REFERENCES

1. Schoeppel SL, Hoppe RT, Dorfman RF, et al. Hodgkin's disease in homosexual men with generalized lymphadenopathy. Ann Intern Med 1985; 102:68-70.

2. Kaplan LD, Rainer C, Yeager D, et al. Hodgkin's disease and non-Hodgkin's lymphoma (NHL) in homosexual men [Abstract]. Paris: International conference on AIDS, 1986:42.

3. Biggar RJ, Horm J, Melbye M, Goedert J. Cancer trends among young single men in the SEER registries of the United States [Abstract]. Paris: International Conference on AIDS, 1986:31.

4. Kennedy BJ, Loeb V Jr, Peterson UM, et al. National survey of patterns of care for Hodgkin's disease. Cancer 1985; 56:2547-56.

7.2.3

Other Cancers in HIV-Infected Patients

Paul A. Volberding, M.D.

Given the large population of individuals infected with human immuno-deficiency virus (HIV) in the United States, medical problems including cancers are expected. It may be very difficult to establish a direct relationship of these other cancers to HIV infection, but there is the growing suspicion that some relationship may exist. In addition to Kaposi's sarcoma and B-cell lymphomas, which have been accepted as diagnostic of AIDS, other cancers that have been seen in AIDS risk group members include squamous-cell carcinomas of various sites, malignant melanoma, testicular cancers of all histologies, Hodgkin's disease, and primary hepatocellular carcinoma.[1-4]

With the exception of Hodgkin's disease in homosexual men, minimal direct evidence exists that these other cancers are caused by HIV-induced immune deficiency or that their mode of presentation or response to therapy has changed. Some of these cancers, particularly anal squamous cell carcinomas, malignant melanoma, and testicular malignancies, are known to have been relatively common in young men even before the beginning of the AIDS epidemic. Others, including hepatocellular carcinoma and other squamous cell carcinomas, have been only rarely reported in AIDS risk-group members and may reflect a simultaneous occurrence of two separate diseases, namely HIV infection and a malignancy. Nevertheless, it will be important to monitor AIDS risk populations for cancers because even if not causally related, previous HIV infection may alter the clinical behavior or response to therapy of the secondary malignancies.

If the clinician encounters a malignancy in a patient considered at increased risk for HIV disease, testing for HIV antibodies would be recommended. If negative, further diagnostic and therapeutic strategy can ignore questions of underlying immune deficiency with all that it might imply in terms of risk of unanticipated drug toxicities and complicating infectious diseases. If HIV antibodies are found, these possibilities of adverse outcome should be factored into the treatment plan. In certain cases in which the suspicion of underlying HIV disease is high, less immunotoxic treatment of the cancer should be seriously considered and unusual infections should be anticipated.

REFERENCES

1. Logothetis CJ, Newell GR, Samuels ML. Testicular cancer in homosexual men with cellular immune deficiency: Report of two cases. J Urol 1985; 133:484-6.
2. Robert NJ, Schneiderman H. Hodgkin's disease and the acquired immunodeficiency syndrome. Ann Intern Med 1984; 101:142-3.
3. Schoeppel SL, Hoppe RT, Dorfman RF, et al. Hodgkin's disease in homosexual men with generalized lymphadenopathy. Ann Intern Med 1985; 102:68-70.
4. Ioachim HL, Cooper MC, Hellman GC. Lymphomas in men at high risk for acquired immune deficiency syndrome (AIDS). Cancer 1985; 56:2831-42.

PEDIATRIC

AIDS

EDITOR

A.J. Ammann, M.D.

8.1

Pediatric AIDS

8.1.1   Pediatric AIDS — *Ammann*

8.1.1

Pediatric AIDS

A.J. Ammann, M.D.

■ DEFINITION

As of July 1, 1989, 1681 cases of pediatric AIDS have been reported in the U.S.[22] Seventy-nine percent (1334) of these children had parents with or at risk for AIDS; 12 percent (195) contracted it through HIV-infected blood transfusions or blood components, 6 percent (96) contracted HIV/AIDS presumably through hemophiliac fraction VIII or IX or infected coagulants; and 3 percent (56) belong to no known transmission category.[22] Approximately 1 percent of all AIDS cases reported to the Centers for Disease Control (CDC) as of July 1, 1989, are in children under 13 years of age. Eighty-three percent of these children are under five years old.[35] The largest number of pediatric AIDS cases are seen in the children of a growing transmission group among adults — IV drug-users and their sexual partners.[22] The total number of U.S. pediatric AIDS cases is expected to exceed 3,000 by the end of 1991.[25]

The definition of pediatric AIDS used here is formulated on the basis of epidemiologic, laboratory, and virologic data.[1] It may be established if the patient has

1. a history of a risk factor;
2. laboratory evidence of immunodeficiency; or
3. evidence of infection with human immunodeficiency virus (HIV).

This definition of pediatric AIDS differs from that of the CDC for both adult and pediatric AIDS because it does not require documentation of opportunistic infection or Kaposi's sarcoma.[2] The definition is in keeping with the World Health Organization's classification of primary and secondary immunodeficiency disorders.[3] Children at risk include infants born to mothers who are prostitutes, intravenous drug users, or of Haitian ancestry; infants of mothers whose sexual partners are bisexual, have hemophilia, or are intravenous drug abusers; infants with a history of blood transfusions; and infants who have hemophilia. Risk factors for children in Africa are similar but include exposure to nonsterilized needles.[25] HIV-infected children have also been born to mothers without known risk factors.[26]

The CDC has published a general classification of pediatric AIDS that is useful in epidemiologic studies. The classification emphasizes certain clinical and laboratory features of AIDS[27] (see Table 1).

Patients suspected of having pediatric AIDS should be evaluated with laboratory studies to either demonstrate immunodeficiency and antibody to HIV or to isolate the virus. Other congenital and acquired immunodeficiency disorders must be excluded. It is essential to establish a diagnosis of pediatric AIDS or HIV infection before the onset of opportunistic infection if such complications of AIDS are to be prevented and if an improved long-term prognosis is to be achieved.

TABLE 1. SUMMMARY OF THE CDC CLASSIFICATION OF HIV INFECTION IN CHILDREN UNDER 13 YEARS OF AGE

Class P-0. Indeterminate infection

Class P-1. Asymptomatic infection
  Subclass A. Normal immune function
  Subclass B. Abnormal immune function
  Subclass C. Immune function not tested

Class P-2. Symptomatic infection
  Subclass A. Nonspecific findings
  Subclass B. Progressive neurologic disease
  Subclass C. Lymphoid interstitial pneumonitis
  Subclass D. Secondary infectious diseases
    Category D-1. Specified secondary infectious diseases listed in the CDC surveillance definition for AIDS
    Category D-2. Recurrent serious bacterial infections
    Category D-3. Other specified secondary infectious diseases
  Subclass E. Secondary cancers
    Category E-1. Specified secondary cancers listed in the CDC surveillance definition for AIDS
    Category E-2. Other cancers possibly secondary to HIV infection
  Subclass F. Other diseases possibly due to HIV infection

■ TRANSMISSION

The two primary means through which children acquire HIV infection are maternal transfer of the virus and transmission of the virus through blood products. In addition, HIV may be transmitted through sexual abuse of children or through the sexual activity of teenagers.[7] Based on patient age at the time of AIDS diagnosis, the incubation period is a mean of 17 months with a range of 1 to 86 months.[4] The incubation period of AIDS acquired through blood transfusion is significantly shorter for infants (mean = 24.4 months; range 4 to 82 months) than for adults (mean = 5.5 years).[5] As in adult AIDS cases, direct inoculation of the virus is required.

Several large family studies failed to document transmission of HIV to household members through casual contact.[6] Transmission of the virus by means of breast feeding has been documented.[28] A single case of a mother seroconverting while caring for her infant with AIDS has been reported. She had frequent contact with the infant's diarrheal fluids and blood.[23]

■ GROUPS AT RISK

Recipients of Blood Products. The majority of infants who develop AIDS after receiving blood products were born prematurely and had multiple blood transfusions.[4,8] After a diagnosis of post-transfusion AIDS, it is imperative that the blood bank investigate donors and other recipients of blood products from the infected donor. Because most infected donors are asymptomatic at the time of blood donation, they may donate blood several times before symptoms occur. The risk of receiving infected blood is greater in geographic areas with an increased incidence of AIDS. Screening of blood donors by simply obtaining a history of risk factors is unreliable.

Screening for HIV antibody should significantly reduce the risk of transfusion-associated HIV infection. In a study of 67,190 units of donated blood, approximately 2 per 1000 were HIV-positive by ELISA testing and confirmed by Western blot.[9] Rarely, HIV may be transmitted by an HIV antibody-negative donor.[10] The repeated administration of pooled blood products results in the greatest risk of transmitting the virus — over 90 percent of patients with hemophilia A who have been treated with Factor VIII concentrate have antibody to HIV.[11]

Infants of Mothers at Risk.   Maternal transmission of HIV is the primary cause of pediatric AIDS. The results of screening women for antibody to HIV in various geographic areas indicates that 0.5 percent to 20 percent may be positive.[19] High rates of HIV antibody-positivity in adults are reflected in high rates of positivity in infants caused by maternal transfer of antibody (1 out of 61 infants is found positive in New York City).[24] Experience suggests that approximately 30 percent to 50 percent of these infants are expected to be infected with HIV.[4]

Most cases of pediatric AIDS result from transmission by mothers who are IV drug users.[12,13] Other mothers may be the sexual partners of HIV-infected men. Although mothers of infants with AIDS may be entirely asymptomatic, all those reported in one series had immunologic abnormalities at the time of diagnosis, including abnormal helper/suppressor cell ratios and impaired functional T-cell studies.[1] Fathers who are either IV drug users, bisexuals, or hemophiliacs may transmit HIV to their wives, who subsequently infect their infants.

Many children with pediatric AIDS are of Haitian ancestry.[14] Although it is not entirely clear whether identical risk factors exist for the mothers of these infants, recent studies suggest that HIV is acquired through the same mechanisms as in non-Haitian populations. Other studies suggest that children in Africa also have a high incidence of AIDS.[15] Some controversy exists regarding the accuracy of these retrospective antibody studies, which have been performed on serum samples of children and adults. However, there is general agreement that HIV infection is spread by means of heterosexual transmission, unsterilized needles, and contaminated blood products. These factors result in a high incidence of AIDS among children in Africa.

Not all infants exposed to HIV develop AIDS, as illustrated by the observation that one twin may have AIDS while another remains free of infection. In addition, normal infants may be born following an infected sibling. This uninfected child may be followed by other infected sibling(s). Some family studies indicate that only 25 percent of infants born to mothers at risk for AIDS develop AIDS.[6] In the pediatric age group, predisposing factors associated with the development of AIDS include exposure to the virus in utero, prematurity, multiple blood transfusions, and repeated exposure to infected blood products such as infected Factor VIII concentrate.

■ PATHOPHYSIOLOGY

Based on prospective studies, infants at risk for developing AIDS may be both clinically and immunologically normal at birth.[16] The first observed laboratory abnormality is elevated immunoglobulin levels (primarily IgG and IgM). Functional T-cell abnormalities usually develop before the onset of symptoms. Patients may become symptomatic as early as 1 month of age or as late as 5 years of age.[6] In general, patients who develop AIDS after a blood transfusion have a shorter incubation period than those who are exposed from a maternal source.[4] This may be related to the fact that most infants requiring blood transfusions during the neonatal period are premature, critically ill, or both — all of these are factors that result in immunodeficiency.

The severity of the initial manifestations of HIV infection vary considerably. HIV may be isolated from the peripheral blood of infants. Isolation of the virus is an important diagnostic procedure, since the presence of antibody in an infant less than 6 months of age suspected of having AIDS usually represents passive transfer of maternal IgG antibody.

■ CLINICAL MANIFESTATIONS

Many of the clinical manifestations of pediatric AIDS are similar to those of adult AIDS and represent the consequence of an impaired immune system.[6,12,14] Virtually all of the opportunistic infections that have been observed in adult patients have also been described in pediatric patients. Common opportunistic organisms include *Pneumocystis carinii* (over 70 percent of patients), *Mycobacterium avium intracellulare*, candida infection of the mucous membranes, and other bacterial, viral, or protozoal infection associated with acute and chronic diarrhea. In contrast to HIV-infected adults, pediatric patients have a higher incidence of bacterial infections in the form of otitis media, pneumonia, and sepsis. Also distinct from the adult population is recurrent or chronic parotid and salivary gland enlargement, which may be confused with lymphadenopathy.[1]

Additional clinical features include failure to thrive, weight loss, fever, mild to severe developmental delay, and gradual neurologic deterioration.[20] Abnormal physical findings include lymphadenopathy, hepatosplenomegaly, pulmonary abnormalities, ataxia, blindness, loss of motor milestones, loss of intellectual capacity, and eczematoid skin rashes. Kaposi's sarcoma rarely occurs in children with AIDS.[16] Chronic interstitial pneumonia is a frequent finding in both pediatric and adult AIDS patients and may be due to *Pneumocystis carinii*, cytomegalovirus, or Epstein–Barr virus infection. It may have a distinct morphologic characteristic termed lymphoid interstitial pneumonia, which is more commonly found in pediatric AIDS patients and has been associated with Epstein–Barr virus infection.[17]

It is important to recognize that the spectrum of clinical abnormalities in patients with documented HIV infection may range from no abnormalities to multisystem involvement. In a single study, children who were clinically stable maintained a higher level of neutralizing antibody than did those who deteriorated.[21]

■ DIAGNOSIS

The Spectrum of HIV Disease in Pediatric Patients.   HIV-infected adults who present with symptoms of chronic lymphadenopathy, weight loss, and fever but who lack AIDS-defining opportunistic infections, HIV dementia, severe wasting, or malignancies are categorized as having stages of symptomatic HIV disease. Categorizing pediatric patients in this manner is not useful because progression from mild to severe HIV infection is so rapid in infants. By diagnosing pediatric HIV infection early, the physician can initiate prophylactic therapies that may prevent or delay some of the complications of AIDS. As discussed earlier, a diagnosis of AIDS in children can be established on the basis of all three of the following requirements: (1) the presence of a risk factor associated with AIDS, (2) isolation of HIV or detection of antibody to the virus in children over the age of 6 months, and (3) the presence of immuno-deficiency established by laboratory tests.

Clinically asymptomatic infants who meet these criteria should receive regular medical attention as well as prophylactic therapy (see Treatment).

Laboratory Diagnosis.   Like adults with HIV disease, children display many nonspecific laboratory abnormalities. Leukopenia, lymphopenia, thrombocytosis or thrombocytopenia, and anemia may be observed. Most children with AIDS have depressed helper/suppressor cell ratios, although unlike adults, some children may have normal or increased ratios.[1] Most children have elevated immunoglobulin levels; some may have hypogammaglobulinemia.[12] They exhibit abnormal results on functional studies of immunity, including stimulation of peripheral blood lymphocytes by mitogens or antigens. Infants who have not been exposed to appropriate antigens do not exhibit delayed hypersensitivity to skin testing, so such tests are of little value.

The most important tests for HIV infection are those that measure antibody to HIV, those that isolate the virus from peripheral blood or from tissue biopsy, and tests that detect circulating viral antigens.[29] Isolation of HIV is essential in establishing a diagnosis in an infant younger than six months of age, since transmission of maternal HIV antibody to the infant occurs in utero and infants do not produce IgM antibody to HIV. In infants, HIV antibody-positivity as a consequence of passively-acquired maternal antibody may persist for as long as 10 months. Establishing a diagnosis in infants can be difficult because some become antibody-negative even though virus can be cultured from their blood.[33] Intra blood-brain barrier antibody to HIV has been reported. HIV antigen can be detected in the serum of many HIV-infected infants and in the cerebrospinal fluid (CSF) of children with progressive encephalopathy.[34] Potentially the most sensitive assay for detecting HIV is the polymerase chain reaction (PCR) test.[42] The PCR may prove to be the most useful diagnostic test for HIV infection in infants, since it detects HIV nucleic acid and thus cannot be confounded by the presence of maternal HIV antibodies. However, its sensitivity, specificity, and limitations in clinical situations are not yet clearly defined.[43] Currently, establishing actual HIV infection rather than passive transfer of antibody in an infant is best done using one or more of the following tests: culture for HIV, PCR, p24 antigen, and serial antibody evaluation by Western blotting (look for the appearance of new bands which indicate active HIV infection, as opposed to passive transfer of maternal antibodies).

Other abnormalities include circulating immune complexes, abnormal monocyte function, and diminished cytokine production.[30] Cultures, biopsies, or both are need to identify the many microbial agents that may be isolated, including *Pneumocystis carinii* (over 70 percent of patients), cytomegalovirus (30 percent), Epstein–Barr virus (28 percent), and *Streptococcus pneumoniae* (28 percent). Recent reports document an increasing incidence of congenital syphilis.[46]

Studies to exclude congenital immunodeficiency diseases should be performed in all pediatric patients suspected of having immunodeficiency or HIV disease. The most important of these to identify are adenosine deaminase and purine nucleoside phosphorylase enzyme-activity deficiencies, which are associated with combined B- and T-cell immunodeficiencies.[31] After a child has been diagnosed with HIV infection, studies of the parents should be performed to determine if they may be the source of HIV infection.

■ TREATMENT

Once a diagnosis of pediatric HIV infection is made, the child should be thoroughly examined for treatable infections. Cultures of nasopharynx secretions, urine, and stool should be examined for virus, bacteria, and fungus. Because specific antimicrobial agents are now available for treating many infections, aggressive and repeated attempts should be made to isolate these agents in symptomatic individuals. An open-lung biopsy may be necessary to establish the diagnosis of *Pneumocystis carinii*. Unlike internists, many pediatric immunologists recommend treating *Pneumocystis carinii* pneumonia (PCP) with both pentamidine and trimethoprim-sulfamethoxazole. In patients who cannot tolerate trimethoprim-sulfamethoxazole and who are old enough to use a pediatric nebulizer, prophylactic aerosolized pentamidine may be of benefit.[44]

Multicenter, controlled clinical trials are now evaluating zidovudine (AZT) as therapy in infants and children. Preliminary results are encouraging and suggest that infants (including those with encephalopathy) improve clinically with minimal drug toxicity.[45]

A group of 21 children, aged 14 months to 12 years, were treated with continuous intravenous infusion of AZT (in a dose range of 0.5 to 1.8 mg/kg/hr). All children improved neurologically. Immunologic abnormalities diminished and general well-being improved. Anemia requiring transfusion occurred in 52 percent of the patients.[43]

Oral AZT has also been evaluated in pediatric patients, but additional studies are needed to determine optimal doses. Doses ranged from 160 to 180 mg/m every 6 hours.[47] Anemia and neutropenia are the common dose-limiting toxicities that require withdrawal or reduction of AZT treatment.[44] Because AZT is still considered an experimental drug, reimbursement for treatment is not always available. Many states, however, provide payment through their state medical programs.

Prophylactic therapy is an important component of pediatric HIV disease. Children with HIV infection who have impaired T-cell immunity may also have impaired antibody formation. These children may benefit from monthly intravenous gammaglobulin treatment if they have clinically significant, recurrent infections or show evidence of impaired immunity (i.e., abnormal T4/T8 ratios or impaired nitrogen transformation of lymphocytes). The usual dose is 100 to 200 mg/kg each month.[48] For prophylaxis against PCP, trimethoprim and sulfamethoxazole should also be given to patients who can tolerate the drug.[49] As in adult patients with AIDS, approximately 30 percent of children treated with trimethoprim and sulfamethoxazole develop a maculopapular rash, fever, thrombocytopenia, and bone-marrow suppression. Aerosolized pentamidine for prophylaxis against PCP, extensively studied in adults, is currently under evaluation in children.[44]

Chronic infection, poor appetite, and chronic gastrointestinal-tract disease may necessitate nutritional supplementation for children with AIDS.

The emotional difficulties encountered by patients and their families as a result of both illness and treatment are severe. Families may require the support of physicians, nursing staff, social workers, and community organizations. Support for patients and families may also be needed when they attempt to reintegrate a child with HIV infection back into school, playgroups, and other parts of the community.

■ PROGNOSIS

A mortality rate of 65 percent has been reported in children with AIDS who have already developed opportunistic infections. In one study, 68 percent of over 300 children with AIDS have died.[4] The median survival of children with AIDS is 9.4 months following diagnosis. The mortality rate in children under one year of age (80 percent) is significantly higher than among children over one year of age (55 percent).[4]

■ PREVENTION

Blood transfusion-associated HIV infection is best prevented by screening blood donors and blood products with assays for antibody to HIV. Tests may be improved in the future by combining antibody screening with antigen screening. Heating hemophiliac Factor VIII concentrate (50°C for 30 minutes) substantially reduces or eliminates the risk of transmitting HIV.[32] Other blood products can be made safe only by screening donors for HIV infection.

Because the majority of children with AIDS acquire HIV infection from their mothers, public-health efforts should be directed toward modifying the behavior of sexually-active adolescents and adults — specifically, altering sexual lifestyle, reducing the number of sexual partners, and curtailing intravenous drug-use. Birth control and abortion may be important in preventing the birth of additional affected children. However, some studies indicate that 60 percent to 75 percent of infants born to mothers who have already given birth to one affected child were normal.[6] Routine screening of pregnant women and infants in high-risk areas has not been universally recommended. However, the need to prevent new cases of infected infants and the recent availability of treatment for infants provide strong medical and ethical reasons for encouraging screening tests.

■ IMMUNIZATIONS IN HIV-INFECTED CHILDREN

The Immunization Practices Advisory Committee (ACIP) has published vaccination recommendations for HIV-infected persons.[50] The following summarizes the risks and benefits of immunizing HIV-infected children[36,37] and explains the recommendations for MMR vaccine in symptomatic HIV-infected patients:

"Previously published ACIP statements on immunizing HIV-infected children have recommended vaccinating children with asymptomatic HIV infection, but not those with symptomatic infection. After considering reports of severe measles in symptomatic HIV-infected children, and in the absence of reports of serious or unusual adverse effects of measles, mumps, and rubella (MMR) vaccination in limited studies of symptomatic patients, the committee feels that administration of MMR vaccine should be considered for all HIV-infected children, regardless of symptoms. This approach is consistent with the World Health Organization's recommendation for measles vaccination.

"If the decision to vaccinate is made, symptomatic HIV-infected children should receive MMR vaccine at 15 months, the age currently recommended for vaccination of children without HIV infection and for those with asymptomatic HIV infection. When there is an increased risk of exposure to measles, such as during an outbreak, these children should receive vaccine at younger ages. At such times, infants 6 to 11 months of age should receive monovalent measles vaccine and should be revaccinated with MMR at 12 months of age or older. Children 12 to 24 months of age should receive MMR and do not need revaccination. While recommendations for MMR vaccine have changed, those for other vaccines have not. A summary of the current ACIP recommendations for HIV-infected persons follows. These recommendations apply to adolescents and adults with HIV infection as well as to HIV-infected children."

ACIP recently recommended pneumococcal vaccine for asymptomatic as well as symptomatic HIV-infected persons[51] and suggested that influenza vaccine is "not contraindicated" for asymptomatic HIV-infected patients, although it is not formally recommended.[50]

TABLE 2. CDC RECOMMENDATIONS FOR ROUTINE IMMUNIZATION OF HIV-INFECTED CHILDREN — UNITED STATES, 1989

VACCINE	KNOWN HIV INFECTION	
	ASYMPTOMATIC	SYMPTOMATIC
DTP[1]	yes	yes
OPV[2]	no	no
IPV[3]	yes	yes
MMR[4]	yes	yes[5]
HbCV[6]	yes	yes
Pneumococcal[7]	yes	yes
Influenza[8]	no[9]	yes

Reprinted with permission of CDC, MMWR 1989; 38:205.

1. *DTP = diphtheria and tetanus toxoids and pertussis vaccine, adsorbed. DTP may be used up to the seventh birthday.*
2. *OPV = oral, attenuated poliovirus vaccine; contains poliovirus types 1, 2, and 3.*
3. *IPV = inactivated poliovirus vaccine; contains poliovirus types 1, 2, and 3.*
4. *MMR = live measles, mumps, and rubella virus vaccine.*
5. *Should be considered.*
6. *HbCV =* Haemophilus influenzae *type b conjugate vaccine.*
7. *Pneumococcal polysaccharide vaccine.*
8. *Inactivated influenza virus vaccine.*
9. *Not contraindicated.*

Despite the ACIP recommendations, many pediatric immunologists feel that live virus immunizations should not be given to any HIV-infected children. Because pediatric immunization studies are incomplete, the vaccines' safety in children with progressive immunologic and neurologic deterioration cannot yet be determined.[38-41]

REFERENCES

1. Ammann AJ. The acquired immunodeficiency syndrome in infants and children. Ann Intern Med 1985; 103:734-7.

2. Revision of case definition of acquired immunodeficiency syndrome for national reporting — United States. MMWR 1985; 34:373-5.

3. WHO Tech Rep Ser. Immunodeficiency. 1978; 630:28-71.

4. Rogers MF, Thomas PA, Starcher ET, et al. Acquired immunodeficiency syndrome in children: Report of the Centers for Disease Control National Surveillance, 1982 to 1985. Pediatrics 1987; 79:1008-14.

5. Medley GF, Anderson RM, Cox DR, Billard L. Incubation period of AIDS in patients infected via blood transfusion. Nature 1987; 328:719-21.

6. Thomas PA, Jaffe HW, Spira TJ, et al. Unexplained immunodeficiency in children. JAMA 1984; 252:639-44.

7. Rubenstein A, Bernstein L. The epidemiology of pediatric acquired immune deficiency syndrome. Clin Immunol Immunopath 1986; 40:1511-21.

8. Ammann AJ, Cowan MJ, Wara DW, et al. Acquired immunodeficiency in an infant: Possible transmission by means of blood product administration. Lancet 1983; 1:956-8.

9. Ward JW, Grindon HA, Feorino PM, et al. Laboratory and epidemiologic evaluation of an enzyme immunoassay for antibody to HTLV-III. JAMA 1986; 256:357-61.

10. Centers for Disease Control. Transfusion associated human lymphotropic virus type III infection from a seronegative donor — Colorado. MMWR 1986; 35:389-91.

11. Levine PH. The acquired immunodeficiency syndrome in persons with hemophilia. Ann Intern Med 1985; 103:723-6.

12. Rubinstein A, Sicklick M, Gupta A, et al. Acquired immunodeficiency with reversed T4/TB ratios in infants born to promiscuous and drug addicted mothers. JAMA 1983; 249: 2350-6.

13. Oleske J, Minnefor A, Cooper R, et al. Immune deficiency syndrome in children. JAMA 1983; 249:2345-9.

14. Scott GB, Buck BE, Leterman JG, et al. Acquired immunodeficiency syndrome in infants. N Engl J Med 1984; 310:76-81.

15. Clumeck N, Sonnet J, Taelman H, et al. Acquired immunodeficiency syndrome in African patients. N Engl J Med 1984; 310:492-8.

16. Cowan MJ, Hellmann D, Chudwin D, et al. Maternal transmission of acquired immunodeficiency syndrome. Pediatrics 1984; 73:382-6.

17. Joshi VV, Oleske JM, Minnefor AB, et al. Pathology of suspected acquired immunodeficiency in children: A study of eight cases. Pediatr Pathol 1984; 2:71-87.

18. Rubinstein A, Morecki R, Silverman B, et al. Pulmonary disease in children with acquired immune deficiency and AIDS related complex. J Pediatr 1986; 108:498-503.

19. Landesman S, Minkoff H, Holman S, et al. Serosurvey of human immunodeficiency virus infection in parturients. Implications for human immunodeficiency virus testing programs of pregnant women. JAMA 1987; 258:2701-3.

20. Ultmann MH, Diamond GW, Ruff HA, et al. Developmental abnormalities in children with acquired immunodeficiency syndrome (AIDS): A follow-up study. Int J Neurosci 1987; 32:661-6.

21. Robert-Guroff M, Oleske JM, Connor EM, et al. Relationship between HTLV-III neutralizing antibody and clinical status of pediatric acquired immunodeficiency syndrome (AIDS) and AIDS-related complex cases. Pediatr Res 1987; 21:547-50.

22. Centers for Disease Control. HIV/AIDS surveillance report. July 1989; 8.

23. Apparent transmission of human T-lymphotropic virus type III/lymphadenopathy-associated virus from a child to a mother providing health care. MMWR 1986; 35:76-9.

24. New York Times, January 13, 1988; 1,14.

25. Institute of Medicine, National Academy of Sciences. Confronting AIDS: directions of public health, health care, and research. Washington, D.C.: National Academy Press, 1986; 86.

26. Quinn TC, Mann JM, Curran JW, Piot P. AIDS in Africa: an epidemiologic paradigm. Science 1986; 234:955-63.

27. Classification system for human immunodeficiency virus (HIV) in children under 13 years of age. MMWR 1987; 36:225-30,235-6.

28. Ziegler JB, Cooper DA, Johnson RO, Gold J. Postnatal transmission of AIDS-associated retrovirus from mother to infant. Lancet 1985; 1:896-8.

29. Ammann AJ, Kaminsky L, Cowan M, Levy JA. Antibodies to AIDS associated retrovirus distinguish between pediatric primary and acquired immunodeficiency diseases. JAMA 1985; 253:3116-18.

30. Fauci AS, Macher AM, Lono DL, et al. Acquired immunodeficiency syndrome: Epidemiologic, clinical, immunologic, and therapeutic considerations. Ann Intern Med 1984; 100:92-106.

31. Cowan MJ, Ammann AJ. Immunodeficiency syndromes associated with inherited metabolic disorders. Clin Hematol 1981; 10:139-59.

32. Spire B, Dormont D, Barre-Sinoussi F, et al. Inactivation of lymphadenopathy associated virus by heat, gamma rays, and ultraviolet light. Lancet 1985; 1:188-9.

33. Mok JQ, Giaquinto C, De Rossi A, et al. Infants born to mothers seropositive for human immuno-deficiency virus. Preliminary findings from a multicentre European study. Lancet 1987; 1:1164-8.

34. Epstein LG, Goudsmit J, Paul DA, et al. Expression of human immunodeficiency virus in cerebrospinal fluid of children with progressive encephalopathy. Ann Neurol 1987; 21:397-401.

35. Centers for Disease Control. AIDS weekly surveillance report — United States. October 3, 1988.

36. Immunization of children infected with human immunodeficiency virus - supplementary ACIP statement Immunization Practices Advisory Committee. MMWR 1988; 37:181-3.

37. Measles in HIV-infected children, United States. MMWR 1988; 37:183-6.

38. von Reyn CF, Clements CJ, Mann JM. Human immunodeficiency virus infection and routine childhood immunisation. Lancet 1987; 2:699-72.

39. Onorato IM, Orenstein WA. Immunization of HIV-infected children. J Pediatr 1988; 112:333.

40. Borkowsky W. Immunization of HIV-infected children: Reply. J Pediatr 1988; 112:334.

41. Campbell [sic]. Immunisation for the immunosuppressed child. Arch Dis Child 1988; 63:113-4.

42. Ou CY, Kwok S, Mitchell SW, et al. DNA amplification for direct detection of HIV-1 in DNA of peripheral blood mononuclear cells. Science 1988; 239:295-7.

43. Laure F, Courgnaud V, Rouzioux C, et al. Detection of HIV-1 DNA in infants and children by means of the polymerase chain reaction. Lancet 1988; 2:538-40.

44. Montgomery AB, Debs RJ, Luce JM, et al. Aerosolised pentamidine as sole therapy for *Pneumocystis carinii* pneumonia in patients with acquired immunodeficiency syndrome. Lancet 1987; 2:48-3.

45. Pizzo PA, et al. Effect of continuous intravenous infusion of zidovudine (AZT) in children with sympto-matic HIV infection. N Engl J Med 1988; 319:889-96.

46. Syphilis and congenital syphilis — United States, 1985-1988. MMWR 1988; 37:486-9.

47. Blanche S, Caniglia M, Fischer A, et al. Zidovudine therapy in children with acquired immunodeficiency syndrome. Am J Med 1988; 85(2A):203-7.

48. Immunodeficiency disorders: general considerations. In: Stiehn ER, ed. Immunologic disorders in infants and children. Philadelphia: W. B. Saunders, 1989; 157-95.

49. Wolff LJ. Supportive care for children with cancer. Guidelines of the Children's Cancer Study Group. Use of prophylactic antibiotics. Am J Pediatr Hematol Oncol 1984; 6:267-76.

50. ACIP: General recommendations on immunization. MMWR 1989; 38:205-27.

51. Pneumococcal polysaccharide vaccine. MMWR 1989; 38:64-8,73-6.

9

SYSTEMS OF CARE FOR THE AIDS PATIENT

EDITOR

Paul A. Volberding, M.D.

9.1

Comprehensive Systems of Care

Ambulatory, Inpatient, and Community-Based Care: The SFGH Model

Paul A. Volberding, M.D.

A IDS is a complex, multisystem, terminal disease whose victims include such diverse individuals as infants born to intravenous drug users, homosexual men, and heterosexuals who have acquired the disease as a result of blood transfusion. Moreover, people with AIDS can be minimally symptomatic, can be facing rapid mortality from multiple opportunistic infections and malignancies, or can be suffering any of the gradations of disease between these two extremes. A panoply of human resources is involved in patient care: physicians who are specialists in those organ systems the disease affects, nurse specialists in both the inpatient and outpatient setting, psychiatrists and medical social workers, and personnel of many different community organizations. Given that there is no vaccine against the human immunodeficiency virus, no known cure to date, and an epidemic rate that continues to rise, nearly unlimited demands can be placed on health care systems and community organizations where a high concentration of people with AIDS and people at high risk for AIDS are located.

San Francisco is such an area. In 1983, to meet an increasing demand to provide care for these people, a system for the care of patients with AIDS and ARC was initiated at San Francisco General Hospital (SFGH), a large public hospital owned by the City and County of San Francisco and staffed by the University of California, San Francisco. The components of this health-care system are discussed in this chapter and the other chapters of this section.

■ AMBULATORY CARE

The AIDS Clinic. The AIDS Clinic at SFGH includes physicians, nurse practitioners, and an extensive psychosocial, nursing, and research support staff. The Clinic is open Monday through Friday and all categories of patients, from the "worried well" to those who are dying, are seen. Currently, two clinic sessions are devoted to AIDS clinical trials and another to patients with ARC. Several AIDS clinic sessions are jointly staffed by oncologists and infectious-disease specialists. Two separate clinics concentrate on patients whose predominant problem is cancer or infectious disease.

Nurses and nurse practitioners also play an important role in outpatient management and provide comprehensive and efficient care. Nurse practitioners, for example, handle routine patient care under the immediate supervision of physicians and operating within the specifications of clearly defined protocols. All nursing staff provide education and counseling services, often more effectively than physicians.

In addition to physician and nursing staff, the third essential element in the outpatient care of patients with AIDS is psychiatric and psychosocial support staff. Additionally, social-work professionals are available to provide guidance in such important practical areas as housing, financial, and insurance problems. In order that the overall needs of patients be met, the functions of the involved medical providers are carried out in an integrated fashion. To this end, key representatives of the professional staff meet for discussion on a regular basis.

For hospitals dealing with appreciable numbers of patients with HIV-related disease, ambulatory care is most efficiently delivered in a dedicated AIDS clinic setting. The SFGH outpatient AIDS Clinic brings together various medical subspecialists who evaluate and care for patients with the multiple medical problems of AIDS and HIV disease. The clinic setting takes advantage of the expertise of specialists, while facilitating an interchange among them for the benefit of patients.

■ **INPATIENT CARE**

A centralized nursing staff provides sensitive nursing care at the AIDS inpatient unit at SFGH. It is widely perceived as a near-ideal place in which to be treated because of its state-of-the-art medical care and its expert nursing. In this system, patients with AIDS are cared for in a discrete hospital area by nurses and physicians, as well as a psychosocial support staff trained to cope with the various difficulties anticipated in the care of large numbers of hospitalized AIDS patients. One of the advantages of this dedicated AIDS inpatient unit is that discharge of patients can be efficiently planned and can be integrated with services of the outpatient clinic and community agencies.

■ **COMMUNITY-BASED CARE**

Community-based care is broadly defined as care that occurs at the patient's place of residence, which can supplement or replace the need for similar hospital-based services. For the AIDS patient at home, care includes assistance with basic needs such as shopping, cleaning, meal preparation, and maintenance of personal hygiene. In most cases, some of these services can be provided by the patient or by family, friends, and neighbors; but when such personal resources are nonexistent, these needs must be supplied. In addition, AIDS patients at home at some time may require more sophisticated and specialized nursing interventions. Although these interventions may be necessary only sporadically, a registered nurse will be required when they are. As patients with AIDS become progressively more ill, their care often changes to palliative support in anticipation of death, and at this time a hospice-oriented approach is needed.

The contribution of the San Francisco community agencies to fulfilling these various needs cannot be overstated. The Shanti Project, for example, provides trained volunteer counselors for every newly diagnosed patient with AIDS in the city and also has organized an ongoing series of support groups for patients and their friends. Often AIDS patients will need a place of residence, since many lack financial and social support and are unable to secure and maintain an independent living environment. In cooperation with the City and County of San Francisco, Shanti provides housing units at low cost to persons with AIDS who are in need of emergency or long-term housing. Apartment units are occupied by several patients with AIDS, who can often help care for each other, thus decreasing the need for attendant and homemaking services. Also, when nursing services are required, they are often more efficiently used because of small group settings.

The San Francisco AIDS Foundation provides a telephone hotline and physician referral lists. Their medical–social workers provide financial and social assistance to people with AIDS, and the Foundation also operates a free food bank for patients with diagnosed AIDS. Another important function of the AIDS Foundation is professional and public education.

The Hospice of San Francisco and the Visiting Nurse Association cooperate to deliver complete in-home nursing and attendant care for patients with terminal illness. Specific services for AIDS patients have been made available by these agencies.

This system of care may be unique to San Francisco and not all of its elements will be appropriate or available to all communities. Nevertheless, AIDS brings special challenges to health-care systems. If optimal care is to be given to AIDS patients everywhere, these challenges must be met.

Unique Psychosocial Issues in Symptomatic HIV Disease

Donald I. Abrams, M.D.

An extensive array of psychosocial services are available to people diagnosed with AIDS, but fewer community resources are available for people with symptomatic HIV disease that does not fit the Centers for Disease Control (CDC) surveillance case definition of AIDS. This loose aggregate of HIV-related conditions is informally known as ARC (for AIDS-related complex). The lack of resources available for these people is unfortunate for two reasons: (1) many symptomatic HIV-infected persons are too debilitated to be employed but cannot obtain the public benefits offered to persons with AIDS, and (2) HIV-infected persons live under the constant, long-term stress of expecting a diagnosis of AIDS. This chapter describes the services available to people in San Francisco who have HIV-related symptoms but have not been diagnosed as having AIDS.

Recent progression studies suggest that approximately 50 percent of persons infected with HIV will progress to AIDS within nine years. During that time, most will experience some symptoms of progressive immune exhaustion; a smaller subset will become disabled by constitutional symptoms (e.g., marked fevers, night sweats, persistent diarrhea, weight loss, lethargy, impaired mental status). While persons diagnosed with AIDS are eligible for presumptive disability payments (these usually start about three weeks after application), such entitlements are not automatic for persons lacking an AIDS diagnosis. San Francisco's HIV-infected community is replete with stories of people who have died of HIV infection without a formal diagnosis of AIDS and without receiving disability payments. Folk wisdom claims that Social Security Disability offices must receive two applications from people with ARC before they are accepted. Some never are.

The plight of HIV-infected persons with severe but non-AIDS-defining conditions is compounded by the limited psychosocial resources available. Because of the declining pool of volunteers and funds available from San Francisco's AIDS service organizations and charitable foundations, services and donations are usually limited to people with CDC-defined AIDS diagnoses. Thus debilitated persons with HIV disease may fall through the cracks of existing entitlements and services, ending up on General Assistance with no help in obtaining transportation, food, and emotional/practical support.

In addition to the physical decline that marks long-term HIV infection, most patients also suffer from the anxiety of what they often describe as "waiting for the other shoe to fall." Knowing the likelihood that they will deteriorate and eventually be diagnosed with AIDS, they live under the constant stress of being unable to make long-term plans and wondering if each cold or cough might portend an episode of pneumocystis pneumonia. Now that people are being diagnosed as HIV-infected earlier in the course of disease, the duration of suspense, anxiety, and fear they endure is also extended. However, because their condition does not carry a diagnosis of AIDS, they are often ineligible for the psychological support services offered to people with AIDS.

Many initiatives for dealing with the symptomatic HIV-infected person's plight come out of the affected communities themselves. Groups like San Francisco's Project Inform hold orientations on treatment issues and on working cooperatively with physicians. The University of California-San Francisco's AIDS Health Project runs emotional support groups for people with symptomatic HIV disease and their partners/spouses, and the San Francisco AIDS Foundation provides help with disability and insurance claims. Several of the city's drug rehabilitation programs give priority to persons with HIV disease, symptomatic or not.

Finally, community-based groups are being developed in cities throughout the country to conduct clinical trials with protocols that often include persons with non-AIDS-defined HIV disease. San Francisco's County Community Consortium of Bay Area Health Care Providers brings together community physicians who are actively treating HIV disease. The County Community Consortium conducts clinical trials of drugs, including those available under Investigational New Drug protocols. Other community research initiatives, such as New York's, are run by patient groups with physician supervision. These groups may have access to increased numbers of subjects and therefore be able to gather data faster than hospital-based programs, and many HIV-infected people are active in promoting and participating in them.

The CDC has updated its definition of AIDS several times. In its September 1, 1987, update, severe weight loss, which had previously been viewed as symptomatic of only severe but non-AIDS HIV disease, became diagnostic of AIDS if accompanied by laboratory evidence of HIV infection. It is possible that other markers of HIV disease will eventually be incorporated into the case definition of AIDS, thereby relieving some symptomatic patients of the financial and psychosocial burdens of living without an AIDS diagnosis. There has also been discussion of the Social Security Administration's redefining its disability criteria to include persons with symptomatic, non-AIDS HIV infection. Until one or both institutions alters its definition of what constitutes severely debilitating HIV infection, however, people suffering from non-AIDS HIV infection have far fewer resources than those living with a diagnosis.

9.2

Inpatient Care

Surgery in HIV-Infected Patients

C. Daniel Sooy, M.D., and James R. Arden, M.D.

Three major questions should be addressed when considering surgery in the patient with acquired immunodeficiency syndrome (AIDS) or AIDS-related complex (ARC) and in the healthy seropositive carrier.

First, what are the surgical indications in the patient infected with human immunodeficiency virus (HIV) and what operations are being done commonly in HIV-infected patients? The indications for surgery are no different in this population but are based on a morbidity/benefit ratio that is generally altered by a greatly shortened life expectancy.

Second, but foremost for many operating room personnel, what are appropriate infection control measures to protect the operating room staff from acquiring this disease and to prevent the transmission of opportunistic disease to the immunocompromised patient?

Finally, what are the specific preoperative, intraoperative, and postoperative anesthetic and surgical considerations posed by a patient with AIDS?

■ SURGICAL POPULATION

No long-term prospective study of surgery in the patient with AIDS has appeared to date. Reports of the incidence of AIDS in the surgical population have been restricted in the past by the fact that AIDS patients were operated on because they lacked a diagnosis. More recently, heightened awareness of the syndrome and a clearer definition of its clinical course have permitted us to define a group of patients who come to surgery already having the diagnosis of AIDS. Description of this subgroup of AIDS patients is also facilitated by the fact that concentrations of these patients may be found at certain medical centers.

We reviewed the preoperative evaluations of 10,085 patients who had anesthesia and surgery at San Francisco General Hospital during the eighteen months between January 1985 and June 1986 (Arden JR, Sooy CD: unpublished data). Fifty-nine patients with the diagnosis of AIDS were operated on during this period, an incidence of 0.6 percent. However, the ratio of HIV-seropositive persons to those with AIDS in San Francisco was 8.2:1 at that time (San Francisco Department of Public Health), suggesting that almost five percent of surgical patients may have been infected with HIV at the time of surgery. The most frequently performed procedures were the diagnostic biopsy (16 patients) and the surgical drainage of an abscess (15 patients).

The majority of procedures were performed by the General Surgery Service; however, otolaryngology (ENT) was prominent among the specialties. The otolaryngology procedures performed during this period were diagnostic procedures, primarily direct laryngoscopic biopsies (70 percent). Operations performed by the General Surgery Service were mostly limited interventions (e.g., abscess drainage), although several more extensive procedures were performed, including two pericardiectomies. Emergency and elective operations were performed with approximate equal frequency.

■ PRACTICAL CONSIDERATIONS

When an operation is scheduled, it is the responsibility of the surgeon to inform operating room personnel that a patient has AIDS. However, with the broader application of universal precautions this has become less important. Because of the incidence of cytomegalovirus infection among AIDS patients, pregnant operating room personnel do not work with AIDS patients. Information on infection-control guidelines in the operating room is described elsewhere.

The compromised immune response of AIDS patients and the incomplete description of the transmissibility of AIDS lead to the suggestions that the operating room, or a separate part of the recovery area, be used whenever possible for preoperative and postoperative care. At San Francisco General Hospital, patients are brought from their rooms or from the intensive care unit through the usual route by our patient transport personnel.[1] Patients wear masks only if reverse isolation is felt to be necessary or they have microbacterial infections. Because of the potential for infection by transmissible opportunistic agents (e.g., *Pneumocystis carinii*), AIDS patients in the later stages of the disease are taken directly to the operating room rather than to a holding area.

AIDS patients are treated with the same precautions taken for patients with active hepatitis B or cytomegalovirus.[2,3,4] Because all information to date suggests hepatitis is more transmissible than AIDS, the use of hepatitis B precautions provides an additional margin of safety. Operating room personnel who may be exposed to patient blood or oral secretions that may contain blood wear gloves and a mask. Intravenous lines are inserted, blood samples are collected, and surgical specimens are handled using the same precautions. Instruments are cleaned and sterilized in the usual way except for sharps, which should be sterilized before they are cleaned. No specific AIDS sterility procedures are used, since routine precautions are felt to be effective against other viruses, including hepatitis B. Single-use supplies are used whenever possible and are disposed of in carriers used for contaminated materials. To avoid accidental puncture injury, needles are never recapped after use.

Postoperatively, patients are extubated in the operating room. This minimizes contamination with blood-tinged secretions in areas where hepatitis precautions are not followed. AIDS patients are brought to an area reserved for patients with communicable diseases. A nurse is assigned to the AIDS patient and does not care for another patient at the same time. If the nurse must care for more than one patient, he or she must change gloves and wash hands between patients as well as follow strict universal precautions.

■ PATIENT EVALUATION

Most AIDS patients are young and generally healthy prior to the onset of their disease. Pulmonary and hematologic manifestations of AIDS are of particular concern to the surgeon and the anesthesiologist. Opportunistic pulmonary infections such as *Pneumocystis carinii* or *Toxoplasma gondii* are seen in patients with AIDS and can result in significant respiratory compromise. A history or physical examination suggesting infection should be further evaluated by a chest x-ray and an arterial blood-gas study. The physiologic basis of any abnormal findings may be clarified by pulmonary function tests. Leukopenia can have serious implications in the postoperative period, and platelet disorders (idiopathic thrombocytopenic purpura) and other coagulopathies can be seen in AIDS, which may cause additional intraoperative bleeding. Evaluation of coagulation status should be considered in addition to preoperative blood count.

■ SURGICAL CONSIDERATIONS

No additional infection control precautions are necessary, since the routine of the operating room is already geared to appropriate precautions. Specimens and cultures should have the lab slip on the outside and be placed in a resealable bag.

The operative techniques that should be observed include glasses whenever there is drilling, endoscopy, or chance of aerosolization of secretions. The routine of double gloves should be observed to reduce the incidence of skin contamination when a glove is torn. It is important to have only one operator's hands in the field with one sharp instrument at a given time to minimize inadvertent hand injuries and possible transmission. The number of sharp instruments should be minimized and scissors and staplers should be used whenever possible.

The significance of aerosolization in this setting is unknown. Viral DNA has been recovered from laser plumes.[5] Vapors and laser plumes should be evacuated by high-volume suction machines with built-in scrubbers. Some delay in wound healing has also been noted.

■ ANESTHETIC CONSIDERATIONS

No particular anesthetic agents or techniques are indicated for the AIDS patient. A variety of regional and general anesthetics have been used. The pulmonary infections associated with AIDS may, however, indicate the general anesthetic technique that permits delivery of a high-inspired oxygen concentration.

There is no evidence that HIV can be spread by the respiratory route. Saliva and sputum can, however, contain blood, which can transmit the virus. We use a disposable anesthetic circuit with disposable soda lime and a disposable ventilator filter for patients on respiratory precautions. However, in-line filters along with stop cocks are used on all cases. Sterilization procedures used for active hepatitis are sufficient for reusable anesthetic equipment. Anesthetists should wear protective glasses and gloves. Gowns, hoods, or special isolation equipment is of no proven value for routine patient contact.

REFERENCES

1. Arden J. Anesthetic management of patients with AIDS. Anesthesiology 1986; 64(5):660-1.
2. Recommendations for preventing transmission of infection with human T-lymphotropic virus type III/lymphadenopathy-associated virus in the workplace. MMWR 1985; 34(45):681-6, 691-5.
3. Recommendations for preventing transmission of infection with human T-lymphotropic virus type III/lymphadenopathy-associated virus during invasive procedures. MMWR 1986; 35(14):221-3.
4. Update: Universal precautions for the prevention of transmission of human immunodeficiency virus, hepatitis B, and other bloodborne pathogens in health-care settings. MMWR 1988; 37:377-82, 387-8.
5. Garden JM, O'Banion MK, Shelnitz LS, et al. Papillomavirus in the vapor of carbon dioxide laser-treated verrucae. JAMA 1988; 259:1199-202.

Critical Care for Patients with AIDS

Philip C. Hopewell, M.D., and Richard E. Chaisson, M.D.

The complications of AIDS can involve nearly any organ system, often producing severe dysfunction that may be life-threatening or fatal.[1] Thus, patients with AIDS can require intensive care for a variety of reasons.[2,3] Pulmonary involvement with opportunistic infections (most frequently *Pneumocystis carinii* pneumonia) or Kaposi's sarcoma frequently cause respiratory failure of sufficient severity to require endotracheal intubation and mechanical ventilation. Hypotension and systemic hypoperfusion (shock) may result from bacterial infections, usually originating in the lungs with organisms such as *Streptococcus pneumoniae*, *Haemophilus influenzae*, and *Staphylococcus aureus* associated with septicemia.[4] Shock may also occur because of intravascular volume depletion caused by severe diarrhea and adrenal insufficiency most frequently caused by cytomegalovirus infection.[5] Severe central nervous system dysfunction may be manifested by coma, seizures, or both.[6]

In all patients for whom critical care is being considered, the goals of such care must be defined clearly at the outset and be continuously reviewed during the course of the patient's treatment. This is especially true for patients with AIDS, a disorder that to the best of our knowledge is inevitably fatal. This chapter reviews the pathophysiology and management of the processes that may require critical care for patients with AIDS, and in addition discusses the extremely pertinent ethical issues that must be carefully considered in determining the appropriateness of critical care in this group of patients.[7]

■ RESPIRATORY FAILURE

The most frequent cause of respiratory failure in patients with AIDS is *P. carinii* pneumonia.[3] *P. carinii* pneumonia is nearly exclusively an alveolar-filling process. The organism is not invasive and there is little inflammatory response in the lung interstitium. There is, however, damage to the type I pneumocytes and also presumably a loss of functional surfactant.[8] This combination of effects results in airless small alveoli that cannot serve as a gas-exchanging unit and that therefore are sites of intrapulmonary right-to-left shunting of blood. This, in turn, causes arterial hypoxemia and, because of the increased "stiffness" (loss of compliance) of the lung, an increase in the amount of energy (work) required for breathing. This set of pathologic processes, together with the radiologic findings associated with severe *P. carinii* pneumonia, meet the definition of the adult respiratory distress syndrome (ARDS).[9]

Management of this sort of respiratory failure consists initially of providing supplemental oxygen. As the severity of the process increases, endotracheal intubation and mechanical ventilation may be necessary. Ventilation is best accomplished using tidal volumes of 12 to 15 ml/kg of body weight, often with the addition of positive end-expiratory pressure. Both of these maneuvers are designed to reinflate previously airless alveoli and thereby decrease the amount of intrapulmonary shunting of blood. Careful attention must be paid to fluid management to avoid contributing to the alveolar flooding by over-vigorous administration of fluids. As in any intubated patient, other complicating super-infections must be sought and appropriate measures taken for their treatment and prevention. Detailed guidelines for the management of processes that result in ARDS are available from a number of sources.[9-11]

Of the AIDS-related processes requiring critical care, respiratory failure seems to have the greatest mortality rate. Wachter and coworkers[3] reviewed 86 admissions of AIDS patients to an intensive care unit, of which 58 were for treatment of respiratory failure. Of the 54 patients in whom respiratory failure was caused by *P. carinii* pneumonia, 44 (81 percent) died in the hospital. All four other patients who had infections leading to respiratory failure also died, resulting in an overall in hospital mortality of 49 of 54 (90 percent).

■ HYPOTENSION

Hypotension in a patient with AIDS may be the result of hypovolemia, sepsis, hypoadrenalism, or pump failure. Obviously, appropriate management ultimately depends on the underlying cause. At the outset of treatment, however, the cause may not be apparent and an empiric approach may be necessary. Fluids are the mainstay of therapy and are often the definitive treatment for hypovolemia. Hypotension from adrenal insufficiency also will generally respond to fluids, although if hypoadrenalism is strongly suspected, hydrocortisone in "stress" doses of approximately 300 mg should be given.

Sepsis may not be readily apparent in patients with AIDS but should be suspected when hypotension occurs in conjunction with an apparent bacterial pneumonia or other bacterial infection. As noted earlier, there appears to be an increased frequency of serious bacterial pneumonias associated with sepsis in patients with AIDS.[4] The organisms found most frequently have been *S. pneumoniae*, *H. influenzae*, and *S. aureus*, although bacteremia with a number of other organisms has also been reported. Because confirmation of the septic origin of hypotension must always await culture confirmation, the diagnosis is nearly always inferred and empiric treatment begun before an organism is identified. Broad spectrum antimicrobial coverage that would be effective against the organisms mentioned previously, as well as against aerobic gram-negative organisms, should be started as soon as the diagnosis is suspected. In addition to fluids, vasoactive agents, particularly dopamine, may be necessary. Because of the potential for ARDS associated with sepsis, lung function should be monitored carefully in addition to blood pressure and urine output. The basic principles of management of hypotension from sepsis in AIDS patients are not different from those that apply in non-AIDS patients. These are presented in much more detail in a number of references.[12-15]

In the report by Wachter and associates,[3] eight patients were admitted to intensive-care units because of hypotension and six of these (75 percent) died. The etiology of hypotension in these patients was not specified.

Pump failure is a potential, although apparently rare, cause of hypotension in AIDS patients. Pericarditis and pericardial effusion, including cardiac tamponade and marantic endocarditis, have been reported in AIDS patients, as has congestive cardiomyopathy.[16]

■ CENTRAL NERVOUS SYSTEM DISORDERS

Involvement of the central nervous system is common in patients with AIDS and most frequently causes dementia. Seizures, which on occasion progress to status epilepticus, also occur as a result of toxoplasmosis, central nervous system tuberculosis, central nervous system lymphoma, or other less common pathogens.[6] Status epilepticus may necessitate treatment in an intensive care unit if it cannot be controlled. Accurate diagnosis and specific therapy in addition to anticonvulsant medications are essentials of successful treatment.

■ MISCELLANEOUS DISORDERS

Patients with AIDS are subject to the same disorders as patients who do not have AIDS. Thus, the need for intensive care may not be caused by an AIDS-related disorder per se. Asthma, drug overdose, and trauma, to name but a few conditions, may occur in patients who also have AIDS and may be severe enough to necessitate intensive care.

■ ETHICAL CONSIDERATIONS

Many of the disorders for which intensive care is provided routinely have short-term prognoses no better than that of an AIDS patient with respiratory failure. Nevertheless, the long-term outlook is usually considerably different and influences the approach to care. In the face of the universally fatal outcome of AIDS, patients should be counseled as to what they might expect and presented their options in realistic terms. If possible, this should be done before they are severely ill. They should be informed of the outcome of mechanical ventilation and of the discomfort often attendant to critical care. Appropriate intensive care should be provided if the AIDS patient desires it after being presented the facts, and if, in the judgment of the responsible physician, intensive care would not be futile at least in the short run. There are a number of valid reasons why critical care even with a very small chance for survival may be of benefit to the patient as well as to those concerned about him or her. Often affairs need to be put in order, reconciliations effected, or family contacted. Even a few days under some circumstances would have tremendous value.

On the other hand, patients who decline critical care should understand that they will not be abandoned but that all necessary and possible comfort measures will be taken. Care, in fact, may be equally intense but have goals in keeping with the patient's wishes and prognosis.

REFERENCES

1. Chaisson RE, Volberding PA, Sande MA. AIDS. In: Parillo JE, Masur H, eds. The critically ill immunosuppressed patient: diagnosis and management. Bethesda, Md.: Aspen Press (in press).

2. Rosen MJ, Tow TW, Teirstein AS, et al. Diagnosis of pulmonary complications of the acquired immune deficiency syndrome. Thorax 1985; 40:571-5.

3. Wachter RM, Luce JM, Turner J, et al. Intensive care of patients with the acquired immunodeficiency syndrome: outcome and changing patterns of utilization. Am Rev Resp Dis 1986; 134:891-6.

4. Polsky B, Gold JWM, Whimbey E, et al. Bacterial pneumonia in patients with the acquired immunodeficiency syndrome. Ann Intern Med 1986; 104:38-41.

5. Tapper ML, Rotterdam HZ, Lerner CW, et al. Adrenal necrosis in the acquired immunodeficiency syndrome. Ann Intern Med 1984; 100:239-41.

6. Levy RM, Bredesen DE, Rosenblum ML. Neurological manifestations of the acquired immunodeficiency syndrome (AIDS): experience at UCSF and review of the literature. J Neurosurg 1985; 62:75-95.

7. Steinbrook R, Lo B, Tirpack J, et al. Ethical dilemmas in caring for patients with the acquired immuno-deficiency syndrome. Ann Intern Med 1985; 103:787-90.

8. Hughes WT. *Pneumocystis carinii*. In: Mandel GL, Douglas RG, Bennett JE, eds. Principles and practice of infectious diseases. New York: John Wiley, 1978; 1549-52.

9. Fowler AA, Hamman RF, Good JT, et al. Adult respiratory distress syndrome: risk with common predispositions. Ann Intern Med 1983; 98:593-7.

10. Hopewell PC. Critical care medicine. In: Wyngaarden JB, Smith LH Jr, eds. Cecil textbook of medicine. 16th ed. Philadelphia: W.B. Saunders, 1984:467-80.

11. Hurewitz A, Bergofsky EH. Adult respiratory distress syndrome: physiologic basis of treatment. Med Clin North Am 1981; 65:33.

12. Root RK, Sande MA, eds. Contemporary issues in infectious diseases. Vol. 4. Septic shock. New York: Churchill Livingstone, 1985.

13. Dale DC, Petersdorf RG. Gram negative bacteremia and septic shock. In: Petersdorf RG et al., eds. Harrison's principles of internal medicine. 10th ed. New York: McGraw Hill, 1983:859-64.

14. Parker MM, Parillo JE. Septic shock: hemodynamics and pathogenesis. JAMA 1983; 250:3324-7.

15. Sheagren JN. Treatment of bacteremia. West J Med 1986; 144:219-20.

16. Cohen IS, Anderson DW, Virmani R, et al. Congestive cardiomyopathy in association with the acquired immunodeficiency syndrome. N Engl J Med 1986; 315:628.

9.3

Ambulatory Care Nursing Management

9.3.1

Ambulatory Care Nurses: Education, Screening, and Primary Care

Gayling Gee, R.N., M.S.

A mbulatory nursing care for AIDS patients consists of a spectrum of services including AIDS screening, primary care, and community and professional education.

■ SCREENING

The signs of symptomatic HIV disease include such general symptoms as fevers, night sweats, fatigue, weight loss, cough, shortness of breath, and diarrhea. All are as likely to indicate another disease process as they are HIV infection. The human immunodeficiency virus (HIV) antibody test, developed for screening blood products, is also useful for establishing whether a person is infected with the virus. However, antibody testing alone is not diagnostic for AIDS. The diagnosis of AIDS is established by definitive diagnosis of a specific AIDS indicator disease, or by a positive HIV-antibody test or culture in association with a definitively or presumptively diagnosed indicator disease.[1] In most cases, a complete medical evaluation is necessary for diagnosis.

In the absence of a single, simple diagnostic test or predictive indicator of AIDS, screening and case-finding services are required to differentiate between AIDS and non-AIDS-related symptomatology. Public-health or clinic nurses may play an important role in case finding and in counseling clients about HIV antibody test results. Appropriate centers for such screening and educational activities may include venereal disease clinics, public-health centers, clinics, or physician offices. Screening protocols for nurse practitioners and registered nurses can be developed for evaluating patients with suspicious symptoms.

Establishing a screening clinic allows the nurse to triage patients. The nurse can assess referred individuals according to their risk practices and presenting symptoms and determine whether further evaluation is required. Such a system allows the nurse to educate, demystify AIDS, and reassure patients at low risk of HIV infection. At the same time, symptomatic patients can be promptly and appropriately referred to appropriate health-care providers. A nurse screening clinic can also alert members of the community about where to go for evaluation and referral if they believe they may be HIV-infected.

■ PRIMARY CARE

People with HIV infection often experience insidious physical deterioration and require frequent hospitalizations for acute care. Most of them succumb to their infection within a two-year period. Once a patient has been screened or a diagnostic evaluation has been completed, the person with AIDS or symptomatic HIV infection is assigned to a regular medical provider, either a physician or nurse practitioner, in the ambulatory care clinic. Ideally this provider will follow the patient throughout the illness. Nurses in the ambulatory care unit frequently find that the AIDS patient has a complex set of needs.

Nursing in the ambulatory-care clinic involves:

- educating patients;
- administering chemotherapy or investigational drugs;
- coordinating diagnostic workup, tests, and medical referrals;
- assessing the patient's psychological status, providing emotional support and appropriate referrals;
- assessing the patient's nutritional, neurologic, cutaneous, pulmonary, and GI systems, and implementing appropriate interventions.

If the patient is hospitalized, the ambulatory care nurse coordinates care with the inpatient nursing staff.

The nurse is frequently the first professional to come into contact with the HIV-infected patient and may be the person who takes the patient's history and records his or her chief complaints. Clinical evaluation of the HIV-infected person is discussed in another chapter.

■ EDUCATION

Widespread community education is essential to provide accurate, noninflammatory information to the general population. Its goals are to demystify AIDS and to quell hysteria and fear. Nurses play an important role in this effort. When involved in community education, the nurse should tailor discussions to the needs of the audience and include basic information on the viral etiology of AIDS, modes of transmission, physical effects of the disease, and risk-reduction activities. Such sessions can discuss the fear of contagion and can stress that HIV is not casually transmitted.

Appropriate community organizations to be targeted include social and political groups, ethnic and minority agencies, church groups, school programs, private work sites, labor organizations, and governmental agencies. Both pamphlets and videotape presentations are useful educational tools. Discussions after the presentation can elicit and address that group's specific fears or concerns. The nurse should always discuss AIDS in a positive, nonthreatening, nonjudgmental way, since the goal is to educate. Repeated presentations to the same organization should be considered if the group's first reaction is negative and if the group's concerns have not been resolved. An active, coordinated approach to education can help communities develop a rational approach to the problem of AIDS.

Education targeted to gay and bisexual groups and intravenous drug users is best achieved by collaborating with gay community organizations, substance-abuse programs, and halfway houses. Pamphlets, brochures, and posters should be sensitive to the needs of each group and written in that group's own vocabulary.

Professional education for nurses and allied health professionals is critical if quality care is to be provided. Not all nurses are involved in the care of AIDS patients, but every nurse needs to be aware of issues such as the etiology of AIDS, clinical presentation, treatment options, infection-control guidelines, psychosocial implications of HIV infection, and patient education needs.[2-4]

Public-health nurses and nurse-educators can coordinate the development of comprehensive educational programs through community and professional task forces. These programs can provide educational outreach to high-risk groups and to health-care workers. Local AIDS advisory groups or foundations can provide assistance and cooperation in extending the scope of services.

REFERENCES

1. Revision of the CDC surveillance case definition for acquired immunodeficiency syndrome. Council of State and Territorial Epidemiologists; AIDS Program, Centers for Infectious Diseases. MMWR 1987; 36(Suppl 1):1S-15S.
2. Hospitals stepping up effort to protect staff from AIDS. Am J Nurs 1983; 83:1468.
3. Crovella AC. The person behind the disease. Nursing 1985; 15:42.
4. Graf TM. Unmasking AIDS. Home Healthc Nurse 1984; 2:44-7.

Opportunistic Infections: General Nursing Interventions

Gayling Gee, R.N., M.S.

A cquired immunodeficiency syndrome (AIDS) is caused by a viral infection that impairs the cellular immune system and results in a variety of opportunistic infections (OI). These diseases are specific fungal, viral, protozoal, and bacterial infections that are defined by the Centers for Disease Control (CDC).

Management of the chronic, nonacute problems of AIDS-related OIs is appropriately handled in the outpatient setting, including most diagnostic evaluation and follow-up care. Treatment regimens for most of the OIs are, however, most safely and appropriately initiated and administered in the inpatient setting.

The primary indications for hospitalizing a patient with an OI are acute symptoms of the respiratory, neurologic, and gastrointestinal systems, and inclusion in drug-treatment regimens. Respiratory symptoms include progressive, severe shortness of breath, dyspnea, cough, and hypoxemia. Fever and malaise often accompany respiratory symptoms. Neurologic symptoms — seizures, weakness, paralysis, headaches, stiff neck, photophobia, or dramatic changes in mental status or altered consciousness — may strongly indicate a need for hospitalization. Systemic symptoms, including fevers with orthostasis, and gastrointestinal problems, including diarrhea with dehydration, are also reasons for inpatient care. The role of the ambulatory care nurse is to assess the patient for changes in physical status that may indicate the need for either home-care service referral or hospitalization.

■ RESPIRATORY DISTRESS

Acute respiratory symptoms may be due to *Pneumocystis carinii* pneumonia (PCP), cytomegalovirus (CMV), cryptococcus, or Kaposi's sarcoma (KS).

Outpatient nurses should assess the patient's respiratory status, including chest sounds, color, and nail beds. Chest x-rays and blood-gas studies may be obtained. If further testing is indicated, pulmonary-function tests, gallium scan, and sputum induction or bronchoalveolar lavage may be performed on an outpatient basis. Oxygen therapy may be begun in the clinic or at home. If the patient requires transbronchial biopsy, or intravenous drug treatment, or mechanical ventilation, hospitalization is necessary. In some cases (e.g., if the patient is relatively stable and ventilatory support is not required), oral antibiotic treatment may be begun on an outpatient basis. If outpatient care is begun, the patient's respiratory status, medication history, and adverse reactions to medication must be closely monitored.

■ NEUROLOGIC CHANGES

The patient's neurologic changes may be due to cryptococcal meningitis, toxoplasmosis, CMV meningitis, progressive multifocal leukoencephalopathy, or a central nervous system (CNS) lymphoma. Blood cultures, toxoplasma titers, cryptococcal antigen, lumbar punctures, and computed tomographic (CT) or magnetic resonance imaging (MRI) scans may be obtained on an outpatient basis. Treating acute neurologic changes generally requires hospitalization.

The outpatient nurse should assess the patient for headaches, stiff neck, photophobia, aphasia, ataxia, weakness, paralysis, seizures or dramatic changes in mental status or level of consciousness. Efforts should be made to insure an environment in which the patient with a history of seizure activity or vision loss will be safe from falls or injuries. If appropriate, the patient can be hospitalized for appropriate drug therapy and monitoring.

■ DIARRHEA/GASTROINTESTINAL DYSFUNCTION

Chronic, severe diarrhea may be related to cryptosporidium, *Isospora belli*, cytomegalovirus (causing colitis), or *Mycobacterium avium-intracellulare* (causing MAC). Other causes of gastrointestinal dysfunction include candidiasis, herpes simplex, hairy leukoplakia, and Kaposi's sarcoma. The outpatient evaluation of individuals with gastrointestinal symptoms includes: endoscopy, upper gastrointestinal series, stools for ova and parasitology and culture, and proctoscopy/sigmoidoscopy with biopsy. The persistence of diarrhea, dysphagia, anorexia, or vomiting may result in dehydration and orthostatic hypotension. Weight loss, inadequate intake, and malabsorption may also occur. Fluid replacement and antidiarrheals may be initiated in an outpatient setting for symptomatic relief; hospitalization for therapy, bowel rest, and parenteral nutrition may be indicated.

The ambulatory-care nurse should assess the need for antidiarrheal medication, and when one is given, assess its efficacy. The patient's hydration status, nutrition status, fluid and electrolyte balance, weight, and skin integrity should all be monitored frequently. Careful assessment of the oral cavity is also important to detect mucocutaneous lesions such as herpes simplex, candida, hairy leukoplakia, and Kaposi's sarcoma that may affect eating and swallowing. Outpatient treatment for herpes, candidiasis, and KS may be initiated. Hospitalization may be indicated for treatment of severe symptoms or the OI, or both.

■ SYSTEMIC SYMPTOMS

Although HIV (human immunodeficiency virus) infection is the underlying condition, systemic symptoms may arise from the OIs, including *Mycobacterium avium-intracellulare*, cytomegalovirus, toxoplasmosis, PCP, cryptococcus, herpes simplex, progressive multifocal leukoencephalopathy, and *Candida albicans*. These may be signaled by persistent fevers. Mild fevers (<101°F) can be treated with antipyretics or nonsteroidal antiinflammatory agents on an outpatient basis. Severe fevers (>101°F) with toxicity and hypotension, neutropenia with a granulocyte count of <500, or positive cultures require hospitalization for further evaluation, treatment, or both.

Outpatient nurses can monitor temperatures (or ask patients to keep temperature charts) and assess the need for and the effectiveness of antipyretic drugs. Cooling measures, such as tepid baths, alcohol rubs, or ice packs, can be instituted as needed. Fluid intake should be monitored and encouraged. Lovers, family, and friends should be encouraged to help monitor and manage these measures. Blood pressures should be taken regularly in cases of severe fever. If these fevers persist, the outpatient nurse should arrange for medical evaluation and treatment. More detailed information about nursing interventions can be found elsewhere.[1-18]

REFERENCES

1. Ake JM, Perlstein LM. AIDS: impact on neuroscience nursing practice. J Neurosci Nurs 1987; 19:300-4.
2. Carr GS, Gee G. AIDS and AIDS-related conditions: screening for populations at risk. Nurse Pract 1986; 11:25.
3. Beckham MM, Rudy EB. Acquired immunodeficiency syndrome: impact and implication for the neurological system. J Neurosci Nurs 1986; 18:5-10.
4. Crocker KS. AIDS-related GI-dysfunction: rationale for nutrition support. Crit Care Nurse 1988; 8:43-5.
5. Cummings D. Caring for the HIV-infected adult. Nurs Pract 1988; 13:28-47.
6. Gee G, Moran TA, eds. AIDS: concepts in nursing practice. Baltimore: Williams and Wilkins, 1988.
7. Howes AC. Nursing diagnoses and care plans for ambulatory care patients with AIDS. Top Clin Nurs 1984; 6:61-6.
8. LaCamera DJ, Masur H, Henderson DK. Symposium on infections in the compromised host. The acquired immunodeficiency syndrome. Nurs Clin North Am 1985; 20:241-56.
9. Lillard J, Lotspeich P, Gurich J, Hesse J. Acquired immunodeficiency syndrome (AIDS) in home care: maximizing helpfulness and minimizing hysteria. Home Healthc Nurse 1984; 2:11-4, 16.
10. Jordan KS. Assessment of the person with acquired immunodeficiency syndrome in the emergency department. JEN 1987:13:342-5.
11. Lovejoy NC. The pathophysiology of AIDS. Oncol Nurs Forum 1988; 15:563-71.
12. Robinson L. Acquired immunodeficiency syndrome (AIDS) — an update. Crit Care Nurse 1984; 4:75-83.
13. McArthur JH, McArthur JC. Neurological manifestations of acquired immunodeficiency syndrome. J Neurosci Nurs 1986; 18:242-9.
14. Perlstein LM, Ake JM. AIDS: an overview for the neuroscience nurse. J Neurosci Nurs 1987; 19:296-9.
15. Sunder JA. AIDS: a neurological nursing challenge. Top Clin Nurs 1984; 6:67-71.
16. Pheifer WG, Houseman C. Bereavement and AIDS. A framework for intervention. J Psychosoc Nurs Ment Health Serv 1988; 26:21-6.
17. Saunders JM, Buckingham SL. Suicidal AIDS patients: when the depression turns deadly. Nursing 1988; 18:59-64.
18. Schietinger H. AIDS beyond the hospital. 1. A home care plan for AIDS. Am J Nurs 1986; 86:1021-8.

9.4

Hospice Care

Definition and Standards of Hospice Care

Eileen Lemus, M.A.

Hospice in action is an autonomous, centrally administered program that provides palliative and supportive care to meet the special needs arising out of the physical, psychosocial, spiritual, social, and economic stresses that are experienced during the final stages of illness and during bereavement. It is a coordinated program of home and inpatient care in which an interdisciplinary team treats the terminally ill patient with his or her family as a single unit. Although its focus is on home care, inpatient care is provided when home care is not feasible.

Differences in hospice models exist, based upon the function of the settings in which they are established. One model is the autonomous hospice in a freestanding building that offers inpatient care and services to the family. It may coordinate its programs with existing home care programs in the community or expand its own services to include home care. An autonomous hospice home-care program is totally involved with terminal care and does not provide home care to other kinds of patients.

Another model of hospice care is the hospital-based program in which the hospital may have a defined unit for hospice beds. Still another model is the interdisciplinary hospice team, which provides consultation for terminally ill patients on all units in the hospital. Finally, many home health-care agencies include a hospice program to care for terminally ill patients.

■ STANDARDS

The following standards are published by the National Hospice Association:

NHO Standards of a Hospice Program of Care

1. Appropriate therapy is the goal of hospice care.

2. Palliative care is the most appropriate form of care when cure is no longer possible.

3. The goal of palliative care is the prevention of distress from chronic signs and symptoms.

4. Admission to a hospice program of care is dependent on patient and family needs.

5. Hospice care consists of a blending of professional and nonprofessional services.

6. Hospice care considers all aspects of the lives of patients and their families as valid areas of therapeutic concern.

7. Hospice care is respectful of all patient and family belief systems, and will employ resources to meet the personal philosophic, moral, and religious needs of patients and their families.

8. Hospice care provides continuity of care.

9. A hospice care program considers the patient and the family together as the unit of care.

10. The patient's family is considered to be a central part of the hospice care team.

11. Hospice care programs seek to identify, coordinate, and supervise persons who can give care to patients who do not have a family member available to take on the responsibility of giving care.

12. Hospice care for the family continues into the bereavement period.

13. Care is available 24 hours a day, 7 days a week.

14. Hospice care is provided by an interdisciplinary team.

15. Hospice programs will have structured and informal means of providing support to staff.

16. Hospice programs will be in compliance with the Standards of the National Hospice Organization and the applicable laws and regulations governing the organization and delivery of care to patients and families.

17. The services of the hospice program are coordinated under a central administration.

18. The optimal control of distressful symptoms is an essential part of a hospice care program requiring medical, nursing, and other services of the interdisciplinary team.

19. The hospice care team will have:

    a. a medical director on staff

    b. physicians on staff

    c. a working relationship with the physicians.

20. Based on patients' needs and preferences as determining factors in the setting and location for care, a hospice program provides inpatient care and care in the home setting.

21. Education, training, and evaluation of hospice services is an ongoing activity of a hospice care program.

22. Accurate and current records are kept on all patients.

A Multidisciplinary Team Approach to Case Management

Jeannee Parker Martin, R.N., M.P.H.

As the condition of the person with AIDS deteriorates, intensive care provided by a hospice team is necessary in order for the individual to remain at home. Expertise is required by members of a variety of disciplines to maintain the person with AIDS in the familiar surroundings of the home environment. The six components of the multidisciplinary team that are essential to this care are attendants (homemakers, home health aides), nurses, physicians, social workers, therapists, and volunteers.[1] The patient will ultimately decide, however, who will intervene and how frequently home visits will be made. Although frequent visits by members of all disciplines will be likely, respect for the person's individual routines at home is essential for patient comfort and emotional support during the terminal stages of illness.

Attendants. Because the person with AIDS often lives alone, attendant care is critical if the individual is to remain at home. Complicated infections and severe neurologic changes often make it difficult for the person with AIDS to carry out routine tasks. Many persons with AIDS deteriorate to a point of needing assistance not only with personal care but with all activities of daily living. Because they usually are the team members who spend the most time with the patient, attendants often are present when problems arise. The nurse should be easily accessible to guide the attendant as problems develop.

Nurses. As the case manager, the nurse continuously assesses the physical symptoms of the person with AIDS and provides intervention to keep the individual as comfortable as possible. It is important for the nurse to monitor the person with AIDS on a regular basis, since it is impossible to predict either the physical or the neurologic changes that will occur from day to day. The nurse communicates regularly with the primary physician and other team members to update the treatment plan as the patient's status changes. The nurse will play a vital role in educating caregivers in specific procedures that will keep their loved one comfortable. The level of comprehension, interest, and availability of these caregivers should be assessed continuously. Symptom control, medication regimes, and signs of impending death should be discussed as the patient's status changes to help allay anxieties of the caregivers in the home.

Social Workers. Psychosocial issues related to caring for those with AIDS are diverse and complex. These issues include the stresses associated with the diagnosis of AIDS and a terminal illness, the lack of financial resources, and bereavement concerns related to multiple loss. The social worker's response to each of these concerns may vary depending upon the individual's support system, the availability of financial resources, and the patient's willingness to discuss problems. At the minimum, social services should be made available to each person with AIDS, and directions should be given to assist him in completing unfinished business.

Trained Volunteers.   Volunteers are specially selected and extensively trained; they augment staff services. Volunteers provide such vital services as transportation, companionship, respite care, recreational activities, light housekeeping, and, in general, are sensitive to the needs of families in stressful situations. Church groups and other community organizations often have volunteers who, with proper instruction and supervision, can help keep the person with AIDS at home. Regular outreach programs and special educational forums may be necessary to elicit the involvement of new volunteers.

Rehabilitation Therapists.   Physical, speech, and occupational therapists complement the hospice team by providing the patient with strengthening exercises and by altering the physical environment of the debilitated person. Although they are not required for every individual in the program, the rehabilitation therapists often can assist other team members in implementing a simple plan to reduce the patient's discomfort.

Medical Consultants.   A physician consultant is a necessary component of every hospice team. The consultant should participate in weekly patient care conferences and assist in modifying the care plan on an emergency basis. The physician may be a helpful advocate for the home care team as well as an educator of other physicians in the community about hospice care. As a team member, the physician also can provide needed in-service education on medication regimes and treatment decisions.

Although each team member has distinct responsibilities, the entire team should meet regularly to discuss the status and care plan of the patient. This helps to ensure that others, such as clergy, pharmacists, nutrition counselors, and substance abuse specialists are incorporated into the plan of care as new problems requiring different expertise arise.[1]

REFERENCES

1.   Martin J. The AIDS home care and hospice program: a multidisciplinary approach to caring for persons with AIDS. Am J Hospice Care 1986; 3:35-7.

Financial Considerations

Jeannee Parker Martin, R.N., M.P.H.

M ost persons diagnosed with AIDS, in whichever risk group, are in their mid-30s. In fact, the average age for diagnosis is 36. For many, this means:

- An unstable financial situation;
- Loss of insurance due to loss of their job after an extended period off work due to illness;
- Lovers in a similar situation;
- Family members far away and unable or unwilling to help out.[1]

Often, illness leaves a previously independent individual reliant on public welfare systems for financial assistance. For some, this is difficult. For most people who are terminally ill, however, these bureaucratic systems are challenging to understand and impossible to manage. The person with AIDS or ARC may find himself or herself relying upon the social worker for complete assistance with financial matters, such as filling out forms or identifying new resources for assistance with day-to-day concerns.[2]

All avenues for financial assistance must be explored if the person is to return to the familiar surroundings of his or her home environment. There are many resources in every community at the local, state, and federal levels for the care of an ill or disabled person at home. Many of these existing resources may have been overlooked as the home care plan was developed for the terminally ill person with AIDS. The following list of resources may help every home care team to sustain those with AIDS at home. It is important, however, to use this as a partial guide and identify even more alternatives in local communities.

■ RESOURCES FOR FINANCIAL ASSISTANCE

Medicaid/MediCal. Pays for home visits by nurses, social workers, home health aides, therapists, and some medical supplies or equipment as prescribed by a physician. There are strict guidelines for the type of services to be provided and the number of visits by various disciplines; the patient must have need for skilled nursing intervention and must be income-eligible for these services. Some home health agencies will not accept Medicaid patients because of low rates of reimbursement.

Medicare. Pays for home visits similar to those described above. Patient must be over 65 years of age or have a disabling disease for greater than two years to be eligible. Patients with a diagnosis of AIDS or of disabling ARC for longer than two years are eligible. Reimbursement for Medicare services is higher than Medicaid. Some home health agencies will accept Medicare but not Medicaid patients because of reimbursement restrictions.

Department of Social Services In-Home Support Service Program.   Pays for homemaker (chore service worker) to assist with light housework and personal care up to 8 hours per day to a maximum of 56 hours per week. Usually pays minimum wage. Often a family member or friend can be designated to provide this assistance and collect reimbursement directly from DSS. DSS has homemakers available when family/friends are not available. It often takes up to 30 days for DSS to make assessment and authorize services.

American Cancer Society.   Pays for attendant care services for those with cancer diagnoses (e.g., Kaposi's sarcoma; brain lymphoma). Pays up to a maximum dollar amount per week, varying in different communities depending upon local funding. May have attendants available or may supplement income of attendants from home health agencies, or pay directly to family members or friends. ACS often has transportation services available to and from hospital, clinic, or physician's office.

Meals on Wheels.   Provides two meals per day delivered directly to the home for a nominal fee (usually $4.00 to $6.00 for two meals). M.O.W. is only one of many home-delivered meals programs; many churches and other community organizations have similar programs.

Services for the Blind.   Many communities have special programs for the blind; talking books or large-print books are often available for loan. Assistance with improving mobility or reorganizing the house is often available at no charge. Support groups and one-to-one counselors assist friends/family to cope with changes in patient's eyesight.

Attendants and Volunteers.   Explore church or civic groups that may provide companions or aides in the home. Senior volunteer programs may provide a few hours of respite to a caregiver as the patient's condition worsens. A church group may have volunteers who will donate a few hours per week to cook, clean, or run errands (e.g., to pick up medications at the pharmacy; to take the patient to a clinic appointment).

Private Donations.   Many individuals will be able to pay for small amounts, and sometimes all, of their home care service. Often friends can be identified to contribute small (or large) amounts to help offset the cost of care when round-the-clock care becomes necessary. Sliding scale reimbursement charts will assist the home care team in their discussions with private donors and in their explanations regarding costs of services.

Private Insurance.   Some persons with AIDS will have private insurance coverage. These policies have many different options and may be interpreted differently by each individual who reads them. This often leads to ambiguity in what is actually covered and will later be reimbursed. Few policies cover home or hospice care to the extent that it is needed by those with AIDS. However, many insurance providers are interested and willing to waive certain clauses and replace them with new, more cost-effective services. The average cost per patient day for the AIDS Home Care and Hospice Program in San Francisco is less than $100, as compared with an average cost per day of greater than $1000 in Bay Area hospitals. It is not difficult to convince most private insurance company managers that home and hospice care will save them thousands of dollars if they consider exceptions to their client's existing policy.

Other Alternatives.   Foundations may provide small grants to pay for attendant care or supplies. Some service organizations have taken up collections to start emergency funds for those in crisis; these groups may have money to help pay for a new blanket or radio, a few hours per week of attendant care, or perhaps to assist with the rent payments if the patient's cash has run low. Resources for financial aid usually do not advertise their funds. It is left to the social worker to explore all options and to assist the patient in obtaining such assistance. Once established, these new funding sources may assist many others who desire hospice care at home.

REFERENCES

1. Martin J. Sustaining care of persons with AIDS. In: Durham JD, Cohen FL, eds. The person with AIDS: nursing perspectives. New York: Springer, 1987:161-77.
2. Martin J. Caring for the person with AIDS at home. Caring 1986; 5:12-4, 17-20.

Psychosocial and Spiritual Concerns

Jeannee Parker Martin, R.N., M.P.H.

■ PSYCHOSOCIAL CONCERNS

A variety of psychosocial issues relating to the dying AIDS patient have just begun to be addressed in a systematic manner. These issues include, but are not limited to, the community's response to AIDS; the patient's fears of contagion, disfigurement, and death; the fear of social abandonment and guilt about past sexual behaviors; the lack of traditional support systems; the lack of financial resources; bereavement concerns or multiple loss issues; and the staff's own need for emotional support. The magnitude of these concerns in various communities, and the community's ability to identify and then cope with these issues, are influenced by diverse factors.

Three issues will be addressed in this chapter:

- The lack of traditional support systems;
- Bereavement concerns and multiple loss;
- Staff needs for emotional support[1,2]

The Lack of Traditional Support Systems. Although some patients are in living situations in which strong support systems are available to help provide physical care and emotional support at home, most are not. Many patients' lovers have fled because they, too, are afraid of contracting the illness. Family members may be willing to care for the patient, but are often at a distance. This is of particular concern in large urban settings that have attracted members of the various groups at high risk for AIDS because of acceptance by the community or the availability of health care resources for those with AIDS.[3] In moving to a large metropolitan area, people with AIDS may have left behind their closest support networks. Because the support group is either nonexistent or the people in it are unable to help on a regular basis, the person with AIDS or ARC is often left alone in his or her own home.

Most persons with AIDS, like many terminally ill patients, experience severe physical and mental status changes. The complications of such symptoms as weakness, memory loss, confusion, and diarrhea necessitate assistance with all activities of daily living. When friends and family are unavailable, intense 24-hour assistance will be required by attendants (homemakers/home health aides). If such assistance is not available, it is important to explore alternatives to home care such as residential care facilities, skilled nursing facilities, or rehospitalization.

Bereavement Concerns and Multiple Loss. Never before in hospice care have we dealt with an illness that affects the lives of so many people. Some persons with AIDS have many friends who also have a diagnosis of or who have died from AIDS. They may know twenty or more people who are also trying to cope with the diagnosis of a terminal illness, the issues of death and dying, and the grief for others who have died from AIDS. It is difficult for the most sophisticated psychotherapist to assist a patient in coping with the issues related to just one death. How then, can the person with AIDS be expected to cope with multiple loss and bereavement related to his or her own diagnosis?

It is essential to have social workers and bereavement counselors who are experienced in dealing with the issues of death and dying. Social workers and bereavement counselors may offer one-to-one support to the person with AIDS, the friends, or the family. A grief support group may be helpful for the bereaved and provide a safe place for them to discuss their own fears and concerns about the death of a loved one. A bereavement social (e.g., a potluck dinner) may also aid the survivor by providing a social atmosphere to get acquainted with others in a similar situation.

When social workers or bereavement counselors are not immediately available to provide assistance, it is important to explore other alternatives in the community. A local hospice organization may have counselors (often volunteers) who can provide direct assistance to the person with AIDS, or who can provide training and education to others to provide this support. Church groups often have volunteers who are available to provide emotional support and counseling to members of their community. Other organizations, such as gay and lesbian groups, may be willing to provide counselors knowledgeable in the areas of death and dying, or to provide financial assistance for bereavement training and education of counselors.

Staff Needs for Emotional Support.   Members of the multidisciplinary team also require special support. They often become surrogate family members when relatives and friends are unavailable on a regular basis. Besides traditional hospice care, staff members and volunteers may be relied upon for more routine tasks that family members could otherwise provide. Team members also may experience emotions similar to that of the person with AIDS, such as anger, frustration, fear of contagion, and of death or dying. All of these needs must be addressed through staff support groups, team conferences, time off, and adequate and effective supervision.[1,3]

■ SPIRITUAL CONCERNS

Hospice philosophy supports the individual's right to seek guidance or comfort in the spiritual practices most suited to that person. Many persons with AIDS explore alternatives to traditional western religions or spiritual practices. It is not uncommon to care for individuals whose spiritual beliefs are based upon eastern cultures or religions. Others will find solace in the support provided by therapists, masseurs, or other less traditional sources.

The hospice team assists the individual in obtaining the necessary spiritual guidance directly through available staff members or identified members of the community. Hospice programs or home health agencies often maintain lists of clergy and other spiritual leaders in the community who are experienced in the issues of death and dying.

When Home-Hospice Care Is No Longer Appropriate.   During terminal stages of the person's illness, sensitive hospice care will be essential. Complicated physical problems, multiple psychosocial concerns, and intense spiritual needs can be met by the multidisciplinary team. For some persons with AIDS, however, these needs will be greater than can be cared for at home. Skilled nursing intervention may be necessary around the clock as physical symptoms and neurologic complications increase. The most skilled home care team may be unable to provide care 24 hours per day because of reimbursement restrictions or staffing limitations. Alternatives must be addressed if the person's needs are greater than the team can manage at home. Hospice care can be continued in hospitals, nursing homes, residential care facilities, and inpatient hospice units when home care is no longer appropriate. Although these options are not available for persons with AIDS in many areas around the country, it is important to explore existing models for long-term care in the community. It is necessary to approach health-care leaders and local politicians to lend their support for appropriate and sensitive terminal care to those with AIDS in the community. In this manner, persons diagnosed with AIDS have access to humane treatment and support during all phases of their illness.

REFERENCES

1. Martin J. Sustaining care of persons with AIDS. In: Durham JD, Cohen FL, eds. The person with AIDS: nursing perspectives. New York: Springer, 1987:161-77.
2. O'Neil M. Effective discharge planning for AIDS patients. Coordinator 1985:42-5.
3. Martin J. Caring for the person with AIDS at home. Caring 1986; 5:12-4, 17-20.

Infection-Control Precautions for the Caregiver

Jeannee Parker Martin, R.N., M.P.H.

Precautions for blocking transmission of human immunodeficiency virus (HIV) in the home environment include measures to prevent entry of the virus into the body, as well as disposal or disinfection of substances that may be contaminated with the virus.[1] If the person with AIDS is dependent and unable to manage his or her own secretions and excretions, the caregiver should take certain precautions.[2]

Hand Washing. Thorough hand washing with soap and water is essential in controlling the spread of many infectious organisms. Soap should be available at all times. Hand washing should occur before and after patient care, after contact with contaminated items, and when preparing or eating food. Adequate education of all caregivers in the proper hand washing techniques should be incorporated into the care plan.

Gloves. Intact skin is the body's natural barrier to infectious agents. Gloves provide an additional barrier, especially in the presence of open skin areas, and should be worn in the following situations:

- When handling secretions and excretions;
- When the patient has rectal or genital lesions;
- When the patient has been incontinent or has vomited;
- When handling soiled diapers, linen, or clothing.

Gloves should be worn during contact with blood, which may occur during wound, nose, or mouth care, during phlebotomy, or when caring for a woman during normal menstrual or postpartum bleeding. Hands should be washed after removing gloves. Gloves are not needed for general care or during casual contact, such as bathing of intact skin, assisting with ambulation, or feeding the person with AIDS.

In the absence of running water, gloves should be worn in preference to washing the hands with antiseptic foams alone, since these do not kill or eliminate all infectious organisms.

Soiling. Household detergents can be used to thoroughly clean floors, furniture, and items that do not come into direct contact with mucous membranes or internal organs of the body. Where soiling occurs, hot soapy water should be used to remove excretions before disinfection. A solution of 1 part household bleach (5.25 percent sodium hypochlorite) to 10 parts water will kill HIV and other organisms. This solution can be used to disinfect counters, toilet bowls, or floors. Because applying bleach directly to soiled areas can cause the release of noxious fumes, it is important to clean the area before disinfecting with the bleach solution.

Bedpans and commodes should be cleaned on a regular basis. If only one patient is using the bedpan or commode, cleaning on a regular basis with household detergent is sufficient. If the bedpan or commode is shared, special disinfection precautions are unnecessary unless diarrhea, herpes lesions, or incontinence are present. Then, cleaning and disinfecting with bleach should occur after each use.

If large amounts of soiling are expected, the caregiver may feel most comfortable wearing a smock or protective clothing to keep a uniform clean. However, this is not necessary in order to prevent disease transmission when working in the home of a person with AIDS. If soiling occurs, regular laundering is adequate to clean the caregiver's clothes. One cup of bleach can be added to hot soapy water in the washing machine to disinfect soiled linens.

Sharps.   Sharps should be handled with particular care. Needles should not be recapped or broken because most needlesticks occur when the needle is being resheathed. Needles and other sharp items should be placed in puncture-resistant containers. If laboratory specimens are drawn at home, the samples should be transported to the laboratory in a resealable plastic bag or other container to avoid spills.

Disposal.   Disposable items such as gloves, diapers, underpads, tissues, paper towels, and dressings should be put in a heavy-duty plastic bag, tied shut, then placed in a second plastic bag before discarding. Needles and other sharp items should be placed into puncture-resistant containers. Removal of these items should be in a manner consistent with local regulations for solid waste removal.[2] The normal trash pick-up by the city or county is generally an appropriate and adequate disposal mechanism.

REFERENCES

1. Lusby G, Martin J, Schietinger H. Infection control at home. Am J Hospice Care 1986; 3:24-7.
2. Centers for Disease Control. Recommendations for preventing transmission of infection with HTLV-III/LAV in the workplace. MMWR 1985; 34:681-95.

9.5

Community-Based Psychosocial Support

Community Support Services for HIV-Infected Persons in San Francisco

J.Z. Grover, Ph.D.

E ach community's epidemic of HIV disease differs epidemiologically and institutionally from other communities' epidemics. If there is any general lesson to be learned from San Francisco's experience, it is this. Because of the magnitude of San Francisco's AIDS epidemic, the city responded early with both city- and county-funded programs and coordinated the development of non-government organizations (NGOs). These complement already existing social services and NGOs (for example, the American Cancer Society and the Visiting Nurses Association), many of which extend their aid to people with HIV disease. Communities need to assess the epidemiologic profile of their own epidemic and the levels of existing government and NGO services that may be of use to persons with AIDS (PWAs) and HIV disease and provide support (funds, personnel, etc.) for the development of appropriate new services.

The city and county of San Francisco offer a distinctive model of care for persons with HIV infection. This system stresses integration of care across the spectrum of a patient's medical, housing, legal, and other needs for the duration of his or her lifetime. This chapter discusses those non-medical resources that are made available to all people with HIV infection/AIDS within the city and county of San Francisco. Most of them are available free of charge to people with an AIDS/ARC diagnosis, and some to anyone with HIV infection. Most of the services are city- and county-supported, although some are provided by voluntary organizations receiving no tax support. All of them are designed to help persons with AIDS and other symptomatic HIV-infected individuals remain ambulatory and independent as long as possible.

By the time this chapter is published, new AIDS-related organizations will have identified needed services and begun offering them. Although the majority of San Francisco's community-based AIDS organizations are not coordinated, the bulk of actual services are offered by a few large organizations whose services do not overlap significantly. This is the result of early planning in the HIV epidemic by the private (San Francisco AIDS Foundation, Shanti Project, Hospice of San Francisco) and the public (City and County of San Francisco) sectors to ensure that important services would not be needlessly duplicated.

As the demographic profile of the epidemic has changed, duplications in services, but not in primary clientele, have occurred. Up until 1987, approximately 97 percent of San Francisco's AIDS cases were among gay men, 86 percent of them white.[1] HIV infection and AIDS are now spreading fastest among intravenous drug users (IVDUs) and their sexual partners; in contrast, newly reported cases of HIV infection among gay white men have slowed down significantly.[2] With the increase in HIV infection among IVDUs and their sexual contacts, the need for basic services associated with poverty (shelter, emergency funds, childcare, food) becomes even greater. Community-based AIDS services will continue to proliferate as long as the demographics of the HIV epidemic shift in the direction of populations previously not targeted by the older, predominantly gay and white, AIDS organizations.

■ COUNSELING SERVICES

Counseling services for people with HIV infection, their families, and their friends are available from a variety of organizations.

The University of California San Francisco's AIDS Health Project provides pre- and post-HIV-antibody test counseling and referral for all persons seeking testing through the city and county's anonymous test sites. In addition, the Project conducts free support groups for PWAs, those with symptomatic and asymptomatic HIV infection. It also provides support groups for women affected by the epidemic (i.e., family members, care providers). Free one-hour consultations are available for couples if one or both members are infected. Stress-management groups for persons with symptomatic HIV infection and couples groups for PWAs and their partners are available free (or at low cost) to San Francisco residents.

The Shanti Project provides free peer counseling for San Francisco residents with AIDS and their families or lovers. The voluntary agency, funded by city, county, and private contributions, offers one-to-one emotional support and support groups for PWAs, their lovers and families, health-care providers, and Shanti volunteers. The services are free.

■ EMERGENCY FUNDS

Several privately administered funds are available to pay for PWAs' utility bills, food, housing, and other expenses. Catholic Charities/Archdiocese of San Francisco offers case-by-case payment for unexpected medical expenses; the AIDS Emergency Fund provides funds for other emergency needs.

Food.   A number of privately and publicly funded services make food and meals available at low or no cost to San Francisco's residents with HIV infection.

The American Cancer Society offers free supplies of Ensure (a nutritional supplement) to patients with a diagnosis of Kaposi's sarcoma or AIDS-related lymphoma. Open Hand delivers a low-cost ($4.25/day), nutritious lunch and dinner seven days a week to PWAs and persons with symptomatic HIV disease. The San Francisco AIDS Foundation operates a food bank from which PWAs can select a free bag of groceries each week. The donated items include canned goods, nutritional supplements, juices, toiletries, and pet foods. The Salvation Army makes both food and food vouchers available to PWAs on a case-by-case basis. In addition, four privately run soup kitchens in the city provide free hot meals to a variety of clients, including women and children.

Housing.   Low-cost housing and free housing referrals are available to San Francisco residents with AIDS or other debilitating HIV disease.

The Housing Hotline (which also serves other city and county residents) provides hotel placement for the homeless. Independent Housing Services assists clients in applying for Section 8 (subsidized) housing for the disabled. The San Francisco AIDS Foundation Emergency Housing Program runs a short-term, rent-free shelter program; Catholic Charities' AIDS/ARC Residential Program provides hotel placement for homeless people with AIDS/ARC. Non-AIDS emergency housing is also provided to people with AIDS and ARC through the Episcopal Sanctuary.

People with substance-abuse problems are ineligible for some of the housing options offered in the city, but Baker Place and New Place, both gay/lesbian residential treatment programs, are open to persons with HIV infection, symptomatic or not, who are also being treated for addictions.

The Shanti Project runs a city-funded housing program for people with CDC-defined AIDS. Residents are placed in low-cost permanent housing maintained by the project. Finally, Family Link provides low-cost apartment accommodations for out-of-town families visiting city residents with AIDS.

Funeral Services. The not-for-profit Neptune Society provides low-cost cremation and burial services for citizens of the Bay Area. The School of Mortuary Science provides cremation for indigent citizens. There are also four privately run, low-cost funeral/cremation/burial services in the city, all of which provide services for PWAs.

Home Care. Free homemaker services are available to PWAs through the Shanti Project, Most Holy Redeemer Support Group, and Hospice of San Francisco. Volunteers from these projects cook, clean, shop, launder, and perform other household tasks for PWAs.

Attendant care is available for indigent and homebound patients through the American Cancer Society (if a person has a KS or lymphoma diagnosis), Visiting Nurses Association (VNA)/Hospice of San Francisco, and San Francisco Department of Social Services. Medical equipment such as beds, oxygen equipment, etc. can be rented through the Cancer Society and VNA/Hospice of San Francisco.

Insurance-Benefits Counseling. The San Francisco AIDS Foundation offers persons with symptomatic HIV infection free counseling on employee benefits, health insurance, state and federal disability programs, and other entitlements.

Legal Services. Free legal advice and advocacy is available to people with symptomatic HIV infection through the AIDS Legal Referral Panel of the Bay Area Lawyers for Individual Freedom (BALIF). BALIF will also write simple wills and powers of attorney free of charge for PWAs. The Employment Law Center offers free assistance to persons with HIV infection who face employment and insurance discrimination, while the city of San Francisco's Human Rights Commission processes complaints filed under the city's AIDS Discrimination Ordinance. The National Gay Rights Advocates (NGRA) is a public-interest law group handling discrimination cases on a no-fee basis for people with HIV infection.

■ MULTICULTURAL AIDS SERVICES

According to the World Health Organization, San Francisco has the world's most ethnically diverse and integrated population. Because of this diversity, AIDS outreach must be tailored to communities with different cultures and languages. The large, predominantly white San Francisco AIDS Foundation provides interpreting services and AIDS prevention/education programs to

Asian, American Indian, black, Chicano, Latino, and Pacific Islander communities. Individual cultural groups provide a wider variety of services to their own constituencies: the Asian AIDS Project; the Bay View–Hunters' Point Foundation Multicultural Alliance for the Prevention of AIDS; the Black Coalition on AIDS; the Gay American Indians' AIDS Outreach Program; Instituto Familial de la Raza's Latino AIDS Project; the Kapuna West Inner City Child/ Family AIDS Network; the Mid-City Consortium on AIDS; and the Westside AIDS/ARC Project. Services provided by these agencies include prevention/ education programs, support groups, and individual counseling.

■ SOCIAL SERVICES

In addition to services provided by the City and County Department of Social Services, free social services for persons with HIV infection are available through the SF AIDS Foundation. These include financial counseling and assistance, medical and social case management, information and referral, client advocacy, and discounts on goods and services (e.g., vitamins, nutritional supplements, massage, acupuncture, psychotherapy).

■ TRANSPORTATION

Free transportation to medical appointments is available for PWAs (both ambulatory and nonambulatory) from the Shanti Project. Discounted taxivouchers and Municipal Railway monthly passes are also available to people disabled by HIV infection.

■ WOMEN'S SERVICES

Help with AFDC (Aid to Families with Dependent Children), housing, child welfare, legal and medical assistance, and family counseling are available to women with HIV infection through the San Francisco AIDS Foundation. The UCSF AIDS Health Project provides counseling and support groups for women with HIV disease as well as for their partners. The Bay View–Hunters' Point Foundation also provides counseling and support services. COYOTE and the California Prostitutes' Education Project (CAL-PEP), activist prostitutes' groups, offer AIDS education and support to women in the sex industry. Project AWARE (San Francisco General Hospital) conducts anonymous HIV antibody testing of sexually active San Francisco women, monitors their health, and provides preventive education and referral.

The Women's AIDS Network, a membership group of women health-care workers and health activists, conducts support and education workshops for women and participates in community AIDS-prevention programs.

REFERENCES

1. San Francisco City & County Department of Public Health. AIDS reported cases from 7/81 to 2/28/87.
2. Natural history of HIV infection: San Francisco City Clinic Cohort. San Francisco Epidemiologic Bulletin. 1988:4.

HEALTH
POLICY
ISSUES
RELATED
TO
AIDS

EDITORS

Merle A. Sande, M.D., and J. Louise Gerberding, M.D.

10.1

Economic, Legal, and Political Issues

The Economics of AIDS

Peter S. Arno, Ph.D., and Jesse Green, Ph.D.

The economic aspects of illnesses are generally analyzed in terms of direct and indirect costs. Direct costs encompass personal medical care and non-personal costs. Personal medical care costs include expenditures for hospital services, physician inpatient and outpatient services, drugs, outpatient ancillary services, nursing home, hospice, and home health care. These costs are generally high if hospital and nursing home care predominate in the provision of care. Nonpersonal costs associated with AIDS include funds for research, blood, health education, and support services.

Indirect costs reflect the economic loss to society and are usually measured by lost wages due to morbidity and premature mortality. These costs are high if illness and death occur among young men and women in the peak of their earning power and their ability to contribute to society.

The economic and social costs of HIV disease and AIDS are far-reaching. They involve the people stricken with the disease, their friends and families, the hospitals and physicians providing their care, their employers, private insurance companies, and finally, the local, state, and federal governments.

■ LIFETIME DIRECT COST OF AIDS CARE

AIDS is an expensive illness requiring care at several levels, ranging from intensive inpatient care to home care. From diagnosis to death, the median survival period is estimated to be about one year[1] and may be increasing. During that period, the average patient incurs medical costs that most analysts place between $40,000 and $60,000 (see Table 1). The early impression that AIDS care costs much more than this was created by a Centers for Disease Control (CDC) study[2] that overestimated the cost at $147,000 per case.[3]

A study at San Francisco General Hospital (SFGH) found a much lower lifetime cost of $27,571, which the authors adjusted upward to $41,499 to take account of the short survival time of the patients sampled. More recent studies have estimated lifetime costs that are roughly comparable to those at SFGH (see Table 1.) Many of these studies suffer from methodological limitations, including small sample sizes and lack of generalizability. These drawbacks eventually led the National Center for Health Services Research to commission a large multicity cost of AIDS study that will follow hundreds of patients prospectively. The results of that study, however, will not be available for several years. For policy purposes in the interim, and for projecting future costs, figures in the mid-range of our table have recently been used. For example, Hellinger[4] used a figure of $60,000 to project 1992 costs based on $50,000 for acute care, $5,000 for other care costs, and $5,000 for zidovudine (AZT). Bloom and Carliner used $80,000 as the likely maximum lifetime cost for AIDS care.[5] Joel Hay[24] used a figure of $60,000 to estimate the cost of AIDS in 1987 but projected that these costs would decline to $35,000 by 1991

TABLE 1. LIFETIME DIRECT MEDICAL COSTS OF AIDS

STUDY	LIFETIME COST	CHARGES/ COST	COST IN 1987 DOLLARS
Kaplowitz[8]	$27,264	Charges	$27,264
Hiatt[9]	$35,054	Cost	$35,054
Drucker[10]	$41,484	Charges	$44,222
Eisenhandler[11]	$40,560	Charges	$49,407
Seage[12]	$42,517	Cost	$51,791
Scitovsky[13]	$47,499	Charges	$57,859
Kizer[14]	$57,000	Charges	$60,762
Thomas[15]	$55,655	Charges	$63,896

as less resource-intensive care becomes more widely accepted. Some very sketchy evidence of declining costs between 1985 and 1987 have been reported.[6,7]

Most of these personal medical costs are incurred when AIDS patients are hospitalized. Even low estimates of lifetime hospital use by persons with AIDS (PWAs) involve three to four weeks of inpatient care; higher estimates have ranged to eight weeks. Some of this inpatient care is not medically necessary but occurs because of limited care and housing options outside the hospital, but the exact amount of such unnecessary hospital care has not been quantified.

There is some limited evidence that the cost of AIDS varies by geographic area within the United States,[16] but these comparisons are not conclusive because they do not control for case-mix. The widespread impression that the cost of providing care to intravenous drug users (IVDUs) with AIDS is higher than for gay men has not been borne out in the few studies that addressed this issue.[15] The only factor that has been fairly well established as affecting AIDS costs is the specific diagnosis (e.g., *Pneumocystis carinii* pneumonia costs more to treat than Kaposi's sarcoma). Some reports have indicated that pediatric AIDS care is very expensive because of long hospital stays.[17] This seems to be true of infants but not of older children.[18]

As Fox has noted,[19] contrary to early reports, AIDS is not more expensive than many other life-threatening chronic illnesses, but AIDS's cost pattern is quite different because it is compressed into a relatively short time period and affects mainly young persons. Also, the total direct cost of AIDS is not only a function of the per-case cost but of the number of cases, which has been growing rapidly each year since the epidemic began.

■ TOTAL DIRECT COST OF AIDS: CURRENT AND FUTURE

In January 1986, Hardy et al. estimated the total lifetime cost of the first 10,000 cases of AIDS at $1.47 billion, but as noted above, this was an overestimate. In early 1989, the 100,000th case of AIDS was reported to the CDC and we can now estimate that the total lifetime costs of these 100,000 cases (using Hellinger's figure of $60,000 per case) will be approximately $6 billion.

For any given year, the total direct costs are usually measured by the cost of care delivered during that year (prevalence-based costs) rather than the total lifetime costs of cases diagnosed that year (incidence-based costs). For example, in 1986, the prevalence of AIDS was estimated by the CDC at 31,080 and was projected to grow to 174,000 in 1991.[20] To arrive at a total cost within a given year, AIDS prevalence must be multiplied by the average annual cost of care for PWAs living any part of that year. On such a basis, Green et al. estimated that annual AIDS-related hospital costs in 1986 were approximately $0.6 billion and would grow to $3.5 billion by 1991 (1985 dollars).[21] Scitovsky and Rice's estimates, which included outpatient costs, were $1.1 billion for 1986. Their 1991 projection, in 1991 dollars, is $8.5 billion.[25] These estimates constitute the mid-range of available studies.

A few estimates were much higher. Pascal's[22] intermediate range estimate was $37.6 billion for the lifetime costs (incidence-based) of all cases diagnosed between 1986 and 1991, but both his lifetime cost figure ($94,000) and his case projection (400,000) seem high. Some other extremely high projections for the year 1991 have been made — $40 billion according to insurance industry representatives, who may have been relying on Pascal.[23] Some recent estimates have been considerably lower than earlier projections. Hellinger's 1991 national projection is $4.5 billion (in 1991 dollars) for cases that meet the pre-1987 CDC definition of AIDS, compared with Scitovsky and Rice's $8.5 billion estimate for that year. Even Hellinger's projection of $6 billion, which includes the new case definition, is lower than the frequently cited $8.5 billion figure. A study by Hay et al.[24] recently projected total costs of only $2.2 billion for 1991 (in 1987 dollars). Hay's low estimate is due to small caseload projections and low annual treatment costs ($35,000 per case) and is based on a medical-decision algorithm.

TABLE 2. TOTAL ANNUAL DIRECT MEDICAL COSTS OF AIDS, UNITED STATES (BILLIONS OF DOLLARS)

AUTHOR	YEAR	TOTAL COST	TYPE OF $	ADJUSTED TO 1987 DOLLARS
Green[21]	1986	$0.6	1985	$0.7
Scitovsky[25]	1986	$1.1	1986	$1.2
Hay[24]	1987	$1.5	1987	$1.5
Hellinger[4]	1988	$2.6	1988	$2.4

TABLE 3. PROJECTIONS OF DIRECT MEDICAL CARE COSTS OF AIDS IN THE UNITED STATES, 1991 (BILLIONS OF DOLLARS)

AUTHOR	YEAR	TOTAL COST	TYPE OF $	ADJUSTED TO 1991 DOLLARS
Hay[24]	1991	$2.2	1987	$2.8
Green[21]	1991	$3.5	1985	$5.2
Hellinger[4]	1991	$6.0	1988	$7.2
Scitovsky[25]	1991	$5.5	1984	$8.5

■ INDIRECT COSTS

In order to calculate the indirect costs of AIDS to society, the total number of cases, morbidity and disability due to the disease, and number of resulting deaths must be calculated. It is the number of premature deaths (shorter average life-expectancy) that is the most significant factor in the total indirect costs of AIDS.

Often the figures reflecting the direct costs of illness are the only ones used by hospital administrators, insurance companies, and government officials. However, when large numbers of productive members of society become ill and die, especially its relatively youthful members, society is deprived of the contribution of these people and the indirect costs are high. According to the CDC, 90 percent of all persons with AIDS in the United States are between the ages of 20 and 49.

The indirect costs of an illness are most commonly measured by placing a monetary value on the wages lost due to disability and premature death.[26] The first attempt to calculate the indirect economic costs of AIDS was made by Hardy et al. in 1986.[2] For the first 10,000 cases in the United States, these investigators estimated that 8387 years of work were lost at a cost of $189 million because of disability. An estimated $4.6 billion in future earnings were lost due to premature death. A more comprehensive study with varying assumptions about disease prevalence estimates the total indirect costs for 1986 and 1991 (see Table 4).

TABLE 4. PREVALENCE OF AIDS CASES AND INDIRECT ECONOMIC COSTS: 1986 AND 1991 (IN MILLIONS OF DOLLARS)*

YEAR	PREVALENCE OF AIDS CASES	TOTAL COSTS	MORBIDITY COSTS	MORTALITY COSTS†
1986	31,440	$7,012	$456	$6,556
1991	172,800	$55,595	$3,315	$52,280

Source: Public Health Rep *1987; 102:5-17.*
*   *All estimates are in 1986 current dollars.*
†   *4 percent discount rate.*

■ FINANCING THE COST OF AIDS

By creating the need to care for a growing number of patients with expensive treatment demands, the AIDS epidemic exacerbates problems that already plague our health-care system. Efforts to distribute the burden rationally have been met by resistance from all parties. The private-insurance sector moved quickly and effectively to limit its financial liability by restricting eligibility through the use of HIV-antibody testing and other screening mechanisms. Congress has been unwilling to provide special disability benefits under Medicare. Many AIDS patients are poor and lack health insurance. This causes a critical situation for some health-care providers — especially public hospitals threatened by inadequate reimbursement for care.

Neither the economic costs of AIDS nor the extent of patient care is evenly distributed around the country. Despite the inexorable spread of HIV disease throughout the country, five states — New York, California, Florida, Texas, and New Jersey — still account for nearly 70 percent of the nation's cases.[27] In New York City alone, it has recently been estimated that the provision of necessary health and social services required to deal with the epidemic will require $7 billion dollars from city, state, federal, and private sources over the next four and a half years.[28]

Evidence suggests that in coming years the AIDS caseload will be more evenly distributed throughout the country. The viability of public hospitals that rely heavily on Medicaid funding will be threatened by high levels of unreimbursed care in states with excessively stringent Medicaid eligibility criteria. In a national survey of public and private teaching hospitals, Andrulis et al. demonstrated that 60 percent of AIDS patients are covered by Medicaid in the Northeast, whereas only 15 percent are covered in the South.[16] This has resulted in higher levels of unreimbursed patient care in the South than in any other region of the country. When the AIDS caseload rises, these hospitals will face serious financial difficulties.

Lack of reimbursement could ultimately damage local governments that subsidize indigent care by weakening their ability to provide other public services. Municipal hospitals in parts of the country already hit hard by AIDS have been forced to reallocate resources by cutting back in non-AIDS-related services and programs, a trend sure to continue and to grow with the epidemic.

Who, then, is going to pay the costs? The two principal sources of payment for AIDS hospitalizations are private health insurance and Medicaid. Although the Andrulis study is heavily weighted toward public hospitals where care is more often publicly subsidized than in private voluntary hospitals, the distribution by payer source is striking — 54 percent Medicaid and only 17 percent private insurance, though the insurance industry's own estimates of its share are considerably higher (53 percent).[29]

There is mounting evidence that the proportion of AIDS patients covered by private insurance has declined over time and that payment responsibilities have shifted to the public sector, primarily through Medicaid. For example, between 1983 and 1986 the proportion of AIDS patients covered by Medicaid increased in New York (from 36 percent to 49 percent) and San Francisco (from 19 percent to 30 percent). Evidence of these shifts remains even after controlling for demographic changes due to the increasing proportion of AIDS cases among IVDUs.[30]

Cost-shifting to the public sector may increase in the future. Private health insurers have already been successful in reducing their financial exposure to the epidemic and will undoubtedly grow more vigilant as the economic burden intensifies. Limiting the insurance industry's financial risk in no way reduces the cost of AIDS treatment. It merely shifts the costs to someone else — most often the public sector. At the same time, it aggravates the already-severe problem of the growing pool of uninsured and uninsurable people in this country.

The primary mechanism used by the insurance industry to limit its exposure to AIDS-related claims has been the widespread use of HIV-antibody testing to screen out potential HIV-infected applicants. The industry's unified demand for antibody screening has ramifications beyond the AIDS epidemic. It may in fact open the door to the use of more advanced prognostic tests for insurance underwriting purposes, such as tests to detect heart disease, certain types of cancer, alcoholism, multiple sclerosis, etc.

Given the high costs of medical care, private health insurance is an important shield against poverty for many Americans who become seriously ill. But as the AIDS epidemic illustrates, the shield is only temporary: people too disabled to work lose their health coverage (if they had any) unless they can afford to pay their own premiums. Their alternative is to impoverish themselves to obtain health services through Medicaid or other indigent-care programs. And there are serious questions about the level of access to care for the poor even with Medicaid.

Risk-pooling is one solution put forward to provide insurance, and therefore access to care, for AIDS patients, those at high risk for AIDS (e.g., individuals who are antibody-positive), and others who are unable to obtain insurance coverage. In general, risk pools are state plans that provide health- insurance coverage to people who have been turned down as bad medical risks by private carriers. Insurance companies in each state contribute to a risk pool to defray its expenses.

State risk pools, however, are currently fraught with problems. High premiums, large copayments, and large deductibles limit their accessibility to the general population. Nationwide, only a few thousand people are enrolled, and despite high premiums, most of the pools lose money. As a result of the rapid growth of self-funded insurance plans, there is a shrinking financial base available to subsidize the losses almost all high-risk pools face. Unlike traditional health insurers, self-funded plans are not required to contribute to high-risk pools or pay state premium taxes. In fact, they are not regulated by state insurance departments at all.

It is the largest firms that are the most likely to self-insure: 85 percent of all firms with more than 40,000 employees and 70 percent of firms with 10,000 to 30,000 employees are self-insured.[31] Approximately 50 percent to 60 percent of the nation's covered work force is self-insured.[32] To enable high-risk pools to play an important role in providing access to health care, the financing base should be expanded to include self-insured businesses or wider tax-based revenues (or both). The cost of policies should be lowered to affordable levels.

The movement toward self-insurance has serious implications not only for financing AIDS care, but for health-care financing in general. Because self-insured plans are virtually unregulated, employers may exclude from coverage any condition they choose. While there have been only a few scattered incidents of AIDS exclusion to date, growing costs may encourage employers to shift toward stricter underwriting practices, particularly pre-employment screening procedures and disease-specific exclusion of benefits. Aside from the dangerous consequences of removing the bulk of group health-insurance coverage from the purview of social regulation, the growth of self-insured plans tends to reduce the cross-subsidization of health care by the private sector. As a result, the costs of indigent care increasingly fall on cities, counties, and public hospitals.

In an era when federal policy is shifting responsibilities for domestic social problems to the local level, local government is being asked to bear an increasing cost burden. For example, a very small but growing proportion of AIDS patients have qualified for Medicare. Since qualifying for Medicare as a disabled person requires a two-year waiting period, the vast majority of AIDS patients die before they ever become eligible. Proposals pending before Congress would eliminate the two-year wait for AIDS patients, a move toward increasing federal responsibility for treatment costs. This would reduce the economic impact of AIDS on local governments. A ruling by the Health Care Financing Administration (HCFA), which made AIDS a disability under the Medicaid regulations, has benefited PWAs who lack insurance but it has not been extended to others with symptomatic HIV illnesses that fail to meet the CDC surveillance definition of AIDS.

To the extent that traditional health insurers and self-insured businesses successfully avoid payment for AIDS-related expenses, the financial burden will be shifted to the public sector. The impact will be felt at the federal level through Medicaid and even more extensively at the state and local levels through ever-increasing contributions to Medicaid, indigent-care programs, and faltering public hospitals.

■ ECONOMIC POLICIES AND PROGRAMS

Several major programs have been designed to address the high cost of AIDS by influencing the ways health-care services are organized. The four largest and best-known among these programs are the AIDS Health Services Program of the Robert Wood Johnson Foundation (RWJ), the AIDS Service Demonstration Program of Health Resources and Services Administration (HRSA), the use of Medicaid Home and Community-Based (2176) Waivers for targeting services to PWAs, and New York State's Designated AIDS Center Program. (A description

TABLE 5. PROGRAMS DESIGNED TO INFLUENCE AIDS CARE-DELIVERY MODELS

PROGRAM	SPONSOR	FUNDING SOURCE	AREAS COVERED
AIDS Health Services Program	Robert Wood Johnson Foundation	Grants from private foundations ($33.9 million)	NJ, FL, TX, GA, LA, WA
AIDS Service Demonstration Program	Health Resources and Services Administration	Federal grants ($37.8 million)	NY, FL, GA, MA, NJ, WA, TX, LA, IL, PA, AZ, PR
AIDS-specific Medicaid Home and Community-Based Waivers	Health Care Financing Administration	State and federal Medicaid dollars	NJ, NM
Designated AIDS centers	New York State Department of Health	Medicaid	NY

of some features of these programs is contained in Table 5.) All of them grew out of a single idea, namely, that care can be provided most humanely and cost-effectively in settings outside the hospital. Organizing services around this principle is sometimes referred to as the "continuum model" or the "case-management model." As applied to AIDS in particular, it has also sometimes been called the "San Francisco model" because that city made a concerted effort to apply this principle to the care of PWAs during the early period of the epidemic.[33] All four of the programs mentioned above were inspired by the hope that the continuum model implemented in San Francisco could be replicated in other cities. In order to facilitate this goal, these programs provide funds for case management and other community-based services. They encourage hospitals to form liaisons with community-based organizations that deliver sub-acute services such as home care, meals on wheels, and counseling. There is a great need for these services: there can be little doubt that they improve the quality of life of persons with AIDS, as they would do for any person with a chronic illness or disability. However, whether these programs can also reduce the cost of AIDS care (as it was initially anticipated) is not yet clear.

The cost of care seems to have come down, as noted above, but the contributing factors have not been sorted out. Currently, evaluation studies of the RWJ and HRSA programs are being conducted. These are of national scope and may shed light on the cost-effectiveness issue.

Programs under development emphasize long-range planning or expansion of services. HRSA is sponsoring a new program of grants to assist areas with low AIDS prevalence in developing strategic plans for delivering community-based services to PWAs. Probably the most significant of the new programs is that for early intervention, i.e., providing treatment and services to HIV-infected persons prior to an AIDS diagnosis.

■ POTENTIAL IMPACT OF EARLY INTERVENTION

The prospect of early medical intervention in the course of HIV disease has far-reaching implications for the organization and financing of health care in the United States. Since the number of reported cases of AIDS reflects only a small portion of the HIV-infected population — approximately 10 percent, according to the CDC's estimates[18,34] — the movement of even a fraction of the approximately one million asymptomatic HIV-seropositive individuals into treatment will radically increase demands on the health-care system.[35]

The ability of the public and private sectors to respond to this challenge — by providing adequate HIV testing, counseling, laboratory monitoring, medications, and overall primary health care — will soon depend on the effective coordination of diverse, largely ambulatory services. It will also rest upon the willingness of governmental agencies, nonprofit organizations, and employers to allocate significant resources for activities that have traditionally been very difficult to fund and staff.

The implementation of large-scale early intervention programs must overcome formidable economic barriers. Unlike end-stage treatment costs, the bulk of which are for inpatient care,[25] the enormous economic costs associated with early intervention are largely for ambulatory services. The ambulatory-based model poses vexing questions for reimbursement. Historically, inpatient care has been more comprehensively reimbursed by third-party payers than have outpatient services.[36] Drug expenditures, which loom as a significant component of early intervention costs, are usually even less well reimbursed by third-party insurance mechanisms.

Currently, the price of AZT is temporarily subsidized by the federal government for those without adequate insurance coverage. Without significant price reductions or subsidies, the extraordinarily high price of drugs such as AZT ($8,000 per year for the full dosage) will place them out of reach for all but a small number of people. It is questionable whether the government will continue to subsidize the purchase of AZT or other drugs for individuals without Medicaid or other third-party coverage. Given the large numbers of HIV-infected persons, the high cost of potential drug regimens, and the inadequate financing mechanisms currently available, new ways to pay for treatment must be found.

Some analysts have argued that the introduction of life-prolonging drugs may shift the financial treatment burden from the Medicaid to the Medicare program and thus federalize treatment costs as persons begin to live beyond the two-year qualifying period required for Medicare eligibility as disabled persons.[37] However, it is unlikely that early intervention will lead to a major shift to Medicare. Current eligibility regulations are based on an AIDS diagnosis, not a seropositive blood test. Even if these rules are relaxed, successful drug treatment may paradoxically restrict a person's qualifications for Medicare.

Though individuals receiving early treatment who remain healthy and employed may retain their private insurance coverage, the demands upon Medicaid — the fastest-growing source of reimbursement for AIDS patient services[21,38] — will probably increase. This will occur for at least two reasons: first, drug expenditures account for the bulk of early treatment costs and the majority of private insurance plans do not reimburse for prescription drugs. Moreover, even those individuals with private insurance but inadequate drug coverage may be forced to spend down to become Medicaid-eligible. Second, as larger numbers of uninsured HIV-infected IVDUs, their sexual partners, and children become potential candidates for early treatment, the provision of their medical care is likely to become more dependent on indigent-care pools or Medicaid.

The enormous financial burden of early HIV intervention described above is in part artificial. The bulk of expenditures is tied to the price of pharmacologic agents. Though drug companies have a legitimate need to recoup their investments on experimental pharmaceutical agents, the public also expects to obtain life-saving drugs at reasonable prices. In the case of AZT, which was originally synthesized as an anti-tumor drug at the Detroit Institute for Cancer Research in 1964, the high price does not accurately reflect development or production costs. AZT's patent had, in fact, been in the public domain before the federal government granted Burroughs Wellcome a monopoly in 1985 under the Orphan Drug Act. The ability of Burroughs Wellcome to market the drug without price constraints has led to a quadrupling of its parent company's stock value during the past two years and has generated $113 million dollars in domestic sales in 1988 alone.[39,40]

Incentives to produce drugs for rare diseases under the Orphan Drug Act include an array of tax credits and deductions, an exclusive seven-year license to market the drug, and a variety of research support grants.[41] These fiscal incentives have proven very profitable for some pharmaceutical companies.[42] It is estimated that under the provisions of the Act and current tax laws, drug companies are able to reduce their tax liability on clinical trials by approximately 70 percent of all company expenditures.[43,44] The effect on the consumer and government is to maintain the artificially high cost of many drug therapies. The price of pentamidine, for example, rose from $24.95 per vial in 1984 to $99.45 in 1987 (an increase of 400 percent) once the manufacturer was granted a monopoly under the Orphan Drug Act.[45]

Effective early intervention in HIV disease has the potential for altering the course of the AIDS epidemic. However, the extensive geographic distribution of HIV disease demands that it be treated as a national emergency rather than as a series of local crises. Unless policy-makers, public-health officials, and medical leaders begin to plan for its impact, we face the prospect of being unable to deliver life-sustaining therapy to hundreds of thousands of people who need it.

REFERENCES

1. Rothenberg R, Woelfel M, Stoneburner R, et al. Survival with the acquired immunodeficiency syndrome: experience with 5833 cases in New York City. N Engl J Med 1987; 317:1297-302.

2. Hardy AM, Rauch K, Echenberg D, et al. The economic impact of the first 10,000 cases of acquired immunodeficiency syndrome in the United States. JAMA 1986; 255:209-11.

3. Green J, Oppenheimer G, Leigh M. The $147,000 misunderstanding: overstating the cost of AIDS [Abstract]. V International Conference on AIDS. Montreal, 1989:M.H.O.10.

4. Hellinger FJ. National forecasts of the medical care costs of AIDS: 1988-1992. Inquiry 1988; 25:469-84.

5. Bloom DE, Carliner G. The economic impact of AIDS in the United States. Science 1988; 239:604-10.

6. Kizer KW, Rodriguez J, McHolland GF. An updated quantitative analysis of AIDS in California. California Department of Health Services, April 1987.

7. Seage GR III, Landers S, Barry M, et al. Temporal changes and institutional variation in the cost of treating AIDS [Abstract]. IV International Conference on AIDS. Stockholm, 1988; 2:9517.

8. Kaplowitz LG, Turshen IJ, Myers PS, et al. Medical care costs of patients with acquired immunodeficiency syndrome in Richmond, Va. A quantitative analysis. Arch Intern Med 1988; 148:1793-7.

9. Hiatt RA, Fireman B, Quesenberry C, Selby J. The impact of AIDS on the Kaiser Permanente Medical Care Program (Northern California Region). AIDS-related Issues Staff Paper 4. Washington, D.C.: Office of Technology Assessment, 1988.

10. Drucker E, McMaster P, Wein A, et al. Hospital utilization patterns and charges for the care of inner city AIDS patients: by risk groups, sex, and race/ethnicity [Abstract]. III International Conference on AIDS. Washington, D.C., 1987.

11. Eisenhandler J, Padgug R. Empire Blue Cross and Blue Shield: the first 7,500 AIDS cases [Abstract]. V International Conference on AIDS. Montreal, 1989:W.H.O.7.

12. Seage GR III, Landers S, Barry A, et al. Medical care costs of AIDS in Massachusetts. JAMA 1986; 256:3107-9.

13. Scitovsky AA, Cline M, Lee PR. Medical care costs of patients with AIDS in San Francisco. JAMA 1986; 256:3103-6.

14. Kizer KW, Rodriguez J, McHolland GF. A quantitative analysis of AIDS in California. California Department of Health Services, March, 1986.

15. Thomas EH, Fox DM. The cost of treating persons with AIDS in four hospitals in metropolitan New York in 1985. Health Matrix 1988; 6:15-50.

16. Andrulis DP, Beers VS, Bentley JD, Gage LS. The provision and financing of medical care for AIDS patients in U.S. public and private teaching hospitals. JAMA 1987; 258:1343-6.

17. Hegarty JD, Abrams EJ, Hutchinson VE, et al. The medical care costs of human immunodeficiency virus-infected children in Harlem. JAMA 1988; 260:1901-5.

18. Green J. Hospital utilization by pediatric AIDS cases in New York and California. Presented at the Fifth National Pediatric AIDS Conference, Los Angeles, 6–8 September, 1989.

19. Fox D. The cost of AIDS from conjecture to research. AIDS Public Pol J 1987; 2:25-7.

20. Morgan WM. AIDS Program Center for Infectious Diseases, Centers for Disease Control, personal communication, July 1986.

21. Green J, Singer M, Wintfeld N, et al. Projecting the impact of AIDS on hospitals. Health Aff 1987; 6:19-31.

22. Pascal A. The costs of treating AIDS under Medicaid: 1986–1991. Santa Monica, Calif.: The Rand Corporation, 1986.

23. Schramm CJ. Not just insurance companies. New York Times, June 17, 1987.

24. Hay JW, Osmond DH, Jacobson MA. Projecting the medical costs of AIDS and ARC in the United States. J Acquir Immune Defic Syndr 1988; 1:466-85.

25. Scitovsky AA, Rice DP. Estimates of the direct and indirect costs of acquired immunodeficiency syndrome in the United States, 1985, 1986, and 1991. Public Health Rep 1987; 102:5-17.

26. Rice DP. Estimating the cost of illness. Health Economics Series No. 6. Washington, D.C.: U.S. Government Printing Office, 1966. (PHS publication no. 947-6.)

27. HIV/AIDS Surveillance. Centers for Disease Control, June 1989.

28. Lambert B. New York report on AIDS assails inadequate financing. New York Times, August 1, 1989:B1.

29. Eby C. The share of AIDS medical care costs paid by private insurance in the United States [Abstract]. V International Conference on AIDS. Montreal, 1989:T.H.P.24.

30. Green J, Arno PS. The "Medicaidization" of AIDS [Abstract]. V International Conference on AIDS. Montreal, 1989:T.H.P.16.

31. Johnson and Higgins Health Group. Corporate Health Care Benefits Survey 1986. New York, 1986.

32. McDonnell P, Guttenberg A, Greenberg L, et al. Self-insured health plans. Health Care Financing Rev 1986; 8:1-15.

33. Arno PS. The nonprofit sector's response to the AIDS epidemic: community-based services in San Francisco. Am J Public Health 1986; 1325-30.

34. Human immunodeficiency virus infection in the United States: a review of current knowledge. MMWR 1987; 36(Suppl 6):1S-48S.

35. Arno PS, Shenson D, Seigel NF, et al. The economic and policy implications of early intervention in HIV disease. JAMA 1989; 262:1493-8.

36. Levit KR, Freeland MS. National medical care spending. Health Aff 1988; 7:124-36.

37. Greely HT. AIDS and the health care financing system. Hohn M. Olin Program in Law and Economics, Stanford Law School. Working paper No. 44, July 1988.

38. Roper WL, Winkenwerder W. Making fair decisions about financing care for persons with AIDS. Public Health Rep 1988; 103:305-8.

39. Wellcome PLC 1988 Annual Report.

40. Freudenheim M. Cautious outlook on AIDS drugs. New York Times, April 1, 1988.

41. Orphan Drug Act (P.L. 97-414). 97th Congress. Washington, D.C.: U.S. Government Printing Office, 1983.

42. Waxman HA. The politics of the new drug economics. Business and Health 1988; 5:21-2.

43. 26 USC Sec. 28; 26 CFR Sec. 1.28-1 and 1.28OC-3.

44. Ashbury CH. Orphan drugs: medical versus market value. Indianapolis: D.C. Heath and Co., 1985:164.

45. Steinbrook R. Firm's sharp price increase for AIDS drug attacked. Los Angeles Times, October 31, 1987:32.

Some of the Legal Issues Posed by HIV Disease

Matt Coles, J.D.

This chapter covers several groups of questions on laws that may be applicable to AIDS and HIV infection. The first part focuses on the relationships between health-care providers and patients. The second part covers two additional areas that all health-care providers should know something about.

It isn't possible to say much that is certain about the law as it pertains to HIV infection and AIDS. First, there are at least 156 sets of institutions making up the rules — a legislature, a court system, and at least one administrative agency for each state, the federal government, and the District of Columbia. This isn't unique to AIDS, but with most subjects, sooner or later all the systems begin to follow one or two accepted approaches. This hasn't happened with AIDS yet. Second, law on AIDS is being made very quickly. Although state legislatures were slow to react to the epidemic at first, some of them are making up for lost time now, and there are plenty of cases in the courts. Any answer seemingly certain today could be wrong tomorrow.

This chapter will try to put some common problems in a legal context and suggest some of the approaches legal institutions are likely to take toward them. Most of the references are to more detailed works on AIDS and the law. Because they, too, confront the problems of multiple sources of law and constantly changing rules, they are also rather general. The only way to get a specific answer to a particular problem is to consult someone who knows the appropriate state law.

There is a third problem with AIDS and the law. While courts and legislatures are providing some very specific answers to some questions, others (for example, discrimination in access to health care) haven't been looked at very much.

The surest way to go wrong is to indulge one's inclination toward a desired answer. For example, when health-care workers want to know something about a patient and the governing principle is "need to know," they often decide that the information is needed for "background" or "context," when "need to know" usually means the information is needed to make a specific decision. Typically, one is on safer ground if the arguments for each possible answer are examined critically.

■ CONFIDENTIALITY AND DISCLOSURE

Almost half the states have passed specific laws on the confidentiality of HIV-related information. These statutes tend to be very specific about what can be disclosed, when disclosure can be made, and who is entitled to information.[1] If your state has a statute, it must be followed exactly. The following general discussion applies where there are no specific statutes.

THE DUTY TO KEEP SILENT[2,3]

Who Is Covered.   Almost every court that has ruled on the subject has decided that physicians have a duty to keep confidential all information obtained from a patient during the professional relationship. The duty applies to psychotherapists as well as physicians. If nonphysician health-care workers get confidential information from a physician, it is likely that they have the same obligation not to disclose. If nonphysician health-care workers get confidential information from a patient for treatment or because the patient confides in them, their duty is apt to be the same. The more society regards the workers as "professionals," the more stringent their duty.

Even if health-care workers (including physicians) get information from a patient in a way that clearly has nothing to do with treatment and is not the result of any trust the patient has in the workers as professionals, there may be limits on the workers' right to tell others. Everyone has the obligation not to publicly disclose facts about another person that are private and that most people would want kept private. It is probably wise to assume that most information about AIDS and HIV infection are covered by this obligation. It is not clear how many people one needs to tell for the disclosure to be deemed public.

Type of Information Covered.   Information about a person's medical condition is covered, so HIV status and AIDS-related diagnoses must be kept confidential. Any information obtained by health-care workers to aid in diagnosis and treatment is covered, so information about risky behavior and risk-group status is confidential.

It is also likely that any information obtained because the patient put some special trust in the health-care worker, as well as any information that a reasonable person would find embarrassing to have spread about, is covered.

Because only objectively trivial information is not covered (and any information about AIDS, HIV infection, and risk-group status is not trivial) health-care workers should not pass on information about patients to anyone, except when disclosure is necessary for treatment or when some other rule requires it.

Disclosure Related to Treatment.   There is little law on when the need to disclose information needed for treatment overrides the duty to keep silent in the context of AIDS and HIV infection. The safest course is never to disclose anything about HIV status, AIDS, or membership in a risk group without the patient's express consent. This means that the patient is told what is going to be disclosed, to whom, and the reason for its disclosure. It isn't clear that disclosing information for treatment purposes without consulting the patient violates the duty to keep silent. With routine medical information, it probably does not. A number of states specifically allow nonconsensual disclosure of HIV test results. However, because information about AIDS is not routine, nonconsensual disclosure is always risky if there isn't a specific law allowing it.

Consent will not be the answer if: (1) the patient is incapable of consent and has not given someone a durable medical power of attorney; or (2) the purpose of the disclosure is to safeguard others (such as a surgical team) and the patient refuses consent.

When no one has the capacity to consent, disclosure should be limited to those who truly need to know — that is, only those for whom the information will play a significant role in a decision that has significant consequences for the patient. Before nonconsensual disclosure, be sure that such disclosure is necessary. If universal precautions are being employed, disclosure may not be necessary. When a patient refuses consent, the best strategy is to avoid the disclosure if possible. For example, a policy can state that all those who refuse to be tested or to disclose their status before invasive surgery will be treated as if they were infected. Both the policy and the consequences need to be explained to the patient before consent is requested. When this kind of a policy is not possible, the only alternatives are to avoid circumstances in which the patient represents a threat, or to disclose against the patient's will. Before choosing, health-care workers should find out which alternative presents the greater likelihood of violating local law.

Waivers in General.   Several states have special laws on waivers of the right to confidentiality for AIDS-related information. Sometimes the laws apply only to some types of AIDS-related information, like antibody-test results. Before asking patients to sign waivers and before relying on general waiver forms signed by patients, health-care workers should check the rules in their state.

The difficulty with general waivers, such as those sometimes used by hospitals, is that they do not usually explain the very serious consequences that can follow the disclosure of AIDS-related information. The traditional concept of "informed consent" usually requires only disclosure of the medical consequences of a particular procedure. However, the fact that disclosure of AIDS-related information can have very serious consequences opens the possibility that a patient who signs a general waiver and then suffers some injury as a result of the disclosure of AIDS-related information may have grounds for complaint. Specific written consents coupled with an explanation of the potential psychological and social consequences of disclosure are therefore a good idea. (Conditioning treatment on confidentiality waivers is treated below.)

Insurance Waivers.   Physicians presented with requests for information from insurance companies accompanied by general waivers signed by patients should first check local law to make sure the waivers apply to AIDS-related information. If they do, the waivers amount to an order from patients to turn over the information requested, so physicians are bound to comply. However, calling the patients to make sure they understand the effect of the waiver (which would also give the patients the chance to withdraw the insurance application if they want) is a good idea.

THE DUTY (AND THE RIGHT) TO DISCLOSE[2-4]

There are two circumstances in which health-care workers may have an obligation to disclose AIDS-related information about a patient: (1) where the law requires reporting; and (2) where the law imposes a duty to warn someone who may be placed in peril by the patient. In addition, some states now specifically give some health-care workers the right (but not the obligation) to either notify specific individuals that they may be or may have been put at risk or to report that fact to public-health authorities. Those statutes usually forbid disclosure of the infected person's name.

Reporting Requirements.   Where state or federal law requires a diagnosis or other information to be reported (usually to a public-health agency), that requirement overrides the duty to keep silent. However, before making a report, health-care workers should verify precisely: (1) what triggers an obligation to report (AIDS diagnosis or a positive HIV-antibody test result?); (2) what details must be reported (only the fact of a diagnosis or identifying information about the patient?); (3) who is required to report; and (4) whom the report is to be made to. No health-care workers should report beyond the law's exact requirements because outside of those requirements the duty to keep silent remains.

The Duty to Warn.   No issue has occupied health ethics more in relation to the AIDS epidemic than the "duty to warn." Three cautions are essential before looking at the circumstances in which that duty may arise. First, most states have not yet considered whether a duty to warn exists in the context of AIDS. While all of the recent cases in other contexts have found the duty does exist, it is by no means certain that the trend will continue or that the courts won't find that AIDS presents a special situation with different considerations.

Second, in some circumstances a duty to warn leads some people to think that they should "err on the safe side" and warn if there is any chance the duty may apply. This is not a good idea, because the duty to warn probably takes up where the duty to keep silent leaves off; that is, if there is no obligation to warn, health-care workers probably have an obligation to keep silent. Erring on "the safe side" of the duty to warn could be a violation of the duty to maintain confidentiality.

Finally, those states ruling that a duty to warn exists have usually said that health-care workers are obligated to be as discreet as possible and to attempt to preserve patients' privacy as much as possible. While it may not always be possible to shield a patient's identity, the requirement of discretion probably makes it wise whenever possible not to reveal the patient's name.

This is the duty to warn: When a physician or a psychotherapist determines (or, under the standards of their profession, ought to determine) that a patient presents a serious danger to another person, the physician or therapist has a duty to take reasonable steps to protect the potential victim.

An Identifiable Victim.   The first problem with the duty is identifying the victim. Must the threat be to a specific individual whom the physician knows or is capable of identifying, or can the duty to take some action arise whenever the physician believes there is a risk of harm to some class of persons? One court has found the duty exists as long as there is a foreseeable risk of harm to a class. All other courts have required that the physician be able to identify at least specific potential victims.

Past and Future Exposure.   All the cases decided so far have dealt with the threat of future harm. With AIDS and HIV infection, the duty may also arise when a physician learns that a patient has already exposed another to HIV.

What Triggers the Duty.   The duty to warn is clearest when a physician knows that a person has, is, or will expose another to HIV. Most decided cases have involved psychiatrists, and the courts have said that the duty is imposed both when practitioners conclude that there is a risk and when they ought to conclude that based on the standards of skill and care of their profession. At least one court has said that a therapist cannot simply rely on patients' stating they will not do anything harmful. On the other hand, given the continuing general duty to remain silent, patients' statements about whether or not they have engaged in risky practices, will inform their partners of their risks, or will not engage in risky practices again, cannot be ignored. Probably the safest course is to attempt to get patients to disclose and to agree to refrain from risky behavior, and to disclose only when reasonably sure that patients are not following through on their promises.

What to Do.   Once the duty arises, it is not clear what must be done. If there is a clear duty and the victims are not identified, notifying the public-health department may be all that is possible. On the other hand, in a celebrated case involving a known victim, the therapists did notify the police (who did not act) but the court said they could be found liable because they failed to warn the victim.[5] Some courts have also mentioned warning those likely to tell the victim when the victim cannot be contacted directly.

Who Has the Duty.   Courts have imposed the duty to inform on physicians and psychotherapists. Because the duty depends on a "special relationship" between the health-care worker and the person who poses the threat, it is likely that some professional relationship of trust will be required before the duty arises.

■ CONSENT TO HIV TESTING[1,6,7]

Many states have specific laws on who must obtain a patient's consent to an HIV test and on the form the consent must take. These laws need to be strictly followed.

Where there is no specific law, HIV tests are covered by general principles of "informed consent." Most often, informed consent means that a patient must be told about the medical risks involved in a given procedure. With a blood test, little information is ordinarily required. Because of the possibility that HIV test results may be disclosed to others (for example, where reporting is required, through communication to other health-care workers where allowed, and through an insurance application) and the potentially serious consequences of a disclosure (loss of health-care coverage, dissemination of information to intimate associates or others, such as employers), "informed consent" when applied to an HIV test may mean more than a description of medical risks.

The safest course is to have the patient's physician obtain written consent after describing the nonmedical consequences that could result from a test.

No court has yet ruled that informed consent to any medical procedure requires disclosure of a health-care worker's HIV status. As long as the risk of health-care workers' transmitting HIV to patients appears slight, that is not likely to change. However, continuing pressure to require disclosure of a patient's HIV status before non-emergency surgery could also change this. The question of whether consent to an HIV test can be required as a condition for treatment is considered below.

■ REFUSAL TO TREAT AND DISCRIMINATION IN SERVICES[8,9]

It used to be generally accepted that health-care workers and institutions had no obligation to begin or continue to treat anyone. That is changing. This section describes the reasons why obligations to treat might be imposed on various providers, the kinds of obligations likely to be imposed, and the possible exceptions.

WHO MAY BE OBLIGATED TO TREAT?

Health-Care Workers.   The first inroads on the old rule came in a few cases where a single physician or group practice was the sole provider available. Drawing on fairly ancient principles, one court said that under those circumstances, a physician, like an innkeeper, had a duty not to arbitrarily refuse anyone treatment. Given the low risk of nosocomial transmission of HIV and the diseases related to it, a refusal based on HIV infection alone would probably be found arbitrary in states following this rule.

If health-care providers or group practices were found to be business establishments or public accommodations (some older cases say they are not, a few more recent cases say they are), they would be covered by laws banning discrimination on the basis of disability. Those courts that have ruled on the matter say that AIDS is a disability, and it is likely that most will say the same thing about HIV infection.

Health maintenance organizations (HMOs) and perhaps some "prudent-buyer plans" may have a contractual obligation to provide services to their members. An individual health-care worker's obligations would be set by her or his agreement with the employing plan or HMO. Health-care workers employed by hospitals are usually obliged by the hospital to treat any patient the hospital admits, and hospitals may have less freedom to refuse patients than individual health-care workers do (see below).

Finally, a number of courts have said that once a physician begins treating a critically ill patient, the physician may not end the relationship without giving adequate notice. The safest course is to make some provision for the patient's continued care before terminating the relationship, and this may be required with patients who are critically ill.

Hospitals.   Hospitals are more likely than health-care workers to be the only available provider, so they are more likely to be obliged not to arbitrarily refuse to treat. Hospitals, especially private hospitals, are also more likely to be considered by the courts as "business establishments" and therefore to be subject to antidiscrimination laws. The fact that a hospital may be organized as a nonprofit does not mean it is not a business. It is an institution's function, not its tax status, that determines its obligations under law.

Hospitals are also more likely than individual providers to receive federal funds and therefore to be covered by the federal Rehabilitation Act, which bans disability discrimination and which several courts have said applies to AIDS and HIV infection. If a hospital receives any federal funds (other than simple payment for services), it is covered by the Rehabilitation Act. With one exception, the courts have ruled that receipt of Medicaid or Medicare funds invokes the Act. Under this Act, it doesn't matter if the hospital is considered a business.

Other Health-Care Institutions.   Other health-care institutions, like ambulance services and residential-care facilities, are even more likely than hospitals to be looked upon as "business establishments," and thus to be covered by antidiscrimination laws.

WHAT THE OBLIGATION ENTAILS

Disability discrimination laws don't only ban the refusal to serve; they also require equal treatment. For example, a hospital that provided less staffing on an AIDS ward or that made services available to other patients but not to HIV-infected patients could be in violation.

EXCEPTIONS AND DEFENSES

A person charged with disability discrimination can escape liability under most laws by showing that the disabled person's participation in the activity in question would represent a threat to either the defendant's health or safety or to the health or safety of another. This defense will not work in most health-care settings given the low risk of nosocomial transmission. However, the defense should work when a patient, because of particular opportunistic infections or other factors, represents a threat to others. It should also work when keeping the patient with others would be dangerous to the patient. The defense might also justify a refusal to perform surgery.

However, the defense works only if the threat cannot be rendered insignificant by "reasonable accommodation." So while it might allow a provider to separate HIV-infected patients from others under certain circumstances or allow a surgeon to adopt different procedures, it might not permit an outright refusal to treat.

A physician or institution might be able to refuse to treat by claiming a threat to the safety of the patient if the physician were not competent or the institution were not properly equipped to take the case. However, claims of incompetence or incapacity may be looked at skeptically. Because there is a duty to make reasonable accommodations, such claims will not work if the training or equipment is easily obtained or if similar accommodations have been made for other diseases.

Except where local law creates some obligation to treat indigents (as some states require some hospitals to do), inability to pay is usually a valid reason for refusing to treat. It may not be a justification for terminating a relationship with a patient who is critically ill, however.

■ TREATMENT CONDITIONED ON TESTING OR CONFIDENTIALITY WAIVERS

Can a health-care worker or institution insist that the patient agree to HIV testing or to a waiver of confidentiality before being treated? In states with specific laws on testing or confidentiality, the answer is probably "no" unless the statute specifically allows that.

Where there are no statutes, the answer is less clear. If discrimination laws apply, demands for testing (or disclosure of HIV status) are arguably legitimate for two reasons only: (1) if it can be shown that there is a significant health risk involved in treatment; or (2) if reasonable accommodation will be needed if the patient is infected.

Where discrimination laws don't apply, a provider's ability to insist on a confidentiality waiver will depend on the applicable state's law on privacy rights (or, in the case of treatment that has already begun, on the provider's duty to keep silent). Some states allow patients to give up their right to confidentiality if the waiver is voluntary and intelligent. To qualify, the patient would probably have to be told about the potential consequences and be offered some other option for treatment. Some states may not allow waivers at all.

■ INCAPACITATED PATIENTS AND HEALTH-CARE DECISIONS

WHO DECIDES?

When a patient is incapable of giving consent to medical treatment, who has the power to consent depends both on local law and on what the patient has done in advance.

Many states now have laws providing for durable powers of attorney for health care. These laws allow competent patients to designate a person to make health-care decisions for them when they become incapacitated. However, unless there is a law specifically authorizing "durable" powers of attorney, a power of attorney becomes ineffective when the patient becomes incapacitated.

Once a patient is incapacitated, the holder of a durable power usually has sole authority over health-care decisions, whatever the wishes of relatives. Most states that recognize durable powers give parents, children, spouses, health-care providers, and certain public officials the right to challenge decisions by filing a court petition. However, patients can eliminate that right in their powers of attorney if they wish to.

The courts in every state have the power to appoint a conservator to make health-care decisions for incompetent patients who have not signed durable powers of attorney for health care. Conservatorships are expensive and difficult to manage, so people usually try to avoid them. So far, no state has said that a conservator is always necessary for health-care decisions if patients are incompetent.

For patients who have neither signed a durable power of attorney for health care nor had a conservator appointed, most states (either by court decision or by statute) give the power to make health-care decisions to the closest relative.

WHAT DECISIONS ARE COVERED?

General Care.   With the exception of authority to refuse life-sustaining treatment (see the next section), the person with the right to make decisions generally has the authority to make all health-care decisions for an incompetent patient. A number of states deny conservators and the holders of durable powers-of-attorney the authority to make commitments to mental-health facilities and to consent to electroshock therapy, psychosurgery, abortion, and sterilization. If a commitment to a mental-health facility appears necessary, a conservatorship for that purpose may be the wisest course.

Life-Sustaining Treatment.   Almost every court ruling on the matter has a different answer to the question of whether and when a health-care provider must comply with a patient who refuses life-sustaining treatment. Some say never, some say if the patient is terminally ill, some say that patients always have that right. Since most hospitals and medical societies have debated this issue recently, it should be easy to find out the rules in the applicable state. Most courts say that health-care providers are never required to remove life-sustaining treatment; if the patient insists, providers can insist that they be replaced on the case.

If a patient has a right to refuse life-sustaining treatment, it is likely that the holder of a durable power of attorney or a conservator has the same right. Some of the states permitting durable powers of attorney have made the holder's right to order an end to life-sustaining treatment explicit. However, even where holders do have this power, the laws sometimes require physicians to make a good-faith effort to discover the patient's wishes. Health-care providers regularly involved with AIDS patients should find out what the rules are in their states before the situation presents itself. Conservators often get specific authorization to refuse life-sustaining treatment from the courts that appoint them.

In one narrowly-defined circumstance, some states provide a clear-cut guide. A few states have "natural death" laws, which allow directives to the physician that require him or her to cease life-sustaining procedures once death is imminent. Such directives must be signed more than 14 days after the patient is diagnosed with a terminal disease to be binding.

■ DISCRIMINATION[10-14]

Some people (including former President Reagan's Commission on the Human Immunodeficiency Virus Epidemic) think that people's fear of the consequences of infection with HIV is the greatest problem public-health efforts face in ending the epidemic. Yet every state has laws that probably prohibit most forms of HIV-related discrimination. The problem is not that the laws do not exist but that people don't know about them. As with most civil-rights laws, public awareness is critical. If people don't know about the law, more discrimination occurs (law works because most people obey it without going to court), discrimination doesn't get reported (it won't be if the victims don't know there is a remedy), and most tragically, people try to avoid discrimination by not getting tested for HIV, thus denying themselves access to public health.

LAWS ON DISCRIMINATION

Every state has laws banning at least some form of discrimination against people who are disabled (some states use the term "handicapped"). Since AIDS is a physical condition that usually becomes severely disabling, early in the epidemic lawyers tried to use the disability discrimination laws to fight discrimination against people with AIDS. For the most part, they were successful.

Every state bans employment discrimination against people with disabilities. Most also have laws covering disability discrimination in housing and in business establishments and public accommodations. The federal government currently bans discrimination by federal agencies and by all institutions receiving federal funds (the Rehabilitation Act). The law applies to virtually everything done by anyone covered by it. Congress is again considering the "Americans with Disabilities Act," which would extend the federal law to all employers with 15 or more employees, all business establishments (specifically including health-care providers), and all government operations.

The federal Fair Housing Act bans housing discrimination based on disability in almost all forms of housing.

A number of cities and counties have local ordinances that apply specifically to discrimination against people with AIDS, those who are HIV-infected, or those who may be perceived to be HIV-infected. While these are usually helpful as statements of policy, local civil-rights ordinances must be used carefully (see below).

Insurance is a different matter. For the most part, insurers can discriminate.

WHO DISCRIMINATION LAW PROTECTS

All courts that have ruled on AIDS as a disability have said that it is a handicap, and there is no reason to think their decisions would have been different if the cases had been brought about any other symptomatic stage of HIV infection. Some laws cover conditions that are not currently but may become disabling, and these should protect people with asymptomatic HIV infection. Even where the law does not apply to "future disabling conditions," most laws prohibit discrimination that is based on belief that a person has a disabling condition (even if he or she does not). This should cover most instances of discrimination against people who are HIV-infected but asymptomatic.

Laws banning discrimination that is grounded on the perception (right or wrong) that a person is disabled should also cover most cases of discrimination based on the unconfirmed believe that a person is infected with HIV (for example, a landlord who evicts a tenant upon learning that the tenant uses drugs intravenously because the landlord assumes that all IV drug users are infected with HIV). However, the laws may not work in the reverse situation: if a landlord evicts an HIV-infected person because the landlord assumes that all HIV-infected persons must be gay, that landlord may be acting legally unless the town or state in which the discrimination occurs bans sexual-orientation discrimination.

Most civil-rights laws, either explicitly or implicitly, prohibit discrimination against people associated with people covered by the law, so most laws also ban discrimination against the lovers, friends, and families of HIV-infected people and against those who treat and serve them.

HOW DISCRIMINATION LAW REGULATES BEHAVIOR

The Federal Rehabilitation Act.   The federal Rehabilitation Act applies to all the activities of any federal agency and of those who receive federal financial assistance. If a state or local agency gets federal funds, then everything the agency does is covered, regardless of where the federal funds are actually used. Funding granted to one state agency doesn't generally impose the Act on other state agencies, but if a state department (or, presumably, the state itself) were to receive general funding, everything the department (or state government) does would be covered. The same basic rule applies to private organizations: funding to the entity as a whole covers everything; funding to any part of the facility covers the whole facility.

Federal "funding" covers virtually everything except the simple purchase of goods and services at fair market value. Even things that look like purchasing are covered. As noted above, Medicare and Medicaid are often viewed by health-care providers as simple payment for services. But because they are also viewed as benefit programs, they provide "financial assistance," and therefore the provisions of the Rehabilitation Act for providers apply to them as well as to anyone else receiving federal money.

The Federal Fair Housing Act.   The Fair Housing Act covers almost all real-estate transactions, including sale, rental, and financing. The act has limited exemptions for religious organizations and private clubs (in nonprofit housing, they can limit or give preference to members), and it generally exempts owners of less than three units who don't use brokers and units in buildings that are owner-occupied and that have less than four units.

State and Local Laws.   Most employment laws have a small-employer exemption that doesn't cover employers with less than a certain number of employees. The number is usually five or fifteen.

Most housing and employment laws also have some form of religious-organization exemption, either removing religious organizations entirely from the law, or allowing preferential or exclusive treatment for members of the religion. The religious exemptions usually do not extend to individuals who seek to discriminate on the basis of religious belief. Most housing laws have some form of small-dwelling exemption removing small buildings that are owner-occupied.

Discrimination Law: Content.   In general, disability discrimination laws say that people with disabilities cannot be excluded from or given different treatment in activities covered by the law as long as they qualify by being capable of participating in the activities. If their participation might differ from that of others because of their disability, discrimination law states that they must be allowed to participate if their special needs can be reasonably accommodated. For example, employees with AIDS who must leave work regularly for medical treatment must be accommodated if flexibility in hours won't impose a hardship on the employer. On the other hand, employees who are so sick that they cannot work are no longer qualified under discrimination law.

When the participation of a person with disabilities represents a threat to personal health or safety or the health or safety of others, the laws generally don't apply. However, this defense must be proven about the individual in question and the situation at hand and not applied to possible situations in the future. It is not a defense, for example, to say that eventually most people with AIDS will become so sick that it would be dangerous for them to work with heavy equipment; it must be shown that the individual is now that sick.

Possible job-related contagion could be fought in terms of the health-and-safety defense. However, because the U.S. Supreme Court ruled in a case about tuberculosis that persons who present a significant risk of contagion are not qualified to hold jobs, this issue gets analyzed as a qualification.

Under federal law, persons who are HIV-infected cannot be discriminated against because of possible contagion unless there is a "significant risk" of transmission. Assessment of risk must be based on the best current medical information, with particular deference to the opinions of public-health authorities. Contagion is unlikely to be a serious defense in most employment, housing, and business situations.

MAKING A DISCRIMINATION CLAIM

Most laws allow people who believe they have been discriminated against to file complaints with a government enforcement agency. When the agency is independent of the person accused of discriminating, this is often a quick, relatively cheap way to get a claim resolved. Some agencies have only the power to "mediate." With a recalcitrant discriminator, using such agencies is often a waste of time. Some administrative complaints have to be made to the agency accused, and that is also usually a waste of time. Some administrative agencies have limited powers — for example, the power to cut off funding to an accused, but not the power to force a rehire.

When an agency remedy does not appear likely to be effective, or when a fast order to prevent a discharge or eviction is essential, it may be best to go directly to court. This is not always an option. Some laws require an administrative complaint before a court complaint can be filed. There are usually (but not always) limited exceptions for emergencies. Since court proceedings are usually lengthy and exhausting, an administrative complaint that may provide some relief is usually a good idea.

The Risk with Municipal Laws.   Each level of government in our system has the power to "preempt" action by lower levels on most things. So, for example, Congress can tell state legislatures and city councils not to pass laws on employment benefits, and state legislatures can tell city councils not to pass laws on insurance.

"Preemption" happens in three ways. Sometimes Congress or a legislature is explicit and says that it means or does not mean to preempt the right to make a more local statute or ordinance. Sometimes a legislature does something so comprehensive that courts think it was intended to encompass the field. Sometimes a court will look at an issue (like insurance regulation) and say that it is so important from a national or statewide perspective that local regulation is precluded.

Federal civil-rights laws are generally not "preemptive." However, many state laws are. In addition, in many states, city governments have very limited rights that often do not include the powers to pass civil-rights laws. Unfortunately, local governments sometimes are not sufficiently informed about these limits. Anyone thinking of making an AIDS-related discrimination claim in an area with a local discrimination ordinance should see if there is a state law on disability discrimination or if coverage under a federal law is possible. If a state or federal remedy is available, that should be pursued as well as the local claim, since the local law could ultimately prove ineffective.

A Note on Survival of Claims.   Every state says that some lawsuits "survive" the death of the parties. In most states, HIV-related discrimination claims should survive. In some states, once a person has died, his or her estate may recover only specific tangible losses, like lost wages, but not damages for pain and suffering.

REFERENCES

1. Gostin LO. Public health strategies for confronting AIDS. Legislative and regulatory policy in the United States. JAMA 1989; 261:1621-30.

2. Belitsky R, Solomon RA. Doctors and patients: responsibilities in a confidential relationship. In: Dalton HL, Burris S, eds. AIDS and the law: a guide for the public. New Haven: Yale University Press, 1987:201-9.

3. Barnes M. Confidentiality. In: Rubenfeld AR, ed. AIDS legal guide, 2nd ed. New York: Lambda Legal Defense and Education Fund, 1987; (4)1-15.

4. Association of State and Territorial Health Officials, National Association of County Health Officials and U.S. Conference of Local Health Officers. Guide to public health practice: HIV partner notification strategies. September, 1988.

5. Supreme Court of California. Tarasoff v. Regents of the University of California. California Vol. 17, 3d, 1976:425.

6. Gostin LO. Traditional public health strategies. In: Dalton HL, Burris S, eds. AIDS and the law: a guide for the public. New Haven: Yale University Press, 1987:47-65.

7. Gostin LO, Curran WJ, Clark ME. The case against compulsory casefinding in controlling AIDS — testing, screening and reporting. Am J Law Med 1987; 12:7-53.

8. Banks TL. The right to medical treatment. In: Dalton HL, Burris S, eds. AIDS and the law: a guide for the public. New Haven: Yale University Press, 1987; 175-84.

9. Campbell JM. Access to health related services. In: Rubenfeld AR, ed. AIDS legal guide, 2nd ed. New York: Lambda Legal Defense and Education Fund, 1987; (3)1-9.

10. Leonard AS. AIDS in the workplace. In: Dalton HL, Burris S, eds. AIDS and the law: a guide for the public. New Haven: Yale University Press, 1987:109-25.

11. Rothstein MA. Screening workers for AIDS. In: Dalton HL, Burris S, eds. AIDS and the law: a guide for the public. New Haven: Yale University Press, 1987:126-41.

12. Mandelker DR. Housing issues. In: Dalton HL, Burris S, eds. AIDS and the law: a guide for the public. New Haven: Yale University Press, 1987:142-52.

13. Leonard AS. Employment discrimination. In: Rubenfeld AR, ed. AIDS legal guide, 2nd ed. New York: Lambda Legal Defense and Education Fund, 1987; (2)1-14.

14. Feldman R. Housing and real estate issues. In: Rubenfeld AR, ed. AIDS legal guide, 2nd ed. New York: Lambda Legal Defense and Education Fund, 1987; (8)1-5).

Wills, Competence, and Health and Disability Insurance

Matt Coles, J.D.

■ WILLS AND COMPETENCE[1]

When Wills are Necessary.   Health-care workers are often called upon to witness wills and to testify to patients' competence or incompetence. For these reasons, a short review of estate law is provided here. Many hospitals have their own policies on these matters as well.

Every state has laws that control where people's property goes at their death if they have not executed a will. These are usually called the laws of "intestate succession." These laws commonly distribute property first to spouses and children. If there are none, the estate passes in order of succession to parents, brothers and sisters, and more remote relatives. If there are no relatives, the property usually goes to the state. Not a single state calls for succession to unrelated persons. For gay people, so disproportionately affected by AIDS, the closest "relations" are often not legally related at all. For these persons, wills are essential. It should be part of each primary-care physician's role to mention wills and health-care powers of attorney to patients when discussing long-term prognosis.

Who Can Be Left Property under a Will.   Property can be left to anyone under a will. In some states, provisions must be made for spouses and children. In others, spouses and children must be acknowledged and then property can be left however a person wishes.

Competence.   The capacity a person needs for making a will is different in most states from the capacity for making a contract or doing other things: it is lower. To make a will, a person needs to be capable of knowing: (1) what it is that he or she is doing; (2) what he or she has; and (3) who is going to be affected by the will and their relationship to the person making the will.

Under this standard, persons making wills need to be capable of knowing that they are deciding what will happen to their property after death. They must be able to keep in mind what they own (even if briefly while making the decision). Finally, they must be capable of knowing who would inherit things under the will and the relationship of those inheriting things to the person making the will. They must also be capable of knowing who would get things if there were no will, how the will changes that, and the relationship of those persons to the person making the will. At a minimum, they must be able to understand these things if told and to keep them in mind long enough to decide.

Free Will.   To be valid, a will must be an act of free will. The person making it cannot be coerced with threats or force. A will isn't valid if its maker was fooled into signing it or deceived about its provisions.

Form.   Every state has its own formal requirements for wills. Most states say that if a will was valid where and when it was signed, it remains valid. Therefore, a will made in another state is usually good even after the maker moves.

Some states recognize "holographic" or "olographic" wills, that is, wills written in a person's own handwriting, then signed and dated. These are a great source of needless errors. For example, in states allowing persons to do anything with their property as long as spouses and children are expressly disinherited, holographic wills often fail to explicitly exclude them and they end up taking part of the estate despite the will. However, holographic wills are almost always better than no will at all.

Avoiding Competency and Free Will Problems.   Courts say that they "favor" wills. The competency standards are usually not very rigorous, and most states say that rigorous standards of proof will apply to claims of fraud and duress. Nonetheless, competency and free will are serious concerns for most wills made by people with AIDS.

Any will made during the course of a serious illness invites claims of incompetence or "undue influence" by the person caring for the sick person. Both types of claims are more likely with illnesses like AIDS that cause neurologic problems. "Undue influence" claims are more likely when outsiders do not understand the relationship of a care giver and a decedent (as is often the case with gay relationships). In such circumstances, family members of the decedent often claim that a lover who acted as care giver has no claim on the decedent other than that of an attendant. Any consideration provided in the decedent's will may be contested as the result of "undue influence."

In addition, courts share the prejudices of the rest of society. They are more likely to find a will made in favor of a lover "strange" and evidence of incapacity than they would find a will made in favor of a relative. They are more likely to find that a lover who took care of a dying partner was overbearing and after whatever he or she could get.

While cases overturning wills are unusual and cases that focus on gay relationships are growing rarer, it is a good idea to encourage patients to take some easy steps to minimize the potential for such claims. The rest of this section discusses what health-care workers can do to help reduce the chance of a claim.

Medical Considerations.   If patients are on medication that is apt to reduce their capacity to think clearly, it is best to plan their interviews with lawyers and the signing of their wills for a time when the influence of the medication will be smallest. It is not necessary that a patient be taken off all medication to sign.

If patients are experiencing intermittent problems understanding basic things (like the identity of those around them, or where they are), it is best to try to hold the interview and the signing when they are most lucid. Intermittent problems will not void the will if patients have basic capacity at the time of making the decisions and signing the will.

Encouraging People to Be Honest with Relatives.   Too often the blood relatives of people who die of AIDS only find out that the person had the disease shortly before or immediately after death. Too often, that is also the first time the relatives find out that the person is or was gay. When the surprise, confusion, and homophobia that often go with those two revelations are added to the usual shock that goes with death, the result is sometimes a challenge to competency or free will that otherwise would not have been made. For these reasons, patients should be urged to discuss their diagnosis with anyone likely to be affected by the disposition of their estate.

Being a Witness.   People argue about who makes the best witnesses — those who know the person making the will or those who do not know the person at all. In any case, persons who are going to get anything under the will should not be witnesses. Very often, it is hard to get anyone else to witness on short notice. At most, witnesses may be called on to testify as to the patient's competence (and most often that will not be necessary), so health-care providers should be willing to witness.

Timing.   The longer HIV-infected persons wait to make their wills, the more likely they are to deteriorate and their competency to make wills to be challenged. The longer they wait, the more likely they are to become totally dependent on those taking care of them and the more likely the care givers are to become open to undue-influence claims. Later is always better than never, but people with AIDS should be encouraged to make their wills as soon as possible.

Entirely new wills that change everything and are signed moments before death have been upheld. What beneficiaries thought were notes on scraps of paper have been found to be valid holographic wills. Wills have been approved even when nobody could find the will itself. Patients should be encouraged to make their wills in a timely and careful way, but people should not give up if things are put off until the last minute.

■ GETTING HEALTH AND DISABILITY INSURANCE[2,3]

A Word about "Underwriting."   It is important for health-care providers treating HIV-infected people to know how health and disability insurance policies are underwritten and screened, since these matters have powerful, long-term effects on their patients' health.

With individual and small group insurance policies, companies usually assess individuals' health to decide whether they are good risks. This is called "underwriting." Companies often do not underwrite with large groups, although this is changing. Some companies consider groups over 25 large, while others go as high as 50.

A Word about Information Banks.   Insurance companies share information about people who apply for policies through an information bank called MIB. If a person is ever refused insurance, his or her name will be sent to MIB along with the reason for refusal. If the same individual applies for insurance later through a different company, that company will usually check with MIB. Patients considering an insurance application who are aware that a company may find adverse information in a medical chart should think about not applying or about withdrawing their application for the reasons discussed below.

Persons with AIDS and Symptomatic HIV Infection.   Virtually every insurance company refuses to issue either health or disability insurance that is underwritten to persons with AIDS or symptomatic HIV infection. Coverage under large group policies is possible, but many plans exclude coverage for illnesses that exist at the time the person enters the plan, either for a waiting period (usually three to six months) or permanently.

Asymptomatic Persons with HIV Infection.   Many insurance companies refuse to insure HIV-infected people who are asymptomatic, arguing that they are bad risks. Although it is possible to challenge these refusals on the grounds that companies could simply charge more for the policy or that they ignore similar risks, these cases will be difficult to win because in many states insurance companies may not be subject to disability discrimination statutes, and insurance through employment is immune from most state regulation under federal law. The most important recent issue here is how companies determine a person's HIV status.

Test Results.   Only one state (California) presently prohibits the use of anti-body tests for insurance, and this ban only applies to health insurance. Everywhere else, insurance companies can test. Even California puts no limit on the use of other tests, such as T-cell counts.

Medical Charts.   State laws on confidentiality usually state whether a physician is required or permitted to release antibody test results or other AIDS-related information. Insurance companies always require applicants to sign a release that allows the company complete access to their medical files. If there is no state law on confidentiality or if the law allows a broad release, releases amount to a directive from the patient to the physician to turn over the entire chart — a directive that the health-care worker must obey.

Even when a patient's record does not contain HIV-antibody test results or when state law requires that they not be released, information in a medical chart can alert a company to the fact that an applicant is a member of a "high-risk" group. While a company's right to use that fact alone to deny coverage is questionable (see below), the company can use it to find another reason to deny coverage. Health-care workers should be careful not to include information of doubtful relevance to medical care in the chart. If such information is released to an insurance company, the patient may be able to complain that it was of a private nature, should not have been put in the chart in the first place, and thus should not have been released.

Markers.   Some insurance companies have denied coverage to applicants on the basis of "markers" that they believe identify persons (usually gay men) at risk for HIV infection. The "markers" range from the applicant naming an unrelated person of the same gender as a beneficiary on a life policy (small life-insurance policies often accompany health-insurance plans), the applicant being employed in certain occupations that the companies think are predominately filled with gay men, to residing in certain parts of a city, e.g., San Francisco's Castro district, or ZIP code 94114.

Some state insurance commissions have already said that they take a dim view of this practice, as have some insurance industry trade associations. The markers usually rest on silly stereotypes and crude ideas about who does and does not get infected.

Questions about HIV Status and Risk-Group Membership.   A few states that allow HIV antibody tests for insurance prohibit questions about whether a person has taken the test. There are virtually no limits on questions about health history.

The propriety of questions about sexual orientation and intravenous drug use is not clear. A few states have said that discrimination based on sexual orientation is objectionable, but most have not considered the issue.

■ KEEPING INSURANCE IN EFFECT

The problem with most health insurance is that it is employment-related. Once a person leaves work, he or she loses the insurance. There are several ways to keep it in effect, and health-care workers should be aware of these so that they can advise patients who are still working on how to retain their coverage.

Continuation. Federal law requires employers with 20 or more employees to offer continuation of insurance if the former employee pays the premium (plus a small surcharge). Coverage for 18 months is usually required (unless the employer ceases to offer insurance to all employees), but 36 months of coverage may be available if the former employee later qualifies for some forms of social security benefits. The law doesn't usually apply if the employee is fired for misconduct.

Several eastern states also require that employers make continued insurance available, and these requirements apply in some circumstances where federal law does not. This is particularly important because some large group plans are issued in these states but cover employees all over the country.

Conversion. Many states require that when people leave a group plan, they be given the option to "convert" to individual health policies. Conversion plans are usually not very good. They tend to have poorer coverage, higher premiums, and high deductibles or co-payments. They may be better than nothing, however.

Waiver-of-Premium Benefit. Many disability plans state that when insured members become ill, they are no longer required to pay premiums, even if the disability policy has not yet gone into effect. Usually, the persons insured must claim the benefit early in the disability, so patients should check their policies and be on the alert.

Pre-existing Conditions. Most individual health policies refuse to pay for treatment of conditions that existed at the time the policy was issued. Some group policies do the same, while others deny coverage for a waiting period (usually three months to a year).

If a patient was symptomatic before coverage was issued, a company may refuse to pay any AIDS-related expenses. So far, most companies have not been successful in claiming that infection alone is a pre-existing medical condition. But as medical thinking on AIDS changes and the once-clear demarcations between HIV infection, symptomatic HIV infection, and AIDS give way to the notion that HIV-related disease is a "spectrum" of problems beginning with infection, this could change.

Exclusion or Limitation of Benefits. Many but not all states closely regulate the coverage of health-insurance policies. Attempts so far to entirely exclude AIDS from coverage have not been successful, but it is by no means clear that they will not eventually succeed. Companies may also try to limit the total benefits paid for AIDS-related treatment.

Most insurance policies specifically refuse to pay for experimental treatments. However, not all new treatments are necessarily experimental. The Food and Drug Administration says its own approved drug-labeling regulations are not meant to proscribe medical practice, so if a new treatment is accepted by the local medical community, it may be possible to argue that the treatment is not experimental. Insurance company decisions on this need not be passively accepted.

REFERENCES

1. Weiss HW. Estate planning. In: Rubenfeld AR, ed. AIDS legal guide, 2nd ed. New York: Lambda Legal Defense and Education Fund, 1987; (9):1-5.
2. Scherzer M. Insurance. In: Dalton HL, Burris S, eds. AIDS and the law: a guide for the public. New Haven: Yale University Press, 1987:185-200.
3. Scherzer M. Insurance. In: Rubenfeld AR, ed. AIDS legal guide, 2nd ed. New York: Lambda Legal Defense and Education Fund, 1987; (5):1-8.

Political Issues Related to HIV Disease

Linda M. Udall, M.P.H., and George W. Rutherford, M.D.

Political concerns and decisions affect the HIV epidemic at many different levels. The opinions of political leaders guide public perceptions about individuals and communities affected by the epidemic, influence strategies for preventing HIV disease, control the funding of research, education, and health-care services, and affect the balance between efforts to control HIV disease and other major public-health concerns. AIDS-related legislation has been enacted in every state and the District of Columbia. The federal Health Omnibus Programs Extension Act of 1988 created a National Commission on AIDS to succeed the Presidential Commission created by former President Reagan in 1987. These and other efforts are evidence of a patchwork national strategy to confront HIV disease.[1]

Despite broad educational campaigns nationwide, fear of and open discrimination against persons with HIV infection and AIDS continues.[2] Education alone cannot change such intolerance, so many states and municipalities have enacted legislation that protects persons with HIV infection from discrimination. At the federal level, the Presidential Commission on the HIV Epidemic recommended national antidiscrimination legislation.[3] In spite of public-health and legal professionals' consensus on the importance of such legislation, there remains much political division and debate about what type of federal legislation is appropriate.

Public-health officials and legislative leaders have worked together to develop policies and laws to protect the confidentiality of persons with AIDS and HIV infection[1]; almost half of the states have passed legislation protecting the confidentiality of HIV-related information. Legislation varies widely in the issues addressed and the extent of protection offered. Issues include guaranteeing anonymity for those seeking HIV antibody testing; limiting disclosures of information in medical charts; limiting the use of HIV antibody test results for insurance purposes; and protecting the identity of individuals who provide information for partner notification. The purpose of these measures is to safeguard individual rights and to encourage infected or at-risk persons to seek medical care and counseling. But not all state and federal legislation protects the rights of the infected. Some states have passed laws imposing compulsory screening and subsequent segregation of persons (e.g., prisoners) who test positive for HIV.

Political influence clearly affects the development of AIDS prevention programs. For example, recent studies indicate that needle-exchange programs may be reasonable strategies for preventing HIV transmission among intravenous drug users,[4] but efforts to implement these programs have met with social, legal, and political resistance. Similarly, conservative federal and state legislation has restricted the ability of health educators to develop explicit prevention messages.

Finally, the impact of political opinion on the HIV epidemic is reflected in federal, state, and local funding for research, prevention, and health-care services for persons affected by the epidemic. Competition for resources among various governmental programs, public perceptions of the need for funding, and accessibility (or inaccessibility) of advocacy groups to policy makers all contribute to decisions about allocations to combat HIV disease.[5]

REFERENCES

1. Gostin LO. Public health strategies for confronting AIDS. Legislative and regulatory policy in the United States. JAMA 1989; 261:1621-30.
2. Blendon RJ, Donelan K. Discrimination against people with AIDS: the public's perspective. N Engl J Med 1988; 319:1022-6.
3. Report of the Presidential Commission on the Human Immunodeficiency Virus Epidemic. Washington, D.C.: U.S. Government Printing Office (Document 1988 0-214-701: QL 3), 1988.
4. Osborne J. AIDS prevention: issues and strategies. AIDS 1988; 2(Suppl 1):S229-S233.
5. Blewett N. Political dimensions of AIDS. AIDS 1988; 2(Suppl 1):S235-S238.

AIDS Public-Health Policy

Linda M. Udall, M.P.H., and George W. Rutherford, M.D.

■ SURVEILLANCE

For any disease, public-health strategy and policy decisions must be well grounded in accurate epidemiologic knowledge. With this knowledge, public-health strategy and policy can be formulated to (1) identify the disease-associated risk factors that can be manipulated to lower the incidence of the disease, and (2) determine the most acceptable and cost-effective ways to manipulate them. These data are largely derived from surveillance, the compilation and analysis of reports of a disease.

Surveillance is used to determine the basic distribution of a disease in a population. The reporting of AIDS is legally mandated in most states, most of which use the narrow Centers for Disease Control (CDC) definition of AIDS for reporting purposes.[1] The information to be collected in each case has been standardized by the CDC. Surveillance can be active or passive. Passive surveillance occurs when health departments wait for health-care providers to report cases they have diagnosed. Active surveillance occurs when health-department workers go into the community to review charts and records to ensure that all cases have been reported.[2] In San Francisco, for instance, the surveillance system is active. Laboratory and pathology reports at major hospitals are reviewed weekly, and any disease indicative of AIDS is noted. Each case is then reviewed with the diagnosing physician.

Almost all AIDS cases fit into classic risk groups. However, early in the epidemic before these groups had been identified, a great deal of misunderstanding and fear existed about the disease and the speed with which it spread. With accurate and timely surveillance data, it became clear that AIDS was generally confined to the now recognized incidence groups. These data from epidemiologic studies provided the basis for early intervention and policy decisions. In addition, the first reports of AIDS among hemophiliacs, transfusion recipients, and children of high-risk mothers were made through the existing surveillance systems and led to strategies to control transfusion-associated and perinatal transmission.[3]

■ HIV ANTIBODY TESTING

In 1985, an enzyme-linked immunosorbent assay (ELISA) to detect antibody to human immunodeficiency virus (HIV) was licensed. Because the virus has been cultured from the lymphocytes of between 60 percent and 80 percent of individuals with confirmed positive antibody tests, for public-health policy purposes a positive antibody test is considered synonymous with infection and infection synonymous with infectiousness.

The sensitivity of the HIV ELISA antibody test is equal to the proportion of patients who have positive confirmatory HIV antibody tests, such as the Western blot or immunofluorescence antibody assay (IFA), and the specificity equal to that with negative confirmatory tests. With repeated ELISA tests, the sensitivity and specificity is extremely high, ranging from 95 to over 99 percent.[4,5]

■ SCREENING

The usefulness of a test for screening populations must take into account the prevalence of the disease in the population as well as the specificity of the test. The positive predictive value of any test is the probability of the existence of the disease, given a positive test. No matter how high the accuracy of a test, in a population in which no disease exists, all positive tests will be false positives, and the positive predictive value will be zero. In a population in which everyone has the disease, there will be no false positives; all positive tests will be true positives, and the positive predictive value will be 100 percent.[5]

Because of these factors, before a recommendation for screening is made, it is important to consider not only the accuracy (sensitivity and specificity) of the test but also the prevalence of the disease. The widespread use of screening in populations in which the prevalence of HIV infection is extremely low will result in many people being falsely labeled as positive. Thus, premarital screening of low-risk individuals will identify mostly false positives, although in some situations, the lower predictive value associated with screening low-prevalence populations (such as blood donors) can be tolerated to protect the public health. On the other hand, in populations in which the prevalence of HIV infection is high, the probability of a test result being correct is much higher.

The ELISA was developed and licensed to screen blood donations for HIV infection. When the test was first licensed, health officers were concerned that individuals in high-risk groups would donate blood to obtain a test. Because of the existence of a small percentage of false-negative results, some of these donations from high-risk group members could get into the blood supply. Therefore, alternative test sites were set up so that a person could be tested in a situation that provided complete confidentiality and, in many cases, anonymity. These alternative test locations are now viewed not only as testing facilities per se, but more importantly, as useful sites at which the education and counseling of members of high-incidence groups take place and where risk reduction is encouraged.

Controversy exists about the use of antibody testing outside of blood banks. People in high-incidence groups who are not engaging in activities that transmit the disease feel they have no reason to be tested. Some members of these groups feel that the test would provide them with no useful information and could cause serious psychological trauma. In addition, because they belong to groups historically oppressed, they fear that their names will be placed on a list that will be used to discriminate against them or that a positive test will prevent them from obtaining insurance. On the other hand, others argue that individuals in high-incidence groups who are placing themselves or others at risk of infection should know their antibody status in order to break through their denial and help to limit transmission of the virus.[6]

Screening is a potentially useful tool in assisting in the prevention of perinatal transmission of the disease. Women in high-incidence groups have been advised to be tested so that they can make informed decisions about becoming pregnant or whether to continue or terminate an existing pregnancy.[7,8] Antibody screening may also prove effective for identifying individuals infected through heterosexual contact.[9]

■ INTERVENTION PROGRAMS

The control and eventual eradication of AIDS ultimately depend on eliminating the sexual, parenteral, and vertical transmission of HIV disease. Intervention strategies must be effective at many different levels in order to achieve these goals. To date, a variety of public-health measures have been successful in decreasing transmission of HIV in the United States. These include screening of blood and blood products, intensive education and outreach about AIDS and HIV infection to gay and bisexual men, anonymous HIV antibody testing and counseling programs, and street outreach to other at-risk populations such as intravenous drug users (IVDUs).[11,12,14]

Intervention strategies should strive to protect the public health with as little infringement of individual rights as possible. Most traditional public-health interventions limit individual freedoms to a certain extent. Gostin points out that "[when] the statute infringes on a fundamental right, such as liberty, the state must demonstrate compelling interest and show that the means used are the least-restrictive necessary to accomplish that statutory objective."[10] The law protects the rights of the individual to autonomy and self-determination, but traditionally children, the mentally ill and mentally retarded, and those harboring contagious diseases have been excluded from this protection. Intervention programs must assure that the confidentiality of patient information is protected and that information identifying infected individuals is used for public-health purposes only and not for unauthorized disclosure.

Information and Education.   Several long-term prospective studies report a dramatic decline in the number of gay and bisexual men newly infected with HIV in San Francisco, from 20 percent of study subjects in 1982 to only 3 percent by 1984.[15] This is evidence that prevention messages combined with strong social support can be extraordinarily effective in preventing transmission of HIV. Educational efforts designed to achieve behavior change have had varied success in other at-risk populations. Evidence indicates that they must be tailored to specific at-risk populations' cultural values and normative beliefs, social and political environment, and other influences that affect individual behavior change (including an individual's own perceived risk).

Even when education is done on a one-to-one basis (for example, street outreach programs), changes in behavior are not easy to achieve. For example, education alone has done little to convince drug users to abstain from drug use, reduce needle-sharing practices, or increase use of bleach to clean needles.[16] Evaluation of existing educational interventions and research on new strategies are essential for the future. Such evaluations must assess the qualitative impact (i.e., actual behavior change) that occurs after, but not before, education so that resources can be used for the most appropriate strategies for specific communities. While both population-specific and general AIDS education campaigns are important, these must be combined with a number of other interventions to stop the transmission of HIV infection.[12]

Public-Health Interventions.   While there is as yet no vaccine or cure for HIV disease, remarkable developments have already occurred in caring for and treating persons with HIV infection. With recently available laboratory tests to help stage disease and the newly acquired ability to diagnose and treat certain opportunistic infections (and possibly HIV infection itself before the onset of symptoms), early intervention has become the standard of care. HIV antibody testing is increasingly seen as part of early diagnosis and treatment and less as a tool of behavior change.

Partner notification or contact tracing, a traditional medical surveillance strategy, may have an increasingly important role as part of a comprehensive HIV disease prevention and control program. A voluntary program that ensures confidentiality, implemented in an environment where the necessary support services are available to index patients and their partners, may contribute significantly to preventing HIV transmission and reducing the morbidity and mortality associated with it.[17,18] Contact tracing remains expensive; in high-incidence populations such as San Francisco's gay male communities, it is also logistically difficult. Its impact on population-wide seroincidence or behavior change must therefore be carefully evaluated before committing significant funds to its use.

Isolation has been used in the past to control certain communicable diseases.[13] In most cases, these diseases were short-lived, amenable to treatment, and transmitted through air, food, or water. With HIV infection, none of these characteristics apply. Isolation for control of HIV transmission is not scientifically justified and is logistically impossible.

Biomedical Interventions.   Biomedical interventions that may prove useful in public-health strategies include: (1) the development of an anti-HIV vaccine; (2) the development of nontoxic anti-HIV drugs that not only prolong survival but also decrease viral shedding and infectivity in early HIV disease; and (3) the evaluation of the use of post-exposure anti-HIV drugs (e.g., following needlestick injuries or rapes). At present, post-exposure use of zidovudine (AZT) is unproved; it will take large numbers of exposures and many years of gathering data to establish whether it is effective in preventing HIV disease.

Other examples of current biomedical interventions are blood- and tissue-screening for HIV prior to transfusion or transplantation and heat inactivation of Factors VIII and IX. Treatment-based interventions that control cofactors associated with sexual transmission of HIV also function as HIV prevention programs (e.g., treatment and prevention of sexually transmitted diseases that cause genital ulcers, such as syphilis and chancroid[16,19,20]). Increasingly, such interventions are based less on creating behavior change and more on providing prophylaxis and treatment.

■ PREVENTING PARENTERAL TRANSMISSION

Preventing and slowing transmission of HIV through shared intravenous (IV) injection equipment can be accomplished in several ways: (1) avoiding IV drug use entirely; (2) treating IV drug addiction; (3) stopping the use of shared injection equipment entirely; and (4) stopping the use of shared, unsterilized injection equipment. Preventing drug use (especially IV drug use) and treating IV drug users should be the cornerstones of any control program. Providing ready access to drug treatment removes both susceptible (HIV-uninfected) and infected individuals from the pool transmitting the infection. A narrower form of this strategy provides essentially same-day access to methadone treatment for any heroin user who wants it, thereby trading persistent dependence on methadone and the possibility of some continued IV drug use for decreased frequency of use of needles and, presumably, for decreased exposure to HIV.[21] However, this approach does not address other types of IV drug use common among IVDUs — for example, cocaine and methamphetamines. Treating IV drug use on demand is expensive and may require new facilities in many areas.

Other approaches can decrease exposure to HIV even though IV drug use continues. Ready access to new needles and syringes reduces IVDUs' risk of exposure to infectious needles.[21-23] There are several major problems with this approach: (1) needle/syringe exchange elicits strong negative political reactions; (2) it does not address the social aspect of needle-sharing among IVDUs; and (3) critics have suggested that it may increase IV drug use by making injection equipment more readily available. Recent experience has not borne out this last possibility,[22] however. Another approach is to teach IVDUs to sterilize injection equipment before use.[24] Both needle-exchange and needle-sterilization involve intensive one-on-one health education and condom distribution to prevent both parenteral and sexual transmission of HIV.[21,25]

Since 1985, transfusion- and hemophilia-associated HIV transmission have been controlled through comprehensive screening of blood donations and heat-treating of Factors VIII and IX.[26,27] Although these measures have all but eliminated HIV transmission in blood, a problem remains in notifying persons who have already received infected blood. In San Francisco, a two-tiered approach is used. At the first level, infected donors are identified through ongoing screening, AIDS case reporting, investigation of a transfusion-associated AIDS case, and voluntary reports to the blood bank.[28] Recipients are notified after a donor has been identified as HIV-infected. At the second level, several hospitals have notified all recipients who received blood products between 1979 and 1985 that they may have received HIV-infected blood. They are asked to be tested. In practice, however, this has not been a highly efficient means of identifying infected recipients.[29]

■ PREVENTING VERTICAL TRANSMISSION

Vertically transmitted HIV infection can be slowed by preventing HIV infection in women and their sexual partners and by preventing pregnancy in HIV-infected women. If (as some have suggested) pregnancy may be associated with more rapid progression, then preventing pregnancy may also decrease HIV-related morbidity.[30,31] Counseling and testing at-risk women before they become pregnant requires a broad-based program that coordinates a variety of clinical facilities (e.g., family planning clinics, drug treatment clinics, private physicians' offices, and sexually transmitted disease clinics). While preventing pregnancy among HIV-infected women is the major strategy for preventing vertical transmission of HIV, some studies suggest that the risk of vertical transmission during pregnancy is variable — at its smallest when the mother is still asymptomatic and at its greatest when she is in the later stages of her HIV infection.[32] Thus, if an HIV-infected woman wanting a child became pregnant early in her infection rather than late, her chance of bearing a non-HIV-infected baby would be greatest. Once pregnant, women at risk of infection, and possibly all women in high-prevalence areas, should be urged to be tested. If found to be infected, they should be carefully counseled about their infection and their options for continuing or terminating pregnancy. The emphasis of any program for controlling vertically transmitted HIV infection should be placed on identifying and counseling HIV-infected women before pregnancy occurs.[7,33]

REFERENCES

1. Centers for Disease Control. Revision of the case definition of acquired immunodeficiency syndrome for national reporting — United States. MMWR 1985; 34:1-30, 373-5.
2. Lilienfeld AM. Foundations of epidemiology. New York: Oxford University Press, 1976:112-42.

3. Goedert JJ, Blattner WA. The epidemiology of AIDS and related conditions. In: De Vita VT Jr, Hellman S, Rosenberg SA, eds. AIDS: etiology, diagnosis, treatment, and prevention. Philadelphia: J.B. Lippincott, 1985.

4. Fletcher RH, Fletcher SW, Wagner EH. Clinical epidemiology — the essentials. Baltimore: Williams & Wilkins, 1982:46-56.

5. Centers for Disease Control. Update: Public Health Service workshop on human T-lymphotropic virus type III antibody testing — United States. MMWR 1985:477-8.

6. Centers for Disease Control. Additional recommendations to reduce sexual and drug abuse-related transmission of human T-lymphotropic virus type III/lymphadenopathy-associated virus. MMWR 1986; 35:152-5.

7. Centers for Disease Control. Recommendations for assisting in the prevention of perinatal transmission of human T lymphotropic virus type III/lymphadenopathy-associated virus. MMWR 1985; 34:721-6, 731-2.

8. San Francisco Department of Public Health. Control of perinatally transmitted human T-lymphotropic virus type III/lymphadenopathy-associated virus infection and care of infected mothers, infants, and pre-school-aged children. San Francisco Epidemiologic Bulletin 1986; 2(Suppl 1).

9. Echenberg DF. A new strategy to prevent the spread of AIDS among heterosexuals. JAMA 1985; 2:129-30.

10. Gostin L. Acquired immune deficiency syndrome (AIDS): a review of science, health policy, and law. In: Witt MD, ed. AIDS and patient management: legal, ethical, and social issues. Owing Mills: National Health Publishing, 1986.

11. Osborn JE. AIDS prevention: issues and strategies. AIDS 1988; 2(Suppl 1):S229-S233.

12. Report of the second Public Health Service AIDS Prevention and Control Conference. Public Health Rep 1988; 103(Suppl 1):1-109.

13. Brandt AM. No magic bullet: a social history of venereal disease in the United States since 1880. New York: Oxford University Press, 1985.

14. Coates TJ, Stall RD, Catania JA, Kegeles SM. Behavioral factors in the spread of HIV infection. AIDS 1988; 2(Suppl 1):S239-S246.

15. Hessol NA, Lifson AR, O'Malley PM, et al. Prevalence, incidence, and progression of human immunodeficiency virus infection in homosexual and bisexual men in hepatitis B vaccine trials, 1978-1988. Am J Epidemiol (in press).

16. Cates W, Bowen GS. Education for AIDS prevention: not our only voluntary weapon. Am J Public Health 1989; 79:871-4.

17. World Health Organization. Consensus statement from consultation on partner notification for prevention of HIV transmission. Geneva: World Health Organization, 1989. (WHO/GPA/INF/89.3.)

18. Rutherford GW, Woo JM. Contact tracing and the control of human immunodeficiency virus infection. JAMA 1988; 259:3609-10.

19. Holmberg SD, Horsburgh CR Jr, Ward JW, Jaffe HW. AIDS commentary: biologic factors in the sexual transmission of human immunodeficiency virus. J Infect Dis 1989; 160:116-25.

20. World Health Organization. Consensus statement from consultation on sexually transmitted diseases as a risk factor for HIV transmission. Geneva: World Health Organization, 1989. (WHO/GPA/INF/89.1.)

21. Report of the second Public Health Service AIDS Prevention and Control Conference. Report of the work-group on intravenous drug abuse. Public Health Rep 1988; 103 (Suppl 1):66-71.

22. Buning EC, van Brussel GH, van Santen G. Amsterdam's drug policy and its implications for controlling needle sharing. Natl Inst Drug Abuse Res Monogr Ser 1988; 80:59-74.

23. Stimson GV. Injecting equipment exchange schemes in England and Scotland. Natl Inst Drug Abuse Res Monogr Ser 1988; 80:89-99.

24. Newmeyer JA. Why bleach? Development of a strategy to combat HIV contagion among San Francisco intravenous drug users. Natl Inst Drug Abuse Res Monogr Ser 1988; 80:151-9.

25. Brown LS Jr, Primm BJ. Sexual contacts of intravenous drug abusers: implications for the next spread of the AIDS epidemic. J Natl Med Assoc 1988; 80:651-6.

26. Pindyck J, Waldman A, Zang E, et al. Measures to decrease the risk of acquired immunodeficiency syndrome transmission by blood transfusion. Evidence of volunteer blood donor cooperation. Transfusion 1985; 25:3-9.

27. Survey of non-U.S. hemophilia treatment centers for HIV seroconversions following therapy with heat-treated factor concentrates. MMWR 1987; 36:121-4.

28. Samson S, Busch M, Ward J, et al. Identification of HIV-infected transfusion recipients: the utility of cross-referencing previous donor records with AIDS case reports. Transfusion (in press).

29. Donegan E, Johnson D, Remedios V, Cohen S. Mass notification of transfusion recipients at risk for HIV infection. JAMA 1988; 260:922-3.

30. Mother-to-child transmission of HIV infection. The European Collaborative Study. Lancet 1988; 2:1039-43.

31. Selwyn PA, Schoenbaum EE, Davenny K, et al. Prospective study of human immunodeficiency virus infection and pregnancy outcomes in intravenous drug users. JAMA 1989; 261:1289-94.

32. Piot P, Plummer FA, Mhalu FS, et al. AIDS: an international perspective. Science 1988; 239:573-9.

33. Rutherford GW, Oliva GE, Grossman M, et al. Guidelines for the control of perinatally transmitted human immunodeficiency virus infection and care of infected mothers, infants and children. West J Med 1987; 147:104-8.

Policies Related to Intravenous Drug Use

Richard E. Chaisson, M.D., and Merle A. Sande, M.D.

The epidemic of AIDS and human immunodeficiency virus (HIV) infection in intravenous drug users raises a series of important public-health policy issues concerning the management of drug addiction. The major focus of AIDS control in this risk group is the prevention of HIV transmission from infected to uninfected individuals. This goal requires efforts to keep uninfected drug users or potential drug users from becoming exposed to HIV, and measures to prevent infected drug users from engaging in behaviors that place uninfected persons at risk of transmission. A secondary goal of public preventive policies is to protect infected drug users from additional exposures that might increase the likelihood of developing clinical disease, although such exposures are largely speculative at present.

Based on estimates of seroprevalence from New York, New Jersey, and California, as many as 20 percent to 30 percent of all IV drug users nationwide are infected with HIV.[1-3] Because the prevalence of infection differs by geographic area, the development of effective interventions requires taking into consideration local rates of infection and drug use patterns. Approximately one million persons in the United States are intravenous drug users,[4] and the turnover in this population may be as high as 25 percent per year. Intervention programs will have to take into account both the large numbers and heterogeneous nature of drug users and the flux in drug using populations.

■ PREVENTION OF TRANSMISSION TO UNINFECTED DRUG USERS

For the majority of addicts who are uninfected, prevention of transmission is the most critical aspect of AIDS control. Several important strategies are necessary to halt the spread of HIV in this population.[5] The primary risk behaviors promoting transmission of HIV in IV drug users are sharing of needles, syringes, and other injection paraphernalia and injection in shooting galleries. Clearly, frequent drug injection intensifies these risks. Prevention strategies must specifically focus on these risk behaviors. The primary level of prevention is to divert individuals at risk from using needles. Many persons who ingest drugs by other routes (e.g., smoking, swallowing) may progress to IV use at some future point. Drug treatment programs and educational campaigns that arrest drug use at this stage may prevent exposure to HIV.

Several obstacles make this goal difficult to achieve. First, persons at risk of becoming IV drug users are frequently outside of conventional social and community networks and may be difficult to reach with educational messages. Second, persons at risk may be functionally illiterate and may not respond to print media. In addition, many of these individuals are members of ethnic minorities who may not trust or consider relevant educational information provided by the public health establishment. Finally, even if preventive educational messages do come across to this population, peer pressures to begin IV drug use may exceed the desire for self-preservation. A number of pilot projects are under way that are attempting to reach this particularly vulnerable group.

For drug users who are already injecting but uninfected, prevention of HIV infection begins with the treatment of drug addiction. Methadone remains the primary modality for the treatment of opiate addiction. Acute methadone detoxification and chronic methadone maintenance can be employed to treat addiction and prevent injection. Although compliance with treatment and continued drug injection while on treatment are serious problems connected with the use of methadone, long-term success has been demonstrated in a substantial proportion of addicts treated with this agent.

Availability of approved methadone treatment positions, with drug counseling, medical monitoring, and some vocational training, continues to be a major policy problem. Waiting lists are long for methadone maintenance or detoxification programs in many American cities and entry can take many months. Expansion of treatment positions would reduce delays in initiating therapy and would thereby diminish the risk of infection for addicts at risk. The cost of methadone maintenance, approximately $3,000 per year per slot, is considerably less than the cost of treating AIDS, which is estimated at $40,000 to $150,000 per case (DesJarlais DC and Friedman SR: unpublished data). Unfortunately, public funds for substance-abuse services are generally allocated independently of funds for medical treatment of AIDS patients, and the connection between AIDS prevention and drug treatment may not be appreciated by policy-makers.

Therapeutic residential communities are another modality that may successfully treat drug addiction. These programs rely on peer support, a structured environment, and individual and group therapy to modify behavior in addicts. Such programs are resource intensive and have a higher dropout rate than methadone programs.[6] Ideally, both therapeutic communities and methadone maintenance can be used to treat addicts who wish to stop using drugs. No addict who seeks treatment should be turned away or prevented from beginning therapy promptly.

Despite compelling reasons to do so, many drug users are unable or unwilling to stop injecting drugs. Prevention in these individuals rests with strong and effective education concerning risk behaviors that promote infection. Needle and syringe sharing are the major risks for infection, and addicts who continue to inject *must be told not to share paraphernalia*. Needle sharing is promoted by both cultural norms among drug users and by legal and economic factors that limit the supply of sterile equipment. For example, in most American cities where IV drug use is common, the possession of a needle or syringe for nonmedical purposes is illegal. Consequently, drug addicts are unwilling to carry these items on their persons and will share equipment when they gather to use drugs. Decriminalization of needle and syringe possession may help to prevent sharing of drug paraphernalia. A more controversial step is to provide sterile syringes and needles to addicts directly. This approach is used by health officials in Amsterdam and has been proposed by others.[7] The impact of this strategy on AIDS prevention is unproved at present, although rates of hepatitis B in Amsterdam have not changed since the adoption of the needle program several years ago. Conversely, the prevalence of drug addiction has not increased subsequent to the introduction of free needles, nor has the frequency of needlestick injuries to the general public from carelessly discarded needles. Several public-health agencies in the United States are considering controlled trials of dispensing free needles to addicts on an exchange basis; used equipment would be returned for clean equipment weekly, and serologic monitoring would be carried out to assess efficacy.

Some drug users will continue to share needles and syringes despite the availability of sterile equipment and educational attempts to reduce high-risk behavior. These individuals may be extremely difficult to reach and may be refractory to intervention. However, an attempt to advise such addicts on needle sterilization may be beneficial. A number of commonly available substances, such as household bleach, isopropyl alcohol, and hydrogen peroxide, are known to kill HIV in the laboratory.[8] No epidemiologic evidence exists to suggest that drug users who sterilize used needles are at lower risk of infection than those who do not. Moreover, it is inconceivable that laboratory conditions resulting in viral killing can be faithfully reproduced in the field by addicts sharing drugs and equipment. Nevertheless, addicts who share needles should be informed that needle sterilization with one of these agents may diminish the risk of infection. It should be made clear, however, that cessation of parenteral drug use is the only completely effective method to eliminate the risk of HIV infection due to drug use.

■ MANAGEMENT OF INFECTED IV DRUG USERS

For drug users who are already infected but clinically well, the strategies enumerated above are equally important to prevent spread of the virus. In fact, most infected addicts will be unaware that they carry the virus, and the health professionals who deal with them will be likewise uninformed. Consequently, all addicts should be presumed to be seropositive for public-health purposes.

Some addicts will know their serologic status from alternate-site testing, research screening projects, or clinical screening by a physician. For individuals who are known to be seropositive, more aggressive interventions are appropriate. These individuals should be informed of the likelihood of their transmitting HIV to fellow addicts if they share injection equipment, and should be strongly encouraged to begin or continue drug treatment. Special accommodations should be made for infected users within the substance abuse system. In San Francisco, for example, seropositive addicts are given priority entry into methadone programs and are not required to make copayments for treatment. Tracking systems by public-health departments may be effective in assuring follow-up of seropositive drug users and in encouraging infected persons to be compliant with drug treatment programs. Seropositive addicts should also be educated on risk-reduction methods for other behaviors. In particular, safer-sex guidelines should be taught and reinforced frequently.

Bearing children, particularly for seropositive women, should be discussed in detail. The CDC advises infected women to avoid pregnancy,[9] although this recommendation is not universally accepted. Vigorous family planning efforts to prevent unwanted pregnancies should be directed toward addicts. Early pregnancy detection programs to allow maximum flexibility in managing pregnancy should be part of the overall health care of female addicts.

In addition to posing a hazard to uninfected addicts, continued needle use and sharing by seropositive IV users should be considered dangerous to the infected individual. Several lines of evidence suggest that continued IV use increases the risk of developing illness in infected addicts. One unpublished cohort study of drug users in New York has demonstrated that seropositive addicts have higher rates of nonopportunistic infections, particularly infective endocarditis, than those who are seronegative (DesJarlais DC: unpublished data). Moreover, in New York City from 1978 to 1984, the death rate from community acquired pneumonias in drug addicts increased substantially, suggesting that impaired host responses to nonopportunistic pathogens may occur in persons infected with HIV.[10] Consequently, it is prudent to assume that seropositive addicts are at increased risk of becoming ill from exposures related to IV needle use and should be encouraged to abstain from drug use to prevent morbidity and mortality from such diseases.

■ USE OF ANTIBODY TESTS IN IV DRUG USERS

Much controversy surrounds the application of antibody testing to populations at risk. Mandatory screening of high risk groups serves no compelling public interest and may drive risk-group members away from the health-care system. Voluntary screening of IV drug users and others at increased risk of infection may be a useful adjunct to an AIDS-prevention program. Protection of confidentiality is an absolute prerequisite to antibody testing. This is best done by anonymous testing at alternative sites. When testing is done for clinical evaluation, results should be protected from unauthorized disclosure to anyone other than the medical staff attending the patient. Ancillary personnel in drug treatment programs should not have access to antibody results. In California, unauthorized disclosure of antibody results is a punishable offense.

Screening within drug treatment programs may be useful in several circumstances. First, in areas of low AIDS prevalence among drug users, screening will help assess the degree to which HIV has entered the community and will be useful in developing public-health control measures. Moreover, serial screening will enable authorities to track the growth of the epidemic. Second, in areas of moderate to high AIDS prevalence among drug users, screening may serve a clinical purpose of reinforcing appropriate behaviors among addicts at risk. Under no circumstances, however, should antibody testing be a prerequisite to entry into a drug treatment program or to the provision of clinical care.

REFERENCES

1. Spira TJ, DesJarlais DC, Bokos D, et al. HTLV-III/LAV antibody in intravenous drug users: comparison of high and low risk areas [Abstract]. In: The International Conference on the Acquired Immunodeficiency Syndrome: Abstracts. Philadelphia: American College of Physicians, 1985.

2. Weiss SH, Ginzburg HM, Goedert JJ, et al. Risk for HTLV-III exposure and AIDS among parenteral drug abusers in New Jersey [Abstract]. In: The International Conference on the Acquired Immunodeficiency Syndrome: Abstracts. Philadelphia: American College of Physicians, 1985.

3. Chaisson RE, Onishi R, Moss AR, et al. Prevalence of HTLV-III/LAV infection in heterosexual intravenous drug abusers in San Francisco [Abstract]. Paris: Proceedings of the Second International Conference on the Acquired Immunodeficiency Syndrome, 1986:119.

4. Ginzburg HM, Weiss SH, MacDonald MG, Hubbard RL. HTLV-III exposure among drug users. Cancer Res 1985; 45(Suppl):4605S-4608S.

5. Marmor M, DesJarlais DC, Friedman SR, et al. The epidemic of acquired immunodeficiency syndrome (AIDS) and suggestions for its control in drug abusers. J Substance Abuse Tr 1984; 1:237-47.

6. Simpson DD. Treatment for drug abuse: follow up outcomes and length of time spent. Arch Gen Psych 1981; 38:875-9.

7. Bruning EC, Coutinho RA, Van Brusser GHA, et al. Preventing AIDS in drug addicts in Amsterdam. Lancet 1986; 1:1435.

8. Resnick L, Veren K, Salahuddin SZ, et al. Stability and inactivation of HTLV-III/LAV under clinical and laboratory environments. JAMA 1986; 255:1887-91.

9. Centers for Disease Control. Recommendations for assisting in the prevention of perinatal transmission of human T lymphotropic virus type III/lymphadenopathy-associated virus and acquired immunodeficiency syndrome. MMWR 1985; 34:721-31.

10. DesJarlais DC, Friedman SR, Hopkins W. Risk reduction for AIDS among intravenous drug users. Ann Intern Med 1985; 103:755-9.

Policies Related to Prisoners

Elizabeth Kantor, M.D.

■ PRISON POLICIES, REALITIES

Guidelines for the control of AIDS in jails and prisons differ widely. The U.S. Centers for Disease Control proposed the development of national guidelines for controlling AIDS in prisons in 1986. They were discouraged from preparing more than a draft, however, because of widely divergent approaches and practices and a lack of interest in accepting a standard approach. Correctional institutions welcomed the decision to leave prison AIDS policies in the hands of their local administrators.[1]

In the fall of 1987, the World Health Organization's Special Programme on AIDS held a consultation on prevention and control in prisons; it was attended by specialists from 26 nations. The consensus statement by this group recognized the risks of HIV transmission in prisons and recommended the following general approaches: (1) treatment of prisoners in a manner similar to other members of the community; (2) consideration of compassionate release for prisoners with AIDS; (3) nondiscriminatory practices relating to HIV infection; (4) provision of information on AIDS to staff as well as prisoners; and (5) informed consent and confidentiality in the event of HIV antibody testing.

All these practices could be enacted only if sufficient human and financial resources were available for preventing and treating AIDS without sacrificing other health services and activities.[2,7]

The American Medical Association and former President Reagan issued statements recommending the mandatory HIV testing of all state and federal prisoners, although they have not suggested how identified seropositive prisoners should be handled by the institutions.[3] Sixty percent of state systems responding to the National Institute of Justice survey reported pressure from governors, legislatures, the media, and the public to begin mass-screening programs. Many believed that mass screening would protect inmates and staff from disease.[3,4]

■ SCREENING

As of July 1, 1988, 13 American state prison systems screen entering inmates for HIV antibody.[5] The prison systems that mandate screening have been least affected by the epidemic.[5] Prisons reporting the vast majority of AIDS cases, on the other hand, have not adopted screening programs.[5] In prisons, unlike in the community, fearful inmates, guards, administrators, or health-care staff can demand and establish the quarantine of an individual with AIDS, ARC, or known HIV seropositivity, regardless of that individual's behavior or wishes. Privileges that have been denied to inmates in AIDS quarantine units include access to jobs, use of the law library, group recreation, and visits. Parole decisions have also been made on the basis of an inmate's HIV antibody status.

■ **HOSPITALIZATION OF HIV-INFECTED PRISONERS**

The prisoner with AIDS faces obstacles to care that do not exist in the community. Prison administrators are not financially equipped to provide a level of care equal to that in the community. Fixed institutional budgets have never before been challenged by an epidemic so costly to treat. Moreover, administrators' priorities rarely lean toward providing health care over other institutional functions.

Prisoners requiring transfer to public hospitals often must vie for scarce beds. These hospitals may be far from the urban centers where AIDS is most common, so prisoner-patients may have to rely upon care from a staff with little experience in HIV infection. Prisoners at community hospitals are guarded by correctional officers 24 hours a day. This surveillance adds substantially to hospital expenses, which the prison system is poorly prepared to finance.

■ **SURVIVAL TIME OF HIV-INFECTED PRISONERS**

A review of the first 200 AIDS deaths in the New York State prison system revealed that prisoners matched for risk factor and race survived less than half as long from diagnosis to death as did community AIDS patients. This finding challenges the generally held notion that the health status of the IVDU is better when he or she is in custody.[6]

■ **CONFIDENTIALITY**

In most prisons and jails, the identity of prisoners diagnosed with AIDS is communicated to custodial staff; issues of confidentiality are considered secondary. Few institutions protect patient confidentiality by informing correctional staff of necessary infection-control precautions; instead, they reveal prisoners' diagnoses.

■ **LEGAL ISSUES, CASES, AND PRECEDENT**

Prisoners have a constitutional right to health care that people on the "outside" do not have. Under the Eighth Amendment, inmates are entitled to a "safe and humane environment." This has been further defined as prohibiting "deliberate indifference to serious medical need" (Section 1983, Civil Rights Act of 1964). This standard of care, however, does not usually permit claims of malpractice or negligence.

Several cases have challenged prisons' AIDS policies. Prisoners in New York State claimed that segregating inmates with AIDS denied them social, rehabilitative, and recreational activities and that this denial violated their constitutional rights (*Cordero* v. *Coughlin* 607 F Supp. 9SD NY 1984). The court found that inmates have no constitutional right to freedom from segregation. In Oklahoma, a healthy HIV-seropositive inmate who was isolated alleged that he was denied equal protection (*Powell* v. *Department of Corrections*). Another New York case alleges inadequate and discriminatory medical care and other policies affecting AIDS patients (*Storms* v. *Coughlin*).

Conversely, in Oregon and New Jersey, inmates have filed suits demanding isolation of inmates with ARC or HIV infection from the general prison population.[8] Following a series of decisions that limited the rights of prisoners in cases involving HIV, two 1988 cases in New York and Wisconsin held that the right to privacy included protection against non-consensual disclosure of a prisoner's diagnosis. A third court ruling (in New York) held that the exclusion of a prisoner from a work-furlough program violated the equal protection clause of the Fourteenth Amendment.[9]

No cases have been filed alleging HIV transmission in a correctional institution. In Orange County, Florida, a correctional officer was compensated in an out-of-court settlement after being bitten by a seropositive inmate. The officer's HIV antibody status was not known.[10]

The imprisonment of persons with AIDS and HIV infection who knowingly expose someone to HIV is increasing in the United States. Statutes that create criminal sanctions against those who may transmit the virus or that penalize (or require testing of) persons for real or suspected HIV infection can be grouped into seven categories[11]: (1) mandatory HIV antibody testing of people charged with sex-related offenses or suspected of being drug users; (2) mandatory testing of people convicted of sex-related offenses or intravenous drug use; (3) intentional transmission of HIV to others; (4) increased charges or extended sentences for certain sex-related crimes if the defendant knowingly exposes someone to HIV; (5) mandatory testing as a condition of probation or parole; (6) laws aimed at special populations, such as mental patients, military personnel, prisoners, and persons in the county youth authority; and (7) quasi-criminal quarantine laws to segregate persons who are seropositive and considered "noncompliant."

Although some inmates with AIDS have been considered for early release, others have been held in prolonged custody because of their HIV-related disease or seropositivity. When mandatory HIV antibody screening of all federal prisoners was begun in 1987, U.S. Attorney General Edwin Meese stated that positive antibody status would be considered at parole hearings and might contribute to denying release from custody. In several counties, judges have offered to release prostitutes from custody in exchange for their agreeing to HIV antibody tests.[12] Other judges have sentenced prostitutes and others with known HIV infection to the maximum time in custody in order to protect potential sexual contacts from infection. A law enacted in Florida provides for 120 days of quarantine for "noncompliant" seropositive persons.[11]

In November 1988, California voters overwhelmingly approved an "AIDS" ballot initiative authored by the Sheriff of Los Angeles County, Sherman Block.[13] Proposition 96 provided for criminal and juvenile court-ordered involuntary testing for AIDS, AIDS-related conditions, and other communicable diseases. Anyone charged with certain sex offenses or assaults on peace officers, firefighters, or emergency medical personnel could be involuntarily tested if there was probable cause to believe that bodily fluids were possibly transferred. In addition, the initiative requires medical personnel in correctional facilities to report inmate exposure to such diseases and to notify personnel who come into contact with such inmates. The legislation will probably be challenged in the courts on the grounds that it violates rights to privacy and equal protection and that its provisions are not medically sound. Some medical personnel object to the requirement that they use their skills for non-medical purposes, i.e., collecting evidence rather than providing care.

■ APPENDIX: STATEMENT FROM THE CONSULTATION ON PREVENTION AND CONTROL OF AIDS IN PRISONS (WORLD HEALTH ORGANIZATION, GENEVA, 16–18 NOVEMBER 1987)

A Consultation on Prevention and Control of AIDS in Prisons was convened by the World Health Organization's Special Programme on AIDS from 16-

18 November 1987 in Geneva. A total of 37 specialists from 26 countries participated, including experts in public health, prison and medical administration, prisoner care, occupational health and safety, epidemiology and health policy.

INTRODUCTION

The Consultation addressed four key aspects of prevention and control of human immunodeficiency virus (HIV) infection and AIDS in prisons:

1. general principles regarding the provision of health care in prisons;
2. identification of HIV-infected prisoners and associated informed consent, confidentiality and counseling issues;
3. information and education needs of prison staff, prisoners and their families;
4. management approaches to care for asymptomatic HIV-infected prisoners and for those with AIDS-related complex (ARC) or AIDS.

The Consultation noted that there is a wide variation between and within different countries regarding:

1. the number of HIV-infected persons and persons with AIDS in prisons (generally reflecting the prevalence of HIV infection in the community);
2. the policies and practices adopted by prison administrations to control the spread of HIV infection;
3. the relative importance of the different HIV transmission modes;
4. the proportion of those convicted of crimes who are sentenced to imprisonment.

THE CONSULTATION DEVELOPED THE FOLLOWING CONSENSUS STATEMENT:

A. Control and prevention of HIV infection must be viewed in the context of the need to improve significantly overall hygiene and health facilities in prisons.

B. In many countries there may be substantial numbers of prison inmates who have a history of high-risk behaviours, such as:

- intravenous drug use;
- prostitution.

In addition, situational homosexual behaviour may occur as a consequence of heterosexual deprivation, characteristic of prison conditions. Prison authorities therefore have a special responsibility to inform all prisoners of the risk of HIV infection from such behaviours. Prisons provide an opportunity to inform and educate large numbers of persons who may have engaged, or may be likely to engage, in HIV high-risk behaviours. Many of these persons are unlikely to have received such education in the general community.

C. The general principles adopted by National AIDS Programmes should apply equally to prisons as to the general community. The policies of prison administrations should be developed in close cooperation with health authorities. The responsibility of prisons' medical services to provide independent advice in the interest of prisoners must be recognized. Prison policies should be clearly defined in guidelines available to the general public and should include the following concepts:

1. Prison administrations should recognize their responsibility to minimize HIV transmission in prison (and consequently in the general community when prisoners are released).

2. Prisoners should be treated in a manner similar to other members of the community, with the same right of access to:

    a. educational programs designed to minimize spread of the disease, including up-to-date information on AIDS and preventive measures;

    b. testing for HIV infection (serological testing) on prisoner request, with confidentiality of results, timely pre- and post-test counselling, and support from appropriately trained persons acceptable to the prisoner;

    c. medical, nursing, inpatient and outpatient services of the same quality as those for AIDS patients in the community at large;

    d. information on treatment programs and the freedom to refuse such treatment.

3. In addition, prisoners with AIDS should be considered for compassionate early release to die in dignity and freedom;

4. Prisoners should not be subjected to discriminatory practices relating to HIV infection or AIDS such as involuntary testing, segregation or isolation, except when required for the prisoner's own well-being.

5. All prison staff should receive up-to-date information and education on AIDS prevention and control in prisons, as part of broader training in occupational health and hygiene. Information on AIDS should include recognition of possible AIDS-associated conditions and guidance on the most humane management of HIV-infected prisoners.

D. Homosexual acts, intravenous drug abuse and violence may exist in prisons in some countries to varying degrees. Prison authorities have the responsibility to ensure the safety of prisoners and staff, and to ensure that the risk of HIV spread within prison is minimized. In this regard, prison authorities are urged to implement appropriate staff and inmate education and drug-user rehabilitation programmes. Careful consideration should be given to making condoms available in the interest of disease prevention. It is also recognized that, within some lower-security correctional facilities, the practicability of making sterile needles available is worthy of further study.

E. Decisions regarding testing and/or screening should be considered in the context of informed consent, the ability to maintain confidentiality and the provision of positive assistance to affected individuals.

F. The WHO projections for growth in HIV infection and the numbers of ARC and AIDS cases suggest that in the coming years prison and health authorities will need to devote considerable additional human and financial resources to the management of AIDS in prisons. This should not be at the expense of other health-related activities in prisons. Rather, AIDS prevention and control programmes in prisons should be regarded as part of the broader national AIDS control measures and receive resources accordingly.

G. Governments may also wish to review their penal admission policies, particularly where drug abusers are concerned, in the light of the AIDS epidemic and its impact on prisons.

THE CONSULTATION RECOMMENDED THAT:

- the WHO Special Programme on AIDS draws the attention of countries to the consensus statement of this Consultation;

- countries be encouraged to include representation on their National AIDS Committees of prison medical services and prison administrations;

- the Special Programme on AIDS develop guidelines and strategies to evaluate the impact of AIDS prevention and control programs in prisons and include a report on prisons in its annual report on AIDS;

- WHO investigate, at the global level, means of fostering consideration of broader health management issues in prisons.

REFERENCES

1. No AIDS guidelines for prisons issued. CDC AIDS Weekly 1986:2.
2. Statement from the Consultation on Prevention and Control of AIDS in Prisons [Appendix]. Geneva: World Health Organization 1987; Appendix 1.
3. National policy on AIDS control. Chicago: American Medical Association, 1987.
4. Hammett TM. AIDS in correctional facilities: issues and options. 3rd ed. (prepublication copy). U.S. Department of Justice/National Institute of Justice, 1988.
5. Greenspan J. 1988 Survey. National Prison Project Journal. Summer, 1988.
6. Gido RL, Gaunay W. Update: acquired immune deficiency syndrome: a demographic profile of New York State inmate mortalities 1981-1986. NY State Commission of Correction, 1987.
7. WHO consensus statement on AIDS in prisons. Geneva, 16–18 November 1987.
8. Vaid U. AIDS in prison. American Civil Liberties Union National Prison Project Journal 1985; 6:1-5.
9. The Exchange. National Lawyers Guild. Issue 9. November, 1988.
10. Out of court settlement for jailer who claims AIDS risk. CDC AIDS Weekly 1986 (February 10):16.
11. Vermeulen M. The criminalization of the AIDS epidemic. The Exchange. National Lawyers Guild, San Francisco. Issue 8. July, 1988.
12. Prostitutes given shorter terms for AIDS tests. CDC AIDS Weekly 1986 (March 10):7.
13. Health and safety code section 199.95-199.98. AIDS public safety and testing disclosure (initiative statute).

10.2

Infection-Control Guidelines:
Health-Care Workers

10.2.1

General Approach to HIV Infection Control in Hospitals and Clinics

J. Louise Gerberding, M.D., and Merle A. Sande, M.D.

Human immunodeficiency virus (HIV) is transmitted by sexual contact with an infected partner, by inoculation with infected blood or blood products, and by perinatal transmission from infected mothers to their offspring. No evidence exists that the virus is transmitted by air, fecal-oral exposure, exposure to contaminated surfaces, or casual contact with an infected individual. The risk to health-care workers exposed to patients infected with HIV has been evaluated in several epidemiologic studies.[1-9,19] The risk from discrete parenteral exposure via needlestick inoculation with HIV-infected blood is approximately 0.4 percent and the risk from mucous membrane inoculation from open skin lesions is at least 10-fold lower. The cumulative professional risk to health-care workers repeatedly exposed over prolonged periods of time has not been completely assessed. Infection-control practices designed to minimize exposure to the virus in the health-care environment are imperative.[10-15]

A rational approach to infection control for HIV should be consistent with available epidemiologic evidence on the virus's transmissibility. The mechanisms of HIV transmission are similar to those of hepatitis B, but the hepatitis B virus is much more contagious.[16-18] Therefore, infection-control practices designed to prevent hepatitis B infection will also prevent HIV infection as well as infection with other blood-borne pathogens.

Current recommendations for preventing transmission of blood-borne pathogens are based on regarding the blood and other body fluids of all patients as potentially contaminated with contagious pathogens. These universal blood and body fluid precautions should be used regardless of whether infection has been diagnosed in a patient.

When this approach to infection control is adopted, screening for evidence of asymptomatic infection is neither necessary nor advocated in most health-care settings.[10] The federal Occupational Safety and Health Administration has created standards for safety in the health-care environment that are based on the concept of universal precautions. It is likely that most health-care institutions will utilize this infection-control strategy in the near future.

REFERENCES

1. Hirsch MS, Wormser GP, Schooley RT, et al. Risk of nosocomial infection with human T-cell lymphotropic virus III (HTLV-III). N Engl J Med 1985; 312:1-4.
2. Gerberding JL, Bryant-LeBlanc CE, Nelson K, et al. Risk of transmitting the human immunodeficiency virus, hepatitis B virus, and cytomegalovirus to health care workers exposed to patients with AIDS and AIDS-related conditions. J Infect Dis 1987; 156:1-8.
3. Weiss SH, Saxinger WC, Rechtman D, et al. HTLV-III infection among health care workers: association with needlestick injuries. JAMA 1985; 254:2089-93.

4. McCray E, Cooperative Needlestick Surveillance Group. Occupational risk of the acquired immunodeficiency syndrome among health care workers. N Engl J Med 1986; 314:1127-32.

5. Henderson DK, Saah AJ, Zak BJ, et al. Risk of nosocomial infection with human T cell lymphotropic virus type III/lymphadenopathy associated virus in a large cohort of intensively exposed health care workers. Ann Intern Med 1986; 104:644-7.

6. Kuhls TL, Viker S, Parris NB, et al. A prospective cohort study of the occupational risk of AIDS and AIDS-related infections in health care personnel. Clin Res 1986; 34:124A. abstract.

7. Gerberding JL, Bryant-LeBlanc CE, Greenspan D, et al. Risk to dentists from exposure to patients infected with the AIDS virus. New Orleans: Twenty-sixth Interscience Congress on Antimicrobial Agents and Chemotherapy, 1986:283.

8. Klein RS, Phelan J, Friedland GH, et al. Prevalence of antibodies to HTLV III/LAV among dental professionals. New Orleans: Twenty-sixth Interscience Congress on Antimicrobial Agents and Chemotherapy, 1986:283.

9. Flynn NM, Pollet SM, Van Horne JR, et al. Absence of HIV antibody among dental professionals exposed to infected patients. West J Med 1987; 146:439-42.

10. Gerberding JL, University of California—San Francisco Task Force on AIDS. Recommended infection-control policies for patients with human immunodeficiency virus infection: an update. N Engl J Med 1986; 315:1562-4.

11. Centers for Disease Control. Recommendations for prevention of HIV transmission in health-care settings. MMWR 1987; 36(Suppl 2):1S-18S.

12. Centers for Disease Control. 1988 Agent summary statement for human immunodeficiency virus and report on laboratory-acquired infection with human immunodeficiency virus. MMWR 1988; 37(Suppl 4):1S-22S.

13. Centers for Disease Control. Recommendations for preventing possible transmission of human T lymphotropic virus type III/lymphadenopathy-associated virus during invasive procedures. MMWR 1986; 35:221-3.

14. Centers for Disease Control. Recommended infection-control practices for dentistry. MMWR 1986; 35:237-42.

15. Centers for Disease Control. Update: human immunodeficiency virus infections in health-care workers exposed to blood of infected patients. MMWR 1987; 36:285-9.

16. Gerberding JL, Hopewell PC, Kaminsky LS, Sande MA. Transmission of hepatitis B without transmission of AIDS by accidental needlestick. N Engl J Med 1985; 312:56-7.

17. West DJ. The risk of hepatitis B infection among health professionals in the United States. Am J Med Sci 1984; 287:26-33.

18. Werner BJ, Grady GF. Accidental hepatitis B surface antigen positive inoculations: use of e antigen to estimate infectivity. Ann Intern Med 1982; 97:367-9.

19. Centers for Disease Control. Update: acquired immunodeficiency syndrome and human immunodeficiency virus infection among health-care workers. MMWR 1988; 37:229-34, 239.

Exposures to HIV in Patients and Laboratory Specimens

J. Louise Gerberding, M.D., and Merle A. Sande, M.D.

The universal blood and body fluid precautions outlined here summarize the current Centers for Disease Control (CDC) infection-control guidelines and the guidelines developed by the University of California, San Francisco, Task Force on AIDS for health-care workers with occupational exposures to HIV-infected patients or laboratory specimens.[1-4] These guidelines are consistent with standard infection-control practices appropriate for all patients, regardless of the probability of their being infected with HIV, hepatitis B, or other blood-borne pathogens. The following practices should be routinely employed by all health-care workers in treating all patients.

Handwashing. Careful handwashing with soap and water is an essential component of infection control. It should be performed before and after each patient contact and any time that contamination with potentially infective materials occurs.

Gloves. The use of disposable protective gloves is recommended if direct exposure to infected blood, secretions, excretions, other body fluids, or tissue specimens is anticipated. Gloves may provide an extra margin of safety by preventing direct contact with body fluids, but they are no substitute for handwashing and needlestick precautions. Health-care workers with open skin lesions, weeping dermatitis, or cutaneous wounds should be excused from patient-care activities until their condition resolves. Double-gloving should be employed when invasive surgical procedures are performed.

Gowns. Gowns or other protective garments should be worn when clothing is likely to be contaminated with blood, secretions, excretions, or other body fluids. Contaminated clothing or gowns should not be worn outside of patient-care or laboratory areas.

Masks and Goggles. Masks and protective eyewear should be used when splashes of saliva, respiratory secretions, or other body fluids can occur. Masks and goggles are routinely recommended for airway manipulations and endoscopic or dental procedures. The use of masks is also prudent in the presence of coughing patients suspected of having *Mycobacterium tuberculosis* infection or other respiratory infection until these infections are excluded as a diagnosis or rendered noncontagious by treatment. Patients with contagious pulmonary diseases should be assigned private rooms and should wear masks when leaving their hospital rooms.

Precautions for Preventing Needlestick Injuries. Needlestick injury is the most important source of nosocomial HIV infection. To prevent it, needles and other sharp instruments should be disposed of in puncture-resistant containers immediately after use. Needles should not be resheathed or otherwise manipulated. Needles should never be placed on beds, furniture, or in waste cans. Disposal containers should be located in emergency-room trauma rooms, on code-blue carts, in operating-room suites, and in other areas where needles are used. In the rare situation when needle recapping is necessary, a single-handed method (e.g., in which the needle cap is placed in a bracket, not held in one hand) or a recapping shield device (e.g., in which a shield device protects the hand holding the needle cap) should be used.

Laundry.   Linens and hospital garments should be placed in impervious bags and laundered using standard hospital procedures. Double-bagging is not necessary unless the outside of the bag is contaminated.

Waste Disposal.   Contaminated disposable items should be placed in waterproof bags and disposed of in accordance with local ordinances. Items saturated with body fluids, laboratory specimens, human and animal tissues, fluid-filled containers, and needles and other sharps should be decontaminated before disposal.

Sterilization and Disinfection.   Germicides that are registered by the U.S. Environmental Protection Agency as "sterilants" can be used for sterilization and high-level disinfection. Germicides that are "hospital disinfectants" and are mycobactericidal may also be used for high-level disinfection. These germicides are effective in killing HIV when used in appropriate concentrations for the recommended period.

All instruments should be cleaned before sterilization. Surgical instruments should be decontaminated (e.g., by soaking in an appropriate germicidal solution) after use and then sterilized.

Environmental Contamination.   Environmental surfaces and fomites should be washed and disinfected with a hospital disinfectant that is mycobactericidal. A freshly made solution of 1:100 dilution of 5.25 percent sodium hypochlorite (household bleach) is an effective germicide. A 1:10 dilution should be used for heavily contaminated items. Spills should be cleaned up before disinfection.

REFERENCES

1. Recommendations for prevention of HIV transmission in health-care settings. MMWR 1987(Suppl 2); 36:1S-18S.
2. Gerberding JL, University of California—San Francisco Task Force on AIDS. Recommended infection-control policies for patients with human immunodeficiency virus infection: an update. N Engl J Med 1986; 315:1562-4.
3. Acquired immunodeficiency syndrome (AIDS): precautions for clinical and laboratory staffs. MMWR 1982; 31:577-80.
4. 1988 agent summary statement for human immunodeficiency virus and report on laboratory-acquired infection with human immunodeficiency virus. MMWR 1988(Suppl 4); 37:1S-22S.

HIV and Operating Room Personnel

J. Louise Gerberding, M.D., and Merle A. Sande, M.D.

Operating room personnel, including physicians, anesthetists, nurses, housekeepers, and other assistants, should follow universal blood and body-fluid precautions.[1,2] These guidelines are designed to minimize exposure to pathogens, including blood-borne organisms such as the human immuno-deficiency virus (HIV), hepatitis B virus, and cytomegalovirus.

Preoperative testing of patients for infection-control purposes remains controversial and most authorities do not recommend it as a routine procedure. Selective pre-procedure testing for elective cases has been implemented in some institutions.[2] Identifying and labeling patients infected with HIV has not been proven effective in lowering the incidence of intraoperative exposures, and at least one study indicates the effect is not likely to be great if standard infection-control practices are already being followed.[5]

Surgeons and others in the operating room should be particularly conscientious about following the guidelines for needlestick precautions. New suture techniques (including the use of instruments instead of fingers for closing wounds, safer methods for passing instruments from person to person, and alternative approaches that minimize the use of sharps) are being evaluated as infection-control strategies. Double-gloving has been shown to prevent cutaneous hand exposures and is recommended by most authorities.[5] Increased use of waterproof gowns, boots, sleeves, and aprons is recommended. In addition, face shields that prevent facial and mucous membrane contamination are strongly advised in most operating room theaters.

Individuals sustaining accidental percutaneous injuries or splashes of potentially infected materials into mucous membranes should follow the recommended guidelines for treatment of accidental exposures.

Surgeons and other health-care workers with HIV infection or other blood-borne infections (such as hepatitis B) should be particularly careful to avoid accidental inoculation of infected materials into patients.[3,4] Blind suturing, use of steel wires and other hardware, and oral surgical procedures are believed to pose theoretical risks of HIV transmission. Extreme caution or even voluntary exclusion from cases where these procedures are required has been suggested by some authorities. Double-gloving may provide an additional increment of protection and is recommended. If a patient is accidentally exposed to blood or other body fluids from an infected health-care worker, the guidelines for treatment of accidental exposures should be followed.

REFERENCES

1. Recommendations for prevention of HIV transmission in health-care settings. MMWR 1987; 36(Suppl 2):1S-18S.
2. Gerberding JL, University of California—San Francisco Task Force on AIDS. Recommended infection-control policies for patients with human immunodeficiency virus infection: an update. N Engl J Med 1986; 315:1562-4.

3. Update: evaluation of human T lymphotropic virus type III/lymphadenopathy-associated virus infection in health care personnel — United States. MMWR 1985; 34:575-8.

4. Recommendations for preventing possible transmission of human T lymphotropic virus type III/lymphadenopathy-associated virus during invasive procedures. MMWR 1986; 35:221-3.

5. Gerberding JL, Littell C, Brown A, et al. Predictors of intraoperative blood exposures [Abstract]. V International Conference on AIDS. Montreal, 1989; M.D.O.14.

HIV and Delivery Room Personnel

Moses Grossman, M.D.

Universal blood and body-fluid precautions should be followed by all health-care workers in the delivery room, including physicians, anesthetists, nurses, housekeepers, and other assistants. Infection-control guidelines are designed to minimize exposure to most pathogens, including such blood-borne organisms as the human immunodeficiency virus (HIV), hepatitis B virus, and cytomegalovirus. In the delivery room, potentially infected fluids include blood of either maternal or fetal origin, amniotic fluid, the placenta, and membranes.

Mothers may be identified as having AIDS, as being seropositive for antibodies to HIV, as belonging to a high-risk group (e.g., an intravenous drug user or sexual contact of a person with AIDS or ARC) for HIV infection, or as having an unknown HIV status. All personnel who are likely to be exposed to blood or other body fluids from an infected or high-risk mother should be especially careful to follow universal precautions. Those exposed to a splash of potentially infectious material (e.g., during rupture of membranes or complicated deliveries) should also wear a mask and protective eyewear. Delivery room personnel should be conscientious about following guidelines for needle-stick precautions. The use of double gloves has not been proven to reduce the risk of transmission of blood-borne pathogens, but it is recommended elsewhere in this text. Individuals sustaining accidental percutaneous injuries or splashes of potentially infected materials into mucous membranes should follow the recommended guidelines for treatment of accidental exposures.

Contaminated linens and disposables, as well as blood and amniotic-fluid specimens, should be handled according to infection-control procedures. This includes handling placentas that may be routed for pathological examination.

The choice of a location for delivery (labor room versus delivery room) should be determined principally by obstetrical issues, but consideration should also be given to limiting contamination only to a single site (labor room). The labor room, delivery room, and all nondisposable instruments should be disinfected according to the hospital's infection-control guidelines.

HIV and Pathologists, Persons Performing Necropsies, and Morticians

J. Louise Gerberding, M.D., and Merle A. Sande, M.D.

Persons providing postmortem care to bodies infected with the human immunodeficiency virus (HIV) may have occupational exposure to infected body fluids. HIV transmission as a result of this type of occupational exposure has not been documented.

Potentially transmissible pathogens are not always diagnosed before death. All body fluids, tissues, secretions, and excretions in the pathology suite should therefore be regarded as potentially infectious. Universal blood and body-fluid precautions designed to prevent exposure to body fluids should be employed routinely by all personnel. These measures include wearing gloves during direct contact with body fluids, masks and protective eyewear when splash or splatter of body fluids is possible, and protective garments when clothing is likely to become contaminated.[1]

Disposable needles and other sharp instruments should be discarded in impervious plastic containers. Reusable equipment should be thoroughly washed and then decontaminated with a mycobactericidal germicide.

Precautions for preventing accidental exposures, including needlestick injuries, should be strictly enforced. Personnel sustaining accidental percutaneous exposures should follow the guidelines recommended for accidental exposures.

REFERENCES

1. Acquired immunodeficiency syndrome (AIDS): precautions for health care workers and allied professionals. MMWR 1983; 32:450-2.

HIV and Ophthalmologists, Opticians, and Ophthalmologic Care Providers

J. Louise Gerberding, M.D., and Merle A. Sande, M.D.

Human immunodeficiency virus (HIV) has rarely been isolated from tears,[1] and then only in extremely low concentration. There is currently no documented case of transmission of HIV by exposure to tears. It is therefore unlikely that occupational exposure to tears poses a risk of acquiring HIV.

Universal blood and body-fluid precautions designed to prevent direct contact with body fluids should be followed by all health-care workers, including ophthalmologists, opticians, and others performing ocular examinations.[2] Adherence to these guidelines will prevent transmission of all blood-borne and ocular pathogens, including hepatitis B virus, cytomegalovirus, herpes viruses, and HIV.

Hands should be washed with soap and water before and after contact with each patient. Gloves are recommended when direct contact with ocular tissues, tears, and other body fluids is anticipated. Gloves should be worn when there are cuts, scratches, or dermatologic lesions on the hands.

Instruments that come into direct contact with the eye, such as tonometers, should be cleaned and disinfected with a 5- to 10-minute exposure to one of the following solutions: (1) a fresh solution of 3 percent hydrogen peroxide; or (2) a fresh solution of sodium hypochlorite diluted 1:10; or (3) 70 percent ethanol; or (4) 70 percent isopropanol. The instrument should be thoroughly rinsed in tap water and dried before reuse.

Disinfection of trial contact lenses should be performed between each fitting. Hard lenses can be disinfected with a commercially available contact-lens disinfection system that is currently approved for soft contact lenses. Most hard lenses can also be disinfected by heat treatment (78–80°C for 10 minutes). Rigid gas-permeable lenses should be disinfected with the hydrogen peroxide system discussed above. Soft contact lenses used for fittings can be disinfected by heat or the above-mentioned hydrogen peroxide system. Surgical instruments should be cleaned and sterilized in accordance with existing standards.

Precautions for prevention of accidental needlestick exposure and injury from sharp objects should also be followed. Needles and other disposable sharp items should be placed in impervious containers and should not be manipulated in any way before disposal.

Individuals sustaining accidental parenteral or mucous membrane inoculations with potentially infected materials should follow the guidelines for treatment of accidental exposures.

REFERENCES

1. Fugikawa LA, Salahuddin SZ, Palestine AG, et al. Isolation of human T lymphotropic virus type III from the tears of a patient with the acquired immune deficiency syndrome. Lancet 1985; 2:529-30.
2. Centers for Disease Control. Recommendations for preventing possible transmission of human T-lymphotropic virus type III/lymphadenopathy-associated virus from tears. MMWR 1985; 34:533-4.

HIV and Otolaryngologists

C. Daniel Sooy, M.D.

■ RECOMMENDATIONS FOR THE HEAD AND NECK EXAM

Otolaryngologists and other health-care workers involved in treating head and neck problems are concerned about their risk of contracting HIV and what appropriate infection-control measures should be taken.[1] The secretions and body fluids commonly encountered in the head and neck from which live HIV has been cultured or antibodies to the virus have been found are listed in Table 1.

TABLE 1. HIV OR ANTIBODY ISOLATED FROM BODY FLUIDS AND SECRETIONS COMMONLY ENCOUNTERED IN THE HEAD AND NECK

SECRETION	ANTIBODY PRESENT	VIRUS CULTURED
Middle-ear effusion†	+	+
Cerumen†	+	−
Tears[2]	n/a	+
Nasal mucus	*	*
Saliva[3-5]	+	+
Pus	*	*
Blood[6]	+	+

* *Secretions known to contain leukocytes and immunoglobulins that would probably test positive.*
† *Sooy, Evans, Levy: unpublished data.*

Appropriate precautions include wearing gloves to avoid contact with blood or secretions and wearing glasses or other protective eyewear when there is a chance of aerosolization.

The universal blood and body-fluid precautions recommended by the CDC for health-care workers for prevention of transmission of HIV are the same as those for hepatitis B virus[7-9] and should be routinely employed for all patients regardless of the probability of infection. Specific office procedures recommended for otolaryngologists and other practitioners working in the area of the head and neck include the following.

- All instruments should be out at the start of the examination to avoid shuffling through drawers with contaminated hands or gloves.
- Gloves should be used for oral and indirect mirror examinations.

- Glasses (or other protective eyewear) and masks (or a protective face-shield) should be used for indirect exams when there is a chance of splash or aerosolization by cough or gag.

- After use, all instruments should be placed in a virucidal solution on the examination table to facilitate cleanup (2 percent glutaraldehyde [for fiberoptic or rust-prone instruments] or hypochlorite as bleach, 1:10 in water).

REFERENCES

1. Sooy CD, Gerberding JL, Kaplan MJ. The risk for otolaryngologists who treat patients with AIDS and AIDS virus infection: report of an in-progress study. Laryngoscope 1987; 97:430-4.

2. Fujikawa LS, Palestine AG, Nussenblatt RB, et al. Isolation of human T-lymphotropic virus type III from the tears of a patient with acquired immunodeficiency syndrome. Lancet 1985; 2:529-30.

3. Groopman JE, Salahuddin SZ, Sarngadharan MG, et al. HTLV-III in saliva of people with AIDS related complex and healthy homosexual men at risk for AIDS. Science 1984; 226:447-8.

4. Ho DD, Byington R, Schooley RT, et al. Infrequency of isolation of HTLV-III virus from saliva in AIDS. N Engl J Med 1985; 313:1606.

5. Levy JA, Kaminsky LS, Morror WJW, et al. Infection by the retrovirus associated with the acquired immunodeficiency syndrome: clinical, biological, and molecular features. Ann Intern Med 1985; 103:694-9.

6. Ho DD, Schooley RT, Rota TR, et al. HTLV-III in the semen and blood of a healthy homosexual man. Science 1984; 226:447-8.

7. Update: evaluation of human T-lymphotropic virus type III/lymphadenopathy-associated virus infection in health care personnel — United States. MMWR 1985; 34:575-8.

8. Recommendations: actions for prevention of transmission of infection with human lymphotropic virus III (HTLV-III)/ lymphadenopathy-associated virus (LAV) during invasive procedures. MMWR 1986; 35:221-3.

9. Update: universal precautions for prevention of transmission of human immunodeficiency virus, hepatitis B virus, and other bloodborne pathogens in health-care settings. MMWR 1988; 37:377-82, 387-8.

HIV and Psychiatric Facilities

J. Louise Gerberding, M.D., and Merle A. Sande, M.D.

U niversal blood and body-fluid precautions for health-care workers in hospitals and clinics should be followed while providing care to psychiatric patients.[1,2] These procedures are designed to reduce exposure to infectious organisms, including blood-borne pathogens such as the human immunodeficiency virus (HIV), hepatitis B virus, and cytomegalovirus. These procedures should be used when providing care to all patients regardless of the probability of HIV infection.

Special infection-control practices may be necessary for uncooperative patients whose behavior cannot be monitored or controlled. Isolation may be indicated for assaultive patients who bite and scratch. Isolation may also be indicated for patients with poor personal hygiene.

In some settings, such as large chronic-care institutions, patients' sexual behavior may be difficult to regulate. Sexually active patients with sexually transmitted diseases such as HIV infection and hepatitis B virus infection may need to be housed away from uninfected patients to protect the latter. Identifying infected patients may require screening for evidence of HIV infection and hepatitis B infection. The decision to screen must carefully weigh the legal rights of high-risk patients against the need to protect other patients. The development of screening programs and housing procedures should therefore proceed only after consultation with medical and legal experts.

Cooperative psychiatric patients with HIV infection may share living quarters, bathroom facilities, and dining facilities with other patients. Infection-control guidelines for household members living with HIV-infected persons should be followed. Patients with additional infections that can be transmitted to health-care workers or other patients should be placed on infection-control precautions appropriate for that pathogen.

REFERENCES

1. Recommendations for preventing transmission of infection with human T lymphotropic virus type III/lymphadenopathy-associated virus in the workplace. MMWR 1985; 34:682-95.

2. Gerberding JL, University of California—San Francisco Task Force on AIDS. Recommended infection-control policies for patients with human immunodeficiency virus infection: an update. N Engl J Med 1986; 315:1562-4.

Accidental Parenteral or Mucous Membrane Exposure to HIV

J. Louise Gerberding, M.D., and Merle A. Sande, M.D.

The risk of acquiring human immunodeficiency virus (HIV) infection after a needlestick or mucous membrane splash from an infected patient is less than 1 percent.[1,2] Exposures that have been associated with occupational HIV transmission include needlestick injuries, mucocutaneous inoculation with infected blood (especially deep intramuscular inoculations or injections), and prolonged or extensive cutaneous contact with infected blood.[2,3] Workers sustaining parenteral or mucous membrane exposure to blood or other body fluids and those with cutaneous exposure to large amounts of blood or prolonged contact with blood (especially when the area of contact is chapped, abraded, or afflicted with dermatitis) should be evaluated and hepatitis prophylaxis administered when indicated. A detailed exposure history defining the route and severity of exposure should be obtained.

The Centers for Disease Control (CDC) recommends that the source patient of an accidental exposure should be assessed clinically and epidemiologically to determine the probability of HIV infection.[2] If HIV infection is suspected, the patient should be asked to consent to a serologic test for evidence of HIV antibody. If the source patient has AIDS or other evidence of HIV infection, refuses to submit to testing, or has a positive antibody test, the CDC recommends that the health-care worker be evaluated as soon after exposure as possible for serologic evidence of HIV infection. If seronegative, retesting after six weeks and periodically thereafter for at least six months is recommended to determine whether transmission has occurred. If the source patient is unknown, decisions regarding appropriate follow-up should be made individually, based on the type and suspected source of the exposure.

The advantages of screening for HIV antibody after occupational exposure include: (1) identifying infection early in the course of the disease; (2) allaying fears in exposed health-care workers; and (3) providing documentation of infection (or lack of infection) for medical–legal purposes. Health-care workers who choose not to undergo testing are strongly advised to have baseline sera banked so that documentation of pre-exposure status can be made should the individual subsequently develop HIV infection. Health-care workers concerned about the confidentiality of any test results recorded in their employee health file may be reluctant to report accidental exposures. Methods for confidential charting should be developed in accordance with local needs and workers' compensation program requirements.

Post-exposure counseling should include a discussion of infection risks, strategies to prevent similar accidents in the future, safer sex, and other recommendations to prevent transmission to others. Indications for follow-up should be explained. Some centers are evaluating the use of zidovudine (AZT) as a post-exposure chemoprophylactic drug for seriously exposed health-care workers. Preliminary animal data with other retroviruses suggest that AZT could have some efficacy as a prophylactic drug. However, experience with AZT is limited in humans, even for short courses; neither efficacy nor toxicity is likely to be established in the near future. Dose, duration, and long-term sequelae for AZT chemoprophylaxis are unknown. Health-care workers who elect AZT therapy after serious HIV exposures are most likely to benefit when therapy begins as soon as possible (ideally less than a 24-hour delay). The CDC, National Institutes of Health, and other agencies are developing strategies for systematic evaluation.

REFERENCES

1. Update: acquired immunodeficiency syndrome and human immunodeficiency virus infection among health-care workers. MMWR 1988; 37:229-34, 239.
2. Recommendations for preventing transmission of infection with human T-lymphotropic virus type III/lymphadenopathy-associated virus in the workplace. MMWR 1985; 34:681-95.
3. Update: human immunodeficiency virus infections in health-care workers exposed to blood of infected patients. MMWR 1987; 36:285-9.
4. Henderson DK, Gerberding JL. Post-exposure zidovudine chemoprophylaxis for health-care workers experiencing occupational exposures to HIV. J Infect Dis (in press).

Care Providers Infected with HIV

J. Louise Gerberding, M.D., and Merle A. Sande, M.D.

Currently, no evidence exists that health-care workers infected with the human immunodeficiency virus (HIV) have transmitted the virus to their patients. Transmission is possible only when a portal of entry (such as an open skin wound or surgical incision) is directly contaminated with blood or serous fluid from an infected health-care worker.

To minimize the risk of transmission, health-care workers with HIV infection should rigorously adhere to universal blood and body-fluid precautions.[1,2]

The Centers for Disease Control has recommended that all health-care workers wear gloves for direct contact with mucous membranes or nonintact skin of all patients. Health-care workers with open or exudative skin lesions or weeping dermatitis should be excused from direct patient care and from handling patient-care equipment until the condition resolves.[2]

Competent health-care workers with HIV infection do not need to be restricted from work unless they have evidence of other infections or illnesses that would restrict any health-care provider's work. Special guidelines for health-care workers who perform invasive procedures are not necessary if universal infection-control practices are strictly followed.[3]

Some health-care workers with HIV infection may have immunologic abnormalities that put them at risk for acquiring other infectious diseases. Such health-care workers should be advised of exposure risks from patients with transmissible infections. They should adhere to existing infection-control guidelines to minimize exposures. The need for changes in work assignment should be evaluated by the employee and the employee's personal physician; consultation with the employee's supervisor and the employee health service should be obtained when appropriate.

An employee's HIV status is confidential medical information. Every effort should be made to protect his or her privacy. All health-care workers should be informed of the mechanisms of HIV transmission and be reassured that HIV is not transmitted by casual contact.

REFERENCES

1. Recommendations for preventing transmission of infection with human T-lymphotropic virus type III/lymphadenopathy-associated virus in the workplace. MMWR 1985; 34:681-95.
2. Gerberding JL, University of California–San Francisco Task Force on AIDS. Recommended infection-control policies for patients with human immunodeficiency virus infection: an update. N Engl J Med 1986; 315:1562-4.
3. Recommendations for preventing possible transmission of human T lymphotropic virus type III/lymphadenopathy-associated virus during invasive procedures. MMWR 1986; 35:221-3.

HIV and Cardiopulmonary Resuscitation (CPR) Providers

J. Louise Gerberding, M.D., and Merle A. Sande, M.D.

There is no documentation that any infectious illness can be transmitted to an individual performing mouth-to-mouth resuscitation. However, mouth-to-mouth ventilation could conceivably expose the rescuer to pathogens present in saliva, including hepatitis B virus, herpes simplex virus, human immunodeficiency virus (HIV), and Epstein–Barr virus. The potential for such exposures is likely to be higher for rescuers performing cardiopulmonary resuscitation (CPR) on hospitalized patients, since the prevalence of many oral infections is higher in the hospital than in the community.

Infection-control guidelines for individuals performing cardiopulmonary resuscitation are designed to minimize unnecessary exposure to saliva and respiratory secretions.[1] These guidelines should be followed for all patients, regardless of the likelihood of infection.[1,2]

1. Appropriate equipment for initiating artificial ventilation, such as self-inflating bags, should be readily available in hospitals, clinics, and rescue vehicles. Such equipment should be present at the bedside of any patient at high risk for cardiopulmonary arrest. Health-care providers should be adequately instructed in the proper use of ventilatory devices.

2. Protective devices such as plastic mouth guards should be provided to firefighters, police officers, and other rescue personnel who may not have immediate access to ventilation bags. These devices have not been proven to be effective in eliminating exposure to saliva but are likely to reduce the amount of exposure when used properly.

3. Rescuers with known exposure to infected saliva should be evaluated by a clinician and offered prophylactic treatment for hepatitis B or other diagnosed pathogens (including TB, meningococcus, etc.) known to be present in the source patient's saliva when such treatment is available and appropriate.

REFERENCES

1. Centers for Disease Control. Recommendations for preventing transmission of infection with human T-lymphotropic virus type III/lymphadenopathy-associated virus in the workplace. MMWR 1985; 34:681-95.
2. Gerberding JL, University of California–San Francisco Task Force on AIDS. Recommended infection-control policies for patients with human immunodeficiency virus infection: an update. N Engl J Med 1986; 315:1562-4.

HIV and Paramedics and Emergency Medical Technicians

J. Louise Gerberding, M.D., and Merle A. Sande, M.D.

There is no evidence of human immunodeficiency virus (HIV) transmission to paramedics or other emergency personnel following occupational exposure to patients infected with the virus. However, paramedics and other emergency personnel are known to be at risk for acquiring hepatitis B virus (HBV) infection. Use of universal blood and body-fluid precautions can prevent transmission of common pathogens, including blood-borne organisms such as HIV, HBV, and cytomegalovirus. These practices should be employed even in the emergency setting.

Like HBV infection, HIV infection cannot be diagnosed with certainty from the patient's appearance, medical history, or physical examination — particularly in the emergency setting. Recommended infection-control guidelines should therefore be employed for all patients, regardless of the probability of HIV infection.

Paramedics and other emergency personnel should be trained to use the recommended infection-control practices for health-care workers. In addition to the guidelines for prevention of exposure to blood-borne infections, guidelines for cardiopulmonary resuscitation and prevention of accidental exposures should be employed.

Ambulances and rescue vehicles should be equipped with disposable gloves and needle-disposal containers. Equipment for ventilatory support should be readily available to avoid the need for mouth-to-mouth resuscitation.

Equipment that is contaminated with body fluids should be cleaned and disinfected according to standard procedures. Contaminated surfaces should also be cleaned and disinfected.

HIV and Cardiopulmonary Resuscitation (CPR) Training

J. Louise Gerberding, M.D., and Merle A. Sande, M.D.

S tandard training in CPR involves the use of manikins. During performance of mouth-to-manikin ventilation, the manikin may become contaminated with saliva. Pathogens in the saliva may be transmitted during mouth-to-manikin contact or during the finger-sweep maneuver. Pathogens that may be present in saliva include hepatitis B virus, herpes simplex virus, human immunodeficiency virus (HIV), cytomegalovirus, Epstein–Barr virus, and various oral bacteria.

Despite the large number of persons participating in CPR training, only two cases of transmission of an infectious agent from contact with a manikin have been reported. Two women apparently acquired herpes simplex virus infections after exposure to saliva during manikin training; one developed herpes labialis and the other ocular herpes, presumably after inoculating her eye with a contaminated finger.[1] In contrast, 18 trainees exposed to saliva from a highly contagious individual with hepatitis B infection (e antigen positive) during manikin training were studied prospectively for six months and none developed evidence of hepatitis B infection.[2]

HIV is infrequently cultured from saliva and is known to be much less transmissible than hepatitis B. In addition, participants in CPR training have a low prevalence of HIV infection. It is therefore extremely unlikely that CPR training imposes a risk of acquiring AIDS.

The following infection-control guidelines for cardiopulmonary resuscitation training were developed by the University of California, San Francisco, AIDS Task Force. These guidelines are intended to minimize exposure during the manikin phase of CPR training to pathogens, including herpes simplex virus, hepatitis B virus, HIV, and other infectious oral, facial, cutaneous, and respiratory pathogens.[3]

■ PARTICIPANTS

Individuals with any of the following conditions should simulate ventilation during the manikin phase of CPR training:

- weeping or exudative lesions on the hands, face, or oral mucous membranes;
- hepatitis B infection;
- oral or circumoral herpes simplex infection;
- upper-respiratory infection;
- HIV infection;
- recent exposure to any infectious process.

■ TWO-PERSON CPR

During training for two-person CPR, there is not time to decontaminate the manikin between rescuers. Therefore, the student taking over ventilation after switching must simulate ventilation and not blow into the manikin.

■ FINGER SWEEP

When the finger-sweep maneuver is performed in the obstructed-airway procedure, contamination of the rescuer's hand with saliva may occur. Handwashing should therefore be performed after this maneuver.

■ DECONTAMINATION

Between students, the manikin's face and mouth should be cleaned and decontaminated with a gauze pad soaked in a freshly made solution of household bleach (1:10 dilution of 5.25 percent sodium hypochlorite). Surfaces should remain in contact with the bleach for at least 30 seconds. Surfaces should then be rinsed with a water-soaked pad and wiped dry.

REFERENCES

1. Mannis MJ, Wendel RT. Transmission of herpes simplex during CPR training. Ann Ophthalmol 1984; 16:64-6.
2. Glaser JB, Nadler JP. Hepatitis B virus in a cardiopulmonary resuscitation training course. Risk of transmission from a surface antigen-positive participant. Arch Intern Med 1985; 145:1653-5.
3. Infection control policy for decontaminating CPR manikins. Infection Control Policy Manual, San Francisco General Hospital.

HIV Antibody Testing and Guidelines for Dialysis Units

Patricia Schoenfeld, M.D.

■ HIV ANTIBODY TESTING

The common practice of using blood transfusions in many end-stage renal disease (ESRD) patients for transplantation and for clinical purposes, as well as the presence of other high-risk groups in the dialysis population, has resulted in concern and debate regarding the need for routine serologic testing of all patients in dialysis facilities. The incidence of HIV antibody positivity in the ESRD population is not known with certainty; however, the results of screening in a group of dialysis facilities in the Chicago area reported by Peterman et al.[1] have shown that the incidence of antibody to human immunodeficiency virus (HIV) using Western blot confirmation was 0.7 percent. There was a high percentage of false positives, since 25 of the 520 patients (4.8 percent) had initial reactivity to the screening enzyme immunoassay (ELISA) tests. This false positivity may be related to blood transfusion, since the number of transfusions was greater in the positive group than in the ELISA-negative patients. Another report of antibody screening from a smaller facility of 79 patients[2] found only one patient whose test results were weakly positive. Further testing will be necessary to determine if the incidence of HIV antibody in ESRD patients is different from that in the general population and if antibody positive patients are largely restricted to already identified high-risk groups.

The use of routine testing for HIV antibody in dialyzed patients, either acute or chronic, remains a controversial issue. Some facilities have begun routine screening of all new and existing patients primarily because of concern regarding the possible transmission of the virus during dialysis treatment and because of widespread fear stemming from the grave prognosis of the disease. Currently, no evidence exists that HIV has been transmitted in a dialysis setting other than from the use of blood transfusions. In the Chicago group of dialysis facilities tested for HIV antibody,[1] no evidence was found for transmission of HIV in the dialysis centers. Data from the Centers for Disease Control (CDC) and other investigators regarding the infectivity of HIV indicates that it would be extremely unlikely for patients or staff to become infected during the course of routine dialysis treatment when customary precautions for prevention of hepatitis B are used.[3,4]

The National Association of Patients on Hemodialysis and Transplantation sponsored a national consensus conference of experts, who concluded that routine screening of ESRD patients was not necessary for infection control, although it was recognized that screening on a research basis was indicated to define the incidence of HIV exposure among renal patients. It is clearly appropriate to screen all transplant donors to the extent possible within the time constraints imposed by organ preservation, and this is now being done by most transplant programs. The use of routine screening should be preceded by careful consideration of the following issues.

1. No testing should be done before adequate counseling services are in place.

2. Policies on treatment of positive patients should be established.

3. If HIV antibody positive patients are to be excluded from the program, adequate arrangements for care of these patients must be established.

4. Screened individuals must be notified that screening is being done, and informed consent obtained in those states where it is required by law.

5. Positive results must be communicated to the patient.

6. High quality laboratory methods should be used to exclude false positives (i.e., Western blot confirmation of ELISA positives).

■ GUIDELINES FOR DIALYSIS OF PATIENTS WITH HIV DISEASE

Identification.   For purposes of infection control, patients who are antibody positive, have AIDS-related complex (ARC), or clinical AIDS should be dialyzed according to the following guidelines.

Modality.   Peritoneal dialysis is the preferred modality for these patients because it minimizes exposure to blood and needles, and it encourages the use of home dialysis. However, in those patients who are hospitalized for clinical AIDS, or who have acute renal failure, it is recognized that hemodialysis will be the preferred mode of treatment. It must be recognized that the modality of dialysis should not be determined solely by concern regarding transmission of HIV, but should be selected according to the medical and social needs of the individual patient. The CDC has published the following recommendations for choice of infection-control strategies when hemodialysis treatment is selected.[4]

1. Ultraconservative: separate area, separate machine.

2. Very conservative: designated area, separate machine.

3. Conservative: separate machine.

The use of a separate machine, along with proper blood precautions and conventional cleaning and disinfection procedures, is a conservative and effective approach for dialysis of patients with AIDS. This approach does not restrict the use of space or limit sharing of equipment, since the machine can be sterilized and reused for other patients as needed.

Equipment and Supplies.   The risk of disease transmission for AIDS as well as for hepatitis B is not associated with the internal fluid circuits of the delivery system. Hepatitis may be spread by contamination of frequently touched surfaces as well as other environmental areas of the dialysis center; however, all data to date show that HIV has not been transmitted by this type of contact. HIV can only be acquired by intimate sexual contact and through the injection of contaminated blood products. Thus, the environmental risks of HIV transmission in the dialysis setting are limited to the use of contaminated blood or exposure to needlestick from an infected patient. Surveys in health workers, however, have shown that the incidence of HIV transmission via needlestick is extremely low, and cases reported to date have included the accidental injection of large volumes of blood or infected tissue.[5]

Routine sanitation, disinfection, and sterilization procedures currently recommended by the CDC for prevention of hepatitis in dialysis units are adequate control measures for the treatment of AIDS patients.[3] No additional environmental control steps have been recommended for the treatment of these patients.

1. When peritoneal dialysis is used in the center, the used peritoneal dialysate bags can be disposed of in the same fashion as other solid waste associated with peritoneal dialysis. In the home, bags of used dialysate should be handled with a disposable glove and the contents carefully poured down the toilet. Empty bags should be double-wrapped and discarded in the conventional trash system.

2. Nondisposable supplies such as blood-pressure cuffs should be restricted to individual patients. Other nondisposables that can be sterilized between use should be so processed between patients.

3. Hemodialyzers may be reused safely.

4. Cleaning and disinfection of dialysis machines, other equipment, and environmental surfaces that are frequently touched by staff members and patients should be performed using conventional intermediate- and high-level disinfectants such as those approved for use in hospitals by the U.S. Environmental Protection Agency.

■ BLOOD PRECAUTIONS AND ASEPTIC TECHNIQUES

The use of gloves, gowns, and handwashing techniques as previously published by the CDC for the prevention of hepatitis B in dialysis facilities should be followed when treating patients with AIDS.[3] The extraordinary use of protective clothing, face shields, or goggles is not warranted during routine dialysis procedures.

REFERENCES

1. Peterman TA, Lang GR, Mikos NJ, et al. HTLV-III/LAV infection in hemodialysis patients. JAMA 1986; 255:2324-6.
2. Poole CL, Johnston DO, Freer C, et al. HTLV-III studies in ESRD patients [Abstract]. National Kidney Foundation Meeting, 1985:A15.
3. Hepatitis control measures for hepatitis B in dialysis centers. Viral hepatitis: investigation and control series. November 1977. HEW publication no. (CDC) 78-8358.
4. Favero MS. Recommended precautions for patients undergoing hemodialysis who have AIDS or non-A, non-B hepatitis. Infect Control 1985; 6:301-5.
5. McCray E, The Cooperative Needlestick Surveillance Group. Occupational risk of the acquired immunodeficiency syndrome among health care workers. N Engl J Med 1986; 314:1127-32.

HIV in Dental Offices and Clinics

Deborah Greenspan, B.D.S.

R outine dental care involves exposure to saliva and blood, and thus the possibility of exposure to infection with human immunodeficiency virus (HIV). Preliminary results of studies on the transmission of HIV to dental personnel have failed to demonstrate transmission of the virus.[1,2] The Council on Dental Therapeutics of the American Dental Association has published an article on AIDS and the dental professional[3] and the CDC has published its recommendations for infection-control measures in dental practices.[4] The following procedures should be adopted for all patients,[5] regardless of diagnosis.

■ OFFICE PROCEDURES

Protective clothing and gloves should be worn for all examinations. Masks and glasses, or a protective face-shield, should also be worn during all procedures. Gloves should be worn once and then discarded. They should not be washed.

■ STERILIZATION

Measures must be taken to prevent transmission of all infectious agents. Disposable items should be used if possible. All instruments and other items that come into contact with the mouth and are not destroyed after use should be sterilized. Steam autoclaves, chemical vapor sterilizers, or dry-heat units should be used. The dry-heat sterilizer is the least expensive but has a long sterilizing cycle. Instruments must be separated in order to ensure adequate sterilization. All units should be checked routinely to ensure their effectiveness. Routine sterilization of handpieces is desirable. The care of ultrasonic scalers and handpieces is described in detail in the CDC recommendations.[2] Where sterilization is not possible, cold solutions should be used as disinfectants.[6,7] Glutaraldehyde solutions are suitable for this purpose. Cold solutions must be changed in accordance with the manufacturers' recommendations in order to maintain their effectiveness. Tables 1 and 2 present a guide to the chemical agents used for disinfection.

TABLE 1. CHEMICAL AGENTS FOR DISINFECTION AND STERILIZATION*

PRODUCTS ACCEPTED	CHEMICAL CLASSIFICATION	DISINFECTANT	STERILANT
ProMed Brand Wescodyne-D	Iodophors, 1% available iodine	Diluted according to manufacturer's instructions, 10 min.	
Household bleach	Sodium hypochlorite	Diluted 1:5 to 1:100 10 to 30 min.	
Omni II	o-phenylphenol 9.0% and o-benzyl-p-chlorophenol 1.0%	Diluted 1:32 10 min. at room temperature	
Sporicidin	Glutaraldehyde 2%, alkaline with phenolic buffer	Diluted 1:16, 10 min. at room temperature	Full strength, 6 3/4 hrs. at room temperature
Glutarex	Glutaraldehyde 2%, neutral	Full strength, 10 min. at room temperature	Full strength, 10 hrs. at room temperature
Banicide, Sterall, Wavicide	Glutaraldehyde 2%, acidic potentiated with non-ionic ethoxylates of linear alcohols	Diluted 1:2, 10 min. at room temperature	Full strength, 1 hr., 60°C; 4 hrs., 40 to 50°C; 10 hrs. at room temperature
Exspor	Chlorine dioxide	2 min. at room temperature	6 hrs. at room temperature
Centra†, Cidex 7, CoeCide, K-Cide 10†, Maxicide†, Omnicide, ProCide†, Saslow Professional†, Sporex, Steril-Ize, Vitacide	Glutaraldehyde 2%, alkaline	Full strength, 10 min. at room temperature	Full strength, 10 hrs. at room temperature

*   *Reprinted with permission from the* Calif Dent Assoc J *1985; 13:64-7.*
†   *Available as regular (14-day activity) or long life (28-day activity).*

TABLE 2. STERILIZATION AND DISINFECTION OF DENTAL INSTRUMENTS, MATERIALS, AND SOME COMMONLY USED ITEMS*

CODES: A = *Effective and preferred method*
B = *Effective and acceptable method*
C = *Effective method, but risk of instrument damage*
D = *Ineffective method, risk of instrument damage*
1 = *Confirm with manufacturer*
2 = *Discard*
3 = *Iodophor*
4 = *Chlorine solution*

	STEAM AUTO-CLAVE	DRY-HEAT OVEN	CHEMICAL VAPOR	ETHYLENE OXIDE	CHEMICAL DISINFECT/ STERILIZE
Angle Attachments (1)	B	B	B	A	B
Burs carbon steel	C	A	A	A	C
Steel	B	A	A	A	B
Tungs-carbide	B	A	B	A	B
Endo instruments					
Stainless-steel handles	A	A	A	A	B
Nonstainless metal handles	D	A	A	A	D
Stainless plastic handles	C	C	C	A	B
Fluoride gel trays					
Heat resist.	A	D	C	A	C
Nonheat resist. (2)	D	D	C	A	C
Hand instruments					
Carbon steel	C	A	A	A	C
Stainless steel	A	A	A	A	B
Handpieces					
Autoclave	A	C	C	A	D
Contraangle	C	C	C	A	B
Nonauto clav. (3)	C	C	C	A	B
Prophy angle	B	B	B	B	B
Impression Trays					
Aluminum metal, chrome-plated	A	A	A	A	B
Custom acrylic	D	D	D	A	B
Plastic (2)	D	D	D	A	B
Instrument packs	A	B (small)	A	A (small)	D
Instrument trays	B	B	B	A	D
Needles, disposable	DISCARD — DO NOT REUSE				

continued on next page

continued from previous page

TABLE 2. STERILIZATION AND DISINFECTION OF DENTAL INSTRUMENTS, MATERIALS, AND SOME COMMONLY USED ITEMS*

	STEAM AUTO-CLAVE	DRY-HEAT OVEN	CHEMICAL VAPOR	ETHYLENE OXIDE	CHEMICAL DISINFECT/STERILIZE
Polishing wheels/disks					
Garnet/cuttle	D	C	C	A	D
Rag	A	C	B	A	D
Rubber	B	C	C	A	B
Prostheses removable (4)	C	C	C	B	B
General items					
Stainless steel	A	A	A	A	B
Rubber	B	C	C	A	B
Plastic	C	C	C	A	B
Carbon steel	C	A	A	A	C

* *Reprinted with permission from the* Calif Dent Assoc J *1985; 13:64-7.*

Surfaces that may have come into contact with blood or saliva should be disinfected. Diluted sodium hypochlorite (1:10 to 1:100 of household bleach, strength dependent upon the amount of material present on the surface) and iodophore solutions are suitable for wiping down exposed surfaces.[4]

Needles should not be recapped, but should be placed along with other sharp items in puncture-resistant containers, which are then sealed in plastic disposal bags. All waste material should be placed in plastic bags, sealed, and handled according to the local requirements.

■ IMPRESSIONS

Impressions may be disinfected in iodophore solutions before pouring the models. Most impression materials will tolerate this procedure.[8]

■ DENTAL TREATMENT

The risk of contracting or spreading HIV through dental treatment is very low or nonexistent. The denial of treatment to known HIV carriers will only encourage patients to seek care elsewhere and to lie about their medical history. All patients, whether they are AIDS patients or asymptomatic HIV carriers, should have access to dental treatment.

REFERENCES

1. Gerberding JL, Nelson K, Greenspan D, et al. Risk to dentists from occupational exposure to human immunodeficiency virus (HIV): follow-up [Abstract]. Washington, D.C.: Twenty-seventh Interscience Conference on Antimicrobial Agents and Chemotherapy, 1987.

2. Klein RS, Phelan J, Friedland GH, et al. Prevalence of antibodies to HTLV-III/LAV among dental professionals [Abstract]. New Orleans: Twenty-sixth Interscience Conference on Antimicrobial Agents and Chemotherapy, 1986:283.

3. Infection control in the dental office: a realistic approach. J Am Dent Assoc 1986; 112:458-68.

4. Centers for Disease Control. Recommended infection control practices for dentistry. MMWR 1986; 35:237-42.

5. Greenspan D, Pindborg JJ, Greenspan JS, Schiodt M. AIDS and the dental team. Copenhagen: Munksgaard, 1986:76-9.

6. Molinari JA. Surface disinfection and disinfectants. Calif Dental Assoc J 1985; 13:74-8.

7. Mitchell EW. Chemical disinfecting/sterilizing agents. Calif Dental Assoc J 1985; 13:64-7.

8. Schaefer ME. Infection control in dental laboratory procedures. Calif Dental Assoc J 1985; 13:81-4.

10.3

Infection-Control Guidelines: Nonmedical Work Environment

General Precautions in the Nonmedical Work Environment

J. Louise Gerberding, M.D., and Merle A. Sande, M.D.

The human immunodeficiency virus (HIV) is transmitted by sexual contact with infected partners, by direct inoculation with infected blood or blood products, and by perinatal transmission from infected mothers to their off-spring. There is no evidence that the virus can be transmitted by casual contact with infected persons in the nonmedical work environment, including offices, stores, schools, and factories. The virus is not transmitted by the airborne route, by objects touched by infected individuals, or by contaminated surfaces.

Persons with HIV may continue to work and to use telephones, bathroom facilities, dining facilities, and other office equipment. Good personal hygiene should be maintained by all employees.

Environmental surfaces or equipment contaminated with blood should be cleaned with soap and water and disinfected with a commercially available solution or a 1:100 dilution of 5.25 percent sodium hypochlorite (household bleach). A 1:10 dilution should be used for heavily contaminated items.

Health-care workers in the work environment should follow the guidelines for infection control in the hospital environment. Employees who participate in CPR (cardiopulmonary resuscitation) training should follow the infection-control guidelines for CPR training.

HIV and Personal Service Workers

J. Louise Gerberding, M.D., and Merle A. Sande, M.D.

There is no evidence of human immunodeficiency virus (HIV) transmission to personal service workers such as barbers, cosmetologists, manicurists, and massage therapists from occupational exposure to clients infected with the virus. There is also no evidence of HIV transmission from personal service workers with HIV infection to their clients. Transmission of the virus requires both a portal of entry, such as cutaneous wounds, mucous membranes, or other interruptions in the skin, and access of blood or other body fluids from one individual to open tissue of another.

The following infection-control guidelines for personal service workers are designed to prevent exposures that could result in HIV transmission by these routes.[1]

Personal Hygiene.   Personal service workers should practice good personal hygiene. Individuals with exudative skin lesions or weeping dermatitis should avoid direct contact with clients until the condition resolves. Hands should be washed before and after contact with each client.

Needles and Other Sharp Instruments.   Infection-control guidelines designed to protect health-care workers from needlestick and other accidental exposures should be followed by personal service workers. Needles and other instruments used for acupuncture, tattooing, ear piercing, and other procedures that penetrate the skin should be disposed of or washed and sterilized before reuse. Instruments that may be contaminated with blood, such as razors, should be cleaned and sterilized or disposed of immediately after use. Impervious containers should be used for disposal of needles, razors, and other sharp objects.

Disinfection and Sterilization.   Disposable wastes should be placed in impervious containers. Contaminated reusable equipment not intended to penetrate the skin should be washed and disinfected according to standard procedures.

REFERENCES

1.   Centers for Disease Control. Recommendations for preventing transmission of infection with human T-lymphotropic virus type III/lymphadenopathy-associated virus in the workplace. MMWR 1985; 34:681-95.

10.3.3

HIV and Public Safety Workers

J. Louise Gerberding, M.D., and Merle A. Sande, M.D.

The human immunodeficiency virus (HIV) is transmitted by sexual contact with an infected partner, by direct inoculation with infected blood products, and by perinatal transmission from infected mothers to their offspring. There is no evidence that the virus can be transmitted by casual contact with infected individuals.

The risk to public safety workers (firefighters, police officers, rescuers, and others) who have direct contact with individuals infected with HIV has not been systematically evaluated. However, the risk to health-care workers and close household contacts of patients with AIDS and ARC has been extensively evaluated and is known to be extremely low. Fewer than 1 percent of individuals who have been percutaneously inoculated with blood during accidental needlestick injuries have acquired the virus. Mucous membrane contact with blood has been implicated as a possible route of transmission in only one health-care provider. Prolonged cutaneous contact and cutaneous contact with a large amount of blood in two other workers with dermatologic lesions may have served as portals of entry for the virus.[1] Public safety workers are therefore unlikely to be at high risk for infection with HIV.

Public safety workers should be instructed in standard infection-control procedures. Handwashing should be performed after contact with all persons. If contact with blood or body fluids is anticipated, disposable gloves should be worn. Gloves or protective dressings should be worn if cuts, scratches, or other dermatologic lesions are present on the hands. Recommended infection-control guidelines for cardiopulmonary resuscitation should be followed. If percutaneous or mucous membrane inoculations with potentially infected materials occur, the guidelines for health-care workers with accidental exposures should be followed.

REFERENCES

1. Update: Human immunodeficiency virus infections in health care workers exposed to blood of infected patients. MMWR 1987; 36:285-9.

HIV and Food Handlers

J. Louise Gerberding, M.D., and Merle A. Sande, M.D.

There is no epidemiologic evidence to suggest that the human immunodeficiency virus (HIV) is transmissible by exposure to foods or beverages. Infection-control guidelines for food handlers (such as cooks, waiters, bartenders, and caterers) are therefore based on standard hygienic practices.[1] Foods should be prepared and served in accordance with existing standards.

Food handlers with exudative cutaneous lesions or weeping dermatitis should not work until the lesions have resolved. Food handlers sustaining accidental injuries such as cuts or abrasions that may cause contamination of food with blood or other body fluids should also be excused from work until the wounds heal. Contaminated or potentially contaminated foods should be discarded.

Food handlers with HIV infection may safely work provided that standard hygienic practices are employed and that other infections or illnesses requiring work restriction are not currently present.

REFERENCES

1. Centers for Disease Control. Recommendations for preventing transmission of infection with human T lymphotropic virus type III/lymphadenopathy-associated virus in the workplace. MMWR 1985; 34:681-95.

10.4

Infection-Control Guidelines: Blood and Blood Products

HIV and Blood Transfusion

Elizabeth Donegan, M.D.

Maximum safety in blood transfusion requires that all aspects of blood collection, processing, and transfusion be performed to eliminate infection. Laboratory tests for HIV are unlikely to ever detect all units of contaminated blood. Blood collection must continue to rely in part upon deferral of donors at risk for HIV infection. Blood should be transfused only if it is absolutely needed and then only if it is not considered potentially infective. This chapter discusses donor selection and handling and testing of blood and its transfusion.

■ BLOOD-DONOR SELECTION

Voluntary deferral by persons at risk for HIV infection remains necessary because laboratory tests alone cannot ensure a maximally safe blood supply. The following individuals are currently asked to refrain from donating:

- those with clinical symptoms of HIV infection (AIDS or symptomatic HIV disease);
- those who have a positive HIV antibody test;
- males who have had sex with other males one or more times since 1977;
- those who are now or have ever been intravenous (IV) drug users;
- those who have emigrated to the United States from Central Africa or Haiti since 1977 or who have had sexual contact with a resident of these countries;
- those hemophiliacs who have received clotting factor concentrates;
- those who are sexual partners, male or female, of any of the above categories;
- those men or women who have been prostitutes any time since 1977, or have been sexual partners within the last six months with anyone of either sex who was a prostitute.

Self-deferral criteria must be explained to potential donors in a non-judgmental way in language clearly understandable to the donor. Information about HIV infection must be available in waiting areas. Locations where HIV testing is available should be advertised to discourage individuals from donating blood in order to obtain free HIV testing. Since some high-risk donors are pressured by others to donate, donors must be given the opportunity to confidentially indicate that they do not wish their blood used for transfusion. Medical history-taking areas should be private in order to promote open discussion. A means of recontacting the collection facility after donation is necessary so that the donor, "with no questions asked," can request that his or her donation be discarded. Prior to collection, both arms of the donor must be inspected for needle tracks. Donors who test positive for antibody to HIV must be contacted and their names placed on permanent deferral lists. To ensure the donor's privacy, the reason for permanent deferral should not be indicated.

Despite the implementation of these measures, some high-risk persons continue to donate. Interviews with donors who test antibody-positive reveal the following.

- The majority admit to belonging to a group at risk for HIV infection.
- Donors commonly believe they are not HIV-infected.
- Some donors want free HIV testing and others feel peer pressure to donate but do not wish to admit risk behavior to others.
- Some donors are unaware of their risk for HIV infection at the time of donation.[1,2]

Blood-collection facilities must continue to develop effective methods of educating potential donors about the risks for HIV infection and its transmission in blood.

■ BLOOD-DONOR TESTING FOR HIV ANTIBODY AND p24 ANTIGEN

Anti-HIV laboratory testing became available in March, 1985, and by July 1, 1985, it was required by the American Association of Blood Banks. Since 1986, the Joint Commission of Accreditation has required that all blood used for transfusion be tested for HIV antibody. Since anti-HIV screening of blood donations began, there have been few reports of HIV transmission by transfusion.[3,4] Screening tests for HIV antibody used by blood facilities are more than 99 percent sensitive and specific.[5] Particularly because these screening tests are used on a population with an expected low prevalence of HIV seropositivity, all positive tests should be confirmed in order to eliminate potential false-positive results before confidentially notifying the donor.

Despite the excellent performance of these assays, some HIV-contaminated blood continues to be transfused. False-negative test results occur through laboratory error or test failure[5,6,7] and because some donors recently infected with HIV-1 have not as yet made antibody (the so-called "window period").[3] No persistently antibody-negative HIV-1-infected blood donors have been identified, although such a possibility exists.[8] The risk of HIV transmission by blood transfusion is currently estimated to be between 1:28,000 and 1:100,000 per unit transfused.[3,4,10] p24 antigen tests as a supplement to antibody tests have not detected HIV-antigen-positive but seronegative donors; more than 750,000 blood donors have been screened using the p24 HIV-antigen test and no antigen-positive seronegative donors were detected. The Food and Drug Administration, after reviewing these results, decided against recommending that the p24 antigen test be implemented for routine screening of blood donors.[11]

■ DONOR NOTIFICATION OF POSITIVE HIV TESTS

Donors who repeatedly test positive on an HIV-1 antibody test by enzyme-linked immunoassay (ELISA) should have these results confirmed by additional tests. ELISA results can be confirmed using reagents from another ELISA test derived from a different cell line, by Western blot, or by radioimmunoprecipitation or immunofluorescence HIV tests. Positive donors should be notified confidentially and referred for physician evaluation. Active-duty military personnel who donate blood at military installations must sign a statement giving consent for antibody-positive HIV-1 test results to be revealed to military doctors.

Blood found to be repeatedly HIV-1 antibody-positive by ELISA but negative or indeterminate on confirmatory tests will not be transfused. If repeatedly ELISA-positive and confirmed negative or indeterminate again after six months, the donor is notified and permanently deferred.[12]

■ HIV-2 AND HTLV-I/II

HIV-2 infection is rarely reported in the United States. There have been no reports of it in blood donors. Blood banks do not currently test for HIV-2, although HIV-1 antibody ELISA tests will give positive results in the presence of HIV-2 42 percent to 92 percent of the time.[9]

It was recently recognized that between one in one thousand and one in four thousand blood donors are infected with HTLV-I/II.[13,14] As of July 1, 1989, the American Association of Blood Banks requires that all donations be tested for HTLV-I/II.

REFERENCES

1. Cleary PD, Singer E, Rogers TF, et al. Sociodemographic and behavioral characteristics of HIV antibody-positive donors. Am J Public Health 1988; 78:953-7.
2. Perkins HA, Samson S, Busch MP. How well has self-exclusion worked? Transfusion 1988; 28:601-2.
3. Ward JW, Holmberg SD, Allen JR, et al. Transmission of human immunodeficiency virus (HIV) by blood transfusions screened as negative for HIV antibody. N Engl J Med 1988; 318:473-7.
4. Cohen ND, Muñoz A, Reitz BA, et al. Transmission of retroviruses by transfusion of screened blood in patients undergoing cardiac surgery. N Engl J Med 1989; 320:1172-6.
5. Taylor RN, Przybyszewski VA. Summary of the Centers for Disease Control human immunodeficiency virus (HIV) performance evaluation surveys for 1985 and 1986. AJCP 1988; 89:1-13.
6. Update: serologic testing for antibody to human immunodeficiency virus. MMWR 1988; 36:833-45.
7. Lampe AS, Pieterse-Bruins HJ, Egter van Wissekerke JC. Wearing gloves as cause of false-negative HIV tests. Lancet 1988; 2:1140-1.
8. Imagawa DT, Lee MH, Wolinsky SM, et al. Human immunodeficiency virus type 1 infection in homosexual men who remain seronegative for prolonged periods. N Engl J Med 1989; 320:1458-62.
9. AIDS due to HIV-2 infection — New Jersey. MMWR 1988; 37:33-5.
10. Kleinman S, Secord K. Risk of human immunodeficiency virus (HIV) transmission by anti-HIV negative blood. Estimates using the lookback methodology. Transfusion 1988; 28:499-501.
11. FDA advisory committee recommends against the use of HIV antigen test for blood screening. Blood Bank Week 1989; 6:1-6.
12. Food and Drug Administration. General biological products standards, additional standards for human blood and blood products; test for antibody to human immunodeficiency virus (HIV). Fed Regist 1988; 53:111-7.
13. Transfusion Safety Study Group. Antibody to HTLV I/II among blood donors in four cities of the United States [Abstract]. V International Conference on AIDS. Montreal, 1989; Th.A.P.32.
14. Williams AE, Fang CT, Slamon DJ, et al. Seroprevalence and epidemiological correlates of HTLV-I infection in U.S. blood donors. Science 1988; 240:643-6.

HIV and Hemophilia Patients

The National Hemophilia Foundation

*T*he National Hemophilia Foundation's Medical and Scientific Advisory Council made the following recommendations concerning AIDS and the treatment of hemophilia (revised January, 1989). — E. Donegan.

■ I RECOMMENDATIONS FOR PHYSICIANS TREATING PATIENTS WITH HEMOPHILIA

A. Human Immunodeficiency Virus (HIV). There is accumulating evidence that improved viral-depleting processes have resulted in Factor VIII products with substantially reduced risk for transmission of human immunodeficiency virus. Products that are heated in aqueous solution (pasteurized), and detergent-solvent treated, monoclonal antibody purified, heated in suspension in organic media, or dry heated at high temperatures for long periods of time are preferred products of treatment of Hemophilia A for substantially reduced risk of HIV transmission.

B. Hepatitis. Preliminary available data suggest that some improved methods of viral inactivation may result in a reduced risk of hepatitis transmission. These products are those that are heated in aqueous solution (pasteurized), detergent-solvent treated, or monoclonal antibody purified. Products heated in suspension in organic media or dry heated at high temperatures for long periods of time may not be as efficient in attenuating or eliminating hepatitis viruses as the products mentioned in the previous sentence. It is recognized that these data are extraordinarily preliminary and more clinical data are urgently needed.

When feasible, another alternative may be the use of cryoprecipitate prepared from a single, well-screened and repeatedly tested donor, or from a small number of such donors.

C. The data concerning the effectiveness of different viral-depleting processes with respect to hepatitis viruses (per I. B., above) are based upon emerging preliminary data which may lead to modification of these recommendations in the future. When choosing the appropriate products for their patients with hemophilia, treaters will need to continue to exercise their best judgment based on their assessment of emerging data. Further, additional data are essential to provide for a better understanding about the safety of blood products. Pharmaceutical companies are urged to increase the number of patients enrolled in carefully controlled post-licensure studies.

D. For patients with severe Factor IX deficiency, we continue to recommend the use of viral-attenuated Factor IX concentrate. As they exist and/or may be developed and subsequently approved by the Food and Drug Administration, preferred techniques should be similar to those described in section I. A., above.

For patients with mild or moderate Factor IX deficiency, when feasible, another alternative would be the use of fresh frozen plasma prepared from a single, well-screened and repeatedly tested donor or from a small number of such donors. It is recognized, however, that there are some circumstances in which viral-attenuated Factor IX may be the more appropriate therapy.

E.   Desmopressin (DDAVP) should be used whenever possible with mild or moderate hemophilia A. When desmopressin does not provide adequate treatment, these patients should be treated as per section I. A. and B., above.

F.   Most persons with von Willebrand's Disease are appropriately treated with infusions of desmopressin (DDAVP) or cryoprecipitate from carefully selected and tested donors. Those affected with uncommon variants of von Willebrand's Disease may require cryoprecipitate. The severely affected persons might be treated with Factor VIII preparations heated in an aqueous solution (pasteurized). Careful consideration of this option for moderately affected patients may be appropriate when confidence in the viral safety of available cryoprecipitate is lacking.

G.   It is emphasized that hepatitis B vaccination is essential for patients with hemophilia and it is recommended that this be done at birth or diagnosis.

H.   All elective surgical procedures should be evaluated with respect to the advantages or disadvantages of a delay, although recent developments in donor screening and in virus inactivation indicate that such surgery can be undertaken when necessary.

I.   Patients should continue treating bleeding episodes with clotting factor as prescribed by their physicians, as the risks of withholding treatment far outweigh the risks of treatment. Health care providers should educate patients to use appropriate doses of clotting factor to minimize over-usage and contain costs.

J.   With the advent of possibly effective treatment for HIV infection and AIDS, physicians are also referred to appropriate NHF Medical Bulletins such as #49 (April 16, 1987); "Measurement of HIV Antibody in Persons with Hemophilia"; #52 (May 15, 1987), "AZT Information Sheet"; #61 (December 10, 1987) "Drug Therapy for AIDS and HIV Infection."

K.   There are other complex issues that must be considered in regard to the impact of possible HIV transmission on the lifestyles of persons with hemophilia. For detailed consideration of these issues, the physician is referred to the following NHF publications: "AIDS and Hemophilia: Your Questions Answered"; "Intimacy, Sexuality and Hemophilia"; "Recommendations for Providing Education to Students with AIDS"; "Let's Talk about Sex" and "What Women Should Know about HIV Infection, AIDS and Hemophilia."

L.   We recognize that patient education, psychosocial support and financial counseling are necessary components of comprehensive hemophilia care. For patients with HIV infection, the need for these services is greatly increased.

■ **II   RECOMMENDATIONS TO CONCENTRATE MANUFACTURERS**

A. Every effort should be made to exclude donors who might transmit AIDS.

   1.   We recommend the continued HIV antibody testing of all blood and plasma donors. At the same time we urge that actions continue to be

taken by blood and plasma collection facilities and other agencies so that HIV testing is available to members of high-risk groups apart from that carried out for blood and plasma donors.

2. Blood plasma donations should not be obtained from prospective donors who are members of groups who are at higher risk of contracting AIDS. Such groups include: male homosexuals and bisexuals, (any male who has engaged in sexual activity with another male), intravenous drug users, those who have resided where AIDS is endemic, and sexual partners of persons with hemophilia or of persons in the other risk groups previously enumerated. This effort should make use of educational materials and questionnaires in a discreet and sensitive manner.

3. Prospective blood donors should be excluded if they have symptoms associated with HIV infection. Assessment of these symptoms should be done as recommended by the Food and Drug Administration, Office of Biologics (December 14, 1984).

4. Manufacturers should continue to avoid using plasma obtained from donor centers that draw from population groups in which there is a relatively high incidence of hepatitis and AIDS. This would include prison populations.

B. Concentrate manufacturers should not purchase recovered plasma for coagulation factor production from blood centers that do not meet criteria listed in II. A.

C. Manufacturers should continue efforts towards the production of purer and safer coagulation factor concentrates. Manufacturers should work towards the development of safer products for treatment of hemophilia B. As these materials are ready for clinical use, the necessary governmental review processes should be carried out as expeditiously as possible.

D. Manufacturers should assess the potential risks of other retroviruses and other infectious agents which may be contained in blood products. Research should be continued to safeguard patients with hemophilia from the potential risks of these infectious agents.

■ III RECOMMENDATIONS TO REGIONAL AND COMMUNITY BLOOD CENTERS

A. The production of cryoprecipitate should adhere to criteria detailed in II. A., above.

■ GLOSSARY TO MASAC RECOMMENDATIONS

Detergent — Solvent. Factor VIII concentrates manufactured using Tri-N-Butyl Phosphate (TNBP) with cholate, Tween 80 or Triton-X-100 (all detergents) to inactivate lipid enveloped potential viral contaminants. A TNBP-cholate concentrate (SD-AHF) is currently produced by the New York Blood Center and marketed through the American Red Cross.

Dry-Heated. Factor VIII or IX concentrates heated under conditions to inactivate potential viral contaminants. Currently available products include Proplex SX-T and Proplex T (Hyland) and Koate HT and Konyne HT (Cutter). Temperatures for heating vary from 60°C to 68°C and times vary from 72 to 153 hours.

Heated in Aqueous Solution (pasteurized).   Factor VIII concentrates heated for 10 hours at 60°C in solution in the presence of stabilizers such as sucrose or neutral amino acids. Products include Humate-P (distributed by Armour; manufactured by Behringwerke) and Koate-HS (Cutter).

Monoclonal Antibody Purified.   Factor VIII concentrate purified using mouse monoclonal antibody on an affinity matrix. Viral attenuation is augmented by a dry-heating step after lyophilization, Monoclate, (Armour). Proposed products of this type employ detergent-solvent processes in lieu of heating, Hemofil M (Hyland, not yet approved) and AHF-M (American Red Cross, not yet approved).

Suspension Heated in an Organic Solvent.   Factor VIII or IX concentrates heated for 20 hours at 60°C in a suspension of heptane. Examples are Profilate Heat Treated (wet method) (Alpha) and Profilnine Heat Treated (wet method) (Alpha).

TABLE 1.   TABLE OF AVAILABLE FACTOR VIII PRODUCTS AS PER MASAC RECOMMENDATIONS*

METHOD OF VIRAL INACTIVATION	PRODUCT	MANUFACTURER
a. Solvent detergent (TNBP-cholate)	Coagulation factor VIII-SD	NY Blood Center
b. Monoclonal antibody		
1. Dry heat (30 hr, 60°C)	Monoclate	Armour
2. Detergent-solvent	Hemofil M† AHF-M†	Hyland American Red Cross
c. Heated in aqueous solution (pasteurized, 10 hr, 60°C)	Humate P Koate HS	Armour Cutter
d. Suspension-heated in an organic solvent (20 hr, 60°C)	Profilate heat treated (wet method)	Alpha
e. Dry heat (72 hr, 68°C)	Koate HT	Cutter

*   Compiled by the National Hemophilia Foundation, February 19, 1988.
†   Not yet FDA-approved. The listing of this trade name is not to be construed as an offer to sell.

TABLE 2.   TABLE OF AVAILABLE FACTOR IX PRODUCTS AS PER MASAC RECOMMENDATIONS*

METHOD OF VIRAL INACTIVATION	PRODUCT	MANUFACTURER
a. Dry heat (72 hr, 68°C)	Konyne HT	Cutter
Dry heat (144–153 hr, 60°C)	Proplex T	Hyland
Dry heat (144–153 hr, 60°C)	Proplex SX-T	Hyland
b. Suspension heated in an organic solvent (20 hr, 60°C)	Profilnine heat treated (wet method)	Alpha

*   Compiled by the National Hemophilia Foundation, February 19, 1988.

10.5

Infection-Control Guidelines: Facilities for Youth and Educational Institutions

10.5.1   HIV and Youth Facilities and Educational Institutions — *Grossman*

HIV and Youth Facilities
and Educational Institutions

Moses Grossman, M.D.

■ CHILD-CARE FACILITIES AND PRESCHOOLS

Placement.   The placement of an HIV-infected child in any child-care facility, preschool program, or grade school raises serious questions. (1) Is the child at increased risk from being in this particular environment? (2) What is the risk/benefit ratio for the child? (3) Are other children at risk when exposed to the infected child? (4) What are the legal and ethical responsibilities and liabilities of the operators of the child-care facility?

To be able to answer these questions, several important pieces of information are needed. These are: (1) the age of the child; (2) whether the youngster is toilet-trained; (3) whether the youngster's behavior is within normal limits for his or her age; (4) the clinical and immunologic status of the child's infection[1]; (5) the characteristics of the other children in the facility; and (6) the likelihood or possibility of sexual activity between the HIV-infected child and other youngsters.

Generally, the benefits of a good educational setting outweigh the risks to the child.[2] Furthermore, there is no evidence that HIV can be transmitted by casual contact or by ordinary activities in child-care facilities, day-care centers, or preschools.[4,5] Thus, the children are not a hazard to other children or school personnel.

Attendance.   Deciding whether children infected with HIV should be encouraged or allowed to attend day-care centers or preschool programs should be based upon two considerations: (1) Will infected children be a source of infection to other children and the personnel of the center? (2) Are children infected with HIV at risk of acquiring a serious infection?

The susceptibility of infected children depends on their immune and clinical status as well as on their developmental status. Children who are not yet toilet-trained (usually those younger than 3 years old) and those who are not capable of learning sanitary habits are at greater risk of acquiring common infections; these infections may become more serious for them than for normal children. This risk declines for children older than 3 years.

Children who are known to have an HIV infection should be reviewed individually by both their physician and a day-care center official before enrollment. For many of the children and their families, day-care center attendance is very important. Its benefit should be weighed against the risks to the child. The final decision depends on the child's age and clinical status — i.e., level of immunosuppression, neurologic status, and behavior.

Education.   If an HIV-infected child attends a day-care center or preschool, it is important to have an AIDS educational program for staff and parents.

▪ GRADE SCHOOLS AND HIGH SCHOOLS

Attendance   After years of debate, it is now widely accepted that HIV-infected children can usually participate in regular classroom instruction. There is no evidence that HIV is transmitted by casual contact or by any kind of activity that takes place in the classroom, gymnasium, or playing field.[4,5] Thus, the students are not a hazard to others.

Risk of Infection.   As in younger students, there is concern that the HIV-infected student may be at risk of acquiring a serious infection while at school. The risk of infection depends upon students' immune and clinical status. For most HIV-infected school-age children, the benefits of an unrestricted setting and the educational experience outweigh the risk of acquiring a potentially harmful infection.[2]

We believe that each child of school age known to be infected with HIV should be reviewed individually by a knowledgeable group of health professionals in consultation with school authorities. This group can then recommend the most appropriate placement for the student's benefit. For the vast majority of students, placement in the regular classroom can be recommended. Because the clinical and immunologic status of the student changes, placement recommendations should be reviewed annually or at other appropriate intervals.

Education.   Each school district should provide an educational program for school personnel, parents, and students about sexually transmitted diseases, including AIDS. Furthermore, when appropriate, students need to be educated about preventing sexually transmitted diseases, including AIDS.

▪ CONFIDENTIALITY

The child's and family's privacy should be respected by all concerned. Disclosure that an HIV-infected child attends the day-care center, preschool, grade school, or high school may result in the child's rejection, isolation, or both, producing serious emotional stress. Thus, information about the child's status should be treated with utmost confidentiality. If the child's immune system is seriously impaired, one or two people at the center or school should know this. The purpose of such notification is twofold: The child will need to be excused from school requirements for immunization with live virus vaccines and the school will need to notify the family of any exposures to varicella, herpes, or other infections so that suitable prophylactic measures can be taken. The parents of other children attending the center or school should not know the HIV status of the child in question.

▪ COLLEGES AND UNIVERSITIES

Attendance and Participation.   HIV infections are not transmitted by casual contact or any activity likely to be included in a college curriculum. Thus, enrollment and participation in all activities should be limited only by the student's own clinical and immune status, which the student should discuss with his or her personal physician. There is no reason to notify any university official of the student's HIV status. However, if the student seeks medical care through the student health service, that service should be apprised of the patient's infection and maintain confidentiality of the medical record.

Education and Counseling.   Colleges and universities should organize educational campaigns about AIDS and HIV infection. This is best done through the health-education branch of the student health service. Personal protection and safer-sex practices should be stressed. Additionally, the student health service should make counselors available for students who may have HIV infections and need support and advice. The student's privacy should be respected by all concerned; antibody status should be treated with utmost confidentiality.

■ HIV AND FOSTER HOMES

In our society, parents bear the ultimate moral and legal responsibility for protecting their children's health. In order to carry out this responsibility, they need all relevant information about their foster child's health status. In the case of children infected with HIV, foster parents need to know that the foster child has an HIV infection and could become seriously immunodeficient.[2]

In the course of daily living in the home, the infected youngster is not expected to endanger others[4,5]; however, the youngster himself might be threatened by everyday infections that pose little hazard to normal children. Foster parents should know what circumstances call for medical care for their youngster. Furthermore, HIV-infected children should not receive certain live-virus vaccines. Foster-parent awareness of this fact affords the youngster extra protection, since health providers change and medical record keeping for foster children is often poor.

Foster-Home Placement.   The circumstances that lead to a child's HIV infection (such as maternal HIV disease) may necessitate foster placement of the child. As indicated above and elsewhere,[2] foster parents should be informed if a child has an HIV infection or may become immunocompromised. Whenever possible, a medical foster home should be secured, because an additional burden will be placed on the foster parents and additional compensation is needed. Foster parents will also need education about HIV infection and support in dealing with the anxieties and misinformation that abound concerning HIV infection. These should be provided by the child's social worker and health-care provider.

Foster parents can have other children living in their home without fear of infection, since HIV is not transmitted by casual contact.[4,5] If the HIV-infected child has clinical AIDS, the burden of care may become so heavy that the number of children the foster parents are able to care for must be limited. In addition, their compensation may need to be increased further.

Education.   In dealing with the foster child's education, foster parents should follow the guidelines suggested above for day-care centers, preschools, and schools.

■ ADOLESCENT DETENTION CENTERS AND GROUP HOMES

The principal difference between the adolescent detention home and other settings for children and youths is the possibility that sexual activity might take place between youngsters housed in these facilities. Operators of detention homes are concerned about the ethical and legal liability they might incur if a youngster contracts an HIV infection while residing in their institution.

With the exception of sexual contacts, intravenous drug use, and tattooing, all other activities that youngsters might engage in at such centers and group homes would not pose a hazard for the transmission of HIV infection.[4,5]

Testing Adolescents for HIV Infection.   Education and counseling of all adolescents, but most particularly those engaged in high-risk behavior, are of the utmost importance. Routine HIV testing is not useful. Testing is indicated on clinical grounds only when there is suspicion of clinical disease. Testing may be used as part of counseling. If treatment of asymptomatic infection proves to be beneficial, then there may be wider indications for testing.

Education.   It is particularly important for each adolescent detention center and group home to conduct an educational program for its staff and resident youths about sexuality, sexually transmitted diseases, and HIV infection in particular. The staff should also be trained to establish policies and procedures that reduce the likelihood of sexual encounters between youngsters in the center.

Confidentiality.   On occasion, the center director and staff may become aware of a youth infected with HIV. Such information needs to be treated with the utmost confidentiality. The health-care provider responsible for the youngster needs to be informed so that suitable precautions can be taken in protecting the infected youngster. Infections such as chickenpox or herpes (usually considered to be minor in adolescents) may need more aggressive treatment in HIV-infected, immunocompromised youths. The health-care provider's information about a youngster's HIV infection need not be passed on to the center director or other nonmedical staff. If the youngster's immune status dictates that he be housed in a single room rather than a dormitory to avoid acquiring infections, such recommendations should be made by the director of health services and accepted by the center director on the grounds that the youngster is immunocompromised. HIV infection need not be specified.

■ DISINFECTION IN ANY SETTING

Even though HIV is not transmitted by casual contact, AIDS has drawn attention to the importance of blood, body fluids, and secretions in transmitting the infection. Many other infectious agents, including hepatitis virus, can also be present in such fluids.[3] Housekeeping personnel should be instructed in handling and disinfecting such secretions. Household bleach (1:100 parts water) is a suitable disinfectant.

REFERENCES

1.   Rogers MF. AIDS in children: a review of the clinical, epidemiologic and public health aspects. Pediatr Infect Dis 1985; 4:230-6.

2.   Centers for Disease Control. Education and foster care of children infected with human T-lymphotropic virus type III/lymphadenopathy-associated virus. MMWR 1985; 34:517-21.

3.   Task Force on Pediatric AIDS. Pediatric guidelines for infection control of human immunodeficiency virus (acquired immunodeficiency virus) in hospitals, medical offices, schools, and other settings. Pediatrics 1988; 82:801-7.

4.   Friedland GH, Saltzman BR, Rogers MF, et al. Lack of transmission of HTLV-III infection to household contacts of patients with AIDS or AIDS-related complex with oral candidiasis. N Engl J Med 1986; 314:344-9.

5.   Kaplan JE, Oleske JM, Getchel JK, et al. Evidence against transmission of HTLV-III/LAV in families of children with AIDS. Pediatr Infect Dis 1985; 4:468-71.

10.6

Infection-Control Guidelines: Miscellaneous

Precautions for Persons with HIV Infection Living in the Community

J. Louise Gerberding, M.D., and Merle A. Sande, M.D.

The human immunodeficiency virus (HIV) is not transmitted by casual contact with infected persons. Individuals with HIV infection may safely share household and public facilities with others. Common sense hygienic practices should be employed to prevent further exposure to HIV as well as to other potentially contagious pathogens.

Individuals with HIV infection who have impaired immune systems should exercise additional precautions in the home to avoid exposure to opportunistic pathogens. Guidelines for minimizing exposure to these pathogens have been developed.[1]

Pets. Certain birds may harbor *Chlamydia psittaci*, *Histoplasma capsulatum*, or *Cryptococcus neoformans*, so contact with birds and bird cages should be avoided. Cat litter boxes may be contaminated with *Toxoplasma gondii*; direct exposure and inhalation of cat litter should also be avoided. Tropical fish tanks may be contaminated with mycobacterial organisms. Gloves should be worn when cleaning fish tanks or when handling fish.

Foods. Organically grown foods fertilized with human or animal feces should not be eaten unless thoroughly cooked. Organically grown fruits may be eaten if peeled and washed. Organic lettuce should be avoided.

Unpasteurized milk and milk products such as yogurts and cheeses may be contaminated with various species of salmonella, brucella, and listeria. These foods should not be included in the diet.

Household Molds. Damp environments such as showers and hot tubs promote the growth of fungi. These areas should be cleaned and disinfected with a 1:100 dilution of household bleach (5.25 percent sodium hypochlorite). The inside of refrigerators should be cleaned with soap and water. Spoiled food should be disposed of promptly.

REFERENCES

1. Lusby G, Schietinger H, San Francisco General Hospital Medical Special Care Unit, San Francisco Bay Area Association for Practitioners of Infection Control AIDS Resource Group. Infection precautions for people with AIDS living in the community. Infection control policy manual, San Francisco General Hospital.

Household Contacts of Persons Infected with HIV

J. Louise Gerberding, M.D., and Merle A. Sande, M.D.

The human immunodeficiency virus (HIV) is transmitted by sexual contact with infected partners, by direct inoculation of infected blood products, and by perinatal transmission from infected mothers to their offspring. There is no evidence of risk to close household contacts of persons infected with the virus.

Infection-control guidelines for people living with AIDS patients and other individuals infected with HIV have been established.[1] These guidelines are based on common sense hygienic practices designed to reduce exposure to most infectious agents transmissible in the home.

Individuals who provide medical care to patients in the home environment should follow the infection-control guidelines for health-care workers in the hospital environment.

Personal Hygiene.   Good personal hygiene should be maintained. This includes regular bathing and handwashing after contact with body fluids and after using bathroom facilities. Coughing individuals should cough into tissues or handkerchiefs.

Shared Utensils.   Dishes and other utensils should not be shared while eating. Separate dishes are not necessary, but dishes should be cleaned with hot soapy water after use.

Toothbrushes, razors, enema equipment, and other implements potentially contaminated with body fluids should not be shared.

Towels and washcloths should not be shared between individuals without first being laundered.

Kitchen and bathroom facilities may be shared. Normal sanitary procedures are adequate to prevent transmission of HIV in these environments.

Food Preparation.   Individuals with HIV infection may safely prepare food for others provided they wash their hands before beginning. Utensils used to sample food while cooking should not be reused in food preparation without first being washed.

Cleaning and Disinfection.   Kitchen surfaces should be cleaned with scouring powder to remove food particles. Sponges used to clean bathrooms or floors should not be used to clean kitchen areas. The kitchen sink should not be used for disposal of mop water.

Bathroom floors should be cleaned at least once a week. Spills or soilage should be cleaned up immediately. Showers, sinks, toilets, and tubs should be disinfected with a 1:100 dilution of household bleach (5.25 percent sodium hypochlorite).

Waste Disposal.   No special precautions for household trash disposal are necessary. Lined trash containers should be used for potentially contaminated items, such as dressings, diapers, and tissues. Trash should be placed in sturdy bags; double-bagging is unnecessary unless the bag is visibly soiled.

REFERENCES

1. Lusby G, Schietinger H, the San Francisco General Hospital Medical Special Care Unit, San Francisco Bay Area Association for Practitioners of Infection Control AIDS Resource Group. Infection precautions for people with AIDS living in the community. Infection control policy manual, San Francisco General Hospital.

11

PUBLIC
EDUCATION
AND
PREVENTION
STRATEGIES

EDITOR

P.T. Cohen, M.D., Ph.D.

11.1

Public Education and Prevention Strategies

Educational Strategies to Prevent AIDS: Rationale

Karen S. Heller, M.A.

■ RATIONALE

A frank and forthright approach is needed in all communications about AIDS to increase understanding of how HIV (human immunodeficiency virus) is and is not transmitted and to motivate responsible actions to prevent its further spread. In the absence of a vaccine, education is the most promising, socially acceptable strategy for preventing HIV transmission.

Surveys indicate that public awareness of AIDS is high. Most people now know that HIV is transmitted through sexual intercourse, infected blood transfusions, and sharing contaminated needles during intravenous drug use.[1-3,18,19,40] However, many people still believe that HIV also can be contracted by donating blood or through casual contact. Among teenagers, the misunderstanding about how HIV is transmitted has been compounded by ignorance about sexuality in general.[4-6,18,19,26,40,41] Although more than half of American teens are estimated to be sexually active, about one-third of these do not use contraception or do so inconsistently.[27,45] As a result, high rates of pregnancy and of sexually transmitted diseases (STDs) occur in this age group. This has led many health officials to call for mandatory AIDS education in public schools.[27,29] According to a Gallup poll conducted in April 1988, 99 percent of the general public and 94 percent of public-school parents support instruction about AIDS in the classroom, although they differ about at what grade to begin such instruction. Eighty-one percent of the parents thought school classes should include discussions about safer sex as a way to prevent HIV transmission[20] (AIDS education of adolescents is presented elsewhere).

Formal evaluations of various AIDS-preventive education methods were rarely conducted during the early years of the epidemic. Only recently have they begun to receive attention.[42] However, several types of evidence indirectly demonstrate the effectiveness of education and information in altering HIV-related high-risk behaviors. The rates of seroconversion among gay men in San Francisco[30] and New York City have dramatically declined. Although this could be interpreted as a "saturation" phenomenon, many health experts attribute it to behavior changes made as a result of the sustained education gay men received in those cities over the past several years. Surveys show that since 1982, gay men have greatly reduced their average number of sexual contacts and have modified their sexual practices.[8,9,21,30-33,42] Other evidence comes from reports of STD clinics in San Francisco and other cities worldwide, which show that rates of rectal gonorrhea among men fell dramatically between 1980 and 1984.[10-14] In addition, syphilis cases dropped 36 percent in San Francisco during the first half of 1987, compared with a rise in incidence elsewhere in

California; this drop has been attributed to the impact of the city's AIDS education program.[34]

Although gay men in urban centers have significantly reduced their risk of HIV infection, some may have difficulty maintaining safer-sex practices without relapse.[21] A recent study of 453 gay men in San Francisco showed a 59 percent decline in high-risk sex between 1984 and 1987, but 15.7 percent of the subjects also acknowledged at least one relapse into unsafe sexual practices during that period.[22] In areas where HIV prevalence is high, even occasional relapse is cause for concern. Stall and Ekstrand suggest that in designing interventions, AIDS educators should differentiate between the kind of motivation that may be needed for initiating behavior changes and the motivation needed to maintain them. A mix of techniques may be needed to encourage both the adoption and longterm adherence to safer-sex practices.[23]

Among heterosexuals, knowledge about AIDS does not necessarily correlate with effective behavior changes to reduce risk of HIV transmission, even when people recognize their vulnerability to infection.[18,38] In recent years, sharp rises in STDs among heterosexuals, particularly in black and Latino inner-city populations, signal that heterosexual HIV transmission also may increase.[39] Much of the AIDS education directed to inner-city populations is being targeted to intravenous drug users (IVDUs) and their sexual partners (many of whom are heterosexual, bisexual, and/or come from racial and ethnic minority groups).

Evidence is accumulating that education and outreach to IVDUs is having some effect. They are now more knowledgeable about their risks for HIV infection, they have reduced sharing needles, or at least have begun to disinfect their needles and syringes.[15-17,35,43-45] However, educational efforts have been less successful in motivating IVDUs and their sexual partners to use condoms.[36] In large cities where intravenous drug use is high among blacks and Latinos, AIDS prevention programs must address cultural attitudes, as these may influence drug users' practices.[37]

A variety of community groups and public health agencies have become involved in education projects for IVDUs, prostitutes, adolescents, and others at high risk for HIV infection. Because 42 percent of reported cases of AIDS have occurred among nonwhites in the United States, racial and ethnic minority groups are increasingly involved in developing culturally sensitive AIDS education programs and materials for their communities. A discussion of issues related to AIDS education among blacks, Latinos, and IVDUs is presented elsewhere.

Besides helping to prevent HIV transmission, AIDS information and education can be used to influence attitudes toward people infected with HIV. One study of knowledge, attitudes, and beliefs about AIDS among adults in San Francisco, New York, and London showed that increased knowledge about AIDS correlated with decreased fear and lessened homophobia.[7] Although knowledge about AIDS increased significantly in all three cities from 1985 to 1987, people in New York remained less knowledgeable and more fearful towards homosexuals and people with AIDS.[46] The authors concluded that public education campaigns about AIDS must go beyond presenting the facts of transmission to address sociocultural and subcultural attitudes and beliefs.

Displaced fear and confusion about how HIV is spread fuel discrimination against HIV-infected people. They also handicap the development and use of appropriate, effective prevention policies. Most knowledgeable medical experts reject coercive measures, such as quarantine or mandatory testing to detect

HIV antibodies, as unjustifiable on scientific and practical grounds. Controversy about the proper roles of law and government versus informed, voluntary change arises in many areas of public-health policy, such as efforts to control cigarette smoking, seat-belt use, alcohol abuse, and other activities associated with high morbidity and mortality. Controversy is especially acute with respect to AIDS because in the United States, HIV has been transmitted primarily through practices widely condemned in the society at large. Moreover, to date, AIDS has primarily afflicted individuals already stigmatized by reasons of sexual preference, drug use, race, or ethnicity. (A discussion of some of the ways in which this stigma has colored federal approaches to AIDS education may be found elsewhere.)

REFERENCES

1. Blake SM, Arkin E. Summary of national public opinion polls on AIDS [Abstract]. IV International Conference on AIDS. Stockholm, 1988; 1:9094.

2. Judin JP, Teahan C, Tseng W-S. Cross-ethnic attitudes and knowledge about AIDS in Hawaii [Abstract]. IV International Conference on AIDS. Stockholm, 1988:1:9119.

3. Gallup G, Gallup A. Surge in awareness of how AIDS is spread. San Francisco Chronicle. November 28, 1988.

4. Price JH, Desmond S, Kukulka G. High school students' perceptions and misperceptions of AIDS. J Sch Health 1985; 55:7-9.

5. AIDS education survey in SF schools. Focus 1986; 1:4.

6. High school attitudes on AIDS are surveyed. CDC AIDS Weekly. May 26, 1986:5.

7. Temoshok L, Sweet DM, Zich J. A three city comparison of the public's knowledge and attitudes about AIDS. Psychology and Health: An International Journal, 1987; 1:43-60.

8. McKusick L, Horstman W, Coates TJ. AIDS and sexual behavior reported by gay men in San Francisco. Am J Public Health 1985; 75:493-6.

9. McKusick L, Wiley JA, Coates TJ, et al. Reported changes in the sexual behavior of men at risk for AIDS, San Francisco, 1982–84 — the AIDS behavioral research project. Public Hlth Rep 1985; 100:622-9.

10. Declining rates of rectal and pharyngeal gonorrhea among males — New York City. MMWR 1984; 3:295-7.

11. Schechter MT, Jeffries E, Constance P, et al. Changes in sexual behavior and fear of AIDS. Lancet 1984; 1:1293.

12. Judson FN. Fear of AIDS and gonorrhea rates in homosexual men. Lancet 1983; 2:159-60.

13. Echenberg DF. A new strategy to prevent the spread of AIDS among heterosexuals. JAMA 1985; 154:2129-30.

14. Waller IVD, Hindley DJ, Adler MW, Meldrum JT. Gonorrhea in homosexual men and media coverage of the acquired immunodeficiency syndrome in London 1982–83. Br Med J 1984; 289:1041.

15. Des Jarlais DC, Friedman SR, Hopkins W. Risk reduction for the acquired immune deficiency syndrome among intravenous drug users. Ann Intern Med 1985; 103:755-9.

16. Marmor M, Des Jarlais DC, Friedman SR, et al. The epidemic of acquired immunodeficiency syndrome and suggestions for its control in drug abusers. J Subst Abuse Tr 1984; 1:237-47.

17. Watters JK. Preventing human immunodeficiency virus contagion among intravenous drug users: The impact of street-based education on risk behavior [Abstract]. III International Conference on AIDS. Washington, D.C., 1987; 60.

18. Helgerson SD, Petersen LR. Acquired immunodeficiency syndrome and secondary school students: their knowledge is limited and they want to learn more. Pediatrics 1988; 81:350-5.

19. Teenagers and Sex. San Francisco Chronicle. October 26, 1988.

20. Parents say yes to AIDS education. San Francisco Chronicle. August 26, 1988:4.

21. Stall R, Coates TJ, Hoff C. Behavioral risk reduction for HIV infection among gay and bisexual men: a review of results from the United States. Amer Psych 1988; 43:878-85.

22. Garcia D. SF gays relapsing into unsafe sex. San Francisco Chronicle. March 11, 1988:A-3.

23. Stall R, Ekstrand M. Implications of relapse from safe sex. Focus 1989; 4:3.

24. Morgan WM, Curran JW. Acquired immunodeficiency syndrome: Current and future trends. Public Hlth Rep 1986; 101:459-65.

25. Institute of Medicine, National Academy of Sciences. Confronting AIDS: Directions for public health, health care, and research. Washington, D.C.: National Academy Press; 1986.

26. Konetzny TK, Konetzny AH, Pifer LL. Knowledge and attitudes of Memphis parochial school adolescents about the acquired immune deficiency syndrome. J Tenn Med Assoc 1987; 80:529-32.

27. San Francisco expert urges mandatory AIDS education. San Francisco Examiner. July 29, 1987:A-5.

28. AIDS educational plan unveiled in Washington. San Francisco Chronicle. March 17, 1987:1, 22.

29. States that require AIDS education in school triple in six months. New York Times. December 4, 1987:B-5.

30. Winkelstein W Jr, Samuel M, Padian NS, et al. The San Francisco men's health study: III. Reduction in human immunodeficiency virus transmission among homosexual/bisexual men, 1982–86. Am J Public Health 1987; 77:685-9.

31. Solomon MZ, DeJong W. Recent sexually transmitted disease prevention efforts and their implications for AIDS health education. Health Educ Q 1986; 13:301-6.

32. Research and Decisions Corporation. A report on: designing an effective AIDS prevention campaign strategy for San Francisco: results from the second probability sample of an urban gay male community. San Francisco: San Francisco AIDS Foundation, 1985.

33. Martin JL. The impact of AIDS on gay male sexual behavior patterns in New York City. Am J Public Health 1987; 77:578-81.

34. City's AIDS education cited in 36 percent drop in syphilis cases. San Francisco Examiner. September 16, 1987:B-4.

35. Krieger L. Education is key to slowing spread of AIDS in drug users. San Francisco Examiner. June 16, 1988:A-1, A-15.

36. Flynn N, Jain S, Bailey V, et al. Characteristics and stated AIDS risk behavior of IV drug users attending drug treatment programs in a medium-sized U.S. city [Abstract]. IV International Conference on AIDS. Stockholm, 1988; 1:8006.

37. Schilling RF, Schinke SP, Nichols SE, et al. Developing strategies for AIDS prevention research with black and Hispanic drug users. Public Health Rep 1989; 104:2-11.

38. Zonana VF. Non-gays see, ignore AIDS peril, study says. Los Angeles Times. Jan 25, 1989.

39. Leary WE. Sharp rise in rare sex-related diseases. New York Times. July 14, 1988:B-9.

40. Teen survey. AIDS myths are believed by teens. San Francisco Examiner. February 10, 1988:4(Z-1).

41. Kegeles SM, Adler NE, Irwin CE Jr. Sexually active adolescents and condoms: changes over one year in knowledge, attitudes and use. Am J Public Health 1988; 78:460-1.

42. Becker MH, Joseph JG. AIDS and behavioral change to reduce risk: a review. Am J Public Health 1988; 78:394-410.

43. Friedman SR, Des Jarlais DC, Sotheran JL. AIDS health education for intravenous drug users. Health Educ Q 1986; 13:383-93.

44. Ginzburg HM, French J, Jackson J, et al. Health education and knowledge assessment of HTLV-III diseases among intravenous drug users. Health Educ Q 1986; 13:373-82.

45. Chaisson RE, Moss AR, Onishi R, et al. Human immunodeficiency virus infection in heterosexual intravenous drug users in San Francisco. Am J Public Health 1987; 77:169-72.

46. Temoshok L, Sweet DM, Moulton JM, et al. AIDS in the public's mind: changes over time in London, New York, and San Francisco [Abstract]. IV International Conference on AIDS. Stockholm, 1988; 1:9099.

Educational Form, Content, and Language Issues

Karen S. Heller, M.A.

Health communications are most effective when they are framed in the cultural values, language, idioms, and imagery of their intended audience.[1,7-9,17] However, health educators and others have caused controversy when they have used explicit language and imagery appropriate to intravenous drug users (IVDUs) or gay men but offensive to mainstream conventions of taste, propriety, or morality.[2-4,10-13,15,18]

The form and content of AIDS educational materials, particularly those paid for by public funds, have frequently been the focus of debate: should medical or moral considerations govern AIDS-prevention strategies and messages?[3,12,14] In 1985, for example, the California State AIDS Office banned organizations from using state funds to distribute several AIDS-prevention pamphlets that it said bordered on "pornography." The office set up an AIDS Materials Review Committee to provide guidelines for printed materials funded through tax revenues.[10] Subsequently, state contracts specified that slang or explicitly worded materials would not be approved. Federal interagency conflict about federally-produced AIDS-prevention materials has delayed and sometimes muzzled clear communication about AIDS risks and prevention.[17] In October 1987, U.S. Senator Jesse Helms labelled a graphically illustrated comic book designed by the Gay Men's Health Crisis (GMHC) in New York "obscene." The comic book demonstrated safer sex practices for gay men.[2] However offensive such material may be to members of Congress, it can help high-risk gay men to adopt safer sexual practices. An evaluation of GMHC's sexually explicit, erotic videos found that compared with lectures or inexplicit material intended for a general audience, the videos were more effective in motivating changes to low- or no-risk sexual practices.[18]

During the first few years of the epidemic, prudish editorial standards and ambiguously worded public health communications may have obscured how HIV is and is not transmitted.[5,6] Such vagueness may have increased public anxiety about both the disease and the populations in which HIV infection was most prevalent. The emphasis on "risk groups" in early press reports and health communications may have reinforced the general public's tendency to view AIDS as a disease of "them" (not "us") as well as the complacency of people who perceived themselves to be outside risk-group "borders." In 1987, the major television networks initially resisted broadcasting the Centers for Disease Control's public-service announcements about AIDS during prime-time hours.[19] Their reluctance both reflected and reinforced imaginary barriers between "the general public" and those at high risk for AIDS. The news media also continued to use overly general descriptions about AIDS risk-related behaviors (e.g., allusions to "intimate contact" and "bodily fluids") that did not specify the types of contacts and fluids most likely to transmit HIV.[5,6] However, as reporters and editors have become more knowledgeable about AIDS and its social and political impact, the major media generally have begun to present risk-related information in frank detail, if not in "street" language.

Health education research suggests that messages targeted to well-defined population segments best promote risk awareness in those groups.[1,7-9,16] The report of the President's Commission on the Epidemic of HIV Infection acknowledged that different population segments have unique educational needs with respect to HIV infection, and because of this, "the educational response to the epidemic needs to acknowledge the eclectic nature of our society and effectively match the proper educational approach with a receptive target population."[20] This effort requires significant input from members of the targeted population so that educational programs and materials are "relevant, appropriate in language, and effectively reach the intended audience."[20]

However, targeted information may fail to reach people engaging in high-risk activities who do not identify themselves with the social profile of a given risk group. For example, AIDS messages developed for gay men may be ignored by women or by men who occasionally engage in homosexual acts but still identify themselves as heterosexual. Recognizing that IVDUs and all sexually active people may potentially be at risk for HIV infection, AIDS organizations, public-health authorities, and the press now tend to emphasize that it is what you do and how you do it, not who you are, that is central to AIDS prevention. This approach reinforces the fact that HIV infection and AIDS do not derive from personal or group characteristics (sexual orientation, race, ethnicity, or national origin) but rather from specific actions that increase the likelihood of exposure to HIV. Prevention messages, therefore, now emphasize avoiding or modifying specific risk-related activities, not avoiding or isolating people at risk for HIV infection or those already infected with the virus.

In their reports, the National Academy of Sciences panel and the U.S. Surgeon General stressed providing people with realistic options for protecting themselves and others against HIV transmission. They also emphasized the importance of using sexually explicit, easily understood language tailored to various audiences in all communications.[21,22] These reports also reflect the frustration of many health professionals and AIDS service groups with the prejudice and prudery that handicap clear communication about AIDS risks and seriously jeopardize efforts to control further spread of the virus.

Guidelines for informing adolescents and intravenous drug users about AIDS and guidelines for safer sex may be found elsewhere.

REFERENCES

1. Richards ND. Methods and effectiveness of health education: the past, present, and future of social scientific involvement. Soc Sci Med 1975; 9:141-56.
2. Altman D. AIDS in the mind of America. The social, political, and psychological impact of a new epidemic. Garden City, N.Y.: Anchor Press/Doubleday, 1986.
3. Institute of Medicine, National Academy of Sciences. Mobilizing against AIDS: the unfinished story of a virus. Cambridge, Mass.: Harvard University Press, 1986:144.
4. Kirp D. AIDS crisis. San Francisco Examiner. February 26, 1986:A-11.
5. Leff L, Adolph J. AIDS and the family paper. Columbia J Rev. March/April 1986:11, 13.
6. Diamond E, Bellitto CM. The great verbal coverup: prudish editing blurs the facts on AIDS. Wash J Rev. March 1986:38-42.
7. Williams LS. AIDS risk reduction: a community health education intervention for minority high risk group members. Health Educ Q 1986; 13:407-21.
8. Siegel K, Grodsky PB, Herman A. AIDS risk reduction guidelines: a review and analysis. J Community Health 1986; 11:233-43.
9. Ad Hoc Working Group of the American Public Health Association. Criteria for the development of health promotion and education programs. Am J Public Health 1987; 77:89-92.

10. Kell G. Foundation blasts state for opposing graphic AIDS pamphlets. San Francisco Examiner. September 16, 1987:B-6.

11. Breakstone L, Krikorian G. State GOP infighting over AIDS. San Francisco Examiner. September 28, 1987:A-1, A-6.

12. Sirica C. The bitter fight over U.S. plan to battle AIDS. San Francisco Chronicle. September 28, 1987:A-1.

13. Lawrence J. Senate's AIDS vote rings "death knell," critic says. San Francisco Examiner. October 15, 1987:A-2.

14. Evans R, Novak R. More AIDS feuding. San Francisco Examiner. September 14, 1987:A-12.

15. Getlin J. Attack on "safe sex" rules stirs AIDS debate. Los Angeles Times. April 29, 1988:1, 30.

16. Becker MH, Joseph JG. AIDS and behavioral change to reduce risk: a review. Am J Public Health 1988; 78:394-410.

17. D'Eramo JE, Quadland MC, Shattls W, et al. The "800 men" project: a systematic evaluation of AIDS prevention programs demonstrating the efficacy of erotic, sexually explicit safer sex education on gay and bisexual men at risk for AIDS [Abstract]. IV International Conference on AIDS. Stockholm, 1988; 1:8086.

18. Shilts R. The politics of prevention. San Francisco Chronicle. February 20, 1989:A-4.

19. Education in AIDS criticized in study. New York Times. December 20, 1988.

20. Report of the Presidential Commission on the Human Immunodeficiency Virus Epidemic. Washington, D.C.: 1988 (June 24):86.

21. Institute of Medicine, National Academy of Sciences. Confronting AIDS: directions for public health, health care, and research. Washington, D.C.: National Academy Press; 1986.

22. U.S. Public Health Service. Surgeon General's report on acquired immune deficiency syndrome. Washington, D.C.: October 1986.

Funding AIDS Education and Conflicts about Approaches

Karen S. Heller, M.A.

I n the United States, public understanding of AIDS and efforts to halt its spread have been profoundly influenced by its epidemiology. Early news reports described the disease as a "gay plague."[1] Some gay leaders at first feared that developing educational materials identifying the risks of specific homosexual practices would intensify homophobia in the general population and create a backlash against hard-won gay rights. Nevertheless, gay organizations were first in informing gay men and others at high risk about AIDS. The first brochures on safer sex were developed by gay organizations in Houston and San Francisco.[1] To date, most educational materials and programs about AIDS have been developed by community-based, often gay-related, organizations in association with state and local health departments.

Community-based groups have had to assume responsibility for AIDS education partly by default: under the Reagan administration, the federal government was slow to provide leadership or funding for prevention and sought to decentralize many health programs. In fiscal year 1984, for example, less than 4 percent of the federal AIDS budget was allocated to information and public affairs.[2] With a cumulative total of 270,000 AIDS cases projected by 1991,[3,4,23] the government faced mounting pressure to commit more funds to AIDS prevention and education. Congress appropriated more funds for AIDS than the administration requested each fiscal year from 1982 through 1988.[5]

State expenditures on AIDS, excluding federal funds, increased 15-fold to $156.3 million between 1984 and 1988. However, state-level per-person expenditure for AIDS education averaged $.65, below the level recommended by the Institute of Medicine.[6] Some states support AIDS activities indirectly by shifting resources, often from sexually transmitted disease (STD) programs, a problematic solution in view of the rise in STD cases.[7]

AIDS education efforts during the Reagan administration were hampered by a lack of coordination and leadership, delays in creating and implementing a comprehensive plan, and major dissension among officials in various federal agencies about what approaches to recommend for risk reduction.[8-10] For some observers, President Reagan's declaration on November 1, 1988, that October was AIDS Awareness Month was emblematic of the sluggish response to the epidemic by his administration.[5] By fiscal year 1989, however, federal funding for AIDS education and prevention increased to $370 million (out of a total AIDS budget of $1.5 billion).

Despite statements by health agency officials that education was a crucial AIDS prevention strategy,[11,12] the Reagan administration impeded effective and timely federal response out of fear of appearing to condone homosexuality or drug use. The administration also feared offending conservative political constituencies through explicit discussions of sexual and drug-use practices.[1] Concerns about what messages to convey and what language to use contributed to a one-year delay in mailing a Centers for Disease Control pamphlet on AIDS to every U.S. household[10,13,14] and a two-and-one-half-year delay in distributing a pamphlet produced by the National Institute on Alcohol and Drug Abuse (NIDA) to inform sexual partners of intravenous drug users (IVDUs) about their high risk for HIV infection.[15] In a report to the White House in October 1986, U.S. Surgeon General C. Everett Koop urged frank discussion of all types of sexual expression as part of AIDS education programs for both children and adults.[16] Although the Surgeon General and the Public Health Service[17] supported disseminating information about sexual abstinence or monogamy along with material on condoms and other safe-sex practices for people who are sexually active outside of marriage, other members of the Reagan administration actively opposed this approach.[18]

The comprehensive federal AIDS education plan, announced by the Department of Health and Human Services (DHHS) in March 1987, was drafted after months of debate between the Public Health Service and the Department of Education on what emphasis to give condom use versus abstinence before and fidelity after marriage in federally-sponsored AIDS prevention programs. The DHHS plan ultimately stated that federally-sponsored AIDS information should encourage "responsible" sexual behavior based on fidelity and commitment, "placing sexuality within the context of marriage" and encouraging abstinence among teenagers.[19]

The debate about federally supported approaches to AIDS prevention was carried to Congress in October 1987. The Senate and the House of Representatives overwhelmingly passed an appropriations bill amendment introduced by U.S. Senator Jesse Helms prohibiting federal funding for educational materials that "promote or encourage homosexual activities." Funded education materials were mandated to emphasize "abstinence from sexual activity outside of a sexually monogamous marriage."[20] Although the final legislation was further amended so as not to "be construed to prohibit description of methods to reduce the risk of HIV transmission,"[20] AIDS educators feared that the Helms amendment would limit state and local agencies' ability to use federal money to produce effective educational materials for the people at greatest risk for the disease.[21]

By April 1988, when the Senate passed a similar Helms amendment attached to the AIDS Research and Information Act (S1220), some states already had curtailed educational efforts targeted to gay men.[22] The impact of the second Helms amendment was later muted, however, by an amendment introduced by U.S. Senator Edward Kennedy, which provided that "nothing shall restrict the ability of the education program to provide accurate information on reducing the risk of HIV infection."

Educational strategies to prevent AIDS are being developed within political and social milieux that influence their form, content, and ultimately, their effectiveness. As Dennis Altman pointed out, in this society there is a fine line between education and control: "the demand to disseminate information leads almost inevitably to demands to enforce certain standards."[1] This, in turn, leads to continuing debate about what information should be communicated to whom, by whom, and how, and whose standards should be used in deciding the appropriateness of information for each audience.

President Bush, while elected with major support from the same conservative constituencies that supported Reagan, has given some indications that his administration may take a more coordinated and "kinder, gentler" approach to AIDS-related issues.[24] Unlike Reagan, Bush fully endorsed the recommendations of the President's Commission on HIV and before his election expressed support for legislation banning discrimination against people infected with HIV or those with AIDS.[24] He also announced plans to establish a national AIDS program within the Public Health Service to coordinate and consolidate AIDS funding, now spread among 23 of its agencies. Such a plan could make HIV research and prevention efforts more effective. Calling AIDS the "highest public-health priority" of his administration, President Bush requested an increase of $313 million in AIDS funding for fiscal year 1990 to $1.38 billion.[25] Similar in many respects to the $1.6 billion requested by Reagan before he left office, Bush's request disappointed AIDS activists, who plan to lobby Congress once again for appropriation increases to levels more in keeping with what federal agencies say they need.

REFERENCES

1. Altman D. AIDS in the mind of America: the social, political, and psychological impact of a new epidemic. Garden City, NY: Anchor Press/Doubleday, 1986.
2. United States Congress. Office of Technology Assessment. Review of the Public Health Service's response to AIDS. OTA-TM-H-24. Washington, D.C.: February 1985.
3. Coolfont report: a PHS plan for prevention and control of AIDS and AIDS virus. Public Health Rep 1986; 101; 341-8.
4. Morgan WM, Curran JW. Acquired immunodeficiency syndrome: current and future trends. Public Health Rep 1986; 101:459-65.
5. Beyond the Bay: curtains close on the Reagan AIDS era. San Francisco Sentinel. February 9, 1989.
6. Rowe MJ, Ryan CC. Comparing state-only expenditures for AIDS. Am J Public Health 1988; 78:424-9.
7. Leary WE. Sharp rise in rare sex-related diseases. New York Times. July 14, 1988:B-9.
8. Boffey PM. Panel of experts finds absence of leadership in battle against AIDS. New York Times. June 2, 1988.
9. Newquist J. GAO raps Reagan on AIDS response. Bay Area Reporter. December 29, 1988.
10. Crewdson J. U.S. to send everyone AIDS prevention brochure. San Francisco Examiner. January 27, 1988:A-4.
11. Curran JW. The epidemiology and prevention of the acquired immunodeficiency syndrome. Ann Intern Med 1985; 103:657-62.
12. Sex education could help battle AIDS. CDC AIDS Weekly. February 20, 1986:10.
13. Breakstone L, Krikorian G. State GOP infighting over AIDS. San Francisco Examiner. September 28, 1987:A-1, A-6.
14. U.S. planning to mail AIDS advisory to all. New York Times. May 5, 1988:A-11.
15. Shilts R. The politics of prevention. San Francisco Chronicle. February 20, 1989:A-4.
16. U.S. Public Health Service. Surgeon General's report on acquired immune deficiency syndrome. Washington, D.C.: October 1986.
17. U.S. Public Health Service. What you should know about AIDS. America responds to AIDS. Washington, D.C.: 1987.
18. U.S. Department of Education. AIDS and the education of our children: a guide for parents and teachers. Washington, D.C.: 1987.
19. AIDS educational plan unveiled in Washington. San Francisco Chronicle. March 17, 1987:1,22.
20. Cranston eases restrictions by Helms on language in federal AIDS pamphlets. San Francisco Examiner. January 7, 1988:A-2.
21. Lawrence J. Senate's AIDS vote rings "death knell," critic says. San Francisco Examiner. October 15, 1987:A-2.
22. O'Loughlin R. Senate passes AIDS bill with Helms ban on funds. Bay Area Reporter. May 5, 1988:1, 19.
23. Institute of Medicine, National Academy of Sciences. Confronting AIDS: directions for public health, health care, and research. Washington, D.C.: National Academy Press, 1986.
24. White A. Lobbyists waiting to see Bush policy on rights, AIDS. Bay Area Reporter. February 2, 1989.
25. Connally M. AIDS plan similar to Reagan's. San Francisco Examiner. February 10, 1989:1.

Safe Sex, Safer Sex, and Prevention of HIV Infection

P.T. Cohen, M.D., Ph.D.

"Safer sex" is a term for sexual practices that have a lower probability of passing human immunodeficiency virus (HIV) from one sexual partner to the other during sexual activity. The term "safe sex" was initially used to describe such practices, but recent evidence indicates that very few practices are completely free from risk. Thus the term "safer sex" has been adopted.

Evidence suggests that some practices are relatively safe, whereas others are unsafe and carry greater risk of transmitting the virus. This evidence is derived from (1) epidemiologic studies correlating HIV infection with some sexual practices and lack of infection with others[1-8,20]; (2) experimental studies directly evaluating conditions that prevent survival and transmission of HIV[9-13]; and (3) inferences from knowledge about the presence and infectivity of virus in specific body fluids and tissue.[14-19,21-23]

There is currently no cure for HIV infection. Education and behavior modification are the only practical preventive strategies for limiting the spread of infection at present. Clinicians and other health workers have a major responsibility to disseminate information about safer sex to individuals at risk for acquiring HIV, since preventing the spread of the virus is the most powerful strategy currently available for combating HIV disease.

Target audiences for safer-sex information include a number of recognizable groups:

- all adolescents and young adults;
- infected individuals and their sexual partners;
- residents of areas with a high prevalence of HIV infection;
- high-risk individuals, including:
    - intravenous drug users;
    - hemophiliacs;
    - gay men;
    - bisexual men;
    - individuals with multiple sexual partners;
    - male and female prostitutes; and
- sexual partners of high-risk individuals.

Practitioners and clinicians should encourage frank, open-ended discussions of sexual practices in relation to sexually transmitted diseases in general, and HIV disease in particular. To achieve maximum participation and interest, the tone and setting of the discussion should imply confidentiality, respect for personal privacy, and tolerance of different values, mores, and lifestyles. Practitioners often have no personal experience with specific sexual practices being discussed. Honesty about matters unknown and a willingness to exchange information should help to generate respect and trust.

Discussion of safer sex should be initiated by the practitioner if the topic does not arise spontaneously. In many geographic and social settings, individuals may be unwilling to acknowledge and discuss personal practices that put them at risk, even with a practitioner whom they respect. Accordingly, they should not be made to feel that they are required to openly acknowledge specific personal practices, lifestyles, or membership in a risk group in order to enter into or participate in this discussion. To introduce the subject to such individuals, a statement might be made such as "There is some useful information about how AIDS is spread, and how it can be prevented. I think everyone should be aware of it, and I want to discuss it with you. You can help spread this information by talking about it with people you know."

Written handout materials and educational sessions by health workers other than the examining clinician can reinforce the clinician's statements.

Other approaches to disseminating this information include using informed members of groups at risk; enlisting support from respected public figures; promoting educational activities by organizations, institutions, and mass media; and identifying existing resources (from community groups, schools, churches, government, etc.) that may serve as sources of accurate information and counseling.

■ PRINCIPLES AND EVIDENCE UNDERLYING SAFER-SEX GUIDELINES

Sexual activity with many different partners carries a high risk for HIV infection. Although much remains to be learned about the mechanisms of transmission, it seems clear on both strong epidemiological and theoretical grounds that contact with many different individuals creates increased opportunities for becoming infected with HIV. Thus, whatever the risk for specific sexual practices, it is multiplied when many different contacts are involved.

Clearly, one sexual partner must be infected and the other uninfected with HIV if primary transmission is to occur. If partners in a monogamous sexual relationship are tested for HIV antibody and both are positive or negative, then no transmission will occur as long as both remain monogamous. On theoretical grounds, there is reason for concern that an HIV-infected individual may be harmed by exposure to foreign antigens and non-HIV infections. This is based on in vitro experiments consistent with the concept that antigenic stimulation may activate HIV from a latent state or potentiate its pathologic activity.[24,25] Thus, a practical extension of this concept is that exposure to antigenic stimulation by a partner's infections or body fluids may be detrimental and should be limited through the use of condoms or other safer sex practices.

One suggested procedure assuring safer sex requires that all individuals be tested for HIV antibody, enter into monogamous sexual relationships, and practice only the safest sexual practices if one partner is HIV seropositive and the other HIV seronegative.[27] While this theoretically sound formulation may work well for some couples, it is limited by the impossibility of stable monogamous relationships for a substantial portion of the population. In addition, applying the HIV antibody test to populations where HIV infection is rare will mean that a positive test result is most likely to be a false-positive result. If testing of low-risk populations is widespread, there will be many false-positive test results. In the absence of guaranteed confidentiality — a condition difficult to achieve except by anonymous testing and notification — individuals with both false- and true-positive results may face significant harmful economic, social, psychological, and emotional consequences. It is at least a debatable matter whether the benefits of such widespread testing outweigh the harm that could possibly result. This problem has been thoughtfully reviewed.[28]

One set of authors advises that carefully choosing a sexual partner is the most important behavior.[53] They calculate that the chances of becoming infected with HIV from a single sexual encounter with a partner who has no risk factors and has tested negatively for HIV is 1 in 500 million, and decreases to 1 in 5 billion if a condom is used. They contrast this with an estimated chance of 1 in 500 of becoming infected from a single sexual encounter with an HIV-positive person. This latter estimate may create a false sense of security and suggest a much lower risk than is really the case, since reports exist of transmission of the virus with very few encounters (or after only one). The estimates are derived by making several unproved assumptions about the risk of sexual transmission. Further, although carefully choosing a sexual partner seems sensible, it is fraught with practical limitations — one of which is the requirement that a prospective partner will relate an accurate history of high-risk behavior.

In the most common case, individuals do not know the HIV status of their potential sexual partners. Obviously, the chance that potential partners will be infected with HIV is greatest if they belong to groups known to be at risk for HIV infection. These include individuals who have had multiple sexual partners, have shared needles for injecting intravenous drugs, are gay or bisexual men, have hemophilia, have had blood product transfusions before blood was routinely screened for HIV (i.e., before 1986), or have had sexual relationships with members of any of these risk groups.

In general, practices that cause the transfer of genital secretions and blood from one sexual partner to another are unsafe. It is more difficult to isolate the virus from saliva and tears than from semen and blood.[14,15] Presumably this is because of the virus's affinity for lymphocytes, which are less numerous in saliva and tears.[16-18] Saliva and tears, therefore, are much less likely to transmit HIV than semen or blood.

Infection is very unlikely to occur if body fluids containing the virus contact only the partner's intact skin. Theoretically, there is a small risk for inoculating virus into the bloodstream through open cuts or wounds in the mouth, on the skin, or through infected body fluid contacting an area such as the conjunctiva of the eyes. Absorption and inoculation of the blood might conceivably occur in these cases. If transmission of HIV occurs at all by these routes, however, it must be a rare occurrence. This conclusion is based on the large number of health workers who have had cutaneous exposures while caring for AIDS patients and who nevertheless have not become HIV seropositive.

However, cutaneous exposure and absorption may explain seroconversion to HIV-positive status in a mother caring for an infant with transfusion-related AIDS[29] and in three health workers exposed to blood from HIV-positive individuals.[30] The mother, who did not wear protective gloves or take special precautions, was exposed daily to diarrheal secretions from her infant. The health workers' skin was in contact with blood from HIV-positive individuals; routes of infection may have included chapped hands, dermatitis of the earlobe, and facial acne. These reports underscore the potential for infection via cutaneous exposure and strongly indicate that mucocutaneous contact with body fluids from HIV-infected persons cannot be considered completely safe, particularly when there are breaks in or disruption of the seronegative person's normal, mucocutaneous barrier.

Evidence indicates that the most efficient mechanism of HIV transmission is inoculation of the virus into a person's bloodstream, as occurs when an intravenous drug user "shoots up" with a needle contaminated with infected blood, or when a blood transfusion introduces blood contaminated with the virus.

HIV also seems able to efficiently cause infection when the virus comes in contact with the rectal mucosa. There is strong epidemiologic evidence that anal receptive sex carries a very high risk for the receptive partner.[8,20] HIV has been shown to infect cells of the rectal mucosa.[21] There is also evidence of ultrastructural cellular abnormalities in the rectal mucosal cells of AIDS patients.[32] Thus, direct inoculation of these cells seems a plausible mechanism for transmission. Alternatively, HIV infection might occur when small breaks or tears in the rectal mucosa allow inoculation of the virus directly into the bloodstream. This mechanism has been proposed in the past to explain rectal transmission of hepatitis B virus.[31] "Fisting" (penetration of the anus with the hand) is epidemiologically associated with HIV infection in homosexual men, perhaps by causing tears in the rectal mucosa.

Epidemiologic data indicate that the practice of anal douching is also associated with HIV infection.[8] One purely speculative interpretation for these data is that douching irritates and inflames the rectal mucosa, damaging capillaries and allowing entry of HIV into the bloodstream during subsequent sexual contacts. No data exist on the relationship, if any, between vaginal douching and risk of HIV infection.

Transmission of HIV infection from male to female during vaginal intercourse is strongly supported by case reports and epidemiologic data.[32-35] Presumably, semen is the vehicle for transmission.

Transmission of HIV infection from female to male during vaginal intercourse has been reported in individual cases[36] and is supported by epidemiologic evidence.[32-35] HIV has been isolated from cervical biopsy specimens and HIV antigen has been identified in monocyte-macrophage and endothelial cells of the submucosa of the cervix.[22] Thus, cervical cells may be the initial site of infection in male-to-female transmission. Sloughing of these infected cells into genital secretions may account for transmission to male partners and to neonates.

Female-to-male transmission of HIV during vaginal intercourse had been less certain, and even controversial, until recently.[37-40] There is now general agreement, however, that vaginal intercourse between an infected female and an uninfected male should be considered unsafe and carries a high risk for transmitting infection. Seronegative male partners of infected spouses engaging in unprotected vaginal intercourse over two years have seroconverted.[41] Although the site of inoculation of the male remains uncertain, most speculative mechanisms have involved ulcers, sores, or breaks in penile skin and inflamed urethral mucosa as sites of HIV entry from vaginal secretions into the male bloodstream.[41,54,55]

If body fluids containing the HIV are ingested orally, the virus is probably inactivated by digestive enzymes and acid in the stomach. Epidemiologic data from male homosexuals has consistently failed to link HIV infection with ingestion of semen.[42-45] Oral ingestion of semen is nevertheless considered to be unsafe because of the possibility that some virus might enter the bloodstream through small tears or wounds in the lining of the mouth, stomach, or gastrointestinal tract. A case of seroconversion that may have resulted from orogenital contact has been reported.[56]

Similarly, the true risk from ingestion of female genital secretions is uncertain, but the practice is assumed to be high-risk in the absence of sufficient epidemiologic data to the contrary. There is one well-described case report of HIV transmission between two lesbians.[46] In this report, an intravenous drug user with lymphadenopathy apparently infected her partner. The sexual practices between these women were often traumatic, resulting in bleeding in the vagina, and involved digital and oral contact with the partner's vagina, as well as oral contact with the anus.

Since menstrual blood and other secretions may contain HIV, it had been suggested that around the time of menses, women who are infected may be more capable of transmitting HIV through their genital secretions. However, isolation of HIV from the cervical secretions does not necessarily correlate with menses, and cervical secretions yielded HIV isolates at times when serum was negative, and vice versa.[23,47] These data are consistent with the idea that viral shedding in genital secretions may occur at any time during the menstrual cycle of HIV-infected women, and that the virus shed from the cervix may arise from locally infected cervical cells.

HIV probably does not pass through condoms. Thus, condoms may provide an effective barrier to HIV transmission and to the transmission of other sexually transmitted diseases.[58] This theory has been evaluated experimentally, using infectious HIV particles cultivated in tissue culture.[12] Four milliliters of a solution containing 1 million infectious virus particles per milliliter were placed inside a condom fitted over the plunger of a syringe. A solution of medium suitable for cultivating the virus was then repeatedly moved in and out of the barrel of the syringe by moving the condom-covered plunger. After the plunger was removed, the condom's distal end was covered with tissue culture media for 30 minutes on ice. The outer surface of the condom was then assayed for virus particles, and none could be demonstrated.

Condoms tested were commercial products: Trojan ENZ (latex); Trojan ENZ lubricated (latex); Fourex lubricated (natural lambskin); Ramses Extra lubricated and with added spermicide (latex); and Skinless Skin lubricated (synthetic).[12]

Similar barrier experiments have been conducted for herpes viruses[10,11] and the hepatitis B virus.[48] In the hepatitis B study, HBsAg particles did penetrate natural membrane condoms.[48] Though these particles were far smaller than the HIV (44 nm vs. 125 nm, respectively), caution would dictate that synthetic (latex) condoms be used because they are not penetrated by the hepatitis B virus.[13,57]

There is also some epidemiologic evidence for the efficacy of condoms in decreasing (though not completely eliminating) risk of HIV transmission. In one study, sexually active heterosexual AIDS patients and their spouses were followed prospectively for 12- to 36-month periods from the time of AIDS diagnosis. Of the spouses who were seronegative at enrollment into the study, 14 did not use condoms. Twelve of these became HIV positive during the follow-up period. Of 10 spouses who were seronegative at enrollment and who used condoms consistently, only 1 seroconverted during the follow-up period.[35] In a different study, however, 17 percent (3 of 18) of seronegative partners using condoms seroconverted during an 18-month (median) follow-up of couples.[41]

In another study, 568 prostitutes from seven urban areas in the United States were interviewed and their HIV serologic status determined. Of 22 prostitutes whose partners always used condoms, none were HIV positive, while 11 percent of the remaining 546 prostitutes whose partners did not use condoms were seropositive.[49] However, in the group as a whole, intravenous drug use seemed to be the most significant factor in acquiring HIV infection.

In West Germany, licensed prostitutes have an HIV-positive prevalence rate of 1 percent, compared with a 20 percent prevalence rate among unlicensed prostitutes. This difference has been attributed to the frequent use of condoms by partners of licensed prostitutes, although their low intravenous drug use and the demographics of their clientele may also be responsible.[50] HIV-seropositive status among prostitutes in Kinshasa, Zaire, was inversely correlated to their partners' use of condoms.[51]

Obviously, condoms must be used properly to provide a barrier that prevents transmission.[58] Instruction about safer sex should emphasize that to avoid breaks and tears, condoms must not be allowed to dry out or age unreasonably long, must be applied carefully, must not be subject to unreasonable trauma during use, must remain on the penis until withdrawal, and must fit so as not to leak from the base. Further, a new condom must be used for each act of intercourse.

Spermicidal contraceptive jellies and vaginal foams may have some ability to inactivate HIV. Nonoxynol-9, a nonionic surfactant, is a chemical ingredient of several commercial spermicides. It has been shown to inactivate the HIV in vitro at concentrations of 0.05 percent. Commercial spermicidal products contain concentrations of nonoxynol-9 in the 1 percent to 5 percent range.[52] Inactivation was observed in laboratory experiments when isolated human blood lymphocytes infected with HIV were grown in culture media in the presence of nonoxynol-9 and control solutions. No experiments or epidemiologic data exist, however, to prove that nonoxynol-9 is effective in preventing transmission of the HIV during intercourse. Therefore, it is important to stress that use of such a product should be an adjunct to, not a substitute for, safer sexual practices.

■ RISK ESTIMATES OF SEXUAL PRACTICES AND RECOMMENDATIONS FOR CONDOM USE

Based on the current understanding of transmission of HIV during sexual activity, the following list estimates the risk of various sexual practices.

SAFER — PROBABLY NO RISK FOR HIV TRANSMISSION

- abstention from sexual contact;
- monogamous relationship, partners both uninfected;
- self masturbation;
- masturbation with partner (if no cuts on hand of either partner);
- touching, massaging, hugging, stroking; and
- dry kissing (social kissing).

LOW BUT REAL RISK FOR HIV TRANSMISSION

- anal or vaginal sex with proper use of intact condom;
- wet kissing (French kissing);
- fellatio interruptus (sucking partner's penis and stopping before ejaculation); and

- urine contact (exclusive of contact with mouth, rectum, or cuts or breaks in skin).

POSSIBLY UNSAFE, THOUGH PROOF IS LACKING

- fellatio (sucking partner's penis, ingesting semen);
- cunnilingus (oral contact with female genitals — risk may be greater during menses when blood present or if sores in mouth); and
- sharing sex toys and implements.

UNSAFE — HIGH RISK FOR TRANSMITTING HIV

- numerous sexual partners;
- unprotected anal receptive sex with infected partner;
- unprotected anal penetration with the hand (fisting);
- anal douching in combination with anal sex;
- oral–anal contact (rimming); and
- unprotected (without condom) vaginal intercourse with infected partner.

EFFECTIVE AND PROPER USE OF CONDOMS

Proper condom use can decrease, though not completely eliminate, the risk of transmission of HIV infection and other sexually transmitted diseases. The Centers for Disease Control has published the following recommendations for proper use of condoms[58]:

1. Latex condoms should be used because they offer greater protection against viral sexually transmitted disease (STD) than natural membrane condoms.[57]

2. Condoms should be stored in a cool, dry place out of direct sunlight.

3. Condoms in damaged packages or those that show obvious signs of age (e.g., those that are brittle, sticky, or discolored) should not be used. They cannot be relied upon to prevent infection.

4. Condoms should be handled with care to prevent puncture.

5. The condom should be put on before any genital contact to prevent exposure to fluids that may contain infectious agents. Hold the tip of the condom and unroll it onto the erect penis, leaving space at the tip to collect semen, yet assuring that no air is trapped in the tip of the condom.

6. Adequate lubrication should be used. If exogenous lubrication is needed, only water-based lubricants should be used. Petroleum- or oil-based lubricants (such as petroleum jelly, cooking oils, shortening, and lotions) should not be used since they weaken the latex.

7. Use of condoms containing spermicides may provide some additional protection against STD. However, vaginal use of spermicides along with condoms is likely to provide greater protection.

8. If a condom breaks, it should be replaced immediately. If ejaculation occurs after condom breakage, the immediate use of spermicide has

been suggested. However, the protective value of post-ejaculation application of spermicide in reducing the risk of STD transmission is unknown.

9. After ejaculation, care should be taken so that the condom does not slip off the penis before withdrawal; the base of the condom should be held while withdrawing. The penis should be withdrawn while still erect.

10. Condoms should never be reused.

Besides unsafe sexual practices, intravenous drug use with needle sharing carries a high risk for transmission of HIV and should be avoided.

It also seems prudent to advise that personal objects such as toothbrushes, razors, and nail clippers are theoretically capable of inoculating small amounts of blood from one person to another. These items should not be shared in households or environments where they will be used by individuals who are known to be infected with HIV or who are at high risk for HIV infection. Evidence for transmission of HIV by sharing such personal objects has been sought but not found; these possible modes of transmission are therefore likely to be very low risk.[59]

Finally, some individuals have the impression that people who look, feel, and seem well cannot be infected, and thus cannot transmit the virus. As a result, they make decisions about who is at high risk based on irrelevant subjective factors, such as personality, cleanliness, morals, or personal values. It is important to convey that individuals are considered at high risk because recently or in the past they engaged in practices that carry a high risk for infection with HIV, or because medical evaluation has demonstrated that they are infected. It must be understood that an individual who is at high risk or known to be infected is not necessarily immoral, bad, unclean, or unpleasant. Similarly, a person who is decent, attractive, neat, and personable may be infected or at high risk.

REFERENCES

1. Melbye M, Biggar RJ, Ebbesen P, et al. Seroepidemiology of HTLV-III antibody in Danish homosexual men: prevalence, transmission, and disease outcome. Br Med J 1984; 289:573-5.
2. Goedert JJ, Sarngadharan MG, Biggar RJ, et al. Determinants of retrovirus (HTLV-III) antibody and immunodeficiency conditions in homosexual men. Lancet 1984; 2:711-6.
3. Blattner WA, Biggar RJ, Weiss SH, et al. Epidemiology of human T-lymphotropic virus type III and the risk of the acquired immunodeficiency syndrome. Ann Intern Med 1985; 103; 665-70.
4. Jaffe HW, Choi K, Thomas PA, et al. National case-control study of Kaposi's sarcoma and *Pneumocystis carinii* pneumonia in homosexual men: Part 1. Epidemiologic results. Ann Intern Med 1983; 99:145-51.
5. Darrow WW, O'Malley P, Jaffe HW, et al. Risk factors for HTLV-III seroconversion in a cohort of homosexual male clinic patients [Abstract]. Atlanta: International Conference on Acquired Immunodeficiency Syndrome, 1985; 24.
6. Marmor M, Friedman-Kien AE, Zolla-Pazner S, et al. Kaposi's sarcoma in homosexual men. A seroepidemiologic case-control study. Ann Intern Med 1984; 100:809-15.
7. Stevens CE, Taylor PE, Zang EA, et al. Human T-cell lymphotropic virus type III infection in a cohort of homosexual men in New York City. JAMA 1986; 255:2167-72.
8. Moss AR, Osmond D, Bacchetti P, et al. Risk factors for AIDS and HIV seropositivity in homosexual men. Am J Epidemiol 1987; 125:1035-47.
9. Additional recommendations to reduce sexual and drug abuse related transmission of human T-lymphotropic virus type III/ lymphadenopathy virus. MMWR 1986; 35:152-5.
10. Judson FN, Bodin GF, Levin MH, et al. In vitro tests demonstrate condoms provide an effective barrier against chlamydia trachomatis and herpes simplex virus. Seattle: Program of the International Society for STD Research, 1983:176. abstract.

11. Conant MA, Spicer DW, Smith CD. Herpes simplex virus transmission: Condom studies. Sex Transm Dis 1984; 11:94-5.

12. Conant MA, Hardy D, Sernatinger J, et al. Condoms prevent transmission of AIDS-associated retrovirus. JAMA 1986; 255:1706.

13. Minuk GY, Bohme CE, Bowen TJ, et al. Condoms and the prevention of AIDS. JAMA 1986; 256:1442-3.

14. Ho DD, Schooley RT, Rota TR, et al. HTLV-III in the semen and blood of a healthy homosexual man. Science 1984; 226:451-3.

15. Zagury D, Bernard J, Leibowitch J, et al. HTLV-III in cells cultured from semen of two patients with AIDS. Science 1984; 226:449-51.

16. Groopman JE, Salahuddin SZ, Sarngadharan MG, et al. HTLV-III in saliva of people with AIDS related complex and healthy homosexual men at risk for AIDS. Science 1984; 226:447-8.

17. Levy JA, Kaminsky LS, Morrow WJW, et al. Infection by the retrovirus associated with the acquired immunodeficiency syndrome. Ann Intern Med 1985; 103:694-9.

18. Ho DD, Byington RE, Schooley RT, et al. Infrequency of isolation of HTLV-III virus from saliva in AIDS. N Engl J Med 1985; 313:1606.

19. Wofsy C, Cohen J, Hauer LB, et al. Isolation of AIDS associated retrovirus from genital secretions of women with antibodies to the virus. Lancet 1986; 1:527-9.

20. Winkelstein W, Lyman DM, Padion N, et al. Sexual practices and risk of infection by the human immunodeficiency virus. JAMA 1987; 257:321-5.

21. Nelson JA, Wiley CA, Reynolds-Kohler C, et al. Human immunodeficiency virus detected in bowel epithelium from patients with gastrointestinal symptoms. Lancet 1988; 1(8580):259-62.

22. Pomerantz RJ, de la Monte S, Donegan SP, et al. Human immunodeficiency virus (HIV) infection of the uterine cervix. Ann Intern Med 1988; 108:321-7.

23. Vogt MW, Witt DJ, Craven DE, et al. Isolation patterns of human immunodeficiency virus from cervical secretions during the menstrual cycle of women at risk for the acquired immunodeficiency syndrome. Ann Intern Med 1987; 106:380-2.

24. Gendelman HF, Leonard J, Weck K, et al. Herpesviral transactivation of the human immunodeficiency virus (HIV) by long terminal repeat sequence [Abstract]. Washington, D.C.: III International Conference on Acquired Immunodeficiency Syndrome, 1987:13.

25. Luciw P, Tong-Sarksen SE, Matija Peterlin B. T-cell activation increases gene expression directed by the HIV LTR: Implications for pathogenesis in AIDS [Abstract]. Washington, D.C.: III International Conference on Acquired Immunodeficiency Syndrome, 1987:6.

26. Shattock AG, Finlay H, Hillary IB. Short Reports: possible reactivation of hepatitis D with chronic delta antigenaemia by human immunodeficiency virus. Br Med J 1987; 294:1656-7.

27. Goedert JJ. What is safe sex? Suggested standards linked to testing for human immunodeficiency virus. N Engl J Med 1987; 316:1339-42.

28. Meyer KB, Pauker SG. Screening for HIV: Can we afford the false positive rate? N Engl J Med 1987; 317:238-41.

29. Centers for Disease Control. Apparent transmission of HTLV-III/LAV from a child to a mother providing health care. MMWR 1986; 35:76-9.

30. Centers for Disease Control. Update: human immunodeficiency virus infections in health-care workers exposed to blood of infected patients. MMWR 1987; 36:285-96.

31. Reiner NE, Judson FN, Bond WW, et al. Asymptomatic rectal mucosal lesions and hepatitis B surface antigen at sites of sexual contact in homosexual men with persistent hepatitis B virus infection. Ann Intern Med 1982; 96:170-3.

32. Bruneval P, Leport C, Tricottet V, et al. Marqueurs ultrastructuraux au cours de l'infection par le virus LAV/HTLV-III: etude de la muqueuse rectale chez 16 patients. Gastroenterol Clin Biol 1986; 10:328-33.

32. Centers for Disease Control. Heterosexual transmission of human T lymphotropic virus type III/lymphadenopathy associated virus. MMWR 1985; 34:561-3.

33. Lederman MM. Transmission of the acquired immunodeficiency syndrome through heterosexual activity. Ann Intern Med 1986; 104:115-7.

34. Melbye M, Njelesani EK, Bayley A, et al. Evidence for heterosexual transmission and clinical manifestations of human immunodeficiency virus infection and related conditions in Lusaka, Zambia. Lancet 1986; 2:1113-5.

35. Fischl MA, Dickinson GM, Scott GB, et al. Evaluation of heterosexual partners, children, and household contacts of adults with AIDS. JAMA 1987; 257:640-4.

36. Calabrese DO, Gopalakrishna KV. Transmission of HTLV-III infection from man to woman to man. N Engl J Med 1986; 314:987.

37. Redfield RR, Markham PD, Salhuddin SZ, et al. Heterosexually acquired HTLV-III/LAV disease (AIDS-related complex and AIDS): Epidemiologic evidence for female-to-male transmission. JAMA 1985; 254:2094-6.

38. Schultz S, Milberg JA, Kristal AR, Stoneburner RL. Female-to-male transmission of HTLV-III. JAMA 1986; 255:1704.

39. Wykoff RF. Female-to-male transmission of HTLV-III. JAMA 1986; 255:1704-5.

40. Redfield RR, Wright DC, Sakahuddin SZ, et al. Female-to-male transmission of HTLV-III. JAMA 1986; 255:1705-6.

41. Fischl MA, Dickinson GM, Segal A, et al. Heterosexual transmission of human immunodeficiency virus (HIV): Relationship of sexual practice to seroconversion [Abstract]. Washington, D.C.: III International Conference on Acquired Immunodeficiency Syndrome, 1987:178.

42. Kingsley LA, Detels R, Kaslow R, et al. Risk factors for seroconversion to human immunodeficiency virus among male homosexuals. Lancet 1987; 1:345-9.

43. Jeffries E, Willoughby B, Boyko WJ, et al. The Vancouver lymphadenopathy-AIDS study II: Sero-epidemiology of HTLV-III antibody. Can Med Assoc J 1985; 132: 1373-7.

44. Scheuter MT, Boyko WJ, Douglas B, et al. Can HTLV-III be transmitted orally? Lancet 1986; 1:379.

45. Lyman D, Winkelstein W, Ascher M, Levy JA. Minimal risk of transmission of AIDS-associated retrovirus infection by oral-genital contact. JAMA 1986; 255:1703.

46. Marmor M, Weiss LR, Lyden M, et al. Possible female-to-female transmission of human immunodeficiency virus. Ann Intern Med 1986; 105:969.

47. Markus WV, Witt DJ, Craven DE, et al. Isolation patterns of the human immunodeficiency virus from cervical secretions during the menstrual cycle of women at risk for the acquired immunodeficiency syndrome. Ann Intern Med 1987; 106:380-2.

48. Minuk GY, Bohme CE, Bowen TJ. Condoms and hepatitis B virus infection. Ann Intern Med 1986; 104:584.

49. Centers for Disease Control. Antibody to human immunodeficiency virus in female prostitutes. MMWR 1987; 36:157-61.

50. Smith GL, Smith KF. Lack of HIV infection and condom use in licensed prostitutes. Lancet 1986; 2:1392.

51. Mann J, Quinn TC, Piot P, et al. Condom use and HIV infection among prostitutes in Zaire. N Engl J Med 1987; 316:345.

52. Hicks DR, Martin LS, Getchell JP, et al. Inactivation of HTLV-III/LAV infected cultures of normal human lymphocytes by nonoxynol-9 in vitro. Lancet 1985; 2:1422-3.

53. Hearst N, Hulley SB. Preventing the heterosexual spread of AIDS. JAMA 1988; 259:2428-32.

54. Piot P, Plummer FA, Mhalu FS, et al. AIDS: an international perspective. Science 1988; 239:573-9.

55. Cameron DW, D'Costa LJ, Karsira P, et al. Genital ulcer disease and transmission of human immunodeficiency virus (HIV) in Nairobi. [Abstract]. Abstracts of the Twenty-seventh Interscience Conference on Antimicrobial Agents and Chemotherapy. 1987(Oct); 683.

56. Mayer KH, DeGruttola V. Human immunodeficiency virus and oral intercourse. Ann Intern Med 1987; 107:428-9.

57. Van de Perre P, Jacobs D, Sprecher-Goldberger S. The latex condom, an efficient barrier against sexual transmission of AIDS-related viruses. AIDS 1987; 1:49-52.

58. Centers for Disease Control. Condoms for prevention of sexually transmitted diseases. MMWR 1988; 37:133-7.

59. Friedland GH, Saltzman BR, Rogers MF, et al. Lack of transmission of HTLV-III/LAV infection to household contacts of patients with AIDS or AIDS-related complex with oral candidiasis. N Engl J Med 1986; 314:344-9.

Education and Intravenous Drug Use

P.T. Cohen, M.D., Ph.D.

■ IMPORTANCE OF PREVENTION

S pread of human immunodeficiency virus (HIV) infections from individuals infected through intravenous drug abuse is a serious public health concern. Intravenous drug users are a major reservoir for HIV, representing roughly 17 percent of United States AIDS cases.[1-5]

The presumed mechanism for spread of HIV infection among intravenous drug users is by inoculation of the victim with traces of blood contaminating a needle or other paraphernalia used previously by an infected individual. Sexual transmission is presumably a second, less significant route of transmission within this group.

Intravenous drug users may be the most important potential source from which HIV infections may spread to individuals who are not homosexual or bisexual men. This spread may occur by several routes.

First, women infected with HIV before or during pregnancy may pass the infection to their children. CDC statistics from 1981 to 1988 showed that 56 percent of the 1344 pediatric AIDS cases were in children whose mothers either used intravenous drugs or had sexual contact with intravenous drug users.[2] Another CDC study found that 60 percent of the children had at least one parent who used intravenous drugs.[3]

Second, non-drug-using heterosexual individuals may acquire HIV infection as a sexually transmitted disease. The frequency of such sexual contact is probably much higher than can be accounted for by social and marital sexual encounters, since prostitution is a method by which some male homosexual and female heterosexual intravenous drug users earn money to support their drug habits.

Finally, both habitual and occasional (so called "casual" or "recreational") users of intravenous drugs may be infected with HIV by sharing contaminated needles and apparatus.

No cure or effective treatment exists for HIV infection, and no realistic strategic alternative to education and behavior modification exists for prevention of spread of HIV.

Thus, in addition to the obvious ethical and humane considerations that make prevention of illness desirable, preventing the spread of HIV infection among and from intravenous drug users is necessary for practical reasons. Failure to do so will greatly increase the prevalence of HIV infections in the general population, and the social and financial cost of caring for infected individuals.

The practice of sharing needles is common among all groups of intravenous drug users evaluated. If no intervention occurs, it can be anticipated that the prevalence of HIV infection in intravenous drug users will continue to rise.[6] In some areas, such as New York and New Jersey, there is already a high prevalence (approaching 60 percent) of HIV infection among intravenous drug users.[5,7] In other areas, such as Northern California, the prevalence of HIV infection among intravenous drug users is still relatively low, estimated at 10 percent of individuals tested San Francisco.[8] Thus, there is opportunity in these geographic areas to intervene at an earlier stage to abort further spread.

■ EDUCATION AS A PREVENTIVE STRATEGY

Education about the relationship between intravenous drug use and AIDS will hopefully modify behavior of occasional users, potential experimenters such as adolescents and teenagers, and many intravenous drug users who are receptive.

The most desirable goal for a preventive educational strategy should be to convince individuals to stop using intravenous drugs and enter a treatment program. Short of achieving this, educational efforts should be directed at modifying the behavior that leads to HIV transmission during intravenous drug use. Accordingly, lesser goals should be to convince intravenous users to use sterile needles and apparatus and avoid sharing these or to use alternative nonintravenous routes to administer drugs.

AIDS risk reduction among intravenous drug users has been discussed in several articles.[9,10] The authors report some evidence that education can modify the behavior of intravenous drug addicts. This consists of the observation of increased efforts by addicts to obtain new needles because of fear of AIDS. The most material demonstration of this trend is the street sale of "good" needles with the pitch that their use will prevent AIDS. At least some of the "good" needles are not new but rather are resealed in packages using heat sealing machines purchased in hardware stores. However, the existence of a market for the sealed packages is apparently a recent phenomenon arising since the emergence of AIDS, and it suggests that addicts may hear and act on information about the disease.

■ DISSEMINATION OF INFORMATION

It is crucial to achieve the widest possible dissemination of information about how to prevent spread of HIV infections among and from intravenous drug users. Information should be aimed at individuals known to be infected or who are from high risk groups, so that they may help prevent spread to their associates, as well as at individuals who may be tempted to experiment with intravenous drugs. The target population for educational information is thus quite large, and should include:

- all adolescents and young adults;
- infected individuals and their sexual partners;
- residents of areas with high prevalence of HIV infection;
- high-risk individuals, including:
  - intravenous drug users;
  - hemophiliacs;
  - gay men;
  - bisexual men;

- individuals with multiple sexual partners;
- prostitutes; and
- sexual partners of high-risk individuals.

For specific outreach to addicts, information should be made readily available at drug treatment centers, hospital emergency rooms, clinics, prisons and jails, and in areas known to be frequented by addicts.

Clinicians and health workers should raise the issue of needle sharing and safer sex and discuss the alternatives whenever patients or clients are suspected of being intravenous drug users. Such suspicion may arise because of specific medical problems (overdose, endocarditis, withdrawal symptoms and signs, unexplained abcesses) or physical findings (fresh needle marks, scars over veins). Medical histories should include a question about intravenous drug use. Obviously, ideas will be communicated more effectively if the tone of the discussion is private, dignified, and suggests concern for the user, than if an angry, threatening, and dogmatic lecture is delivered.

To achieve maximum participation and interest, the tone and setting of the discussion should imply confidentiality, respect for personal privacy, and tolerance of different values, mores, and lifestyles. An attitude of genuine concern for the welfare of the individuals at risk will result in greater credibility for the clinician than an attitude of indifferent and aloof professionalism. Practitioners usually have no personal experience with the day-to-day lifestyle and practices of intravenous drug users. Honesty about matters unknown and a willingness to exchange information will lead to greater respect and trust than will expounding pontifically and moralistically.

A discussion of safer sex and needle sharing should be initiated by the practitioner if the subject does not arise spontaneously. In many geographic and social settings, individuals may be unwilling to acknowledge and discuss personal practices that place them at risk, even with a practitioner whom they respect. Accordingly, they should be made to feel that they are not required to openly acknowledge specific personal practices, lifestyles, or membership in a risk group in order to enter into and participate in the discussion. Introducing the subject of intravenous drug use to individuals who do not acknowledge being members of risk groups might be done with statements such as "There is some useful information about how AIDS is spread, and how it can be prevented. I think everyone should be aware of it, and I wanted to discuss it with you. You can help spread this information by talking about it to people you know."

Written materials to hand out, and education by health workers other than the examining clinician can reinforce and supplement the clinician's statements. Members of minority ethnic or racial groups may respond best to information framed in a perspective reflecting their particular concerns and prepared or delivered by a member of their own group.

Other approaches to dissemination of this information include providing handouts listing salient points (example handouts are presented in the paper by Marmor et al.,[10]); enlisting public support from visible and respected individuals such as musicians, celebrities, and athletes; promoting educational activities by organizations, institutions, and mass media; and identifying resources (from community groups, schools, churches, government, etc.) that may already exist as sources of additional accurate information and counseling. Reformed intravenous drug users know the lifestyle and the manipulative patterns of intravenous drug users; they are often effective in communicating with drug users and thus can be a particularly valuable asset in disseminating information about HIV transmission to these individuals.

■ SALIENT POINTS TO COMMUNICATE

Educational efforts should communicate the following points to persons at risk about the relationship between intravenous drug use and HIV disease:

1. Seek help to discontinue intravenous drug use. Intravenous drug use carries many health risks. HIV disease is one such risk.

2. Intravenous drug users transmit human immunodeficiency virus (HIV, the virus that causes AIDS) to one another by sharing contaminated needles and apparatus. If you use intravenous drugs, don't share needles, syringes, and other apparatus with anyone. If you continue to shoot drugs, use your own clean apparatus. Don't rent, borrow, or share apparatus.

3. Intravenous drug users also transmit HIV to one another through sexual relations. The virus can be spread from men to women and from women to men during sexual activity. Learn about and practice safe sex.

4. If you become infected with HIV, you risk infecting your lovers and your children. Pregnant women who are infected may pass the infection to the incubating fetus.

5. You can't tell whether someone is infected with HIV, the AIDS virus, by how they look and feel. People may look and feel well and yet carry the virus in their blood, so don't assume that some people are not infectious.

6. Some "new" needles sold on the street are not new, but are repackaged. Inspect packaging carefully for signs of rebagging and don't use rebagged needles because they may not be clean.

7. HIV is inactivated under laboratory conditions by the following treatments. These may kill virus present on needles and other apparatus under street conditions:

    -   soaking in 10 percent household bleach (1 part bleach to 10 parts water) for 1 minute
    -   soaking in 70 percent ethyl alcohol for 1 minute.

In San Francisco, the Mid City Consortium to Combat AIDS is informing IV drug users about a rapid disinfection procedure to kill any HIV remaining in syringes and needles. The procedure uses undiluted bleach because drug users can easily obtain it and may not take the time to prepare a diluted solution. The procedure consists of two steps:

1. Draw up a syringe full of bleach (or the above bleach solution) and flush the syringe. Repeat the drawing up and flushing step with more bleach or bleach solution.

2. Draw up water in the syringe and flush out the bleach. Repeat this step with more water, two or more times.

Intravenous drug users frequently use tap water to prepare solutions for injection. However, tap water may contain infectious organisms other than

HIV. Therefore, if possible, sterile (boiled) water should be used for this cleaning procedure and to prepare any solutions used for intravenous injection.

Be sure to emphasize to IV drug users that bleach and ethyl alcohol will kill HIV only on needles, syringes, and other apparatus, and NOT in the body. *These substances should not be swallowed or injected.*

HIV is NOT inactivated by simply allowing the apparatus to dry out.

The procedures for killing HIV are based on several published studies.[11-16] They are presented because it is unrealistic to suppose that all intravenous drug users will stop using drugs or sharing needles. Clearly the only guaranteed method of avoiding HIV infections and other complications of intravenous drug use is to stop using intravenous drugs.

Along with education about needle sharing, it is important to stress that unsafe sex with infected individuals carries a high risk for transmission of human immunodeficiency virus (HIV).

Involvement in policy making is yet another way for clinicians and health workers to work to control the spread of HIV disease. Clearly, renewed efforts are in order to eradicate the social and economic conditions that generate and nurture drug abuse. The existence of a substantial population of intravenous drug users serving as a reservoir and vehicle for transmission of AIDS and other infectious diseases is but one of the hidden costs of neglecting such fundamental problems in this and other societies.

REFERENCES

1. Centers for Disease Control. Update: acquired immunodeficiency syndrome — United States. MMWR 1986; 35:17-21.

2. Centers for Disease Control. AIDS and human immunodeficiency virus infection in the United States — 1988 update. MMWR 1989; 38(Suppl 4):19S.

3. AIDS cases attributed to heterosexual contacts, January 28, 1987. Personal communication with Ann Hardy, CDC.

4. Spira TJ, Des Jarlais DC, Bokos D, et al. HTLV III/LAV antibodies in intravenous drug abusers. [Abstract]. Atlanta: International Conference on Acquired Immunodeficiency Syndrome, 1985.

5. Weiss SH, Ginzburg HM, Goedert JJ, et al. Risk for HTLV-III exposure and AIDS among parenteral drug abusers in New Jersey [Abstract]. Atlanta: International Conference on Acquired Immunodeficiency Syndrome, 1985.

6. Levy N, Carlson JR, Hinrichs S, et al. The prevalence of HTLV-III/LAV antibodies among intravenous drug users attending treatment programs in California. N Engl J Med 1986; 314:446.

7. Novick D, Kreek MJ, Des Jarlais DC, et al. Abstract of clinical research findings: therapeutic and historical aspects. In: Harris LS, ed. Problems of drug dependence, 1985. Proceedings of the 47th Annual Scientific Meeting, The Committee on Problems of Drug Dependence, Inc. NIDA Research Monograph 67. Washington, D.C.: NIDA, 1986; 318.

8. Chaisson RE, Moss AR, Onishi R, Osmond D, Carlson JR. Human immunodeficiency virus infection in heterosexual drug users in San Francisco. Am J Public Health 1987; 77:169-72.

9. Des Jarlais DC, Friedman SR, Hopkins W. Risk reduction for the acquired immunodeficiency syndrome among intravenous drug users. Ann Intern Med 1985; 103:755-9.

10. Marmor M, Des Jarlais DC, Friedman SR, et al. The epidemic of acquired immunodeficiency syndrome (AIDS) and suggestions for its control in drug abusers. J Substance Abuse Tr 1984; 1:237-47.

11. Martin LS, McDougal JS, Loskoski SL. Disinfection and inactivation of the human T-lymphotropic virus type III/lymphadenopathy associated virus. J Infect Dis 1985; 152:400-3.

12. Centers for Disease Control. Recommended infection control practices for dentistry. MMWR 1986; 35:237-42.

13. Resnick L, Veren K, Salahuddin SZ, et al. Stability and inactivation of HTLV III/LAV under clinical and laboratory environments. JAMA 1986; 255:1887-91.

14. Barre-Sinoussi F, Nugeyre MT, Chermann JC. Resistance of the AIDS virus at room temperature. Lancet 1985; 2:721-2.

15. Spire B, Dormont D, Barre-Sinoussi F, Montagnier L. Inactivation of lymphadenopathy associated virus by heat, gamma rays, and ultraviolet light. Lancet 1985; 1:188-9.

16. Spire B, Barre-Sinoussi F, Montagnier L, Chermann JC. Inactivation of lymphadenopathy associated virus by chemical disinfectants. Lancet 1984; 2:899-901.

Issues and Strategies for AIDS Education among Latinos

Ernesto O. Hinojos, M.P.H.

A IDS prevention, education, and outreach programs are essential to limit the spread of AIDS and HIV infection in the Latino community. The myths that AIDS only affects gay white men and that AIDS is transmitted casually are as common among this group as elsewhere; accurate AIDS information is the best antidote. Intravenous drug use is a factor in 36 percent of male and 80 percent of female Latino AIDS cases. Factual AIDS information will lessen AIDS hysteria and assist Latinos in adopting preventative behaviors that will help curb infectivity in this population.

■ INCIDENCE AND PREVALENCE

Census data show that 14.6 million Latinos reside in the United States. If we assume that this figure is undercounted by about 5 percent, we can safely say there are 20 million Latinos in the United States, or 9 percent of the total U.S. population.[1] According to the Centers for Disease Control report from June 1, 1981, through July 4, 1988, of the 66,464 cases of AIDS reported nationally, Latinos accounted for 13 percent (8,467) of the total. Of the cases among Latinos, 52 percent (4,431) were among homosexual/bisexual men; 36 percent (3,062) were among intravenous-drug-using heterosexual men; 9.6 percent (821) were among women; and 2.4 percent (202) were among Latino children under 13 years of age. Table 1 lists AIDS cases in U.S. resident Latino men by exposure category.[2] Table 2 lists AIDS cases in U.S. resident Latinas by exposure category. The tabulated material listed below is more exhaustive, but less recent, than the figures given above.

TABLE 1. LATINO AIDS CASES, 7/81 TO 7/88

	NUMBER	PERCENT
Homosexual or bisexual men without IVDU*	3907	52.1
Heterosexual men with IVDU	2596	34.6
Homosexual or bisexual men	524	7.0
Men with coagulation disorder	39	0.5
Heterosexual men whose sex partners had IVDU*	29	0.4
Heterosexual men born in certain countries†	4	0.0

continued on next page

continued from previous page

TABLE 1. LATINO AIDS CASES, 7/81 TO 7/88

	NUMBER	PERCENT
Heterosexual men whose sex partners were born in certain countries†	1	0.0
Transfusion recipients	65	0.9
Undetermined	322	4.2

* *IVDU = intravenous drug use.*

† *Countries (e.g., Haiti, Central African countries) in which heterosexual transmission is believed to play a major role, although precise means of transmission have not been fully defined.*

TABLE 2. LATINA AIDS CASES, 7/81 TO 7/88

	NUMBER	PERCENT
Women with IVDU*	425	51.8
Women whose male sex partners had IVDU*	233	28.4
Women whose male sex partners were bisexual	25	3.0
Women whose male sex partners had hemophilia	1	0.1
Women born in certain countries†	3	0.4
Women whose male sex partners were HIV-positive transfusion recipients	2	0.2
Women whose male sex partners had HIV infection by undetermined means	15	1.8
Women whose male sex partners had unspecified type of high risk	4	0.5
Transfusion recipients	41	5.0
Undetermined	71	8.6

* *IVDU = intravenous drug use.*

† *Countries (e.g., Haiti, Central African countries) in which heterosexual transmission is believed to play a major role, although precise means of transmission have not been fully defined.*

Latinas represent 22 percent of the female AIDS cases in the United States. Nationally, of the Latina women who have AIDS, 53 percent are IV drug users, 28 percent are the sexual partners of men in AIDS risk groups, and 10 percent received HIV-infected blood transfusions. Auerbach and colleagues estimate that among Latinas with AIDS, the actual percentages in the categories "sexual partners of men at risk" and "IV drug users" are slightly higher.[3]

■ DOES AIDS PREVENTION WORK?

AIDS prevention education has had a substantial impact upon gay men and has caused widespread behavioral changes in many parts of the country. In San

Francisco, this is evident from the dramatic decrease in rates of rectal gonorrhea in gay men.[7] Reported cases for 1985 were half the number reported in 1984, and less than one-third the number reported in 1983 (San Francisco Department of Public Health, 1986, unpublished data).

Research conducted by the San Francisco AIDS Foundation in 1985 and by the San Francisco Department of Public Health (in an ongoing study) showed that a majority of gay and bisexual men in San Francisco have discontinued unsafe sexual behaviors such as anal intercourse without a condom and ingestion of semen.[6,8]

Studies of gay and bisexual men have generally included those men most likely to respond to educational programs: (1) men with moderate to high incomes and college education and (2) access to health care. Numerous studies have determined that a respondent's knowledge of health risk is correlated with these two variables. Latinos are not in the same social strata to benefit from health education approaches that have worked in the gay community. Strategies need to be specific to the target group. The following are target groups in the Latino community that are at high risk for exposure to HIV:

- Latino gay/bisexual men;
- heterosexual intravenous drug users (male/female);
- partners of intravenous drug users (male/female);
- teens; and
- general population (to reduce fear about casual contagion).

If an AIDS prevention program for Latinos is appropriately designed and implemented, major risk activities can be reduced, thereby reducing HIV infection in this population. In some areas of the U.S. (e.g., San Francisco), the number of Latino AIDS cases is still relatively low; the implementation of appropriate AIDS prevention programs can help keep the figures that way by preventing further HIV exposure.

■ EFFECT OF ATTITUDES AND VALUES

The Latino population is as diverse as the Anglo population. An understanding of the demographic characteristics of this population and its socioeconomic and cultural differences is critical to the development of effective educational and intervention strategies. The following attitudes and values may prevent Latinos from accepting AIDS prevention messages:

- unwillingness to discuss drug use or to admit that a family member may have alcohol or drug problems;
- unwillingness to discuss human sexuality in the family context;
- unwillingness to discuss homosexuality/bisexuality;
- lack of acceptance of gay lifestyle: "Homosexuality does not exist among Latinos"; and
- lack of support and training among Latinas for negotiating sexual activity with partners.

■ INTRAVENOUS DRUG USE

Low income, low educational attainment, and lower self-esteem make it difficult to reach Latino IVDUs. Brochures dense with words may be difficult for this population, and motivation to read them correspondingly low. Materials for IVDUs are difficult to distribute, since, obviously, the population is not centrally situated. To develop appropriate messages and to understand where to distribute materials, interviews with professionals working with Latino IVDUs and other research into their social behavior patterns is necessary. Other approaches may include methadone maintenance programs and outpatient drug rehabilitation programs, interviews with nonprofit agencies working with Latino IVDUs, and county hospitals. Research such as interviews with Latino IVDUs may provide one with some idea of how many Latino IVDUs are in treatment. This baseline information is necessary in designing effective intervention.

■ DEMOGRAPHIC FACTORS

Key demographic factors to consider when planning preventative education for Latinos are national origin, geography, income, education, and language.

■ EFFECT OF NATIONAL ORIGIN

The breakdown by national origin of the United States Latino population is shown in Table 3.[1]

TABLE 3. NATIONAL ORIGINS OF U.S. LATINOS

Mexican ancestry	66%
Puerto Rican	14%
Central or South American	8%
Cuban	6%
Other Spanish-speaking countries	6%

These figures signify substantial regional differences; therefore, national origin is an important factor to consider in developing materials that are both language-appropriate and culturally sensitive. Many health-education campaigns targeted to Latinos in the past have not been successful, in part because written material in Spanish was geared to people of Mexican ancestry. While this group is the largest of those comprising the U.S. Latino population, materials geared toward this group will not necessarily be meaningful to Latinos with different national origins. Different regions of the United States have Latino populations with different needs. For example, an AIDS educational brochure developed for the Spanish-speaking population of the New York City area should reflect the Spanish vocabulary and language usage familiar to Puerto Ricans; however, the same brochure might not be appropriate for San Francisco, where many Latinos from Central or South America live. These cultures may have words or expressions that are distinctly different.

One successful method utilized by the Latino AIDS project of San Francisco has been their AIDS prevention video "Ojos Que No Ven" ("Eyes that Fail to See"). Using actors of various national origins in the video, various cultures are represented, making it representative and more culturally specific. A "photo novella" in Spanish has also been produced by the Latino AIDS Project to make the same information accessible to those in the Latino population who may not have the opportunity to see the video. The video and photo novella cover topics such as AIDS transmission, sexuality, homosexuality, bisexuality, and intravenous drug use.

■ EFFECT OF LANGUAGE USAGE

How long a Latino has been in the United States affects his or her language familiarity and usage. A Mexican immigrant who has been in the U.S. for a decade will clearly have a much better understanding of the dominant language and culture than a new immigrant. On the other hand, the newer immigrant may have stronger cultural and religious biases about homosexuality, promiscuity, and drug use than a more assimilated person. These factors could affect the presentation of the necessary issues involved in AIDS education.

■ EFFECT OF EDUCATION

In 1980, 46 percent of the U.S. Latino population had graduated from high school, and 20 percent had some college education.[1] Of the Anglo population, 69 percent had completed high school. In major urban centers across the country, there is a much higher high-school dropout rate for Latino than for Anglo youths. The educational level of a population should strongly influence the selection of appropriate media for outreach programs. For example, it is far more effective to use electronic media than traditional newspaper advertising to reach Latinos. Although print ads reach some Latinos, TV and radio ads will be more effective. TV and radio messages reach the maximum number of teenagers, young adults, and seniors.[4] Despite the high cost of producing a TV public-service announcement (PSA) on a limited budget, if such a vehicle reaches many more members of the target population, it may still be the most cost-effective approach.

■ SPECIFIC RECOMMENDATIONS

A demographic sketch of the targeted Latino population should assist the health educator, program planner, or community organizer to prepare appropriate materials and outreach. It is imperative that these programs be sensitive to local cultural factors. This may mean creatively developing new methods of outreach; for example, street theater, which proved very successful in raising the level of awareness about unionization among farmworkers in 1973, may be used to reach illiterate Latinos. Because the Latino population has large numbers of people with limited formal education, printed materials (if used at all) should be written in common vocabulary. Community-outreach workers, who can provide health education in person, along with written materials in a community setting, have been successful educators in the past. Although this method is time- and energy-intensive, it has the potential to greatly increase comprehension and retention of written materials.[5]

In developing AIDS-prevention programs for Latino IVDUs, as is true for other IVDUs, the focus should be on two major routes of transmission: sharing IV drug equipment and sexual transmission. AIDS-prevention campaigns are needed to help drug users reduce needle-sharing. One method is through the use of methadone treatment clinics in Latino communities. This allows face-to-face interaction between the client and counselor, who assists the client in clarifying misinformation and in asking questions. This also solves the problems of illiteracy and language in communicating information.

Since IVDUs not in treatment outnumber those in treatment by a margin of four to one, street outreach programs provide another approach to AIDS prevention. Rehabilitated Latino IVDUs trained in AIDS prevention provide credible sources of AIDS information for IVDUs in the community.

One effective method employed by the San Francisco AIDS Foundation has been "Bleachman." This campaign is a multifaceted AIDS-education effort that uses a "superhero" character, Bleachman, in a wide-scale San Francisco outreach to encourage IVDUs to always clean their needles with bleach before injecting drugs. The campaign uses bilingual billboards, comic brochures, cards displayed on buses, posters, T-shirts, TV public-service announcements, and direct street outreach. The Bleachman hero has proven to be credible, nonjudgmental, and nonthreatening to the IVDU on the street.

Like other male IVDUs, Latino male IVDUs transmit HIV to their female sexual partners. Women infected by their IVDU partners or through their own drug use in turn transmit HIV perinatally to their infants. Besides educating IVDUs about cleaning their equipment, community programs should provide information on safe sexual practices. In addition to information, social support-systems need to be set up to help IVDUs apply the knowledge they have learned. Promotion of condom use needs to be developed for both Latino IVDUs and their sexual partners.

From my experience, I recommend the following guidelines for the development of educational materials and outreach programs for the Latino population:

- Utilize Latino providers and educators when possible and use Latino agencies familiar with the target population. This ensures the credibility and the accessibility of the educator/provider to the audience and increases the receptivity of the target population.

- Develop educational strategies and AIDS education materials with participation and suggestions from the target audience.

- Use educational materials and presentation styles commensurate with the educational levels of the target population; develop materials in conjunction with research on the values and belief systems of the target population to ensure an appropriate approach.

- Provide AIDS training for Latino health professionals and community-agency professionals serving Latinos. These individuals understand the language, cultural, and immigrational differences among Latinos and can therefore more easily provide the appropriate education.

- Use employers, churches, schools, community organizations, and local AIDS organizations as support networks to assist in disseminating AIDS information to the Latino community and to reinforce the appropriate AIDS-prevention message in the community.

- Develop media (TV and radio) messages in different languages and use spokespersons from the target populations. Use a reading level appropriate to the target population when developing printed ads; use culturally relevant language and symbols.

REFERENCES

1. Juarez FN. The Hispanic market in the 1980's. In: The state of Hispanic America, vol. III. Oakland, Calif.: National Hispanic Center for Advanced Studies and Policy Analysis and the National Hispanic University, 1983:13-24.

2. Centers for Disease Control. Weekly surveillance report — United States AIDS Program, December 1, 1986.

3. Auerbach I, Carlson M, Shaw N, et al. Women and AIDS clinical resource guide. San Francisco: San Francisco AIDS Foundation, 1986.

4. Green LW, Kreuter MW, Deeds SG, Patridge KB. Health education planning: a diagnostic approach. Palo Alto, Calif.: Mayfield, 1980.

5. Report of the secretary's task force on black and minority health. Washington, D.C.: U.S. Department of Health and Human Services, August 1985.

6. Self-reported behavioral change among gay and bisexual men — San Francisco. MMWR 1985; 34:613-5.

7. Selik RM, Castro KG, Pappaioanou M. Distribution of AIDS cases by racial/ethnic group and exposure category, U.S., June 1, 1981–July 4, 1988. MMWR CDC Surveillance Summary 1988; 37:1-10.

8. Doll LS, O'Malley P, Pershing A, et al. High-risk behavior and knowledge of HIV antibody status in the San Francisco City Clinic Cohort [Abstract]. IV International Conference on AIDS. Stockholm, 1988:I; 474.

HIV Disease and the African-American Community

Victoria A. Cargill, M.D., and Mark D. Smith, M.D., M.B.A.

HIV disease disproportionately affects blacks in the United States. This chapter will review the epidemiology of HIV among African Americans, clinical issues of particular relevance to black patients, important social issues including the response by various sectors of the black community to the AIDS epidemic, and important policy issues with special relevance for blacks.

■ EPIDEMIOLOGY

Every two hours a black person dies from HIV disease.[1] Since its appearance in 1981, HIV disease has claimed an increasing number of blacks, including celebrities such as designer Willie Smith, entertainer Sylvester, and television newsman Max Robinson. Many members of the African-American community have, however, been slow to accept the magnitude of the epidemic. While skepticism and disbelief slowly yield to awareness and action, the national statistics demonstrate that the incidence of AIDS and HIV-related diseases continues to increase in the black population. The higher seroprevalence rate among blacks virtually guarantees continued HIV disease disproportionate to population size for many years.

The cumulative incidence of AIDS in American blacks is 83.8 cases per 100,000 black persons. While the proportion of AIDS cases in adult white males for 1988 has decreased, the proportion in black males has increased, in part due to the revised AIDS case definition.[2] Black males constitute 12 percent of all U.S. men and 24 percent of adult male AIDS cases. Major risk behaviors in black male adults with AIDS are gay or bisexual behavior (45 percent), intravenous drug use (34 percent), or both (8 percent).[3] AIDS in women increased from 7 percent to 10 percent of all adult cases in 1988; over half (54 percent) are black. Intravenous drug users (IVDUs) and the sexual partners of IVDUs account for 83 percent of the cases among black women. Similarly, black children make up 14 percent of the U.S. child population, but they comprise 55 percent of the pediatric AIDS cases. Of these, 62 percent have mothers who are IVDUs or the sexual partners of IVDUs.[2] The numbers of AIDS cases in adolescents has increased from 283 cases as of August 31, 1988, to 335 as of December 31, 1988.[3] Black teens are disproportionately represented in this cohort; their risk behaviors are similar to black adults'. Intravenous drug use is the leading transmission category in black adolescent AIDS cases, followed by heterosexual and homosexual or bisexual behavior. Data from DiClemente[4] and the Centers for Disease Control (CDC) confirm the need for continued education.[5] In both studies, black teens knew significantly less about AIDS than white teens, although both groups demonstrated a need for a better knowledge base. Finally, sexually-transmitted disease (STD) rates continue to be disproportionately higher in black teens.[6]

■ CLINICAL FEATURES

It is beyond the scope of this chapter to discuss the entire spectrum of clinical manifestations of HIV among blacks. In many respects, of course, diagnosis and management of HIV infection and its sequelae are not affected by the patient's race. Nevertheless, there are several clinical issues worth noting because of epidemiologic or biologic differences between patients of different races.

Tuberculosis.   U.S. morbidity from tuberculosis (TB) declined by an annual average of 5 percent for 32 years until 1985; it then plateaued because of tuberculosis in HIV-infected individuals.[7] TB in HIV-infected patients, as in non-infected patients, is predominantly a reactivation of an earlier infection. Concurrent HIV infection increases the risk of clinical illness among those with previous infection with *Mycobacterium tuberculosis*. One study demonstrated that 15 percent of HIV-positive and PPD-positive persons developed TB over two years, compared to none in an HIV-negative/PPD-positive group.[8]

Several studies have demonstrated higher rates of TB among black AIDS patients. In New York, AIDS patients with TB were more likely to be non-Haitian black, Haitian, or hispanic than AIDS patients without TB.[9] Forty-one percent of these patients were black, compared to 11 percent Haitian and 29 percent hispanic. In a San Francisco study, blacks constituted only 5 percent of AIDS cases without evidence of TB, but 17 percent of TB and AIDS cases.[10] The presence of clinical TB, particularly in the setting of high-risk behaviors, should alert the clinician to the potential for underlying HIV infection, especially in blacks. All patients with active TB should, therefore, be offered HIV testing.[11]

Conversely, TB should be high on the list of suspected pathogens for HIV-infected patients with pulmonary problems, especially black patients. All patients with HIV infection should be tested for TB and receive 12 months of isoniazid prophylaxis if the PPD test reaction is greater than 5 millimeters.

Kaposi's Sarcoma.   Kaposi's sarcoma (KS), seen primarily in homosexual men, is the most frequent of the AIDS-associated malignancies. It appears to be decreasing in frequency, for unknown reasons.[12] KS has been less common in blacks and IVDUs.[13,14] The cause of this apparent discrepancy is unknown. Despite this finding, KS does occur in some black AIDS cases. The lesions of KS in blacks are quite variable and may be subtle. In light-skinned individuals, these lesions are blue to violet; in darker-skinned patients, they may be black. Whatever their color, KS lesions are often nodular and rubbery, as in whites. The lesions may occur on virtually every body surface, as well as in the oral cavity, lungs, and viscera. A high index of suspicion is the key to diagnosis.

Drug Use.   Much of the disproportionate impact of HIV disease on the black community derives from its historically higher rates of illicit drug use.[15] In addition, blacks have repeatedly been shown to have higher rates of HIV infection than white drug users.[16,17] This finding appears to be due to behavioral factors such as intravenous cocaine use (which involves more frequent injection than heroin or methamphetamines), frequency of needle-sharing, and use of shooting galleries.[18] Since black HIV-infected patients are more likely than whites to be (or to have been) users of intravenous drugs, they are more likely to have other medical conditions associated with drug use. These conditions may in turn be exacerbated by concurrent HIV infection (e.g., bacterial pneumonia and sepsis, endocarditis, and hepatitis).

■ PRIMARY-CARE ISSUES

Delivery of Primary Care.   Because of the high percentage of AIDS cases among black women and adolescents, diagnosis and treatment of HIV-related infections often falls to primary-care physicians serving minority populations (e.g., internists, family and general practitioners, gynecologists, and pediatricians). But because these populations have poor primary care in general, patients often appear for treatment at ambulatory-care sites where there may be poor continuity of care and lack of comprehensive care. Facilities such as STD clinics and emergency rooms have an important role to play in preventing and detecting HIV infection and in recognizing HIV-related illnesses. They are not, however, well-equipped to provide the ongoing care needed by HIV-infected individuals.[19] And despite other obstacles (such as high rates of staff turnover) in health centers and other facilities equipped to deal with HIV disease, primary-care physicians cannot relegate the management of HIV to the subspecialist.[20]

Women and Adolescents.   In addition to their clinical needs, HIV-infected patients also pose a great challenge to the educational skills of the physician. Blacks consistently have shown lower knowledge scores and greater misconceptions than whites about AIDS.[3,21,22] Many black women with HIV disease are IVDUs and may have little medical knowledge; their future health problems with HIV infection are commonly less immediate to them than the daily trials and frustrations of poverty and drug use. Differences in values between the health provider and patient may also prove significant. Estimates of the risk of HIV transmission to the fetus range from 21 percent to 50 percent; nevertheless many HIV-infected women become pregnant and refuse abortion despite their knowledge of this risk. Whether due to denial, cultural values, or religious conviction, their behavior sometimes increases their stigmatization by physicians.[23] Providers for women need to be alert to the danger of addressing the risk of HIV in women solely from the perspective of neonatal infection — a tendency that implies that women are not patients but only vectors of disease.[24]

Adolescents also present numerous challenges, in part because they are often sexually active while developing their sense of sexuality and sexual identity. At the same time, they have little sense of their own mortality. Heightened sexual activity, drug experimentation, and the emergence of crack cocaine also have increased the risk of HIV infection in adolescents.[5,25] Associated with the increased use of crack is a growing trend of teenagers exchanging sexual favors for drugs or for money to buy drugs. These adolescents, sometimes called "strawberries," are commonly in or near crackhouses, where they may receive as little as $4 for each (often unsafe) sexual encounter. STD rates among adolescents underscore the need for concern and intervention. Ten- to twenty-year-olds accounted for 40 percent of syphilis cases reported in 1985, but rates for all STDs are higher among black adolescents.[26,27] Seroprevalence data from an overwhelmingly black STD clinic population in Baltimore revealed that 2.9 percent of the females age 15 to 19 were HIV-positive, as were 2 percent of the males.[22] In Ohio, for the first quarter of 1988, 539 cases of gonorrhea were reported in black males aged 10 to 19, compared to 80 cases in white males; a similar discrepancy was seen in females.[28] The need to incorporate AIDS education and prevention in adolescent health care cannot be overstated.

■ CLINICAL TRIALS

Through the National Institute of Allergy and Infectious Diseases (NIAID), AIDS Clinical Trial Groups (ACTG) centers have been established to recruit patients to participate in trials of new and promising therapeutic agents. Subjects recruited to date in these trials do not reflect the increased percentage of AIDS cases in blacks in general, or in black women in particular. Although blacks accounted for almost one of three AIDS cases in 1988, less than 7 percent of the population enrolled in ACTG trials are black.[29,30] Women are excluded unless they are outside the childbearing years or are using some form of birth control, because of uncertainty about possible teratogenic effects of experimental drugs. For black women, this may pose an additional barrier because they may have two to three pregnancies even after their first child is identified as HIV-positive.[31]

The black community's perspective on clinical research is a complex one, conditioned in part by poor blacks' decades of reliance on medical-school teaching hospitals for care as well as by suspicion about being used as "guinea pigs." Such fears would seem to have been justified by revelations about a syphilis study conducted in Tuskegee, Alabama, from 1932 to 1972 by the CDC and the Alabama Department of Health. Black men were recruited by a black nurse to participate in exchange for free rides to the clinic, hot meals, and a promise of burial stipends to their survivors. The men were tested, and if positive, followed without treatment to determine the natural history of syphilis, even after penicillin was available to eradicate the infection. The trial continued until 1972.[32] Although new safeguards exist and research standards have changed, this trial is well-known in many parts of the black community and is often cited as an example of abuse of black research subjects.

Other barriers to participation in clinical trials include limited access to health care, limited medical knowledge, difficulty in understanding the role of clinical trials in testing drug effectiveness, scarcity of minority staffing in research units, and few ACTG sites in inner-city areas. These barriers combine with blacks' relatively poor knowledge about AIDS to continue the underrepresentation of blacks in research. One strategy to overcome this deficit is the NIAID's Community Research Initiative program, which will target hard-to-reach populations by involving community providers such as private physicians, substance-abuse programs, and neighborhood health centers in research.

■ SURVIVAL

The life expectancy of persons with AIDS has continued to increase since 1981. With the advent of therapeutic interventions such as zidovudine (AZT) and aerosolized pentamidine, the average length of survival has increased from 6 months to 15 months. This improvement, however, is not uniformly distributed. Data obtained from New York City suggest that blacks have not experienced this improved survival. Blacks comprised 30 percent of the AIDS cases in this cohort. Unlike whites, 8.5 percent of whom died at the time of AIDS diagnosis, 14.1 percent of the black AIDS patients died at the time of diagnosis. Life-table analyses further underscore the differential survival, as black women IVDUs with *Pneumocystis carinii* pneumonia (PCP) had the least favorable survival in the cohort.[33]

PCP is consistently associated with marked immune dysfunction and, moreover, symptoms similar to those of AIDS are relatively common among HIV-seronegative IVDUs and are often ascribed to cocaine use, "drug sickness," or drug withdrawal; this obscures the association between HIV exposure and current or future health status.[13] Also, the poorer survival may reflect generic differences such as delayed presentation for care, which accounts for inferior health status for blacks in general.[35] (For instance, blacks have lower survival rates for colon-rectal cancer and breast cancer than whites. In both of these cancers, decreased survival is associated with more advanced disease at presentation.[36,37]) Continued education efforts to alert blacks to the early signs and symptoms of HIV infection, as well as provision for increased testing in the inner city may help decrease the lag time. Testing without a link to medical care is unlikely to make a difference.[38]

■ COMMUNITY RESPONSE

Compared to the gay white community, the black community has not responded to the AIDS crisis as wholeheartedly. The lack of volunteerism that has been the hallmark of gay white service organizations has placed additional strain on black AIDS service and education agencies. With increased attention focused on AIDS in blacks, there has been an increase in these community-based organizations. The majority of these are grassroots efforts that developed from the community need or perception of the impending crisis. The National Coalition of Black Lesbians and Gays (NCBLG) is one organization that took a front-line approach to the problem. This group sponsored the first national AIDS in the Black Community Conference, in Washington, D.C., in 1986. At the time this conference was organized to focus attention on the problem of AIDS in the black community, Jeff Levi, then executive director of the National Gay and Lesbian Task Force, was quoted as stating that over the 1981–1986 period, the $500 million to $600 million poured into AIDS research by the federal government was matched by the gay and lesbian community in private contributions.[38] Such an outpouring of funds has not been seen in the black community, where the percentage of those who live below the poverty level, who are unemployed, or single women heads of households exceed the white percentages by severalfold. This reality forces black service agencies to be more dependent upon grants than white-identified agencies, which in turn slows the pace of agency development, maturation and growth. As an example, the first National AIDS Network "NAN Multicultural Notes" (on AIDS service and education) was not published until July 1987, almost one year after the first AIDS in Minorities conference sponsored by the NCBLG. This newsletter discusses issues of education and service for black Americans as well as other ethnic minorities. (It was initially made possible by grants from Burroughs-Wellcome Co. and Apple Computer.[40])

Any discussion of the black community's response to AIDS would be incomplete without including the National Minority AIDS Council (NMAC), whose leadership helped focus national attention on AIDS in blacks. Its efforts continue to link and support local black community AIDS services. NMAC is made up of local minority-oriented AIDS organizations and agencies, such as

BEBASHI (Blacks Educating Blacks About Sexual Health Issues) in Philadelphia, Kupona Network in Chicago, POCCAN (People of Color Against AIDS Network) in Seattle, and the Minority AIDS Project in Los Angeles. NMAC has worked with the National Urban League not only to increase awareness but also to encourage those community-based organizations working to diminish the HIV emergency in minority communities.

The response from the black church has been mixed. A few leaders, such as the Rev. Carl Bean of the Minority AIDS Project and the Rev. Harrold Burris of Washington, D.C., have repeatedly pointed to the need for greater education in the church. The fundamentalist nature of many black religions, combined with the view of some that AIDS is a punishment from God, has blunted the church response.[34,41] Homosexuality, intravenous drug use, and sexual promiscuity are difficult subjects to tackle even without superimposed moral and religious overtones. The epidemic therefore confronts black clergy with the dilemma of providing AIDS education to their congregations without committing ecclesiastical suicide. Controversial interventions to decrease the transmission of HIV, such as provision of needles and abortion, may reinforce the schism within and between black clergy and their congregations, unless a more public-health oriented view of the epidemic is taken.

■ POLICY ISSUES

Education.   AIDS has presented the biggest challenge to our scientific, public-health, and health-care communities in many decades. Broad HIV-related policy issues are confounded by social, religious, political, and ethical considerations at a community level. Blacks have experienced unequal access to medical care, lower living standards, higher unemployment, alcoholism, intravenous drug use, and overall mortality rates since the time of slavery. The addition of HIV disease has yielded predictable results; poorer survival and delayed presentation for care are part of this legacy. The CDC has urged improved AIDS education for minorities, stressing the need for cultural sensitivity and relevance. AIDS education, however, must be further tailored to address the specific behaviors of those at risk and to urge alternatives to those behaviors that cannot or will not be changed. Many black community-based organizations provide this education but are dependent upon federal grants to survive, due to the lack of private donations. Because Senate bill S1220 was amended under conservative pressure to prohibit federal funding for organizations that "promote or encourage" homosexual sexual relations (the "Helms amendment"), those at greatest risk may receive incomplete information.[42]

Unlike white men with AIDS, over 30 percent of black males with AIDS report bisexual behavior, which also places women and their subsequent children at risk. It is the authors' impression that black gay men are also more likely to engage in high-risk practices and to have anonymous sexual contacts. By day, bisexual black men maintain a straight facade, but they may also engage in sex with men picked up in bars, baths, or bookstores. Some of these men may travel to other cities to avoid detection. Moreover, engaging in this behavior may not be perceived as homosexual, bisexual, or high risk.[43] Our constricted views of appropriate AIDS education must be revised in light of such behavior if the epidemic is to be slowed.

Abortion.   HIV can be vertically transmitted to the fetus[44,45]; the capacity of both symptomatic and asymptomatic pregnant women to transmit HIV to their children has ominous implications for the health of America's future generations. This is particularly an issue for blacks, as over half of U.S. AIDS cases in children are black.

Black women are placed at risk through intravenous drug use, as sexual partners of IVDUs, or as sexual partners of bisexual men. Maternal infection is often discovered incidentally after the birth of an HIV-positive infant or with the development of opportunistic infections during pregnancy. Currently available data are insufficient to resolve questions about the role of pregnancy in accelerating HIV-related disease. Nevertheless, the impact of HIV on the course of pregnancy has been significant. Of the pregnancy-associated deaths due to AIDS in the U.S. from 1981 to 1988, the majority were black or hispanic women. Half of these women were IVDUs and the majority died of PCP.[46]

Despite the widespread recognition of perinatal HIV transmission, the current political climate concerning reproductive rights has allowed little open discussion about induced abortion as an option to HIV-infected pregnant women.[47]

The current controversy therefore threatens to worsen the epidemic both by restricting broad discussion of the options and by erecting social and economic barriers to abortion, particularly for poor women — the very population most exposed to HIV. Because of the restrictions imposed by the Helms amendment and the summary prohibition of Federal support for making clean needles available to IVDUs, many women at high risk can receive neither explicit sexual information for their partners nor clean works if the agency they use for service receives federal funds. In epicenters there are already homes such as Hale House (New York City) and Grandma's House (Washington, D.C.) to care for infected neonates, who are often not enrolled in foster care because of illness or lack of interested foster parents. The emergence of grandmothers as the surviving relative who cares for the infected or uninfected children is already common in East Coast centers. What support, if any, will these abortion and education policies include for these women, who often live on fixed incomes? These children are also often without resources or have Medicaid as the only source of health coverage. The country's failure to develop a comprehensive and realistic plan to interrupt the spreading wave of HIV infection among minority women assures us that hundreds or thousands of women and their children will suffer years from now.

■ CONCLUSION

Although the AIDS epidemic was recognized many years ago by the scientific, public-health, and gay communities, it is only recently that it has been recognized in the African-American community. HIV infection is clinically similar in blacks and whites, but epidemiologic differences increase the likelihood of certain clinical presentations in blacks. Many traditional black organizations, such as churches, have been slow to respond, but other, new organizations have grown up to provide culturally-sensitive education and patient services. The AIDS-minority connection is a sensitive one, both for minority communities (because it highlights behaviors such as drug use that do not portray them in their best light) and for the country as a whole (because the extent of the epidemic among minorities is exacerbated by the general inequalities that minorities suffer). Because poverty among black AIDS patients is common, HIV infection, which is usually of paramount concern to the patient's physician, may be but one of many pressing issues to the patient. Physicians caring for large numbers of HIV-infected black patients need to examine several factors that influence their ability to provide good care: the makeup of their staffs, the accessibility of their services, and the provision of ancillary services such as child care and transportation. They may also need to examine and confront some of their own attitudes towards patients from different backgrounds, some of whom live in a world apart from their own.

REFERENCES

1. Parsons A. Black leaders, groups act to confront the AIDS threat. Baltimore Sun. November 28, 1987:12A.

2. AIDS and human immunodeficiency virus infection in the United States: 1988 update. MMWR 1989; 38(Suppl 4):1-38.

3. Miller G. Continuing jeopardy: children and AIDS. A staff report of the Select Committee on Children, Youth, and Families. U.S. House of Representatives Select Committee on Children, Youth, and Families. 100th Congress, 2nd Session. September 1988.

4. DiClemente RJ, Boyer CB, Morales ES. Minorities and AIDS: knowledge, attitudes, and misconceptions among black and Latino adolescents. Am J Public Health 1988; 78:55-7.

5. HIV-related beliefs, knowledge, and behaviors among high school students. MMWR 1988; 37:717-21.

6. Crack and resurgence of syphilis spreading AIDS among the poor. New York Times. August 29, 1988:A-1.

7. Diagnosis and management of mycobacterial infection and disease in persons with human T-lymphotropic virus type III/lymphadenopathy-associated virus infection. MMWR 1986; 35:448-52.

8. Selwyn PA, Hartel D, Lewis VA, et al. A prospective study of the risk of tuberculosis among intravenous drug users with human immunodeficiency virus infection. N Engl J Med 1989; 320:545-50.

9. Tuberculosis and acquired immunodeficiency syndrome — New York City. MMWR 1987; 36:785-90, 795.

10. Chaisson RE, Schechter GF, Theuer CP, et al. Tuberculosis in patients with the acquired immunodeficiency syndrome. Clinical features, response to therapy, and survival. Am Rev Resp Dis 1987; 136:570-4.

11. A strategic plan for the elimination of tuberculosis in the United States. MMWR 1989; 38:269-72.

12. Mitsuyasu R. Kaposi's sarcoma in the acquired immunodeficiency syndrome. Infect Dis Clin N Am 1988; 2:541.

13. Safai B, Johnson KG, Myskowski PL, et al. The natural history of Kaposi's sarcoma in the acquired immunodeficiency syndrome. Ann Intern Med 1985; 103:744-50.

14. Epidemiologic aspects of the current outbreak of Kaposi's sarcoma and opportunistic infections. N Engl J Med 1982; 306:248-52.

15. Kozel NJ, Adams EH. Epidemiology of drug abuse: an overview. Science 1986; 234:970-4.

16. Robert-Guroff M, Weiss SH, Giron JA, et al. Prevalence of antibodies to HTLV-I, -II, and -III in intravenous drug abusers from an AIDS endemic region. JAMA 1986; 255:3133-7.

17. Chaisson RE, Moss AR, Onishi R, et al. Human immunodeficiency virus infection in heterosexual intravenous drug users in San Francisco. Am J Public Health 1987; 77:169-72.

18. Chaisson RE, Bacchetti P, Osmond D, et al. Cocaine use and HIV infection in intravenous drug users in San Francisco. JAMA 1989; 261:561-5.

19. Northfelt DW, Hayward RA, Shapiro MF. The acquired immunodeficiency syndrome is a primary care disease. Ann Intern Med 1988; 109:773-5.

20. Smith MD. AIDS: roles for black physicians. J Natl Med Assoc 1987; 79:917-8.

21. Thomas SB. Knowledge and attitudes towards AIDS. A survey of inner-city black residents in selected public housing units, black churches and black college freshmen. Unpublished manuscript, University of Maryland, 1987.

22. Cargill VA, Gayle JB, Klonoff EA. AIDS in minorities: knowledge, attitudes and sexual practices. Clin Res 1988; 36:721A. abstract.

23. Kelly JA, St Lawrence JS, Smith S Jr, et al. Stigmatization of AIDS patients by physicians. Am J Public Health 1987; 77:789-91.

24. Wofsy CB. Human immunodeficiency virus infection in women. JAMA 1987; 257:2074-6.

25. Hein K. AIDS in adolescents: a rationale for concern. NY State J Med 1987; 87:290-5.

26. Centers for Population Options. The facts: AIDS, adolescents and the human immunodeficiency virus. Washington, DC, April 1989.

27. Quinn TC, Glasser D, Cannon RO, et al. Human immunodeficiency virus infection among patients attending clinics for sexually transmitted diseases. N Engl J Med 1988; 318:197-203.

28. Ohio statewide gonorrhea data, January 1, 1988 to March 1, 1988. Pinckney L, personal communication.

29. Rogers DE. Federal spending on AIDS — how much is enough? N Engl J Med 1989; 320:1623-4.

30. Stokes LB. Keynote address. AIDS in the minority community: where do we go from here? May 6, 1989. Cleveland, Ohio.

31. Scott GB, Fischl MA, Klinas N, et al. Mothers of infants with the acquired immunodeficiency syndrome. Evidence for both symptomatic and asymptomatic carriers. JAMA 1985; 253:363-6.

32. Jones RH. Bad blood. New York: The Free Press, 1981.

33. Rothenberg R, Woelfel M, Stoneburner R, et al. Survival with the acquired immunodeficiency syndrome. Experience with 5833 cases in New York City. N Engl J Med 1987; 317:1297-302.

34. Des Jarlais DC, Friedman SR, Hopkins W. Risk reduction for the acquired immunodeficiency syndrome among intravenous drug users. Ann Intern Med 1985; 103:755-9.

35. Heckler MM. Report of the Secretary's task force on black and minority health. U.S. Department of Health and Human Services, August, 1985.

36. Bassett MT, Krieger N. Social class and black-white differences in breast cancer survival. Am J Public Health 1986; 76:1400-3.

37. Krain LS. Racial and socioeconomic factors in colon cancer mortality. Oncology 1972; 26:335-44.

38. Lambert B. U.S. urges treatment for millions with the AIDS virus. New York Times. July 9, 1989:12.

39. Gerald G. AIDS and the black community. Equal Time. Jun 15, 1986:75.

40. National AIDS Network. NAN Multicultural notes on AIDS service and education. June/July, 1987.

41. Chandler R. Believer's views differ in doctrine, sex, afterlife, public policy. Los Angeles Times. July 26, 1986; PEII:4-5.

42. Roover J. After fiery debate, Senate passes AIDS bill. Congress Quart 1988; April 30:1167.

43. Mays VM, Cochran SD. Acquired immunodeficiency syndrome and black Americans: special psychosocial issues. Public Health Rep 1987; 102:224-31.

44. Sprecher S, Soumenkoff G, Puissant F, Degueldre M. Vertical transmission of HIV in 15-week fetus. Lancet 1986; 2:288-9.

45. Lapointe N, Michaud J, Pekovic D, et al. Transplacental transmission of HTLV-III virus. N Engl J Med 1985; 312:1325-6.

46. Koonin LM, Ellerbrock TV, Atrash HK, et al. Pregnancy-associated deaths due to AIDS in the United States. JAMA 1989; 261:1306-9.

47. Grimes DA. The CDC and abortion in HIV-positive women. JAMA 1987; 258:1176.

AIDS Education for Adolescents in High School

Marcia Quackenbush, M.S.

Teenagers are at risk for HIV infection, either through unprotected sexual intercourse or sharing needles for IV drug or other use.[1,2,6]

About half of U.S. teenagers are currently sexually active; by age 17, 57 percent have had intercourse.[3] Unprotected intercourse is common in this group and reported rates of sexually transmitted diseases (STDs) continue to be high.[4,7,8] Each year, one in seven teenagers is diagnosed with an STD.[9] There are over one million teen pregnancies in the U.S. annually.[10] Even teenagers from conservative backgrounds are often sexually active: a recent poll of teenagers involved in fundamentalist churches showed that 43 percent had had sexual intercourse by age 18.[11]

The amount of needle use and needle sharing among teenagers cannot be described accurately, since no national statistics are kept, but we know that over 1 percent of high school students have reported using heroin, which is usually injected. Several million teenagers have used other opiates, amphetamines, barbiturates or cocaine,[5] all of which may be injected. Needles may also be used for injecting steroids, for piercing ears, tattooing, or other purposes. Risk of exposure to HIV is associated with needle sharing in any of these circumstances.

The use of alcohol or noninjected drugs (also high among teens) is also a risk factor for HIV infection because such drugs may cloud judgment and impair resolve, making sexual- or needle-risk behaviors more likely. In a 1987 survey, 66.4 percent of high school seniors had used alcohol within the past month and 56.6 percent had used illicit drugs at some point in their lives.[12]

Some studies suggest that crack cocaine poses a risk of HIV infection because of the multiple sexual encounters common among users. HIV seropositivity among nonintravenous crack users is comparable to that found in the intravenous-drug-using population.[30]

For some time, there has been limited epidemiologic evidence of HIV infection among teens. About 0.5 percent of total U.S. AIDS cases have been among 13- to 19-year-olds. Though it may appear from such figures that the overall risk of AIDS for teenagers is low, the fact that the disease has an average incubation period of 9.8 years[13] makes it clear that many individuals diagnosed in their twenties (21 percent of total U.S. cases) were infected as teens. Recent statistics reinforce these disturbing conclusions. In New York City, 20 percent of all reported AIDS cases are among persons 13 to 21 years of age.[14]

Early in our efforts to promote school-based AIDS education, we often heard the argument "AIDS is primarily a disease of gay men, and our students do not fall into that category." The likelihood that many gay youths will go unidentified in schools and other youth programs has been well addressed elsewhere.[15,16] There are many reasons gay or lesbian teenagers choose to hide their sexual orientation and many administrative policies and social prejudices that lead to gay students being overlooked. Most schools have gay students in attendance.

We have ample and convincing data that HIV is not a "gay" disease. IV drug use plays a significant role in the spread of HIV, and bidirectional (male-to-female, female-to-male) heterosexual transmission is well documented and increasing. Among adolescents, heterosexual HIV transmission is significantly greater than among adults: nationally (excluding New York City), teenagers are heterosexually infected at twice the rate of adults; in New York City, at three times the adult rate.[14]

We are no longer looking at the possibility of teenagers becoming HIV-infected. This is now a fact, and the potential for further spread is enormous. It is essential that young people be informed of the risks of transmission and of the methods to protect them from infection.

All schools and communities should implement AIDS education for young people. We should remember that teenagers who do not currently have HIV-related risks may face such risks later and can therefore benefit from AIDS preventive education now. Surveys show that teenagers are quite eager to receive AIDS education in school settings.[6,17,18] The Centers for Disease Control's (CDC) anonymous questionnaire, administered to students in grades 9 through 12 in 6 cities of 24 different states, indicates that "almost all respondents believed students their age should be taught about AIDS in school (range, 89.0 percent to 96.8 percent).[29]

■ CONCEPTS

Guidelines have been developed by both the CDC[19] and a student advocacy organization[20] suggesting appropriate AIDS-related concepts for schools to present to children and teenagers. These should be reviewed by schools or individuals developing AIDS curricula.

There are four essential concepts for teenagers to understand about AIDS:

1. **AIDS/HIV Infection Is a Viral Disease, Not a Gay Disease.** It is caused by a pathogen, not by a particular lifestyle.

2. **AIDS/HIV Infection Is Not Easily Transmitted, and It Is Not Transmitted by Casual Contact.** An individual will not contract HIV infection in the normal course of daily contact with friends and acquaintances. This is important to emphasize, since the CDC survey of high-schoolers' beliefs and knowledge about HIV infection indicates that many students continue to believe that "HIV infection may be acquired from giving blood, using public toilets, or having a blood test or from mosquito and other insect bites."[29]

3. **Under the Proper Circumstances, Anyone Can Contract AIDS/HIV Infection.** Most commonly, HIV is transmitted through unprotected sexual intercourse (vaginal, anal, or oral); the sharing of needles for IV drug or other purposes; or from an infected woman to her fetus or newborn.

4. **You Can Protect Yourself from AIDS/HIV Infection.** First, do not use drugs and do not share needles for drug use, tattooing, ear piercing, or any other reason. Second, abstain from sexual intercourse, or have intercourse with only one lifetime partner who does not use IV drugs and has had sex with no one but you, or, if you do choose to be sexually active, use safer-sex techniques, including condoms, to avoid infection.

Students should also understand that HIV has a long incubation period and that most people currently infected do not feel or appear ill and do not know that they are infected.

The meaning of "safer sex" should also be explained, including how condoms are used and where they can be purchased. If this material is too controversial for the classroom setting, students should be offered referral to sources where they can obtain this information.

■ BEHAVIOR CHANGE

The ultimate goal of AIDS education is behavior change. If teens are knowledgeable about AIDS, they can protect themselves by abstaining from sexual intercourse and IV drug use or they can practice safer-sex techniques and avoid needle-sharing (if they use IV drugs).

Unfortunately, existing studies on teenagers' sexual behavior are not encouraging. In a study of 860 Massachusetts teenagers, for example,[17] 70 percent reported being sexually active but only 15 percent of the sexually active youths reported taking steps to protect themselves from sexual transmission of HIV. Further, only 20 percent of that 15 percent had taken effective precautions (i.e., abstaining from some sexual activities or using condoms).

A recently reported San Francisco study explored adolescent attitudes and behaviors concerning condom use.[21] Many of the subjects had participated in school-based AIDS education programs and had been exposed to intensive AIDS education in the general community during the period of the study. Though these teens perceived that condoms prevented STDs and that such prevention was important, they did not intend to use condoms or increase their condom use.

These results are consistent with other studies on the impact of sexuality and health education on teen sexual activity. Though sex education correlates positively with increased knowledge and decreased misinformation about sexuality, changes in sexual behavior have not been shown,[22,23] even with otherwise exemplary programs.[24]

Evidence from successful drug-abuse and smoking-prevention programs suggests that these discouraging results in modifying teenagers' sexual behavior reflect an error also being made in most AIDS education programs — AIDS information is being presented out of context and so it has less impact than information presented in a comprehensive, integrated format. An isolated unit on AIDS has little influence on students, but students accept lessons on HIV prevention that are related to broader curricula. The message "Protect yourself from AIDS" has significantly more meaning when set in a comprehensive health program that spans a student's full school career (kindergarten through twelfth grade). Such programs teach skills related to health promotion and building self-esteem, help students develop decision-making abilities and refusal skills (so they can say "no" when appropriate), and encourage a sense of responsibility to the well-being of the larger community.

■ DIRECTIONS FOR SUCCESS

Some established, successful drug-abuse and smoking-prevention programs provide a useful model for AIDS preventive education. Overall, studies have found that classes that only emphasize the hazards of these activities have little effect. However, programs that help students develop decision-making and refusal skills have been effective. Some models use charismatic older students to teach these skills to younger ones.[25]

■ A COLLABORATIVE EFFORT

AIDS education for young people works best as a collaborative community effort involving schools (school boards, administration, teachers, counselors, nurses, and other staff), public health departments, churches and temples, and community organizations. Physicians and medical clinics can also play a role. Special attention has been given recently to the importance of parental involvement in AIDS education for youths. Programs now exist to help parents learn how to better communicate with their children about AIDS and related issues.[26,27] The San Francisco AIDS Foundation has produced materials for a parent-education program, including a video, "Talking with Teens, with Jane Curtin," and a manual with suggestions for facilitating a workshop for parents, "The Parent-Teen AIDS Education Program: Talking With Teens." Information can be obtained from San Francisco AIDS Foundation, P.O. Box 6182, San Francisco CA 94101-6182.

■ MATERIALS

Support materials for AIDS education for young people, especially those focused on school-based programs, have increased in number recently. These include curricula, textbooks, teaching guides, audiovisual materials, and trainings for teachers. Two excellent catalogues through which such materials can be ordered are:

"Educating About AIDS" Network Publications
ETR Associates
P.O. Box 1830
Santa Cruz, CA 95061-1830
(408) 438-4060

"AIDS Educator"
San Francisco AIDS Foundation
P.O. Box 6182
San Francisco, CA 94101-6182
(415) 861-3397

In addition, two national organizations offer regularly updated reviews of current materials. (The SIECUS report is not limited to materials for adolescents.)

"AIDS and Adolescents: Resources for Educators"
Education Department
Center for Population Options
1012 14th Street N.W.
Washington, D.C. 20005
(202) 347-5700

"AIDS and Safer Sex Education: An Annotated Bibliography of Print and Audio-Visual Materials for Sale"
SIECUS (Sex Information and Education Council of the U.S.)
New York University
32 Washington Place
New York, NY 10003
(212) 673-3850

The CDC has added an "AIDS School Health Education Subfile" to its "Combined Health Information Database" (CHID). This excellent document contains descriptions of programs, curricula, guidelines, policies, regulations and materials relevant to school-based AIDS education. It can be searched by computer, although the CDC also makes hard copies of the database available upon request. For further information, contact:

Centers for Disease Control
Center for Health Promotion and Education
Division of Health Education
Attn: AIDS School Health Education Subfile
Atlanta, GA 30333
(404) 639-3492 or (404) 639-3824

■ RECOMMENDATIONS

It is clear that schools have a major role to play in providing AIDS prevention education. Many districts now use guidelines and materials to carry out this task, and some states have mandated AIDS education in public school settings.

For schools that already have an AIDS-education program in place, we offer the following recommendations:

1. Continue to review and evaluate current programs. Share honest and critical assessments of both successes and failures with colleagues to help build the most effective programs possible. Revise programs as necessary.

2. Continue to utilize community support and resources — or, if these don't exist, make efforts to build them so that AIDS education can be carried out in cooperation with the larger community.

3. Offer regular inservices and training to teachers providing AIDS education, keeping them updated on AIDS information; share new studies about adolescent beliefs and behaviors related to AIDS; and bring in new approaches to teaching that may have a greater impact on decreasing student risk behavior. Help keep teachers inspired in their tasks.

4. Establish or continue to support a regular AIDS education committee that collects and reviews information relevant to AIDS prevention in the schools, reports on this information to school boards and administrators, and assists in the planning of teacher inservices.

5. Carry out general AIDS information training for all school personnel, including teachers who might not teach about AIDS directly, as students may bring questions or concerns to anyone at the school with whom they have developed trust (e.g., administrative and support staff, counselors, cafeteria workers, nurses and health officers, or janitorial staff). All school personnel should support young people's efforts to be informed and to make wise AIDS prevention choices.

Schools or districts beginning the task of planning AIDS education should set up an advisory group (consisting, perhaps, of a school administrator, a teacher, a parent representative, a student, someone from the local health department, and a school health professional) to review some of the available materials and literature. It is important to move expeditiously in this effort. Pilot programs can be developed, parents informed of AIDS education plans, and the program broadened to include more students. AIDS education must be offered to students across several grades — a "senior assembly" the week before graduation offers too little, too late. Middle-school students are developmentally ready to learn about AIDS, and carefully designed programs can also be offered to students in elementary schools (for suggestions about AIDS education with younger children, see[19,20,27,28]). A public-relations effort may be needed to gain community and parent support for broad-based AIDS education programs reaching into the elementary grades.

REFERENCES

1. Haffner D. AIDS and adolescents: the time for prevention is now. Washington, D.C.: The Center for Population Options, 1986.
2. Quackenbush M. Educating youth about AIDS. Focus: A Review of AIDS Research 1987; 2:1-3.
3. Louis Harris and Associates. American teens speak: sex, myths, TV, and birth control. New York: Planned Parenthood Federation of America, 1986.
4. Bell TA, Holmes KK. Age-specific risks of syphilis, gonorrhea, and hospitalized pelvic inflammatory disease in sexually experienced U.S. women. Sex Transm Dis 1984; 11:291-5.
5. Johnston L, O'Malley P, Bachman J. Use of licit and illicit drugs by America's high school students 1975–1984. Washington, D.C.: U.S. Department of Health and Human Services publication no. (ADM)85-1394, 1985.
6. DiClemente R, Zorn J, Temoshok L. Adolescents and AIDS: a survey of knowledge, attitudes and beliefs about AIDS in San Francisco. Am J Pub Health 1986; 76:1443-5.
7. O'Reilly KR, Aral SO. Adolescence and sexual behavior. Trends and implications for STD. J Adolesc Health Care 1985; 6:262-70.
8. Cates W Jr, Rauh JL. Adolescents and sexually transmitted diseases: an expanding problem. J Adolesc Health Care 1985; 6:257-61.
9. Lumier R, Cook S. Healthy sex. New York: Simon & Schuster, 1983.
10. Hayes C. Risking the future: adolescent sexuality, pregnancy and childbearing. Vol 1: Report by the Panel on Adolescent Pregnancy and Childbearing of the National Research Council. Washington, D.C.: National Academy Press, 1987.
11. "Church sex survey: religious youths fool around too." San Francisco Chronicle. February 2, 1988.
12. Johnston L, O'Malley P, Bachman J. National trends in drug use and related factors among high school students and young adults, 1975-1986. U.S. Department of Health and Human Services publication no. (ADM)87-1535. Rockville, Md.: National Institute on Drug Abuse, 1987.
13. Bacchetti P, Moss AR. Incubation period of AIDS in San Francisco. Nature 1989; 338:251-3.
14. "Stockholm speakers on adolescents and AIDS: catch them before they catch it." JAMA 1988; 260:757-8.
15. Martin AD. AIDS prevention and education with gay and lesbian youth. In: Quackenbush M, Nelson M, Clark K, eds. The AIDS challenge. Santa Cruz, Calif.: Network Publication, 1988:379-95.
16. Martin AD. Learning to hide: the socialization of the gay adolescent. In: Feinstein SC, Looney JG, Schwartzberg A, Sorosky A, eds. Adolescent psychiatry: developmental and clinical studies 1982; 10:52-65.
17. Strunin L, Hingson R. Acquired immunodeficiency syndrome and adolescents: knowledge, beliefs, attitudes and behaviors. Pediatrics 1987; 79:825-8.
18. Helgerson SD, Petersen LR. Acquired immunodeficiency syndrome and secondary school students: their knowledge is limited and they want to learn more. Pediatrics 1988; 81:350-5.
19. Guidelines for effective school health education to prevent the spread of AIDS. MMWR 1988; 37(Suppl S-2); 1-14.
20. Davidson, Devon. National Coalition of Advocates for Students: guidelines for selecting teaching materials. In: Quackenbush M, Nelson M, Clark K, eds. The AIDS challenge: prevention education for young people. Santa Cruz, Calif.: Network Publications, 1988; 447-61.
21. Kegeles SM, Adler NE, Irwin CE Jr. Sexually active adolescents and condoms: changes over one year in knowledge, attitudes and use. Am J Public Health 1988; 78:460-1.
22. Kirby D. Sexuality education: a more realistic view of its effects. J Sch Health 1985; 55:421-4.
23. Zelnik M, Kim YJ. Sex education and its association with teenage sexual activity, pregnancy and contraceptive use. Fam Plann Perspect 1982; 14:117-26.
24. Kirby D. Sexuality education: an evaluation of programs and their effects. Santa Cruz, Calif.: Network Publications, 1984.
25. Brown LK, Fritz GK. AIDS education in the schools: a literature review as a guide for curriculum planning. Clin Pediatr (Phila.) 1988; 27:311-6.

26. AIDS Education at Home and School — PTAs Respond to the Need. Chicago: The National PTA, 1988.
27. Quackenbush M, Villarreal SF. "Does AIDS hurt?" Educating young children about AIDS. Santa Cruz, Calif.: Network Publications, 1988.
28. Post J, McPherson C. Into adolescence: learning about AIDS. Santa Cruz, Calif.: Network Publications, 1988.
29. HIV-related beliefs, knowledge, and behaviors among high school students. MMWR 1988; 37:717-21.
30. Sterk C. Cocaine and HIV seropositivity. Lancet 1988; 1:1052-3.

AIDS Education in Prisoners

Elizabeth Kantor, M.D.

■ THE POWER OF ATTITUDE VERSUS FACT IN PRISONS AND JAILS

Prisons, more than most institutions, tend to base infection control upon fear and popular sentiment rather than medical knowledge and fact. The fears are primarily those of correctional staff and inmates who are uninformed about proper precautions for avoiding infection. They may also be suspicious of what seems simple advice regarding infection prevention.

In an environment where staff and residents already are polarized by their divergent life styles, frank hostility, and conflicting roles and interests, the scene is set for unbridled AIDS hysteria. Ignorance of the illness is common and fear is a natural response. In jails and prisons, the response to inmates with known or suspected HIV disease is often based upon this fear, and many institutions have policies of inmate isolation and segregation that are not practiced in the community setting.

In Michigan, the correctional officers union exacted an agreement from the Department of Corrections stating they would be notified of all AIDS cases in the prison. Officers in other states have demanded that all inmates be tested for AIDS antibody. Some have refused to work with possible AIDS patients.

Almost all state and federal prisons have or are developing AIDS educational programs for staff, as are a slightly smaller percentage of city and county jail systems. Fewer prisons have educational programs available or planned for inmates. Education is recognized by most institutions to be the major factor in controlling AIDS as well as in reducing staff and inmate hysteria. Educational programs are recognized to have reduced fears among the large majority of staff and inmates to whom they have been provided.[1]

REFERENCES

1. Hammett TM. AIDS in correctional facilities. Rockville, Md.: U.S. Department of Justice, 1986.

ETHICAL ISSUES RELATED TO AIDS

EDITOR

Molly Cooke, M.D.

12.1

Ethical Issues Related to AIDS

Health-Care Workers and AIDS: An Ethical Overview

Molly Cooke, M.D.

■ **MORAL VALUES OF PROVIDERS**

Resistance to providing health care to HIV-infected individuals is very common.[1,2] The most frequent rationales offered for this resistance include:

1. other institutions have more expertise in managing HIV complications and can serve the patient better;

2. care of HIV patients creates a risk for providers and unaffected patients;

3. care of HIV-infected individuals is under-reimbursed and may be difficult because of the poor social support system and disorganized lifestyles of some of the patients;

4. admission of patients with HIV disease may change the character of admitting hospitals and threaten established referral patterns.[3]

These seemingly disinterested formulations may have little to do with the real mechanism of resistance, which is more deeply rooted psychologically and may arise from symbolic issues stirred by the illness and by providers' alienation from the lifestyle of their patients.[4,5,9,10]

Doctors, nurses, and other health-care providers bring their own sets of moral values to their work, and it has been demonstrated that these moral values have the potential to influence health-care decisions.[6] A physician's impression of an individual patient's value to society and the possibly self-inflicted nature of his disease may vie with his or her knowledge of natural history and prognosis while selecting therapeutic options at the bedside. Ill people seek help and expect that the advice they receive will reflect the physician's best professional opinion. A particular danger posed by the influence of these moral values in treatment decisions is that they vary markedly from physician to physician.[7] Patients are not prepared and should not be expected to screen their health-care providers for biases, personality quirks, and moral values that may be prejudicial. This places upon the physician the burden of identifying for himself or herself areas of bias and strongly held moral opinion, and then guarding against their undue influence while caring for patients.

■ **RISK TO PROVIDERS**

The recognition that HIV disease is a communicable illness that poses some risk to health-care workers has augmented the stigma associated with the illness and has provoked some physicians and hospitals to avoid the care of patients. These evasions, commonly rationalized as efforts to secure care in the most experienced facilities, continue to occur as more hospitals grapple with their responses to their first AIDS patients. We now know that the risk of occupational transmission of HIV is a function of significant inoculation with body fluids, particularly blood, containing the virus. The risk of seroconversion is approximately 0.4 percent after a needlestick when the needle is known to have been used on an HIV-positive patient.[8,13,14] Although it is reasonable to anticipate the rare case of occupational HIV infection, the risk of acquiring it appears to be considerably below that of acquiring lethal hepatitis B in an occupational setting.

■ CONCEPTS OF PROFESSIONAL OBLIGATION

Physicians have found it difficult to identify their obligations.[15-19] One school of thought holds that doctors have a categorical obligation to care for any patient whose illness falls within their competence. A second camp argues that physicians are obliged only to ensure that the health-care needs of patients are met but that physicians are under no individual obligations to provide the care themselves. This latter, contractual formulation of professional responsibility affords physicians broad latitude in selecting or declining patients on the basis of perceived risk to the provider. However, the former categorical model also admits adjustment in the treatment plan in response to high risk to the provider.[20]

The risk of HIV transmission associated with some occupational exposures, particularly needlestick, is becoming known. Other exposures remain less clear. The variety and types of occupational exposures, the lack of hard data, and individual psychological difference in perception of threat make it very difficult to develop a consensus on occupational risk. In turn, this lack of consensus about risk has led to marked differences of opinion about the physician's obligation to treat HIV-infected patients. Further exploration and discussion of the obligation of health-care workers, involving surgeons, pathologists, obstetricians, internists, and nurses are clearly required. Modification of the treatment plan of an HIV-seropositive patient may be appropriate in order to protect health-care staff when a consensus is established on the significance of the risk posed to the health-care worker and the benefit to health-care providers is of a magnitude to justify the loss of benefit to the patient.[21,22]

■ INSTITUTIONAL ETHICS

The individual health-care worker deals with risk and responsibility in the context of an organization, clinic, hospital, or medical school.[23] These institutions have obligations beyond ensuring that employees provide appropriate care to patients. Institutional responsibilities include a vigorous and effective infection-control program, comprehensive and innovative attention to benefits for employees who might become infected on the job,[24] and provision of psychological support and other services as they are needed to cope with burnout. The obligation of professionals to care for people with HIV infection does not turn on whether this activity is completely safe.[11,12] Epidemic illness has been a central part of the experience of physicians from the beginning of medicine. Exposure to communicable diseases remains a risk inherent in the health-care professions despite the fact that antibiotics and successful immunization campaigns have diminished this risk somewhat over the past 40 years. The commitment of health-care workers to care for sick patients must not be so tenuous that anxiety can disrupt it.

REFERENCES

1. Whalen JP. Participation of medical students in the care of patients with AIDS. J Med Educ 1987; 62:53-4.

2. Link RN, Feingold AR, Charap MH, et al. Concerns of medical and pediatric house officers about acquiring AIDS from their patients. Am J Public Health 1988; 78:455-9.

3. Cooke M. Ethical issues in the care of patients with AIDS. Qual Rev Bull 1986; 12:343-6.

4. Mathews WC, Booth MW, Turner JD, Kessler L. Physicians' attitudes toward homosexuality — survey of a California County Medical Society. West J Med 1986; 144:106-10.

5. Wachter RM. The impact of the acquired immunodeficiency syndrome on medical residency training. N Engl J Med 1986; 314:177-80.

6. Eisenberg JM. Sociologic influences on decision-making by clinicians. Ann Intern Med 1979; 90:957-67.

7. Pearlman RA, Inui TS, Carter WB. Variability in physician bioethical decision-making. Ann Intern Med 1982; 97:420-5.

8. Henderson DK, Saah AJ, Zak BJ, et al. Risk of nosocomial infection with human T-cell lymphotropic virus type III/lymphadenopathy-associated virus in a large cohort of intensively exposed health care workers. Ann Intern Med 1986; 104:644-7.

9. Richardson JL, Lochner T, McGuigan K, Levine AM. Physician attitudes and experience regarding the care of patients with acquired immunodeficiency syndrome (AIDS) and related disorders (ARC). Med Care 1987; 25:675-85.

10. Kelly JA, St. Lawrence JS, Smith S Jr, et al. Stigmatization of AIDS patients by physicians. Am J Public Health 1987; 77:789-91.

11. Jonsen A. Ethics and AIDS. Bull Am Coll Surg 1985; 70:16-8.

12. Jonsen AR, Cooke M, Koenig B. AIDS and ethics. Issues in Science and Technology 1986; 2:56-65.

13. Update: acquired immunodeficiency syndrome and human immunodeficiency virus infection among health-care workers. MMWR 1988; 37:229-34, 239.

14. Marcus R. Surveillance of health care workers exposed to blood from patients infected with the human immunodeficiency virus. N Engl J Med 1988; 319:1118-23.

15. Zuger A, Miles SH. Physicians, AIDS, and occupational risk. Historic traditions and ethical obligations. JAMA 1987; 258:1924-8.

16. Annas GJ. Not saints, but healers: the legal duties of health care professionals in the AIDS epidemic. Am J Public Health 1988; 78:844-9.

17. Freedman B. Health professions, codes, and the right to refuse to treat HIV-infectious patients. Hastings Cent Rep 1988; 18(2, Suppl):20-5.

18. Ethical issues involved in the growing AIDS crisis. Council on Ethical and Judicial Affairs. JAMA 1988; 259:1360-1.

19. Fox DM. The politics of physicians' responsibility in epidemics: a note on history. Hastings Cent Rep 1988; 18(2, Suppl):5-10.

20. Arras JD. The fragile web of responsibility: AIDS and the duty to treat. Hastings Cent Rep 1988; 18(2, Suppl):10-20.

21. Emanuel EJ. Do physicians have an obligation to treat patients with AIDS? N Engl J Med 1988; 318:1686-90.

22. Hagen MD, Meyer KB, Pauker SG. Routine preoperative screening for HIV. Does the risk to the surgeon outweigh the risk to the patient? JAMA 1988; 259:1357-9.

23. Friedland G. AIDS and compassion. JAMA 1988; 259:2898-9.

24. Brennan TA. The acquired immunodeficiency syndrome (AIDS) as an occupational disease. Ann Intern Med 1987; 107:581-3.

Ethical Issues in Treating Competent AIDS Patients: Decisions to Limit Treatment

Molly Cooke, M.D.

■ INTENSIVE CARE AND MECHANICAL VENTILATION

Initiating any therapy in a competent patient requires that the treatment offers the likelihood of benefit in excess of burden and that the patient desires the intervention. No currently available therapy can cure the viral infection in patients with HIV disease. However, short-term benefits of many treatments, including intubation and mechanical ventilation, may be substantial. Early data from San Francisco General Hospital demonstrated that patients with pneumocystis pneumonia who require intubation in the first several days of hospitalization had a 13 percent chance of leaving the hospital and having months of a partial remission.[1] A more recent study suggests that survival under the same conditions may now approximate 50 percent.[4] We know that the costs of treatment in physical suffering, fear, loss of autonomy, and dollars are borne by all patients treated, but we cannot know the value of the additional weeks or months of life to them or their survivors.

Any dogma ("all patients with respiratory failure should be intubated and mechanically ventilated," or "no patients with AIDS are admitted to the ICU") will serve some patients badly. We do not currently have guidance other than the preference of the patient to decide when aggressive intervention is appropriate in the face of low but real chances for success. It is critical that we collect detailed information about the outcome of specific interventions so that our benefits-and-burdens discussions can be as informed as possible.[5]

Patients with HIV infection want to discuss life-sustaining treatment, including ICU hospitalization and mechanical ventilation, with their physicians. In a study of 118 men with AIDS at San Francisco General Hospital, 73 percent wanted to hold such discussions, although only one-third had done so.[2] Study respondents recognized that these discussions were emotionally difficult. Forty-four percent reported anxiety and 40 percent reported sadness, but these dysphoric reactions did not diminish patients' interest in participating in decision-making. In addition, even this intelligent, well-informed patient population had important misconceptions about the efficacy of intubation and mechanical ventilation. Thus, discussing options in later care serves the dual purpose of recognizing the importance of patient preferences and of furthering the accurate education of the individual.

HIV-infected individuals from certain risk groups and social backgrounds have had vast second-hand experience with these issues. Many gay men in San Francisco start discussions about late care with their physicians. Cultural, racial, and educational differences may make these discussions more difficult for practitioners dealing with individuals who have acquired HIV through intravenous drug use or heterosexual intercourse. However, establishing the patient's preference is no less important when working with members of these groups. Sensitive confrontation of the issues must be combined with a stated and demonstrated commitment to the patient to overcome many patients' previous experiences of medical settings as hostile and punitive.

■ "DO NOT RESUSCITATE" ORDERS

Physicians are often reluctant to discuss options in care, especially terminal care, for fear that these discussions will depress the patient, make him or her anxious, or undermine his or her confidence in the physician's efforts to provide care.[6] Our study of the attitudes of people with AIDS conducted in the AIDS Clinic at San Francisco General Hospital reveals that this reluctance is unfounded.[2] Seventy-eight percent of respondents had formed opinions about intubation, mechanical ventilation, and cardiopulmonary resuscitation (CPR). Fifty-five percent of patients wanted ICU care, and 46 percent wanted CPR. They had often discussed their feelings with friends and family but had seldom done so with their physicians. Respondents stated that they would appreciate a chance to discuss code status with their physicians.

Discussing code status obviously requires great sensitivity on the part of the physician. It may be more comfortable and effective to do it at a time when the patient is feeling relatively well and is an outpatient. Like other patients, patients with HIV infection find it difficult to make very important decisions about their lives when they are feeling acutely ill. In the study cited above, 69 percent of respondents preferred to discuss options in later care while they were outpatients. The support and, if appropriate, actual participation of friends and family in the discussion can be most helpful. Health-care providers should recognize that strong ambivalence usually complicates patients' consideration of their code status. They should be prepared for patients to occasionally change their minds. Nine percent of respondents in the San Francisco General study reported changing their minds about life-sustaining treatment.

In some situations, life-sustaining treatment may be clearly futile. The patient with progressive pneumocystis pneumonia despite three weeks of therapy with trimethoprim sulfa and pentamidine will not benefit from intensive care, mechanical ventilation, or CPR. Neither the law nor ethical considerations oblige the physician to offer these interventions in circumstances of manifest futility.[3]

REFERENCES

1. Wachter RM, Luce JM, Turner J, et al. Intensive care for patients with the acquired immunodeficiency syndrome — outcome and changing patterns of utilization. Am Rev Resp Dis 1986; 134:891-6.

2. Steinbrook R, Lo B, Moulton J, et al. Preferences of homosexual men with AIDS for life-sustaining treatment. N Engl J Med 1986; 314:457-60.

3. Steinbrook R, Lo B, Tirpack J, et al. Ethical dilemmas in caring for patients with the acquired immunodeficiency syndrome. Ann Intern Med 1985; 103:787-90.

4. Fahrner R, Clement MJ, Kline A, Cohen JB. Helping young people face death: resuscitation status and outcome in first episode pneumocystis pneumonia (PCP) [Abstract]. III International Conference on AIDS. Washington, D.C., 1987; 154.

5. Raviglione MC, Battan R, Taranta A. Cardiopulmonary resuscitation in patients with the acquired immunodeficiency syndrome. A prospective study. Arch Intern Med 1988; 148:2602-5.

6. Wachter RM, Cooke M, Hopewell P, Luce JM. Attitudes of medical residents regarding intensive care for patients with the acquired immunodeficiency syndrome. Arch Intern Med 1988; 148:149-52.

Ethical Issues in Treating Incompetent AIDS Patients

Molly Cooke, M.D.

■ COMPETENCE

Only a competent patient can accept or reject treatment. Competence is a legal concept implying the ability to understand one's situation, the benefits of treatment, and the risks of refusal.[1] Psychiatric disorders and organic brain syndromes do not preclude competence. Disturbances of affect may complicate assessment of patient preference, but they do not necessarily affect competence. In other words, schizophrenic, demented, or depressed patients may be competent to refuse treatment.[1] The law presumes competence unless the patient has been declared incompetent by the courts. Non-emergency medical therapies cannot be administered to patients whose competence is in question. State laws vary in the breadth of authorization for emergency treatment when the patient refuses and competence is uncertain. Because of the potential for great harm to the patient whose refusal of indicated treatment is accepted, it is prudent to have at least two qualified examiners assess competence in uncertain situations before treatment is withheld.

HIV-related infections may affect competence. The patient's expressed preferences about care made while still competent — particularly preferences about limiting aggressive, technologically-oriented terminal care — have been recognized by the courts as relevant to medical decisions made after the patient has become incompetent.[2] For this reason, it is particularly important that practitioners caring for patients with HIV infection discuss options in late AIDS care. For practical reasons, patients' friends and family should also be made aware of these preferences.

■ ADVANCE DIRECTIVES

It is impossible to specify all clinical possibilities and to elicit the patient's preferences for each potential situation. Unfortunately, encephalopathy or incapacitating debility often manifest themselves in AIDS patients before the major therapeutic options become clear. In California, this problem has been addressed by legislation that sets forth a simple procedure for designating a durable power of attorney for health care.[3] This permits patients to appoint someone to speak as their proxy in the event that they become unable to participate in their own health-care decision-making. The spokesman with durable power (who is not permitted to be a health-care provider involved in the patient's clinical management) is protected by California law from suits arising out of discharging these responsibilities. Besides the clear benefit of having a spokesman who knows the patient's wishes assist physicians in their decisions about treatment, the durable power of attorney can provide clarification when different individuals or groups (lovers, friends, parents, spouses) claim to speak for the uncomprehending patient.[4] Physicians caring for people with HIV infection should encourage them to designate a proxy spokesman in case they become incompetent. Despite the sophistication of the HIV-infected population at San Francisco General Hospital, only 28 percent of a sample of 118 men had executed a durable power of attorney.[5]

Many times decisions must be made on behalf of patients who have not designated a legal surrogate. In these situations, if medical care is not altogether futile, the preferences of customary surrogates (e.g., parents, spouses) are relevant. Physicians usually work with spouses and members of the biological family. However, they should identify the individual or individuals best able to characterize the patient's own prior preferences. In the case of gay and bisexual men, the lover or gay friends may be better able to meet this test than family members, who may not have seen the patient for years. Case law recognizes the legitimacy of proxy preferences expressed by non-family members.

■ BURDENS AND BENEFITS

Unfortunately, many patients are admitted to the hospital unable to express their wishes, without a previous documented discussion, and without a legally designated or conventionally recognized proxy. The less that is known about what a patient desires, the greater the opportunity for confusion and conflict. In the past, a distinction has been made between "usual" and "aggressive" or "heroic" care, with the implication that the former is obligatory and the latter discretionary. This is arbitrary and unsatisfactory.[6] The President's Commission for the Study of Ethical Problems in Medicine proposed an analysis for the benefit and burdens of any intervention. It considers the application of that intervention discretionary, if not contraindicated, when the discernible burden outweighs the potential for benefit.[7] In this analysis, intravenous hydration and tube alimentation are not inherently different from intubation and mechanical ventilation. Because this system replaces dogma ("hydration must be guaranteed") with thoughtful consideration and requires that the benefit and burden of each intervention be weighed on a case-by-case basis, it may introduce new uncertainties. If helpful interventions are more frequently administered and inappropriately burdensome ones are more frequently withheld, this extra uncertainty and effort are justified.

REFERENCES

1. Nelson LJ. The law, professional responsibility, and decisions to forego treatment. Qual Rev Bull 1986; 12:8-15.

2. Jonsen AR. What is extraordinary life support? Medical Staff Conference, University of California, San Francisco. West J Med 1984; 141:358-63.

3. Steinbrook R, Lo B. Decision making for incompetent patients by designated proxy — California's new law. N Engl J Med 1984; 310:1598-1601.

4. Cooke M. Ethical issues in the care of patients with AIDS. Qual Rev Bull 1986; 12:343-6.

5. Steinbrook R, Lo B, Moulton J, et al. Preferences of homosexual men with AIDS for life-sustaining treatment. N Engl J Med 1986; 314:457-60.

6. Wanzer SH, Adelstein SJ, Cranford RE, et al. The physician's responsibility toward hopelessly ill patients. N Engl J Med 1984; 310:955-9.

7. President's Commission for the Study of Ethical Problems in Medicine and Biomedical and Behavioral Research. Washington, D.C.: U.S. Government Printing Office, 1983.

Ethical Issues in the Use of the HIV Antibody Test

Molly Cooke, M.D.

■ ETHICAL PRINCIPLES IN THE USE OF THE HIV ANTIBODY TEST

Complex ethical principles underlie testing for antibody to HIV.[1,2] Although many clinicians have argued that the test should be handled like any other test ordered strictly at the physician's discretion, the reactions of the patient, the health-care community, and society at large to a positive HIV test should remind us to be cautious in "normalizing" it. The practitioner should be guided by three considerations in HIV testing: the concern for the quality of the information obtained; a presumption that well-informed patients can make their own best risk–benefit determinations; and the recognition that in our society, the individual's personal integrity and authority should only be violated when there is manifest and significant benefit to others and then only by the least intrusive means. In specific circumstances, these considerations may come into conflict and individuals of different temperament and background will give precedence to different concerns. Although the temptation is to sacrifice one "right" for another, solutions to ethical dilemmas are possible that recognize the merits or benefits of various strategies and seek to reconcile them.

The quality of information resulting from an HIV test is a function of its predictive value. Predictive value is central to the use of tests in all areas of medicine and underlies their ethical application as well as their clinical interpretation. Some tests are intrinsically inaccurate (low sensitivity, low specificity, or both) and perform badly in all populations. Even tests with excellent performance characteristics, such as the test for antibody to HIV,[3,4] may produce unreliable results in low-prevalence populations,[5] particularly when performed by inexperienced personnel and without adequate protocols for confirming positive results. This must be clearly understood if patients who request antibody testing are to be appropriately counseled.

The principle of informed consent is well recognized, if imperfectly implemented, in American medicine. We recognize that patients must be informed of the implications of and alternatives to a proposed procedure before their consent is meaningful and that informed patients may decline indicated and recommended procedures. Some physicians object to the placement of HIV testing under the constraint of informed consent because no other blood test is handled this way. This argument trivializes the impact of HIV testing. Because most of the benefits of determining an individual's antibody status depend on that individual's understanding of the meaning of the test, HIV testing only by informed consent serves the goals of increasing patient autonomy and providing maximal medical benefit. When HIV antibody testing is performed without informed consent and counseling, much potential benefit is lost.[6,7]

Respect for individual liberties is fundamental to our society, but we recognize that one person exercising his or her freedom should not limit the liberty of others. The converse of this principle is that in protecting the general good we should not be more burdensome than necessary. Therefore, the questions that must be asked of the interventions intended to promote the public good are these:

- Will the intervention actually increase public health or safety? Only a material and substantial increase in general safety justifies compromise of individual liberty.

- Is the proposed intervention the one least intrusive that accomplishes the desired increase in the general good? The liberty of one person should not be compromised more than is necessary to protect others.

■ QUALITY OF TEST RESULTS IN LOW-PREVALENCE POPULATIONS

Individuals proposing or requesting HIV antibody testing need to know the probability that a given test accurately reflects their antibody status. This concept is referred to as predictive value. In a low-prevalence population, positive predictive value is low; many more positive tests are false-positive than are true-positive. This is fundamental to any ethical analysis of broad-based screening (e.g, universal, pre-employment, or premarital screening). Persons who are told that they have a positive HIV antibody test may suffer significant psychological and social consequences and often are not easily reassured that their test results were in error. Any program that inevitably produces this kind of burden must produce a greater benefit in order to be justifiable.[8] Screening in blood banks is an example of antibody-test use in a low-prevalence population where the benefit of protecting the blood supply offsets the cost or burden of false-positive tests.

■ QUALITY OF TEST RESULTS IN HIGH-PREVALENCE POPULATIONS

Testing in high-prevalence populations produces dramatically different results. In San Francisco, it has been estimated that approximately 50 percent of sexually active homosexual men have antibody to HIV. Therefore, if 100 men from this risk group request testing, 50 percent of them will have the antibody, and a test that is conservatively 95 percent sensitive will detect antibody in 47.5 individuals (true positive). The incidence of false-negatives will be 2.5. Of the 50 men who do not have the antibody, a test that is 99 percent specific will give a negative result in 49.5 individuals (true negative) and a false-positive determination in 0.5 individuals. Therefore, the predictive value of a positive test is 47.5 divided by 48, or 98.95 percent. The predictive value of a negative test is 49.5 divided by 52, or 95 percent.

Clearly, the quality of the information obtained by using a test with good performance characteristics in a high-prevalence population is virtually unimpeachable. The ethical questions here revolve around the risks and benefits of individuals knowing their antibody status. Although people determined to be antibody-negative may be considerably relieved, there are negative psychological repercussions to knowing that they are antibody-positive. In addition, there are potential social and economic consequences, such as the loss of health insurance.[7]

Patients whose behaviors have put them at risk for HIV infection should be counseled about their risk and strongly encouraged to be tested. They should be advised to consider how they would feel about both a positive and a negative test result before they are tested. Ideally, the motivation to reduce risk behaviors is not materially affected by testing, but behavior change is difficult and incompletely understood.[9] Often people report that finding they are antibody-negative has helped them avoid risky behaviors associated with infection. People with positive tests are often motivated to reduce their risk behaviors out of concern for their sexual partners and other contacts. Medical considerations include prophylactic and antiviral therapies. Their availability now makes early determination of HIV infection important in planning infected individuals' medical management.

■ HIV ANTIBODY SCREENING AS AN ADJUNCT TO INFECTION-CONTROL PROCEDURES

Some clinicians and hospital administrators argue that HIV antibody screening should take place when patients are admitted to the hospital in the interest of protecting staff against occupational transmission. However, recommended infection-control procedures for routine care and invasive procedures do not depend on determination of antibody status.[10] A stratified infection-control procedure could produce either unacceptably casual attitudes toward the possible transmission of serious infection from antibody-negative patients or the use of inappropriate and ineffective measures to prevent transmissions from antibody-positive patients, or both. Thus, screening hospitalized patients to protect staff does not produce the increase in safety that would justify the intrusion of testing.

■ AUTONOMY AND CONSENT IN HIV ANTIBODY TESTING

Antibody testing of appropriate patients under the doctrine of informed consent serves two principles of ethical medicine: providing high-quality medical care and maintaining the patient's autonomy. Thus, consensual antibody testing is always the ideal. In many states, it is the only avenue to testing permitted by law. In some instances, the question of non-consensual antibody testing does arise, however (e.g., forced testing of sex offenders or other alleged or convicted criminals, source patients in needlestick accidents, demented or incapacitated patients, and patients whose medical care is made contingent on acceding to a request for testing). People who refuse to give their consent should be distinguished from those unable to give consent and attention should be given to the beneficiary of possible testing, whether it is the patient, a specific injured individual, or the general public.

REFERENCES

1. Lo B, Steinbrook RL, Cooke M, et al. Voluntary screening for human immunodeficiency virus (HIV) infection. Weighing the benefits and harms. Ann Intern Med 1989; 110:727-33.
2. Rhame FS, Maki DG. The case for wider use of testing for HIV infection. N Engl J Med 1989; 320:1248-54.
3. Burke DS, Brundage JF, Redfield RR, et al. Measure of the false positive rate in a screening program for human immunodeficiency virus infections. N Engl J Med 1988; 319:961-4.

4. MacDonald KL, Jackson JB, Bowman RJ, et al. Performance characteristics of serologic tests for human immunodeficiency virus type 1 (HIV-1) antibody among Minnesota blood donors. Public health and clinical implications. Ann Intern Med 1989; 110:617-21.

5. Meyer KB, Pauker SG. Screening for HIV: Can we afford the false positive rate? N Engl J Med 1987; 317:238-41.

6. Henry K, Maki M, Crossley K. Analysis of the use of HIV antibody testing in a Minnesota hospital. JAMA 1988; 259:229-32.

7. Sherer R. Physician use of the HIV antibody test. The need for consent, counseling, confidentiality, and caution. JAMA 1988; 259:264-5.

8. Cleary PD, Barry MJ, Mayer KH, et al. Compulsory premarital screening for the human immunodeficiency virus. Technical and public health considerations. JAMA 1987; 258:1757-62.

9. Becker MH, Joseph JG. AIDS and behavioral change to reduce risk. A review. Am J Public Health 1988; 78:394-410.

10. Recommendations for prevention of HIV transmission in health-care settings. MMWR 1987; 36(Suppl 2):1S-18S.

Ethical Issues in
AIDS Research

Molly Cooke, M.D.

■ ACCESS TO RESEARCH PROTOCOLS

Many of the ethical dilemmas in AIDS research stem from conflict between the scientific and therapeutic purposes that research is thought to serve.[1,7] The question of the patient's access to research protocols and experimental treatments has generated considerable controversy.

The arguments for making experimental treatments universally available outside of research protocols are powerful. First, no treatment is available through community physicians that is effective in eliminating HIV or correcting the underlying immunodeficiency. Second, the inclusion and exclusion criteria essential for achieving population homogeneity in randomized clinical trials precludes many ill patients from receiving experimental and possibly effective treatment. Third, many patients who, in fact, meet selection criteria are excluded on grounds such as distance from a research center or prior recruitment of an adequate number of patients. Fourth, until an effective standard of care intervention is demonstrated, some enrolled patients will receive placebo and cannot hope to profit immediately from participation. Finally, even if a drug currently being tested proves to be efficacious, the tempo of end-stage HIV disease is such that patients who are currently sick may be dead before the drug's efficacy can be conclusively demonstrated.

Arguments against making experimental drugs universally available are based on considerations of minimizing harm to individual patients, maximizing the general good, and justice. Experience with apparently promising therapies, both in treating HIV and other diseases, has shown that many are actually harmful. Determining harm and benefit is fastest when therapies are tested in carefully designed and executed clinical trials that use control groups. Given that only finite resources are available to treat an epidemic that is massive in scale, it is critical that both benefit and harm be quickly assessed. Finally, many experimental agents are not available in unlimited supply. If only some people can receive experimental therapies, it is important that they receive them under circumstances that maximize the benefits for all people with HIV disease — i.e., in carefully designed clinical trials.

The arguments for and against universal availability of experimental drugs are not always in conflict. Many people do not want therapies of unclear benefit and possible harm, recognizing that their immune status makes them particularly susceptible to drug toxicities. If a particular therapy is readily available, patients who want to participate in a clinical trial can be randomized and other patients reluctant to participate but eager for treatment can be treated off-protocol.

■ INFORMED CONSENT

The major obstacle to informed consent in research is patients' lack of familiarity with the conventions and assumptions underlying the design of randomized clinical trials.[2] A placebo-controlled randomized clinical trial admits in its design that the experimental intervention may be worse than no treatment at all. This concept requires careful explanation so that participants can enter a study aware that they may incur harm.

Many people are drawn to clinical trials in the hope that they will receive the active agent, so the odds that they will receive placebo instead must be carefully explained. Participation in protocols also limits the participants' freedom in important respects; it constrains them to attend follow-up appointments at specified intervals, to have certain tests performed, and often to avoid over-the-counter and prescription drugs that are not administered as part of the research protocol. Informed patients can then accept or refuse these limitations.

INFORMED CONSENT AND THE ISSUE OF CONFIDENTIALITY

All participants in clinical trials suffer some loss of privacy when their experience in the protocol is summarized and disseminated. Often this occurs in the aggregate, but it is not uncommon for individual summaries or photographs to be included in published and oral reports. The use of even the most nonspecific clinical descriptors such as age, sex, and extent of disease is troubling to some patients. Detailed records required in the conduct of research protocols expose the participant to the risk of a massive invasion of privacy should confidentiality be lost either through carelessness or maliciousness in the conduct of the study or through legal maneuvers such as subpoena. The special challenge of informed consent in HIV disease research is to make such risks clear.[3]

■ CONFIDENTIALITY

Precautions to ensure confidentiality are usual in medical research, but HIV disease, particularly its epidemiology, has raised especially troubling issues. The lifestyles and behaviors associated with a large majority of AIDS patients are stigmatized. Currently, approximately 85 percent of cases are associated with homosexuality or intravenous drug use. Even if the epidemiology of the disease changes to become more like other sexually transmitted diseases (e.g., associated primarily with heterosexual activity), the illness will continue to carry the double stigma associated with sexual incontinence and incurable mortal illness. To the extent that participation in a research project labels the study subject as HIV-infected or as having indulged in a risk behavior, it exposes that subject to the risk of further stigmatization and to potential psychological, social, and economic consequences.

Second, the nature of the information sought in epidemiologic research is often highly sensitive. Investigation of HIV disease typically includes questions about sexual preference, number of sexual partners, mechanics of intercourse and other aspects of sexual practice, and the use of illicit drugs, especially parenteral use. For these reasons, both clinical research on HIV disease and epidemiologic investigation raise particular concerns about confidentiality.

Political assaults on the confidentiality of HIV disease research are another area of concern. While the typical consent form reads, "I understand that information obtained in this study will not be given to anyone without my permission unless required by law," subjects perceive this promise as an adequate guarantee. They find it difficult to anticipate any reason why an outside party would take any particular interest in the individual information uncovered by the research. In the case of HIV disease, however, subjects and investigators have always been aware that efforts might be made to obtain the names and details of medical and social histories of people at risk or infected. Several special precautions have been taken by investigators to protect the confidentiality of participants in HIV disease research, including minimizing the use of identifiers, centralizing study records (often under lock and key), and minimizing or eliminating duplicate records.[4] Some investigators have also eliminated the consent-form phrase "unless required by law." Such provisions probably do not provide protection against subpoena. Special statutory protection exists for some forms of sensitive research; whether more would be adequate in the face of severe public-health or political pressure is unclear.[5]

The question of confidentiality will probably be further complicated as public-health measures to control the epidemic change.[6] Currently in many states AIDS is a reportable disease but HIV viral and antibody positivity are not reportable. Because patients with AIDS represent a relatively small proportion of the total exposed population, public-health authorities are likely to increasingly favor reporting of the infected but not clinically affected population. If HIV viral and antibody positivity become reportable, a clear conflict will develop between the legal obligation of investigators to identify study subjects in these categories and their ethical obligation to maximize confidentiality. This tension could create an insuperable impediment to effective epidemiologic research.

REFERENCES

1. Levine C. Has AIDS changed the ethics of human subjects research? Law Med Health Care 1988; 16:167-73.
2. Schafer A. The ethics of the randomized clinical trial. N Engl J Med 1982; 307:719-24.
3. Purtilo R, Sonnabend J, Purtilo D. Confidentiality, informed consent and untoward social consequences in research on a "new killer disease" (AIDS). Clin Res 1983; 31:462-72.
4. Bayer R, Levine C, Murray TH. Guidelines for confidentiality in research on AIDS. IRB: a review of human subjects research, 1984; 6:1-7.
5. Boruch RF. Should private agencies maintain federal research data? IRB: a review of human subjects research, 1984; 6:89.
6. Novick A. At risk for AIDS: confidentiality in research and surveillance. IRB: a review of human subjects research, 1984; 6:10-1.
7. Appelbaum PS, Roth LH, Lidz CW, et al. False hopes and best data: consent to research and the therapeutic misconception. Hastings Cent Rep 1987; 17:20-4.

Ethical Aspects of AIDS-Related Public Health Interventions

Molly Cooke, M.D.

■ CONTACT TRACING

The causative agent of AIDS was identified in 1983 and shortly thereafter the development of the antibody test permitted detection of the virus in asymptomatic individuals. However, the obligation to report has remained linked to the Centers for Disease Control's (CDC) surveillance definition of AIDS rather than to HIV-antibody positivity. This public-policy decision can be seen as the result of a number of social considerations, including a wish to avoid inhibiting voluntary HIV antibody testing, concern about creating a databank of infected individuals who could potentially be exposed to adverse social consequences, uncertainty about the long-term implications of a positive test, and lack of effective interventions for persons with asymptomatic HIV infection. These considerations are not static; for example, zidovudine (AZT) and other antiviral drugs may prove beneficial to people with asymptomatic infection. The existence of useful therapies and increasing moderation in the public's and politicians' attitudes toward those with AIDS are factors in current public health interest in mandatory reporting and contact tracing.

Where contact tracing has been used, preliminary experience suggests that contacted partners accept voluntary testing and modify their risk behaviors.[5-8] Ideally, index cases will notify their contacts, but if they fail to do so, a tension arises between the patients' right to confidentiality and the rights and safety of their sexual contacts. Contact tracing is mandated by law in the case of syphilis, but there is not a strict analogy between the two diseases, since a completely effective treatment is available for syphilis. For conditions other than syphilis, standard ethics would support preserving confidentiality.[2] The relative inefficiency of sexual intercourse as a mode of transmission raises the possibility that many seropositive individuals might have seronegative partners who could reduce their risk if notified. This has increased interest in contact tracing. Any notification scheme must attempt to maximize respect for the rights and sensibilities of the index case through the process of contact tracing.[1,9,10]

■ RESTRICTED EMPLOYMENT, SCHOOLING, AND QUARANTINE

Concern about the transmission of AIDS has led to proposals to restrict schooling and employment, and even to quarantine. In general, these proposals reflect unwarranted fear and ignorance about transmission of HIV infection and would not succeed in containing it. Interventions that are demonstrably ineffective cannot be considered ethical. Such proposed restrictions are particularly nonsensical when limited to patients with diagnosed AIDS because at most they represent only 5 percent to 10 percent of infected (and presumably infectious) persons. Transmission in schools and workplaces will not occur unless sexual activity or needle use also occurs there. Therefore, no benefit will result from excluding AIDS patients or HIV antibody-positive people from these settings. Finally, quarantine is not a feasible proposal because to succeed it would require: (1) perfectly executed, repetitive universal screening; (2) commitment to quarantine all people who test positive; (3) completely accurate test results; and (4) logistical support for housing hundreds of thousands — if not millions — of people.[3] If quarantine were imperfect, its arguable benefits would be severely compromised or lost. Because the harm involved in quarantine is incalculable, the benefits would have to be similarly large. As the four conditions above cannot be met, the deficits of quarantine greatly outweigh the benefits and the strategy is therefore unjustifiable.[4]

REFERENCES

1. Echenberg DF. A new strategy to prevent the spread of AIDS among heterosexuals. JAMA 1985; 254:2129-30.

2. Perkins HS, Jonsen AR. Conflicting duties to patients — the case of a sexually active hepatitis B carrier. Ann Intern Med 1981; 94:523-30.

3. Bayer R, Levine C, Wolf SM. HIV antibody screening — an ethical framework for evaluating proposed procedures. JAMA 1986; 256:1768-74.

4. Jonsen AR, Cooke M, Koenig BA. AIDS and ethics. Issues in Science and Technology 1986; 2:56-65.

5. Wykoff RF, Heath CW Jr, Hollis SL, et al. Contact tracing to identify human immunodeficiency virus infection in a rural community. JAMA 1988; 259:3563-6.

6. Rutherford GW, Woo JM. Contact tracing and the control of human immunodeficiency virus infection. JAMA 1988; 259:3609-10.

7. Potterat JJ, Spenser NE, Woodhouse DE, Muth JB. Partner notification in the control of human immunodeficiency virus infection. Am J Public Health 1989; 79:874-6.

8. Partner notification for preventing human immunodeficiency virus (HIV) infection — Colorado, Idaho, South Carolina, Virginia. MMWR 1988; 37:393-6, 401-2.

9. Brennan TA. AIDS and the limits of confidentiality. The physician's duty to warn contacts of seropositive individuals. J Gen Int Med 1989; 4:242-6.

10. Lo B, Steinbrook RL, Cooke M, et al. Voluntary screening for human immunodeficiency virus (HIV) infection. Weighing the benefits and harms. Ann Intern Med 1989; 110:727-33.

Resource Allocation and Cost of Care

Molly Cooke, M.D.

The final issues of great ethical importance in HIV infection are how and by whom care for HIV-infected patients will be funded. The cost of HIV disease care has attracted considerable attention. It will probably continue to do so as the number of persons infected rises and the epidemic shifts into populations with few financial and social resources.

Private insurers are not enthusiastic about accepting responsibility for high-risk populations[1-9]; at the same time, the cost of public care (projected as $4.3 billion in 1992[10]) may sap the will of politicians and the public to provide needed care. Decisions about the appropriate level of financial support for treating HIV disease must avoid short-sighted solutions that favor cost savings over service to stigmatized and often disenfranchised populations.[11]

REFERENCES

1. Oppenheimer GM, Padgug RA. AIDS: the risks to insurers, the threat to equity. Hastings Cent Rep 1986; 16:18-22.
2. Hummel RF. AIDS, public policy, and insurance. AIDS and public policy journal, 1987; 2:1.
3. Blaine JH. AIDS: regulatory issues for life and health insurers. AIDS and public policy journal, 1987; 2:2-10.
4. Oppenheimer GM, Padgug RA. AIDS and health insurance: social and ethical issues. AIDS and public policy journal, 1987; 2:11-4.
5. Iuculano RP. D.C. Act 6-170: the five-year ban on risk-based pricing for AIDS. AIDS and public policy journal, 1987; 2:15-8.
6. Scherzer M. AIDS and insurance: the case against HIV antibody testing. AIDS and public policy journal, 1987; 2:19-24.
7. Fox DM. The cost of AIDS from conjecture to research. AIDS and public policy journal, 1987; 2:25-7.
8. Childress JF. An ethical framework for assessing policies to screen antibodies to HIV. AIDS and public policy journal, 1987; 2:28-31.
9. American Council of Life Insurers. White paper: the acquired immunodeficiency syndrome and HTLV-III testing. AIDS and public policy journal, 1987; 2:32-3.
10. Winkenwerder W, Kessler AR, Stolec RM. Federal spending for illness caused by the human immunodeficiency virus. N Engl J Med 1989; 320:1598-603.
11. Rogers DE. Federal spending on AIDS — how much is enough? N Engl J Med 1989; 320:1623-4.

INDEX

C

Finances, 9.4.3:1-3
of care costs, 12.1.7:1
emergency funds, 9.5.1:2
patient resources, 9.1.1:2, 9.4.2:1, 9.4.3.1-3

Fine-needle aspiration, of lymph nodes, 4.1.4:5-6

"Fisting," 1.2.3:2, 11.1.4:3-4

Florida
and heterosexual distribution, 1.2.4:2
and prisoners, 10.1.7:3
and tuberculosis, 6.2.2:1, 3-4

Fluid abnormalities, 5.9.2:1-2

Focal airspace consolidation, 5.5.2:2

Focal and segmental glomerulosclerosis (FSGS), 5.9.1:2-3

Folinic acid, 6.5.6:11, 13

Folliculitis, 5.3.1:2-3

Food, 10.6.1:1
for persons with AIDS, 9.5.1:1
proper handling of, 4.2.2:8

Food and Drug Administration, 4.2.2:7
and AZT, 4.2.5:1
and blood-donor screening, 10.4.1:2
and GLQ-223, 4.2.4:3
and hemophiliacs, 10.4.2:2-3
and HIV testing, 2.1.2:4-6
and pentamidine, 6.5.4:11
and peptide T, 4.2.4:1

Food handlers, 10.3.4:1, 10.6.2:1

Foscarnet, 4.2.4:2
and cytomegalovirus, 6.4.8:2
and cytomegalovirus retinitis, 5.11.1:4
and herpes simplex virus, 5.2.1:4; 6.4.2:12, 14

Foster homes, 10.5.1:3

Fourteenth Amendment, 10.1.7:3

France
and immune thrombocytopenic purpura, 5.8.1:10
toxoplasmosis in, 6.5.6:1, 8

Free will, 10.1.3:1

Funding, 10.1.4:2

Funeral services, 9.5.1:3

Fungal encephalitis, 5.4.2:2

Fungal infections, 5.3.1:9-12, 6.3.2:1-5
aspergillosis, 6.3.1:1-3
and hearing loss, 5.12.1:4
and hyponatremia, 5.9.2:1
pulmonary, 5.5.2:4
and radiography, 5.15.1:3

G

gag gene, 3.1.1:2, 3.1.6:2, 3.1.7:1-2, 4, 3.2.2:2, 3.2.5:6

gag protein, 3.1.7:2-3, 3.1.8:1

Gallbladder, and salmonella, 6.1.1:2-3

Gallium citrate lung scans, 5.5.3:1-2

Gallium scannings, 5.15.1:1-2
and Kaposi's sarcoma, 7.1.3:8
and pneumocystis pneumonia, 6.5.2:4

Ganciclovir, and cytomegalovirus, 6.4.6:2-3, 6.4.8:1-3

Gastrointestinal bleeding, 5.10.7:1-3, 5.10.9:1

Gastrointestinal dysfunction, causes of, 9.3.2:2

Gastrointestinal infection, 6.4.6:1-2

Gastrointestinal Kaposi's sarcoma, 5.10.9:1-4, 7.1.3:7-8, 10

Gastrointestinal procedures, precautions for, 5.10.1:2

Gastrointestinal symptoms, in persons with AIDS, 5.10.1:1-2

Gay lymph-node syndrome, 4.1.3:1

Gay Men's Health Crisis (GMHC), 11.1.2:1

Gene amplification, 1.2.9:2

Genitalia, of patient, 4.2.1:6

Genome structure, of HIV, 3.1.6:1-3

Gingivostomatitis, 6.4.2:3-4

Gloves, 10.2.2:1, 10.2.3:1, 10.2.4:1, 10.2.5:1, 10.2.6:1, 10.2.7:1-2, 10.2.10:1, 10.2.12:1, 10.2.14:3, 10.2.15:1, 10.3.3:1, 10.6.2:1
at home, 9.4.5:1
in surgery, 9.2.1:3

Glycosylation, inhibitors of, 3.2.5:6

GLQ-223, 4.2.4:3-4

Gonorrhea, 1.2.4:1, 11.1.7:3-4
in Africa, 1.1.4:5
and anorectal disease, 5.10.10:1
declining rate of, 1.2.3:1
and education, 11.1.1:1-2
and HIV risk factor, 1.2.3:2, 1.2.4:1
in San Francisco, 1.1.7:6

Gowns, 10.2.2:1, 10.2.14:3

gp41, 3.1.2:2, 3.1.7:3
and HIV testing, 2.1.2:4

gp160, 3.1.2:1-3, 3.1.1:3, 4.1.2:3

gp120, 3.1.2:1-2, 3.1.5:2, 3.1.7:3-4, 3.2.5:2-3, 4.1.2:3, 4.2.3:3

Grade schools, 10.5.1:2

Grandma's House, 11.1.7:7

Group homes, 10.5.1:3-4

Growth factor theory, of Kaposi's sarcoma, 7.1.3:2-3

Gummatous syphilis, 6.6.1:3

Gynecological disorders, 4.2.9:3-4

H

Haemophilus influenzae b vaccine, 4.2.3:3

Hairy leukoplakia, 5.2.1:2, 5.2.3:1-2, 5.10.4:1, 5.12.1:6-7, 6.4.9:2
and AIDS, 5.2.3:2
and thrush, 6.2.3:3